Frequently Used Emergency Drugs

These drugs are usually stocked on "code" or "crash" carts in acute care settin This list is only representative, since modifications are necessary in specialized intensive care units or emergency rooms.

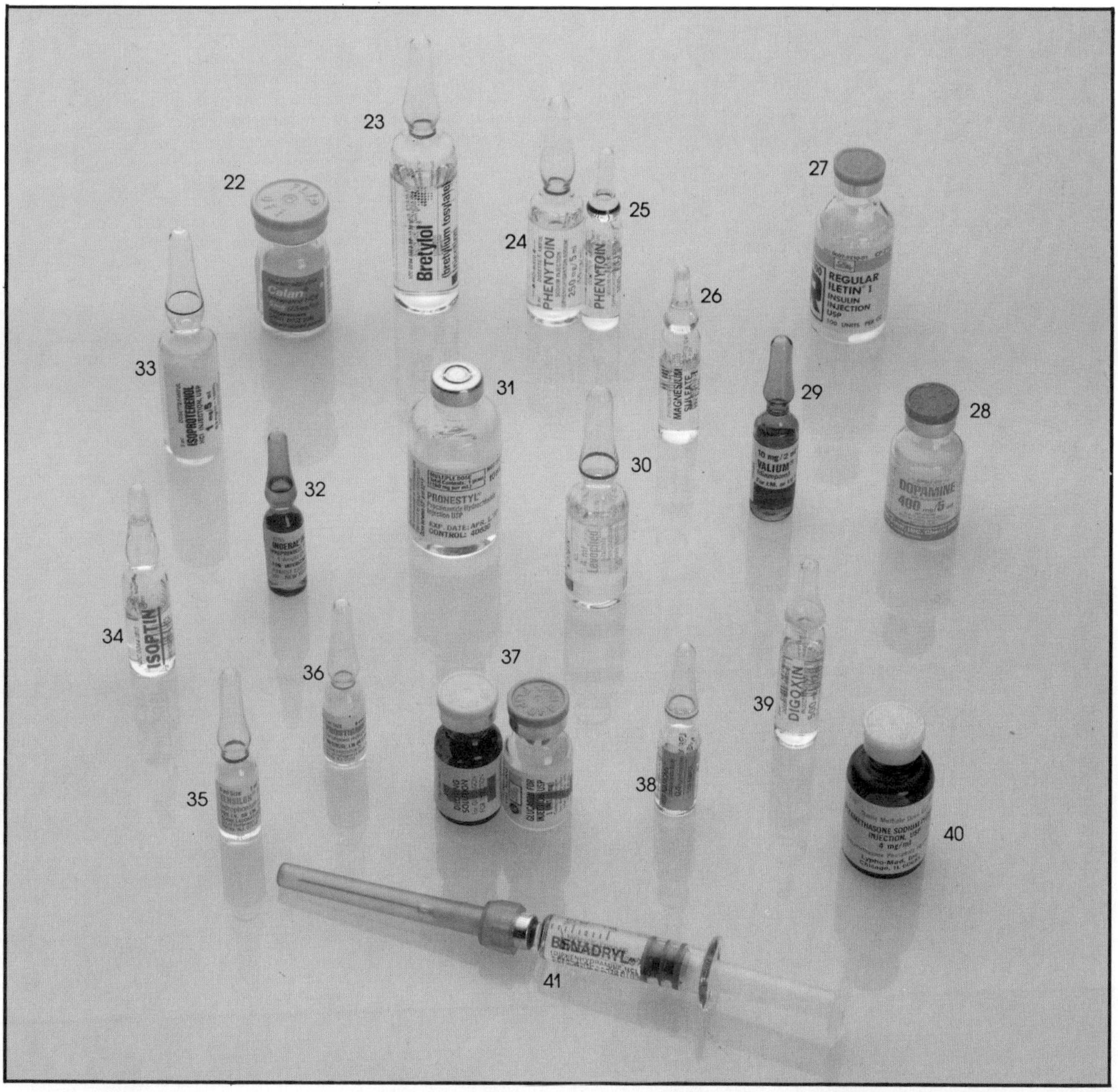

22. **Calan** (verapamil hydrochloride) 5 mg; 2 ml vial *Searle Pharmaceuticals, Inc.*
23. **Bretylol** (bretylium tosylate) 50 mg/ml; 10 ml ampule *Arnar-Stone*
24. **Phenytoin** (diphenylhydantoin sodium) 250 mg/5 ml; 5 ml ampule *Elkins-Sinn, Inc.*
25. **Phenytoin** (diphenylhydantoin sodium) 100 mg/2 ml; 2 ml ampule *Elkins-Sinn, Inc.*
26. **Magnesium sulfate** injection, 50%, 1 g/2 ml; 2 ml ampule *Elkins-Sinn, Inc.*
27. **Regular Iletin I** (insulin) injection, 100 units per ml; 10 ml vial *Eli Lilly and Company*
28. **Dopamine** 400 mg/5 ml; 5 ml vial *Elkins-Sinn, Inc.*
29. **Valium** (diazepam) 10 mg/2 ml; 2 ml ampule *Hoffmann-LaRoche, Inc.*
30. **Levophed Bitartrate** (brand of norepinephrine bitartrate injection formerly called Levarterenol Bitartrate); 4 ml ampule *Sterling Drug Company*
31. **Pronestyl** (procainamide hydrochloride) injection; 10 ml vial *E. R. Squibb & Sons, Inc.*
32. **Inderal** (propranolol hydrochloride) injectable, 1 mg/ml; 1 ml ampule *Ayerst Laboratories*
33. **Isoproterenol** 1 mg/5 ml; 5 ml ampule *Elkins-Sinn, Inc.*
34. **Isoptin** (verapamil hydrochloride) 5 mg/2 ml; 2 ml ampule *Knoll Pharmaceutical Company*
35. **Tensilon** (edrophonium chloride) 10 mg/ml; 1 ml ampule *Roche Laboratories*
36. **Prostigmin** 1:2000 (neostigmine methylsulfate) 1 ml ampule *Roche Laboratories*
37. **Glucagon** for injection, with diluting solution; two 1 ml vials *Eli Lilly and Company*
38. **Narcan** (naloxone hydrochloride) injection, 0.4 mg/ml; 1 ml ampule *Du Pont Pharmaceuticals, Inc.*
39. **Digoxin** 500 mcg/2 ml; 2 ml ampule *Elkins-Sinn, Inc.*
40. **Dexamethasone sodium phosphate** 4 mg/ml; 5 ml vial *Lypho-Med, Inc.*
41. **Benadryl** (diphenhydramine hydrochloride) 50 mg/ml; 1 ml syringe *Parke-Davis*

NURSING PHARMACOLOGY

A Comprehensive Approach to Drug Therapy

SANDRA COLEMAN WARDELL, RN, BSN, M.Ed.

Middlesex County College
Edison, New Jersey

LORRAINE BETZ BOUSARD, RN, MA

Dominican College
Orangeburg, New York

Wadsworth Health Sciences Division
Monterey, California
A division of Wadsworth, Inc.

Wadsworth Health Sciences Division
A division of Wadsworth, Inc.

Printed in the United States of America

10 9 8 7 6 5 4 3 2 1

Library of Congress Cataloging in Publication Data

Wardell, Sandra C.
Nursing pharmacology.

Includes index.
1. Pharmacology. 2. Chemotherapy. 3. Nursing.
I. Bousard, Lorraine B. II. Title. [DNLM: 1. Drug Therapy—nurses' instruction. 2. Pharmacology—nurses' instruction. QV 4 W265n]
RM300.W37 1985 615'.1 85-622

ISBN 0-534-01338-4

Sponsoring Editor: James Keating
Production Services Coordinators: Marlene Thom, David Hoyt
Production: Greg Hubit Bookworks
Manuscript Editor: Debra Myson-Etherington
Typesetting: Graphic Typesetting Service
Printer and Binder: The Maple-Vail Book Manufacturing Group

Front endpaper photographs produced by E. J. Quigley Associates, Gwynedd Valley, Pennsylvania 19437. Photographer, Michael Joniec. Drugs supplied through the courtesy of Jerry Meyer, Jefferson Hospital, Philadelphia, Pennsylvania.

The selection and dosage of drugs presented in this book are in accord with standards accepted at the time of publication. The authors and publisher have made every effort to provide accurate information. However, research, clinical practice, and government regulations often change the accepted standard in this field. Before administering any drug, the reader is advised to check the manufacturer's product information sheet for the most up-to-date recommendations on dosage, precautions, and contraindications. This is especially important in the case of drugs that are new or seldom used.

CONTRIBUTORS

Anna Cardinale
(digitalis and the cardiac glycosides)

Formerly of Seton Hall University
South Orange, New Jersey

Joyce Timm Cohen, RN, MA
(tetracyclines, chloramphenicols)

Dominican College
Orangeburg, New York

Maureen Cribben Creegan, MEd, RN, CCRN
(penicillins, cephalosporins, aminoglycosides)

Nurse Study Associates
West Nyack, New York
and Mount Sinai Medical Center
New York

Joy Lent Davis, RN, GNP
(active immunizing and diagnostic agents, passive immunizing and immunosuppressive agents)

Formerly of Rutgers University
College of Nursing
Newark, New Jersey

Marie T. DiGennaro, RN, BS, MA, JD
(antiarrhythmic agents)

Formerly of Rutgers University
College of Nursing
Newark, New Jersey

Alayne Araman Fitzpatrick, BSN, MSN
(antidiabetic and hypoglycemic agents, antineoplastic agents)

Mercy College
Dobbs Ferry, New York

Elizabeth Jane Forbes, RN, CMSEd, MSN, EdD
(stool softeners and laxatives)

Thomas Jefferson University
Philadelphia, Pennsylvania

Karen Davis Frank, RN, MA
(antipsychotic agents, antidepressants, antianxiety agents)

Englewood Hospital
Englewood, New Jersey

Evelyn Hart
(gonadotropic hormones, oral contraceptives)

Late of Rutgers University
College of Nursing
Newark, New Jersey

CONTENTS

See opening page of each chapter for detailed contents listing.

PART XV ANTINEOPLASTIC AGENTS 943

PART XVI DIGESTIVE SYSTEM AGENTS 965

PART XVII OPHTHALMIC AND OTIC AGENTS 1013

PART XVIII IMMUNOLOGIC AGENTS 1047

PREFACE

Purpose

THE NEED FOR health professionals to have ready access to a single, comprehensive source of drug information has never been more evident than it is today. This book fills that need by presenting essential pharmacological content—history, theory, practice, and calculation of dosages and solutions—in a thorough and systematic manner. Moreover, the drug monographs—numbering over one thousand—provide precise and complete information including extensive nursing management content. The student and the practitioner will find all essential pharmacological information in this text.

Organization of the Text

Although this book is designed primarily for the nursing student, it will meet the needs of health care practitioners in all settings. With this purpose in mind, we enlisted the help of colleagues with expertise in many specific areas within the drug monographs. The book is organized into sections that present historical and theoretical information in a manner that is concise and yet considerably more detailed than most other books in the field.

Part I is designed to orient the reader to the historical development of pharmacotherapeutics as a significant adjunct to other treatments. Included are important concepts related to interdisciplinary functions and responsibilities, regulatory and legal statutes and problems, and drug abuse.

Part II presents detailed content on pharmacotherapeutics, including all relevant theory underlying the various kinds of untoward drug reactions.

Part III is devoted to the calculation of dosages and solutions—an area that has generally been given only superficial attention in pharmacology textbooks. We have divided this content into three very detailed chapters, each of which includes a pretest and practice exercises. Thus, readers who successfully complete a pretest may omit that chapter.

In Part IV, the various routes and procedures for administering medications are presented. Techniques for administration are presented in a step-by-step "critical element" format and are reinforced by illustrations. The coverage is sufficiently thorough so that even a beginning student will be able to master techniques of administration without consulting a separate procedures book. Another feature in this section is the chapter detailing the various drug packaging techniques and dosage forms.

Following these four parts are the drug monographs, organized into fourteen major sections. Because many modern drugs have more than one physiological action, these drugs are cross-referenced, with the complete monograph appearing in the chapter related to their most common use. The drug monographs contain the most current available information, including such important details as extent of protein binding, distribution to various body sites and fluids, and laboratory test and drug interactions. Each major monograph concludes with a section on nursing management, including planning, administration, evaluation, and client teaching factors.

Acknowledgments

We would like to thank the following people for their significant contributions to this book by graciously sharing with us their expertise. Jeanne Von Oesen, RN, BSN, compiled the combination drugs for several chapters, at a time when we were in most need of assistance in order to meet publishing deadlines. Cyrus Ettinger, RP, and Mary Beth Van Strander, RP, BS, helped on numerous occasions by providing valuable literature, reviewing manuscript, and opening their libraries for our use. Our typists, Lisa Brodhead and Eileen Carlson, met their challenges with skill and dedication. We thank them for the many hours they spent at their keyboards.

We are proud to include in Chapters 21 and 22 contributions by the late Evelyn Hart. Evelyn, an unusually skilled and compassionate nurse practitioner, was an inspiration to her students and colleagues. Her contributions to this book represent only a small part of her substantial professional legacies. Nonetheless, we are pleased and proud to have this opportunity to share her work with our readers.

The years of research, writing, and rewriting that preceded publication of this book would have been in vain were it not for the skill and dedication of the publishing and production staff. The editing and design are, we have discovered, crucial to a finished product that is attractive, clear, and appealing to the reader. For their many months of toil and dedication, we thank Jim Keating, Marlene Thom, and Greg Hubit. To the many others who shared in the monumental task of editing and designing, we extend our grateful thanks for persevering!

Last but not least, we would like to thank our families for so patiently sharing us with this undertaking.

Sandra C. Wardell
Lorraine B. Bousard

PART I

ORIENTATION TO PHARMACOLOGY

MEDICATIONS ARE AN essential part of the treatment commonly prescribed today for most physical and mental diseases. As a member of the health team, a nurse has a vital function to perform in the administration of medicinal agents.

To understand present-day attitudes toward drugs, it is helpful to be aware of the evolution of ideas about sickness and health over the course of history. It is also useful to know the important individuals and events that figure in the history of pharmacology. From such understanding, the future direction of pharmacotherapeutics can to some extent be predicted. Chapter 1 traces these developments.

Chapter 2 outlines the roles and functions of the pharmacist, the physician, and the nurse. A primary responsibility of the nurse is administering medications, and observing clients' reactions to drugs. This information must be shared with the other members of the health team so that drug therapy can be appropriately adjusted.

Chapter 3 deals with **pharmacognosy,** the study of the sources of drugs. Knowledge of the plant, animal, mineral, and synthetic origins of drugs is important in understanding their nature, properties, and uses.

In the second half of Part I, the perspective is expanded to include the concerns of society about the use of drugs. Chapter 4 describes the methods used to control drug production and administration in the United States. Chapter 5 presents legal aspects of drug administration, and Chapter 6 deals with drug abuse and the implications of this behavior for the health team and the larger society.

Chapter 1

History of Pharmacotherapeutics

THE HISTORY OF pharmacology properly belongs within the history of human culture. Attitudes toward illness and ways of using medicinal agents are intimately related to social conditions, religious beliefs, and contemporary views about the nature of human beings and the world. Many groups have considered illness the work of evil spirits; the first pharmacists were therefore priests and shamans. Some individuals today still believe that spiritual leaders can cure disease. Understanding the source of such attitudes can help medical personnel meet the health care needs of society. This chapter traces the evolution of attitudes toward medicine and drugs and describes important historical advances in pharmacology. It also attempts to indicate the future direction of the field.

PREHISTORIC PERIOD (APPROXIMATELY 1,000,000 B.C.–4000 B.C.)

From the dim beginnings of the species to the dawn of history, human beings were essentially at the mercy of nature. During the Stone Age, they learned only by trial and error to distinguish edible, usually sweet-tasting, substances from poisonous, usually bitter-tasting, ones. They believed that the harmful life crises, such as hunger, disease, illness, and death, were caused by evil spirits, and they developed fetishes—beliefs in the magical powers of certain objects—to protect themselves from them. The evil spirit in an individual with a minor illness was often "driven out" with massage or various herbs. But the evil spirit in an individual with a major debilitating illness, such as a fracture or a psychosis, was sometimes "driven away" by killing the individual. The other members of the group were thus protected from an additional burden. Elements of nature, such as the sun, the wind, and some inanimate objects, like stones, were considered neither evil nor good, but neutral or benign.

During the Neolithic period, or New Stone Age, small villages began to develop as primitive people domesticated certain plants and animals and became food producers. Hunters learned to kill prey more easily by dipping their spears or arrows into solutions made from poisonous plants such as digitalis, which is used today as a heart medication.

People began to believe that some of the fetishes and neutral objects were possessed by benevolent spirits. At the same time, since disease and injury were believed to be caused by supernatural evil spirits, they turned to certain individuals who seemed to have supernatural powers for controlling disease. These people were called medicine men or shamans; they combined the functions of doctor, pharmacist, and priest. To treat illness they used herbs, foul-tasting solutions, changes in diet, exorcism, bleeding, and various rituals, including human sacrifice. They often attempted to drive out the evil spirit by giving a "medicine" that caused either diuresis—increased discharge of urine—or catharsis—evacuation of the bowels.

As the shaman's power increased, taboos developed. A taboo is a prohibition against touching or using a particular object or performing a particular act. Breaking taboos was believed to cause disease or injury. Many taboos were irrational, but some of them evolved, over time, into the rudiments of sanitary codes. The shaman's knowledge and rituals were taught to selected individuals who would become the next generation of shamans. Primitive people's traditions, beliefs, and customs were passed on orally, and their *folklore* about various herbs, plants, and poisons represented the beginning of pharmacology.

ANCIENT PERIOD (4000 B.C.–A.D. 500)

With the development of irrigation and the invention of writing, a new era began. Irrigation ensured a continuous supply of food and allowed populations to grow dramatically. The invention of writing meant that people no longer had to rely on folklore to receive the wisdom of the previous generation or to pass on their own.

Mesopotamia

The various Mesopotamian tribes worshipped and sought help from several benevolent deities and appeased the gods of evil through homage, praise, and sacrifice. For spiritual, moral, and physical aid, the people initially turned to the head of their group, the priest or priestess who served not only as spiritual leader but also as judge, physician, pharmacist, and, sometimes, surgeon. As the population grew, the leader's tasks came to be performed by different individuals. The role of physician-pharmacist began to be separate from that of priest. Surgical procedures, such as setting fractured bones and performing craniotomies, were often performed by barbers. Dysentery and typhoid were widespread and, like diseases of the "organs," were treated with herbs, mineral solutions, and physical therapy.

In the 18th century B.C., Hammurabi consolidated the Babylonian empire and organized its laws into a uniform code. The Code of Hammurabi contains the first known regulations of the conduct of physicians and surgeons. It stated not only the fees that should be obtained for various services, but also the penalty that should be paid if a surgeon killed a patient or destroyed a body part. Since surgery is performed with the hands, the penalty was that the surgeon's offending hand should be cut off.

Egypt

The ancient Egyptians also believed that disease was caused by evil spirits. Their medicine contained elements of magic and religion and was administered by priests. Treatments included various rituals and charms, as well as potions containing herbs, minerals, and poisons to purge the devil from the body. The practice of **polypharmacy,** the combination of several ingredients in one prescription, started with the early Egyptians.

With the advent of writing, the priest-physicians began to record their observations, diagnoses, and remedies. The most noteworthy of these records are the Ebers Medical Papyrus, written in about 1500 B.C., and the Edwin Smith Surgical Papyrus, dating from the 17th century B.C. The Ebers Papyrus is a collection of prescriptions delineating ingredients, precise dosage, and method of administration for numerous remedies. Substances in the prescriptions include vinegar, honey, castor oil, opium, iron, magnesia, putrified meat, animal fat, ground bones, and animal excreta. Most of the medications were given as powders, either pressed into a pill, dissolved in liquid, or made into a suppository. The Smith Surgical Papyrus contains descriptions of external injuries and ailments, such as skin lesions and fractured bones, along with recommendations for surgical procedures and various spells and rituals.

Gradually two classes of physicians developed in Egypt. The priest-physicians, with their magical spells and rituals, treated the masses, and the more knowledgeable physicians treated the wealthy. The latter group developed a more rational approach to medicine and used a variety of diets and drugs in their therapy. Some of them even specialized in specific body parts, such as the eyes, the abdomen, or the bowels.

When the Egyptians were conquered by the Greeks and, later, by the Romans, their medical knowledge and techniques were borrowed and incorporated into the conquering cultures.

The Hebrews

The Hebrews were influenced by the health practices of both the Egyptians and the Babylonians. They believed not only that sickness was the will of God, or Yahweh, but that health was restored and maintained by him as well, so their priests were physicians and pharmacists. The will of Yahweh was often revealed to the priests and prophets in dreams. They sought his favor by offering him the first fruits of their harvest, sacrificial animals, and, during the early years, occasionally human sacrifices. The Hebrews adhered to a number of sanitary laws, probably the earliest in existence, that were revealed to their prophets and recorded in the Biblical books of Leviticus and Numbers. These laws prescribed (1) bathing in many religious ceremonies; (2) the proper treatment of certain foods considered clean and others considered unclean; (3) the correct disposal of excreta; and (4) the isolation of individuals with certain diseases, such as leprosy.

Epilepsy, tumors, diphtheria, and various skin conditions are among the diseases described in the Old Testament. There are also references to the treatment of disease with drugs, such as parts of plants and ointments. The Talmud, the compilation of Jewish oral law and tradition, also contains references to various diseases, to surgery, and to some medications.

Greece

Little is known of prehistoric Greece, since few artifacts of the period have been found, but, by the fifth century B.C., Greek culture was highly advanced. The Greeks had many gods resembling human beings in form and in attributes. In their mythology, the god of disease, pestilence, healing, and prophecy was Apollo. His son Asclepius (or Aesculapius in Latin) was a healer and was called the god of medicine. Greek priests became specialized into various cults, including the cult of Asclepius. An ill person seeking treatment could go to one of Asclepius' outdoor temples and spend a night there, during which the proper treatment would be revealed to the priest in a dream. The remedies in this mystical-religious cult included fasting, special diets, drugs, physiotherapy, various charms, and complex rituals.

A group of secular physicians also emerged in Greece, most notably *Hippocrates* (c. 460–c. 377 B.C.), the "Father of Medicine." Hippocrates rejected superstition and magico-religious explanations of disease, believing that medicine could be placed on a scientific plane. He emphasized (1) careful observation of the patient; (2) the power of the body to heal itself; (3) a natural climate of fresh air, sunshine, and hydrotherapy; (4) proper diet; and (5) physical exercise and gymnastics. Occasionally he would also treat disease with herbs, drugs, and surgery.

Hippocrates had a large following of physicians who later expanded his rational view of diagnosis and treatment. A series of more than 60 Greek medical texts, called the Hippocratic Collection, has been found, covering topics such as epidemics, epilepsy, and reduction of fractures. More than 400 drugs are mentioned that were administered as pills, powders, suppositories, ointments, and lotions. The Hippocratic oath, exemplifying Hippocrates' moral and ethical commitment to the service of healing the sick, is still recited at graduation at many medical schools.

An indirect contributor to pharmacology was the Greek philosopher *Theophrastus* (c. 372–c. 287 B.C.). He classified plants into trees, shrubs, and herbs and systematically described their structure. His work was later used by physician-pharmacists to identify and describe medicinal herbs and plants.

When Greece fell under Roman domination in about 200 B.C., the Romans, who had limited knowledge of medicine and pharmacy, welcomed the Greek physicians as slaves and, later, as free men. Therefore, Greek medicine continued to flourish. *Dioscorides,* who lived in the first century A.D., was a Greek physician who traveled with the Roman army. He collected information on nearly 600 medicinal plants and wrote the first series of drug books, called *De Materia Medica.* Previously, drugs had been classified according to the diseases for which they could be used, but Dioscorides classified nearly 1000 drugs according to the ingredients in each and the method for preparing them. Included were opium and arsenic, which was used as a caustic agent—that is, one that burns, corrodes, or destroys living tissue.

Another notable Roman physician of Greek parentage was *Galen* (c.130–c. 200). He compiled all known medical knowledge into more than 80 books and added the results of his own anatomical research as well. His works in medicine and pharmacy were used for several centuries. Galen believed that, since disease is contrary to nature, it should be treated by counteracting its signs and symptoms. He also supported Hippocrates' belief in supporting nature through the use of personal hygiene, fresh air, wholesome diet, and exercise. Hippocrates used very few medications, but Galen advocated polypharmacy. The preparations included in his 30 pharmacology books are still called *galenicals.*

MEDIEVAL PERIOD (500–1500)

The downfall of Rome took with it the status of medicine. There were only a few respected physicians and most of them were slaves. Since only the very wealthy lived in decent homes, disease, illness, and ignorance were rampant during the Dark Ages (500–1100). The masses reverted to superstitions and supernatural beliefs about health and illness, which was considered a punishment for sins. They wore charms to prevent illness and sought treatment from priests and monks, who, besides performing religious rituals, prescribed fresh air, sleep, wholesome food, and some herbs, particularly cathartics.

An exceptional physician of this era was *Paul of Aegina,* who is thought to have lived during the seventh century. Although most surgery was performed by barbers, this Greek-born physician was familiar with some advances in surgery. His seven-volume medical history, entitled *On Medicine,* describes the use of ligatures in surgery, treatment of aneurysms, and techniques for tracheotomy, lithotomy, tonsillectomy, and mastectomy.

During the medieval period, many Greek and Roman texts were translated by Arab scholars, so the knowledge of medicine and pharmacology accumulated by earlier civilizations was not lost. Among the prominent physicians of the Arab culture was *Rhazes* (865–925), a Persian who served as chief physician at the Baghdad hospital. He wrote more than 140 papers on medicine and was the first to recognize the difference between measles and smallpox. He also described the use of animal gut for sutures and introduced the use of mercurical ointment.

Avicenna (980–1037) was also a Persian physician and philosopher serving in the Arabic courts. His *Canon of Medicine* was translated into several languages after his death. Based on Greek medical knowledge, the *Canon* also contained a number of Egyptian medicinal remedies. Mercury, alcohol, and sulfuric acid were among the substances included in prescriptions. The Crusades of the 11th, 12th, and 13th centuries brought the medical knowledge of the Arabs to Europe, along with a variety of drug ingredients, such as sugar, opium, and spices.

During the latter part of the Middle Ages, Western civilization experienced recurrent episodes of deadly infections, including dysentery, smallpox, and bubonic plague. Although magic and rituals were still accepted treatments, the use of drugs containing many obnoxious ingredients—animal excreta, toads, ground rats, and the viscera of animals or humans—was becoming widespread. The greatest therapeutic value was thought to derive from the most foul-tasting and foul-smelling remedies. It was also believed that a substance similar in appearance to the affected body organ would relieve the ailment. This belief was called the *theory of similars* and the remedies were called *signatures.*

Apothecary shops specializing in the preparation and sale of drugs were becoming commonplace. However, pharmacy was not to become a respected science until the development of chemistry and other sciences. Alchemy, the forerunner of chemistry, was introduced into Europe by the Arabs in the 12th century. Alchemists sought to transform one substance into another, primarily base metals into gold and silver. Although their attempts failed, the alchemists did discover several valuable substances, such as arsenic, plaster of paris, barium sulfide, bismuth, and phosphorus. They also designed many of the essential tools of chemistry, such as a crude measuring balance and the distilling flask. Some respected scholars of the Renaissance era, including *Paracelsus,* were enthusiastic alchemists. (See Figure 1-1.)

The advent of printing in the mid-15th century signaled another advance for medicine, as well as for all fields of learning. Works previously hand-copied at great cost and often containing errors could now be reproduced accurately and inexpensively. Writings and drawings about the materia medica—the materials used for medicines—could be made available not only to scholars but, eventually, to the common people.

RENAISSANCE PERIOD (1500–1600)

The transitional period from medieval to modern times, called the Renaissance, brought not only cultural and artistic development but a resurgence of medical knowledge and pharmacology as well (Table 1-1). As people began to turn away from the authority of the Roman Catholic Church, secular physicians increased in number. The use of superstitions and religious rituals to treat disease was slowly replaced by rational remedies. Recognition and diagnosis of different

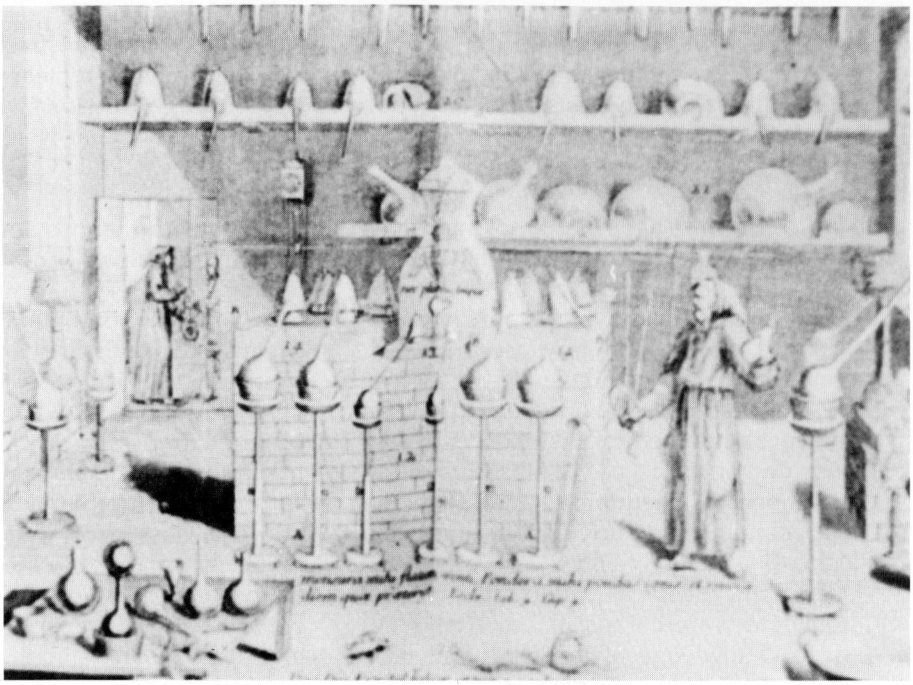

FIGURE 1-1 A 16th century alchemist compounding a drug. (From H. von Braunschweig, *Liber de arte distillandi,* Strasbourg, 1512.)

TABLE 1-1 Major Medical Advances During the Renaissance (1500–1600)

Individual	Contribution	Comment
Paracelsus (1493–1541)	Used mercury for treating syphilis Popularized use of specific medicinal agents for specific diseases	He disagreed with the common practice of polypharmacy.
Leonardo da Vinci (1452–1519)	Made anatomical studies and drawings	He did more than 1500 anatomical sketches.
Andreas Vesalius (1514–64)	Published anatomical atlas, *De Humani Corporis Fabrica*	He called attention to numerous errors in Galen's work.
Ambroise Paré (1517–90)	Used ligatures to stop surgical bleeding	He advocated using only clean dressings on wounds rather than the traditional hot oils or irritating pastes.
Valerius Cordus (d. 1544)	Studied medicinal plants—the first pharmacopeia in Germany, the *Dispensatorium,* was based on his work	

diseases were improving, and drugs were being evaluated for their effectiveness against specific ailments.

Precolonial North and South America

During the time of the Renaissance, Europeans were discovering and exploring the Americas, and some medicinal agents were brought back from the native cultures. Most of the peoples of the Western Hemisphere had animistic religions—beliefs in the permeation of the natural world by spirits—and relied on shamanistic medicine for treatment of disease.

The Incas of Peru believed that illness was caused by angry gods, so they sought treatment from priests. Among the North American tribes, the role of physician was filled by the medicine man, who used trancelike states, ventriloquism, dances, and other rituals, along with a variety of plants and herbs, to treat illnesses. Some of these practices still exist today—in some cultures, for example, garlic is used to ward off evil spirits.

THE AGE OF SCIENTIFIC DISCOVERY (1600–1850)

The observations and impressions of Renaissance study were gradually replaced by systematic scientific inquiry and new theories. Some saw the human body as a machine that became sick due to "tension in the fibers"; others regarded it as a chemical laboratory that became diseased when the "chemicals stopped fermenting." Polypharmacy was still advocated and a few new therapeutic substances were imported from South America, notably dried cinchona bark and the dried rhizome and roots of ipecacuanha, often called ipecac. A number of significant advances in medicine and pharmacology occurred during this period (Table 1-2). Experimentation with crude drugs resulted in the identification of a number of active principles. From crude opium came *morphine* in 1803, *codeine* in 1832, and *papaverine* in 1848; from ipecac came *emetine* in 1817; from cinchona came *quinine* in 1820; from belladonna came *atropine* in 1831; and from the nux vomica bean came *strychnine* in 1817.

North America

The early settlers in North America had to struggle for survival during the 17th century. Hygiene was not a priority and there were few sanitary measures. Medicines imported from Europe were still considered superior to the herbs and medicinal agents that Americans were growing in their family gardens. During the first half of the 18th century, some apothecaries were established, but the clergy continued to play a major role in medical care. Apothecaries, grocers, and even postal clerks sold the latest patent drugs from Europe, such as Daffy's Elixir and Turlington's Balsam. (At that time, a patent drug was one that listed its ingredients on the label.) Unscrupulous individuals began to fill the medicine bottles with their own concoctions and sell them as "patented" drugs from Europe or as their own "secret family cure-alls." Many of these products were ordered by mail through catalogs by the unsuspecting public.

The few practicing physicians in the colonies learned medicine by apprenticeship; there were no trained nurses. The frequent disease epidemics soon created a need for central locations where victims could be properly treated. Consequently, the first hospital in colonial America was founded in New Orleans in 1737. Soon hospitals were established in other cities: Philadelphia in 1756, New York in 1776, and Boston in 1821. Moreover, the first medical college in North America was established in 1765 and the U.S. College of Pharmacy was founded in Philadelphia in 1821.

During the early 1800s, a number of scientific advances were recorded. American physicians popularized the use of gaseous anesthetic agents (see Figure 1-2) and proudly heralded "man's triumph over pain." Table 1-3 lists the principal advances in pharmacology achieved during this period.

THE BIRTH OF MODERN PHARMACOLOGY (1850–1900)

During the latter half of the 19th century, the scientific advances of the previous era developed into specific methods of diagnosing and treating illness (see Table 1–4). New advances in

TABLE 1-2 Major Medical Advances (1600–1850)

Individual	Contribution	Comment
Galileo Galilei (1564–1642)	Made discoveries in physics and astronomy Constructed first astronomical telescope—1609 Invented compound microscope—1610	He is considered the founder of experimental science.
Robert Boyle (1627–91)	Invented air pump Discovered what is now known as Boyle's law Studied specific gravity and devised color tests for acidity and alkalinity of substances	His experiments and tests were used to identify medicinal agents in later centuries.
Gasparo Aselli (1581–1626)	Identified lymphatic circulation	His followers studied and described this circulation.
Anton van Leeuwenhoek (1632–1723)	Refined compound microscope Studied plant and animal structures	His experiments led to the identification of medicinal agents by microscopic analysis.
Joseph Priestly (1733–1804)	Discovered oxygen—1774	Karl Scheele conducted experiments on air in 1771–72, but his work was published after Priestley's.
Antoine Laurent Lavoisier (1743–94)	Discovered the nature of combustion and the role of oxygen in respiration Showed that chemical reactions can be expressed as equations	He is considered the "Father of Chemistry."
Edward Jenner (1749–1823)	Concluded that individuals who had cowpox were protected against smallpox Performed the first inoculation against smallpox—1796	Despite his work, the cause of communicable diseases was not discovered until the next century.
Matthias Jakob Schleiden (1804–81)	Propagated the cell theory for both plants and animals	The theory that plants and animals were composed of living cells was not proven until better microscopic techniques were developed a few decades later.
Sir Humphry Davy (1778–1829)	Conducted experiments with nitrous oxide—1799	Horace Wells publicized its use.
Thomas Sydenham (1624–89)	Credited with the beginning of epidemiology	He used Laudanum (tincture of opium) to treat dysentery and restored the ancient belief in the body's ability to heal itself.

TABLE 1-2 ***Continued***

Individual	Contribution	Comment
F. Anton Mesmer (1734–1815)	Used hypnotism successfully for treating hysteria	"Mesmerism" (hypnotism) was also used for surgical anesthesia.
Samuel Hahnemann (1755–1843)	Founded homeopathy	He used small doses of only one drug to create symptoms similar to those of the offending disease (called the *simile rule*).
Giovanni Morgagni (1682–1771)	Founded the study of pathology	He concluded that each disease has its seat in body organs.
Gabriel Pravaz (1791–1853)	Invented the hypodermic syringe	His invention increased use of parenteral routes of drug administration.
Sir James Y. Simpson (1811–1870)	First used chloroform for childbirth (1847)	Chloroform was also called *sweet whiskey.*

medicine were disseminated quickly because of progress in transportation and communications. As the invention of the power press (1822), the rotary press (1846), and the linotype (1886) made printed material cheaper and more abundant, scientific books and journals became widely available. Knowledge about medical advances traveled even more quickly with the invention of the steam locomotive (1804), the steamboat (1807), the telegraph (1836), the cable car (1858), the bicycle (1865), the telephone (1876), and the automobile engine (1885). Medical knowledge spread so rapidly that urban physicians began to concentrate on specific areas of interest and thus became *specialists.*

A number of medicinal agents were discovered and introduced into therapeutic use at this time, including *aspirin, silver nitrate, diphtheria antitoxin,* and *epinephrine.* Once it became clear that certain drugs, such as arsenic and digitalis, were highly toxic, researchers became interested in the fate of drugs after they were administered and began to study drug detoxification and excretion.

By 1815, the branch of pharmacology dealing with the preparation of medicinal agents from natural substances had been named *pharmacognosy.* As the distinction between crude medicinal

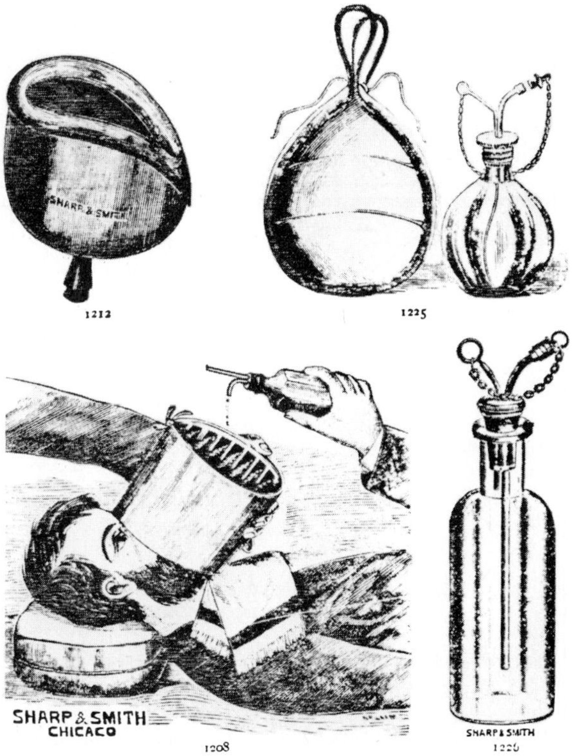

FIGURE 1-2 Some early anesthetic devices. (From *Sharp and Smith Medical Supply Catalog,* 1888.)

TABLE 1-3 Major Pharmacological Advances in North America (1600–1850)

Individual	Contribution	Comment
Zabdiel Boylston (1679–1766)	Performed first vaccination for smallpox in the colonies	A major smallpox epidemic occurred in the Boston area in 1721.
Thomas Addis Emmet (1764–1827)	Introduced improvements in gynecological treatment	He repaired vaginal and uterine lacerations and disorders.
William Withering 1741–99)	Used crude digitalis to treat congestive heart failure	
William Proctor, Jr. (1817–74)	Appointed first professor of pharmacy at the U.S. College of Pharmacy in Philadelphia	He is often called the "Father of American Pharmacy."
Lyman Spalding (1775–1821)	Proposed the first United States drug compendium (printed in 1820)	The *U.S. Pharmacopeia* was a response to the hazards of unconventional remedies; after 1850, pharmacists as well as physicians assisted in each five-year revision.
Crawford W. Long (1815–78) William T. Morton (1819–68)	First used ether for anesthesia	The use of ether spread quickly through America and Europe.

TABLE 1-4 Major Medical Advances (1850–1900)

Individual	Contribution	Comment
	In the study of the human body:	
Hugo De Vries (1848–1935)	Developed theory of genes	
Gregor Johann Mendel (1822–84)	Discovered and formulated principles of heredity	His experiments were performed on garden peas and other vegetables.
Claude Bernard (1813–78)	Developed principles of experimental research in physiology	His work centered on digestive processes and the vasomotor mechanism.
	In diagnosis:	
Hermann L. F. von Helmholtz (1821–94)	Invented ophthalmoscope—1851	He also explained lens accommodation in the eye.
Manuel Patricio Rodriguez Garcia (1805–1906)	Invented laryngoscope—1855	

TABLE 1-4 ***Continued***

Individual	Contribution	Comment
Chevalier Jackson (1865–1958)	Adapted bronchoscope for surgical use—1903	
Karl August Wunderlich (1815–77)	Made advances in clinical thermometry	He developed fever charts.
Wilhelm Conrad Roentgen (1845–1923)	Discovered x-rays—1895	"X" stands for unknown (unknown rays).
	In pathology:	
Rudolf Virchow (1821–1902)	Founded cellular pathology	He was the first to regard pathology as abnormal physiology in the cells (previously regarded as abnormality in organs or tissues or both).
Louis Pasteur (1822–95)	Introduced germ theory; founded bacteriology	He studied diseases in wine, food, animals, and human beings.
Robert Koch (1843–1910)	Identified a microbial disease (anthrax) for the first time—1876	He developed techniques of bacteriological culture and discovered several disease-causing organisms.
	In surgery:	
James Marion Sims (1813–83)	Introduced improvements in gynecological treatment	He repaired vesico-vaginal fistulas (between the bladder and vaginal tract), a complication of childbirth.
Joseph Lister (1827–1912)	Founded antiseptic surgery	He demonstrated the value of carbolic acid and heat sterilization of instruments in decreasing postoperative infections.
Theodor Billroth (1829–94)	Improved techniques in abdominal surgery	He resected esophagus—1881; excised complete larynx—1874; perfected stomach resection.
Charles McBurney (1845–1913)	Improved techniques for appendectomy	
	In therapeutics:	
Paul Ehrlich (1854–1915)	Made contributions in chemotherapy	He searched for drugs that would be effective against pathogens without affecting the body's cells; he discovered salvarsan for the treatment of syphilis.
Sigmund Freud (1856–1939)	Founded psychoanalysis; used the therapeutic dialogue to treat mental illness	His work revolutionized the concept of mental illness.

agents and pure active principles became increasingly important, pharmacognosy developed rapidly in the latter half of the 19th century.

Since the isolation of morphine and other alkaloids earlier in the century, researchers began comparing one substance to another. These *comparative studies* resulted in several new drug discoveries—including *salvarsan,* used for treating syphilis.

The greatest contribution to medical progress during this time was Pasteur's *germ theory,* which led to the identification of a number of disease-causing microbes (Table 1-5).

Pharmacotherapeutics in the United States

Although health care in the United States had not essentially improved since the early 1800s, some progress was made. The invention of the hypodermic syringe and the discovery of cocaine made regional anesthesia possible. *James Leonard Corning* was the first to inject large nerves with cocaine; by the end of the century, anesthetic agents were becoming popular. Antiseptics too, especially phenol, potassium permanganate, and iodine, became more popular. In fact, the effectiveness of present-day germicides is often compared to phenol by means of a rating called the *phenol coefficient.* The early antiseptic agents were so caustic to normal tissue, however, that following Lister's demonstrations of their usefulness, research was directed at finding less irritating substances.

John Jacob Abel (1857–1938) founded the first department of pharmacology in the United States, at the University of Michigan, and became the first full-time professor of pharmacology in this country. Educated in physiology, medicine, chemistry, and pharmacology in Europe and in the United States, he was professor of pharmacology at Johns Hopkins University from 1893 to 1932. He conducted research on the chemical composition of animal tissues, isolating epinephrine, insulin, and blood amino acids, and studied the toxic and therapeutic effects of various substances. He is often called the "Father of American Pharmacology."

Meanwhile, the sale of worthless and often dangerous products called *nostrums* was thriving—in fact, charlatans reaped fortunes from nostrums that were patented or trademarked. These conditions prompted the American Pharmaceutical Association to publish the *National Formulary* in 1888, establishing standards for the medically accepted drugs not listed in the *United States Pharmacopeia.*

THE DEVELOPMENT OF MODERN PHARMACOLOGY (1900–1950)

In an attempt to control the threat to the public posed by quackery, the United States enacted many laws during the first half of the 20th century aimed at controlling the pharmaceutical industry and other aspects of drug use. (See

TABLE 1-5 Major Disease-Causing Microbes Identified Between 1850 and 1900

Microbe	Year	Discoverer
Anthrax	1876	Robert Koch
Typhoid bacillus	1880	Karl J. Eberth and Robert Koch
Tuberculosis bacillus	1882	Robert Koch
Cholera bacillus	1883	Robert Koch
Diphtheria bacillus	1884	Edwin Klebs and Friedrich Loffler
Tetanus bacillus	1884	Arthur Nicolaier

Chapters 2 through 5 for descriptions of these laws.) Many advances in drug therapy were also made during the first half of the 20th century (see Table 1–6), some by accident, such as the discovery of penicillin, others by careful scientific research into physiology, disease prevention, and drug analysis and synthesis. The major advances in pharmacology were in the drug classifications of vitamins, hormones, and antibiotics.

The World Wars

Several advances in pharmacotherapeutics were spurred by the world wars. The American physician and chemist *Henry D. Dakin* (1880–1952) found that a 0.5% solution of sodium hypochlorite, later called *Dakin's Solution,* was an effective topical antiseptic solution for treating wounds. During World War I, there were no antibiotics, few effective analgesics, and little or no blood available for transfusions. During World War II, blood banks were established and *Edwin J. Cohn* and his associates at Harvard University fractionalized the various blood components so that each part could be used for specific conditions—for example, serum albumin for shock. These accomplishments helped to decrease the war mortality.

Malaria was a threat to the Allied soldiers in the Pacific, especially since the Japanese had cut off the supply of cultivated cinchona, the source of quinine, growing in Java. Working diligently to produce synthetic antimalarial agents, biochemists developed chloroquine, quinacrine, and primacrine.

Because of the rapid discovery of new drugs, the need for expensive specialized equipment to produce them, and the demand for massive quantities of them during World War II, the compounding and the production of drugs was taken over by large companies. Furthermore, by the end of World War II, the study of drugs was divided into five distinct areas:

1. *Pharmacognosy*—The study of sources of drugs, plant, animal, mineral, and synthetic
2. *Pharmacology*—The study of all aspects of the effects of drugs on living tissues, including experimental, comparative, and clinical pharmacology
3. *Pharmacodynamics*—The study of the action, fate, and excretion of drugs
4. *Pharmacotherapeutics*—The study of the medical uses of drugs to treat or prevent diseases
5. *Toxicology*—The study of the harmful effects of drugs

THE AGE OF SYNTHETIC DRUGS (1950–PRESENT)

Advances made in chemistry and biochemistry during the first half of the 20th century paved the way for the production of many kinds of synthetic drugs. Synthetic antihistamines, psychotherapeutic agents, particularly tranquilizers, cancer chemotherapeutic agents, diuretics, and cardiovascular agents now account for a large proportion of prescribed drugs. The search for more effective and less toxic drugs to treat inflammatory diseases, for example, has resulted in the discovery of a number of synthetic compounds that can be used in place of aspirin.

Even the natural processes of pregnancy and childbirth have been altered with drugs since 1950. There are now agents to assist women in becoming pregnant, as well as products to prevent pregnancy. In fact, *oral contraceptives* are a multimillion-dollar industry in the United States. There is even an immune globulin, called Rho-Gam (first used in 1968), which prevents Rh-negative mothers from rejecting Rh-positive fetuses.

Regulation of Medicinal Agents

Some of the drugs released in the United States since 1950 have been found to be health hazards. The constant use of antibiotics has caused drug-resistant mutations to appear in some pathogens (called a mutagenic effect), necessitating an ongoing search for newer and more effective antibiotics. Some drugs, such as thalidomide, have caused malformations in the fetuses of pregnant women (teratogenic effect), while others are suspected of causing cancer (carcinogenic effect).

The federal Food and Drug Administration (FDA) now requires more extensive testing of drugs before they can be used by the public. Consequently, the number of drugs released each

TABLE 1-6 Major Advances in Pharmacotherapeutics (1900–1950)

Individual	Contribution	Comment
Karl Landsteiner (1868–1943)	Discovered human blood groups—1900	He won the 1930 Nobel Prize in Physiology and Medicine.
Sir Frederick G. Hopkins (1861–1947)	Discovered that vitamins are essential to health—1906	He is considered the founder of experimental nutritional chemistry; his work mainly concerned vitamins A and B, carbohydrate metabolism, and muscular activity.
Christian Eijkman (1858–1930)	Discovered that beriberi is caused by a thiamine deficiency Discovered other vitamins	He isolated rice polishings as a nutritive substance that would prevent beriberi. He shared with Hopkins the 1929 Nobel Prize in Physiology and Medicine.
Paul Ehrlich (1854–1915)	Popularized the use of intravenous injection—1910	He administered salvarsan intravenously for syphilis.
Elmer V. McCollum and Marguerite Davis; Thomas B. Osborne (1859–1929) and Lafayette B. Mendel (1872–1935)	Discovered the fat-soluble accessory food factor vitamin A—1913	The two teams identified vitamin A as a "substance in butter, eggs and cod liver oil, but not in plain lard."
Edward C. Kendall (1886–1972)	Isolated thyroxine—1914	Thyroid extract had been used since 1891 but Kendall isolated the crystalline form.
Sir Frederick G. Banting (1891–1941)	Isolated insulin—1921	It was extracted from a fetal pancreas.
Charles H. Best (1899–1978)	Injected insulin into a 14-year-old diabetic—1922	
John J. Abel (1857–1938)	Introduced crystalline insulin—1926	
Edgar Allen (1892–1943) and Edward A. Doisy (b. 1893)	Isolated female sex hormone estrogen—1923	Using rats, they developed a method (bioassay) of determining the amount of "ovarian extract" present.
Edward A. Doisy (b. 1893)	Isolated female sex hormone "theelin"—1929; later called estrol.	
Sir Alexander Fleming (1881–1955)	Discovered penicillin—1928	He noted lack of staphylococci in culture contaminated with the mold penicillium.
Sir Howard W. Florey (1898–1968) and Ernst B. Chain (b. 1906)	Isolated a crude penicillin mixture—1938	Florey, Chain, and Fleming shared the 1945 Nobel Prize in Physiology and Medicine.

TABLE 1-6 *Continued*

Individual	Contribution	Comment
Adolph F. J. Butenandt (b. 1903)	Identified and isolated the first male sex hormone androsterone—1931	
Adolph F. J. Butenandt (b. 1903)	Isolated female sex hormone progesterone—1933	He was awarded a Nobel Prize in 1939, but the German government prevented his acceptance.
Henrick Dam (b. 1895)	Identified coagulation vitamin (vitamin K)—1934	His research showed it to be a blood-clotting substance.
Edward A. Doisy (b. 1893)	Isolated two forms of vitamin K	The two men shared the 1943 Nobel Prize in Physiology and Medicine.
Gerhard Domagk (1895–1964) and coworkers	Discovered efficacy of Prontosil against infections—1935	An azo dye with a sulfonamide group in its structure, Prontosil was originally synthesized by Paul Gelmo in 1908; Domagk's work led to the discovery of sulfa drugs. He was awarded the 1939 Nobel Prize in Physiology and Medicine but the German government prevented his acceptance.
Edward C. Kendall (1886–1972) and coworkers; and	Prepared cortisone by partial synthesis—1935	He also studied other hormones of the adrenal cortex (e.g., ACTH).
Philip S. Hench (1896–1965)	Studied effects of ACTH and cortisone on rheumatic fever and rheumatoid arthritis	He and Kendall were colleagues.
Tadeus Reichstein (b. 1897)	Identified the structure of several adrenocorticosteroids, including cortisone, cortisol, and corticosterone—1943	Kendall, Hench, and Reichstein shared the 1950 Nobel Prize in Physiology and Medicine.
Merrit and Putnam	Introduced phenytoin (Dilantin)—1938	This synthetic anticonvulsant is used in the treatment of epilepsy.
Eislef and Schaumann	Isolated meperidine hydrochloride (Demerol)—1939	Today it is a commonly used synthetic narcotic.
Karl Landsteiner (1868–1943) and Alexander S. Wiener	Identified the Rh factor—1940	
Selman A. Waksman (1888–1973) and coworkers	Discovered streptomycin (first aminoglycoside antibiotic)—1944	Derived from *streptomyces griseus,* it was the first drug found to be effective against tuberculosis; Waksman was awarded the 1952 Nobel Prize in Physiology and Medicine.
R. P. Ahlquist	Discovered adrenergic receptors—the autonomic nerve sites that release epinephrine and norepinephrine—1948	He classified receptor sites as alpha and beta types.

year has decreased considerably. Besides evaluating new drugs more carefully, the FDA has also been examining the older remedies and has begun to classify them as "effective," "probably effective," "possibly effective," and "having little or no effect." The first *Drug Efficacy Study Report*, published in 1971, resulted in the removal of some products from the market (see Chapter 4).

Other protective actions taken by the FDA include (1) the establishment of U.S. Recommended Daily Allowances (RDA) for 19 essential vitamins and minerals; (2) the classification as drugs of those vitamins, foods, and food supplements containing more than three times the RDA; (3) the requirement of a prescription for more than 400 IU of Vitamin A and more than 10,000 IU of Vitamin D; and (4) the recall of all "diet drugs" containing amphetamines. These rules went into effect in 1973. In 1976, the U.S. Supreme Court ruled that states must allow pharmacists to advertise their drug prices.

New Dimensions in Pharmacology

During the first half of the 20th century, drugs were primarily checked for their content, strength, purity, and safety. But since 1950, as the techniques of analyzing medicinal agents have grown more sophisticated, other aspects have been investigated. Not only is the dosage considered but also the amount that reaches the circulating blood—the *bioavailable dose*. These studies then led to investigations into the movement, or kinetics, of drugs through the body, from absorption to excretion. Consequently the field of *pharmacokinetics* developed. (Part II covers this subject in detail.)

The search for new synthetic agents for specific diseases has also become more sophisticated. Some research laboratories are using computers to discover the properties of potential medicinal substances rather than using the older, time-consuming methods. Drugs have been designed not only for the prevention and treatment of illness but also for the diagnosis of disease. Several radiopaque substances have been created to outline specific body parts on x-rays. Radioactive drugs are also being used in diagnosing illness. The College of Pharmacy at the University of New Mexico has been studying techniques for detecting all forms of human cancer through *nuclear pharmacy*.

One of the most recent innovations in pharmacology involves *genetic engineering* for the production of drugs. The human gene for insulin, for example, can be introduced into certain bacteria that multiply rapidly, producing large quantities of insulin. Insulin produced by this method is now being used in clinical trials on human subjects. Similar possibilities exist for the production of many other drugs including interferon, which is still scarce and extremely expensive to produce.

REFERENCES

American Medical Association. 1911, 1921, 1936. *Nostrum and Quackery*, vols. I, II, III.

Anderson, A. W. 1957. *Plants in the bible*. New York: Philosophical Library.

Bethea, O. W. 1940. *Materia medica: Drug administration and prescription writing*, 5th ed. Philadelphia: F. A. Davis.

Dietz, L. D. and Lehozky, A. R. 1967. *History of modern nursing*, 2nd ed. Philadelphia: F. A. Davis.

Goodman, L. S. and Gilman, A. 1980. *The Pharmacological Basis of Therapeutics*, 6th ed. New York: Macmillan.

Hamilton, S. W. 1944. *The history of American mental hospitals: One hundred years of American psychiatry*. New York: Columbia University Press.

La Wall, C. H. 1927. *Four thousand years of pharmacy*. Philadelphia: Lippincott.

Nutting, M. A., and Dock, L. L. 1935. *A history of nursing*. New York: Putnam's.

Sonnedecker, G., ed. 1963. *History of pharmacy*, 3rd ed. Philadelphia: Lippincott.

Young, J. H. 1967. *The medical messiahs: A social history of health quackery in twentieth century America*. Princeton: Princeton University Press.

Chapter 2

Pharmacology and the Health Team

FROM ITS HUMBLE beginnings, *pharmacology* has grown into a broad field of knowledge concerned with chemical agents, or drugs, that affect the biological functioning of living organisms. The field includes the study of the history of drugs, their natural and synthetic sources, their biological and chemical properties, and desirable and undesirable actions of various drugs on living processes. These major subdivisions of pharmacology are introduced in this chapter.

All members of the health team need to have some knowledge of the different aspects of pharmacology, but the emphasis varies according to the individual's role in the use of drugs. The traditional role of the *pharmacist* has been to prepare, compound, and dispense drugs; however, pharmacists' comprehensive knowledge of drugs is beginning to be more fully utilized by other members of the health team. The *physician* prescribes medicinal agents and must therefore know the biochemical and physiological effects of given amounts of various drugs. As the individual who administers medicinal agents and who is frequently present to see their effects, both desired and undesired, the *nurse* needs to have in-depth knowledge not only of the biochemical and physiological changes to expect, but also of the specific techniques of administration and of possible adverse reactions. As the primary client educator, the nurse must also be prepared to instruct the client in self-administration as well as in the expected action and possible adverse effects of medicinal agents.

MAJOR SUBDIVISIONS OF PHARMACY

As described in Chapter 1, people originally learned by trial and error that various parts of plants, when prepared in specific ways, were useful in treating or curing illnesses. Historically, these substances were collected, dried, prepared, and administered by an individual who often fulfilled the functions of pharmacist, priest, and physician. As civilizations expanded and diversified, these functions came to be performed by different individuals. Some of the older terms used in pharmacology have broader definitions than the more specific ones of modern-day invention.

The ancient term **apothecary** is from the Greek word *apotheke* meaning storehouse, a place where the ingredients of drugs were stored, prepared, and given out. The term was originally applied to the prescriber of drugs, but, as the roles of physician and pharmacist began to separate, it came to apply only to the individual who stored, compounded, and dispensed drugs. It is sometimes used as a synonym for the terms *pharmacy* or *pharmacist*, or *drug store* or *druggist*.

The **apothecary system** is the system of weights and measures developed by apothecaries so they would have a common system of measuring drug ingredients. It is still used by some members of the health team and is described in Chapter 10.

Literally, **materia medica** means the materials used in medicine and the term originally indicated all the knowledge available about drugs. Books on materia medica, the forerunners of today's official books on drugs, called pharmacopeias, usually included the drug's name, physical properties, therapeutic action, uses, method of preparing or compounding or both, average dose, and adverse effects if known. Later the term came to be restricted to medicinal agents only; today it is seldom used.

Therapeutics is the branch of medical science dealing with the remedial treatment of disease. Historically, the emphasis was on drugs but therapeutics actually comprises all measures used in the treatment, cure, and prevention of illness, including nutrition, rest, hygiene, and psychotherapy.

By the 13th century, the distinction between physicians and pharmacists was growing, but pharmacy did not become an independent profession until the 19th century. As scientific knowledge about pharmacology expanded, the field began to be subdivided into specialties. Much of the leadership for these divisions came from the newly developed profession of pharmacy.

The term **pharmacy** is probably derived from the Greek word *pharmakevein*, meaning to practice witchcraft, to use medicines, or both. Today, the term refers to the art and science (or the profession) of preparing, compounding, and dispensing drugs. The technical aspects of pharmacy include the following:

1. *Metrology*—The study of weights and measures (see Chapter 10)
2. *Posology*—The study of drug dosages (see Chapter 11)
3. Methods of manufacturing, compounding, and dispensing drugs (including medicinal agents, poisons, and dressings)

Pharmacy is also used to mean a drugstore. Due to the influence of alchemists during the latter part of the Middle Ages, pharmacies in European countries are sometimes called chemist's shops.

The oldest branch of pharmacology is **pharmacognosy,** originally the study of the natural sources of drugs—plants, animals, and minerals. As the allied fields of botany and chemistry grew, pharmacognosy expanded to include the active constituents of naturally occurring drugs and, later, synthetic agents.

Pharmacotherapeutics is the branch of medical therapeutics concerned with drug therapy—the use of medicinal agents in treating, curing, and preventing illness. During the 20th century, this branch was expanded to include agents that assist in the diagnosis of disease.

When **pharmacodynamics** first developed in the late 19th century, it concerned the action of drugs. Today it also includes the changes drugs undergo from absorption to excretion. Using knowledge and investigative techniques from other sciences—bacteriology, biochemistry, pathology, and physiology—researchers in pharmacodynamics identify and describe the interrelationships between the physical and chemical properties of drugs, on the one hand, and the living cells and tissue responding to them, on the other. The field also includes the development of new synthetic medicinal agents through the correlation of alterations in the chemical structure of a drug with its resulting action.

Pharmacokinetics is a relatively new branch of pharmacology, originally a part of pharmacodynamics, concerned with the rates at which drugs are absorbed, distributed, stored, metabolized, and excreted. Because it includes the study of all the variables affecting the rate at which drugs are processed, some health team members use the term *pharmacokinetics* interchangeably with the older term *pharmacodynamics.*

People have been interested in the study of the effects of poisons, such as hemlock, poisonous mushrooms, and strychnine, since ancient times, not least because of their use in homicide and suicide. The initial development of **toxicology** was related to criminology. It expanded as people began to identify and study poisonous plants and to develop pesticides. Furthermore, certain medicinal agents were found to be poisonous to the body if given in too large a dosage; their poisonous or noxious signs and symptoms were called *toxic effects.* Today toxicology is concerned with the study of the noxious effects not only of natural and synthetic chemical agents, including drugs, but also of hazardous industrial and environmental chemicals as well.

As knowledge of drug action developed, it was discovered that some clients did not have the expected response to a particular medicinal agent. Unusual responses to a drug's normal dosage have been termed *idiosyncrasies* and include an overdose response, an underdose response, a completely different response, and entirely different symptoms. It was determined that many of these idiosyncrasies were inherited and the field of **pharmacogenetics** was founded in the 20th century to study genetically determined variations in drug response.

Comparative pharmacology is the study of the effects of drugs on various animals and on human beings. Since the beginning of the 20th century, all new drugs have been tested extensively on animals before being released for use on humans. However, since the human response to a drug is often different from that of an animal, it is advisable for health professionals to study the literature of comparative pharmacology carefully.

The branch of pharmacology that deals with the potential uses of a drug for human beings is called **clinical pharmacology.** Research is aimed at discovering new uses for known drugs, as well as at determining the possibilities of new chemicals (see Chapter 4).

THE PHARMACIST

A pharmacist prepares, compounds, and dispenses medications. To be licensed in pharmacy, an individual must (1) graduate from an accredited school of pharmacy, (2) complete a year-long internship in a retail pharmacy, in a hospital, or in the pharmaceutical industry, and (3) pass a state board examination in the state where the individual intends to practice. The professional education lasts from five to six years. Some schools of pharmacy are graduate schools. Besides supportive courses in chemistry, botany, and other sciences, the curricular emphasis is on the various aspects of pharmacology—pharmacokinetics, pharmacotherapeutics, pharmacognosy, toxicology, and technical and commercial aspects of pharmacy.

The professional opportunities for a pharmacist are not restricted to a retail pharmacy or hospital. Some pharmacists are hired for federal or state government services, including the military, the Food and Drug Administration, the United States Public Health Service, the Treasury Department's Narcotic Bureau, and various health departments. The pharmaceutical industry needs pharmacists in all stages of drug manufacture, from research to sales.

Each state has its own laws governing the practice of pharmacy. The state board of pharmacy administers and enforces the pharmacy laws. Other laws regulating the practice of pharmacy include the federal Food, Drug and Cosmetic Act, the Lee-Wheeler Act, postal regulations, patent and copyright laws, animal anticruelty laws, the Controlled Substances Act, the federal Caustic Poison Act, and local commercial and zoning laws.

Preparing and Compounding Drugs

In the past, the pharmacist prepared all medicinal agents and other drugs. Today most drugs are prepared by pharmaceutical manufacturers, and drugs are purchased by the pharmacist in specific dosages. Drugs that deteriorate rapidly, however, are purchased in a dried, powdered state ready for reconstitution by the pharmacist, usually by the addition of a specified amount of fluid. Moreover, products not compounded by pharmaceutical companies are still compounded by the pharmacist.

The pharmacist is also responsible for storing drugs properly and ensuring their potency by disposing of outdated medicines. Protecting medications from microbial contamination is another responsibility of the pharmacist, since all medicinal agents are aseptically treated when they are prepared.

Dispensing Drugs

Dispensing over-the-counter and prescription drugs involves more than giving out the designated amount of a medication in a specified form. To safeguard the client, the pharmacist will call the physician if (1) part of the prescription is illegible; (2) the dosage is inappropriate; (3) the medication interacts with other drugs the client is taking; or (4) there are other problems known to the pharmacist, such as allergies or inappropriate dosage form.

After the prescription order is filled, the medication container is labeled (Figure 2-1). If the drug must be prescribed by a licensed physician, as opposed to over-the-counter drugs, the symbol (or legend) *Rx* will appear on the label, or a statement such as the following: "Caution: To be dispensed only by prescription of a physician, dentist, or veterinarian."

The label should include the following information:

1. Client's name
2. Physician's name
3. Identification number of the prescription
4. Directions for taking the medication (amount and frequency)
5. Date prescription is filled
6. Name, address, and phone number of the pharmacy
7. Name of the proprietor or chief pharmacist

The name and strength of the drug may also appear on the label.

Other data will appear on the label as necessary. There may be instructions to the client, such as "shake well," "refrigerate," or "for external use only." Or there may be a warning or precaution, such as "keep out of the reach of chil-

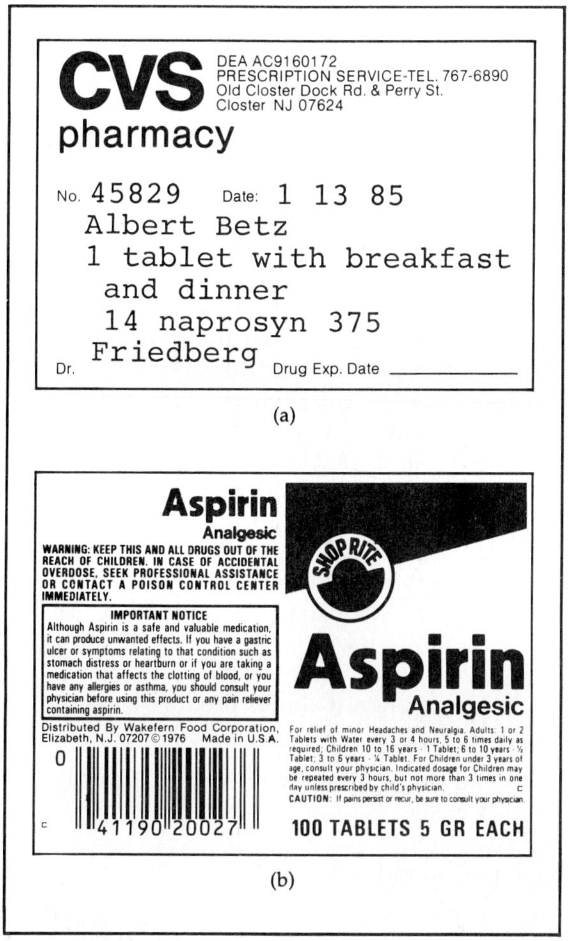

FIGURE 2-1 (*a*) Sample of prescription drug label (manufacturer); (*b*) Sample of over-the-counter drug label (manufacturer).

dren," "may be habit-forming," or "may cause unfavorable reactions—see your physician."

The federal Food and Drug Administration requires that over-the-counter drugs contain the following information on the label:

1. Name, strength, and dosage form of drug
2. Directions for use in all conditions for which the drug is used
3. Recommended dosage and frequency of administration for different ages and physical conditions
4. Route or method of administration
5. Specific directions, if any, such as "shake well" or "take after meals"
6. Maximum time the drug can be taken safely
7. Warnings, if any, about its use by children and in illness

Maintaining Control Records

Federal and state government agencies require pharmacists to keep records on narcotics, barbiturates, poisons, syringes, needles, and other medicinal products. Many of these products must be stored in single or double-locked areas and inventories must be rigorously maintained. As the products are dispensed, the following information must be recorded:

1. Name and address of client
2. Type, dosage, and quantity of product
3. Prescribing physician's name and narcotic number for certain substances
4. Signature of dispenser

Additional records must be maintained on the disposition of outdated products and wasted substances. If a glass container of phenobarbital elixir is accidentally dropped and broken, for example, this incident must be recorded and a witness must sign that the elixir was disposed of properly.

Records on Clients

Pharmacists working in drugstores and other community locations keep prescription records, particularly on clients who use their services frequently. The records often include the following information:

1. Name, address, and phone number of client
2. Client's chronic illnesses or allergies or both
3. Filling date; drug name, strength, dosage form; quantity of medication dispensed; and directions for use
4. Name or initials of the dispenser, the identification number, and sometimes the price
5. Any adverse reactions the client may have had

The pharmacist is likely to be the first health professional to realize that a potentially suicidal client is stockpiling medications from more than one physician. The pharmacist may also be the first to identify a drug abuser. Other potential problems can be recognized, such as a drug being taken over too long a period of time, in which case the physician and other members of the health team are notified. The health team should keep the pharmacist informed of a client's chronic illnesses, allergies, and adverse reactions to medications so that he or she can assist in identifying potential hazards.

The Pharmacist as a Source of Drug Information

Pharmacists are an excellent source of current information on prescription and over-the-counter drugs, including adverse effects, drug interactions, incompatibilities, new medicinal agents, and revisions in regulations. When a nurse is to administer an experimental drug, information on the medication can be obtained from the pharmacist. Pharmacists are valuable members of hospitals' and clinics' patient care committees for the information they can contribute about medication problems and for their evaluation of current drug literature. The pharmacist can also provide assistance when there is doubt about a medication. Furthermore, because of their background in botany, plant chemistry, and pharmacognosy, pharmacists are the most knowledgeable members of the health team in identifying accidentally ingested poisonous plant materials and the nature of such plants' active principles.

THE PHYSICIAN

The primary function of the physician in pharmacology is to prescribe medications for the diagnosis, treatment, cure, and prevention of illness. Most medical students receive a bachelor's degree in a program emphasizing anatomy, chemistry, physics, and other sciences. They then attend medical school, usually for four years. The curriculum in medical school emphasizes anatomy, physiology, biochemistry, pathology, therapeutics, pharmacology, and the application of pharmacotherapeutics. After completing a specified amount of time, usually twelve months, as *interns* in supervised clinical programs in internal medicine, surgery, pediatrics, and obstetrics, they take the state licensing examination. Newly licensed physicians can gain additional training as *residents* in certain areas of specialization. Although not yet licensed, interns may prescribe drugs if the orders are countersigned by licensed physicians; legally the countersigner accepts responsibility for the prescription. A medical student cannot order drugs.

Prescriptions

The word *prescription* comes from the Latin *prescriptio,* meaning "that which is written before" a treatment is given. The term can include other forms of therapeutics, such as diet, but it is usually restricted to drug therapy. A prescription is the order written by a licensed physician to a pharmacist for a specific medication for a client.

Until recently, prescriptions were written only in Latin, but now they are written in English, with some Latin abbreviations still used. Dosages are often written in metric measurements, although the apothecary and household systems are sometimes used. (See Chapter 10 for an explanation of the three systems.)

A prescription includes the following parts:

1. Date
2. Name and address of client, and age if client is a child
3. Superscription—R_x
4. Inscription—body of order
   a. Basis
   b. Adjuvant
   c. Corrective
   d. Vehicle
5. Subscription—instructions to the pharmacist
6. Signatura—instructions for the client
7. Physician's signature and DEA number when required

The **superscription** consists of the symbol R_x. The letter *R* is an abbreviation for the Latin word *recipe,* meaning "take thou." It is believed that the upstroke through the R represents a prayer to the god Jupiter, whose symbol is *v.* The R_x symbol is used for all drugs that require a prescription, and sometimes for drugs that can be sold over-the-counter.

The **inscription** consists of the name and amount of each medicinal agent. When the desired agent is available from a manufacturer, the inscription is called *precompounded.* Occasionally, a prescription must be compounded by the pharmacist; this type of inscription is called *extemporaneous, magistral,* or *compounded.* The inscription may consist of one or more of the following parts:

- *Basis*—The chief active medicinal agent
- *Adjuvant*—A medicinal agent that aids the action of the chief ingredient—for example, by aiding absorption or by increasing the action
- *Corrective*—An agent that modifies an undesirable effect of the basis or adjuvant, such as an unpleasant taste
- *Vehicle*—An agent that facilitates the administration of the other ingredients, such as a solvent for a solution, a base for an ointment, or a means of diluting the ingredients

The ingredients of a compounded inscription are written in the order given above. If there is more than one active medicinal agent, the most important or the most potent agent is written first. The total amount of each ingredient is given, along with its symbol of measure in the apothecary system; for example, five grains is written gr $\overline{\text{v}}$ and two fluid ounces is written fl. oz. ii. When the metric system is used, a line may be substituted for the period in order to avoid confusion:

Aspirin	6.0 g	Aspirin	6/0 g
Phenacetin	3.0 g	Phenacetin	3/0 g

The **subscription** consists of the instructions to the pharmacist. Some well-known Latin abbreviations, such as m which means mix, are still used, but otherwise most subscriptions are written in English. Since most pharmacists do not have the equipment to make compressed tablets, most powders are placed in capsules. The number of capsules required will be stated in the subscription—for example, "Mix and put (or divide) into 20 capsules" or "Make into 15 doses." Table 2-1 shows some abbreviations commonly used in the subscription portion of a prescription.

TABLE 2-1 Abbreviations for Instructions to the Pharmacist

Latin Word or Abbreviation	Meaning
add	add
aq bull (aqua bulliens)	boiling water
aq dest (aqua destillata)	distilled water
bulli	boil
chart (chartas)	powder
div	divide
et	and
filtra	filter
ft (fiat or fiant)	let there be made
m (misce)	mix
m et div in	mix and divide into
no (numero)	in number
pone	put
solve	dissolve
tere simul	rub together (refers to ointments)

The directions to the client is called the **signatura,** often abbreviated Sig or simply S. The term comes from the Latin word *signa,* meaning to "label" or "mark" the medication. The term *transcription* is sometimes used instead of *signatura* so that there is no confusion with the last element of a prescription, the physician's signature.

The client's instructions consist of the amount of medication to be taken, the frequency of administration, and any other directions or information, such as "for external use only," "poison," and "use to moisten dressings." The pharmacist uses prepared labels with little room for instructions, so the directions are kept as short as possible.

The instructions to the client are written in English since the signatura is to be quoted verbatim on the medication label. However, some physicians do use the Latin abbreviations to save time—for example, "1 tab tid pc" instead of "One tablet three times a day after meals." The pharmacist must interpret the abbreviation and write the instructions in English. Tables 2-2, 2-3, and 2-4 show some of the abbreviations commonly used in prescriptions and drug orders.

A prescription cannot be filled unless the *physician's signature* is included. When prescription blanks printed with the physician's name and address are used, it is not necessary for the full signature to appear unless it is a prescription for a narcotic. The federal Narcotic Law requires that the physician's full signature be written in ink or indelible pencil on all narcotic prescriptions, along with the prescriber's address and narcotic registry number.

TABLE 2-2 Abbreviations for Drug Preparations

Abbreviation	Meaning
ad lib	freely, as desired
$\bar{c}$	with
cap	capsule
elix	elixir
ext	extract
fl ext	fluid extract
inf	infusion
ol	oil
pulv	powder
qs	as much as necessary or required
qs ad ____	as much as necessary up to ____
$\bar{s}$	without
sol	solution
sp, Sp	spirit
supp	suppository
tab	tablet
tr, tinct	tincture
ung	ointment

Drug Orders

Drug orders are written by physicians for nurses to follow in hospitals and other community agencies and consist of the following:

1. Client's full name and location (either address or hosptial room number)
2. Name of drug
3. Dosage
4. Route or method of administration
5. Frequency of administration
6. Physician's signature

The name of the medication is written out, but Latin abbreviations are sometimes used to indicate the desired preparation. For example, the cathartic cascara is available as a tablet (abbreviated tab), a fluid extract (abbreviated fl ext), and an elixir (abbreviated elix). Latin abbreviations are also used to indicate the desired method and frequency of administration (see Tables 2-2, 2-3, and 2-4). Consequently, the Latin symbols must be memorized by nurses and other health professionals in order to interpret drug orders.

The dosage of drugs in drug orders, as in prescriptions, is written in the metric, the apothecary, or the household system of measurement. Since medication doses are sometimes written in one system and the drug is available in another system of measuring dosage, the nurse must be

TABLE 2-3 Abbreviations for Route and Location of Drug Administration

Abbreviation	Meaning
(H)	hypodermic (into subcutaneous tissue)
inhal	inhalation into respiratory tract
IM	intramuscular
ID or intraderm	intradermal
IV	intravenous
MM	mucous membrane
OD or R eye	right eye
OS or L eye	left eye
OU	both eyes
po	by mouth
PR, per rectum, or R	by rectum
SC, subc, or SQ	subcutaneous
SL	sublingual
topic	topical (apply to the skin)
ureth	urethral
vag	vaginal

TABLE 2-4 Abbreviations for Frequency and Time of Drug Administration

Abbreviation	Meaning
ac	before meals
bid	twice a day
hs	hour of sleep (bedtime)
pc	after meals
prn	when required, as needed (repeated doses)
qh	every hour
qid	four times a day
q2h, q3h, etc.	every two hours, every three hours, etc.
qd	every day
sos	one dose if necessary
stat	immediately
tid	three times a day

able to convert from one system to another (see Chapter 10).

As with prescriptions, the physician's signature must appear on the drug order. If this is omitted, it is not a legal drug order.

The Physician as a Source of Drug Information

Because of their education in pathology and therapeutics, physicians are excellent sources of information on the uses of drugs in various pathological states. The prescribing physician should be consulted whenever there is a question concerning therapeutic indications for a drug.

THE NURSE

Responsibility for the administration of medications belongs primarily to the nurse, who must not only be proficient in the techniques of administering drugs but also be able to teach the procedures to clients and their families when necessary. Since the nurse is with the client for longer periods of time than any other health professional, the continuous assessment of the client's response to a medication is part of his or her role as well.

Registered nurses must receive either a diploma from a hospital school of nursing or an associate or bachelor's degree from a college of nursing before they can take the state's licensing examination. Supportive course work emphasizes the behavioral and physical sciences; nursing courses emphasize nursing care in health and illness. In addition to a general overview of the subject, the pharmacology course covers metrology (the conversion of systems of weights and measures), posology (the calculation of dosage), the techniques of drug administration by various routes, drug therapy in healthy and diseased states, and assessment of desired and adverse drug responses. Baccalaureate programs also contain extensive course work in the various aspects of teaching clients and families.

In some localities, licensed practical nurses are allowed to administer medications. Their programs, which last from 12 to 18 months, include course work in pharmacology similar to that received by registered nurses, although it is not as comprehensive.

The nurse is subject to the federal and state laws regulating nursing and the administration of medications, such as the Harrison Narcotic Act and the federal Food, Drug and Cosmetic Act (see Chapters 4 and 5). Each state has its own set of laws governing nursing, often called the state's nurse practice act. A copy of a state's nurse practice act can be obtained by writing to the state's board of nursing, which enforces and administers the law.

Drug Administration

Once a drug has been prescribed by a physician and dispensed by a pharmacist, it is usually administered by a nurse. Since most drug orders contain Latin abbreviations, the order must first be translated. Table 2-5 shows some examples of such translations.

The commonly used abbreviations should be memorized (see Tables 2-3 and 2-4). To prevent an inaccurate translation, especially when infrequently used symbols appear, a comprehensive table of abbreviations should be available at all times. The nurse must also be able to convert dosages among the three measurement systems.

Although most medications are given orally, some are administered topically, to the skin or to a mucuous membrane, and others are given parenterally. Specific descriptions of the routes of administration are given in Part IV.

Continuous Assessment

Historically, physician-priests diagnosed clients and observed their responses to drugs. Physicians today assess clients to diagnose illness and to determine the effectiveness of the therapeutic prescription. Nurses not only assess clients to determine appropriate nursing care but also monitor responses to physician-prescribed therapeutics, including drug therapy. Since nurses spend more time with clients than do other health professionals, it is appropriate that they make continuous assessments that provide data for other health professionals. The observations of desired and untoward responses to medications

TABLE 2-5 Examples of Translations of Drug Orders

Drug Order	Translation
Aspirin gr x po q4h prn	Give 10 grains of aspirin by mouth every four hours as needed.
Maalox 30 ml po qid between meals	Give 30 milliliters of Maalox by mouth four times a day between meals (often at 10 A.M., 2 P.M., 6 P.M. and 10 P.M.).
Regular insulin 15 U sq $\frac{1}{2}$h ac	Give 15 units of regular insulin subcutaneously one-half hour before meals.
Vitamin B_{12} 1000 mcg IM qd	Give 1000 micrograms of vitamin B_{12} intramuscularly once each day (usually at 10 A.M.).

require monitoring that cannot be achieved during the physician's brief contacts with clients. The nurse's assessments are used to modify nursing care appropriately and to provide accurate data for other health professionals.

Untoward drug effects are described in Chapter 8. When an adverse response is noted, the physician should be notified immediately so that alterations in the client's drug therapy can be made.

The Nurse as Health Teacher

Providing accurate information to the public about health care is an increasingly important aspect of the nurse's role. Teaching clients and their families about drug therapy is part of this role. Hospitalized clients should be told pertinent information about the drugs they are receiving, including the desired effects of the medication. When clients are required to self-medicate, such as when they are discharged from a hospital, they and their families should be given detailed information about the medication. Nurses also have the opportunity to provide information about drug therapy when their own families, friends, or neighbors are medicating themselves with over-the-counter or prescription drugs.

There are times when giving instructions about a medication is the prerogative of another health team member. If a client is receiving an experimental drug or is unaware of his or her diagnosis, the physician is responsible for providing the client with this background information first. Other times, a client does not want his or her family to be aware of the diagnosis or prescribed drug therapy. Collaboration with other members of the health team is often necessary to protect the client.

Content of teaching plan

Most clients, particularly those who are administering their own medications, should be given the following information about their drugs:

1. Purpose—for example, antibiotics destroy pathogens; antihistamines prevent allergic responses; antihypertensive agents reduce blood pressure.

2. Measures that will promote the desired therapeutic response—for example, if the medication is a cathartic or laxative, adequate fluids (2 quarts per day) should be taken.

3. Method and frequency of administration—for example, antacids should be taken between, not during, meals; most antibiotics should be taken around-the-clock, since a certain blood level must be maintained.

4. Technique for administering the medication, if necessary, along with supervised practice—for example, insulin is administered by subcutaneous injection, vitamin B_{12} by intramuscular injection.

5. Duration of administration, if necessary—for example, antibiotics are to be taken until they are all gone, not until the symptoms subside.

6. Storage factors, if necessary—for example, some drugs need to be refrigerated; others may be destroyed by light so they must be kept in a dark place, such as a kitchen cupboard; still others may be destroyed by moisture so they should not be kept in the bathroom or kitchen.

7. Potential adverse responses, if necessary—for example, phenothiazine tranquilizers may cause an increase in the blood sugar of diabetic clients; if this occurs, the physician should be contacted for readjustment of the hypoglycemic agent.

8. Drug and food interactions—for example, absorption of oral iron preparations is enhanced by citrus juices (vitamin C) but decreased by milk (calcium phosphate); phenothiazine tranquilizers should not be taken with barbiturates, narcotics, or antihistamines except under the guidance of a physician.

9. Nonharmful side effects—for example, some drugs may cause changes in the color of urine or stool.

10. Measures that will prevent undesirable side effects—for example, some drugs should be taken with meals to prevent irritation of the stomach lining; others may cause constipation unless there are adequate fluids and bulk in the diet; some drugs cause drowsiness and clients therefore should not drive a car or operate heavy machinery while taking them.

Informed clients, who understand the purpose of their medication, are more apt to take their drugs willingly and responsibly. They are also less apt to abuse their medications by, for example, giving the drug to a friend for similar symptoms, discontinuing the drug when their symptoms disappear, taking more than the prescribed dosage, or taking the drug at the wrong time.

It is important that clients be advised of the major adverse responses they may have to a drug and what action they should take if such a response occurs. For example, clients who receive an anticoagulant drug, such as warfarin, should watch for the presence of blood in the urine or for bleeding in the mouth or under the skin. If these symptoms occur, they should discontinue the drug and call the prescribing physician immediately. Clients should also be informed of the nonharmful side effects of some medications—for example, black stools caused by orally administered iron preparations—so they will not be alarmed when the symptom occurs.

Parameters for teaching

Before a teaching plan is prepared, it is important to have some knowledge of the client and the client's home situation. In addition to the usual teaching factors, such as intellectual ability, vocabulary, and motivation to learn, the following items should be explored with the client:

1. Attitude toward drugs
2. Knowledge about the medication and other drugs
3. Ability to administer the medication
4. Ability to store the medication properly
5. Forgetfulness
6. Presence of children
7. Ability to pay for the medication

Attitude toward drugs in general can affect the individual's ability to administer the medication properly. Individuals who resist taking any form of medication need to know the purpose of the medication and the reasons for taking it on time. Individuals who abuse medications by adjusting the dosage or the frequency of administration need to understand why the drug must be taken a certain way.

If the client's previous knowledge about drugs, particularly the prescribed medication, is limited, a comprehensive teaching plan should be prepared, but if the client has previous knowledge, the teaching plan might consist of a review. If the client has misinformation about the medication, the errors should be corrected.

Sometimes a client who knows how to administer a medication is hampered by his or her physical condition. If failing vision might cause the client to take the wrong medication or the wrong dosage, measures to compensate for this disability must be explored, such as having a family member or friend identify the drug or the dosage or keeping the medication in a specific place away from other drugs. If a client's manual dexterity is limited by arthritis or other ailments, suppositories and injections may be difficult to administer. A friend or neighbor may be instructed, and the client's ability to use one of the various self-help aids, such as an automatic injector, may be explored. If a child-proof container is too difficult for an elderly client to open, a nonchild-proof container can be requested from the pharmacist when the drug is dispensed.

Because medications will deteriorate if they are not properly stored, it should be ascertained that the client has appropriate storage facilities. An individual living in a rooming house may not own a refrigerator; a person who owns a refrigerator may not be able to pay the electric bill; a wheelchair-bound client may not have a reachable cupboard. Alternatives for these individuals should be explored and identified.

Some clients, particularly the elderly and the mentally retarded, may be inclined to forget to take their medication. It can be suggested to them that they associate taking their medicine with a routine daily activity, such as meals for a drug taken three times a day. A prominently hung calendar can be marked as a reminder for medications that are taken daily or every other day.

The possibility of children being present in the client's home should be considered so that appropriate storage measures can be taken. Even though a client does not have children, grandchildren may visit periodically or the client may babysit for other children.

Some clients postpone having a prescription refilled or periodically skip a dose in order to save money. The importance of taking the medication regularly should be emphasized and alternative methods of paying for the drugs should be explored. A social worker might be notified to help determine whether the client is eligible for prescription coverage or reduced cost under a federal or state plan. Occasionally, medications can be paid for by a local organization or obtained without charge from a clinic.

The Nurse as a Source of Drug Information

Because of their educational preparation and experience, registered nurses are the best source of information on the administration of medications, the various aspects of teaching clients about drugs, and the assessment of desired and adverse responses. Some clients have difficulty taking drugs in certain forms or by particular routes. For example, swallowing tablets is difficult for some individuals and receiving injections is very frightening for others. The nurse can bring these difficulties to the attention of the prescribing physician so that alternatives can be considered.

Nurses are very knowledgeable about the aspects of a drug that will need to be explained to a client. They are also skilled at identifying clients' attitudes toward drugs, their potential for abusing their medications, and possible difficulties in administering their own drugs. These factors should be discussed with the physician and other members of the health team when necessary.

Identifying a client's responses to drugs is the responsibility of the nurse, the physician, and the pharmacist, but the nurse is in a better position than the others to observe subtle changes in response. Such changes should be discussed with the physician so that appropriate adjustments in the drug therapy can be made.

OVERLAP OF ROLES

The roles of various members of the health team in drug therapy are not always distinct and separate. Occasionally the physician must dispense drugs, particularly in rural areas. Sometimes the nurse compounds medicinal agents, and sometimes the physician or hospital pharmacist administers a medication. Since each member of the health team is legally responsible for his or her own actions, any questions that arise should be directed to the team member who usually performs that function. Therefore, professional collaboration is necessary to ensure safe and effective drug therapy for clients.

REFERENCES

Books

Deno, R. A. 1959. *The profession of pharmacy.* 2nd ed. Philadelphia: Lippincott.

Martin, E. W., ed. 1971. *Dispensing of medicine.* 7th ed. St. Louis: C. V. Mosby.

Martin, E. W., ed. 1978. *Hazards of medication: A manual on drug interaction, contraindications and adverse reactions with other prescribing and drug information.* 2nd ed. Philadelphia: Lippincott.

Osol, A., ed. 1980. *Remington's practice of pharmacy.* 16th ed. Easton, Pa.: Mack Publishing Company.

Articles

Armstrong, B. and others. 1976. "Fatal drug reactions in patients admitted to surgical surfaces." *American Journal of Surgery* 132:643–45.

Blackwell, B. 1973. "Drug therapy: Patient compliance." *New England Journal of Medicine* 289:249–251.

Lambert, M. L., Jr. 1975. "Drug and diet interactions." *American Journal of Nursing* 75:402.

Porter, J., and Jick, H. 1977. "Drug-related deaths among inpatients." *Journal of the American Medical Association* 237:879-81.

Rodman, M. J. 1974. "Dangers of unsupervised medication." *RN* 37:51.

Chapter 3

Pharmacognosy: Sources of Drugs

HISTORICALLY, MOST SUBSTANCES used as medicinal agents were derived from the various parts of plants—roots, stems, leaves, or flowers—although occasionally parts of animals and even some minerals were found to be useful. Today, many drugs are prepared synthetically in the laboratory; they have two advantages over crude, natural drugs. Since they are mass-produced, they are often less expensive than their natural counterparts. And, because the synthetic products are made under carefully controlled circumstances, they consist of pure chemicals without unwanted additives.

Familiarity with the physical and chemical properties of medicinal agents helps the nurse and physician to understand the responses their clients have to medications. Knowledge of pharmacognosy is also helpful to the nurse in understanding the special storage requirements of certain drugs and the interactions of some drugs with particular nutrients or with other drugs. This chapter will not only identify some of the physical and chemical properties of medicinal agents, but also indicate some of the measures that should be considered when medications are administered.

PLANT SOURCES

Plants are an age-old source of drugs. To kill their prey, African hunters dipped their spears into a poisonous solution prepared from the seeds of the *Strophanthus Kombé.* The active ingredient of this solution is known today to be one of the digitalis preparations, a cardiotonic. Opium, the juice of the unripe seeds of the opium poppy, *Papaver somniferum,* was known to have medicinal properties and to produce a euphoric state at least as early as the third century B.C. and is mentioned in the writings of Theophrastus. In fact, the word *opium* is derived from the Greek word for juice.

Drugs prepared by drying the leaves, roots, seeds, or other parts of plants contain substances other than the desired, active ingredient and are consequently called **crude drugs.** The health of medicinal plants, like all plants, is affected by the amount of water and nutrients they receive. Their condition in turn affects the amount of active ingredient they contain. Crude drugs are therefore less reliable than the isolated, pure active ingredient, called the **active principle** or **constituent,** that causes the desired therapeutic effect. When the separate active principle is administered, it is more potent and consequently given in smaller doses. For example, 1 mg of digitoxin administered orally has the same therapeutic effect as 1000 mg of crude digitalis leaf. The client receiving the pure active principle of a plant needs to be watched closely for signs and symptoms of overdose.

The pharmacologically active constituents of plants are grouped according to their chemical and physical properties and include alkaloids, glycosides, saponin, oils, resins, gums, organic acids, and tannins. Table 3-1 outlines the characteristics of each class of constituents and the implications of those characteristics for the medicinal use of the substance.

ANIMAL SOURCES

Plants were the chief source of drugs throughout history, but parts of animals were also used to some extent. The Chinese used the dried skin of the common toad to treat toothaches and bleeding gums. It was discovered much later that it contained the local hemostatic agent epinephrine. Powdered toad skin was also used in Europe during the Middle Ages to treat dropsy. Widespread use of animals as a source of drugs did not occur until the 20th century, when developments in physiology, biochemistry, and immunology made it possible. Serums had been introduced by Pasteur, Koch, Jenner, and others during the 1800s, but other discoveries—for example, thyroxin, discovered in 1914, insulin, 1921, and estrogen, 1923—were impossible without the technology of the 1900s.

Several potent drugs have been extracted from the organs of animals and found useful in treating human beings. Vitamin A is found in the liver of saltwater fish; insulin can be obtained from the pancreas of cattle and pigs; the hormone ACTH can be extracted from the anterior pituitary gland of cattle, pigs, and sheep.

The major drugs obtained from animals, including humans, are (1) hormones, (2) some

TABLE 3-1 Pharmacologically Active Constituents of Plants

Active Constituent	Characteristics	Implications
Alkaloids	Complex nitrogenous compounds (carbon, hydrogen, nitrogen, and oxygen)	
	Most are crystalline solids with bitter taste; they rarely appear as liquids.	Have fluids ready *before* administering the drug so that client doesn't have to hold drug in mouth.
	Effect is rapid and potent. (They are often synthesized chemically in laboratory.)	There is a danger of poisoning: observe client closely for signs and symptoms of overdose. Administer small doses.
	They dissolve poorly in water. Most combine with acids to form salts. They dissolve easily in water as a hydrochloride or sulfate, but sulfates are less soluble.	Their hydrochlorides and sulfates are used for injection; that is, morphine sulfate, *not* morphine, is injected.
	Names end in *-ine.* Examples: atropine, morphine, nicotine, papaverine, pilocarpine, quinine	Do not confuse with *non*-alkaloid drugs with same ending, such as epinephrine, procaine.
Glycosides	Combination of an aglycone and a sugar or sugar derivative. Aglycone (or genin) is a complex alcohol or phenol and produces the therapeutic effect.	
	Sugar element may aid the aglycones in entering the body cells.	
	The aglycone is separated from the sugar by acid or enzymatic hydrolysis.	Aqueous solution should be stored in alkali-free, hard glass ampules or phosphate-buffered solutions.
	Gastrointestinal secretions can inactivate glycosides to varying degrees.	Some are absorbed irregularly and poorly from the gastrointestinal tract and are therefore dangerous—for example, *Strophanthus,* squill, ouabain (digitalis glycosides).
	Names of official glycosides end in *-in.* Examples: digitoxin, santonin, salicin The most frequently used are digitalis glycosides.	
Saponins	Glycosides that resemble soap; they lower surface tension	In solution they tend to froth upon shaking.
	Many cause lysis of red blood cells and are powerful toxins.	
	Example: quassia	
Oils	Highly viscous liquids that are insoluble in water	

TABLE 3-1 ***Continued***

Active Constituent	Characteristics	Implications
Fixed oils	They are extracted from seeds or fruits of plants.	
	They are hydrolyzed (separated) by lipase in the intestines to form fatty acids and glycerin. Heat tends to decompose the oil.	Store in dark containers in a cool location.
	They feel greasy and don't evaporate easily.	They can be used on the skin as emollients.
	Example of food: olive oil Example of medicine: castor oil Example of vehicle used to dissolve other drugs: sesame oil	They tend to stain clothing.
Volatile oils	Obtained from the whole plant or its flowers, fruit, or seeds, they are also called *essential oils.*	
	They evaporate easily and seldom leave stains.	
	They have a particular odor—the aroma of the plant—and are usually colorless.	They are used as flavorings or for their odor.
	They rarely appear as liquids, usually as crystalline solids.	They tend to be irritating and mildly stimulating, with some antiseptic effect.
	Not soluble in water, they dissolve easily in alcohol, ether, and chloroform.	They are often dissolved in alcohol.
	Examples: oil of clove, peppermint, spearmint	
Resins	Solid brittle substance obtained from the sap of trees	
	Not soluble in water, they do dissolve in alcohol, ether, and various oils.	
	They are local irritants; for example, podophyllum is a constituent of belladonna and cascara.	When used as cathartics, they are harsh irritants to the small intestine and tend to produce large quantities of watery stools; they can cause considerable colic.
	Balsams are resins with benzoic acid or cinnamic acid added.	May be used on wounds for their stimulating, mildly antiseptic effect.
	Examples: balsam of Peru, Benzoin	
Gums	Complex sugars (heterosaccharides) obtained from the stems of plants as an exudate	

TABLE 3-1 *Continued*

Active Constituent	Characteristics	Implications
	Some will swell when water is added and form a gelatinlike substance called mucilage, a thick, viscid, adhesive liquid.	They make useful suspensions and emulsions that soothe irritated skin and mucous membranes.
	In the gastrointestinal tract, some will attract water (hydrophillic colloids) and cause a laxative effect.	
	Examples from nature: agar, psyllium seeds Synthetic example: methylcellulose	These are mild laxatives that add watery bulk to the stool.
Organic acids	Exist in plants as potassium and calcium salts; may be combined with a base such as an alkaloid	
	Examples: malic acid, citric acid	
Tannins	Complex substances present in many plants and the bark of some trees	
	They form insoluble complexes with alkaloids, glycosides, and several heavy metals.	They have been used as an antidote in poisoning when alkaloids, glycosides, or some heavy metals have been swallowed.
	Some have little or no action on the unbroken skin but an astringent action on mucous membranes of the gastrointestinal tract.	They may interfere with the absorbent action of activated charcoal and can cause constipation.
	They precipitate proteins when applied to abrasions, forming a mechanically protective film on the skin.	They have been used in the treatment of burns.
	Example: tannic acid	

vitamins, (3) some enzymes, and (4) antibiotics. (Some vitamins, enzymes, and antibiotics are derived from plants.) Some animal products are used extensively in medicine for applications other than drug therapy. For example, surgical dressings are sometimes made from wool and silk fibers (although most surgical dressings are made of cotton fibers and cotton wool), and animal substances are sometimes used to add form or flavor to medicinal agents. Table 3-2 indicates the characteristics of each group of agents and the implications for their use.

MINERAL SOURCES

Some valuable drugs are obtained from free elements or their compounds. Some of these inorganic chemicals were used therapeutically as antiseptics during the 19th century, such as iodine, discovered by Courtois in 1811 and used by a French surgeon in 1839. Various clays have been used as a traditional treatment for diarrhea for centuries. One remedy called for the powdering

TABLE 3-2 Pharmacological Substances Derived from Animals

Agents	Characteristics	Implications
Hormones	Metabolically active principles secreted by endocrine glands of mammals	
	Hormones are amino acids or steroids with diverse chemical structures. They include:	When taken orally, protein substances are inactivated by digestive enzymes; therefore they are given parenterally.
	Adrenalin—derived from adrenal glands or prepared synthetically	Foreign protein substances in the body can cause allergic and other adverse reactions.
	Androgens—steroidal male sex hormones found in urine or prepared partially by synthesis	Protein substances can deteriorate rapidly, particularly if proper storage is not maintained. Pharmaceutical directions for storage should be carefully followed and a substance should not be used if it changes color, shows other signs of deterioration, or is past its expiration date.
	Corticosteroids—steroids derived from adrenal cortex, though some are prepared synthetically	
	Corticotropins—polypeptides produced by pituitary gland	
	Estrogens—steroidal female sex hormones found in urine or ovaries	
	Gonadotropins—water-soluble glycoproteins produced by pituitary gland	
	Insulin—two polypeptide chains linked by two disulphides, produced by the isles of Langerhans in the pancreas	
	Oxytocin—octapeptide produced by pituitary gland	
	Thyrotropin—protein and carbohydrate produced by pituitary gland	
	Thyroxin—iodine compound produced by pituitary gland	
	Vasopressin—octapeptide produced by pituitary gland	
	Hormones are used for:	
	Replacement therapy when the function governed by a hormone is deficient—for example, insulin for regulating blood sugar levels	Since it is difficult to determine the exact amount needed, the client must be observed closely for a lack of hormonal response or for excessive activity.
	Short-term stimulation—for example, oxytocin for strengthening uterine contractions during labor	Some hormones may cause rapid excessive activity and require close observation.
	Therapeutic effect other than the direct endocrine response—for example, glucocorticosteroids for their antiinflammatory action	Prolonged therapeutic use may cause irreversible atrophy of the endocrine gland that produces that hormone, or disruption of other parts of the endocrine system, or both.

TABLE 3-2 *Continued*

Agents	Characteristics	Implications
		Therapeutic use may also require high doses, which could cause severe adverse responses.
Vitamins	Necessary for normal growth and the maintenance of health: they regulate metabolic processes.	
	They are not active as they exist but become active when transformed into other substances.	Therapeutic responses may not occur unless all other chemicals required for the transformation are present.
	They are obtained from both plants and animals.	
	Vitamins have diverse chemical structures and include both simple and complex substances. They differ considerably in physical properties; for example, vitamins A, D, E, and K are oil soluble, but vitamins C and the vitamin B complex are water soluble.	Each vitamin has its own characteristics and must be learned as a separate substance. Some interact with other nutrients and therefore must be given when that nutrient is not present; for example, iron interacts with calcium phosphate and so should not be given with milk.
	Vitamins are given when: They are lacking in the diet	Observe the client for deficiencies, usually a generalized response; for example, signs and symptoms of scurvy indicate a vitamin C deficiency. If lacking in the diet, they can usually be administered orally.
	The body is unable to absorb and/or process the vitamin.	It may be necessary to administer parenterally and/or with other substances.
Enzymes	Proteins or protein-containing substances that act as catalysts: they must be present for various chemical reactions to occur in the body.	(See implications of use of protein substances under Hormones, above.)
	They are obtained from living plants and animals but will continue to exert their catalytic effect when isolated.	
	They are colloidal substances that influence the rate of chemical reactions.	
	They are soluble in water and dilute alcohol and salt solutions, and are precipitated by acetone and concentrated alcohol.	
	Enzymes operate most effectively between 35 and 40°C (95–104°F)	They may be ineffective when administered to clients whose body temperature is below 35°C (95°F) or above 40°C (104°F).
	They are destroyed by heat and the ultraviolet rays of sunlight.	Protect enzymes from sunlight and other forms of ultraviolet light.

TABLE 3-2 *Continued*

Agents	Characteristics	Implications
	Each enzyme works best in a particular pH range.	Read pharmaceutical directions for proper pH; a slight alteration in client's pH may be required (for example, topically) by adding a nonharmful acid or alkaline substance.
	In order to function, some enzymes require the presence of a nonprotein substance called a *coenzyme.*	Some enzymes will not have the desired therapeutic effect unless their coenzymes are also administered.
	Examples: *Pepsin*—proteolytic enzyme used as a digestant	
	Hyaluronidase—enzyme that increases the subcutaneous tissue's ability to absorb fluid; used in clysis therapy	This enzyme has been used to decrease the size of myocardial infarctions.
	Trypsin—proteolytic enzyme used topically for debridement of necrotic tissue	When taken internally, it inactivates the antidiuretic hormone vasopressin.
Antibiotics (The term was originally limited to those substances produced by microorganisms; however, it has now been broadened to include synthetically produced chemical substances and substances from higher plants.)	Chemical substances capable of destroying and/or interfering with the life processes of microorganisms	
	The microorganisms that produce antibiotics are mostly from the following genuses: *Bacillus* *Cephalosporium* (fungus) *Micromonospora* *Penicillium* (fungus) *Streptomyces*	A client with an allergic reaction to one antibiotic may have the same response to other antibiotics from the same genus.
	Many deteriorate rapidly in heat or sunlight and/or when in aqueous solution.	Carefully observe pharmaceutical directions for storage. Dispose of reconstituted solutions when indicated; for example, some deteriorate within four hours of reconstitution. Label all reconstituted solutions with date and time.
	Antibiotics may cause an imbalance in normal body flora by destroying and/or inhibiting one or more of the normally present microorganisms, thereby allowing other flora microorganisms to flourish, such as the yeastlike organism *Candida albicans.*	They may cause diarrhea and other gastrointestinal disturbances, particularly with prolonged use.
	With the exception of broad spectrum antibiotics, which destroy and/or inhibit many pathogens, each antibiotic works only against specific pathogens.	Obtain a culture and determine the sensitivity of the pathogen before starting antibiotic therapy.

TABLE 3-2 *Continued*

Agents	Characteristics	Implications
Other animal substances:		
Beeswax	The melted and purified honeycomb of certain bees	It is used in plasters and ointments.
	It is insoluble in water, but soluble in warm fixed and volatile oils.	It cannot be washed off but can be removed by rubbing with a warm washcloth. Apply sparingly so that it can be removed and reapplied as necessary.
Lanolin	Purified fatty substance prepared from the wool of certain sheep	It is used as an emollient base for creams and ointments.
	It is insoluble in water, but soluble in ether and chloroform.	It can be removed by rubbing with a clean dressing containing small quantities of ether.
Gelatin	Gel-forming protein prepared from the tissues and bones of certain animals—boiling water converts insoluble collagens into soluble gelatin.	It is used in pastes and suppositories and as the covering for capsules.
	It is translucent and colorless or pale yellow.	
	Insoluble in cold water, it dissolves in hot water and will form a gel when cooled.	Capsules made of gelatin can be dissolved by placing them in hot water. Allow the solution to cool to 100°F before administering orally or through a feeding tube; flush feeding tube with at least 50 ml of warm water. If medicinal agent in capsule will be destroyed by heat, break capsule open with a file.
Honey	Saccharine secretion deposited by worker bees in a honeycomb	It is used as a vehicle for oral medicinal agents.
	It is a clear, thick, syrupy liquid but becomes granular and opaque over time.	Note expiration date of agents containing honey and dispose of the medication when expired.
	It contains sucrose, dextrin, formic acid, volatile oil, wax, and pollen grains.	Do not use with infants who have a sucrose intolerance: it may cause a mild allergic reaction.
	Medicines made with honey cause more of a laxative effect than do medicines prepared with a syrup vehicle.	It may cause diarrhea, particularly in infants; do not use with clients who already have diarrhea.

of the bowls of old clay pipes. The principal ingredients of such pipes would be kaolin and activated charcoal, both of which are used today to treat diarrhea.

Medicinal agents made from mineral sources contain few impurities and are relatively stable substances capable of keeping for prolonged periods of time. The expiration date on minerals prepared as liquids usually applies to the liquid vehicle, which, when it deteriorates—for example, by evaporation—makes the agent too concentrated for medicinal use. Minerals tend to precipitate out of solution, so many liquid mineral agents must be shaken well before using.

BIOLOGIC AGENTS

Biologic agents are medicinal products derived from living plants and animals. Technically, this category of agents includes the following:

1. Vaccines—made from bacteria, viruses, and rickettsiae
2. Immune serums
3. Human blood and blood by-products

Hormones, vitamins, and antibiotics are not included, according to the definition of biologics set forth by the Public Health Service. Vaccines, toxins, toxoids, and tuberculin agents are produced from plants; serums, antitoxins, and globulin are derived from animals.

Most biologic agents are used to provide immunity against a disease to individuals who do not have a natural or innate resistance to that disease. Individuals are said to have obtained or **acquired** immunity when they have antibodies against a specific disease. When specific antibodies are introduced (injected) into the body, the resulting immunity is called **acquired passive immunity**. When specific antigens are introduced into the body, forcing the body actively to produce its own antibodies, the resulting immunity is called **active immunity** and can be either a naturally acquired active immunity or an artificially acquired active immunity. The former is developed by actual contact with the disease, the latter by injection with a pharmaceutical preparation. (See Part XVII for further discussion of immunity.)

All biologics contain proteins and must be gathered, prepared, stored, prescribed, and administered carefully. They tend to deteriorate rapidly and must be stored in specific ways—for example, at specific temperatures. Most biologics must be injected because they are inactivated by digestive enzymes. Clients must be carefully observed for allergic and other adverse reactions to these protein substances. Table 3-3 outlines the characteristics of each group of biologic agents and the implications for their use.

SYNTHETIC AGENTS

Unlike natural substances, synthetic drugs are artificially produced by combining two or more compounds or elements. Some drugs, such as caffeine, epinephrine, and penicillin, can be made either synthetically or from natural substances. Synthetic drugs are pure chemicals and so do not cause the unwanted pharmacodynamic changes that natural substances sometimes produce due to adulterations. They also have a consistent potency, tend to be more stable, and are generally cheaper to produce. Consequently, synthetically produced drugs are becoming more and more common.

Synthetic agents may be either partially synthetic or totally synthetic. When a derivative of a natural substance is combined with a pure chemical, the end product is only partially synthetic. Many tranquilizers and chemotherapeutic agents are totally synthetic. The field of chemistry is so advanced that a minor alteration in a known agent's chemical structure can create a completely new drug, perhaps one with fewer adverse effects. Some pharmaceutical firms are now attempting to design new pharmacotherapeutic agents by programming computers with all the known information about specific drugs and making minor alterations in chemical formulae on the computer. This technique eliminates the lengthy and haphazard trial-and-error method used for discovering new agents in the past.

REFERENCES

Claus, E. P., and others. 1970. *Pharmacognosy.* 6th ed. Philadelphia: Lea and Febiger.

Trease, G. E., and Evans, W. C. 1972. *Pharmacognosy.* 10th ed. Baltimore: Williams & Wilkins.

TABLE 3-3 Biologic Agents

Agents	Characteristics	Implications
Vaccines	Contain living, attenuated, or killed viruses, bacteria, or rickettsiae	When used for inoculations, they stimulate antibody formation. Use disposable syringes when administering.
	They confer an active immunity after a prescribed number of injections.	A booster may be required after a period of time.
	Viruses and rickettsiae for vaccines are often grown in living chick or duck embryos.	Individuals who are allergic to eggs could have an allergic reaction to these vaccines.
	Bacterial vaccines are suspensions of attenuated or killed organisms in normal saline or other vehicles.	Rotate or shake gently before withdrawing the desired amount into a syringe.
	Vaccines may cause a temporary fever.	Inform client of potential response, which is usually treated with aspirin.
Other antigens	Used to determine hypersensitivity or allergy to specific antigen, or occurrence of previous infection They are prepared from plants and animals. Examples: pollens, tuberculins	Inject minute quantity of antigen intradermally. Client has positive reaction if erythema with a wheal is present within 24 to 72 hours.
Toxoids and toxins	Contain modified or inactivated poisonous bacterial waste products	
	Toxoids are toxins that are modified to reduce or eliminate toxic properties. They are used to stimulate the body's production of antibodies against the toxins. Example: tetanus toxoid	
	Toxins are often unmodified by-products of bacterial growth.	Minute quantities of toxins are used as diagnostic tools to determine whether the client already has antibodies against the disease. A positive reaction indicates the individual probably had the disease at one time. Example: Schick test for diphtheria Toxins are also used to prepare antitoxins.

TABLE 3-3 ***Continued***

Agents	Characteristics	Implications
Antitoxins	Contain toxin antibodies	They are used either as a cure for the disease or as a means of producing passive immunity.
	Most are produced by injecting horses with the disease toxin and then extracting the horse's serum.	Individuals who are allergic to horse serum may have an allergic reaction to these antitoxins.
Antivenins	Contain venin antibodies (Venoms are poisonous excretions produced by animals, such as snakes and spiders.)	They are used as an antidote to a particular venom after a client has been bitten. It is important to know the exact identity of the animal—for example, copperhead snake—since each venom has its own antivenin.
Other antiserums	Contain antibodies against specific bacteria or viruses They are prepared in a manner similar to that used for antitoxins.	They are used as either a cure for the disease or as a means of producing passive immunity. Example: antiserums against certain influenzas
Immune globulins	Contain antibodies against specific diseases	They provide immediate artificial passive immunity.
	They are obtained from the blood of a human being who has survived the specific disease.	Allergic reactions are less common than with preparations from animal sources.
	They contain several antibodies.	They are useful against several diseases other than the one for which they are injected.
Human blood and blood by-products:		
Whole human blood (500 ml/unit)	Contains many potential antigens	It must be carefully matched with client's blood in order to avoid allergic reactions.
	Blood cells and other elements will precipitate upon standing.	Rotate gently to suspend the cells and elements before administering.
	It is stored at temperatures between 1° and 10°C.	It may cause adverse responses if given at this temperature: administer with a blood warmer.
	Nonrefrigerated blood tends to contain bacterial growth after two hours.	Administer complete transfusion in two hours or less.

TABLE 3-3 *Continued*

Agents	Characteristics	Implications
	Whole blood contains an anticoagulant	If anticoagulant is citrate ion, use blood within 21 days; if anticoagulant is heparin, use blood within 48 hours.
	RBCs (red blood cells) are hemolyzed by dextrose solutions.	Use IV isotonic saline solutions before and after transfusion.
	RBCs are relatively large and fragile.	Administer through a large IV lumen—that is, 18-gauge IV catheter. Bags are used instead of bottles: handle gently.
Packed blood cells (250–300 ml/unit)		Volume is determined by the hematocrit of the donor.
	Contains all but the serum of human blood and is therefore viscous	Prepare within six days after the blood is drawn.
		Administer through a large IV lumen and handle bag gently.
		The use of a blood pump may be required to ensure that packed cells are transfused within two hours.
		Use IV isotonic saline solutions before and after transfusion.
Platelets (approximately 30 ml/pack)	Consists primarily of the tiny, clear, disk-shaped bodies called thrombocytes (platelet pack)	Match with client's blood in order to prevent allergic reactions.
	Prepared from fresh whole blood	*See* implications under Whole human blood, above.
Albumin (25 g/100 ml)		Other concentrations are also available.
	Contains most of the protein found in human blood	
	It is treated with heat to destroy any hepatitis virus present.	Cross-matching is not required.
	It assists in the maintenance of the blood's osmotic pressure.	It is used as a plasma expander to treat shock; it is also used to treat hypoalbuminemia.
Plasma protein fraction (100 ml of solution contains 4.5–5.5 g of protein)	Contains alpha, beta, and gamma globulins	Gamma globulin contains most of the immune antibodies and is often used to prevent certain infections.
Fibrinogen	Protein substance obtained from frozen human blood	

TABLE 3-3 ***Continued***

Agents	Characteristics	Implications
	When in solution, it converts into fibrin in the presence of thrombin.	It is used to control bleeding, such as in afibrino-genemia of pregnancy.
Thrombin	Protein substance prepared from the prothrombin of pigs by adding thromboplastin and calcium	It is used to control localized bleeding.
	Prepared as a powder, it is then reconstituted into a solution; the solution deteriorates rapidly.	Use solution within a few hours.
Antihemophilic factors	Prepared promptly from human plasma and then frozen or changed into a solid	They are used to prevent and treat bleeding episodes in hemophiliacs.
Plasma (200–250 ml/unit)		Volume depends on the hematocrit of the donor.
	Serum is removed from fresh whole blood when packed cells are prepared.	Cross-matching is not required but it may be done to prevent adverse reactions.
	It contains albumin, other plasma proteins, and the coagulation factors.	It is used as a plasma expander and to treat bleeding episodes—for example, in hemophiliacs.
		It is used to prepare other plasma products.
	It may be stored as fresh frozen plasma for two years.	Plasma is often available when cross-matched blood can not be obtained. It is often used in emergencies.
Interferons (experimental substance)	One unit is able to protect one-half of a cell culture plate from a virus.	They are measured in units of activity. They may prove to be effective against viral infections and possibly even some forms of cancer.
	Three types have been isolated: from WBCs—produced in tiny quantities from fibroblasts—extracted from the foreskin of circumcised infants from T-lymphocytes	Available now only for experimental use, they will continue to be extremely expensive—$150 a day—until they can be mass-produced. This is immune interferon.
	Interferons are species specific.	They must be obtained from human blood.
	They are technically difficult to isolate.	They contain numerous impurities depending on technique used.

TABLE 3-3 ***Continued***

Agents	Characteristics	Implications
Synthetic blood	Two forms are under experimentation:	They have been released for limited clinical use.
	one prepared from animal blood	
	one prepared synthetically	This form may be given to clients whose religion prevents the use of human or animal blood—for example, Jehovah's Witnesses.

Chapter 4

The Regulation and Control of Medicinal Agents

DRUGS ARE CONTROLLED by laws and regulations from the time the raw materials are collected to the time the final products are administered. Laws regulate drugs in current use, poisons, unlawful drugs, and the development of new therapeutic agents.

Drugs must meet the minimum requirements of purity, potency, and quality set forth in established *drug standards,* which provide guidelines for the pharmaceutical industry and protection for the public. Drugs are tested by their manufacturers and by government inspectors from the Food and Drug Administration to ensure that they meet the standards, which are listed in official drug books called *compendia.*

The Food and Drug Administration also carefully controls the development of new agents, regulating the phases of testing and approving the release of new products. Health team members are often involved in prescribing, dispensing, or administering experimental drugs; they should be aware of the information available on these substances and understand the techniques and procedures used to evaluate them.

This chapter describes the various laws and regulations that apply to medicinal agents in each phase of production and use. The potentially hazardous substances regulated by the comprehensive Drug Abuse Prevention and Control Act are discussed in Chapter 6.

THE STANDARDIZATION OF DRUGS

In order to protect the public from impure drugs of poor quality and questionable potency, the federal and state governments have enacted legislation designed to standardize the ingredients in medicinal agents. To ensure adherence to these strict standards, drugs are evaluated at all stages of production by a variety of scientific techniques.

The Food and Drug Administration

The federal *Food and Drug Administration (FDA),* a branch of the Department of Health and Human Services with headquarters in Washington, D.C., administers most of the federal laws concerned with the pharmaceutical industry, the major one of which in effect today is the Pure Food, Drug and Cosmetic Act. The FDA maintains several district chemical and microanalytical laboratories; it also operates the National Center for Drug Analysis in St. Louis, Missouri. The FDA is primarily concerned with the interstate commerce of drugs and drug ingredients, since each state has its own laws as well. Inspectors are stationed in the field throughout the United States and also work with customs officers at ports of entry. The FDA is authorized to see that the pharmaceutical industry observes all of the minimum standards set for drugs.

Compendia

Every country has its own list, or *compendium,* of officially accepted drugs, called a *pharmacopeia,* containing the standards for each drug's identity, strength, quality, and purity. The accepted techniques of evaluation are often included as well.

In the United States, the Pure Food and Drug Act of 1906 designated the *United States Pharmacopeia* (U.S.P.) and the *National Formulary* (N.F.) as the official compendia. These books contain the following information on each official drug:

1. Source
2. Physical properties—for example, solubility
3. Chemical properties—for example, composition of the drug
4. Method(s) of chemical and/or biological assay
5. Usual dose and method(s) of administration
6. Major therapeutic use(s)
7. Other related information—for example, storage factors

All medicinal agents appearing in the U.S.P. or N.F. must meet the minimum standards or requirements listed. These volumes are currently revised every five years and supplements are issued when necessary. In general, the U.S.P. lists drugs with only one active principle and the N.F. lists drugs compounded from more than one active principle. These two sources are now published together as a single volume, which is abbreviated U.S.P. The U.S. *Homeopathic Pharmacopeia* was also accepted as an official reference in the 1906 legislation.

The U.S.P. is published in Spanish as well as English, and the Spanish version has been accepted by Puerto Rico and the Philippines. Several Central and South American countries use it as their official compendium as well.

In the United States, drugs listed in the U.S.P. are called *official drugs.* Medicinal agents that have been accepted for forthcoming publication in this compendia but do not appear in the current issues are called *unofficial drugs.* A great number of medicinal agents have never appeared in the U.S.P. and are called *nonofficial drugs.* Many are relatively new and require further testing of their therapeutic value before they will be considered for inclusion.

Other Regulations

Even though a drug does not have official status, it must still meet rigid minimum standards before the FDA will allow it to be used. Many of the techniques that are to be used in analyzing drugs are listed in the U.S.P. Other methods for drug analysis are listed in the FDA's Food and Drug Technical Bulletin #1, entitled *Microscopic-Analytical Methods in Food and Drug Control.*

All new drugs must be analyzed and tested on animals before they are used on humans. New agents must also be tested clinically on humans under controlled conditions before they are released for general use, as described later in this chapter.

In 1962, legislation was passed mandating that the *therapeutic index* of new drugs be high enough to warrant their use; otherwise they would not be allowed to reach the public. Therapeutic index refers to the relationship between the desired and undesired effects of a particular drug and is measured as the ratio of toxic dose to therapeutic dose. The closer the ratio is to 1.0, the more dangerous the drug. Drugs marketed before 1962 are also being evaluated for their *therapeutic effectiveness.* Some drugs have been taken off the market entirely by the FDA because they have been deemed either ineffective or of little therapeutic value.

Biologic agents are regulated by a different part of HEW—namely, the Division of Biologic Standards (DBS) of the National Institutes of Health. Responsibility for biologic agents was given to HEW by the 1902 Virus Law and the present Public Health Service Act. The DBS issues specific standards for biologic agents as well as regulations designed to protect the public from poor quality and contaminated products.

Crude medicinal ingredients are often prepared and stored by individuals who are neither pharmacologists nor pharmacists. These agents are then mass-produced by machines. Consequently, the pharmaceutical industry and the regulating agencies must inspect each phase of drug production carefully to ensure the maintenance of minimum standards.

THE PREPARATION OF DRUGS

The raw materials for most drugs are derived from wild or cultivated plants found all over the world. Many of the wild plants are collected by local individuals and brought to a designated area. For example, podophyllum and white pine are gathered in sections of the Blue Ridge Mountains and brought to a collection station at Asheville, North Carolina. The quality of the plants varies according to the environmental conditions under which they grew and the time they were harvested. If the plant parts are harvested at the wrong time, the amount of active principle they contain will be low and the quality and appearance of the substance will be be affected. Cultivated plants are usually harvested by skilled botanists, but wild plants are often collected by individuals with less education in botany.

The plant parts are dried to remove enough moisture to prevent chemical changes and the growth of bacteria and mold. The heat must be carefully regulated so that it is high enough to vaporize the moisture but low enough not to affect the constituents. Unwanted substances, such as dirt, sand, excess plant parts, and other adulterants are removed; this phase is called *garbling.* The material is then packaged for transportation and storage. During each of these processes, the plant material is carefully examined to determine its quality.

Proper packaging and storage help to preserve the substances, which are sold in various forms, such as bags of seeds, bundles of roots, bales of compacted leaves, and containers of coarsely ground powder. If the bales are not packed hard, excessive moisture is absorbed and destructive changes occur. Even the presence of light can cause deterioration of some substances. Many packages are kept at 65°C or lower to destroy insects. The plant material is often stored in metal or amber glass containers that are airtight, moistureproof, lightproof, and rodentproof.

Drugs derived from animal sources are prepared from wild or domestic animals. Fish, such as cod and halibut, are purchased from fishermen. Hogs, sheep, cows, and other animals are raised under specified environmental conditions and then purchased from slaughterhouses. When possible, insects are attracted to a designated area by supplying them with food and shelter; bees are maintained and propagated this way. Every drug ingredient from an animal source is processed and purified in a different way according to set standards. Most biologic drug materials are stored at temperatures between 2° and 10°C to preserve their quality.

The raw material is transported to a designated area and stored until it is purchased by a pharmaceutical company. The manufacturer evaluates the substance to confirm its identity and determine its purity and quality. The FDA may analyze substances when they are brought into the country or transported from state to state.

Any unwanted changes in the drug substances or any undesired additions to them are called **drug adulterations**. The most common adulterations today are (1) substandard active principles, (2) the presence of microorganisms, and (3) deterioration of the ingredients due to moisture, heat, light, insects, or aging. **Admixture,** or the accidental or careless addition of an unwanted substance, is also a problem, although some admixture frequently occurs, such as the inclusion of stems with digitalis leaves. The amount of unwanted substance must not exceed a designated limit.

There are two forms of illegal drug adulterations—namely, the *substitution* of an entirely different substance for the product and the *sophistication* of the product by the addition of inferior material or a counterfeit substance with the intent to defraud. For example, the addition of a material similar in appearance to the original substance in an attempt to expand it is a fraudulent act. Substitution and sophistication were common during the latter half of the 19th century, but the 1906 Pure Food and Drug Act stopped these practices by stipulating that drug materials could be examined by government inspectors. The development of better chemical techniques to evaluate drugs facilitated the enforcement of the law.

THE MANUFACTURE OF ACTIVE PRINCIPLES

Depending on the nature of the chemicals, various manufacturing techniques are used to separate active principles from crude substances. Some active principles are extracted by the use of solvents; others are isolated by physically removing the unwanted elements by centrifuging or various chemical techniques. Once the active principle is separated and purified, flavoring and other nonactive agents are added and the substance is mixed. The mixture is then sent through a tablet press, placed in capsules, or prepared in some other drug form, and finally packaged and labeled for shipment. Aseptic technique is observed at all times.

Drug companies must observe rigid quality control throughout the entire manufacturing process, guarding against adulteration, contamination by microorganisms, unacceptable variations in potency, and mislabeling. Government inspectors also evaluate the various phases of the manufacturing process to ensure that specific official standards are maintained.

METHODS OF EVALUATING DRUGS

For centuries, the only means of evaluating drugs was macroscopic: measurement of weight and volume and evaluation of certain physical properties. Microscopic examination of drugs began in the 19th century and chemical and biological evaluation was developed in the 20th century. Today there are even more advanced techniques available for evaluating medicinal agents, such as chromatography.

Macroscopic evaluation refers to the examination of drugs for their appearance, color, distinctive markings, shape, size, odor, taste, feel, and sometimes the sound made when vegetative fibers are broken or "snapped." Since this method relies on the sense organs, it is often referred to as **organoleptic** evaluation.

The *apothecary system* of weights and measures was developed to facilitate macroscopic evaluation of drugs. This system of determining dry weight and liquid volume provided an accurate method of measurement for growers, buyers, and compounders of medicinal ingredients, as well as a way of determining equivalencies of drugs. Today the more accurate metric system is used for most medicinal agents.

Some drugs, particularly the alkaloids and oils, both fixed and volatile, are evaluated by their *physical properties*, including solubility, specific gravity, melting and solidification points, optical rotation, and refraction index. Every substance has its own physical characteristics that help investigators identify it and assess its purity.

Microscopic evaluation is used to identify the active principles of powdered drugs and to recognize the presence of various adulterations. Special microscopes and a variety of reagents are required to evaluate particular physical and chemical properties. Many drugs can now be identified by the form and structure of their crystals; this technique is called crystallography.

Neither macroscopic nor microscopic evaluation provides an indication of a drug's potency. Potency can be determined by **chemical assay** for some drugs and **biological assay** for others. Chemical analysis is used whenever possible because it permits accurate identification of the amount of each ingredient present. The amount of active principle present in a given weight of the material depends on the manufacturing method used to extract it from the crude drug. The purer the extraction, the more potent the drug. If the drug is too pure, a suitable admixture, such as sucrose, is added to the drug, so that a given quantity of the drug has a standard potency.

Not all medicinal agents can be analyzed chemically, either because the active ingredients cannot be isolated or because there is no known means of chemically evaluating them. Biological assay or **bioassay** is necessary to analyze and standardize these agents' pharmacologic activity. Standardization is achieved by determining the amount required to produce a specific effect on a living animal or on a suitable excised animal organ. Microorganisms, frogs, rats, mice, guinea pigs, pigeons, rabbits, and dogs are the most frequently used laboratory animals. The potency of drugs tested by bioassay is measured in *units of activity* or by a U.S.P. reference standard. For example, powdered digitalis leaf contains several glycosides. When it is manufactured, 100 mg of the substance must contain one U.S.P. digitalis unit. If the powdered digitalis is too potent, an admixture of lactose, starch, or another suitable diluting agent is mixed with it until the U.S.P. reference standard is met. Other medicinal agents whose potency is measured in units include some antibiotics, insulin, and heparin—for example, 40 units of NPH insulin in each milliliter of solution.

Chemical assays are preferable to bioassays because they are more definitive in determining potency and because they are often less expensive. Consequently, drugs that are chemically analyzed are usually less expensive than those that are bioassayed.

NEW MEDICINAL AGENTS

Pharmaceutical companies maintain research laboratories that screen thousands of potential agents each year for evidence of physiologic activity. Very few of these agents ever show enough promise to warrant development.

The Testing Process

Step A—Screening

A potential agent is chemically and biologically tested to determine (1) its chemical formula and properties; (2) its potential use and effect on humans; and (3) its potential toxic effects. When the substance is examined in a test tube, or chemically, it is called **in vitro** testing, and when it is tested in the living tissue of animals, it is called **in vivo** testing.

Since the acceptance of the therapeutic index regulation, the development of new synthetic agents with a high therapeutic value and low level of toxicity has been facilitated by the use of computers in some research laboratories. Some potential agents with therapeutic abilities are accepted for further development despite the indication that they will be highly toxic in humans; some chemotherapeutic agents for the treatment of cancer fall into this category.

Step B—Preclinical evaluation

Promising agents are then systematically screened in more than one species of test animal for the following factors:

1. Mechanism(s) of action(s), including the dosage required to produce a specific effect
2. Bioavailability (biological availability)—how much of the substance is free to act rather than stored in fat, bound in protein, or otherwise rendered unavailable
3. Rates and routes of absorption
4. Distribution—which body organs accumulate the substance and at what rate
5. Excretion—how the substance is excreted and at what rate
6. Metabolism—how the substance is changed or detoxified
7. Toxicity, acute and chronic, including the substance's ability to cause either mutation of cells and/or cancer (long-term toxicity is investigated later)
8. Other pertinent data, depending on the substance—for example, drug interactions

The FDA issues general guidelines for testing drugs in animals. Extensive toxicity studies are done to determine the safety of the substance for use in humans. The therapeutic index and other techniques are used in reporting the safety of experimental substances. Levels of effectiveness and toxicity are reported for each of the potential routes of administration: oral, subcutaneous, intramuscular, intravenous, topical, intraperitoneal, and so on. The animals' adverse responses are also examined.

The *preclinical research reports* are then prepared; they include all the information obtained thus far. Since animals do not have the same physiology as humans, the reports are carefully studied by experts to determine the efficacy of trying the substance on humans.

Step C—Clinical evaluation

If a substance has been determined to be safe enough for a controlled, limited trial on humans, certain forms are completed and submitted to the FDA, including the *Notice of Claimed Investigational Exception for a New Drug* (IND). The IND includes the known information on the substance as well as a description of proposed clinical studies. Each investigator must also submit forms indicating his or her competence to undertake the clinical testing. Each volunteer subject must sign an informed consent for the clinical study to be conducted on him or her. The guidelines for conducting clinical studies were published in 1970 by the FDA.

Clinical investigation of a new agent has four phases. The volunteer may either be healthy or have a specific illness for which the agent may be effective. The studies may be conducted in clinics, hospitals, nursing homes, or other institutions—for example, prisons—or in physicians' private practices. Periodic progress reports are required by the FDA and studies may be discontinued at any point at which an investigator or the FDA considers it "unsafe to continue."

Phase I—Initial evaluation of agent Depending on the substance, the agent is tested on one or more healthy subjects to determine its effect and toxicity in humans, as well as the degree of human tolerance for it. These tests provide the following information about the drug:

1. Rates of absorption (by route)
2. Drug blood/serum levels in relation to dosage
3. Amount of toxicity to various body organs or systems
4. Excretion factors
5. Biotransformation factors
6. Distribution factors
7. Any adverse responses

Phase II—Expanded evaluation of agent A small number of diseased subjects, or healthy subjects in some cases, is then tested. Information similar to that in Phase I is collected. If the FDA considers the agent potentially therapeutic and relatively safe, the agent will be released for Phase III testing.

Phase III—Clinical trials In general, 1000 subjects or fewer are used. The investigator assists selected physicians who treat clients with the disease for which the agent may be effective. A control group of subjects may also be included. The physicians compare the agent's effectiveness with that of the standard drugs in use for the illness. The volunteers are closely observed for adverse responses as well as favorable ones. *If the substance was not clinically tested in children, the drug label must indicate that it is not recommended for pediatric use.*

When these studies are completed, a *new drug application* (NDA) form is completed and submitted to the FDA. By this time, the long-term or chronic toxicity studies in animals have been completed and are included in the report. After studying the reports, the FDA determines whether the drug is therapeutic and relatively safe. If so, it approves the NDA and allows the product to be released for Phase IV use. The FDA must also approve the information to be included on the drug package insert provided by the pharmaceutical company.

Phase IV—Clinical evaluation of a newly marketed agent The chronic toxicity of the new agent in humans is still not known. It is now released to many physicians for the treatment of clients and careful note is taken of all adverse reactions, which are then reported to the FDA. Rare side effects and chronic toxicity data are tabulated and reported. Since 1970, the FDA has had the authority to withdraw an agent under the principle of "imminent hazard" if a potential or actual problem is believed to exist.

Administering New Medicinal Agents

Nurses, physicians, and pharmacists are involved with new agents in Phase IV and sometimes Phase III of clinical studies. Legally, they must obtain as much information on the new product as possible before they prescribe, dispense, or administer it. During Phase III, the physician and pharmacist receive information from the drug's investigator on the data collected in Phases I and II. During Phase IV, a drug package insert is available. Before administering these new agents, the nurse can obtain the available data from the pharmacist or physician or both.

Since the clinical trials of Phase III essentially concern the agent's therapeutic effectiveness, as well as the adverse reactions it may produce, the nurse and physician should collaborate when assessing the client's responses. The physician has specific forms to complete; the nurse should carefully note the client's responses in his or her record. The information available from the investigator will help direct attention to potential adverse responses, therapeutic responses, and other pertinent observations. Certain groups of drugs tend to cause similar adverse responses, for which clients should be particularly assessed. Table 4-1 shows some examples of frequently encountered adverse responses to drug groups.

Since the physician has the primary responsibility for new agents in clinical trials, he or she must obtain the consent from the subject. If the nurse is not present when the consent is signed, the physician should inform the nurse about the discussion so that the client receives consistent information. The client's questions should be directed to the physician.

LAWS GOVERNING MEDICINAL AGENTS

At the beginning of the 20th century, the American public was essentially unprotected from hazardous drugs and fraudulent sales and advertising practices. In 1906, in response to complaints, Congress passed the *Pure Food and Drug Act,* which not only recognized the U.S.P. and the N.F. as the official American drug compendia, but also prohibited drug adulterations and false or misleading labeling. The law required that all drugs transported between states be labeled with the type and amount of their contents.

In most cases, however, the actual safety of drugs was not subjected to legislation until 1937, when sulfanilamide elixir caused more than 100 deaths. The federal *Food, Drug and Cosmetic Act* was passed in 1938 and required that all new drugs be tested on animals for toxicity before being used on humans. It also required more precise labeling of medicinal agents. This law also stated that the U.S.P. and N.F. standards must be followed.

The 1938 Act has been amended several times. The *Durham-Humphrey Amendment* of 1951 required that all prescription drugs be labeled "Caution: Federal law prohibits dispensing without a prescription." Labels on over-the-counter drugs (OTC) were to contain information on the

TABLE 4-1 Examples of Frequently Encountered Adverse Responses

Drug Group	Adverse Responses
Antineoplastic agents	Leukopenia, resulting in an inability to fight infections—for example, upper respiratory infections, infected cuts
Barbiturates	Respiratory depression; cause tolerance; may require increasingly large doses to produce the same response over a period of time
CNS depressants	Respiratory depression, coma, slurred speech, seizures, cardiovascular collapse
Iodides	Skin reactions—rashes, urticaria, pruritus
Opiates	Respiratory depression, addiction, pulmonary edema, coma, depressed sensorium
Penicillins	Allergic reactions—hives, urticaria, gastrointestinal disturbances when taken orally
Phenothiazines	Orthostatic hypotension, cardiovascular disturbances
Salicylates (aspirin)	Gastrointestinal bleeding
Sulfonamides	Allergic reactions—skin reactions, rash, pruritus, urticaria
Tranquilizers	Cause tolerance; may require increasingly large doses to produce the same response over a period of time

use of the drug and such warnings as "See a physician if cough lasts more than a few days."

Within another ten years it became apparent that tests for acute toxicity did not sufficiently protect the public from agents with long-term toxicity. For example, the tranquilizer and hypnotic thalidomide was tested for effectiveness and toxicity between 1953 and 1957 in Europe and was shown to be very effective and to have little toxicity in animals and humans. It was prescribed for thousands of pregnant women in Europe. Following its usual procedure, the FDA released this product to only a few physicians in the United States for investigational purposes. By 1961 the long-term toxicity and teratogenic effects of thalidomide were recognized. In the United States, the FDA was able to recall the product quickly, but in Europe, the product's popularity prevented the rapid cessation of its use. Thousands of European children were born with deformities as a result.

The *Kefauver-Harris Act* and the *Drug Efficacy Study Implementation* of 1962 corrected some of the oversights in the Food, Drug and Cosmetic Act. The new act called for (1) long-term toxicity studies in animals, (2) clinical testing in humans, (3) evidence of therapeutic effectiveness, and (4) further regulation of prescription advertisements. Old drugs as well as new agents were to be tested. If an old drug was found to have little or no therapeutic value or demonstrated evidence of unwanted toxicity, or both, the FDA was empowered to remove it from the market. The FDA was given the responsibility for regulating and implementing the necessary procedures and in 1967 that agency formed a special staff to evaluate clinical investigators. In the 1970s they began to require that all clinical subjects for new agents be followed for five years. In 1970 the FDA published its guidelines for clinical studies, entitled *Description of an Adequately and Well-Controlled Clinical Investigation*. Other FDA regulations are still being formulated to increase protection from harmful agents.

The *Animal Welfare Act* was passed in 1966 and amended in 1976. It empowers the U.S. Department of Agriculture to regulate the treatment of laboratory animals and set standards for their feeding, shelter, sanitation, health care, and transportation. Testing medicinal agents on unhealthy or poorly treated laboratory animals can alter research findings, so many drug investigators are now using accredited laboratories that are evaluated by the American Association for Accreditation of Laboratory Animal Care in Joliet, Illinois.

The *Comprehensive Drug Abuse Prevention and Control Act* (Controlled Substances Act) of 1970 replaced the Harrison Narcotic Act and its various amendments. The regulation of controlled substances is under the authority of the Federal Bureau of Narcotics and Dangerous Drugs, a bureau of the Department of Justice (see Chapter 6).

The *Public Health Service Act* replaced the Virus Law of 1902 and stipulates that biologic agents be controlled and regulated by the Division of Biologic Standards, part of HEW's National Institutes of Health. Each biologic agent must meet specific standards regarding its source, production, storage, and marketing.

The *Lea-Wheeler Act* is administered by the Federal Trade Commission (FTC) and, along with other laws, regulates the interstate advertisement of medicinal agents, including over-the-counter drugs. Various consumer groups have helped control false or misleading advertising by bringing it to the attention of the FTC.

Postal regulations must be observed when certain medicinal agents are mailed, such as poisons, and other regulations apply to the use of the mail for advertising.

In addition, every state has its own *state laws* controlling various aspects of drug preparation, manufacture, distribution, and administration. The individuals who are involved with medicinal agents—pharmacist, physician, and nurse—are licensed by the states, and facilities where drugs are dispensed or used, such as pharmacies and hospitals, may be inspected or evaluated by state agents. Advertising for drugs that are produced and marketed within a given state are also controlled by state laws.

REFERENCES

Books

Beyer, K. H. 1978. *Discovery, development and delivery of new drugs.* Jamaica, N.Y.: Spectrum.

Blake, J. B., and others. 1970. *Safeguarding the public: Historical aspects of medicinal drug control.* Baltimore: Johns Hopkins University Press.

Claus, E. P., and others. 1970. *Pharmacognosy.* 6th ed. Philadelphia: Lea and Febiger.

FDA/HEW. 1977. *General considerations for the clinical evaluation of drugs.* Washington, D.C.: U.S. Government Printing Office.

Hemelt, M. D., and Macket, M. E. 1978. *Dynamics of law in nursing and health care.* Reston, Va.: Reston Publishing Co.

Martin, E. W. 1978. *Hazards of medication.* 2nd ed. Philadelphia: Lippincott.

Siegler, P. E., and Moyer, J. H. 1967. *Pharmacologic techniques in drug evaluation.* Chicago: Year Book.

Articles

Barron, B. A., and Bukanty, S. C. 1967. "The evaluation of new drugs." *Annual of International Medicine* I19:547–56.

Kelsey, F. O. 1978. "Biomedical monitoring." *Journal of Clinical Pharmacology* I8:3–9.

Chapter 5

Legal Aspects of Drug Administration

WHETHER NURSES HAVE had technical training or professional preparation, they are viewed by the public and by courts of law as safe and competent health practitioners. To function effectively and safely, nurses must demonstrate technical expertise and must also be well versed in the legal aspects of their work. No court will accept lack of knowledge as an excuse for failure to perform safely. Nurses are held liable not only for their own actions or omissions but also for those of the health team members to whom they delegate tasks.

All states have laws defining the practice of pharmacy and the specific functions of health professionals regarding drugs. Although these laws may vary in certain details from state to state, the basic activities concerning drug preparation and handling are clearly defined in all states.

COMPOUNDING, DISPENSING, PRESCRIBING, AND ADMINISTERING DRUGS

The licensed pharmacist is the person legally designated to compound, dispense, and sell drugs and other chemicals within the limits of federal and state regulations. The term *compounding* means the mixing together of drugs or chemicals into a form suitable for dosage. Although most compounding of commonly used drugs is done by the pharmaceutical manufacturers, the independent or hospital pharmacist may need to compound drugs to fill a physician's prescription. *Dispensing* is giving out or distributing drugs or chemicals. In a few states, the pharmacy laws specifically authorize nurses to dispense drugs in certain instances, as in emergency rooms or outpatient clinics. Unless the state law specifically authorizes them to dispense drugs, which is the exception rather than the rule, nurses may not remove a drug from the pharmacy stock supply and dispense it to a client, even if they are following the physician's order.

The state pharmacy statutes do exempt certain persons from the provisions of the law in the following circumstances:

1. Physicians may compound and dispense drugs for their patients when a licensed pharmacist is not available.
2. Nurses may administer single doses of a drug to a client while carrying out the verbal or written order of a physician.

Until recently, physicians were the only health professionals legally permitted to *prescribe* medications—that is, to order specific drugs for use by a client. However, changes in state nursing practice acts are beginning to reflect the rapidly expanding roles of nurses in the health care system. In at least eleven states,[1] nurse practice acts have been revised to include conditions under which nurses may prescribe drugs. The restrictions in individual states range from permitting nurse prescriptions in emergencies only to allowing prescriptions for noncontrolled substances by certified nurse practitioners. Physicians' assistants are also permitted to prescribe certain drugs in states where they are licensed to practice.

State laws vary greatly in their definitions of nursing practice. Some states define the practice of nursing in general terms, but most states distinguish between professional and practical nursing. In all cases, however, state practice acts clearly authorize nurses to administer medications prescribed by licensed physicians. The following definitions for professional and practical nursing come from the New York State practice act:

> Sec. 6902: Definition of the Practice of Nursing
> 1. The practice of the profession of nursing as a *registered professional nurse* is defined as diagnosing and treating human responses to actual or potential health problems through such services as case-finding, health teaching, health counseling, and provision of care supportive to or restorative of life and well-being, and executing medical regimens prescribed by a licensed or otherwise legally authorized physician or dentist. A nursing regimen shall be consistent with and shall not vary [from] any existing medical regimen.
> 2. The practice of nursing as a *licensed practical nurse* is defined as performing tasks and responsibilities within the framework of case-finding,

[1]The states that currently permit qualified nurses to prescribe selected drugs include Alaska, Arizona, California, Idaho, Maine, Nevada, New Hampshire, New Mexico, North Carolina, South Dakota, and Washington.

> health teaching, health counseling, and provision of supportive and restorative care under the direction of a registered professional nurse or licensed or otherwise legally authorized physician or dentist.

In this example, both professional and practical nurses are clearly authorized to administer medications upon the orders of licensed physicians. Apart from the obvious necessity of being familiar with the scope of practice defined by the state practice acts, the nurse must also be aware of legal doctrine and precedent as they relate to the administration of medications.

MALPRACTICE AND NEGLIGENCE

Malpractice is the term used for careless, illegal, or immoral acts related to the practice of a profession, or failure to perform the acts that any reasonable person would perform in similar circumstances. Because a jury composed of persons who are not health professionals has no background for determining malpractice, the law uses the prevailing standard of care as the basis for the jury's determination of guilt or innocence. The standard of care is determined by the testimony of practitioners whose backgrounds and experiences are similar to that of the defendant. The defendant's performance is then measured against the prevailing standard of care. If the jury finds the defendant guilty of malpractice, it must also determine that harm was caused to the patient as a direct result of the negligent act and, moreover, that harm could have been prevented by simple foresight.

In administering medications, for example, the standard of care is clearly defined as giving the right drug to the right client in the right dosage at the right time by the right route. To achieve this standard consistently, nurses are expected to follow certain procedures in preparing and administering drugs. If the nurse does not check the order with the drug container and gives 2 g of a drug instead of 0.2 g, the nurse has not met the standard of care. Furthermore, the nurse knows that an incorrect dose can cause harm to a client—in other words, the nurse has the knowledge to *foresee* the consequences of an incorrect drug dose. If the overdose in this instance actually causes harm or death to the client, the nurse is clearly guilty of malpractice under the law. There have been, in fact, a number of court cases in which nurses have been found guilty of malpractice because of medication errors.

Roles and functions of health care practitioners are changing so rapidly, however, that the overlapping boundaries between nursing and medical practice can lead to situations in which the standard of care is not so easily determined. Consider the following case. A physician does a cutdown and begins an intravenous infusion in a client's leg. Twelve hours later the nurse notes swelling of the leg and notifies the physician, who examines the client and decides that the swelling is a normal reaction to the cutdown and the infusion should be continued. Another five hours pass and the staff nurse asks her charge nurse to examine the client. When they call the physician, he asks whether there has been a great change in the client's leg in the last five hours. The nurse says the change is not great, so the physician orders the infusion to be continued. Another seven hours pass, and another staff nurse observes the leg to be edematous and slightly red. She notifies the charge nurse, but this time the physician is not called. After another seven hours, a third staff nurse notes that the leg is more edematous and her charge nurse tells her to notify the physician. (In later testimony, the physician said he was told only that the client's leg was "still edematous," but the staff nurse testified that she used the phrase "increasing edema.") The physician, in any case, orders the infusion to be continued. Within the next three hours, the charge nurse observes increasing swelling that now extends above the knee, but the infusion is not discontinued. One and a half hours later, the charge nurse calls the physician, who arrives in another hour and removes the infusion. By this time the client's leg is swollen to twice its normal size.

The physician testified later that it is the nurse's duty either to notify the doctor or to discontinue an infusion when swelling reaches a critical point. The nurses testified that the nurse's duty is to notify the physician when swelling occurs at an infusion site, but that an infusion should not be discontinued without a doctor's order.[2] When there is such conflicting testimony on the standard of care, the jury must decide which standard it will use in determining liability. This case, which occurred in 1963, illustrates several characteristics of the standard of care. First, conflicting standards may be used by different health professionals, all of them expert practitioners. Second, the standard of care is not static but changes constantly with new techniques in health care and with the expanding functions of health care professionals. The prudent nurse in 1983 would, in all probability, take responsibility for discontinuing an infusion that was so obviously infiltrated. Third, testimony relating to the standard of care is not confined to local professionals. If the local standard of care is below the norm for other areas, the practitioner is not excused from liability because he or she conformed to the lower standard. Professional testimony relating to prudent standards of care can be obtained from any practitioner in any part of the country—hence the need for continuing education and exposure for all health professionals.

The recent expansion of the nurse's roles and functions has distinct legal implications related to the standard of care. In some states, the nurse practice acts have not been revised to recognize functions that were once within the sole province of medical practice but have now been taken over by nursing. In these states, therefore, the new functions are not legally sanctioned. If a lawsuit for malpractice against a nurse relates to one of these "illegal" functions, the nurse is judged according to the prevailing standard of care for *physicians* who would normally perform that function.

In at least 33 states, however, nurse practice acts have been revised to reflect the independent decisions that are characteristic of contemporary nursing practice. In such situations, nurses are not only expected to function under their traditionally high professional standards of care; they also have a legal mandate to apply their knowledge in making independent nursing diagnoses and in taking appropriate actions related to the client's welfare. If a client is unable to take a medication in the form prescribed by the physician, for example, it is the nurse's responsibility to collaborate with the pharmacist in obtaining an appropriate dosage form. In this instance, the nurse's knowledge indicates that the client's need for the medication is the overriding concern, and immediate collaboration with the pharmacist is a matter of sound professional judgment.

[2]See N. Hershey, "Standard of care," *American Journal of Nursing*, September 1964.

THE DOCTRINE OF *RESPONDEAT SUPERIOR*

According to the legal concept known as *respondeat superior,* an employer is responsible for the acts of his or her employees while they are engaged in service to the employer. This concept evolved from the old master-servant relationship, in which it was implicit that the servant was under the control of the master and performing a service for the master. An employee ("servant") need not be compensated or under written contract for this doctrine to apply. For example, even though a nurse may be employed by a hospital, the nurse can be called upon to serve a physician during a procedure on a patient within that hospital. If the nurse's action results in harm to the patient, the physician may be held liable under the doctrine of *respondeat superior,* because the nurse (servant) was at that time engaged in the physician's (master's) business.

Health agencies may also be held liable for negligent acts committed by any of their employees. Even though health professionals are viewed more and more as independent practitioners, agencies are expected to hire people who can give appropriate care to clients. This means that the employer has an obligation not only to screen prospective employees carefully, but also to provide a proper setting, safe equipment, and any instruction necessary for adapting to changing procedures and regulations.

The doctrine of *respondeat superior* does not exempt the practitioner from personal liability. For example, if a staff nurse administers a drug from a vial containing an outdated medicine, and the client has an untoward reaction to the drug, the nurse can be held negligent. The hospital in which the harmful act was committed, however, can also be held liable for negligence because it occurred during the course of the nurse's service to the employer. Following are descriptions of several other situations concerning drug administration where the nurse's familiarity with legal responsibilities is particularly important.

CONTROLLED SUBSTANCES

The *Controlled Substances Act* of 1970 replaced all previous legislation dealing with narcotics, depressants, stimulants, and hallucinogens. Since the law requires complete record keeping for all controlled drugs, nurses must be meticulous in their handling and administration of these drugs.[3] The drugs and records are always stored in a double-locked area, and only authorized persons have access to the supply. Only licensed nurses may sign for a controlled drug. In addition, the supply is checked by two nurses either daily or at every shift change. If a dose of a controlled drug is discarded, for any reason, the control sheet must be signed by two nurses, namely, the discarder and a witness: every dose of a controlled drug must be accounted for. The law also includes strict policies on orders for controlled substances. These policies limit the number of hours or days that an order can be effective; when the time limit expires, the physician must write a new order for the drug. For example, all prn orders for narcotic drugs must be rewritten after 72 hours.

Similar prescription time limits have been extended to a number of other substances. For example, in many agencies, antibiotic orders are effective for a period of only five days. The nurse may not administer the drug on the sixth day unless the physician writes a new order. Similarly, heparin and other anticoagulants must be reordered every 24 hours in many agencies. Although state and federal laws do not specifically mandate expiration times on orders of noncontrolled drugs, hospitals often institute such regulations in order to safeguard their patients from unnecessary doses of potent drugs.

[3]See Chapter 6 for a list of these drugs.

In addition to the federal Controlled Substances Act, most states have laws that further define the dispensing, prescription, and sale of controlled drugs. In almost every state, unlawful use, possession, or sale of these drugs is a crime, but the criminal penalties imposed vary widely from state to state. The nurse must be familiar with state law governing controlled substances, as well as with the specific procedures of his or her agency concerning the handling and administration of these drugs.

EXPERIMENTAL DRUGS

Any drug that is administered before it has been thoroughly tested and approved for general medical use by the federal Food and Drug Administration is considered experimental or investigational. Since these drugs have not yet been approved for widespread use, information about them will not be available in the standard sources of drug information. However, the nurse who administers the drug must be aware of all *known* information concerning the drug action, dosage, and side effects. This data is usually packaged with the drug by the manufacturer and will be available from the dispensing pharmacist.

The client must be told all the known facts about the drug and must give written consent to the "experiment." If this condition has not been met, the nurse should not administer even a single dose of the experimental drug. If the client suffers harm, the nurse could become a defendant in a criminal lawsuit.

TELEPHONE AND VERBAL ORDERS

In most client care situations, medication needs are anticipated by standing or prn orders, or both. There are times, however, when the physician is not physically available to write an order for a drug that is needed immediately, such as in emergencies or when a client's condition changes suddenly. The physician may then give a telephone order. When taking a telephone order from a physician, the nurse should immediately write

Telephone order:	1/12/85 @ 10:30 A.M. Give aspirin gr X q4h prn for temp above 101° F.	T.O. Dr. Mack / S. Smith, R.N. / J. Mack, M.D.
Verbal order:	1/12/85 @ 3:45 P.M. Give Tigan 200 mg IM stat	V.O. Dr. Brenner / L. Jones, R.N.
Verbal order:	1/12/85 @ 6:50 P.M. Lasix 40 mg IV stat	V.O. Dr. Brenner / L. Jones, R.N.

FIGURE 5-1 Examples of recording stat, telephone, and verbal orders.

the order in the nurse's notes as stated and repeat it to the physician, including drug name, route of administration, dosage, and time of administration. Some agencies permit the nurse to write the order directly on the physician's order sheet, indicating that it is a telephone order. The telephone order must be verified and signed by the physician as soon as possible, but always within 24 hours.

In emergency situations, the physician often calls out "stat" drug orders verbally to the nurse. The drugs may be administered by the nurse or the physician, but in either case certain safeguards must be employed. The nurse should immediately repeat the drug name, dosage, and route of administration, and quickly prepare the medication according to established procedure. When the drug is brought to the client for administration, the nurse should again repeat the drug name, dosage, and route, no matter who administers it. In addition, the nurse should bring the drug container to the bedside as a final safeguard. The importance of these precautions cannot be overemphasized. In one emergency situation, two nurses were found negligent when a client was given epinephrine instead of procaine. One nurse handed the drug vial to a second nurse who administered the medication, but neither nurse read the label on the container. If a nurse gives a physician a syringe containing the wrong medication, the nurse is clearly in error. The nurse should record stat medications on the client's chart as soon as possible, and have the physician countersign the orders before leaving the unit. See Figure 5-1. In all instances in which the nurse accepts any verbal medication order, the physician must confirm that order in writing within 24 hours.

QUESTIONING MEDICATION ORDERS

There are two potential circumstances in which a nurse may need to question a physician's medication order. The first instance concerns an order that is illegible or incomplete; in this case the nurse must contact the prescribing physician to clarify exactly what was intended. Since the state pharmacy statutes specify the information that must be included in a prescription, an order that is illegible or incomplete is unlawful and cannot be dispensed or administered until it is clarified. If the nurse guesses and the client suffers harm because the wrong drug or dosage is given, the nurse bears full legal responsibility.

The second instance concerns an order that the nurse judges to be inaccurate for any reason, such as quantity of dosage, route of administration, or action of the drug. The nurse's first action should be to consult the prescribing physician to determine whether the order is in fact correct as written or stated. If the drug order is obviously incorrect, the physician usually acknowledges the error and modifies the prescription accordingly. Suppose, however, that the physician insists on having the drug administered as originally prescribed. A logical resolution is to request that the prescribing physician, rather than the nurse, administer the medication. If the nurse believes that potential harm to the client may result from the medication, however, the nurse has a definite professional responsibility to report the problem immediately to a superior who has the authority to intervene. A nurse's *inaction* is no more legally defensible than is an incorrect action.

RECORD KEEPING

The client's chart is a written document that can be used as legal evidence in a court of law. Every clinical agency has its own specific format and regulations for record keeping, and has a right to expect all of its professional employees to adhere to its established charting procedures. Although charts vary widely in design from agency to agency, there are general principles in common use for the charting of medications.

1. Any drug allergies the client may have are determined at the initial interview with the nurse or physician. A red allergy alert sticker is completed and attached to the cover of the client's chart. In addition, the drug allergy is noted in the patient's medication Kardex.
2. When physicians' drug orders are transcribed to a medication Kardex, the Kardex cards become a part of the legal record. There can therefore be no erasures or pencil notations. If the nurses use their initials for verifying drug dosages administered, the nurses' full names and corresponding initials must be entered in the designated space on the medication Kardex. A medication Kardex has special sections for preoperative medications, prn and stat medications, and daily and around-the-clock medications. Some agencies require that prn, stat, and preoperative medication doses be entered in the nurses' notes as well as in the medication Kardex.
3. Many agencies use *flow sheets* for certain drugs whose time of administration and dosage are dependent on the results of laboratory tests. For example, when heparin is administered intravenously, the dosage is modified continuously according to changes in the client's partial thromboplastin time. The flow sheet has sections for the date, the time, the partial thromboplastin time, and the dose of heparin administered. Flow sheets are also used when administering doses of regular insulin, which are dependent on the results of the client's urine tests for sugar and acetone.
4. The important points to remember when charting medications are: (a) all doses must be recorded immediately following administration; (b) effects of the drug on the client must be accurately and promptly recorded, whether desirable or undesirable; and (c) all drug doses withheld for any reason must be recorded. Failure to record pertinent data about medications is as indefensible as an error in dosage, route, or drug used.
5. Information on the chart cannot be released to anyone other than the client, the client's immediate family, and the health team members caring for that client, without the written consent of the client. However, when a lawsuit for negligence goes to trial, the contents of the chart must be available to both plaintiff and defendant. The entries on that chart then become very important in determining whether the prevailing standard of care was met. Therefore, agency policies on charting must be scrupulously observed; moreover, the nurse must regularly record assessments of the client's reaction to drug therapy. The absence of pertinent data on a chart does not free the nurse from liability; rather, it tends to be interpreted as failure to meet the prudent standard of care.

DISPOSAL OF EQUIPMENT

The importance of proper handling and disposal of medication equipment cannot be overemphasized. The prevalence of drug abuse in recent years gives credence to the strict policies instituted by health care agencies for disposal of syringes and needles and for storing and dispensing habit-forming drugs. Used syringes and needles should never be left at the client's bedside; nor should they be discarded in a wastebasket. Appropriate receptacles for both must be available in a locked or supervised area. Many agencies have designed systems for keeping accurate counts of all syringes, needles, and drug containers. Recording all medication supplies dispensed to individual units, and ensuring that used supplies are returned to a central department for recounting, will help to prevent drugs and related equipment from reaching drug abusers.

CONCLUSION

The contemporary nurse is often subject to conflicting demands from three distinct sources of authority: the hospital administration, the physician, and the nursing hierarchy. All three lines of authority demand compliance with policies and directives, but at the same time nurses are expected to think critically and make independent professional judgments. It is not surprising, then, that nurses often have trouble deciding to whom they owe their first allegiance. Ideally the demands and goals of the three lines of authority should never be in conflict; in reality, though, the reverse is often true. In resolving such dilemmas, it must be recognized that the nurse's primary responsibility is always to act in the client's interest, even when that action may conflict with hospital policy or physician's orders. The American Nurses Association's Standards of Practice provide the basis for the nurse's ethical decisions on behalf of the client; the state's nurse practice act defines legal responsibilities. Nurses must be familiar with both if they are to practice as responsible professionals.

REFERENCES

Bullough, B., ed. 1975. *The law and the expanding nursing role.* New York: Appleton-Century-Crofts.

Creighton, H. 1981. *Law every nurse should know.* 4th ed. Philadelphia: Saunders.

Fenner, K. 1980. *Ethics and law in nursing: Professional perspectives.* New York: Van Nostrand Reinhold.

Health Law Center and C. J. Streiff. 1975. *Nursing and the law.* 2nd ed. Rockville, Md.: Aspen Systems.

Hemelt, M., and Macket, M. 1978. *Dynamics of law in nursing and health care.* Reston, Va.: Reston Publishing Co.

Murchison, I., Nichols, T., and Hanson, R. 1978. *Accountability in the nursing process.* St. Louis: C. V. Mosby.

"Nurses notes as legal evidence." 1979. *Regan Report on Nursing Law* 20:2.

Rothman, D., and Rothman, N. 1977. *The professional nurse and the law.* Boston: Little, Brown.

Rozovsky, L. 1979. "Legal rules for Nurses' Notes." *Dimensions in Health Service* 56:22.

Chapter 6

Drug Abuse

HISTORICAL PERSPECTIVE

A realistic approach to contemporary drug abuse can be gained by putting the problem in historical perspective. Raw opium, hashish from the hemp plant, cocaine from coca leaves, alcohol, and other natural drugs have been known and available to human beings for centuries. In many cultures, the use of these drugs was limited to rituals associated with religion, such as attempts to contact spirits, or with rites of passage, such as puberty. Certain groups still practice this limited use of drugs; for example, some Mexican Indians consume certain mushrooms for their hallucinogenic effect during religious rituals. Other groups use certain drugs to produce desirable physical or mental qualities; the people of the Andes Mountains credit their strength and endurance to the regular consumption of coca leaves.

Opium was used for medicinal purposes by the ancient Egyptians and Greeks, and later found its way to Europe and the American colonies. Many people were no doubt addicted to opium even in ancient times, but we have no way of knowing to what extent. It should be remembered, however, that the drug was ingested orally in teas, or mixed with other ingredients, and was therefore much less potent than the concentrated forms available today.

Opium became a focus of worldwide attention in the 19th century when China attempted to enforce its ban on the importing of Indian opium. The ensuing Opium War with Great Britain and other Western powers ended with China's agreeing to ease its foreign trade restrictions and to legalize opium importation. When large numbers of Chinese emigrated to the United States, they brought the practice of opium smoking with them. The drug was traded without restriction on a worldwide basis and addiction was widespread. At about the same time, the hypodermic needle and syringe were invented, and morphine, produced from opium in 1803, was administered hypodermically on a large scale to Civil War soldiers. By the 20th century, use of raw opium, morphine, and heroin was extensive. The drugs were not only freely available in any store, but compound medicines and even soft drinks contained opiates (see Figure 6-1). It has been estimated that there were at least one million opiate addicts in the United States alone at the beginning of this century. This widespread abuse led to the passage of the Harrison Narcotic Act of 1914, the first piece of legislation that addressed the problem of narcotic drug availability. However, no provisions were included for the rehabilitation of the addicts, so those who were unable to withdraw from opiates on their own were forced to obtain their drugs from the underworld. The Harrison Narcotic Act represents the beginning of the legal regulation of drug use, but the legal ramifications of illicit drug use are separate and distinct from the psychological, physical, and sociological dimensions of the current drug abuse problem.

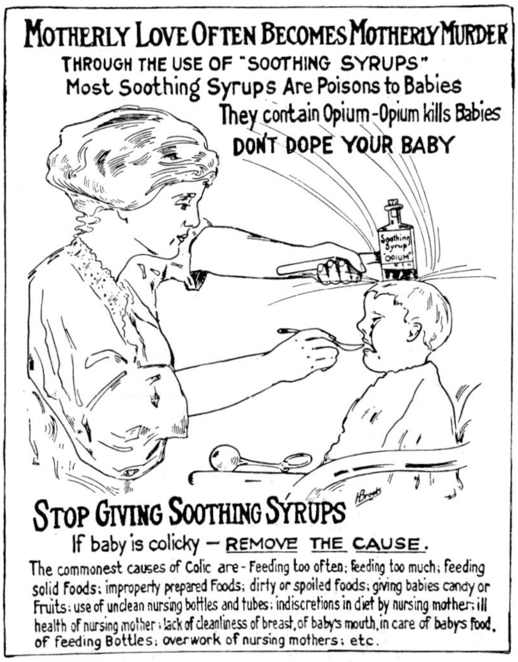

FIGURE 6-1 Sample of a type of poster prevalent in the early 20th century, when opium addiction was widespread. (From *Michigan Public Health Magazine,* October, 1918.)

The extent to which drug use is condoned in any society is related to that society's view of human nature and the universe. Just as opium smoking enhances those personal qualities—calm, reserve, detachment—prized in Oriental cultures, so alcohol consumption releases inhibitions and enhances the aggressive behavior seemingly valued in some Western cultures. What is widely tolerated and even encouraged in one culture may be abhorrent in another. In the foregoing example, it is notable that both drugs have well-known potential for abuse, but most persons in each culture are able to limit their use of the drug to nonaddictive levels. The dominant cultural group, then, dictates not only which drugs are socially acceptable, but in what situations and in what quantities they are to be used. It follows that those persons in any society who become physically or psychologically addicted to drugs are in violation of some part of the dominant social codes. Among the reasons for turning to drugs in the first place may be an inability to fulfill the expectations of the dominant social group, and a tendency to withdraw from its demands and sanctions through drug use.

DRUG DEPENDENCE IN CONTEMPORARY SOCIETY

The underlying causes of present-day addiction are complex, hotly disputed and beyond the scope of this chapter. What is pertinent here, however, is the fact that drug dependence is generally recognized by health professionals to be an illness with both physical and psychological components. The addict's overwhelming craving for the drug, which often leads to repeated relapses after withdrawal, is a product of psychosocial factors and physical need.

Recent research indicates that mood-altering drugs, including marijuana, have a direct effect on specific areas of the brain or on the synaptic chemical activities that occur during the transmission of impulses between neurons. Drug stimulation of the pleasure-seeking centers of the brain, for example, results in the characteristic "high" described by drug users. In other words, this basic neurophysiological alteration, which occurs with even the initial drug dose, acts as a primary physical stimulus or reinforcer and may itself be the basis for drug dependence.

The other major reinforcer related to drug addiction is the entire psychosocial context in which drugs are abused. Within the last two decades the use of mood-altering drugs by the respectable mainstream of society has become quite acceptable and even encouraged. The widespread availability of these drugs, coupled with increasing instabilities in the family and community, creates a social setting that supports drug use, particularly among adolescents and young adults who are in a vulnerable stage of growth and development.

Habitual drug use in adolescents affects the physiological processes that are crucial to physical and psychosocial development. Because of impaired memory, interference with abstract reasoning, inability to make independent moral judgments, listlessness, and an inability to sustain relationships with peers and adults, the teenage drug user is incapable of mastering the tasks necessary for developing into an independent, industrious, and self-fulfilled adult. The confusion and aimlessness characteristic of the habitual adolescent drug user often progress to overt psychotic episodes and sometimes to chronic psychosis. Whether or not overt psychotic behavior develops, the young drug abuser becomes an individual without goals, without meaningful relationships, incapable of concentrating on academic or occupational pursuits. These symptoms are often referred to as the *amotivational syndrome*. The user substitutes drug-seeking behavior for all others and is usually alienated from family relationships. Until now, the greatest number of drug abusers have been under the age of 25. Recent changes in social attitudes toward greater permissiveness and acceptance of formerly deviant behavior, however, suggest that the incidence of drug abuse will rise among those over 25 as well. The implications for communities, the workplace, and society are ominous, since few other conditions result in the destructive behavior characteristic of the drug addict.

The term *addiction* has been defined by the World Health Organization as including physical or psychological dependence, tolerance, and an uncontrollable desire to continue taking the drug. *Physical dependence* is confirmed by the presence of withdrawal symptoms when the drug is withheld; intense physical symptoms, specific for each class of drugs, are described later in the chapter. *Psychological dependence* is defined as a condition that requires continued use of a drug to achieve pleasurable feelings or to avoid uncomfortable feelings. The World Health Organization is emphatic in stating that *all* drugs of abuse are characterized by psychological dependence in varying degrees. This observation is of major importance in understanding the behavior associated with drug abuse, particularly for drugs such as marijuana, cocaine, and tobacco that do not usually lead to profound physical dependence. Since the fact that psychological dependence is a characteristic of all drugs of abuse is not generally recognized by most people, it does not serve as a deterrent to the initial drug experience.

Tolerance refers to the individual's need for ever-increasing amounts of the drug to produce the desired physical and psychological effects. Tolerance is based on physiological adaptations to the drug in specific organs. For some drugs, the brain reacts by altering the production and release of substances needed for normal transmission of impulses between neurons. For other drugs, the liver reacts by accelerating its metabolism of the drugs. Some drugs cause reactions in both brain and liver; drugs causing these major chemical changes can lead to tolerance within a few weeks.

Addiction should be differentiated from drug *abuse,* which is a broad term relating to the self-administration (without medical supervision) of a drug or other chemical substance. Abuse may result in *habituation* when the substance becomes a routine substitute for healthier patterns of coping. (*Physical dependence* and *psychological dependence* are now the preferred terms for describing addiction.) Common habit-forming substances in contemporary society include caffeine, nicotine, and alcohol; although generally condoned, these substances are certainly not without potentially harmful effects and can lead to physical dependence. Alcohol is a leading cause of death (just after heart disease and cancer) and is currently thought to be responsible for more than half of all the automobile accidents in the United States—grim testimony to the effects of abusing a legal and socially sanctioned drug. When one considers the incredible variety of nonprescription drugs available to the consumer, coupled with those that are freely prescribed by physicians, the potential for *legal* drug abuse is staggering.

PATTERNS OF DRUG USE

According to recent statistics, approximately 65% of American high school seniors have used illicit drugs at least once. The most commonly used illicit drug is marijuana (60%)—more than 10% of high school students are using it on a daily basis. Other illicit drugs used at some time by more than 10% of the students include, in descending order of frequency, stimulants, hallucinogens, tranquilizers, cocaine, sedatives, PCP, and opiates. The two legal drugs, alcohol and nicotine (cigarettes), have been used at least once by 94% and 74% of high school students, respectively. In general the prevalence of drug use, with the exception of cigarettes, is higher in males than in females: 17% of females smoke regularly as opposed to 15% of males. For this age group, the drugs that have shown the greatest increase in popularity in the 1980s are marijuana, cocaine, and alcohol.[1]

In the past, drug availability and abuse were associated primarily with ghetto neighborhoods in large metropolitan centers. Now, however, drug abuse is prevalent in all segments of society, and recent evidence suggests that the reliable predictors of drug use relate to knowledge of drugs and their availability, the extent of drug use in the family and among friends, and early experience with legal drugs (alcohol and cigarettes).

The most widely available illicit drug is marijuana—90% of high school seniors say that marijuana is fairly easy to obtain. In fact, almost every high school student not only has access to marijuana but probably is friendly with someone who uses it regularly. Moreover, there has been much publicity about the supposedly innocuous effects of marijuana as opposed to alcohol or other drugs, whereas very little attention has been given to research evidence substantiating the multiple risks to health associated with frequent use of marijuana. If knowledge

[1]For more detailed statistics, see Johnston, Bachman, and O'Malley, *1979 highlights: Drugs and the nation's high school students* (Washington, D.C.: National Institute of Drug Abuse, Department of Health, Education, and Welfare, 1979).

and availability of a drug are one predictor of its use, marijuana abuse is likely to continue escalating if present drug enforcement policies are perpetuated.

Regarding drug use in families, a recent study (Rittenhouse, 1980) documented the fact that mothers who smoke cigarettes and drink alcohol have a higher percentage of children who use marijuana than mothers who abstain from both. Youngsters who have an older sibling who uses a drug are likely to use the same drug. It seems obvious that the widespread use of psychotropic drugs in all age groups, whether medically prescribed or not, provides a socially sanctioned model for young people.

Finally, the use of alcohol and cigarettes among young people seems to be closely related to the use of other drugs at a later date. Youngsters who smoke cigarettes are far more likely to use alcohol and marijuana than youngsters who do not smoke. The percentage of young people who go on to use other drugs such as cocaine, hallucinogens, and heroin is much higher among the cigarette smokers. It would seem, then, that early use of the legal drugs provides a training ground for future use of illicit drugs.

IMPLICATIONS FOR NURSING

The statistics on drug abuse, particularly among young people, suggest a great need for more intensive drug education programs, as well as for greatly improved recreational and other support systems for adolescents and families. Drug education programs in schools seldom dispense the kind of information young people need. And since teachers and parents are often uncomfortable in addressing the problem, these programs are usually superficial in their approach. Everyone needs to be taught that *all* mood-altering drugs are not only psychologically addictive but interfere with normal neurological activities in the brain. When an area such as the hypothalamus is affected, hormonal functions are disrupted. Moreover, the effects do not disappear as soon as the drug use is stopped; rather, it may take many weeks or months for organ systems to return to normal physiological functioning. The active ingredient in marijuana, for example, can be retained in the body's fatty tissues for as long as six months following the last dose.

Teachers should be kept informed of the latest research on addictive drugs—if for no other reason than to answer students' questions with factual and straightforward responses. All nurses, particularly the school nurse and the community health nurse, can be key sources of information for teachers, parents, and students.

Early detection and crisis intervention are professional nursing functions that can have a significant impact on drug abuse. Given the effect of addiction and drug-seeking behavior on addicts and families alike, the need for assessment and intervention at all levels is clear. The nurse's assessment skills can be used to identify subtle changes in psychological and physiological functions that may suggest marijuana abuse. Adolescents are particularly vulnerable because of the rapid developmental changes that normally occur in this age group. In planning intervention and collaborating with other professionals, the nurse must recognize that comprehensive support and treatment are necessary if the client is to modify the behavior associated with drug taking. Thus nurses must become familiar with all the local services for treating drug abusers and providing support to their families.

Moreover, the nursing profession needs to become more active in initiating and supporting legislation that would deal more effectively with the drug abuse problem. The rate of relapse among treated drug abusers is very high, suggesting that many present methods of treatment are inadequate. Drug treatment agencies with a higher success rate must be supported with appropriate funding and enlarged to provide the range of treatment so desperately needed by addicts and their families.

TYPES OF ABUSED DRUGS

Drugs with abuse potential fall into three major categories: (1) stimulants, (2) hallucinogens, and (3) sedatives and narcotics (central nervous system depressants). All individual drugs have a wide range of both desirable and undesirable effects; actual drug actions are dependent on the personality and physical condition of the user.

Stimulants

The stimulant drugs include cocaine and the amphetamines, which cause sleeplessness, euphoria, and heightened alertness. *Cocaine,* which is usually inhaled as a white powder, produces an intense euphoria in addiction-prone people. The euphoria lasts a very short time, and often leads to more frequent doses at short intervals. After such a "binge," the user may experience intense anxiety, fear, hallucinations, and paranoid delusions, and, as a result, may become aggressive and violent. There is no evidence of direct physical dependence on cocaine—that is, there is no withdrawal sickness—but continued cocaine use does result in psychological dependence to the point that the user may become preoccupied with obtaining the drug at any cost. The cocaine addict experiences deterioration of the nasal mucosa and perforation of the nasal septum after prolonged use, and may also exhibit signs of nervous system irritability, including muscle twitching and convulsions.

Cocaine has recently become increasingly popular among the middle and upper classes. It is much more expensive than heroin in the underworld market, so it is seldom used by the addict whose drug source is the street peddler. The narcotic addict, however, will sometimes use cocaine intravenously in conjunction with opiates in order to experience the intense euphoria of cocaine without the unpleasant aftereffects.

The effects of the *amphetamines* on the central nervous system are similar to those of cocaine. The user's physical activity increases markedly; at first, it may be purposeful but later it tends to deteriorate into disorganized or repetitive acts. Amphetamines also reduce appetite and many people have inadvertently become addicted to these drugs after taking them for weight loss. Many others who use amphetamines habitually to eliminate fatigue—for example, truck drivers and college students—have become dependent on them.

There is some difference of opinion about the physical addiction potential of amphetamines. When the drug is abruptly withdrawn, the user sleeps for long periods over several days. Profound depression and exhaustion follow and have led to suicide in unsupervised individuals. This phenomenon is interpreted by some researchers as evidence of physical dependence. Because amphetamines have a high potential for abuse, the FDA has restricted the prescription of amphetamines to the treatment of narcolepsy and hyperkinesis only. Amphetamine labels no longer contain a prescribing indication for weight loss and fatigue. Canada has similar restrictions.

Hallucinogenic Agents

Until fairly recently, hallucinogens were used by relatively isolated groups of primitive people, who ingested them during religious rituals. The "consciousness-expanding" properties of these drugs include vivid and colorful hallucinations, both visual and olfactory, and heightened perceptions of one's surroundings. They provide an escape from reality and, in many cases, result in bizarre and self-destructive behavior. The drugs in this category include *mescaline, psilocybin, DMT, STP,* and *LSD. Marijuana,* although actually a nonnarcotic sedative, also causes heightened visual, auditory, and olfactory perceptions, and is used socially in much the same way as the hallucinogens. It is a much less potent drug than the other hallucinogens, but, as with all drugs, its action depends on the personality of the user; it is known to have precipitated psychotic episodes in vulnerable individuals. The other hallucinogens occur naturally in certain cacti or mushrooms, or, in the case of LSD, in a fungus growth found on grain. They are also prepared synthetically but their only legitimate use is in very carefully supervised medical research.

The oral ingestion of hallucinogenic substances is often followed by a brief period of nausea, vomiting, diarrhea, and abdominal cramps. Within a few hours, these unpleasant effects are replaced by vivid hallucinations of intense color, beauty, and clarity, and heightened perceptions of the environment. One can easily understand the effect of such experiences on people with a mystical religious orientation.

The effects of LSD, however, range from these general hallucinatory experiences to severe psychotic episodes characterized by panic, paranoid delusions, and delirium, and sometimes resulting in accidental suicide. The "bad trip," or psychotic episode, can occur in users who have previously taken LSD many times with only pleasurable results. There have also been many incidents of "flashback," a delayed reaction to an

LSD experience, sometimes many months after the last dose. Furthermore, there is increasing scientific evidence of chromosome damage in LSD users.

Physical dependence on the hallucinogenic drugs does not seem to occur, but psychological dependence is common. One of the greatest potential hazards of LSD is its ingestion by unsuspecting people, as may occur when the drug is placed in food or drink at a party. The resultant hallucinations can cause mass chaos and panic and may unleash some individuals' latent psychoses, with disastrous consequences.

One of the newer drugs to appear on the street is PCP (phencycline). Its general effects are similar to those of LSD, but its potential for producing a "bad trip" is at least five times greater than any other hallucinogen. The delusions and severe excitability seen in users are often a prelude to respiratory depression and coma. Latent psychoses are intensified by PCP, and the long-term effects include severe depression and flashbacks. The raw chemicals of this drug are highly combustible and its illegal manufacture in home laboratories has resulted in some explosions.

Psychodepressants

This category of drugs contains many substances that are chemically unrelated to each other, but that produce similar physiological effects. (See Part VII for detailed information on therapeutic uses of these drugs.) There is cross-tolerance among almost all the drugs in this category, so that the physiological actions of two or more of these substances taken together can have disastrous, if not fatal, effects on the user.

Of all the sedative drugs, there are only two that seem to cause no physical dependence; they are marijuana and the bromides. Marijuana is probably the most widely used illicit drug among young people today. It is usually smoked in a social context, accompanied by much merriment and laughter. Its range of effects depends greatly on the personality of the user but includes euphoria, release of inhibitions, altered perceptions of time and space, periods of excitability, and, sometimes, hallucinations. Despite these "consciousness-expanding" properties, it also has depressant effects on the central nervous system, resulting in impaired motor performance, judgment, and decision-making—in other words, symptoms similar to those of alcohol intoxication. Psychic dependence and mild tolerance to marijuana do occur, but there is no withdrawal sickness when its use is abruptly terminated.

The latest reports from international drug researchers indicate that marijuana is a powerful drug with many risks to the user's health. The drug can exacerbate the symptoms in patients with disorders such as diabetes, cardiovascular disease, and epilepsy. The effects of marijuana may be intensified by interactions with alcohol, tobacco, and other drugs. Marijuana can damage the lungs, the reproductive system, and the immune system. It has also been responsible for causing acute psychotic reactions and chronic psychoses. There is no doubt that a significant number of individuals go on to abuse other drugs after their first experience with marijuana.

The bromides will accumulate in the body with prolonged use and cause severe toxic symptoms similar to those of barbiturate toxicity. Because there is no physical dependence, however, the treatment for chronic or acute toxicity consists of immediate cessation of the drug. Addiction-prone individuals use the bromides for their sedative effects, which include a generalized indifference to the problems in their lives.

The sedative drugs that cause definite physical dependence include *alcohol, barbiturates, paraldehyde, methaqualone, chloral hydrate, propoxyphene* (Darvon), and the major *tranquilizers.* The chronic abuse of all these drugs results in varying degrees of constant intoxication, depending on the personality of the user and the amount of drug consumed. The symptoms of abuse include loss of motor control, confusion, slurred speech, and muscle tremors. When toxic drug levels are reached, respiratory depression and coma result. Addiction-prone individuals use these drugs to experience mild euphoria and a release of inhibitions. The general loss of emotional control sometimes results in physically aggressive behavior, but the user's motor coordination is so impaired that these attempts at violence are usually easily subdued.

Because tolerance to these drugs does develop, a danger lies in the user's increasing the dosage to toxic levels, resulting in coma and death. Another danger occurs when barbiturates are used with other sedatives, including alcohol. The potentiating effect of one drug on the other can cause a fatal central nervous system depression.

The withdrawal illness from barbiturate, alcohol, and other sedative drug abuse is an especially dangerous one and must be managed carefully. Abrupt withdrawal results in initial calm, followed by nausea, weakness, tremors, and postural hypotension; it then progresses to delirium and convulsions by the third day. If untreated, these symptoms may result in vascular collapse and death. With medical supervision, a long-acting barbiturate is substituted for the addicting drug, and the dosage is gradually decreased, by about 10% daily, until it can be safely withdrawn.

Glue and other inhalants are used for their intoxicating effects, similar to those of alcohol, caused by central nervous system depression. The effects are of short duration, and actual permanent physical damage is usually the result of overdose, which can lead to liver damage, paralysis, respiratory depression, and coma.

Narcotics

Included in the category narcotics are the *opiates* and their synthetic equivalents, the *morphines, morphinones, meperidines,* and *methadone.* (See Chapter 27 for information on specific drugs.) The narcotics act as central nervous system depressants but also cause euphoria; they are used by addicts for their mood-elevating effects. Medically, the narcotics are the most potent analgesics available, and, although the search for an equally potent nonaddicting analgesic continues, none has yet been discovered.

The opiate user experiences a feeling of intense pleasure from his first narcotic dose. Although the extent of this pleasurable sensation varies according to underlying personality differences, it seems to be absent in some individuals, particularly in acutely ill patients who are receiving medically-prescribed doses. In fact, for these people, the first contact with a narcotic may be very unpleasant, resulting in nausea and restlessness along with analgesia. The intense pleasure experienced by addiction-prone persons makes a vivid impression, and the desire to recapture this "high" is what leads to repeated doses and eventual addiction. As tolerance develops and drug intake is increased, the pleasurable sensation gradually disappears, and the addict's motivation in continuing narcotic use is primarily to avoid withdrawal sickness. Of course, the tranquility, detachment from reality, and general contentment resulting from narcotic use are also powerful motivators for continued use by people who, in an undrugged state, have difficulty coping with life's vicissitudes.

Withdrawal sickness from abrupt cessation of chronic narcotic use is a most unpleasant and frightening experience, but it is seldom life threatening. However, medically unsupervised withdrawal is inhumane and dangerous, because there is always the chance that the addict combined narcotics with barbiturates, in which case withdrawal could be fatal. Most of the deaths related to narcotic abuse occur from inadvertent overdose; the percentage of pure drug in the illicit preparations varies widely and the addict may unknowingly inject a much stronger preparation than he or she has used in the past. Allergic reaction is another cause of death. The first-time user may be allergic to the narcotic itself; the addict may be allergic to one of the ingredients used to dilute the drug. Deaths from bacterial endocarditis and hepatitis are fairly common; they are, of course, the result of injecting the drugs with nonsterile equipment.

Slang usage and street terms for commonly abused drugs are shown in Table 6-1. The characteristics of these drugs are listed in Table 6-2; all these drugs cause psychological dependence.

TREATMENT OF ADDICTION

The short-term goal of all treatment of drug dependence is to wean the addict from drugs—usually by hospitalizing the addict and substituting doses of a related drug in gradually decreasing amounts so that withdrawal illness is minimized. The long-term goal of total rehabilitation is often difficult to achieve, particularly in *opiate* addicts. Since the psychosocial problems related to the addict's strong psychological dependence on drugs develop over a long period of time, one cannot expect resolution of these personality problems to take any less time. Realistically we must classify drug dependence as a chronic disease in which we expect to see repeated remissions and exacerbations over a long period

TABLE 6-1 Street Terms for Commonly Abused Drugs

Drug	Street Terms
Stimulants	
Amphetamines:	
Benzedrine	Hearts, bennies, cartwheels, speed, crank
Methamphetamine	Meth, splash
Cocaine	Coke, big C, candy, snow, blow, nose candy
Hallucinogens	
LSD	Acid, blotter, cube, zen, sugar, blue heaven, window pane
Dimethyltryptamine	DMT
Mescaline	Peyote
PCP	Angel dust, crystal, hog, peace pill, rocket fuel, cyclones
Psilocybin	Magic mushroom
Inhalants (glue, solvents, aerosols)	Gunk
Psychodepressants	
Meprobamate	Mother's little helper
Tetrahydrocannabinal	THC
Marijuana (cannabis, hashish)	Pot, grass, hash, joint, Mary Jane, weed, gold, reefer, goof butt
Alcohol	Juice, grog, booze
Methaqualone	Love drug, ludes, quads, soaps
Amyl nitrite, butyl nitrite	Poppers, snappers (Locker Room, Rush—brand names)
Barbiturates:	Peanuts, pink ladies, barbs, candy, dolls, downers
Amobarbital, amytal	Blue angels, blue birds, blue bullets, blue dolls, blue tips, blues
Phenobarbital	Phennies
Nembutal	Yellow dolls, yellow jackets, yellows, nebbies, nemmies, abbots, blockbusters
Tuinal	Tootsies, trees, tuies, gorilla pills
Seconal	F-40's, reds, red dolls, red bullets, seccies, seggies
Combinations:	
Dexamyl	Christmas trees, hearts, purple hearts
Any barbiturate and alcohol	Geronimo
Seconal and amobarbital	Double trouble, rainbows, reds and blues
Chloral hydrate and alcohol	Mickey Finn
Opiates	
Heroin	Horse, H, junk, scag, smack, dope, hard stuff

TABLE 6-2 Characteristics of Commonly Abused Drugs

Drug	Physical Dependence	Tolerance	Withdrawal Symptoms	Duration of Withdrawal	Possibility of Lethal Overdose?	Illegal in U.S.?
Stimulants						
Cocaine	none	no	no	—	yes	no
Amphetamines	little	yes	yes	3–5 days	yes	no
Hallucinogens						
Mescaline	none	yes*	probably not	—	yes	yes
Peyote	none	yes*	probably not	—	yes	yes
Psilocybin	none	yes*	probably not	—	yes	yes
DMT	none	yes*	probably not	—	yes	yes
LSD	none	yes*	probably not	—	yes	yes
PCP	none	yes*	yes	unknown	yes	no
Psychodepressants						
Marijuana	little	yes†	no	—	unknown	yes‡
Bromides	none	no	no	—	yes	no
Alcohol	yes	yes	yes	5–10 days	yes	no
Barbiturates	yes	yes	yes	5–10 days	yes	no
Paraldehyde	yes	yes	yes	5–10 days	yes	no
Methaqualone	yes	yes	yes	5–10 days	yes	no
Chloral hydrate	yes	yes	yes	5–10 days	yes	no
Propoxyphene	yes	yes	yes	5–10 days	yes	no
Tranquilizers	yes	yes	yes	5–10 days	yes	no
Inhalants	little	possibly	no	—	yes	no
Opiates (narcotics)						
Opium	yes	yes	yes	3–6 days	yes	no
Heroin	yes	yes	yes	3–6 days	yes	yes
Morphine	yes	yes	yes	3–6 days	yes	no
Methadone	yes	yes	yes	3–6 days	yes	no
LAAM	yes	yes	yes	3–6 days	yes	no

* In habitual users.
† At high doses.
‡ See text for exceptions.

of time; first-treatment cure is thus the exception rather than the rule. The relapse rate among young narcotic addicts is especially high, but the percentage of long remissions and cures increases with the advancing age of addicts. In any case, the most successful treatment programs focus on long-term therapy aimed at some degree of personality restructuring. In the federal narcotic rehabilitation programs, the addict is confined for a minimum of four to six months for intensive therapy and is supervised for three years after discharge. The California program for addicts, which provides a similar pattern of treatment, has an encouraging success rate. Many addicts relapse several times before achieving complete abstinence from drugs; some never achieve lifelong abstinence.

Methadone Treatment

Methadone treatment programs for heroin addicts have become very popular in recent years. The treatment consists of substituting a daily oral dose of **methadone**, a long-acting synthetic, to replace the heroin. Except for weekends, clients must be physically present at the methadone clinic to receive daily doses, which are free or very inexpensive. The most effective programs also provide counseling services and psychotherapy. Methadone programs are of debatable value for several reasons. First, they do not cure addiction; they merely substitute one addicting drug for another. Second, methadone itself is now being found on the streets for resale. Third, cases of primary dependence on methadone are appearing. Fourth, the chance for long-term success in treating addicts seems to depend on confinement for at least four months after the addicting drug is withdrawn. Since addicts on methadone maintenance usually remain in the same social milieu in which they became addicted, their chances of quitting drugs are indeed slim. It was originally thought that because methadone blocks the euphoric effects of heroin, the addict who converted to methadone would cease to crave any drug and could then be weaned from drugs by gradually reducing the methadone dosage. Experience has shown that, generally speaking, treatment of the heroin addict means methadone maintenance for life.

Although methadone addicts are able to lead productive and crime-free lives, their life-styles almost always involve the use of other drugs, including alcohol and barbiturates. The chief benefits of methadone maintenance lie in the addict's release from an expensive dependence on the underworld—resulting in reduction of crime and freedom from the devastating effects of needle use.

LAAM Treatment

A new synthetic called **LAAM** (levo-alpha-acetylmethadol) is being tested in selected clinics by the National Institute of Drug Abuse. LAAM has all the properties of methadone, including physical dependence, but its effects last for 72 hours. This long-term effect frees addicts from daily clinic visits and allows them to lead a more normal life because the daily ritual of drug taking is modified. It also means that methadone clinics using LAAM could treat three times as many addicts as they now do.

Transitional Treatment

A new approach to the treatment of narcotic dependence involves a four-phase effort to wean the addict from both psychological and physical drug dependence. In stage 1, the addict is placed on daily doses of methadone as a substitute for the illicit narcotic. Because addicts are assured a steady supply of methadone, their other drug-taking behavior can be modified—that is, their energies are no longer geared to obtaining drugs from illicit sources in an effort to prevent the agony of withdrawal.

Stage 2 involves the gradual substitution of LAAM for methadone. Because LAAM is effective for 72 hours, addicts need to be medicated only every third day. The psychological bonus to this stage is the interruption of the daily ritual of drug taking. Not only is the addict's psychological dependence on the drug modified, but there is no need to take a weekend supply home from the treatment center. Thus there is less danger of LAAM appearing on the street as a primary source of addiction.

Stage 3, detoxification, is the most difficult stage because of the addict's fear of the pain of withdrawal. **Clonidine**, now being used in clinical trials to block the withdrawal symptoms related to detoxification, acts by stimulating the brain to suppress the symptoms of withdrawal. When the narcotic drug is abruptly discontinued, the addict is given controlled doses of clonidine every four to six hours. Because careful observation is necessary, this stage of treatment is best accomplished at an inpatient facility. The clonidine is gradually reduced after the eighth to tenth day; the entire phase of treatment lasts about two weeks.

Stage 4 is geared toward preventing relapse, which occurs in 30 to 70% of clients. **Naltrexone**, a narcotic antagonist used for the addicts most vulnerable to relapse, acts by binding to opiate receptor cells, thereby inhibiting the binding of other opiates to these cells. Naltrexone itself has no narcotic activity. If an opiate drug is taken during naltrexone treatment, therefore, the client will not experience the euphoria or other effects of opiates. Thus drug dependence is reduced and there is evidence that clients treated with a single daily dose of naltrexone are less apt to relapse. This phase of treatment is usually limited to a six-month period—the length of time it takes for a return to normal physiological function after chronic opiate use. Other narcotic antagonists, *bupernorphine* and *oxilorphan,* are currently being tested. *Cyclazocine* and *naloxone* are used less often, since they have a shorter duration of action.

The importance of a *comprehensive* treatment program cannot be overemphasized. Without concomitant intervention relating to personality and social factors, the pharmacological approach alone has little hope of reducing the high relapse rate among addicts.

Self-Help Organizations

Self-help groups, such as Odyssey House and Phoenix House, claim a reasonable degree of success in long-term remission and cure. These programs are operated by nongovernmental groups and are staffed largely by former drug abusers. The addict can relate readily to staff members who are thoroughly familiar with the drug subculture and who have themselves been cured of drug dependence. These programs, which rely extensively on group therapy and rehabilitation, are successful for addicts who remain in the supportive environment. The relapse rate for those who leave the group prematurely is as high as that for any other treatment program. The powerful physical and psychological craving for opiates in particular accounts for the high relapse rate among addicts, even after relatively long periods of abstinence. Without extensive restructuring of the addict's life-style, the chances for even short-term remission are very slight. When addicts are confined in a closely supervised facility for the initial stages of treatment, however, their contact with the street drug subculture is broken. If this confinement is combined with intensive rehabilitation efforts at all levels, a long-term remission is indeed possible. Under no circumstances is it advisable to attempt abrupt withdrawal on an outpatient basis.

Even though many addicts insist that they first became addicted via medical prescription, actual medical addiction is quite rare. For patients in need of short-term analgesia after painful procedures, therefore, opiates may be administered as needed without fear of physical or psychological dependence. In cases of terminal illness, where opiates are administered over longer time periods, the resultant dependence is entirely justified. The small number of people who have become addicted for medical reasons alone can generally be cured after the initial withdrawal treatment. The term *drug addiction,* with all its psychological, sociological, and legal implications, relates to those whose craving for drugs becomes so powerful that it dominates their lives.

Treatment of Alcoholism

As with opiates, long-term abstinence from alcohol by the addicted individual is difficult to achieve and the relapse rate is high. Initial detoxification is easily managed with the aid of *benzodiazepines,* such as Valium. After detoxification the addict is sometimes given *disulfiram,* which causes violent symptoms when even a small amount of alcohol is ingested. The symptoms include headache, nausea and vomiting, sweating, palpitations, hypotension, chest pain, blurred vision, and confusion. The physical reaction to the disulfiram-alcohol combination is so severe, in fact, that many clients refuse to take disulfiram at all. Disulfiram is not a cure for alcoholism and should be used only as a temporary measure encouraging the addict's compliance with a comprehensive treatment program. Alcoholism continues to be as difficult to treat as is opiate addiction. Self-help groups such as Alcoholics Anonymous (AA) are moderately successful in preventing relapse because they deal with the complex psychosocial forces that shape addictive behavior. But, as with Phoenix House and other groups, long-term abstinence depends on the addict's continued close contact with the treatment milieu.

LEGISLATION TO CONTROL DRUG ABUSE

International Activities

International recognition of the drug abuse problem dates back to the beginning of the 20th century when addiction to opiates was widespread. The League of Nations, and later the

United Nations, have addressed the problem by promoting the exchange of information on the worldwide production and traffic in narcotic drugs. In 1961 the nations participating in the World Health Organization agreed on many important measures related to drug abuse, including a commitment to eliminate the traffic and use of marijuana by 1985. International activities concerning drug abuse have dealt primarily with scientific study and information sharing. The controls imposed by individual nations on drug use and traffic, however, bear testimony to the international recognition that drug abuse has serious individual and social consequences.

National Legislation

From the Harrison Narcotic Act in 1914 to 1970, the federal government passed at least ten laws in response to specific problems concerning illicit drug traffic and abuse. Virtually all the provisions of these early laws were incorporated into the Comprehensive Drug Abuse Prevention and Control Act of 1970, which became effective in 1971 and is usually referred to as the Controlled Substances Act. This section summarizes the main provisions of the Controlled Substances Act and then reviews earlier laws directed to drug abuse.

Comprehensive Drug Abuse Prevention and Control Act of 1970 This legislation deals with the handling of controlled substances at every level, including importing and exporting, manufacture, distribution in health agencies, and individual prescription. Practitioners legally permitted to dispense and prescribe controlled substances must register with the Drug Enforcement Agency (formerly the federal Bureau of Narcotics and Dangerous Drugs), which is a division of the Department of Justice. Registered practitioners, which include health care agencies, must keep accurate inventory records on all controlled substances and must record all doses dispensed or discarded. Moreover, theftproof storage and handling by agencies and individual practitioners is mandated by this law. The controlled drugs included in the law are divided into five categories called *schedules* (Table 6-3).

Schedule I lists drugs that have no legitimate medical use in the United States—LSD, heroin, marijuana, and many others that find their way to the streets through illegal channels. *Schedule II* includes the more potent narcotics (natural and synthetic) as well as most amphetamines and methamphetamines. *Schedule III* includes the potent codeine combination preparations, paregoric, the potent barbiturate drugs, some nonbarbiturate hypnotics, and the remainder of the amphetamines and methamphetamines. *Schedule IV* includes the rest of the barbiturates and barbiturate combination drugs, chloral hydrate, paraldehyde, and the tranquilizers. *Schedule V* includes the preparations containing very small amounts of opiates, such as cough syrups with codeine.

Each schedule has its own set of restrictions relating to the use of the drugs and refilling of prescriptions. Prescriptions for drugs in Schedule II, for example, may not be refilled; those in Schedule IV may be refilled no more than five times in a six-month period. The law specifies that any violation of its provisions for manufacture, distribution, and dispensation of controlled drugs is subject to fines, imprisonment, and revocation of license.

Harrison Narcotic Act (1914) This tax law required anyone involved in handling opium, coca leaves, and their derivatives to register for a license and pay tax on the drugs. It was designed not so much to secure revenue as to control the widespread traffic in opium.

Narcotic Drug Import and Export Act (1922) This law limited the amount of opium and coca imported to that needed for medical purposes only.

Narcotic Hospital Law (1929) This law provided for federal hospital facilities for treating narcotics addicts. Two facilities were established—one in Lexington, Kentucky, and one in Fort Worth, Texas, which is now under the jurisdiction of the federal Bureau of Prisons. The hospital in Kentucky conducted research on new drugs and on the treatment of addiction in both voluntary and court-committed clients.

Narcotic Information Act (1930) This act provided rewards for information leading to the arrest of narcotics laws violators.

Marijuana Tax Act (1937) This act put the same restrictions on marijuana that the Harrison Act of 1914 placed on opiates and coca.

Narcotic Transportation Act (1939) This act gave the federal government the power to confiscate any vehicle or vessel used for the transport of illegally acquired drugs.

Opium Poppy Control Act (1942) This law prohibited the growth of the opium poppy in the United States.

Durham-Humphrey Law (1952) This law imposed controls on barbiturates and related drugs by limiting the number of times prescriptions could be refilled. It also categorized drugs into two groups: those that could safely be sold without a prescription (over-the-counter drugs) and those requiring a medical prescription.

Narcotic Control Act (1956) This law made the possession of heroin and marijuana illegal; a few researchers were allowed small quantities, however.

Drug Abuse Control Amendments (1965) This law gave the federal government the power to control the manufacture and sale of barbiturates, amphetamines, and many other drugs considered potentially dangerous.

Narcotic Addict Rehabilitation Act (1966) This law provides for the rehabilitation of addicts in appropriate treatment facilities, including long-term supervision by community agencies. Addicts may voluntarily commit themselves for treat-

TABLE 6-3 Controlled Substances

Schedule I (C-I): No accepted medical use; high abuse potential; illegal	**Schedule II (C-II):** Medical use with restrictions; high abuse potential; R_x only—no refills	**Schedule III (C-III):** Accepted medical use; moderate abuse potential; R_x—refill 5 times in 6 months	**Schedule IV (C-IV):** Accepted medical use; less abuse potential; R_x—refill 5 times in 6 months	**Schedule V (C-V):** Accepted medical use; low abuse potential; R_x for most
Heroin and opium derivatives	Raw opium	Paregoric	Barbital	Cheracol syrup with codeine[2]
LSD	Morphine	Nalorphine	Chloral hydrate	Phenergan with codeine[2]
Mescaline	Apomorphine	Acetaminophen with codeine	Paraldehyde	Robitussin with codeine[2]
Peyote	Oxymorphone	APC with codeine	Phenobarbital	Elixir terpin hydrate with codeine[2]
Psilocybin	Levomethorphan	ASA with codeine	Pemoline	Cidicol syrup with ethylmorphine[3]
THC	Fentanyl	Dihydrocodeinone	Benzphetamine	Donnagel-PG (opium)[3]
Marijuana[1]	Anileridine	Ethylmorphine	Diethylpropion	Lomotil (diphenoxylate)[4]
	Methadone	Aprobarbital	Fenfluramine	
	Codeine	Glutethemide	Phentermine	
	Hydrocodone	Amobarbital	Chlordiazepoxide	
	Cocaine	Pentobarbital	Diazepam	
	Many amphetamines and methamphetamines	Secobarbital	Meprobamate	
	Methaqualone	Butabarbital	Oxazepam	
	Phenmetrazine	Aprobarbital	Propoxyphene	
		Hexobarbital		
		Methprylon		
		Talbutol		
		Chlorphentermine		
		Mazindol		
		Phendimetrazine		
		Phencyclidine		

[1]The National Institute on Drug Abuse is now allowing limited quantities of marijuana to be prescribed only for the treatment of glaucoma or for nausea associated with chemotherapy.

[2]Not more than 200 mg codeine per 100 ml or 100 g.

[3]Not more than 100 mg opium or ethylmorphine per 100 ml or 100 g.

[4]Not more than 2.5 mg diphenoxylate per dosage unit; not less than 0.025 mg atropine per dosage unit.

ment, or they may be committed to a treatment facility by the courts instead of being prosecuted. Addicts who have committed crimes of violence are not eligible, nor are those charged with selling narcotics.

The national *Office for Drug Abuse Prevention* was created in 1972 to assist states in establishing rehabilitation facilities as well as to coordinate research into all aspects of drug abuse.

PERSPECTIVES ON DRUG ABUSE

The inability of current policy and legislation to curb the drug abuse problem suggests that drug addiction is a stubborn disease that resists all current methods of treatment and control. Clearly, continued research into the psychobiological effects of drug abuse is needed and new policies for dealing with the drug abuse epidemic should be considered. The few attempts at educating young people in the consequences of experimentation with drugs have failed to stem the rise in drug use. The Drug Enforcement Agency, although diligent in attempting to curtail supplies of illegal drugs and control trafficking in legal drugs, is hampered by laws that provide meaningful penalties for trafficking in drugs but not for possession. Several states have, in fact, "decriminalized" marijuana.

The evidence on drug abuse suggests that national and international drug policies need to be revised to reflect current scientific knowledge. Educational programs that now emphasize controlled use must be replaced with programs emphasizing the dangers of all drugs, including marijuana and cocaine. Moreover, health professionals and community leaders must take measures to prevent the sale of drug paraphernalia in their communities.

Research should continue to focus on the psychobiological effects of drugs so that educational programs geared toward prevention of drug use will be based on scientific fact. The knowledge that all psychoactive drugs stimulate the pleasure-seeking centers of the brain, for example, explains the addict's craving as well as the need to progress to higher doses and more potent drugs. As tolerance develops, stronger drugs are needed to achieve the pleasurable sensations, and the brain's pleasure center becomes incapable of being stimulated by any other forces. Such scientific data should become the foundation for all prevention and treatment programs.

The latest scientific evidence also suggests that legislation and law enforcement policies need to be strengthened on a national and international scale. Since programs directed at controlling drugs have failed to halt the acceleration in drug abuse, it seems logical in light of the known health and social hazards to call for total prohibition. This means that criminal penalties would be imposed for possession as well as dealing in drugs. Moreover, international cooperation is a necessity to control supplies of illegal drugs at their sources. Certainly epidemic drug abuse is a worldwide problem long recognized by such international organizations as the World Health Organization and the United Nations International Narcotic Control Board.

The mounting evidence on the hazards of drug use suggests that people should no longer be deluded into thinking that experimenting with safe or "soft" drugs is harmless and should therefore be sanctioned. On the contrary, statistics suggest a need for intensive local, state, national, and international efforts aimed at reversing the epidemic of drug abuse. Young people need to understand that there is no known cure for drug addiction. Once they are addicted, the craving for drugs is a life-long affliction.

REFERENCES

Becker, C., Roe, R., and Scott, R. 1974. *Alcohol as a drug*. New York: Krieger.

Blain, J.D., and Julius, D. A., eds. 1977. *Psychodynamics of drug dependence*. Washington, D.C.: U.S. Government Printing Office.

Gardner, E., ed. 1981. *Drug and alcohol abuse: Implications for treatment*. Washington, D.C.: Department of Health and Human Services.

Glatt, M. 1977. *Drug dependence: Current problems and issues*. Baltimore: University Park Press.

Grinspoon, L., and Hedblom, P. 1975. *The speed culture*. Cambridge, Mass.: Harvard University Press.

Handbook on Drug Abuse. 1979. Washington, D.C.: U.S. Government Printing Office.

Hofmann, F. G. 1975. *A handbook on drug and alcohol abuse: The biomedical aspects.* New York: Oxford University Press.

Maurer, D., and Vogel, V. 1973. *Narcotics and narcotic addiction.* Springfield, Ill.: Charles C Thomas.

Nahas, G., and Frick, H., eds. 1981. *Drug abuse in the modern world.* New York: Pergamon Press.

Nahas, G., and Paton, W. 1979. *Marihuana: Biological effects.* New York: Pergamon Press.

Rittenhouse, J. D., ed. 1980. *National survey on drug abuse during the seventies: A social analysis.* Washington, D.C.: U.S. Government Printing Office.

Young, L., and others. 1977. *Recreational drugs.* New York: Macmillan.

PART II

PHARMACO-THERAPEUTICS

MEDICATIONS ARE GIVEN to clients in order to achieve a desired response. The general terms used to indicate these purposes are sometimes used to describe a drug or group of drugs: diagnostic agents, preventative agents, prophylactic agents, and the like.

Diagnostic agents are drugs given during tests or examinations to assist in diagnosing illness. The *contrast media* diagnostic drugs are used to outline a body cavity or organ. Barium sulfate, for example, is a radiopaque substance that is swallowed during a gastrointestinal (GI) series. It is used to fill the stomach and intestines so that defects can be exposed for x-rays. The *immunologic* diagnostic agents, such as the tine test, are used for tuberculosis screening. Other diagnostic agents include betazole hydrochloride (Histalog) for determining alterations in gastric secretions and edrophonium chloride (Tensilon) for the differential diagnosis of myasthenia gravis.

Preventative agents are drugs given to prevent disease or an unwanted state of health. For example, trivalent oral polio vaccine is given to prevent poliomyelitis.

Prophylactic agents are drugs used to prevent a secondary illness. (This term is often used interchangeably with preventative agent.) Antibiotics, for example, can be given prophylactically to victims of influenza (a viral infection) in order to prevent a secondary bacterial infection from invading the weakened client.

Replacement or **substitutive agents** are drugs given to replace deficiencies (replacement agents) or a total lack (substitutive agents) of the normal body substance. These terms are often used interchangeably. Clients who have hypothyroidism are given thyroid preparations to replace their deficiency, for example. Whereas clients with severe diabetes mellitus require insulin to meet their daily needs, the oral hypoglycemic agent acetohexamide (Dymelor) may be all that is necessary for the client with maturity-onset diabetes.

Maintenance agents are drugs given to enhance a normal body function that may be inadequate.[1] For example, dioctyl sodium sulfosuccinate (Colace) is a stool softener that is sometimes given to bedridden clients to help them maintain normal bowel function.

Symptomatic or **palliative agents** are drugs that do not cure the disease or illness but only relieve the client of a specific symptom or group of symptoms. Infectious gastroenteritis may cause nausea and vomiting, for example. An antiemetic agent, such as prochlorperazine (Compazine) or benzquinamide hydrochloride (Emetecon), can be given to relieve the client's distress from these symptoms, but the drug will not cure the infection.

Supportive agents are drugs that assist in maximizing the state of health in an acutely ill client or one with a progressively debilitating illness. These drugs do not cure the disease or illness; nor do they relieve a specific distressing symptom. Vitamin-fortified fluids may be given intravenously to an acutely ill client who is unable to retain fluids, for example, and food supplements high in vitamin, mineral, and protein content may be given to a chronically ill client in order to maintain optimum nutrition. Some health team members use the term *supportive* interchangeably with symptomatic and palliative agents.

Invasive or **chemotherapeutic agents** are drugs given to destroy or inhibit the growth of fast-growing atypical cells (neoplasm) or disease-causing microorganisms. These drugs invade atypical cells and microorganisms and alter or destroy them. Antineoplastic drugs, antibiotics, and antimetabolites are included in this category. Although all drugs are chemical substances given for a therapeutic reason, some health team members reserve the term *chemotherapeutic* for antineoplastic agents. Although drugs are prescribed for a specific purpose, these chemical substances can often cause other responses—for example, the disruption of normal intestinal flora by antibiotics and the adverse effects of antineoplastic agents on other fast-growing cells, such as the mucosa of the gastrointestinal tract. Consequently health team members must be aware of the entire spectrum of drug effects.

Almost all drugs cause more than one pharmacologic effect. The desired drug effects are often accompanied by nonintended effects that may be harmless, beneficial, or hazardous (see figure). A harmless color change in the urine may be

[1]Do not confuse maintenance agents with the term *maintenance dose.* A maintenance dose is the dosage of a drug that is taken daily to replace the amount of drug excreted daily by the body. The dosage maintains the therapeutic blood level in the body, as in digitalized clients.

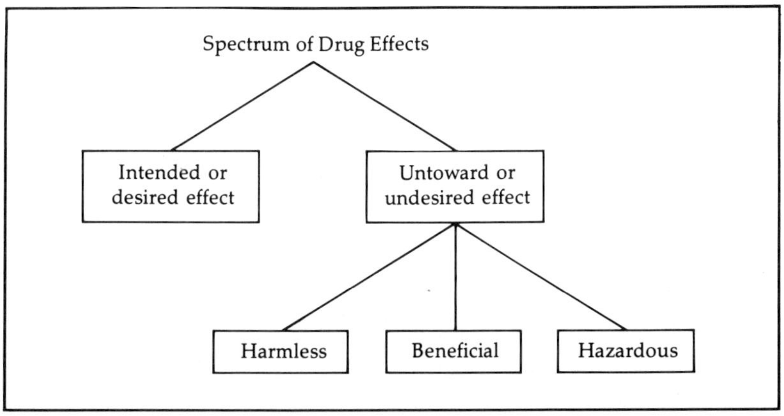

FIGURE II-1

caused by the antibiotic rifampin (Rifadin) and other drugs. Although the desired response to antihistamines, such as diphenhydramine hydrochloride (Benadryl), is suppression of an allergic reaction, these drugs tend to depress the central nervous system and cause drowsiness. The additional sleep may be beneficial to some clients, but this unintended response may be hazardous to others, such as truck drivers. All drugs present hazards in certain situations. If an individual takes an overdose, unknowingly or otherwise, or if the client is unable to metabolize or excrete the drug, there may be toxic effects. Even in normal doses, certain clients may develop toxicity, have an allergic or hypersensitivity reaction, or develop another undesired response. How drugs act and how they are processed in the body are explained in Chapter 7. Untoward or undesired drug effects are presented in Chapter 8.

Chapter 7

Pharmacodynamics

PHARMACODYNAMICS IS THE experimental science that deals with the interactions between drugs and living tissues. It is the study of the mechanisms of drug action, including absorption, distribution, storage, metabolic change, and excretion of drugs in animals and man.

Although medications are given for specific purposes, different individuals have different responses to the same substances, and sometimes the same client responds differently to a drug at different times. Pharmacodynamics is an important field for health team members because it helps to explain these variable responses. It is especially important for nurses to understand the principles of pharmacodynamics, because they are often the first to observe these unexpected changes and must be able to institute appropriate measures when necessary. For example, many diabetics take oral hypoglycemic agents daily. A stress, such as illness, can alter the client's need for insulin. If the signs and symptoms of impending diabetic coma or insulin shock are observed, the nurse must notify the physician and take other appropriate measures as necessary.

DRUG MOVEMENT THROUGH BIOLOGICAL MEMBRANES

The movement of a drug from its site of administration to its sites of action, metabolism, and excretion involves specific characteristics of both the drug and the body's cellular membranes. The water-soluble antibiotic neomycin is so poorly absorbed from the gastrointestinal tract that it must be administered parenterally for a systemic effect to occur. But many other oral drugs are easily able to penetrate the cellular membranes of the intestinal mucosa, enter the bloodstream, and pass through the vessel walls to their sites of action. The methods of drug movement in the body depend on the drug's ability to pass through these cell membranes.

Composition of Cell Membranes

Cell membranes in the body are protein-lipid barriers about 80 to 90 angstroms thick.[1] They are thought to contain an outer layer of protein molecules, a layer of lipid molecules, called the *lipid matrix*, an inner layer of protein molecules, and a number of tiny channels or pores (see Figure 7-1). The proteins provide structural strength and the lipids act as a cellular protector by preventing the passage of undesired substances, such as excessive quantities of water and many water-soluble substances. Water and some lipid-insoluble substances can gain entry into the cell through the minute channels. The diameter of a channel in the average cell is approximately 8 angstroms, but there are channels as large as 40 angstroms in diameter located in the walls of capillaries.

[1] An angstrom is equal to 10^{-10} meter.

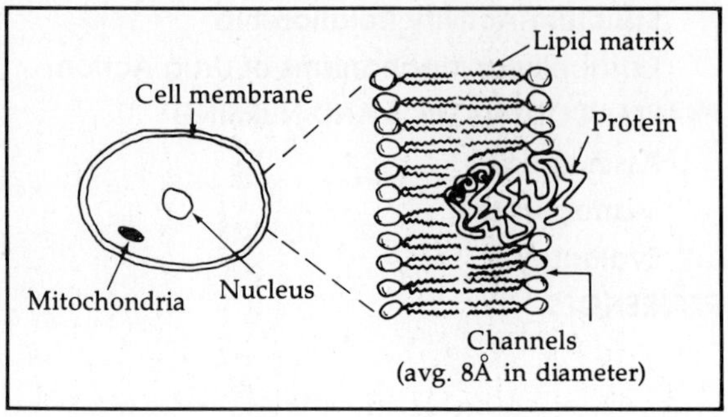

FIGURE 7-1 Composition of cell membranes. Drugs and other substances pass through cell membranes either by diffusion or by an active transport mechanism. The drug movement depends in part on the chemical characteristics of the drug.

Characteristics of Drugs

The process of drug movement across cellular membranes is determined largely by various characteristics of the drug, including its solubility and ionization properties.

Drugs may be soluble in water, soluble in lipids, or both. The degree of *solubility* varies among drugs and can be altered by the drug state. Drugs that are highly soluble in lipids tend to be transported more readily since they can cross the lipid matrix rather freely.

Most drugs are weak acids or weak bases. When a drug is dissolved in body fluids, some of the drug molecules are **ionized** (dissociated into a positively charged or negatively charged portion) and others remain in a *nonionized* or *free* state. Since the nonionized portion is usually more lipid soluble than the ionized part, the nonionized drug molecules may diffuse freely through the cells' lipid material. But if the ionized portion of a drug is small enough, it may still enter the cell by traveling through the tiny channels in the cell membrane. When the ionized part is too large for the channel passage, it may diffuse slowly through the membrane's lipid matrix or it may even be actively transported by the cell membrane.

The degree of drug ionization depends on the pH of the dissolving body fluids and on the drug's dissociation constant. The **drug dissociation constant,** abbreviated pKa, is the pH at which a drug has equal concentrations of ionized and free molecules.

Drugs that are weak bases (pKa of 0 to 4) tend to have equal concentrations of nonionized and ionized drug molecules at a low pH. Consequently, these drugs tend to be more completely dissociated into ions in acidic environments—for example, the stomach—and less ionized in more alkaline environments—for example, the intestines (see Figure 7-2). Since the ionized portion tends to be less lipid soluble and therefore less transportable, weak basic drugs are absorbed better in the intestines than in the stomach.

Drugs that are weak acids (pKa of 2.5 to 10) tend to have equal concentrations of nonionized and ionized drug molecules at higher pH levels. These drugs tend to be more completely dissociated into ions in alkaline environments, and to remain in the free state in acidic body fluids (see Figure 7-3). Salicylic acid (pKa of 3.0) undergoes less ionization in the stomach and is therefore better absorbed in the stomach than in the intestines.

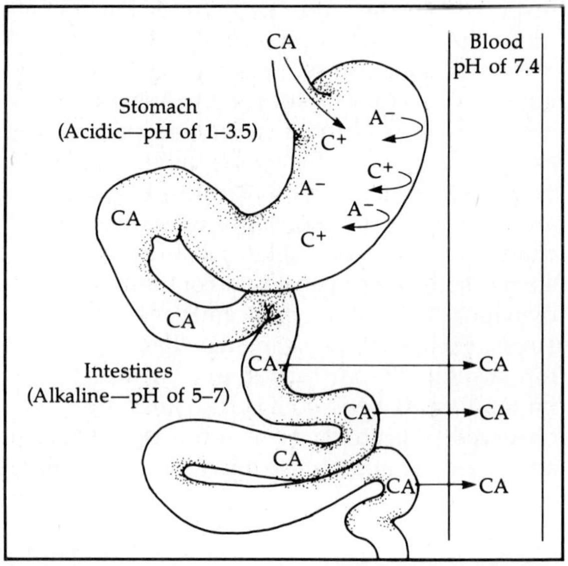

FIGURE 7-2 Ionization of a drug (CA) that is a weak base. (A− = anion, C+ = cation.) Drugs that are weak bases tend to be ionized in the stomach's acid pH and, therefore, are unable to pass through biological membranes. They are absorbed better from the small intestine, since they tend to be in the free state in alkaline environments.

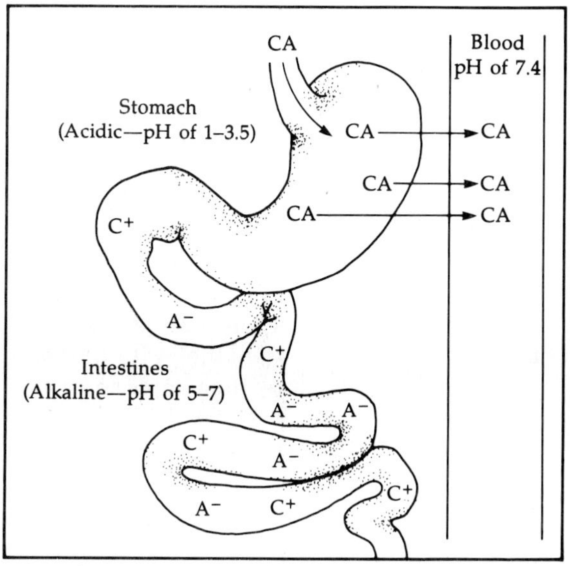

FIGURE 7-3 Ionization of a drug (CA) that is a weak acid. Drugs that are weak acids tend to remain in the free state in the acid environment of the stomach and to become ionized in the alkaline environment of the intestines. Therefore they are absorbed better from the stomach.

Methods of Drug Movement

The solubility and ionization properties of a drug determine not only the rate at which drug molecules move across biological membranes, but also the method of drug movement. There are three basic processes by which drugs cross cellular membranes: passive diffusion, facilitated diffusion, and active transport. Most drugs move via passive diffusion.

Passive diffusion

Diffusion is the passive process by which drugs move from an area of high drug concentration to an area of lower drug concentration. The difference between the drug concentrations on either side of the cell membrane is called the **concentration gradient** or the **diffusion gradient.** Since the blood and lymphatic circulations are constantly moving the absorbed drug molecules away from the site of absorption, the concentration gradient at the absorption site tends to be great and the drug is often absorbed into the blood rapidly.

A drug must reach a minimum level in the circulation, called the **critical concentration,** in order to be moved into the site of action in large enough quantities to create a therapeutic response.

The rate at which a drug diffuses across a biological membrane is determined by many factors, including the following:

1. *The concentration gradient*—The greater the gradient, the faster the rate of diffusion.

2. *The body temperature*—The rate of diffusion at elevated temperatures is greater. Drugs diffuse more rapidly in clients with high fevers and more slowly in clients with severe hypothermia.

3. *The drug's molecular size*—The smaller the drug's molecular size (molecular weight), the faster the diffusion. However, if the drug molecule attracts a water molecule, the larger hydrated drug molecule will diffuse at a slower rate.

4. *The thickness of the cell membrane*—The thinner the cell membrane involved, the faster the diffusion. For example, liver cell membranes tend to be thinner than bone cell membranes and therefore allow diffusion at a faster rate.

Drugs with a high lipid solubility tend to diffuse through the lipid matrix rapidly and those with a low lipid solubility tend to diffuse slowly. Therefore, the greater a drug's lipid solubility, the faster it will diffuse through the matrix. The amount of drug and the rate at which the lipid-soluble drugs diffuse increase dramatically if the drug remains in the free state.

The greater the **pH gradient**—the difference between the pH on either side of the membrane—the greater the diffusion. For example, the pH gradient between the blood, with a pH of 7.4, and the stomach, with a pH of 1, is great. Weak basic drugs that are administered intravenously exist in the blood's pH environment primarily in the nonionized state. These drugs penetrate lipid membranes well and will enter the stomach because of the large pH gradient. In the stomach's pH, these drugs become ionized and are therefore unable to return to the blood for redistribution. This method of drug loss can be acute in clients who have continuous nasogastric suction, because they may not be able to sustain the drug's critical concentration level for a therapeutic response.

Diffusion also occurs through the channels. As water diffuses through the tiny membrane channels, it carries with it molecules of water-soluble drugs that are small enough to pass through the channel with ease. However, the channel walls are thought to be positively charged, and, since like charges repel each other, positively charged ionized drugs diffuse at a much slower rate, if at all.

Facilitated diffusion

Some drugs with little lipid solubility can diffuse through the lipid matrix by combining with a substance that carries them. Glucose enters most cells this way. The "carrier" picks up the drug, carries it into the cell, and then returns to the outer surface of the membrane to pick up another drug molecule (see Figure 7-4). The rate of diffusion depends on the concentration gradient as well as on the amount of carrier available to transport the drug. Facilitated diffusion is said to be *saturable*, because there may be a limited amount of carrier substance available. The carrier is said to be *selective* as well, since it will assist the diffusion of only certain drugs.

Active transport

Drugs that cross cellular membranes by diffusion move passively with the concentration, pressure, electrical, and other gradients. Other drugs move against one or more of these gradients. Their "uphill" movement against a concentration or other gradient *requires energy* and is, therefore, termed *active transport.* This method of passage is *saturable* and *selective,* since specific amounts of certain drugs are moved across membranes this way.

It is believed that drugs are actively transported by *carriers.* As in facilitated diffusion, the carrier picks up the drug on the outer surface of the membrane, carries it to the inside surface, discharges the drug, and then returns to the outside membrane (see Figure 7-5). Unlike facilitated diffusion, active transport of drug molecules has to work against a concentration or other gradient. The energy is probably supplied to the transport system by adenosine triphosphate (ATP). Many sugars, amino acids, and some electrolytes are known to be transported actively.

Pinocytosis and phagocytosis

Some drug molecules, particularly large molecules that have been hydrated or that have a low lipid solubility, may enter cells by the processes of pinocytosis or phagocytosis. **Pinocytosis** occurs when a drug molecule adheres to the cell membrane's outer surface. The membrane surrounds the molecule, along with a small

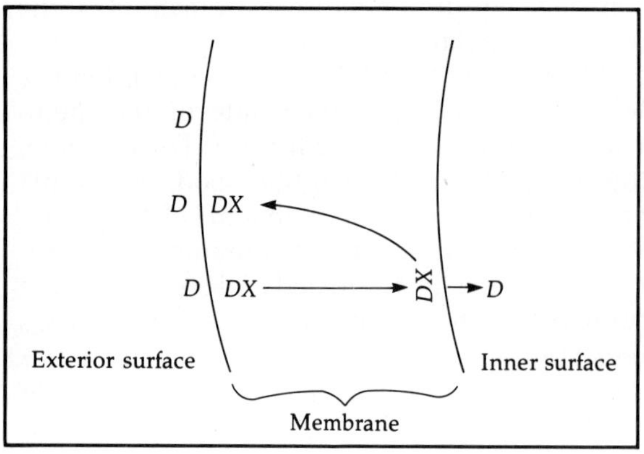

FIGURE 7-4 Facilitated diffusion of drugs. The drug (*D*) is transported by an unknown carrier substance (*X*) to the inner surface of the membrane, where it is released.

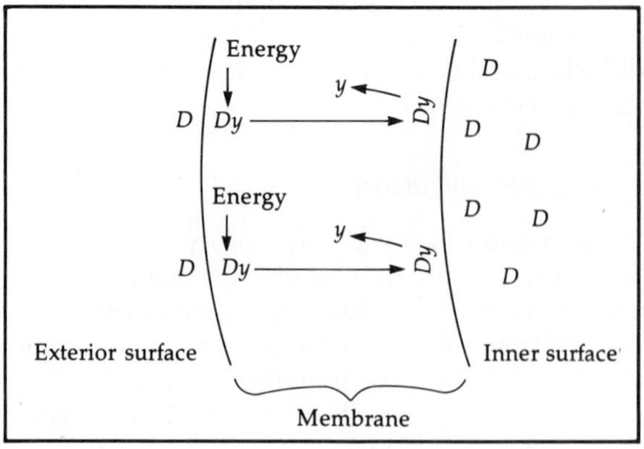

FIGURE 7-5 Active transport of drugs against a concentration gradient. Energy is required for the drug (*D*) to be transported by an unknown carrier (*Y*) to the inner surface of the membrane where the drug is released. This movement is "uphill" against a concentration, pressure, or other gradient.

amount of extracellular fluid, creates a *vacuole,* and moves the engulfed substances into the cell. **Phagocytosis** is similar, but involves the engulfment of a larger area. The engulfed section can contain solid particles as well and is often called a *vesicle.* See Figure 7-6.

Table 7-1 summarizes the various methods of drug movement across cell membranes.

DRUG ABSORPTION

No drug absorption is required when drugs are administered directly into body fluids, such as the blood or spinal fluid. The entire dose of an intravenously administered drug is available to produce an effect. But when a drug intended for systemic effect is administered via any other route, it must be absorbed from the site of administra-

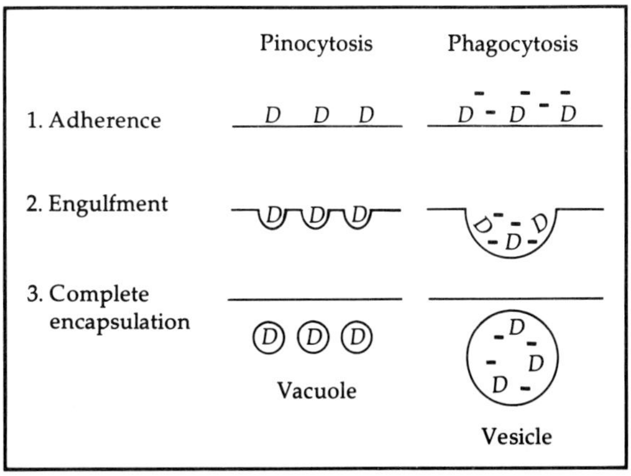

FIGURE 7-6 Pinocytosis and phagocytosis. The drug (*D*) adheres to the cell membrane's outer surface. In pinocytosis, only the drug and a small amount of extracellular fluid are engulfed and then completely encapsulated. In phagocytosis, a larger area, including solid particles, is completely encapsulated.

TABLE 7-1 Summary of the Mechanisms of Drug Movement Across Cell Membranes

Transport Mechanisms	Free or Nonionized Drug Molecules (High Lipid Solubility)	Ionized Drug Molecules (Low Lipid Solubility)
Diffusion and facilitated diffusion through lipid matrix	Readily used	Not used; cannot penetrate lipid matrix
Diffusion through channels	Probably not used	Used by tiny negative ions and very tiny positive ions
Active transport or slow diffusion as determined by pKa and pH gradient	Somewhat used	Used by large ions and hydrated ions that are too large for channels
Pinocytosis*	Probably not used	Used by a few ions, such as hydrated ions
Phagocytosis*	May be used by some very large molecules	May be used by some very large ions

*Although no drugs have been proven to use these mechanisms to cross cellular membranes, they are potential methods by which some drugs may enter cells.

tion into a body fluid, usually the blood, before it can reach its site of action. Sometimes the entire dose is not absorbed. A small quantity of many oral medications is excreted unchanged; therefore the total administered drug dose is not *biologically available to produce a pharmacologic response.*

Bioavailability

The quantity of active drug molecules, or its active metabolites, that actually reaches the circulation ready to cause a pharmacologic response is termed the **bioavailable dose.** Two means of determining drug bioavailability are measuring the blood concentration of a drug and determining the intensity of the pharmacologic response.

Drug absorption—and therefore drug bioavailability—can be altered by certain characteristics of the drug, the method by which the drug is administered, and characteristics of the client who receives the drug. The major altering factors are explained below.

Pharmaceutical Factors

Many bioavailability reports are in vitro studies conducted in "test tubes" rather than in intact organisms. This method of study is conducive to determining many pharmaceutical factors, such as the rate at which a drug dissolves and potential chemical interactions that can occur.

Drugs must be in solution before absorption through a biological membrane can occur. Elixirs, parenteral injections, and other liquid medications are already in a drug form that is conducive to absorption. But pills, tablets, suppositories, and other solid drug forms must first disintegrate and then dissolve in a body fluid, such as the stomach contents, before absorption can begin.

Disintegration is the process by which the active principles are released from the drug form. (See Chapter 12 for a detailed explanation of drug forms.) Binders and other adjuvants can be added by a pharmaceutical company to alter the amount and rate of disintegration. For example, some oral capsules are made with a heavy outer shell intended to preserve the encapsulated medication until it reaches the alkaline environment of the small intestines. Substances called binders are often added to pressed tablets to keep them from "flaking apart" before they are administered. A tablet that has prematurely disintegrated should not be administered to a client because it no longer contains the amount indicated on the container. Suppositories encase a medication in a solid form intended to disintegrate at body temperature. Consequently, suppositories should be removed from the refrigerator, carried on a tray—not held in the hand—and administered to the client immediately. Warm suppositories are difficult to insert because they disintegrate prematurely and lose their shape.

Dissolution is the process in which the drug dissolves and mixes with body fluids. A drug will not be absorbed unless it is soluble in the body fluids at the absorption site. Some drugs dissolve and mix readily, but others do not. A drug's rate and amount of dissolution can be altered by its particle size, its physical state, and the pH of the dissolving fluid. Dissolution rate depends largely on how the drug is manufactured. When drug companies produce a finely divided drug particle, they are ensuring a faster dissolution rate by increasing the surface area of the drug. Conversely, when a slower dissolution rate is preferred, larger particles will be produced.

A drug's physical state—crystalline, hydrated, amorphous, and so on—also influences its solubility in body fluids. Pharmaceutical companies can dramatically alter the absorption rate of penicillin and numerous other antibiotics by changing the physical characteristics of the drug. The crystalline solution of penicillin, potassium penicillin B, is highly soluble and must be administered several times a day; an intramuscular deposit of benzathine penicillin G is absorbed very slowly and the therapeutic effect of one injection will occur for days.

The dissolution of weak acid or base drugs may be changed by adding sodium bicarbonate, sodium citrate, magnesium carbonate, or another suitable buffer to the drug formulation. The pH of the area immediately surrounding buffered aspirin is raised by the added buffer and the dissolution rate is therefore faster than that of plain aspirin. The added buffer does not appreciably increase the pH of the stomach contents, so the slight increase in aspirin absorption from buffered aspirin is due only to the increase in the drug's dissolution.

Although the rate of drug dissolution will seldom alter the drug's clinical effectiveness, it does alter the rate at which the desired therapeutic effect occurs. The generic name of a drug may not vary from one company to another, but generic substitution is not always advisable because the drug formulations may vary and have different rates of dissolution. Toxic effects due to too rapid absorption have been reported when a cheaper generic substitute was taken instead of the prescribed trade-name drug.

Chemical interaction can occur between a drug and other substances, such as nutrients and other drugs, and enhance or prevent drug absorption. Oral iron preparations tend to be more completely absorbed when administered with orange juice and poorly absorbed when given with milk or other dairy products. Drugs that tend to interact adversely with nutrients should be administered at least one hour before or after meals.

Unabsorbable complexes may be formed when drugs are administered with an interacting drug or nutrient. For example, when tetracycline is administered with an antacid, an insoluble chelate is formed and the tetracycline is poorly absorbed. When both drug therapies are required, potential interaction can be avoided by administering the drugs at least one hour apart. Known adverse and desirable chemical interactions are indicated in the individual drug monographs.

Route of Administration

Most drugs are administered orally but other routes are available. Nurses administer drugs via the gastrointestinal, parenteral, and dermal-mucosal routes, and by application to other mucous membranes, such as the respiratory tract and vagina. Since the nature of the different absorbing surfaces varies, the factors that affect absorption vary also. The details of drug absorption through each of these routes are explained in Part IV.

Client Factors

Drug characteristics and the route by which a drug is administered are important factors in determining bioavailability, but it is the characteristics of the individual client that ultimately determine the amount and rate of drug absorption. The absorbing surfaces of different people are never exactly alike. Since in vivo bioavailability studies are usually conducted in animals or "normal, average adults," the data must be viewed as a guideline. The nurses must observe the client for his or her individual therapeutic response to a drug.

The major client factors that may either enhance or decrease the amount and rate of drug absorption are the pH of the client's body fluids, the amount and rate of his or her circulation, and the size and health of the surface area.

The *pH of body fluids* varies from one route of administration to another in the individual. The pH of the fluid in which the drug is dissolved affects the drug's ionization and therefore its absorption. Knowledge of a drug's pKa and of the pH of the dissolving fluid (see Table 7-2) can help one determine the potential rate and amount of drug absorption and therefore the time interval between drug absorption and therapeutic response. The drug monographs list the pKa's that are known.

At times, it may be desirable to change the pH of a body fluid when administering a drug. Antacids are sometimes given to elevate the pH of stomach contents, thereby increasing the absorption of certain weak base drugs or delaying the absorption of certain weak acid drugs. Unless one of these two effects is desired, antacids should not be administered with other medications.

TABLE 7-2 Average pH of Body Fluids

Fluid	Average pH
Stomach contents	1–3.5
Duodenal contents	5–7
Lower ileum contents	8
Plasma	7.35–7.40
Cerebrospinal fluid	7.32–7.35
Urine	4.6–8
Interstitial fluid	7.35
Intracellular fluid	7.0–7.2 (estimated)

The pH gradient between the dissolving body fluid and the circulation can change the drug absorption, a high pH gradient favoring absorption into the circulation and a low pH gradient depressing it. The pH gradients are discussed further in Part IV.

The *circulation* of blood and lymph provides the means by which systemic drugs are distributed. The greater the quantity of blood and lymph circulating in the area of the absorbing site, the greater the drug absorption. For example, the highly vascular pulmonary surface provides a means by which clients can be anesthetized rapidly and asthmatics treated quickly. Intramuscular injections need to be given deep into large muscle masses in clients with peripheral vascular diseases.

The rate at which blood circulates through the absorbing site also affects absorption. Athletes tend to have more rapid circulation than the average individual, so drug concentration gradients are greater in their bodies and drugs are absorbed more quickly. The converse is true of clients who have been bedridden for any length of time.

The amount and rate of circulation to a site can be increased when necessary with such measures as massage, warm compresses, or sitz baths. Each absorbing surface has its own circulatory characteristics; the details of circulatory patterns and the factors that affect circulation are discussed in Part IV.

The *surface area* available for drug absorption and the length of time that the drug remains in contact with the surface will alter the drug's absorption rate. Clients who have had a subtotal gastrectomy or a small bowel resection will have less surface area than the average individual with which to absorb oral medications. Drug absorption is diminished in clients with colitis and other disorders that move intestinal contents through the gastrointestinal tract too quickly. These pathologies and other factors affecting drug absorption are explained in Part IV.

DRUG DISTRIBUTION

Once a drug has been absorbed into the circulation, it is actively or passively distributed from its site of entry to other parts of the body. The rate of distribution depends on the rate of circulation flow. As a drug is being circulated, some of it will be unavailable at the desired site of action due to (1) body barriers that prevent entry to the action site; (2) binding of the drug to circulating proteins, such as albumin; or (3) distribution to tissue storage site.

Drug distribution tends to be uneven in the body. Many drugs pass freely throughout the body's extracellular fluid but have difficulty entering certain fluids, such as cerebral spinal fluid. One of the major factors influencing drug distribution is the drug's ability to move across the cell membrane that encloses the fluid. Drugs with high lipid solubility tend to cross barrier membranes and are therefore distributed more evenly than drugs that are water soluble. Sometimes these body barriers protect a body reservoir from the unwanted effects of a drug; the placental barrier serves this function. Other times the barrier must be crossed for a drug to reach its intended site of action; the blood-brain barrier is sometimes in this category.

Blood-Brain Barriers

Infections and disorders of the brain are difficult to treat with drugs because of the low permeability of brain fluids. Two types of fluids are found in and around the brain: the cerebrospinal fluid (CSF) and the brain's interstitial fluid. Although many large molecular substances, such as some drugs, are able to enter most of the body's interstitial and other extracellular fluids with relative ease, they can seldom pass into the CSF (**blood-CSF barrier**) or the brain's interstitial fluid (**blood-brain barrier**). Both the ependymal surface of the choroid plexus, the structure that secretes CSF, and the brain tissue itself have low drug permeability.

At times it is necessary to treat meningitis by injecting antibiotics directly into the CSF (intrathecally). Since CSF fills the subarachnoid space, the fluid, and therefore the drug, is in contact with large surface areas of the ependyma and the meninges. The frequent administration of drugs directly into the CSF can be painful and may inadvertently cause the introduction of a pathogen into this sterile fluid. Hoping to avoid these problems, many physicians prefer to treat meningitis with high doses of parenterally administered medications.

Several factors influence the ability of a drug to enter the CSF from the blood. If a drug has a high lipid solubility and a low degree of ionization, it will probably be able to penetrate the blood-CSF barrier. Drugs that do not combine with proteins to form large protein-drug molecules also have a greater ability to penetrate the barrier. Amphetamine has these features and is a potent psychomotor stimulant because it can readily enter the CSF.

Pathological factors also influence the ability of drugs to penetrate the CSF. Although the CSF is normally more acidic than plasma, a client with respiratory acidosis (high PCO_2) will have a CSF pH that is similar to that of the plasma. (Because the bicarbonate ion is transported slowly across the blood-CSF barrier, metabolic acidosis and alkalosis have little effect.) Consequently, in respiratory acidosis, weak organic acids, such as phenobarbital and the salicylates, will be transported into the CSF faster than usual. Conversely, weak organic bases will enter the CSF faster when there is respiratory alkalosis. When there is an inflammation or a laceration in the brain, more drugs than usual do enter the CSF.

It is difficult not only to achieve a high drug level in the CSF, but also to maintain it. Spinal fluid is constantly being secreted—about 500 ml daily—in order for the required volume of 135 ml to be maintained. Nearly 15% of the CSF is exchanged hourly with the circulating blood. Consequently, the concentration level of a drug in the CSF drops rapidly. Clients with epilepsy and certain other brain disorders must receive their medication on a q 6 h, q 8 h, or q 12 h schedule, rather than on a qid, tid, or bid schedule, in order to maintain the drug concentration level in the CSF.

Placental Barrier

The placenta is unfortunately a poor barrier against the passage of drugs. Most drugs taken by a pregnant woman are transported through the placenta to the growing fetus. Drugs with a molecular weight of 1000 or less tend to cross the placental barrier by simple diffusion. Most drugs that are lipid soluble and poorly ionized enter the fetus. Even some drugs with a molecular weight greater than 1000 cross the barrier, by active transportation.

Once absorbed, drugs can cause undesirable changes in the fetus, such as fetal distress, teratogenesis, or even fetal death. Large doses of chloral hydrate, for example, have been implicated in cases of fetal death. Drugs that are safe in the mother may be toxic to the fetus, since the fetus (and the neonate) have immature liver enzyme systems with which to metabolize drugs.

Teratogenesis is the production of a deformity in the developing embryo; some drugs have been implicated as causes of teratogenesis. The danger tends to be greater during the first trimester. In most cases the exact cause of the malformation is unknown, but any drug may be implicated and pregnant women should be cautioned against taking any drugs without medical supervision. Table 7-3 lists some drugs that have been implicated in teratogenesis.

Fetal changes and fetal distress have also been attributed to the use of certain drugs during pregnancy (see Table 7-4). Whereas the standard adult dose of streptomycin does not cause toxic effects in the average pregnant woman, in the developing fetus it may cause eighth cranial nerve damage, permanent hearing loss, and other toxic effects. The sulfonylureas—oral hypoglycemic agents—have caused goiters and severe hypoglycemia in fetuses. Even tetracycline has been

TABLE 7-3 Drugs That Have Been Implicated in Teratogenesis

Classification	Drug
Antibiotics	Streptomycin Tetracycline
Antineoplastic agents	Busulfan methotrexate
Antituberculin agent	Isoniazid (INH)
Cathartic	Podophyllum
CNS stimulants	Dextroamphetamine sulfate (Dexedrine)
Expectorant	Potassium iodide
Hormone	Cortisone
Hypoglycemic agent	Tolbutamide (Orinase)
Vitamins	Vitamin A (excessive doses) Vitamin D (excessive doses)

TABLE 7-4 Commonly Prescribed Drugs That May Cause Fetal Changes

Classification	Drugs	Reported Fetal Changes
Antibiotics	Sulfonamides Streptomycin Tetracycline	Liver atrophy, hyperbilirubinemia, anemia Eighth cranial nerve damage, hearing loss Slowed bone growth, discolored teeth
Anticoagulants		Death due to intrauterine hemorrhage
Antidepressants	Lithium carbonate	Goiter
Antihypertensive agents	Reserpine	Respiratory obstruction
Antiinflammatory	Phenylbutazone (Butazolidin)	Goiter
Diuretic	Thiazides	Thrombocytopenia
Hypoglycemic agents	Sulfonylureas	Goiter, hypoglycemia
Hormones	Estrogens	Clitoral enlargement, labial fusion
Tranquilizers	Chlorpromazine	Jaundice
Vitamins (excessive doses)	Vitamin A Vitamin D	Eye damage Hypercalcemia, mental retardation

implicated as a cause of slow bone growth and discolored teeth in the newborn, and neonatal bleeding has been reported when the mother used salicylates during pregnancy. Hyperbilirubinemia, respiratory distress, cyanosis, thrombocytopenia, and even death of the neonate have been reported as resulting from drugs taken during pregnancy.

Fetal distress during labor and delivery has been attributed to the use of certain analgesics and anesthetics (see Table 7-5). If these drugs become necessary, the smallest effective dose possible should be administered and the fetus should be monitored frequently. The fetal heart rate may increase initially but may then be suppressed to a dangerous level (below 80 beats per minute). The physician should be notified immediately if the fetal heart rate falls below 100 beats per minute.

The use of "street drugs" by a pregnant woman can also cause fetal distress (see Table 7-6). Although knowledge about the effects of these drugs on the fetus is limited, it is clear that all drugs are potentially toxic to the fetus and no medications should be taken by pregnant women unless prescribed by a physician.

Drug Storage

As it is distributed throughout the body, a drug may accumulate in body tissues other than the site of action. The drug may have an **affinity** for —that is, be highly attracted to—specific tissues. Depending on the physiochemical factors influencing it, a drug may be bound to proteins, stored in tissues, or dissolved in neutral fat. The drug will be released from the storage sites as its concentration in the blood decreases; therefore, plasma protein binding and other storage mechanisms may alter the duration and intensity of drug action.

Protein binding is usually reversible, particularly when it occurs in the blood. The ionic form of many drugs binds to the serum albumin before globulin binding occurs. This drug-protein complex is too large to pass through many body membranes, including the glomerulus and the liver membranes. A drug held in the circulation is unavailable to the receptor sites and to the pathways of metabolism or excretion, but as the concentration of free drug in the blood decreases, the drug will be released from its protein bond.

TABLE 7-5 Drugs Used During Labor and Delivery That Have Caused Fetal and Neonatal Distress

Drug	Fetal or Neonatal Distress
Anesthetics:	
Cyclopropane Ether Nitrous oxide	Inhibited fetal movement, depressed heart rate, respiratory depression, apnea
Barbiturates:	
Phenobarbital	Respiratory depression, depressed heart rate, hemorrhage
Salicylates	Bleeding
Morphine	Respiratory depression, depressed heart rate

TABLE 7-6 Commonly Abused Street Drugs That May Cause Fetal or Neonatal Distress or Changes

Drug	Fetal or Neonatal Distress or Change
Ethyl alcohol	Alcohol distress syndrome
Heroin	Respiratory depression, neonatal death and initial addiction
Lysergic acid diethylamide (LSD)	Stunted growth
Methadone	Respiratory depression
Nicotine (cigarette smoking)	Underweight neonates
Chloral hydrate	Respiratory depression, death

The amount and strength of protein binding varies from drug to drug. Drugs that are highly bound to plasma albumin and other proteins include (1) the diuretic furosemide (Lasix), about 95%; (2) the anticoagulant warfarin (Coumarin), about 95 to 97%; and (3) the antiinflammatory agent phenylbutazone (Butazolidin), about 98 to 99%. Drugs that are less bound include the barbiturate phenobarbital, which is 40 to 60% bound, and the antiarrhythmic lidocaine, which is 50 to 75% bound.

When these drugs are first administered, the amount of protein binding that will occur must be considered, along with the client's ability to metabolize and excrete the drug. With some drugs, the storage sites must be saturated with a *loading dose* before therapeutic drug levels can be obtained. For example, it is necessary to administer an intravenous loading dose, called an **IV bolus**, of 50 to 100 mg of lidocaine hydrochloride before the drug can exert its antiarrhythmic action. If the normal heart rhythm is not restored in five minutes, a second IV bolus may be required. The preferred administration rate for an IV bolus of lidocaine is 25 mg per minute, but, in most cases, only 2 mg per minute is required to maintain the antiarrhythmic effect. Once the plasma proteins and other distribution sites are initially saturated, the IV bolus will maintain lidocaine's therapeutic blood level for approximately 20 minutes. The nurse must therefore prepare and start the continuous IV lidocaine drip in less than 20 minutes.

Since there is a limited number of protein binding sites available in the body, toxic drug reactions and other adverse effects can result when two drugs are competing for the same sites. The expected amount of protein binding will not occur for one or both of the drugs, so there may be more free drug available to receptor sites. For example, when phenylbutazone is given to a client who is already receiving warfarin, the client will have a potentiated anticoagulant response. Information on drug interactions can be found in the drug monographs.

Tissue storage occurs when drugs bind to tissue proteins and other tissue constituents—phospholipids, mucopolysaccharides, and nucleoproteins. Certain drugs have a special affinity for various tissues, such as the liver, spleen, lungs, muscle, bone, and even hair and nails. The antimalarial agent quinacrine has an affinity for the liver; lead and tetracycline have a special affinity for bone and teeth.

Tissue binding is usually reversible, but the release of a drug accumulated in tissue tends to be much slower than release from plasma proteins. The less vascular tissues, such as bone and teeth, may store the drug for prolonged periods of time, even months.

Drugs with high lipid solubility may accumulate in fat tissue. *Neutral fat storage* is particularly important to consider when treating the obese client. As much as 50% of the obese client's body weight is neutral fat, which provides a large storage area for drugs with high lipid solubility. Since fat tissue has a relatively poor blood supply, fat-accumulated drugs tend to be released slowly. The ultrashort-acting anesthetic thiopental (Pentothal) is highly lipid soluble and is rapidly moved from its desired site of action, the brain, into fat tissue, thus abruptly curtailing its duration of action. However, the low-level drug action, the "hangover" feeling, may last for hours because of the drug's slow release rate from fat and other tissue sites.

Redistribution

The process by which the concentration of a drug is shifted from the initial tissue sites to secondary tissue sites is termed **redistribution**. Although drug metabolism and excretion are the primary means by which drug action is terminated, drug action may also cease when drug concentrations are redistributed away from the action site into storage sites.

As in the case of thiopental and barbiturates, drug molecules that are stored in their active form cause a low-level effect until the drug is metabolized and excreted hours later.

Knowledge of the redistribution patterns of certain chemicals can be very useful. Inorganic lead is distributed in soft tissues and then redistributed into bone, teeth, and hair. Bone deposits are in the form of insoluble lead phosphate and so do not contribute to toxicity. Although chelating agents are now used to treat lead poisoning, the condition was formerly treated by therapy that forced the redistribution of lead into bone through a high phosphate intake. Later the lead was remobilized by altering calcium and phosphate intake in the hope that it would then be eliminated in the urine. If the remobilization was adequately controlled, acute intoxication did not reoccur and the client survived.

Occasionally, an unwanted drug redistribution is precipitated by another drug, a nutrient, an environmental chemical, or a physiological change in the client. If an active drug is unexpectedly released from its storage site, there may be a higher than usual drug concentration at the drug's action site, leading to a potentially toxic response. Conversely, the drug may be redistributed to its sites of metabolism and excretion, creating the need for another loading dose when the drug's distribution returns to normal.

Any alteration in the physiochemical factors in the body that affect membrane permeability, active drug transport, significant shifts in body fluids, or alterations in pH gradients can cause an unexpected drug redistribution. Since several of these alterations can occur during surgery, postoperative clients should be observed for inadequate drug responses and for drug toxicity.

DRUG METABOLISM

Detoxification, biotransformation, and *metabolism* are terms used to indicate the changes a drug undergoes in the body. The term **detoxification** is limited to the conversion of a drug to a less poisonous substance by the body. We now know that some drugs are not changed in the body, and others are changed into more toxic substances. For example, barium sulfate, a contrast medium used for diagnostic x-rays, is insoluble in body fluids and has no biologic action. Pentavalent arsenic compounds, on the other hand, are converted into the more toxic trivalent compounds by the body. All the changes that a drug undergoes in the body cannot be encompassed by the term *detoxification*.

The term **biotransformation** is used to indicate the changes produced in a drug by the body's natural processes, such as oxidation, reduction, and so on. Technically, the term is limited to the natural changes that occur in living tissues, so the term *drug metabolism* is preferred by many health professionals. **Drug metabolism** refers to all the physical and chemical processes and reactions that drugs undergo, both in their initial forms and as ions. The new compounds created during these processes, called **metabolites,** are also included. Technically, *drug metabolism* is the most inclusive term.

Before elimination can occur, most drugs must

be changed into more ionized, less lipid-soluble substances. Since these metabolites have less ability to penetrate cell membranes, the drug is essentially inactivated and converted to substances that can ultimately be eliminated from the body. The body uses several mechanisms to metabolize drugs, but most of them require one or more body enzyme systems.

Enzyme Systems

Although a few drugs are eliminated from the body unchanged, most are affected by the various enzyme systems that act on many normal body functions, including digestion, acid-base balance, and use of energy. If a drug's chemical structure is similar to that of a natural substrate—a substance that is catalyzed by enzymes—the drug is often metabolized by the same enzymes as the natural substrate. There are hundreds of enzymes located throughout the body, but most are found in the intestines, plasma, liver, and kidneys.

Many drugs are altered by enzyme systems, particularly those of the liver, that are intended to metabolize invading foreign substances. Several drug metabolizing enzymes, called the **hepatic microsomal enzyme systems,** are located in the microsomes of the hepatic reticular endothelium. Lipid-soluble drugs penetrate the liver's membranes easily and are acted upon by the microsomal enzymes. There are individual variations in the abilities of the microsomal enzymes to act, and there are marked variations in the rate of drug metabolism from individual to individual. Individual variations in the hepatic microsomal enzyme systems will be explained later in this chapter.

Types of Drug Metabolism

Drugs can undergo a variety of chemical reactions. The resulting metabolites usually have the following characteristics:

1. They are less lipid soluble than the original compound.
2. They are less capable of being transported across lipid membranes and therefore have less biological action.
3. They are more soluble in body fluids.
4. They are more easily eliminated from the body since only lipid-soluble molecules are passively reabsorbed by the kidneys.

The major types of reactions are listed below.

1. *Oxidation* is thought to be catalyzed by the hepatic microsomal enzymes in most cases. However, oxidation can be catalyzed by enzymes located in the mitochondria of liver cells and other tissues.

2. *Deamination* is the oxidation of a drug in such a way that the amino group (NH_3) is removed from the compound, such as occurs when amphetamine is converted to phenylacetone and ammonia.

3. *Sulfoxidation* is the oxidation of a thioether to a sulfoxide. An example is the conversion of a phenothiazine to phenothiazine sulfoxide.

4. *Reduction* of azo- and nitro- compounds is catalyzed by microsomal and other enzyme systems located in the liver and other tissues. An example is the reduction of nitrophenols to aminophenols.

5. *Hydrolysis* of procaine (an ester) and some chlorine esters is catalyzed by enzymes, such as pseudocholinesterase in plasma. An example is the hydrolysis of procaine to diethylaminoethanol and benzoate. Amides are hydrolyzed primarily in the liver.

6. *Methylation,* the transfer of a methyl group to the nitrogen of a variety of amines and to the oxygen of catechols, is catalyzed by enzymes, such as methyltransferases. Examples are the conversion of epinephrine to metanephrine and of niacin to N-methylinicotinamide.

7. *Conjugation* is the joining of two compounds—the drug and a body substance—to produce another compound that is less toxic and that can be eliminated. This chemical reaction is sometimes called a *synthetic reaction* because new compounds are formed. The body substrate that enters the reaction is usually a carbohydrate, an amino acid, acetic acid, or an inorganic sulfate. Microsomal and other enzymes catalyze the combining of the compounds. Examples are the conversion of phenols to sulfates and glucuronides, and of salicylic acid to salicyluric acid.

8. *Glucuronide synthesis* is one of the most common forms of conjugation. The substrate glucuronic acid is transferred to the receptive structure of the drug molecule, which then creates a new compound. The enzyme uridine diphosphate-transglucuronylase (UPD-glucuronic acid) catalyzes the reaction. This form of conjugation occurs with phenols, alcohols, and certain carboxylic acids.

Drug Metabolites

When drugs are metabolized, they often undergo more than one chemical reaction and produce more than one metabolite. Aspirin undergoes hydrolysis to salicylic acid and is then changed to salicyluric acid, gentisic acid, ether glucuronide, and ester glucuronide. The analgesic activity of aspirin occurs before hydrolysis, so the metabolites of aspirin are less biologically active. In fact, most drug metabolites are less active than the original drug, particularly after conjugation.

There are some drug metabolites, however, that are just as active as, or even more active than, the original drug. The oral hypoglycemic agent acetohexamide (Dymelor) is changed to the active metabolite hydroxyhexamide, and when the narcotic codeine is metabolized, about 10% of it is converted to morphine.

A few drugs have little or no biological activity until they are changed to metabolites. It is believed that vitamin D_3 must be metabolized in the liver to its active metabolite before it can transport calcium in the intestines or into the bones. The analgesic phenacetin must be changed to the active metabolite acetaminophen (Tylenol) in order for it to produce its pharmacologic action.

Knowledge of the nature of drug metabolites has led to the effective treatment of some disorders. Parkinson's disease is caused, at least in part, by a deficiency of dopamine, a neuromal transmitter, in the basal ganglia. Dopamine will not cross the blood-brain barrier, but dopamine *precursor,* levodopa, is able to cross the barrier and is converted to dopamine by the enzyme dopa decarboxylase.

The amount of a particular metabolite formed from the original drug is dependent on the amount and activity of the enzymes responsible for its metabolism. If the original, biologically active, drug has poor accessibility to its metabolizing enzyme—that is, has poor lipid solubility—the drug will be metabolized slowly and its duration of action may be prolonged. If the drug has a high accessibility to the enzyme, it will be metabolized and eliminated rapidly. These and other factors influence the metabolism of drugs.

Factors Affecting Drug Metabolism

The major factors that alter an individual's ability to metabolize drugs are age, genetic make-up, pathology, and the presence of enzyme stimulators and inhibitors.

Age

The hepatic microsomal enzyme systems are known to be immature in the neonate. Consequently, infants and young children are unable to metabolize effectively drugs that require these enzymes.

Most drug research conducted by drug companies is done on "normal, healthy adults." It is known that a decline in many of the body's processes occurs after the age of 40, with anatomical, physiological, and biochemical changes occurring. The age of onset and the rate of decline varies, but the changes include a slowing of the basal metabolic rate and a decrease in kidney function. During the aging process, the body's ability to adjust to changes in the regulation of blood glucose is progressively impaired, and there is some indication that the hepatic microsomal enzyme systems are also impaired. Consequently, the elderly tend to metabolize and excrete drugs more slowly than the "normal, healthy adult."

Drugs should be given to infants, children, and the elderly with caution. Drugs that require hepatic microsomal enzyme systems should be avoided in the infant and given in reduced doses to the very young and elderly. A slowing of drug metabolism and excretion may cause toxicity even when the average dose is administered. Toxicity can sometimes be avoided by either decreasing the dose administered or increasing the dosage interval.

Genetics

There is a wide variation in drug metabolism from individual to individual. This fact has led to the establishment of the study of genetic variations in drug therapy, a relatively new field called **pharmacogenetics**. Many of the biochemical functions of living organisms are genetically controlled, including the synthesis of enzymes. Pharmacogenetics involves not only metabolic abnormalities but also the subtle changes in genes that can account for variations in drug metabolism and enzyme deficiencies. For example, some individuals metabolize the antituberculin drug isoniazid rapidly and others metabolize it slowly. This variation is caused by differing amounts of the drug's metabolizing enzyme, acetyl coenzyme A. The therapeutic and adverse effects of isoniazid, procainamide, hydrolazine, and certain other drugs can be altered by the client's "acetylator status."

Clients with an excess of a drug's metabolizing enzyme may require a larger than average drug dose. Toxic and other adverse reactions may occur in clients with a deficiency of a drug metabolizing enzyme. In the latter case, the client can be given a smaller than average dose, the dosage interval can be lengthened, or an alternate drug can be administered.

Pathology

Alterations in the rate at which drugs are metabolized, or in the pathways of metabolism, can be caused by a variety of illnesses. Poor nutritional status may alter the quality of a client's enzyme systems. Since the liver is the primary site of metabolism for many drugs, liver disorders, such as tumors, hepatitis, and cirrhosis, can alter and often decrease the client's ability to metabolize drugs that require the hepatic microsomal enzyme systems.

Enzyme stimulation or induction

Some substances can shorten a drug's duration of action by increasing the rate at which it is metabolized. Evidence indicates that there is more than one method of stimulating drug metabolism. The stimulator may cause increased accessibility to an enzyme or an increased amount of the enzyme, or it may block destruction of the enzyme. Many substances are known to induce the metabolism of one or more drugs, such as rifampin, phenobarbital, nitrous oxide, components of cigarette smoke, phenytoin, and certain insecticides. The long-term consumption of ethyl alcohol in alcoholics stimulates the metabolism of warfarin and other drugs.

When some drugs are administered on a long-term basis, they may stimulate the liver to enhance the drug's metabolic rate as well as the metabolism of other drugs. Prominant among these drugs are phenobarbital (Luminal), pentobarbital (Nembutal), chlorpromazine (Thorazine), and meprobamate (Equanil). Clients taking any one of these drugs develop a tolerance to the medication and periodically require increased doses in order to obtain the same therapeutic effect.

Phenobarbital induces the metabolism of several drugs, including some steroids and estrogen. Women who take oral contraceptives regularly have become pregnant because of concurrent use of barbiturates and other enzyme inducers.

Enzyme inhibition

The duration of drug action is prolonged when a substance inhibits or blocks the enzyme system responsible for the drug's metabolism. Several substances are known to inhibit the metabolism of certain drugs. Since microsomal drug metabolism requires oxygen, carbon monoxide and certain chemicals that are toxic to the liver can act as microsomal enzyme inhibitors.

A toxic drug reaction or other adverse reaction can result from enzyme inhibition. If a client receives a drug that causes inhibition of an enzyme required to metabolize a second drug, concomitant administration of the second drug may result in an adverse reaction due to higher blood levels of the second drug than expected. Several oral anticoagulants and oral antidiabetic agents, as well as some sedatives, are known to inhibit the metabolism of one or more other drugs. Specific drug monographs should be consulted for potential interactions.

Drugs that cause enzyme inhibition can also be used therapeutically. Gout can be treated with allopurinol (Zyloprim), a drug that inhibits the action of xanthine oxidase. The latter is an enzyme required for the biotransformation of hypoxanthine to uric acid. Disulfiram (Antabuse) is an alcohol deterrent sometimes used in the rehabilitation of alcoholics. Alcohol consumed by a client taking disulfiram is incompletely metabolized by the liver and the client's blood level of acetaldehyde rises sharply, resulting in vomiting, flushing, sweating, and weakness.

Drug Metabolism Research

Initial drug research is conducted in animals, but the pathways and rates of drug metabolism in animals can vary from the same processes in human beings. Animal studies are helpful in determining some of the basic rates and methods of drug metabolism, but the results should not be viewed as absolutes for humans.

DRUG EXCRETION

Drugs and their metabolites are usually excreted from the body through the kidneys. Other body structures that assist in drug elimination include the gastrointestinal tract, the liver, the mammary glands, the lacrimal glands, the sweat glands, the respiratory tract, and even the nails and hair. Some of these sites, however, allow drugs to be reabsorbed back into the circulation. The faster a drug is eliminated from the body, the lower the drug concentration will be in the blood and the sooner the drug effects will disappear. Conversely, a drug that is excreted slowly will be retained in the blood at a high concentration, either of the drug itself or of its metabolites, for a longer period of time.

Factors Affecting Drug Excretion

The rate of drug excretion is influenced by the same factors that alter drug distribution, transport through membranes, and rates and types of drug metabolism, as well as by the condition of the eliminating organ.

Although some drugs may be eliminated unchanged, many must be metabolized before they can be excreted in any appreciable amounts. The rate and ability of the kidneys to excrete drugs is affected by the polarity and solubility of a drug. Ionized, water-soluble drugs are excreted easily, but, since many drugs are lipid soluble, they must be changed into ionized, more water-soluble metabolites before they can be readily eliminated.

The drug and its metabolites are usually transported to the site of excretion by the blood. If the blood flow to the excreting organ is hampered—for example, by partial obstruction, low blood pressure or high blood viscosity—the drug will be eliminated slowly. Once at the excretion site, the drug must be actively or passively transported through the structure's membranes, and the factors affecting drug transport through membranes, such as pH, ionization, and concentration gradients, apply.

The condition of the organ also affects excretion. The fewer functioning nephrons and liver cells there are, the slower the drug will be eliminated. Consequently, geriatric clients and infants may have difficulty excreting drugs. Pathological conditions can alter drug excretion dramatically. If the kidneys are damaged by glomerulonephritis or some other kidney disorder, drug elimination via this site will be hampered. If the liver is damaged from hepatitis or other liver disorders, drugs metabolized or excreted into the bile by the liver will be excreted more slowly than usual. Organ damage can cause the active drug concentrations to remain in the blood for prolonged periods of time and result in adverse drug reactions.

Because of their unique characteristics, renal, gastrointestinal, biliary, mammary, and pulmonary excretion are explained separately.

Renal Excretion

Glomerular filtration and tubular secretion are the two processes by which drugs and their metabolites are excreted by the kidneys in the urine. However, the processes of active and passive reabsorption return much of the drug to the blood. The actual rate of excretion is essentially the difference between the amount filtered and secreted minus the amount reabsorbed.

$$\text{Rate of excretion} = \begin{pmatrix}\text{filtration}\\ \text{and}\\ \text{secretion}\end{pmatrix} - \begin{pmatrix}\text{active and}\\ \text{passive}\\ \text{reabsorption}\end{pmatrix}$$

Glomerular filtration is the movement of large quantities of fluid (about 125 ml/min.) from the blood through the glomerular membrane into Bowman's capsule. (See Figure 7-7 for the major features of the nephrons.) Since the glomerular membrane is nearly 25 times more permeable

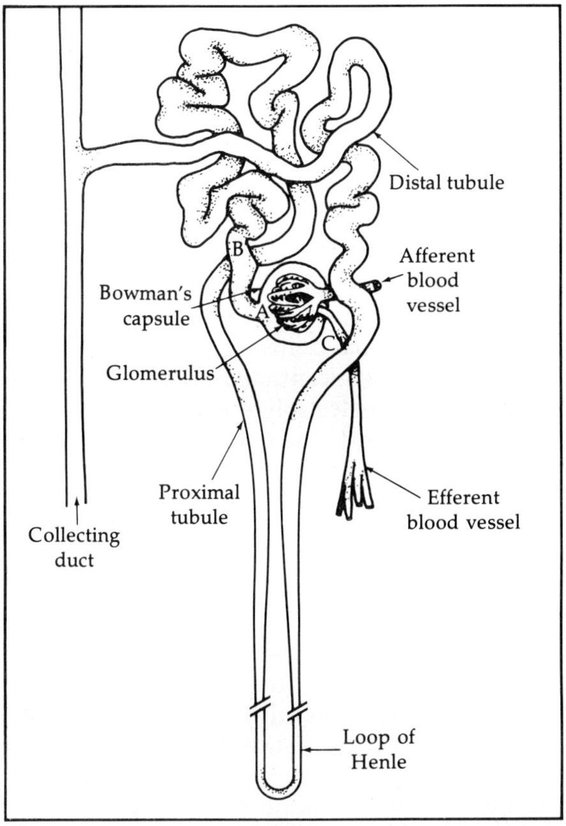

FIGURE 7-7 Major sites of drug movement in the nephrons. Many free, unbound drugs enter the urinary filtrate in Bowman's capsule (A). The proximal tubule (B) is the site of tubular secretion of drugs; most lipid-soluble drug molecules are reabsorbed into the blood (C) before the tubular fluid enters the loop of Henle.

than most other body membranes, large quantities of water, electrolytes, nutrients, and other plasma constituents, including most free drug molecules, are passed through it. But since few, if any, blood cells, proteins, or other large molecular structures are able to penetrate the glomecular membrane, drug molecules that are bound to plasma proteins are not filtered. Consequently, the rate of drug movement into the filtrate depends on the amount of the particular drug's plasma protein binding and the filtration rate of the drug.

Tubular secretion of drugs tends to be an active, carrier-mediated process; it occurs in the proximal tubules. Although there are several systems, the basic mechanism of transport is similar to the active transport of drugs through other body membranes. One system transports acid drugs, such as penicillin, acid metabolites, such as salicylic acid, and other organic acids, such as uric acid. Another system transports basic drugs, such as quinine, basic metabolites, and other organic bases, such as histamine. These two systems are not selective; the drugs must compete with the body's organic acids and bases for transport. There are some selective transport systems, however, for substances such as glucose, vitamins, and some drugs. Some of the drugs that are secreted into the filtrate by these systems may also be transported back into the blood by the same systems.

Reabsorption, particularly of glucose, proteins, water, electrolytes, and most lipid-soluble drug molecules, takes place in the proximal tubules. Only 20% of the filtrate ever reaches the loop of Henle. The rate of reabsorption depends on the drug's solubility and concentration gradient, as well as the pH and pressure gradients between the filtrate and the blood.

Since nonionized drug molecules tend to be lipid soluble, they are easily reabsorbed from the filtrate back into the blood through the tubule's lipid membranes. However, water-soluble, highly ionized drugs and their metabolites are poorly reabsorbed and are therefore excreted in the urine.

The *urinary pH* alters the quantity of drug excreted. Alkaline urine tends to enhance the excretion of weak acidic drugs, such as aspirin, whereas drugs that are weak bases, such as meperidine, tend to be excreted more rapidly in acidic urine.[2]

When drug toxicity or poisoning occurs, the offending drug may be eliminated faster if the urinary pH is altered with another substance. Sodium bicarbonate can be used to alkalinize the urine and acidic substances, such as ascorbic acid (vitamin C) or ammonium chloride, can be used to acidify it. For example, when a child is accidentally poisoned with aspirin, the drug can be excreted faster if an alkaline urine is maintained with appropriate quantities of sodium bicarbonate, and if the child is kept adequately hydrated.

[2]It is important to remember that (1) weak organic bases are more ionized in acidic body fluids; (2) weak organic acids are more ionized in alkaline body fluids; and (3) ionized drug molecules are less lipid soluble and will therefore remain in the urine instead of being reabsorbed.

The urinary output and pH must be monitored frequently so that the urine does not become too alkaline and precipitate the formation of kidney stones.

Although the kidney is the primary organ of excretion for most drugs, some drugs and many drug metabolites are excreted via other organs.

Gastrointestinal Excretion

Drugs that are not absorbed after oral administration are eliminated in the feces. Drugs that have a slow rate of absorption or that form unabsorbable complexes with food or other substances will be eliminated in the feces in relatively large amounts. However, many drugs are well absorbed and only small quantities are left to be eliminated from the gastrointestinal tract unchanged.

Certain drugs or their metabolites may reenter the gastrointestinal tract for ultimate elimination in the feces. Most of these substances either reenter the gastrointestinal tract by passing through the tract's membrane or enter with bile from the gall bladder.

Biliary Excretion

Drugs that are metabolized in the liver may be excreted as metabolites in the bile and, occasionally, as unchanged drug molecules. When the bile enters the gastrointestinal tract, the metabolites may be either reabsorbed or excreted in the feces. The cycle of biliary excretion, entrance into the gastrointestinal tract, and reabsorption into the blood may continue until all of the drug or its metabolites is eliminated in the feces or via the kidneys.

Pulmonary Excretion

The lungs can serve as an organ of drug excretion for gaseous drugs, such as many general anesthetics, and gaseous metabolic end products. The rate of excretion will vary with physiochemical factors, such as the volume of air exchanged, depth of respiration, rate of pulmonary blood flow, and the substance's concentration gradient. Post-surgical clients who had gaseous anesthetics should be encouraged to breathe deeply and turn, so the anesthetics can be excreted faster.

Mammary Excretion

Most lipid-soluble drugs are capable of entering breast milk. Since breast milk is more acidic (pH about 6.5) than plasma, weak basic drugs may be found in higher concentrations in the milk than in the plasma. Conversely, weak acidic drugs tend to be less concentrated in breast milk than in plasma. Nonelectrolyte substances, such as ethyl alcohol, enter the milk and reach the same concentration as in plasma.

When drugs are excreted in the milk of nursing mothers, they may pose a threat to the baby. Many of the drugs taken by lactating mothers do appear in the milk (see Table 7-7). Anthraquinone-type cathartics (cascara) may cause hyperactivity of the infant's gastrointestinal tract, called colic. Other possible infant reactions to drugs include toxicity, blood dyscrasias, lethargy, and allergy. Some drugs, such as atropine and the nicotine in cigarette smoke, may cause a decrease in the amount of milk produced. The breast-fed infant should be observed for adverse drug reactions when the mother must take medications that are excreted in the milk. Alternatively, the mother can be cautioned against breast-feeding.

Other Sites of Excretion

Glands in the body excrete minute quantities of certain drugs and their metabolites. When drugs are excreted via the sweat glands, the skin should be washed twice daily to prevent drug accumulation on the skin. Drugs eliminated by salivary glands are usually swallowed and then reabsorbed through the intestinal mucosa. Lacrimal gland secretions are usually reabsorbed through the nasal mucosa, unless the client's eyes are tearing excessively.

PHARMACOKINETICS

The processes of drug distribution, metabolism, and excretion are continuous and begin soon after

TABLE 7-7 Commonly Used Substances Excreted in Breast Milk

Classification	Examples
Amphetamines	Dextroamphetamine (Dexedrine)
Analgesics	Aspirin Pentazocine (Talwin)
Antibiotics	Ampicillin Cephalexin (Keflex) Erythromycin Streptomycin Tetracycline
Anticoagulants	Bishydroxycoumarin (Dicumarol) Warfarin (Coumadin)
Anticonvulsants	Phenytoin (Dilantin)
Antidiabetic agents	Tolbutamide (Orinase)
Antihistamines	Diphenhydramine (Benadryl)
Barbiturates	Phenobarbital
Caffeine	Coffee Tea
Cathartics and laxatives	Cascara Senna (Senokot)
Diuretics	Furosemide (Lasix) Hydrochlorothiazide (HydroDiuril)
Food supplements	Ferrous sulfate (iron) Folic acid Vitamins A, B, C, D, E, K
Narcotics	Codeine Morphine
Nicotine	(From cigarette smoking)
Oral contraceptives	
Tranquilizers	Chlordiazepoxide (Librium) Diazepam (Valium) Meprobamate (Equinal)

a drug is absorbed or administered intravenously. The rate at which these processes occur affects the drug's concentration in the blood and at the site of action. The onset of drug action, the duration of action, the minimum effective dose, and the maximum safe dose (toxic dose) are affected by the rate at which the drug is absorbed, distributed, metabolized, and excreted. **Pharmacokinetics** is the study of the *rate* at which the processes occur. Knowledge of a drug's pharmacokinetic patterns helps the health team to determine the proper dosage, most adequate route for administration, optimum times for administration, timing of potential toxic reactions, and other aspects of the client's potential response to a drug.

Ideally, one would measure the changes in drug concentration at the drug's site of action. However, most drug action sites are thought to be in tissues, so the more accessible body fluids, particularly the blood and urine, are used to measure drug concentration levels. As with other blood tests, the quantity of drug in the plasma is measured in *milligrams percent* (mg%) or some other measure of concentration.

Phases of Plasma Drug Concentration

When a drug is administered only once, its concentration in the blood will follow the following sequence of events:

1. *Absorption phase*—Plasma concentration climbs as the drug is absorbed. Drugs administered intravenously have no absorption phase.
2. *Peak*—Highest plasma concentration level that the drug dosage permits is achieved.
3. *Distribution phase*—Plasma drug concentration undergoes an initial, relatively rapid drop.
4. *Elimination phase*—Plasma drug concentration undergoes a slow, continuous drop. This phase reflects the processes of metabolism and excretion.

The shape of plasma drug concentration curves (see Figure 7-8) can vary dramatically among drugs, doses administered, methods of administration, and various clients. As described earlier in this chapter, the factors that alter the rate of a drug's absorption, distribution, metabolism, and excretion would be reflected in the drug's plasma concentration curve.

Peak drug concentration level in the blood varies in time and amount depending on the route of administration. As indicated in Figure 7-9, the peak concentration for intravenous medications occurs at the time of administration. Drugs given intramuscularly and subcutaneously peak later; the height of concentration is less for subcutaneously administered drugs.

Basic Pharmacokinetic Principles

The principles of pharmacokinetics are based on a compartment model of the human body. Depending on which body process is being measured, a compartment may consist of the gastrointestinal tract, the blood, the tissues, the urine, any other body compartment or system, or the whole body.

When a drug is moved passively through a membrane, the drug concentration decreases in the first compartment—for example, the gastrointestinal tract—and increases in the second compartment—for example, the blood—until the drug concentrations achieve equilibrium. Ini-

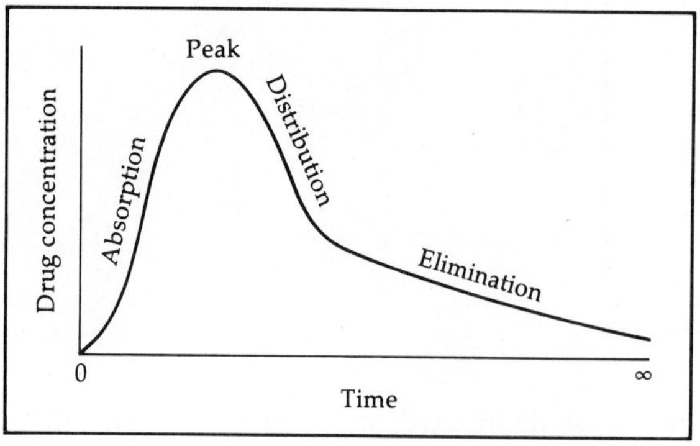

FIGURE 7-8 Example of plasma drug concentration curve. The plasma concentration of a drug administered extravascularly once only reflects the processes of absorption, distribution, and elimination (metabolism and excretion).

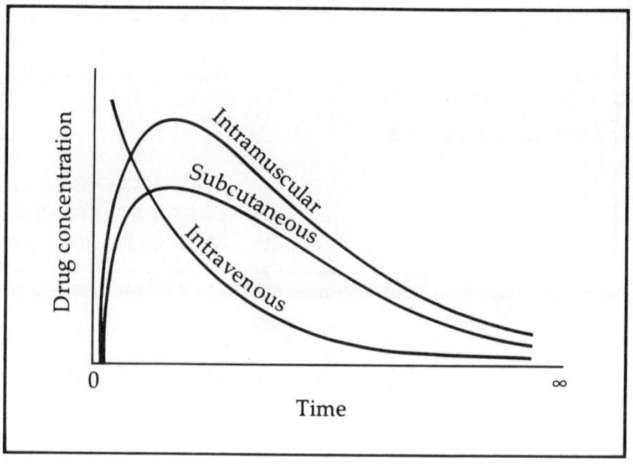

FIGURE 7-9 Example of the variation in plasma drug concentration levels when the same drug dose is administered by three different parenteral routes.

tially, a large amount of drug is moved from the first compartment to the second, but as equilibrium is approached, the net amount moved decreases. Equilibrium between the compartments does not always mean that the concentrations are equal. Drug molecules are still transferred between compartments, but there is no further *net transfer of drug* at the point of equilibrium. The steady rate at which a fractional amount of the total dosage is transferred per unit of time is called the **rate constant** and is expressed as k. This process is called *first-order kinetics* (see Figure 7-10).

At least four drug rate constants should be considered. Figure 7-11 illustrates a basic model of pharmacokinetics in which K_1 to K_4 represent these four constants. Changes in the plasma drug concentrations are the result of (1) the bioavailability at the site of administration; (2) the absorption rate constant; (3) the distribution and redistribution of the drug between the plasma and the tissues; (4) the rate of metabolism; and (5) the rate of excretion, particularly urinary excretion.

The rate constants for many drugs are directly influenced by the drug concentration in each compartment and are said to follow first-order kinetics, as described above. But it must be remembered that some drugs require active transport through a biological membrane and that the systems are saturable. If the drug concentration exceeds the capacity of the available drug carrier, the rate of drug movement will follow *zero-order kinetics*. The rate of drug transport will be determined by the capacity of the system, so that a *constant amount* of the drug is transferred instead of a fractional amount per unit of time. The rate of drug transport will follow first-order kinetics until the carrier capacity is reached, and then it will follow zero-order kinetics (see Figure 7-12).

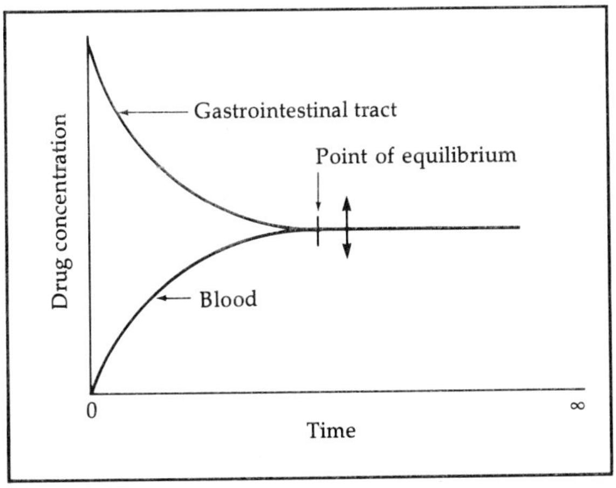

FIGURE 7-10 Example of the rate of movement of a drug passively diffused between two compartments. A constant fraction of the drug concentration in the gastrointestinal tract is moved into the blood and causes the drug concentration in the blood to rise until equilibrium occurs.

Several of the drug metabolizing and excretion processes are capacity-limited systems. Quantities of certain drug metabolizing enzymes in the body are limited, as is the renal secretion process. An unexpected drug accumulation or other untoward effects can occur when (1) a liver pathology has decreased the required drug metabolizing enzyme, (2) kidney pathology has decreased the functioning nephrons, or (3) two drugs are competing for the same enzyme or points of renal secretion.

Knowledge of the limited capacity of tubular secretion can be used beneficially. For example, probenecid is actively secreted and can compete with other acidic drugs that are excreted by tubular secretion. It has been added to penicillin to inhibit penicillin excretion and, therefore, prolong the antibiotic activity.

The kinetics of drug absorption, distribution, metabolism, and excretion are important to know but may be cumbersome to use in clinical situations. A composite picture of a drug's elimination processes—its biological half-life—is more useful in some cases.

Biological Half-Life

The time it takes for 50% of an active drug to be eliminated from the body is called the **biological half-life,** abbreviated $t_{1/2}$. About 75% of the drug is eliminated in two half-lives and about 87.5% in three half-lives, if the drug elimination processes follow first-order kinetics. The plasma drug concentrations will decrease by a constant fractional amount no matter how much drug is administered initially (see Figure 7-13).

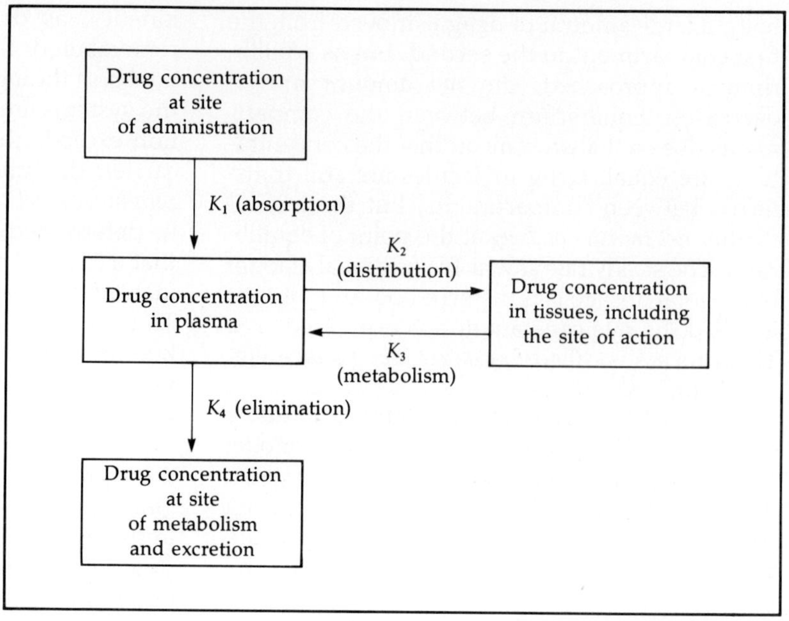

FIGURE 7-11 Basic model of pharmacokinetics.

Drugs that are metabolized and excreted by active transport systems may overload the carrier capacity and a constant amount of drug will then be eliminated. It will take longer for the drug to be removed from the body than if a constant fractional amount (following first-order kinetics) were eliminated. Consequently, the half-life of drugs following zero-order kinetics is dependent on the initial drug concentration. The larger the drug dose, the longer the drug's half-life (see Figure 7-14).

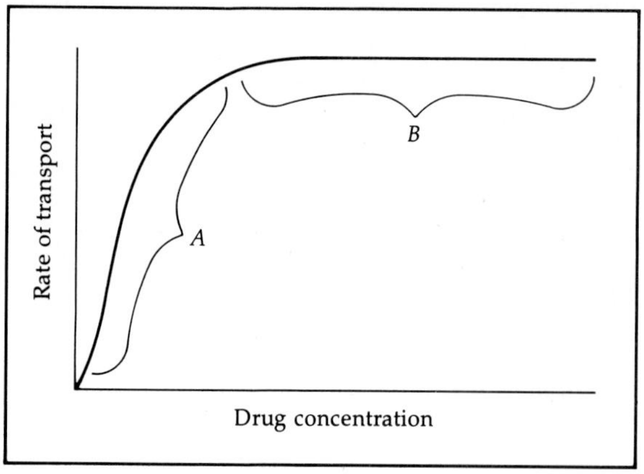

FIGURE 7-12 Drug concentration curve in a capacity-limited system. The rate at which a drug is transferred in this system follows first-order kinetics (*A*) until the system is saturated, at which time it will appear to follow zero-order kinetics (*B*).

Many drugs follow a combination of the two kinetics. When posted in a drug monograph, the drug half-life should be used as an estimate for the recommended dosage. Variations will occur according to the client's state of health and the quantities of drug that are processed by first-order and zero-order kinetics.

The biological half-life of some drugs is comparatively short. Regular insulin administered intravenously has a plasma $t_{1/2}$ of only nine minutes. The drug absorption process is slowed by the use of additives—for example, PZI contains zinc and protamine sulfate so that the insulin will be released into the plasma at a slower rate and the drug's duration of action will be increased. Antibiotics, such as kanamycin ($t_{1/2}$ = two to four hours), are often administered intravenously every six hours in order to sustain the antibiotic effect. The thyroid hormone levothyroxine, on the other hand, has a $t_{1/2}$ of six to seven days and is administered once every one to three weeks.

The biological half-life of a drug can be altered by the client's prescribed dosage, age, and physical status. When low doses of aspirin are taken, the $t_{1/2}$ is only two to four hours, but when high

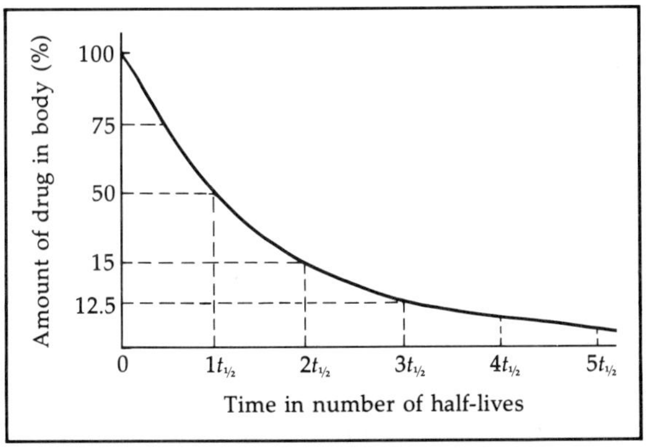

FIGURE 7-13 The biological half-life of a drug that follows first-order kinetics. About 50% of the drug is removed during the first half-life. About 25% remains after two half-lives and 12.5% after three half-lives. The effect of the drug essentially disappears after four or five half-lives.

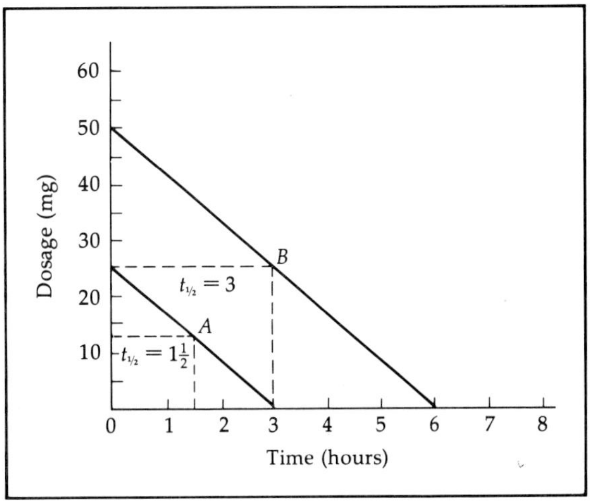

FIGURE 7-14 The biological half-life of a drug that follows zero-order kinetics. When two different dosages are administered, the half-life of the lower dosage is less. Dose *A*, 25 mg, yielded a 1.5-unit half-life; when the dose was doubled (dose *B*), to 50 mg., the half-life became 3 units of time.

doses are taken, the half-life may increase to as much as 30 hours. Aspirin tends to follow zero-order kinetics. The smooth muscle relaxant theophylline has a $t_{1/2}$ of five hours in adults, but a $t_{1/2}$ of three and a half hours in young children. The renal excretion of kanamycin may be prolonged in clients with renal impairment, thereby increasing the drug's duration of action.

Plasma and urine drug concentrations are used to determine a drug's pharmacokinetics, but the site of action for most drugs is the tissues and not the blood. The relationship between the plasma drug concentrations and the drug's effect in the body—as well as the safe drug dose—must be determined.

Drug Dose-Response Parameters

All drugs are ineffective unless a certain blood concentration is reached and maintained. The **minimum effective dose** is the smallest dose that can be given in order to achieve the desired effect. *Dose-response* experiments are conducted to determine the minimum effective plasma drug concentration that corresponds to the desired therapeutic effect. The same type of experiments can determine other drug dose-response parameters (see Figure 7-15), including the following:

1. *Onset of action* is the time required to achieve the minimum effective plasma drug concentration following administration of a particular dosage form—tablet, spansule, and so on—or administration by a particular route—subcutaneous, intramuscular, and so on.

2. *Duration of action* is the length of time the plasma concentration remains above the minimum effective level for therapeutic response.

3. *Toxic dose* is the quantity of drug that, if exceeded, will result in the onset of toxic or other untoward effects. It is the maximum safe dose that can be administered without exceeding a toxic plasma drug concentration.

4. *Therapeutic range* is the plasma drug concentration between the minimum effective concentration and the toxic drug concentration. The objective of drug therapy is to maintain a relatively consistent plasma drug concentration within the therapeutic range.

Antacids, antinausea agents, laxatives, and headache remedies are often taken once and not repeated, unless the symptoms return, but many drugs are administered regularly in order to sustain a desired therapeutic effect, sometimes for the remainder of the client's life.

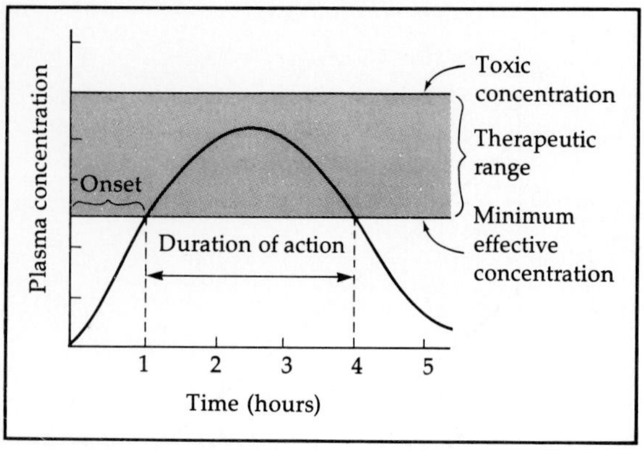

FIGURE 7-15 Example of the plasma drug concentration following oral administration. The onset of this drug's action is one hour and the duration of effect is three hours; total time is actually four hours from the time of drug administration.

Multiple Dosage Regimes

Whereas antibiotics may be prescribed for a relatively short period of time—ten days or two weeks—many drugs require repetitive administration to maintain the plasma drug concentration level over prolonged periods of time. The therapeutic range of some drugs is wide and of others, quite narrow. If the plasma drug concentration falls below the drug's minimum effective level for a period of time, the client's original symptoms will return, but if the drug's toxic level is exceeded, untoward reactions will occur. Digoxin, theophylline, and procainamide have narrow therapeutic ranges and clients taking these drugs need to be observed frequently following hospitalization.

Some drugs achieve plasma concentrations within the therapeutic range following the administration of the first dose, but others must accumulate in the body and require several doses to reach the therapeutic range (see curve *A* in Figure 7-16). To shorten the time required for therapeutic response to occur, a *loading dose* may be administered, followed by a daily *maintenance dose* to maintain the drug concentration within the therapeutic range. For example, the loading dose for the antiarrhythmic lidocaine is about 100 mg (1 mg/kg) via IV bolus; then a continuous IV drip of 3 mg/minute is started. The initial loading dose of digoxin—also called the "digitalizing dose"—may be 0.25 to 0.5 mg IV, followed by 0.25 mg IV every six hours until the total loading dose of 10 mcg/kg is administered. A maintenance dose of 0.125 to 0.25 mg is usually given orally to keep the client free of congestive heart failure symptoms. Figure 7-16 shows the effect of different dosage regimes on the plasma drug concentrations.

Applying Pharmacokinetic Data

Knowledge of the pharmacokinetics of a drug gives the health team guidelines for providing effective drug therapy for their clients. The data assists the physician in selecting the appropriate dosage form, dose, route of administration, and frequency of administration, and assists the nurse in performing all aspects of his or her role more effectively.

Drug administration can be more effective when the nurse is aware of the specific parameters of a drug. For example, the duration of the antiarrhythmic effect of an IV bolus of lidocaine is 10 to 20 minutes, so after the bolus is administered, the nurse has only 10 to 20 minutes to prepare and hang the continuous IV lidocaine drip. In order to maintain the desired response without toxicity, all intravenous drugs with a narrow therapeutic range should be administered through an IV pump or with memory tubing and the client should be monitored continuously. The IV rate, blood pressure, heart rate, and heart rhythm of a client on the adrenergic stimulant norepinephrine (Levophed) should be monitored every five minutes, since there are great individual variations in the therapeutic range and since the blood pressure effects disappear within one to two minutes after the IV is discontinued.

The *optimum times* for drug administration are prescribed by the physician, but there are times when the nurse may need to know whether an order for four times a day should be on a qid or a q6h sequence. In general, most antibiotics need to be administered around the clock, not qid. A q8h, q6h, or q4h interval of drug administration will sustain the desired steady state within the therapeutic range, whereas a tid or qid sequence will not. When in doubt, the nurse should consult the pharmacokinetic data in the drug monograph.

The erratic administration of a drug may result

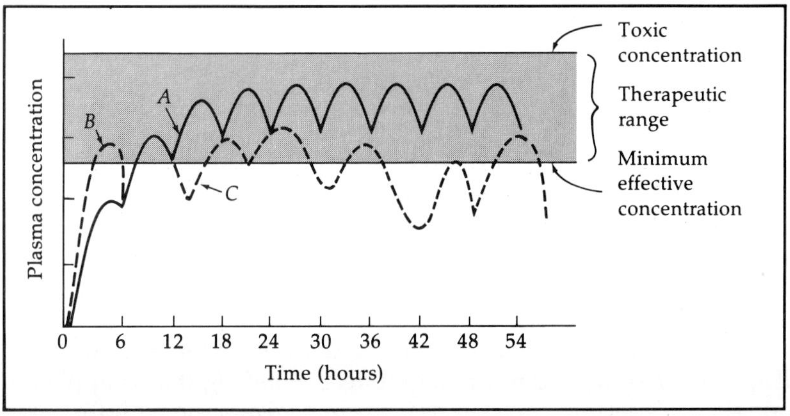

FIGURE 7-16 Example of the changes in the plasma drug concentrations when different dosage regimes are followed. When equal doses are administered consistently every six hours, a "steady-state" plasma drug concentration will eventually be achieved (curve *A*). Sometimes a loading dose (curve *B*) is administered to achieve the desired therapeutic response more quickly. But if the drug is administered at erratic time intervals, a steady-state drug concentration within the therapeutic range will not occur (Curve C).

in noneffective plasma concentration, as illustrated by curve C in Figure 7-16. Note that the client received the third drug dose two hours after the prescribed time, which lowered the plasma concentration below the minimum effective level. Many drugs cannot be administered on an erratic schedule or the result will be noneffective drug therapy. Clients who self-administer their drugs should be informed of the necessity of maintaining a rigid drug time sequence.

The *timing of expected response and of potential toxic reactions* can be anticipated when one is aware of the time required for the drug to achieve the minimum plasma concentration (onset) and the peak plasma level. Clients who are frightened or in pain, particularly children, often ask the nurse, "When will my pain disappear?" after being given an analgesic. The nurse who knows the pharmacokinetics of the analgesic can answer this and other questions. The onset of action of meperidine, after oral administration, is 15 minutes, of aspirin, 30 minutes, of pentazocine (Talwin), 15 to 30 minutes. Parenteral administration (IM or SC) shortens the onset for most analgesics—for meperidine, to 10 minutes, for pentazocine, 10 to 20 minutes, for codeine, 5 to 10 minutes. By the time the drug level peaks, the client should be comfortable and may even be sleeping. It should be remembered that the peak plasma drug level for IV analgesics is immediate but the duration of action is often shortened—the duration of pentazocine is two to three hours, of meperidine, only two hours—therefore necessitating drug administration q2–3h.

If a toxic drug reaction occurs, it will often coincide with the drug's peak plasma concentration, particularly for drugs with a narrow therapeutic range. One of the dangers of drugs administered by IV bolus is the potential for an immediate toxic reaction. When a loading dose is being administered, the client should be assessed for potential toxic drug reaction, particularly during and following the last divided dose. This is the time when the plasma drug concentrations may unexpectedly exceed the toxic level. Visual disturbances and impaired cardiac conduction are frequently the first toxic symptoms to appear after a client is digitalized with digoxin. The physician should be notified immediately so that corrective action can be started.

Client education about drugs can be more effective when the nurse is aware of the particular drug's pharmacokinetic parameters. Clients should be informed of the necessity of maintaining a strict time sequence for taking their drugs, as well as the reasons for not altering the drug dose or schedule unless the physician is consulted. Although the alteration of some drug regimens is not life threatening, the alteration of others is, and the clients should be made aware of this. Propranolol (Inderal) is prescribed for several arrhythmias and is sometimes used to prevent angina attacks. Following oral administration, its onset of action is 30 minutes. It reaches its peak plasma level in 60 to 90 minutes and its duration of action is about 6 hours. Clients and their families should be informed that the symptoms of toxicity—hypotension, bradycardica, paresthesia, disorientation—will appear 60 to 90 minutes after drug administration. They need to be taught how to assess these symptoms, what to do if they occur, and that medical assistance should be sought immediately. The plasma half-life of propranolol is variable (3.4 to 6 hours) and prolonged use causes physiological dependence on the drug. Clients taking this drug should be informed that abrupt withdrawal can cause serious consequences, which can be avoided by slow reduction of dosage by the physician.

The above examples suggest only a few of the ways in which nursing uses drug pharmacokinetic data to provide more effective drug therapy. The specific data can be found in comprehensive drug monographs.

After a drug has been absorbed and distributed to its site of action, the therapeutic effects occur. The next section deals with the theories of drug action.

DRUG ACTION

Although their meanings are slightly different, the terms *drug action* and *drug effect* are often used synonymously. Since the literature does distinguish between them a basic understanding of the specific meaning of each is important. Most drugs interact with the body's cells to produce a response in a client. Only the initial drug-cell interaction is called **drug action**. **Drug effect** refers to the chemical and physiological response of the body to the initial drug contact.

The Location of Drug Action

Until more knowledge is available about cellular physiology and the action of drugs, the specific sites of drug-cell interaction will remain a mystery. However, the effects of medicinal agents are often referred to as either local or systemic.

When a drug primarily affects the tissues with which it comes into contact, the effect is called **local**. A local anesthetic prevents the transmission of pain impulses from the immediate area but does not render the client unconscious. For example, procaine may be injected into the area surrounding a wound that requires suturing in order to anesthetize the immediate area. The term *topical* is sometimes used to indicate the local effect of a drug that is applied to the skin or a mucous membrane with the intention of creating an effect in a distant organ, but **topical** should only be used to indicate the *application* of a medicinal agent to the skin or mucous membrane and not its intended location of action.

Percutaneous is the term used to indicate the topical administration of a drug intended for systemic action. The cardiac drug nitroglycerin can be administered topically as an ointment and will be absorbed percutaneously.

After being absorbed into the body's fluids, a drug with a **systemic** effect (1) circulates throughout the body, (2) interacts with the body's cells, fluids, or other constituents, and (3) creates its effect. When the drug exerts its effect on most of the body, it is said to have a *general systemic effect*. When the drug interacts with particular sites within the body, where it produces a more specific effect, it is said to have a *selective effect*. For example, thyrotropin has an affinity for the thyroid gland and has a stimulating effect on it, but it has little or no effect on the rest of the body.

Ideally, all medicinal agents would have a selective action and create only the single desired effect. However, most drugs create more than one effect. For example, aspirin not only relieves pain but also decreases fever (antipyresis) and inflammation and has an anticoagulant effect by prolonging the prothrombin time. In addition, aspirin can also cause undesired effects, such as gastrointestinal irritation and acid-base imbalance.

Critical Concentration for Drug Action

Drugs that are taken for their systemic effect reach their sites of action by passing through the body's fluids. When the fluid around the site has a sufficient drug concentration, the action and, therefore, the effects of the drug will occur. This minimum drug concentration is termed the **critical concentration**. For most drugs, only a low concentration is required before the effects occur, but for others, such as some general anesthetics, relatively high concentrations are needed.

Mechanisms of Drug Action

Some drugs seem to create their therapeutic effect by means that are external to the cell, but most drugs act directly on the cell. Too little is currently known about cellular biochemistry to explain the exact mechanism(s) by which drugs act on the cells. However, it is believed that some aspect of cellular chemistry and physiology is directly changed by the drug. There are several theories of the mechanisms of drug action, and, although it does not explain everything, the drug-receptor interaction theory is widely accepted.

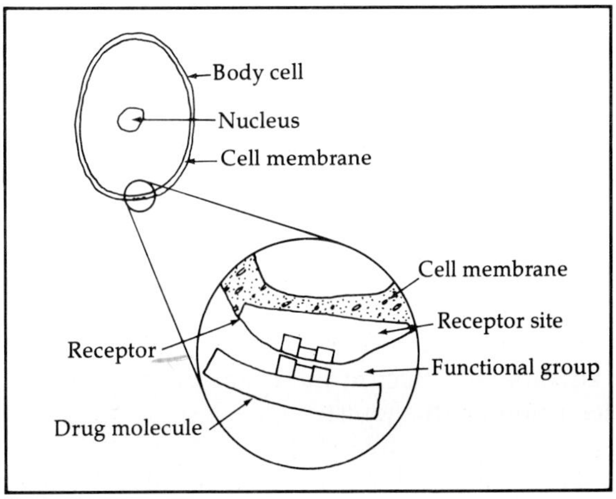

FIGURE 7-17 Drug-receptor interaction theory of drug action. The drug's functional group matches the receptor site on the cell, interacts with it, and initiates drug action.

Drug-Receptor Interaction Theory

It is believed that many drugs interact with the component of the cell called the **receptor**, which may be part of the cell's surface membrane or a component within the cell. The receptor is thought to have a chemically reactive area that is capable of combining with some aspect of the drug's chemical structure. The specific reactive area in the cell is referred to as the *receptor site* or the *locus of action.*

The receptors are generally believed to be chemical groups that take part in some aspect of the cell's metabolism, such as cellular oxidation or enzyme activity. These chemical groups include the amino, carboxyl, sulfhydryl, and phosphate groups.

It is also thought that an aspect of the drug's chemical structure must complement the cell's receptor in order for the drug to interact at the receptor site. The drug's complementary area is termed its **functional group(s)** and may be a basic nitrogen atom, an amide group, or a phenolic group. Figure 7-17 shows the main features of the drug-receptor interaction model. The specific mechanisms of many receptor site-functional group interactions are only speculative at this time, but progress has occurred in identifying the nature of some receptor sites.

The following terms are used in the drug-receptor theory to describe and explain the action of drugs at receptor sites:

1. *Affinity*—Drugs that are attracted to specific receptor sites are said to have an affinity for those receptors.

2. *Agonist*—A drug that combines with a receptor, interacts, and produces a response is called an agonist.

3. *Antagonist*—A drug that combines with a receptor and inhibits the action of an agonist is an antagonist. Antagonists do not initiate an effect; they only prevent a response from occurring. There are two types:
   - (a) *Competitive antagonist*—If the inhibition caused by the antagonist drug can be overcome by large quantities of the agonist, the antagonist is said to be competitive. The agonist and antagonist are both competing for the same receptor and are able to displace each other at the receptor site.
   - (b) *Noncompetitive antagonist*—If the inhibiting effect of an antagonist cannot be overcome by large quantities of an agonist, the antagonist is said to be noncompetitive.

4. *Blocker* or *inhibitor*—Drugs that are antagonists are also called blockers or inhibitors; the terms are used interchangeably.

5. *Competitive inhibition* or *blocking*—These terms describe the action of a competitive antagonist.

6. *Efficacy*—When a drug is capable of initiating an effect—a biochemical or physiological change in the body—it is said to have efficacy. Only agonists have efficacy. Although antagonists do not initiate a drug action, they can have a therapeutic effect in the client by preventing the action of an agonist.

There are probably many types of receptors in the body. The receptor sites in the nervous system, called **neuroeffectors,** have undergone the most research. They are classified according to the efficacy of specific agonists on the receptor site and the effect, or lack of effect, of specific antagonists. Nerves release chemical substances, called **neurohumoral transmitters**, to carry impulses across most synapses and neuroeffector junctions. The impulse is stopped when the transmitter substance is destroyed or inactivated by an enzyme produced in the area, usually from the impulse receiver side of the gap. An agonist may stimulate the action of a neurotransmitter, whereas an antagonist may block it. For example, nicotine mimics the effects of acetylcholine, the transmitter of cholinergic nerve fibers, at nicotine receptors. The poison curare competes with acetylcholine and thereby blocks the transmitter action of acetylcholine to striated muscle fibers. Thus, nicotine stimulates striated muscle action, and curare blocks it.

Structure-Activity Relationship

The drug-receptor interaction theory posits that the drug's functional group structure must match up with the receptor site for the drug action to occur. Therefore, the chemical structure of a drug is directly related to its effects and even slight variations in the structure of the molecule may cause loss of drug action. It has also been discovered that two drugs with entirely different chemical structures can cause the same or similar action. For example, the curare alkaloid tubocurarine has a chemical structure similar to that of curare. But, whereas curare causes paralysis of skeletal muscles and, ultimately, death due to paralysis of the respiratory muscles, tubocurarine is a valuable muscle relaxant used in surgery. Similarly, the more refined digitoxin has a cardiac activity similar to that of digitalis leaf. It is hoped that discoveries about structure-activity relationships will provide us with more specific and safer drugs.

Extracellular Mechanisms of Drug Action

Drugs that do not interact directly with the cells follow various laws of physics or chemistry when creating their therapeutic effect. Many drugs that alter gastrointestinal functioning and acid-base balance operate by external mechanisms, including the following:

1. *Adsorption*—The process of taking up dissolved or suspended substances, such as bacteria and their toxins, moisture, or gases, is called adsorption. When *adsorbents* are taken orally, they do not discriminate between noxious and desired substances, such as enzymes. Examples are activated charcoal and kaolin.

2. *Alteration of osmosis*—Certain drugs change the osmolarity of various body fluids and therefore alter the distribution of fluids in body compartments. Electrolytes by themselves are unable to promote the redistribution of the body fluids into any one body compartment. However, there are solutes that cannot permeate membranes and can therefore cause the osmotic pressure to rise in the compartment in which they have been injected. Water will then be redistributed from other areas of the body into the altered compartment. For example, when osmotic diuretics such as urea and mannitol are injected into the blood stream, they will cause a fluid shift from the body tissues into the plasma; the body can then eliminate the drug and fluid through the kidneys.

3. *Normalization of pH*—Normalization refers to the process of neutralizing a natural body substance's acid or alkaline quality. For example, the antacid aluminum hydroxide can be given to neutralize the stomach's hydrochloric acid.

The normal pH of the blood is 7.35 to 7.45. When a client develops acidosis (pH below 7.35) or alkalosis (pH above 7.45), it is possible to normalize the blood's pH with drugs that will make the blood more alkaline, such as sodium bicarbonate, or more acidic, such as intravenous ammonium chloride.[3]

4. *Mechanical protection*—Some drugs coat the body part to which they are applied and thereby provide mechanical protection to the underlying cells from air, fluid, and other irritants. Examples are demulcents and emollients. When *mechanical protector* is used as a drug category, it refers only to topically applied drugs that provide protection but are insoluble and chemically inert, such as collodian and petrolatum gauze.

5. *Precipitation* and *chelation*—The process of separating a substance from a solution by the action of a reagent, forming insoluble solid particles, is called *precipitation*. However, *chelation* is the term preferred for chemical precipitation. A *chelate* is the chemical compound formed when a metallic ion is firmly bound to a ring of a receptive chemical substance, called a *chelating agent*. For example, tannic acid will chemically bond with many heavy metals, such as arsenic, and alkaloids, such as strychnine, thereby preventing the heavy metal poisons from being absorbed. Provided the poison is still in the stomach, tannic acid is a useful antidote for some poisons.

Unwanted chelating can also occur. When oral tetracycline is given with certain cations, such as calcium, iron, or aluminum, a chelate will be formed and the tetracycline will not be absorbed. Tetracycline should therefore not be given with milk, milk by-products, or antacids, but should be administered alone between meals.

PHARMACODYNAMICS AND NURSING

Knowledge of the principles of pharmacodynamics—drug absorption, drug distribution, drug metabolism, drug excretion, pharmacokinetics, and drug action—helps the nurse monitor drug therapy more effectively. Historically, the nurse has had to rely on experience to recognize problems in drug therapy. But with an understanding of the pharmacodynamic principles, the nurse can assess clients more prudently, predict potential problems, and institute appropriate nursing measure(s) to maximize desired responses while anticipating and thereby minimizing untoward reactions.

Assessment

The health history—data about the client and his or her family and environment—is collected at an initial interview and is correlated with prescribed drug orders and the pharmacodynamic data about the drugs. The factors that may alter the client's drug dose, such as age, body weight, and renal or liver pathology, are considered in determining the relative safety of the drug dose. Other safety factors, such as a history of drug allergy in the client or his or her family, or drug-drug interactions, should be considered as well. The physician should be notified of any discrepancy between the nurse's data and the prescribed drug *before* the first dose is administered.

Management

Correlations between drug data—expected peak drug concentrations, biological half-lives, and rates of absorption and elimination—and client data—condition of absorbing site, condition of the circulatory system, liver or kidney pathology, potential drug tolerance, and possible client noncompliance—are used to determine the appropriate drug form, route, and time sequence. For example, the client may be unable to swallow a capsule; the drug form could be changed to a liquid if available. If the client has been bedridden for a prolonged period, the intravenous or oral route is often more effective than the intramuscular route. A q6h or a q8h time sequence instead of a 10-A.M., 2-P.M., 6-P.M., 10-P.M. schedule may be required to maintain a consistent drug plasma level. If a client's daily activities preclude a regular schedule of drug administration, a long-acting spansule drug form or a drug deposit should be considered. The physician

[3]Alkalosis is seldom corrected with acidic drugs since these drugs tend to perpetuate the depletion of needed electrolytes, such as potassium.

should be notified of potential alterations in dosage form, route of administration, or time sequence.

Evaluation

The most accurate method of evaluating the effects of a drug on a given client is to correlate the client's response with the actual plasma concentration level. The therapeutic range for certain antibiotics, antiarrhythmic agents, anticonvulsants, and cardiac glycosides is well established, but the tests require specific, expensive equipment. Consequently, measurements of plasma drug concentrations are used primarily in emergency situations. Assessment of a client's therapeutic response, failure to respond, and untoward reactions are often left to the nurse. Although a hospitalized client is observed continuously, particular attention should be given to the client's response to a drug. Does the client have the appropriate response? When the drug is administered only during the day, does the therapeutic response subside during the night? Are there any side effects? Do the side effects and other untoward responses outweigh the therapeutic response? Correlations between the expected pharmacodynamics of a drug and the client's actual response help the health team determine what alterations, if any, should be made in the drug therapy.

REFERENCES

Books

Benet, L. Z., ed. 1976. *The effects of disease states on drug pharmacokinetics.* Washington, D.C.: American Pharmaceutical Association.

Curry, S. H. 1980. *Drug disposition and pharmacokinetics.* 3rd ed. Boston: Blackwell Scientific Publications.

Ditlert, L. W., and Di Santo, A. R. 1975. *The bioavailability of drug products.* Washington, D.C.: American Pharmaceutical Association.

Goldstein, A. 1974. *Principles of drug action: The basis of pharmacology.* 2d ed. New York: Wiley.

Goodman, L. S., and Gilman, A. 1980. *The pharmacologic basis of therapeutics.* 6th ed. New York: Macmillan.

LaDu, B. N., and others. 1971. *Fundamentals of drug metabolism and drug distributions.* Baltimore: Williams & Wilkins.

Levine, R. R. 1978. *Pharmacology: Drug actions and reactions.* 2nd ed. Boston: Little, Brown.

Martin, E. W. 1978. *Hazards of medication.* 2nd ed. Philadelphia: Lippincott.

Notari, R. E., and others. 1975. *Biopharmaceutics and pharmacokinetics: An introduction.* 2nd ed. New York: Marcel Dekker.

Wilson, C. O., and others. eds. 1971. *Textbook of organic medicinal and pharmaceutical chemistry.* 6th ed. Philadelphia: Lippincott.

Articles

Azarnoff, D. I. 1970. Application of metabolic data to the evaluation of drugs. *Journal of the American Medical Association* 211:1691.

Jacob, J. T., and Plun, E. M. 1970. Factors affecting the dissolution rate of medications from tablets. *Journal of Pharmacy Science* 15:171–88.

O'Brien, T. E. 1974. Excretion of drugs in human milk. *American Journal of Hospital Pharmacy* 31:844–54.

Sapeika, B. A. 1960. The passage of drugs across the placenta. *South African Medical Journal* 34:49–55.

U.S. Food and Drug Administration. 1974. Human drugs: procedures for establishing a bioequivalence requirement. *Federal Registry.* Washington, D.C.: Government Printing Office.

Chapter 8

Untoward Drug Reactions

THE NATURE OF ADVERSE AND OTHER UNTOWARD REACTIONS

A cause-and-effect relationship cannot always be established between a drug and an adverse drug reaction (ADR). Therefore the Food and Drug Administration coined the term *adverse drug experience* to indicate all adverse reactions, whether caused by a drug or not, that occur during drug therapy. The adverse reactions can result from contact with other offending chemicals in the environment such as food additives or from an undiagnosed disease process. For example, a report to the FDA may indicate that a skin rash developed during the course of treatment with a particular antibiotic, but the rash may have been due to an allergy to tomatoes, an irritation from contact with an insecticide, or an undiagnosed skin infection. The development of a gastrointestinal irritation may be blamed on an orally administered medication, when in fact the symptoms are related to emotional stress or anxiety about the disease for which the drug was prescribed.

But when there is strong evidence that there is a relationship between the reaction and the drug, the term *untoward drug reaction* is used. An **untoward drug reaction** is any response to a drug other than the desired response. Drug interactions, harmless reactions, minor adverse reactions, and adverse reactions are all types of untoward drug reactions. An **adverse drug reaction** is an untoward reaction that has the potential for causing temporary loss of functioning, permanent damage, or death. ADRs are often classified according to the type of effect that occurs.

The Classification of Adverse Drug Reactions

An adverse drug reaction can be directly related to the desired action of a drug: the drug may cause too much of the desired therapeutic action. These hyperdrug responses have been reported in the literature for many years and are termed **toxic effects**. A toxic effect may be due to excessive intake, inadequate drug distribution, a drug sensitivity, or inadequate metabolism or excretion of the drug. Causative factors include the particular drug form, the client's genetic makeup and pathology, and interference by other drugs, chemicals, or diseases.

Many drugs will cause toxic reactions in all clients if the dosage is sufficiently high. Some individuals will demonstrate toxic effects at lower dosages than other clients. It has been determined that body weight has a direct relationship to dosage-related toxic reactions, so the recommended dosage of many drugs is now indicated in units per kilogram of body weight. Other client characteristics such as sex and age are also related, and some drugs have recommended dosages for infants and children. Most drugs do not have recommended dosages for the elderly. As explained in Chapter 7, some clients accumulate drugs until toxicity is observed, due to an inability adequately to metabolize or excrete them. Serum drug level measurements are useful in adjusting dosages and avoiding toxicity.

Some drugs tend to require increasingly higher dosages over time in order for the client to sustain the desired physical or psychological effect, due to the phenomenon of **drug tolerance**. Other drugs may cause withdrawal symptoms when they are abruptly discontinued because they create physical dependence.

The amphetamines, CNS depressants, hallucinogens, and narcotics may lead to drug tolerance or to physical or psychic dependence. Appropriate warnings are placed on the labels of these drugs, and their use is carefully controlled by the government.

Certain drugs will cause toxic or other adverse effects only after they have been taken for prolonged periods of time. For example, the prolonged use of ergotamine will cause chronic ergotism with intermittent claudication, numbness, and cold, cyanotic extremities. The specific causes are unknown, but it is believed that biochemical or immunologic mechanisms are involved. Prolonged use of a drug may directly or indirectly alter DNA synthesis, disrupt a cellular enzyme system, alter antibody characteristics, or cause changes in some other biochemical process. Various drugs, industrial pollutants, pesticides, certain food additives, and various other chemicals have been implicated as causative agents in certain blood dyscrasias, hepatic diseases, and forms of cancer. Drugs that are classified as carcinogenic agents include hormones, cytotoxic antineoplastics, nitrites, and excesses of vitamins. Further research is required to determine specific effects of prolonged exposure in human beings, since most of the studies to date have been conducted on animals.

Many lay people use the term *side effect* to indicate any response other than the intended drug action, and, indeed, the older definitions of *side effect* included all untoward effects except toxicity. But as the field of pharmacodynamics developed, the term has come to be replaced by more specific designations, such as *secondary effect, allergy* and *hypersensitivity,* and *idiosyncrasy.*

In some cases, an untoward reaction may consist of signs and symptoms that are related to the drug's action but not necessarily to its intended action. Most drugs create more than one action and the **secondary actions** or **secondary effects** may be responsible for the untoward reaction. For example, many anesthetic agents cause hypotension, and, in some cases, cardiovascular collapse can occur.

Some clients may have a major or minor **allergic reaction** to a drug. Allergic reactions are rather common, particularly with certain drugs, such as the penicillins. Since allergic and other hypersensitivity drug reactions are complex, they are described in detail later in the chapter.

Genetically inherited factors may alter a client's response to a drug and cause a drug-induced illness. The relatively new field of *pharmacogenetics* has increased our understanding of genetic factors in drug reactions. Sometimes a client reacts to a drug in an unexpected manner; this reaction is called an **idiosyncratic reaction.** Idiosyncrasies are rare and some are due to unusual enzyme deficiencies, such as glucose-6-phosphate dehydrogenase (G-6-PD). Clients with this deficiency can develop severe blood dyscrasias when certain drugs are taken.

Adverse drug reactions, then, are classified as follows:

1. Extension of primary effect
   (a) Accumulation
   (b) Toxicity
2. Drug tolerance/dependence
3. Secondary effect
4. Hypersensitivity (allergic reaction)
5. Idiosyncratic reaction

Characteristics of Untoward Drug Reactions

Although some untoward drug reactions are harmless, they can cause the client unnecessary alarm. Changes in the color or characteristics of feces and urine can occur with some drugs (see Tables 8-1, 8-2, and 8-3). Clients should be warned about these changes and informed that they are harmless side effects. However, other urinary and fecal color changes can be dangerous and demand medical attention. Untoward drug reactions can produce *local* or *systemic* symptoms. Although most local reactions are confined to a limited area, serious systemic reactions can follow, so clients with local reactions should be closely observed.

Many drug reactions are *acute* and have a rapid onset, but some can develop into *chronic* problems. If detected and treated early, most acute reactions will not cause permanent damage and will disappear once the causative agent is discontinued. Whereas the vast majority of drug reactions are *minor,* some are *major* and require quick action. The sooner a drug reaction is detected, the smaller are the chances of severe consequences occurring. The more nurses know about untoward drug reactions, the greater their opportunity to detect reactions early and to decrease mortality and morbidity from drug-induced reactions.

Minor adverse reactions include the following:

1. Abdominal cramps
2. Anorexia
3. Dizziness
4. Drowsiness or excessive sleeping
5. Euphoria
6. Excessive hunger
7. Fatigue
8. Headache
9. Indigestion
10. Loose stools or mild diarrhea
11. Mild skin irritations, rashes, and photosensitivity
12. Nausea or vomiting
13. Secondary infections when mild and localized—for example, vaginitis
14. Weakness

TABLE 8-1 Harmless Fecal Color Changes Caused by Drugs

Drug	Color Changes
Aluminum hydroxide and other antacids	White spots
Barium	Black or very dark brown
Bismuth	Whitish or clay colored
Iron	Black
Rifampin (antitubercular agent)	Reddish-orange*

* Rifampin therapy also causes the urine, saliva, sputum, sweat, and tears to turn reddish-orange.

Major adverse reactions include the following:

1. Allergy—anaphylaxis, serum sickness, drug fever
2. Bleeding or hemorrhage
3. Blood dyscrasias
4. Cardiovascular reactions—arrhythmias, heart failure, hypotension
5. Fluid and electrolyte imbalances—hyperkalemia, hypokalemia
6. Impaired senses—hearing loss, vision loss
7. Kidney reactions—necrosis
8. Liver disorders—obstructive jaundice
9. Neurologic reactions—coma, convulsions, disorientation, depression
10. Respiratory depression
11. Severe cutaneous reactions and photosensitivity
12. Supra infections

Preventing Severe Adverse Reactions

I. Establishing a data base
   A. Obtain from the client a list of all drugs taken and consult drug monographs for complete descriptions of them.

TABLE 8-2 Harmful Fecal Color Changes Caused by Drugs

Drug	Color Change	Cause
Phenylbutazone (Butazoladin)	Black	High intestinal bleeding
Salicylates	Black	High intestinal bleeding
Warfarin (Coumadin)	Black or red streaks	High and low intestinal bleeding

B. Obtain a description of all drug allergies/hypersensitivities and list the drug, method taken, nature of reaction, and relationship of reaction to the time the drug was started.
For example: Oral penicillin—hives—occurred three days after taking drug

C. Obtain a history of all drugs taken that are in the same category as the newly prescribed drug and list any untoward effects.
For example: Antibiotics—has taken sulfa once and streptomycin once without adverse reaction

D. Obtain a family history of adverse drug reactions.
For example:
- Mother—penicillin (hives)
  aspirin (pruritis)
- Father—none known
- Sibling—penicillin (drug fever)

E. Obtain a personal and family history of potential immune or hypersensitivity conditions, including asthma, eczema, psoriasis, hay fever, dermatitis, anaphylaxis—for example, from bee stings, known enzyme deficiencies—for example, G-6-PD, and photosensitivity.

F. Obtain history of liver and kidney diseases or injuries and determine presence or absence of diabetes.
For example: Hepatitis three years ago with no residual damage

G. Assess function of the hepatic, renal, cardiovascular, pulmonary, and gastrointestinal systems.

H. If hospitalized, check CBC, urinalysis, and liver function tests for abnormality.
For example:
Elevated eosinophil count
RBCs and WBCs in urine
Elevated BUN or bilirubin

II. Assessments

A. Determine the potential effect the prescribed drug dosage will have on the client.
1. Determine the effects of primary action and adequacy of the affected body systems to tolerate the drug.
2. Determine the effects of secondary action and adequacy of the affected body systems to tolerate the drug.

B. Determine the client's state of health and ability to process the drug.
1. Determine client's ability to absorb and distribute the drug, as well as the appropriateness of the route of administration.
For example:
Amount of protein binding that occurs with this drug
Presence of vomiting or diarrhea
2. Determine the adequacy of the body to metabolize and eliminate the prescribed drug dosage.

C. Determine potential toxic reactions the client may manifest.

D. Determine potential immune hypersensitivity reactions the client may manifest.

III. Management

A. Assess client as necessary for therapeutic response and the indication of toxic drug reactions.

B. Assess client as necessary for drug immune/hypersensitivity reactions.

TABLE 8-3 Harmless Urine Color Changes Caused by Drugs

Classification	Drug	Color Change
Anticoagulant	Warfarin (Coumadin)	Orange
Anticonvulsant	Phenytoin (Dilantin)	
Antidepressant	Amitriptyline (Elavil)	Bluish-green
Antiinfective	Furazolidone (Furoxone)	Orange-brown
Antimalaria agent	Quinine	Brownish to blackish
Cathartic	Cascara sagrada	Reddish (in alkaline urine)
Diagnostic agent	Azurisin (Diagnex Blue) Phenolsulfonphthalein (PSP)	Bluish-green/ Reddish (in alkaline urine)
Sulfonamides	Sulfisoxazole (Gantrisin)	Brownish or rusty-yellow
Phenothiazines	Chlorpromazine (Thorazine)	Reddish-brown
Urinary antiseptics	Methylene blue	Bluish-green
	Nitrofurantoin (Furadantin)	Brownish or rusty yellow

C. When necessary, observe client closely for at least one half-hour after administering agents that may cause anaphylaxis.
D. Notify physician when untoward effects first appear and obtain alternative prescription when necessary.
E. List and explain to clients the symptoms for which medical advice should be sought and the importance of immediate medical attention.
F. List and explain to clients potential side effects and other minor untoward drug reactions. Indicate what should be done, if anything.
For example: Color change in urine or stool is expected and is not harmful. Drug may cause dizziness and decrease reflex time; do not drive a car or operate other heavy machinery.

ALLERGIC AND HYPERSENSITIVITY REACTIONS

Because they are foreign substances, drugs can evoke antigen-antibody responses in reactive clients. Most antigens are complex protein molecules, but there are only a few protein-based drugs—for example, insulin. However, some nonprotein drugs, which are usually nonantigenic, can evoke an immune reaction in individuals who are overly sensitive to the drug. **Hypersensitivity** is a broad term indicating excessive reaction to a foreign substance. The term **allergy** is used to indicate the state of hypersensitivity in which obvious signs and symptoms occur, such as those seen in anaphylaxis, asthmatic attacks, and allergic rhinitis. An *idiosyncratic reaction* to a drug is now assumed to be a form of hypersensitivity.

Antigens

Any drug that has the capacity to create a hypersensitivity response is an antigen. Although only a few drugs are true antigens in the sense that they cause the formation of antibodies, some drugs or their metabolites may induce a hypersensitivity reaction. Many drugs form a loose bond with tissue or blood proteins; in certain individuals, drug molecules may combine with a body protein in such a way as to modify the protein. The altered *drug-protein complex* is then perceived by the body as an antigen and antibodies are produced. A normally nonantigenic drug molecule that forms a drug-protein complex is called a **hapten**. Since, in this case, the immune system is evoked against a body protein, hapten-type sensitivities are called **autoimmune** responses.

Antibodies

The body responds to an antigen by producing antibodies within cells or tissues (*cellular immunity*) or specific antibodies that circulate in the body fluids (*humoral immunity*). Most antibodies are large protein molecules called globulins, and, since they produce immunity against infections, they are called **immunoglobulins**. They are classified in various ways according to their biological behavior and their molecular size and structure. Immunoglobulins can be identified by their unique polypeptide chains and are referred to as immunoglobulin alpha, delta, epsilon, gamma, and mu (IgA, IgD, IgE, IgG, and IgM, respectively). Serum contains high concentrations of IgG, the bacterial antibody, but low concentrations of IgA. IgA is present in high concentrations in respiratory, gastrointestinal, and other body secretions. Small amounts of IgE and IgD circulate in the serum. IgE plays an active role in asthma, urticaria, and other allergic reactions. Both IgA and IgE seem to have an active role in drug hypersensitivities.

Antibodies are classified according to their characteristics during an antigen-antibody reaction. **Precipitins** are those antibodies that cause the formation of an insoluble complex when they combine with an antigen—that is, precipitation occurs. **Agglutinins** are those antibodies that attach to the surface of an antigen or antigen-containing cell—that is, agglutination occurs. **Reagins** are antibodies that react with antigens to initiate a sequence of events that may ultimately cause cell lysis, the release of histamines, and various other responses. Reagins are responsible for several allergic reactions, particularly genetically-related hypersensitivity responses called *atopic reactions*.

Antibodies that circulate in the serum and other body fluids can be identified by laboratory testing. These **humoral antibodies** frequently cause the *rapid onset* of an allergic reaction. The precipitin antibodies are present in hypersensitivity reactions that occur within the first few hours of contact with an allergen, and they may cause life-threatening reactions, such as anaphylaxis. Although reagin antibodies may be found in plasma, the related allergic reactions may occur several hours or even days following contact with the allergen.

Cellular antibodies are found in and on cells and tissues. Since they are less accessible to identification by testing, less is known about them. Skin testing can be used to determine if a client has a cellular hypersensitivity, but it is nonspecific and can be unreliable. Cellular hypersensitivity to drugs is frequently responsible for reactions that are delayed for as long as two weeks; the range of reaction time is a few days to several months. Consequently, cellular hypersensitivity is sometimes said to cause *delayed reactions*. Many idiosyncratic drug reactions, including contact dermatitis, have been attributed to cellular antibodies.

GENERALIZED HYPERSENSITIVITY REACTIONS

Although most drug hypersensitivity reactions tend to be confined to a particular body system—for example, dermatomucosal reactions, pulmonary reactions, and so on—they may affect several systems. There are two forms of drug hypersensitivity that cause a generalized tissue response: anaphylactic-type reactions and serum sickness-type reactions.

Anaphylaxis (Anaphylactic Reaction)

Anaphylaxis is an abrupt, generalized, life-threatening, immunologic tissue response. With the first exposure to the offending drug, the body produces humoral, precipitin immunoglobins (IgE), and when the drug is administered a second time, the body responds immediately. If the drug is administered parenterally, the initial response is often a pruritic urticaria starting at the injection site and spreading rapidly throughout the body. Histamine is released and causes contraction of smooth muscle, an increase in capillary permeability, and profound vasospasm. The onset of symptoms can occur within minutes of administration, or it may be delayed for as long as 30 minutes. If symptoms are untreated, death occurs from asphyxia, circulatory collapse, or convulsions. It is possible for death to occur within five to ten minutes. Fortunately, anaphylactic reactions are rare. Careful history taking and drug skin testing help to prevent their occurrence.

Causative agents The most common causative agents are penicillin and its derivatives, corticotropins, iodides, mercurial diuretics, salicylates, and vaccines. Drugs containing horse serum and the venom of wasps, bees, and other insects are also causative agents.

Clinical picture If the causative is administered parenterally, there may initially be erythema and edema at the injection site. The client may complain of anxiety, restlessness, a pounding headache, throbbing in the ears, sneezing or itching in the throat. If the causative is administered orally, the initial response may take 30 minutes to appear, but *a few minutes later* the client may complain of the sensation of suffocation. A generalized pruritic urticaria, laryngeal edema, bronchial spasms, dyspnea, hypotension, cyanosis, a rapid, thready pulse, and incontinence may occur. Loss of consciousness, asphyxia, cardiovascular collapse, and convulsions soon follow.

Treatment The treatment depends on the severity of the symptoms. Epinephrine is lifesaving, particularly when bronchospasm is present; 1 ml of 1:1000 epinephrine solution is administered parenterally every five to ten minutes as necessary. An open airway is maintained and oxygen therapy is given. A tracheostomy may be required in severe cases. Since histamine causes the excessive production of mucous secretions, frequent but gentle suctioning is required. Defibrillation, external cardiac massage, IV drips to maintain blood pressure, and other lifesaving measures may be required. Antihistamines and corticosteroids are of some benefit as the client recovers.

Nursing management Any time a common causative agent is administered, the client should be closely observed for at least 30 minutes. If anaphylactic symptoms occur, epinephrine should be administered immediately as indicated by agency protocol. The client should be in a supine position with legs elevated to counteract the shock.

Serum sickness

Serum sickness is a generalized allergic reaction characterized by dermal eruptions, edema, fever, lymphadenopathy, and joint pains. Initially, the client has no circulating antibodies against the offending drug but develops humoral precipitins after several days of drug therapy. When there are enough antibodies present to interact with the remaining antigen, the immunologic reaction occurs. Once it appears, the disorder is self-limiting in two or three days and is usually less serious than anaphylaxis. Although skin testing may be of little value in preventing the reaction, a careful history of drug allergies and idiosyncrasies is helpful in identifying potentially reactive clients. Clients who develop a serum sickness reaction have circulating antibodies against the drug and must be cautioned against ever taking the drug a second time, since anaphylaxis may occur.

Causative agents Drugs produced from horse serum, such as tetanus antitoxin and diphtheria antitoxin, were the first drugs known to produce serum sickness—hence the name. Barbiturates, digitalis glucosides, insulin, iodine, isoniazid, mercurial diuretics, penicillin, salicylates, streptomycin, and sulfonamides may cause this reaction.

Clinical picture If the drug was administered parenterally, there may initially be erythema and severe pruritus, particularly at the site of injection, followed by generalized urticarial reaction. The rash may progress and begin to look like vasculitis or even erythema multiforme. The lymph nodes that drain the injection site become enlarged and the client may complain of joint pains. In more severe cases, a high fever (105°F) may develop and last a week or more. The spleen may become enlarged and there may be wheals in the larynx and bronchi, causing dyspnea and other respiratory symptoms. In rare cases, kidney failure occurs, particularly glomerulonephritis. The Davidsohn differential Heterophil test distinguishes serum sickness from infectious mononucleosis.

Treatment If the reaction is mild, antihistamines or ephedrine may control it. Salicylates are effective for relieving the joint pains and controlling fever. Epinephrine, antihistamines, or corticosteroids may be required in severe cases.

Nursing management Inform clients who receive vaccines to notify their physicians if itching or rash occurs within two weeks. Measures to alleviate pruritus, such as cool baths, may be required. Soft gloves, mittens, or socks on hands are helpful to prevent scratching injuries to the dermis. Cool baths, forced fluids, and other measures may be necessary to reduce the fever.

DERMATOMUCOSAL REACTIONS

Drug-induced disorders of the skin and mucous membranes usually appear as a rash, urticaria, or pruritus. Although the drug reactions are usually confined to the skin and mucous membranes, internal organs can be involved.

Most dermatomucosal drug reactions are thought to be caused by drug hypersensitivity, but other mechanisms may be involved. Individuals who have a family or personal history of anaphylaxis, asthma, hay fever, chronic sinusitis, serum sickness, or eczema should be carefully observed for potential drug reactions. It is also known that clients suffering from certain pathological processes, particularly those involving the liver, are susceptible. For example, clients with mononucleosis tend to have a high incidence of cutaneous reactions to drugs that are metabolized by the liver. Because they are foreign to the body, all drugs can be potential causative agents, but some drugs cause cutaneous reactions more frequently than others (see Table 8-4).

Dermatomucosal drug reactions can occur within minutes of contact with the offending agent, or the reaction may occur several weeks after the termination of the drug therapy. In general, clients who react within the first hour of drug therapy are having *allergic reaction* due to preexisting circulating antibodies against the drug. If an anaphylactic reaction occurs, it needs to be treated aggressively. *Delayed reactions,* which occur several days after contact with the causative agent, are usually less severe than acute drug reactions. The *toxic effects* of a drug can occur at any time. Unless the drug has caused permanent damage to the organs that metabolize or excrete it, toxic skin reactions will disappear after the drug's blood concentration has dropped, either from decreasing dosage or withdrawing the drug entirely.

TABLE 8-4 Drugs That Frequently Cause Dermatomucosal Reactions

Category	Drug
Antibiotics	Penicillin Sulfonamides Tetracyclines Streptomycin
Barbiturates	Phenobarbital
Diuretics	Thiazides
Heavy metals	Gold Mercury Arsenicals
Immunizing agents	Diphtheria and tetanus toxoids Pertussis vaccine Salk polio vaccine Measles vaccine
Narcotics	Codeine Morphine
Oral hypoglycemic agents	Tolbutamide
	Chlorpropamide
Salicylates	Aspirin

Anyone who has had a prior urticarial reaction to a drug should be observed closely, since anaphylaxis may develop.Some of the general terms used to describe drug-induced dermatomucosal reaction are as follows:

- *Bulla* (bullae)—A fluid-filled elevated area of the skin greater than 0.5 cm in diameter
- *Erythema* (rash)—Reddening of the skin caused by cutaneous vasodilatation
- *Macule*—A flat, circumscribed area of color change in the skin, either brown, due to increased pigmentation from the melanocytes, or red, due to cutaneous vasodilatation
- *Papule*—An elevated lesion on the skin less than 0.5 cm in diameter, filled with cells, fluid, or metabolic deposits
- *Plaque*—A large, flat-topped, slightly elevated, spot on the skin, usually caused by thickening of one or more skin layers

- *Vesicle*—A fluid-filled, elevated area of the skin less than 0.5 cm in diameter
- *Wheal*—An irregularly shaped, plaque-like elevation of the skin caused by fluid in the upper aspect of the dermis

Since dermatomucosal reactions to drugs occur abruptly, a drug reaction should be suspected in any suddenly appearing rash. If the drug is continued, the reaction may become severe or internal organs may become involved. Most dermatomucosal reactions are of three types: eczema, purpura, or a combination of erythema and bullae. In this section, the relatively minor drug-induced cutaneous reactions are described first. The life-threatening skin reactions are described in detail so that health team members can be knowledgeable in identifying suspicious rashes early. Some drugs (photosensitizers) will not produce a cutaneous reaction unless the client is exposed to a second stimulus containing ultraviolet rays. These photosensitivity reactions are explained last.

Non-fatal Dermatomucosal Reactions

Drug Eruption

The term frequently used for the most common drug-induced cutaneous reaction is **drug eruption**. A drug eruption is caused by hypersensitivity to a drug and, in most cases, the skin is the only organ involved. This classical, non-life-threatening disorder is manifested by an erythematous, generalized, macular or papular rash, which is bilaterally symmetrical.

Pruritus may accompany the rash. The onset of this cutaneous reaction is usually abrupt and may occur within 24 hours of initiating drug therapy or as long as two weeks following discontinuation of the treatment. Once the offending agent is identified and discontinued, the rash may last one week. If the drug is readministered, the rash will usually reoccur.

A **scarlatiniform rash** has a similar appearance to the rash of scarlet fever, a diffuse, pink-red flush of the skin with a "goose flesh" character and feel. When used in the context of drug-induced reactions, the term refers to the same rash as that described in *drug eruption*.

Exanthematous rash has a similar appearance to the rash seen in viral exanthema, a discrete, nonpruritic, nondesquamative rash. When used in the context of induced reactions, the term refers to the same rash as that described in *drug eruption*.

Pruritus (itching)

Pruritus is an unpleasant, irritating sensation arising from the skin, causing the desire to scratch or rub the area. *Itch nerve endings* located in the lower aspect of the epidermis and at the dermal-epidermal junction may be stimulated by irritating drugs and other substances that damage the skin, such as antibiotics; by drugs that cause excessive dryness to the stratum corneum, such as narcotics; and by the retention of sweat, such as is caused by occlusive dressings. Some drug hypersensitivity reactions can cause pruritus without an erythema or skin lesion.

Scratching can cause cutaneous vasodilatation (erythema) and damage to the epidermis. Unfortunately, once the client scratches the affected area, cutaneous vasodilatation occurs and intensifies the itch sensation. Consequently, an itch-scratch-itch cycle is elicited and must be relieved in order to prevent further damage to the skin.

When possible, the causative agent is identified and removed. The local application of cold—for example, cold compresses—will cause cutaneous vasoconstriction and thereby relieve the itch-scratch-itch cycle. Dry skin can be relieved by oily lotions or baths. The itch nerve endings can be calmed by the use of antipruritic local anesthetic lotions, creams, or ointments. At times, topical corticosteroids may be required to reduce the inflammation.

Vasculitis (Allergic cutaneous vasculitis)

Vasculitis is a cutaneous vascular reaction in which there are marked changes in the vessel walls with lesions that are elevated and palpable. Plasma, blood cells, and even whole blood escape into the surrounding dermis and cause a purplish-red discoloration of the skin called **purpura**. Vasculitis is usually caused by a drug hypersensitivity.

Erythema nodosum

Erythema nodosum is a form of vasculitis characterized by reddish, tender nodules located deep in the subcutaneous tissue. As the blood cells are reabsorbed, the lesions become flattened and look more like old bruises. The lesions usually occur on the anterior and medial surface of the lower leg. This type of vasculitis occurs more frequently in women and may be due to drug hypersensitivity, such as to oral contraceptives. Treatment consists of removing the offending drug and instituting supportive measures.

Eczema (eczematous dermatitis)

Eczema is a superficial inflammation of the skin characterized by pruritus and edema between the epidermal cells.

Spongiosis In the *acute phase* of spongiosis, erythema is present due to the dilatation of cutaneous blood vessels. As the edema fluid pushes its way around the epidermal cells to the surface, the stratum corneum becomes stretched, porous, and poorly formed, resulting in raised weeping lesions. Tiny vesicles form and, as they break, crusts develop. Since pruritus is present, the client may infect the lesions through scratching, and pustules may develop. This reaction can become chronic. In the *chronic phase*, the affected skin becomes thickened and the skin markings are accentuated (lichenification) due to the repeated rubbing or scratching of the lesions. The skin becomes dry and scaly. Fissures may develop and the skin may become hyper- or hypopigmented. Although it can be produced by other stimuli, several forms of eczema can be caused by drugs and other chemicals. Heredity, metabolic alterations, and immunologic factors can also cause eczematous dermatoses.

Contact dermatitis Contact dermatitis is a form of eczematous dermatitis. When the inflammatory reaction occurs from exposure to an irritant, it is called *primary irritant dermatitis.* Any person whose skin is exposed to a sufficient quantity of an irritant for a long enough period of time will develop this toxic response. Soaps and detergents may cause a dermatitis after prolonged use ("dishpan hands," "scrub hands"). Primary irritants are usually occupation or hobby related, and identification requires extensive history taking. Nurses, pharmacists, physicians, and other health team members are likely candidates for primary irritant dermatitis because of their exposure to drugs and other chemicals.

Allergic contact dermatitis is a hypersensitivity reaction that develops after the first exposure to the substance. It is believed to be caused by the formation of cellular antibodies in response to the absorption of small amounts of antigen through the skin. The length of time required for the skin to become sensitive to the antigen varies widely, from three days to four weeks. Upon subsequent exposure to the antigen, the sensitized skin develops an eczematous dermatitis. Almost all topically applied drugs, including antibiotics and even antihistamines, have been known to cause allergic eczema reaction in certain clients. However, the offending substance may not be the drug itself but an ingredient used in its manufacture, such as a preservative.

The location and configuration of the contact dermatitis provide clues to the identity of the causative agent. For example, if the dermatitis is located in the underarms, it may be due to a deodorant, if under a dressing, a drug, if under adhesive tape, the adhesive, if under a ring, the metal. Since the stratum corneum of the palms of the hands and the soles of the feet is relatively thick and therefore impermeable to antigens, eczema reactions in these locations are usually due to irritants. The acute phase of primary irritant contact dermatitis tends to involve erythema and edema, but the allergic dermatitis response usually includes the formation of tiny vesicles. After the offending agent is identified and removed, if possible, the client is usually treated with systemic corticosteroids and topically applied antipruritic therapy, such as calamine lotion or Burrow's solution. Allergic reactions respond to systemically administered antihistamines. Measures need to be taken to prevent infection or other injuries to the affected skin.

Atopic dermatitis (allergic eczema, neurodermatitis, infantile atopic dermatitis) Atopic dermatitis is an eczematous dermatitis that occurs in certain individuals with a family history of allergic reactions, such as eczema, asthma, or hay fever, and who have a personal history of pruritus. Although the etiology is unknown, it is believed that the client has a hypersensitivity reaction to many substances, including drugs, foods, food additives, and other chemicals or physical factors. The lesions may first appear on the cheeks, scalp, and diaper area in infants, particularly male infants. In children and adults, the lesions commonly appear on the lateral neck surfaces or in the antecubital and popliteal regions, or both.

Although so-called childhood eczema may disappear in adulthood, clients who had it should be carefully observed for drug-induced allergic reactions, including anaphylaxis and serum sickness-type reactions. They tend to have dry skin that may blanch upon stroking (white dermographism), pruritus following minor skin irritations, such as might be caused by exercise or by alterations in temperature or humidity, and a nervous personality, which may be due to intermittent bouts of pruritus. These clients should not receive smallpox vaccinations or come into contact with individuals who have herpes simplex, since they may develop a life-threatening infection with high fever. Penicillin has caused anaphylactic reactions in these clients.

Life-Threatening Dermatomucosal Reactions

Urticaria (hives)

Urticaria is an acute reaction of the skin characterized by the rapid onset of wheals and often accompanied by pruritus. The lesions consist of transient, edematous, slightly reddened elevations of the skin. They are produced by a localized increase in the capillary and venule permeability caused by the release of histamine and histaminelike substances. The affected dermal vessels leak plasma, eosinophils, and circulating antibodies into the surrounding tissue. Urticaria may be caused by allergy or hypersensitivity to several drugs, such as antibiotics, blood transfusions, nutrients, such as eggs and other chemical substances.

Although each individual lesion may last for less than 24 hours, other lesions will appear elsewhere on the body. They may appear in any location but most occur on the trunk. Mucous membranes of the respiratory and gastrointestinal tract may also be involved. In severe cases, edema of the glottis can cause respiratory failure and death. Epinephrine and other lifesaving measures described under *anaphylaxis* may be useful in severe cases. The disorder is self-limiting in less than two weeks if the offending agent is identified and withdrawn.

Angioneurotic edema (giant hives)

Angioneurotic edema is a severe form of urticaria that involves the mucous membranes as well as the skin. When the respiratory tract is affected, the condition may be serious enough to require intubation. Intubation by endotrachial tube, oxygen therapy, the administration of epinephrine, and other lifesaving measures as described under *anaphylaxis* may be essential.

Erythema multiforme (EM syndrome)

Erythema multiforme is an acute syndrome characterized by circular, edematous lesions with central hemorrhagic circles. The lesions are sometimes called *bulls-eye* or *target lesions.* Erythema, edema, urticaria, vesicles, and bullae may also be present. It is thought to be caused by hypersensitivity that produces vascular changes in the skin and results in the seepage of fluid and cells into the dermis. An unidentified necrotizing substance may be released into the area and epidermal necrosis results. The erythema and lesions are bilaterally symmetrical and tend to be more pronounced on the extremities, including the palms of the hand and soles of the feet.

The disorder is often preceded by signs and symptoms of a viral infection—that is, fever, headache, rhinitis, conjunctivitis. Individual lesions remain about two weeks and the duration of the syndrome is three to eight weeks. Since there are no diagnostic laboratory tests, the disorder is diagnosed by clinical appearance and the presence of bull's-eye lesions. Potential causative agents include antibiotics, inoculations, and sunlight. After removal of the causative agent, the client is treated symptomatically, since the disorder is self-limiting and heals without scars.

Stevens-Johnson syndrome

Stevens-Johnson syndrome is a severe, life-threatening form of erythema multiforme characterized by bull's-eye lesions involving not only the skin but the mucous membranes as well. The mucous membrane vesicles and bullae quickly develop into erosions. The membrane lesions are very painful, particularly when they occur in the mouth. Joint pains, high fever, malaise, rapid, weak pulse, and a purulent ocular exudate may accompany the lesions. Although the course of the disorder is similar to that of erythema multiforme, it is more likely to result in death. This disorder may persist for ten weeks. Steroid therapy has been of some benefit, but treatment is primarily symptomatic.

Toxic epidermal necrolysis (TEN syndrome, scalded skin syndrome, Lyell's syndrome)

Toxic epidermal necrolysis is a life-threatening form of toxic erythema. The erythema is tender, bilateral, and symmetrical. Even gentle touching may cause the epidermis to slide off, leaving a reddened, painful dermal covering that resembles a scalding burn. Confusion, fever, conjunctivitis, and bull's-eye lesions (erythema multiforme) may accompany the disorder.

Hypersensitivity to a drug—for example, antibiotics—is believed to be the primary causative factor. It affects women more frequently than men. Toxic epidermal necrolysis in children is especially serious, since their skin lesions often become infected with staphylococcus.

After removing the causative agent, the client is treated with steroids and other supportive measures. Reverse isolation is instituted in order to minimize infection. Although oral nutrition is encouraged, the client has difficulty swallowing, so IV fluids and even hyperalimentation may be necessary. The fluid and electrolyte balance must be carefully monitored, since large quantities of fluids and electrolytes are lost through the denuded skin. Sound nursing management is essential to the survival of the patient.

Staphylococcal scalded skin syndrome (SSSS) This syndrome is toxic epidermal necrolysis that has become infected with staphylococcus. It is usually found in infants and children and is treated with an appropriate antibiotic.

Exfoliative dermatitis (exfoliative erythroderma)

Exfoliative dermatitis is a potentially life-threatening inflammation of the skin characterized by generalized erythema, scaling, and alopecia (loss of hair). The client may have severe pruritus and the skin may peel off in flakes or large sheets. The client loses fluid and proteins through the skin, which is prone to infection. Potential causative agents include antibiotics (penicillin, sulfonamides, tetracyclines), barbiturates, heavy metals (gold, mercury), iodides, nitrates, oral hypoglycemic agents, phenothiazines, and vaccines (measles, pertussis, and diphtheria and tetanus toxoids). Treatment includes topically applied antiinflammatory agents and systemic corticosteroids. Fluid and electrolyte balance must be carefully monitored and corrected, and reverse isolation and other measures can be instituted to prevent infection. Although the etiology is unknown, it is more likely to occur in clients with benign skin disorders like psoriasis. Deaths have been attributed to this reaction.

Photosensitivity Reactions

Photosensitivity reactions include a wide range of exaggerated skin responses after exposure to sunlight and other sources of ultraviolet rays. Although more than 99% of the ultraviolet rays of the sun are blocked by the earth's atmosphere, primarily by the ozone layer, the rays that reach the earth can be dangerous to certain individuals. The skin pigment *melanin* absorbs the ultraviolet rays, thereby preventing them from reaching the cutaneous vasculature and dermal cells. Exposure to ultraviolet rays stimulates two protective skin responses: melanin is produced in larger quantities (tanning) and the skin grows faster and thicker (peeling). Dark-skinned individuals have more protective melanin and therefore have fewer photosensitivity reactions.

Ultraviolet radiation can be divided into short, middle, and long waves (see Figure 8-1), each of which causes a characteristic skin reaction. Although *short rays* seldom reach earth, they are capable of causing severe injury and even cell death. Short rays have been produced artificially for their germicidal effects. Even brief exposure may cause severe conjunctivitis and sunburn in unprotected skin areas. *Middle rays* penetrate the epidermis, enter the dermis, and cause dilatation of cutaneous blood vessels (sunburn reactions) several hours later. The less melanin present, the greater the penetration and therefore the more severe the reaction. These rays are thought to be responsible for skin wrinkling. *Long rays* are believed to be nondestructive in

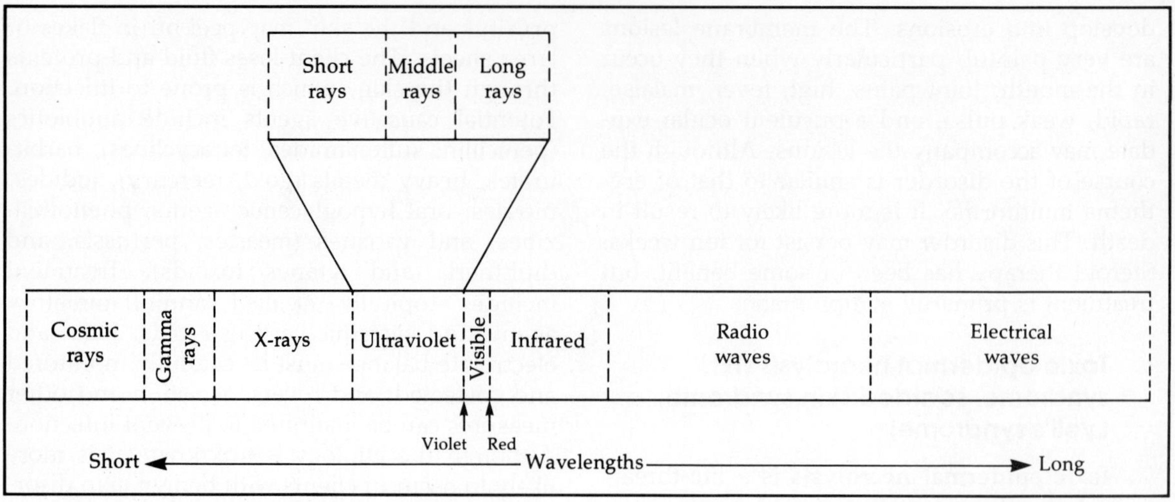

FIGURE 8-1 The electromagnetic spectrum. Ultraviolet radiation can cause a variety of severe dermatomucosal reactions, particularly when the client is taking a photosensitizing drug. Short rays are germicidal and can cause erythema. Middle rays cause sunburn, bullae, and urticarial reactions. Long rays cause little or no damage.

most individuals, but may cause severe reactions in photosensitive clients, in certain disease processes, such as lupus erythematosus and herpes simplex, and in the presence of certain topical or systemic drugs or chemicals or both.

Certain drugs can precipitate erythema, urticaria, bullae, dermatitis, scaling, and skin thickening (see Table 8-5). Most clients taking these drugs have photosensitivity reactions following relatively brief sun exposure, and these reactions probably indicate drug toxicity. The less frequent reactions that occur with drugs not normally associated with photosensitivity reactions probably indicate drug hypersensitivity. The toxic reaction is probably due to the ability of the drug to alter skin resistance to the rays. The hypersensitive reaction may result from the ability of the drug to form a hapten in certain individuals when they are exposed to sunlight, thus causing an antibody-antigen reaction. The severity of these reactions depends on the length of exposure to ultraviolet rays, the initial degree of the client's photosensitivity, and the drug dosage.

GASTROINTESTINAL REACTIONS

Most, if not all, of the drugs that are absorbed from the gastrointestinal tract have the capacity to cause adverse reactions in that system. Nausea, vomiting, and diarrhea are observed most frequently. They are the least life-threatening reactions to drugs, and are often termed *minor drug-induced reactions.* Discontinuation of the offending drug is all that is required to treat the reaction in most cases. When the minor GI reaction is dose related, decreasing the dose or administering the drug with milk may be sufficient. The elderly and clients with preexisting GI disturbances are more likely to experience these minor GI reactions to drugs.

Inflammatory Reactions

Such *inflammatory reactions* as drug-induced esophagitis, stomatitis, colitis, and proctitis have occurred, particularly from the following irritants: alkaloids such as digitoxin, alkylating agents, diuretics, certain cathartics, and potassium supplements. If the medication is continued, the client may develop GI ulcerations and, ultimately, necrosis, so the identification of the causative agent is essential.

Malabsorption syndromes

The oral administration of certain drugs can result in *malabsorption syndromes.* Mineral oil is a primary offender. It prevents the absorption of the lipid-soluble vitamins, and its prolonged use can

TABLE 8-5 Commonly Used Drugs That May Cause Photosensitivity Reactions

Category	Drug
Antibiotics	Tetracylines Sulfonamides Griseofulvin Demeclocycline
Anticonvulsants	Phenytoin
Antimetabolites	5-Fluorouracil Mustards 9-Mercaptopurine
Barbiturates	Phenobarbital
Heavy metals	Gold salts Silver salts
Oral contraceptives	
Oral hypoglycemic agents	Chlorpropamide Tolbutamide
Quinine and its derivatives	Quinidine
Salicylates	Aspirin
Tranquilizers	Phenothiazines
Thiazide diuretics	Chlorothiazide Hydrochlorothiazide

cause dangerously low levels of vitamins A, D, E, and K, particularly in pregnant women.

Parenterally administered drugs that are widely distributed in the body tissues may affect the GI tract as well. The digitalis preparations can stimulate the vomiting center and result in vomiting without nausea. Antimetabolites such as 5-fluorouracil and methotrexate may slow the growth of protective epithelial cells in the GI tract and therefore induce severe vomiting, diarrhea, and anorexia, ultimately leading to malnutrition.

Major Drug-Induced GI Disturbances

Major drug-induced GI disturbances, including ulcerations, necrosis, and hemorrhage, tend to occur in clients with preexisting conditions like inactive ulcers, cancer, hernias (particularly diaphragmatic hernias), colitis, diverticulitis, and hemorrhoids. Individuals with a history of any of these conditions should have their stools tested for occult blood and mucous. Slowly progressing anemia, epigastric pain, abdominal cramps, abdominal tenderness, nausea, and frequent bowel movements are all symptoms of potential underlying major GI drug reactions. These symptoms may occur within the first two days of drug therapy but usually appear in 5 to 14 days.

The primary causes of bleeding are anticoagulants, phenacetin, phenylbutazone (Butazolidin), and ethacrynic acid (Edecrin). Edecrin has caused perforations of gastric ulcers that resulted in life-threatening peritonitis. Corticosteroids, reserpine, salicylates, and potassium supplements have also been associated with GI ulcerations. Susceptible clients receiving these medications should be monitored carefully—that is, a complete blood count taken, stools checked for occult blood—during the first two weeks of drug therapy, and should be monitored at weekly intervals if drug therapy continues.

KIDNEY REACTIONS (NEPHROTOXICITY)

The vast majority of drugs and their metabolites are excreted by the kidneys, along with many other toxic metabolic wastes. Therefore, damage to the kidney from drug action can have far-reaching consequences related to fluid and electrolyte imbalances. When the kidney is damaged, the urinary excretion of drugs is hampered, leading to signs and symptoms of drug toxicity.

When sufficient dosages of some drugs are administered over a prolonged period of time, kidney damage can result in all clients (see Table 8-6). The antifungal agent amphotericin B (Fungizone) elevates the BUN and serum creatinine levels in nearly all clients. The sulfonamides and a few other drugs may cause kidney dysfunction by precipitating in the urinary tract. However, some kidney reactions occur only if the client has a preexisting kidney disorder, or if the client develops an immune or hypersensitivity reaction to the drug.

TABLE 8-6 Commonly Used Drugs That May Cause or Aggravate Kidney Dysfunction (Nephrotoxins)

Category	Drug
Antiinfective agents	Aminoglycosides Amphotericin B Ampicillin Sulfonamides Colistin (Coly-Mycin) Nitrofurantoin (Furadantin) Para-aminosalicylic acid (PAS) Tetracyclines Penicillin Vancomycin (Vancocin)
Diuretics	Acetazolamide (Diamox) Chlorothiazide (Diuril) Furosemide (Lasix) Hydrochlorothiazide (HydroDiuril) Meralluride (Mercuhydrin)
Nonnarctoic analgesics	Phenacetin Acetaminophen (Tylenol)
Heavy metals	Mercury Copper Gold Iron Lead
Electrolytes	Potassium Calcium
Antiinflammatory agents	Salicylates Phenylbutazone (Butazolidin)

Indirect drug-induced kidney reactions may also occur. The primary or secondary effect of a drug may cause an inadequate amount of blood to be delivered through the renal arteries. Vasopressors are the primary offenders. Renal dysfunction may also be precipitated by normally nonnephrotoxic drugs that cause an acid-base imbalance—for example, anesthetics and corticosteroids.

Clients with preexisting kidney disorders should not be given nephrotoxins unless absolutely necessary; when they are prescribed, renal function must be closely monitored. The physician should be notified if the BUN or serum creatinine levels are excessive, if electrolyte imbalance occurs, or if oliguria or proteinuria develops. With the support of renal or peritoneal dialysis, nephrotoxicity reactions are seldom fatal, but they may cause permanent kidney dysfunction. If the offending drug is identified and removed, most kidney dysfunctions are reversible and leave little or no permanent impairment. The treatment is symptomatic and is aimed at maintaining renal artery blood flow, fluid and electrolyte balance, and acid-base balance.

There are four major types of drug-induced kidney reactions: (1) noninflammatory malfunction, called *nephrotic syndrome*; (2) the development of kidney gravel or stones due to precipitation, called *nephrolithiasis*; (3) inflammatory changes, called *nephritis reactions*; and (4) actual *renal shutdown* due to tubular necrosis.

Nephrotic Syndrome (Nephrosis, Ideopathic Nephrotic Syndrome)

Nephrotic syndrome is a noninflammatory malfunction of the nephrons characterized by marked proteinuria, hypoalbuminemia, and edema. Although the exact course of the reaction is unknown, it is believed that nephrotic syndrome results from an immune or a drug hypersensitivity reaction that causes glomerular dysfunction but that may also cause proximal tubular dysfunction (upper nephron nephrosis).

Clinical picture In the course of nephrosis, the permeability of the glomerulus is increased, thereby causing the loss of large quantities of serum proteins, particularly the relatively small albumin molecules, into the filtrate. Since albumin has a primary role in maintaining the blood colloidal osmotic pressure, the loss of plasma albumin and other plasma protein lowers the colloidal osmotic pressure to the point at which large amounts of fluid are permitted to leak into the interstitial and other body spaces. Dependent edema, ascites, plural effusion, pericardial effusion, and fluid in the joint spaces may develop. Blood volume decreases and stimulates the release of aldosterone from the adrenal glands, causing the body to retain sodium and water; this adds to the edematous state. Even when the offending agent is identified and removed, the client may not have a spontaneous remission. The prognosis is generally poor, because the nephrotic syndrome may cause the nephrons to degenerate.

Treatment The treatment includes diuretics to reduce the edema, a high-protein, low-sodium diet, and infusions of albumin. When the urinary output is adequate, corticosteroid therapy may be effective.

Nursing management Appropriate measures are required to prevent injury and infection. Monitoring intake and output, checking body weight and vital signs, and measuring the abdominal girth are all important in determining the progress of the client.

Nephrolithiasis

Nephrolithiasis is related to the high concentration of a drug in the kidney and the solubility characteristics of the drug. Some drugs tend to precipitate in the acidic pH of the urine, causing deposits in the pelvis, ureters, or bladder. The sulfonamides are the primary offenders, although other drugs have been implicated. The level of nonprotein nitrogen in the client's blood may be elevated and renal colic may occur.

Clinical picture The client may have cloudy urine or small, sandlike particles, called gravel, in the urine. He or she may complain of low back pain or pressure. Frequency of urination may develop and hematuria may occur.

Treatment If the causative agent cannot be discontinued, the pH of the urine can be altered as necessary by the ingestion of acid or alkaline foods or medications. Cystoscopy or surgery may be necessary to remove stones.

Nursing management In some cases, precipitation may be prevented by having the client drink at least 8 ounces of water hourly while awake, thereby diluting the drug's urinary concentration. Each voiding of urine should be strained, intake and output recorded, and fluids encouraged. Measures to relieve pain and anxiety should be instituted.

Nephritis Reactions

Nephritis reactions are drug-induced inflammatory responses of the kidney occurring in the glomeruli or the tubules. Local inflammation may occasionally occur, but it is usually due to a preexisting kidney disorder. The onset of symptoms tends to be abrupt, and the symptoms vary according to the severity and location of the inflammation. The prolonged use of certain drugs that are excreted in the urine may cause irritation with resulting inflammation in the glomeruli or tubules. The salicylates, phenacetin, and acetaminophen, as well as other drugs, have been implicated.

Inflammatory responses of the glomerulus tend to be associated with immune reactions in the body, with symptoms occurring within two weeks of the initiation of drug therapy. When the inflammation occurs in the tubules or interstitium, the reaction is due to an idiosyncratic hypersensitivity. Sulfonamides and antibiotics have been implicated in hypersensitivity nephritis reactions.

Clinical picture The initial symptoms consist of dependent edema, along with the presence of albumin, blood, and casts in the urine. When the inflammation is due to a hypersensitivity or immune response, there may be an elevation in the eosinophil cell count. As the inflammation progresses, the urine may become progressively darker, moderate elevation in the BUN and serum creatinine levels may occur, and serum electrolytes may be altered.

Treatment The inflammation tends to subside spontaneously after the offending agent is withdrawn, but, in some cases, the symptoms may progress until renal shutdown occurs. Supportive therapy is given; corticosteroids may be effective.

Nursing management Recording intake and output and weighing the client daily will assist in determining the amount of fluid retention. Bed rest and other measures to promote rest and sleep are important. Dialysis may be required if renal shutdown occurs.

Acute Tubular Necrosis (Acute Renal Shutdown)

Acute tubular necrosis involves massive destruction of the tubules. The epithelial cells of the tubules may be destroyed by the nephrotoxic action of poisons, such as carbon tetrachloride and the heavy metals, or by hypersensitivity reactions. Drugs such as vasopressors have the potential for causing a severe decrease in renal artery blood flow and may cause inadequate oxygenation and nutrition to the kidney, resulting in massive destruction of the tubular epithelium. Even drugs that induce hemolytic anemia can produce tubular destruction by causing the lysed cells to release a vasconstricting substance.

The destroyed epithelial cells separate from the tubular basement membrane and obstruct the nephron, terminating nephron function. If the basement membrane is left intact and if the offending substance can be identified and removed from the body by dialysis, the epithelial cells may regenerate within three weeks.

Clinical picture The symptoms are associated with the inability of the kidney to excrete water, electrolytes, acids, and nonprotein nitrogenous compounds, such as uric acid and creatinine. Hyperkalemia is one of the most difficult problems. The quantity of urine decreases daily, and there are large quantities of albumin, casts, and hemoglobin present. The client may complain of lower back pain.

Treatment The treatment is directed at the resulting edema, elevated potassium levels, azotemia, and metabolic acidosis. Dialysis is the principal method of treatment.

Nursing management Decreasing anxiety, preventing infection, and instituting comfort measures are the main elements of nursing management. Checking weight daily, recording intake and output, and measuring abdominal girth will help the health team determine the quantity of fluid retention.

NEUROLOGIC REACTIONS

Most drugs have the ability to cause adverse neurologic reactions, either directly or indirectly. Certain drug toxicities can directly affect the central nervous system or peripheral nerves. Hypersensitivity reactions can occur with any drug that can penetrate the blood-brain barrier or damage the peripheral nerves. Hypersensitivity and toxicity reactions may cause CNS or peripheral nerve dysfunction and damage by indirect mechanisms as well. Cerebral blood flow can be altered by many drugs, including vasopressors, leading to cerebral ischemia and resulting infarcts. Several other drugs can cause hypertensive crisis and cerebral hemorrhage. Even drugs that alter the fluids, electrolytes, and nutrients supplying the brain have the potential for initiating a neurologic reaction, particularly drugs that alter blood glucose levels. Drugs that severely affect the liver may produce secondary neurologic reactions by creating excessive levels of toxic metabolic end products, such as ammonia, that the liver is unable to process.

Encephalopathy (Cerebral or Cerebellar Syndrome)

The general term **encephalopathy** indicates a dysfunction of the brain. Drug-induced brain dysfunctions may manifest as convulsions, an alteration in the level of consciousness, possibly progressing to coma, behavioral changes, and other abnormal neurologic signs. Although relatively rare, encephalopathy is potentially life threatening. The incidence of drug-induced brain dysfunction is higher in clients with preexisting disorders, such as CVA. Convulsions may result from excessive dosages or from hypersensitivity to several groups of drugs, including the CNS depressants and antibiotics, which are able to penetrate the blood-brain barrier.

The treatment is symptomatic. Anticonvulsants are helpful in some cases. Maintaining an adequate airway is essential during convulsions. Oral suctioning and oxygen therapy are helpful. Seizure precautions should be instituted with all clients who develop drug-induced encephalopathy.

Behavioral Changes

Behavioral changes may include "crying jags," depression, psychoses, agitation, hallucinations, disorientation, and confusion. Once the drug has been eliminated by the body, the symptoms subside spontaneously in most cases. Since clients may not be aware of the changes, they should be protected from emotional and physical traumas.

Extrapyramidal Syndromes

Symptoms of *extrapyramidal syndromes* include tremors or twitching, other involuntary movements, disturbances in posture, and changes in muscle tone that involve the basal ganglia. Several types of motor, sensory, or motor-sensory responses may occur from drug toxicity or hypersensitivity. The most commonly observed alterations are the following:

1. Akinesia—Loss of movement
2. Dyskinesia—Difficulty in making purposeful movements
3. Dystonia—Impairment of muscle tone, usually manifested as twitching
4. Palsy—Inability to move or control one's muscles; may be unilateral, bilateral, or focal
5. Parkinson-type (Parkinsonism)—Fine, slowly spreading tremors, initially seen in the hands, possibly with muscular weakness or rigidity
6. Paresthesia—Abnormal sensations, such as numbness and tingling, usually located in extremities

The primary causative agents are phenothiazines, MAO inhibitors, and some antibiotics. Although drug toxicity may be the cause, extrapyramidal syndromes tend to occur in individuals with hypersensitivity to the drug. Although withdrawal of the offending agent is all that is necessary in most cases, irreversible damage can occur. The anticholinergic agents and antihistamines have been useful in treating phenothiazine-induced extrapyramidal reactions.

Disturbances of Sensory Organs

The *eye* and *ear* may be adversely affected by drug toxicity or hypersensitivity. In many cases, the client may have an adverse reaction to normal dosage levels because of a preexisting condition.

The eyes

Delicate membranes are sensitive to minor variations in pH; consequently, several topical agents may cause a severe inflammatory reaction when administered in the eye. All ocular drugs are adjusted for ocular tolerance and are labeled "for ophthalmic use only." Severe ocular burns that result in blindness can occur when inappropriate and outdated drugs that have become concentrated or altered in some fashion are used. Many cholinergic drugs have a miotic effect and should not be given when there is preexisting acute-angle closure glaucoma. Some cholinergic blockers, such as atropine, may cause a mydriatic effect and should not be given in narrow-angle glaucoma, since they may increase the intraocular pressure. Blurred vision, diplopia, myopia, and retinopathy may occur from a toxic or hypersensitivity reaction to digitalis preparations, certain antibiotics, belladonna, heavy metals, and chlorpromazine. Adverse eye reactions should be treated immediately to prevent permanent damage.

The ear

Nerve, vestibular, or cochlear damage to the ear may result in loss of hearing, dizziness, motion sickness-type reactions, or perception of abnormal sounds (ringing in the ears). If the offending agent is not immediately withdrawn, permanent hearing loss may occur from toxic levels of certain antibiotics—for example, the aminoglycosides, such as garamycin and kanamycin. Hypersensitivity or toxic reactions to salicylates, ethacrynic acid, furosemide, phenylbutazone, and quinidine have been reported. Since permanent damage may occur, clients who are receiving these causative agents should immediately report any alterations in hearing or balance.

CARDIOVASCULAR REACTIONS

Almost all drugs are distributed throughout the body by the cardiovascular system and have the capacity to cause, either directly or indirectly, one or more cardiovascular reactions. Drug toxicity, hypersensitivity reactions, or drug-induced imbalances in body fluids and electrolytes are frequently involved. Clients who have preexisting cardiac diseases, such as coronary artery disease or valvular disease, respiratory disorders, such as emphysema or asthma, kidney diseases, such as nephritis or nephrosis, metabolic disorders, such as hyperthyroidism or diabetes, or vascular disorders, such as hypertension, are more prone to experience adverse cardiovascular responses. Complete cardiovascular collapse may occur as a result of drug-induced immune or hypersensitivity reactions.[1] The heart's electrical conduction system may be adversely affected, resulting in life-threatening arrhythmias, or the myocardial tissue may become ischemic or inflamed following the use of certain drugs. Hypertensive crisis and even damage to the blood vessels can be drug induced.

Potential causative agents include drugs that directly affect the heart or blood vessels; they may cause toxic reactions in these tissues. Vasodilators, vasoconstrictors, bronchodilators, antiarrhythmic agents, and cardiac glycosides cause toxic effects in the cardiovascular system of any client if the dosage is great enough or if the drug is given over a long enough period of time. Clients who have hypersensitivity reactions to these drugs may develop adverse responses with small dosages. Drugs that may cause indirect adverse effects on the cardiovascular system include any agents with the potential for disturbing the fluid and electrolyte balance. Although hypersensitivity reactions may occur, the adverse cardiovascular response is often a toxic effect.

Cardiac Arrhythmias

Cardiac arrhythmias are disturbances in the rate or rhythm of the heart. A sinus rate of less than 60 beats/minute (*sinus bradycardia*) or greater than 100 beats/minute (*sinus tachycardia*) may be caused by many drugs. Since stimulation of the vagus nerve may slow the heart rate, irritation to the vagal center of the brain or a drug-induced stimulation of the vagus induces sinus bradycardia. Although the client is often asymptomatic, syncope and cardiac arrest can occur. The primary causative agents are some general anesthetics and sympathomimetic drugs. Withdrawal of the causative agent is usually adequate, but it may be necessary to block vagal effects in severe cases by administering atropine intravenously.

Sinus tachycardia may result from inhibition of the vagus nerve, stimulation of the cardiac accelerator nerve, or both. The onset is gradual and removal of the offending drug will usually result in a gradual decrease in rate. Occasionally it may be necessary to use sedatives, such as barbiturates, to make the heart rate return to normal. Certain sympathomimetics, such as epinephrine, may cause sinus tachycardia.

Premature contractions (extrasystoles) are beats initiated in cardiac tissue other than the SA node, causing a disturbance in the cardiac rhythm (coupled beats, skipped beats). Supraventricular arrhythmias may arise from the atria (premature atrial contractions—PAC) or from the AV node (premature nodal contractions), but are seldom life threatening. Frequent premature ventricular contractions (PVC or VPC) and ventricular tachycardia tend to create a marked decrease in cardiac output with resulting symptoms. The ventricular arrhythmias may even lead to ventricular fibrillation, which is incompatible with life. These rhythm disturbances may be caused by cardiotonic drugs, such as digitalis, and by drugs that induce electrolyte imbalances, such as diuretics and calcium supplements. Drug-induced supraventricular arrhythmias tend to disappear without treatment once the offending source is

[1]See *anaphylaxis* and *serum sickness response* for further explanation.

removed. However, ventricular arrhythmias frequently require aggressive therapy, such as an antiarrhthymic drug like lidocaine. If the client develops ventricular fibrillation, defibrillation and other lifesaving measures must be instituted immediately. Sometimes even antiarrhythmic drugs induce arrhythmias, particularly when the client is hypersensitive to the drug.

The toxic effects of some drugs may cause the normal wave of electrical stimulation to be slowed or even blocked. Heart block may be caused by drugs that induce an electrolyte imbalance, such as potassium supplements, and by digitalis toxicity. Although the client may be initially asymptomatic, the heart block can progress to a life-threatening form and cause cardiac standstill and syncope. Lifesaving measures, including external cardiac massage and administration of epinephrine, must be instituted immediately.

Cardiac monitoring is necessary to determine the presence of a potentially hazardous arrhythmia. If a drug-induced arrhythmia is suspected, an electrocardiogram should be taken and the client should be transferred to a cardiac care unit.

Myocardial Reactions

Myocardial reactions are usually manifested as myocarditis or myocardial fibrosis, which may lead to necrosis. Although rarely observed, these responses are usually fatal. Drug-induced cardiac tissue responses tend to occur after severe systemic toxic or hypersensitivity reactions. Poisoning with heavy metals, such as lead and antimony, can lead to myocarditis and myocardial fibrosis. Drug toxicity from certain antineoplastic agents and arsenic preparations has been implicated in myocardial reactions. Even the prolonged use of ethyl alcohol has been associated with myocardial fibrosis, undiscovered until an autopsy is performed.

The antineoplastic agent doxorubicin (Adriamycin) can be highly toxic to the myocardium. Acute heart failure that is resistant to standard treatment can occur, particularly in clients who have received 550 mg/m^2 or more. If radiotherapy to the mediastinal area is given concurrently with doxorubicin, only 400 mg/m^2 can precipitate cardiac failure. Early detection is essential but difficult, since few symptoms appear. However, a persistent decrease in the QRS complex voltage is considered an indication for discontinuing the drug.

Vascular Reactions

Hypertensive or *hypotensive vascular states* can result from excessive dosages of drugs with vasoconstricting or vasodilating actions. The toxic effect may be caused by the primary action or a secondary action of the drug. Hypertensive crisis, cerebrovascular hemorrhages, and myocardial infarctions may occur as a result of drug-induced excessive vasoconstriction. Excessive vasodilatations, resulting in severe hypotension, have been induced by the nitrites and the adrenergic blockers. Inflammation and even necrosis of the blood vessels has occurred with the intravenous administration of levarterenol (Levophed). Hypersensitivity to antibiotics, such as penicillins and sulfonamides, has been implicated in necrotic responses.

Toxic vascular reactions usually respond well to the withdrawal of the drug and even to a decrease in dosage. When the drug has a prolonged half-life, it may be necessary to administer the appropriate antidote.[2] Hypersensitivity reactions tend to disappear spontaneously after the offending drug is withdrawn.

BLOOD DYSCRASIAS

Disorders of the hematopoietic system have been attributed to idiosyncratic drug reactions, as well as directly to the action of drugs. Although relatively rare, drug-induced blood dyscrasias are often serious and sometimes fatal if not detected early. Exposure to the causative agent, which may be a drug, a chemical, or radiation, could have occurred several weeks prior to the onset of symptoms or may still be occurring.

Knowledge of the production, life span, and ultimate destruction of blood cells is essential to an understanding of blood dyscrasias. Only a brief summary is presented here. The bone marrow produces *precursor cells* called *erythroblasts* (erythrocytes or RBCs), *granulocytes* (the WBCs

[2]See individual drug monograph for appropriate antidotes.

called lymphocytes), and *thrombocytes* (platelets). Immature granulocytes are called *myeloblasts*. While the normal life span of mature erythrocytes is 120 days, the mature platelets last only 8 to 10 days and the mature granulocytes a mere 1 to 7 days. The reticuloendothelial tissue, particularly that located in the liver and spleen, breaks down and destroys the old and defective blood cells. The hormone *erythropoietin*, which is produced by the kidney in response to an alteration in tissue oxygenation, stimulates the production of erythrocytes. Several enzymes, including glucose-6-phosphate dehydrogenase (G-6-PD), are necessary for the production and proper development of erythrocytes and other blood cells.

Aplastic anemia and hemolytic anemia were the terms first used to describe drug-induced anemia. *Aplastic anemia* is the condition in which the bone marrow fails to produce or release cells to the blood. *Hemolytic anemia* is the condition in which erythrocytes are destroyed rapidly. As the fields of hematology and pharmacotherapeutics developed, more precise terms were devised to describe the disorders; they include *agranulocytosis* (*leukopenia*), *thrombocytopenia*, *megaloblastic anemia*, and *pancytopenia*. Table 8-7 summarizes important facts abut the various blood dyscrasias.

A blood dyscrasia can be caused by a drug-induced abnormality in the production, life span, or destruction of blood cells. Substances that destroy bone marrow are called *myelotoxins*; they may prevent the development of all or most of the precursor cells. High doses of immunosuppressive drugs will cause thrombocytopenia in all clients.

The mechanisms by which drugs cause selective blood dyscrasias are not fully understood. Some individuals have deficiencies of certain enzymes or other blood-forming substances and are unable to produce normal blood cells when they take certain medications. Some protein-bound substances, particularly potent chemical oxidants like arsenic compounds, may destroy or weaken the cell membranes of erythrocytes, resulting in hemolytic anemia. Even weak chemical oxidants like aspirin can cause hemolytic anemia in clients with a G-6-PD deficiency. In most cases, clients recover completely after the causative agents are removed and supportive therapy is instituted. Early detection and treatment can dramatically decrease the mortality and morbidity rates.

The names of the various blood dyscrasias are descriptive of the blood cell(s) involved. The greatest offenders in drug-induced blood dyscrasias are the antineoplastic drugs, antibiotics, heavy metals, such as gold salts, and the phenothiazine tranquilizers. Any client receiving drug therapy with one of these agents should have weekly complete blood counts.

Agranulocytosis

Agranulocytosis is an acute reduction in the number of circulating granulocytes, particularly the neutrophils. This blood dyscrasia is relatively common, with symptoms appearing suddenly. The client is acutely ill and complains of severe oral pain from infected oral and pharyngeal ulcers. The disorder is sometimes called *leukopenia* because neutrophils comprise 50 to 70% of the circulating leukocytes. Since neutrophils are the body's first defense against infection, the client develops severe infections, and, if the disorder is left untreated, the mortality rate is about 50%.

Different drugs interfere in different ways with the production of granulocytes. There may be an alteration in purine or pyrimidine metabolism, or in DNA synthesis, caused by either excessive drug doses or idiosyncratic reactions. Individuals who are sensitive to aminopyrine derivatives, such as the antipyretic dipyrone (PYRD), may develop agranulocytosis when exposed to a chemically related drug.

Clinical picture Initially, the client complains of a sore throat, fatigue, headache, and weakness. Later, ulcerative, oropharyngeal, vaginal, and rectal lesions with little or no exudate develop. If the condition is not detected and treated immediately, the client will experience severe oral pain and dysphagia. High fever and severe chills develop as the infection progresses.

Treatment The causative agent is discontinued, a throat culture obtained, and an appropriate antibiotic administered. Narcotic analgesics, anesthetic lozenges, and other local measures are instituted to control pain. The client is kept on bed rest until the fever subsides, and a high-caloric diet with vitamin supplements is given.

Nursing management Frequent and meticulous oral hygiene with the use of soothing saline gargles or irrigations helps to control the pain and to keep the lesions clean. The fever can be relieved with tepid baths and a high fluid intake. Restricted visiting and reverse isolation may be required to contain certain infections.

Thrombocytopenia

Thrombocytopenia is an acute reduction in the number of circulating platelets. The mechanism is poorly understood, but it is believed that this blood disorder is caused by the direct action of certain drugs. Quantities of blood escape into the tissues and mucous membranes, causing ecchymosis and purpura, the characteristic symptoms of this disorder. Since drug-induced thrombocytopenia is related to depression of platelet production and not to the abnormal destruction of platelets by the spleen, splenectomy is not recommended. The prognosis is good and recovery is rapid after the causative agent is removed.

Clinical picture Initially, there is spontaneous bleeding in the skin, mucous membranes, and internal organs, causing *petechiae* (small lesions) and *ecchymosis* (larger lesions). Small lacerations, intramuscular injections, and venipunctures cause prolonged oozing. Gastrointestinal bleeding and melena may occur. Later, the client will develop epistaxis, hematuria, and intestinal, cerebral, and other internal hemorrhages. The client will have increased capillary fragility, producing ecchymosis when the blood pressure is taken.

Treatment Recovery is usually spontaneous after the causative agent is discontinued. Measures to control bleeding include platelet transfusions and administration of corticosteroids. Stool softeners are used to prevent constipation and subsequent straining that can precipitate an intercranial hermorrhage. Bed rest with padded side rails should be instituted in order to prevent unnecessary trauma.

Pancytopenia

Pancytopenia is a pronounced reduction of all the cellular elements in the blood—that is, erythrocytes, white blood cells, and platelets. The onset of this disorder is often sudden and the client is acutely ill. It is characterized by a waxy pallor of the skin and mucous membranes. The client may have the beginning signs and symptoms of agranulocytosis before bleeding occurs, since the life span of granulocytes is slightly shorter than that of thrombocytes. Although poorly understood, this disorder may be due to an idiosyncratic reaction to a drug, or it may be the direct result of the drug effect in the body. The condition is often fatal.

Clinical picture The initial symptoms include pallor, weakness, fatigue, dyspnea, petechiae, and bleeding from mucous membranes, particularly when the client brushes the teeth. Severe bacterial infections and hemorrhage may occur if the disorder is not detected and the causative agent discontinued.

Treatment Bone marrow reproduction will usually resume after the causative agent is withdrawn. Blood transfusions may be required until the bone marrow becomes active. Corticosteroids and androgens may be used to stimulate bone marrow production. A high-caloric, high-vitamin, *low*-iron diet is beneficial, since high iron levels may result from frequent transfusions. When infection is present, antibiotics will be prescribed.

Nursing management The acute illness occurs abruptly and may cause concern to the client; therefore, emotional support is essential. Visitors should be restricted and reverse isolation should be instituted when necessary. Healing, rest, and sleep should be promoted. Since the client is anorexic, the diet should contain small portions that are attractively prepared.

Aplastic Anemia (Bone Marrow Failure)

Aplastic anemia is a broad term used to indicate suppression or destruction of the bone marrow. The marrow fails to produce or release erythrocytes (anemia), granulocytes (agranulocytosis), thrombocytes (thrombocytopenia), or all three blood constituents (pancytopenia). This disorder is commonly caused by exposure to the poisons in insecticides and weed killers or by prolonged exposure to certain antineoplastic agents, antibiotics, and other drugs. Aplastic anemia is occasionally the result of an idiosyn-

TABLE 8-7 Blood Dyscrasias

Dyscrasia	Blood Findings	Bone Marrow	Other Tests
Agranulocytosis	Leukopenia—less than 3000/mm^3 Neutrophils—0–2% RBCs—normal or slightly decreased	Few or no myelocytes Normal erythropoiesis Normal thrombopoiesis	
Thrombocytopenia	Platelets below 10,000/mm^3; prolonged bleeding time Poor clot retraction Normal coagulation time	Variable	Positive tourniquet test
Pancytopenia (normocytic and normochromic)	RBCs—below 1,000,000/mm^3 WBCs—below 2000/mm^3 Platelets—below 100,000/mm^3	Fatty deterioration Decreased number of all precursor cells	
Aplastic anemia (secondary and normocytic)	Depression of one or more blood cell counts	Decreased number of precursor cells Increased number of lymphocytes	
Megaloblastic anemia (macrocytic)	Macrocytic RBCs with irregularities in size and shape Platelets—normal count or slightly decreased WBCs—depressed count	Hyperplasia Numerous megaloblasts Enlarged neutrophil precursor cells	Elevated serum bilirubin Elevated LDH levels
Hemolytic anemia (normocytic and normochromic)	RBCs—below 1,000,000/mm^3 Elevated reticulocyte count WBCs—normal or slightly elevated count Platelets—normal or slightly decreased count	Hyperplasia	Increased RBC fragility Elevated serum bilirubin Elevated urobilinogen in urine Positive direct Coombs test if immune to reaction Heinz bodies if related to G-6-PD deficiency

Causative Agents	Clinical Findings	Remarks
Antineoplastic agents Heavy metals Phenothiazines Sulfonamides and other antibiotics Radiation Chemicals—benzene	Oral and pharyngeal ulcerations High fever, chills, and rapid pulse	Fatal in one week if untreated
High dosages of immunosuppressive agents Phenothiazines Quinine compounds Salicylates Sulfonamides and other antibiotics Radiation	Generalized petechiae and ecchymosis Prolonged oozing at needle sites Purpura Hematuria Internal bleeding	Spontaneous recovery when causative agent removed
Antineoplastic agents Barbiturates Heavy metals Phenothiazines Sulfonamides, streptomycin, and other antibiotics Radiation	Pallor, weakness Dyspnea Petechiae Hemorrhages	Poor prognosis Severe infections develop
Antihistamines Antineoplastic agents Dilantin and other anticonvulsants Heavy metals Phenothiazines Salicylates Sulfonamides and other antibiotics Excessive radiation Chemicals—insecticides, weed killers, hair dyes	Fatigue Dyspnea Bleeding from oral and nasal mucosa	Infection and/or bleeding likely Poor prognosis
Antineoplastic agents Barbiturates Cephalothin and other antibiotics Dilantin and other anticonvulsants Phenothiazines	Pallor, weakness Angina or chest pain	Good prognosis if causative agent identified and withdrawn Clients with megaloblastic anemia are sometimes inadvertently treated for pernicious anemia instead
Antineoplastic agents Heavy metals Nitrites Phenacetin, salicylates and other analgesics Quinine compounds Sulfonamides and other antibiotics Thiazide diuretics Vitamin K preparations Snake and spider venoms Mushrooms and other vegetable poisons	Weakness Dyspnea Jaundice Splenomegaly Hepatomegaly Hemolytic crisis	Death often due to renal failure

cratic reaction to drugs, but the mechanism is poorly understood. The onset of the disorder is often insidious and difficult to recognize without the blood and bone marrow laboratory results. The client's prognosis is poor unless the disorder is diagnosed early.

Clinical picture The signs and symptoms will vary according to the degree to which each cell type is depressed. Since the platelet count is usually depressed, small ecchymotic areas from minor trauma may be the first indication. As the neutrophils become depressed, the client becomes susceptible to infection. The client will complain of fatigue, dyspnea, and bleeding from the nose and mouth as the anemia progresses. If the disorder is untreated, death usually results from hemorrhage or severe infection.

Treatment The treatment depends on the blood findings and clinical picture. Transfusions of the appropriate cell type are administered until the bone marrow begins to function appropriately. A thorough health history may be required to identify the causative agent. If the bone marrow does not resume functioning after the causative agent is removed, corticosteroids and androgens may be used to stimulate the marrow. Supportive therapy is given as needed.

Nursing management The nursing actions are initially focused on identifying the causative agent and on supportive therapy. Restriction of visitors and reverse isolation may be required to protect the client from infection. Initially, the vital signs are monitored frequently in order to detect and treat internal bleeding immediately. The nursing management is adjusted according to the client's response to therapy.

Megaloblastic Anemia

Megaloblastic anemia is characterized by the presence of megaloblasts in the bone marrow and the presence of irregularly shaped macrocytic erythrocytes in the blood. Although it is usually associated with vitamin B_{12}, vitamin C, and folic acid deficiencies, the disorder may be caused by drugs; however, the mechanism is unknown. The onset is insidious and it may be difficult to identify the causative factor. The clients are often treated for pernicious anemia, since the symptoms are similar. Prognosis is good if the causative agent is identified.

Clinical picture Since the life span of the macrocytic erythrocytes is shortened, the serum bilirubin and urinary urobilinogen are elevated and the client may be jaundiced. Serum iron levels are also elevated. The client will be pale complain of fatigue and weakness. Middle-aged and elderly clients may develop agina and chest pains from the added strain to the heart.

Treatment The causative agent may be difficult to identify, so an extensive health history may be required. The client is treated symptomatically. Oxygen therapy will usually relieve the chest pain. A low-iron diet is prescribed until the serum iron level reaches normal range. If the bone marrow does not resume normal activity after the causative agent is discontinued, corticosteroids and androgens may be prescribed.

Nursing management An extensive health history, including identification of potential offenders in the home, garden, and workplace, must be obtained. The nursing and medical data is correlated in an attempt to identify the causative agent. Measures to promote rest and sleep, along with other supportive therapy, will be required.

Hemolytic Anemia

The blood dyscrasias described above were related to drug-induced disorders of blood cell production, whereas **hemolytic anemia** is an abnormal increase in destruction of circulating erythrocytes. Although the mechanisms are not clearly understood, there seem to be three basic means by which drugs induce hemolytic anemia:

1. Some protein-bound drugs, particularly the potent cellular oxidants, can destroy or weaken the cell membranes to which they are attached, thus causing the erythrocytes to be destroyed prematurely. Toxic dosages of arsenic compounds, certain antineoplastic agents, and other chemical oxidants, or prolonged exposure to them, can cause hemolytic anemia in all clients.

2. Individuals with certain erythrocyte enzyme disorders, such as a deficiency of G-6-PD, are susceptible to hemolytic anemia when relatively weak chemical oxidants like phenacetin, aspirin, and menadione (vitamin K_3) are taken for two or three days.

3. A few individuals are thought to have an immune reaction, in which the drug binds to the erythrocyte and forms a modified protein that the body interprets as an antigen. Antibodies are formed, an antigen-antibody reaction occurs, and the affected erythrocytes agglutinate and are ultimately broken down by the spleen, liver, and other structures.

There are a few substances that will affect blood production and cause blood destruction at the same time. When lead compounds are accidentally ingested, hemolysis and inhibition of heme synthesis occur. Individuals exposed to these compounds develop an anemia that resists standard therapy because their bodies cannot compensate for the hemolysis with increased bone marrow activity. Benzene and trinitrotoluene are two other substances known to cause a simultaneous bone marrow depression and hemolysis.

Clinical picture The rapidity with which the symptoms appear will vary according to the mechanism of hemolysis and to the drug dosage. When there is prolonged exposure to small dosages, the client's hemolytic disorder will be insidious. The initial symptoms include fatigue, weakness, exertional dyspnea, and jaundice. If untreated, hemolytic crisis occurs, often precipitated by infection. Clients with a G-6-PD deficiency or an immune reaction to a drug may develop hemolytic crisis after two or three days of exposure to the offending drug. The crisis is characterized by fever, chills, abdominal pain, backache, malaise, darkened urine (urobilinogen), hematuria, splenomegaly, and hepatomegaly. Ischemia of the renal tubules may lead to renal failure. Clients with a G-6-PD deficiency will have oxidized hemoglobin in their erythrocytes, called Heinz bodies. A positive direct Coombs, negative indirect Coombs, elevated WBC count, and depressed platelets are often found in clients with immune reactions. All clients with hemolytic anemia will have elevated serum bilirubins and urinary urobilinogen due to massive breakdown of erythrocytes.

Treatment A spontaneous recovery will sometimes occur after the chemical oxidant is removed. Blood transfusions, IV fluids, and other supportive measures may be all that is necessary if the disorder is detected early. Once hemolytic crisis occurs, more drastic measures, such as splenectomy and corticosteroid therapy, may be necessary. Narcotics may be required to control the pain.

Nursing management Continuous assessment is necessary if the client is in hemolytic crisis. Maintenance of the client's fluid and electrolyte balance can be vital to survival. Oxygen therapy and measures to promote rest and sleep will lessen the work load on the heart and lungs.

LIVER REACTIONS (HEPATOTOXICITY)

Many drugs are found in high concentrations in liver tissue and some of them can injure the liver or alter the normal liver functions. Altered liver function can be the cause of encephalopathy, endocrine dysfunctions, and dysfunctions of the blood-forming organs.

Drug-induced liver reactions can be caused by drugs that are toxic to all clients when given in high doses, or by a drug hypersensitivity or allergy. When the causative agents are withdrawn, the liver damage is usually reversible, but normalization of liver function may take weeks. If the agent is not identified, the damage may be irreversible and cause a chronic liver disorder or death. Symptoms of liver damage from drug hypersensitivity and allergic reactions may appear during drug therapy, or they may be delayed until months after the drug is discontinued. The hepatotoxic state will generally reappear if the drug is reintroduced at a later date.

There are two basic forms of hepatotoxicity. In **hepatocellular toxicity** the liver cells are damaged or destroyed and the mortality rate is high. Intrahepatic cholestasis—inflammation of the bile ducts—is more common and, although clients are often alarmed by the extensive jaundice, they usually recover spontaneously as soon as the causative agent is removed. The presence of jaundice does not necessarily mean that the causative agent has affected the liver directly. Clients with hemolytic anemia may develop jaundice secondary to the rapid destruction of erythrocytes.

Hepatocellular Toxicity (Necrotic Jaundice, Toxic Hepatitis)

This life-threatening liver reaction resembles viral hepatitis. The offending agent may be inhaled, ingested, injected, or absorbed through the skin. Some drugs actually destroy liver cells, whereas others damage them in such a way as to interfere with the organ's normal ability to metabolize toxic metabolic products. High doses of certain toxic drugs may cause the reaction in anyone, and a drug hypersensitivity may cause it in susceptible individuals. Alcoholism, malnutrition, and pregnancy increase susceptibility to hepatocellular toxicity.

Causative agents The general anesthetic halothane and other halogenated hydrocarbons are the primary offenders, although other drugs, including acetaminophen (Tylenol), salicylates, para-aminosalicylic acid (PAS), chlordiazepoxide (Librium), MAO inhibitors, phenytoin (Dilantin), and the tetracyclines have been implicated.

Clinical picture The initial signs and symptoms usually appear five days to three weeks after drug therapy is instituted and include abrupt nausea, vomiting, anorexia, fever, malaise, and a rash. Liver size may remain within normal limits or the organ may atrophy. If the condition is untreated, neurological signs and symptoms soon develop, similar to those of meningitis (severe headache, tremors, muscular rigidity, and abnormal reflexes). Convulsions, delirium, and stupor will occur. As the serum ammonia levels increase, the client's breath becomes foul smelling (fector hepaticus). When the client's ability to synthesize prothrombin is impaired, bleeding from oral and nasal mucosa, hematuria, and melena may occur. The client usually dies in hepatic coma.

Treatment If the causative agent is identified and withdrawn early, recovery is usually spontaneous, but the longer the delay, the greater the chance of irreversible liver damage, possibly leading to chronic liver disease or death. The treatment is symptomatic, aimed at preventing or correcting metabolic acidosis, dehydration, hypoglycemia, and anemia. Corticosteroids are effective in some clients; antibiotics may be used with caution to prevent infection; and transfusions may be necessary to treat severe anemia.

Nursing Management Continuous assessment is necessary as the client begins to develop neurologic and bleeding symptoms. Maintenance of the fluid and electrolyte balance and promotion of the elimination of ammonia may be vital to the client's survival. Measures to prevent injury to the skin, such as padded side rails and gentle handling, are important as the bleeding tendency increases. A low-protein diet is necessary as the serum ammonia level rises. Measures to promote rest and sleep are essential; the client should be protected from infection from visitors.

Intrahepatic Cholestasis (Cholestatic Jaundice, Hepatocanalicular Jaundice)

The disorder resembles obstructive jaundice. The offending agents cause inflammation of and injury to the tiny bile ducts (bile canaliculus) leading to the terminal bile duct. Occasionally, the portal vessels are inflamed as well. The inflammation hampers the flow of bile and other hepatic excretions and secretions, thus producing the symptoms.

Causative agents The phenothiazines are the primary offenders, but other drugs have been implicated, including chloramphenicol (Chloromycetin), chlordiazepoxide (Librium), meprobamate (Equanil), para-aminosalicylic acid (PAS), and propoxyphene (Darvon).

Clinical picture Progressive jaundice and accompanying pruritus are the most obvious signs. As the serum bilirubin level increases, eosinophilia and fever usually occur. Hepatomegaly is often present and the liver function tests indicate biliary obstruction.

Treatment Once the offending agent has been identified and removed, the reaction usually disappears spontaneously. Symptomatic treatment is given until the liver function tests return to normal. Sedatives and hypnotics are avoided, since they are metabolized by the liver.

Nursing management Meticulous skin care is necessary to remove the irritating skin products and to relieve pruritus. Avoidance of fatigue is essential and bed rest is recommended.

FLUID AND ELECTROLYTE IMBALANCES

A complete explanation of fluid and electrolyte imbalance is beyond the scope of this book. However, hypokalemia and hyperkalemia are frequent complications of drug therapy and are therefore presented here. Hypomagnesemia has been included because this disorder is occurring with greater frequency as hyperalimentation therapy increases.

Alterations in extracellular fluid volume can be caused by excessive IV fluid, diuretics, nephrotoxins, and other drugs. **Hypervolemia** is characterized by an elevated central venous pressure, rales in the lungs, and edema, whereas **hypovolemia** is characterized by a low central venous pressure, a urinary output of less than 30 ml per hour, dry skin and mucous membranes, and a depressed fontanel in infants. Treatment of hypervolemia includes diuretics and a limited fluid intake; treatment of hypovolemia consists of hydration with IV fluids.

Alterations in serum sodium levels can be caused by numerous drugs, including diuretics, antibiotics, corticosteroids, and drugs containing sodium, such as sodium bicarbonate. An excess of sodium, **hypernatremia**, is seldom drug induced; **hyponatremia**, on the other hand, can result from excessive intake of diuretics and is characterized by fatigue, muscle cramps, apprehension, confusion, and diarrhea. When hyponatremia is caused by a diuretic, discontinuation of the drug will usually result in spontaneous recovery. Infusions of 5% dextrose in sodium chloride may be required.

Hypokalemia

Hypokalemia, a deficit in serum potassium, is characterized by muscular weakness and electrocardiographic (EKG) changes. Mild symptoms may appear when the serum potassium level falls below 3.5 mEq/l, but a level below 3 mEq/l is life threatening. Individuals particularly susceptible to hypokalemia include infants, the elderly, the debilitated, and clients who are experiencing prolonged vomiting or diarrhea or are on continuous gastric suctioning.

Causative agents The corticosteroids and several of the diuretics can cause hypokalemia, particularly in susceptible clients. The thiazide diuretics, ethacrynic acid (Edecrin), and furosemide (Lasix) can cause severe hypokalemia, particularly if the client is also taking a digitalis glycoside. Even mildly depressed serum potassium levels can precipitate digitalis toxicity and result in cardiac arrhythmias. The antifungal agent, amphotericin B, enhances the urinary excretion of potassium.

Clinical picture Initially, the client may complain of muscle weakness and orthostatic hypotension. The blood pressure drops gradually and the peripheral pulse pressures decrease as the serum potassium levels decline. On EKG, the T wave flattens or becomes inverted.

Atrial or ventricular arrhythmias occur in digitalized clients, sometimes leading to congestive heart failure. As the gastrointestinal muscles become involved, anorexia, vomiting, abdominal distention, and even paralytic ileus may result.

Treatment Whenever possible, the diuretic or other causative agent is discontinued until the serum potassium level returns to normal. An infusion of 1000 ml of 5% D/W (dextrose in water) with 20 to 40 mEq of potassium chloride is administered, but since rapid infusions of potassium can induce hyperkalemia, the IV rate should not exceed 10 mEq of potassium per hour. In mild cases, orally administered potassium supplements may be adequate.

Nursing management Careful monitoring of the client's response to the potassium infusion is essential. The IV should be administered into a large vein, since potassium is irritating to the vessels and can cause pain.

The urinary output should be monitored and if the output drops below 30 ml per hour, the IV should be slowed to a KVO (keep vein open) rate and the physician notified immediately. All digitalized clients who are taking diuretics should also take a potassium supplement. All clients who are taking potential causative agents should be given a list of potassium-rich foods, such as bananas, citrus juices, dates, and dried apricots, and instructed to eat at least one serving each day in order to prevent hypokalemia.

Hyperkalemia

Hyperkalemia, an excess of serum potassium, is characterized by oliguria and cardiac disturbances. Mild symptoms may appear when the serum potassium level exceeds 5 mEq/l; levels above 7 mEq/l are life threatening. Clients who are particularly susceptible to hyperkalemia include the elderly and clients with impaired renal functioning.

Causative agents Intravenus fluids containing potassium and potassium supplements and drugs containing potassium, such as potassium penicillin, are the primary offenders. Drugs containing potassium may precipitate hyperkalemia in clients with impaired renal function. The potassium-sparing diuretics may also cause hyperkalemia.

Clinical picture Initially, the client may complain of abdominal cramps and diarrhea. As the serum potassium level increases, the client becomes irritable, develops weakness and flaccid paralysis, and may start vomiting. The urinary output decreases progressively until the client becomes anuric. But the most dangerous symptoms are the cardiac disturbances. The T waves become very peaked and the QRS complex widens. Sinus bradycardia develops and the client will have a cardiac arrest if not treated immediately. Only rapid diagnosis and treatment can prevent death.

Treatment All potassium-containing drugs and foods are avoided. Potassium loss is promoted through either dialysis or ion exchange resins (Kayexalate), administered orally or rectally.

Nursing management Regular monitoring of vital signs, urinary output, and serum potassium levels of clients taking potassium drugs is essential to the early detection of hyperkalemia. Once the condition is detected, the client should be moved to an intensive care unit or a dialysis unit with EKG monitoring equipment. Since Kayexalate exchanges sodium ions for potassium ions, hypernatremia may occur, precipitating congestive heart failure or renal failure in susceptible clients. Digitalized clients must be observed frequently during treatment since a too-rapid loss of potassium may precipitate digitalis toxicity.

Hypomagnesemia

Hypomagnesemia—a deficiency of serum magnesium—can precipitate digitalis toxicity. This deficiency is characterized by hyperactive reflexes, twitching, and other signs of neuromuscular irritability. The normal serum magnesium level is between 1.5 and 2.5 mEq/l. Prolonged therapy with thiazide, ethacrynic acid (Edecrin), furosemide (Lasix), metolazone (Zaroxolyn), and other diuretics can cause this condition. Digitalized clients who have had major surgery or prolonged IV therapy, alcoholics, and clients with long-standing diarrhea are prone to having low serum magnesium levels and are therefore susceptible to digitalis toxicity. Infusions of 5% D/W with magnesium sulfate added may be all that is required to treat the client. Intramuscular administration of magnesium sulfate is usually avoided, since it is irritating to muscle tissue and can cause severe pain.

DRUG INTERACTIONS

Some untoward drug reactions are caused by interactions with other drugs, nutrients, or chemicals. The interfering drug or substance, called the **interactant**, causes the action or effect of the *primary drug* to be increased, decreased, or nullified. The primary drug-interactant combination can also result in an effect entirely different from the one intended. The interactant may interfere with the absorption, distribution, metabolism, excretion, or action of the primary drug.

One of the difficulties of identifying the dynamics of a drug interaction is that most drugs cause more than one effect. The classic example is aspirin, which is an analgesic, an antipyretic, and antiinflammatory, and an anticoagulant. When two drugs have the *same or similar effect* in the range of drug effects, they are potential interactants. Clients taking aspirin or other salicylic acid preparations should not take any warfarin derivatives (anticoagulants) or indomethacin (an antiinflammatory) concurrently, since adverse reactions will occur. Knowledge of the complete range of a drug's effects is important in preventing untoward drug reactions.

Clients often require *more than one drug* to treat their illnesses. More than 4% of clients who take five drugs concomitantly develop adverse reactions, and, of the clients who take six to ten drugs, more than 7% develop adverse reactions.[3] Geriatric clients with more than one illness and clients with chronic illnesses, such as cardiac disease or chronic obstructive lung disease, frequently require multiple drug therapies and should be observed for potential drug interactions.

Occasionally, two drugs that are known to interact may be administered together intentionally. For example, probenecid interferes with the renal excretion of penicillin, and, though now used infrequently, the administration of the two drugs together causes the duration of effect of the penicillin to be prolonged. Some drug preparations contain a drug intended to decrease the side effects of the primary drug. For example, Tedral contains 130 mg theophylline, 24 mg ephedrine, and 8 mg phenobarbital. The bronchodilators (theophylline and ephedrine) are effective in treating bronchial asthma but cause unpleasant side effects, such as insomnia, nervousness, and irritability. The small amount of barbiturate, a central nervous system depressant, is added to decrease these undesired side effects.

Responses to Drug Interactions

Although an interactant may not cause an untoward drug reaction when given alone, it can cause changes in client responses to the primary drugs. The interactant may (1) increase the action of the primary drug; (2) antagonize the client's response; (3) prevent any response; or (4) result in a totally different response.

A number of terms are used to indicate the overall effect that occurs in drug interactions. The following terms are used to indicate a combined effect that is *greater than* the expected client response when a drug is given alone.

1. *Addition*—The combined effect of two similar drugs that act on the same receptors is called **addition**. Since the drugs are often close congeners,[4] their combined effect is related to the *summation* of effects produced by each when given alone. It is called *addition* because the effect of the interactant adds to the effect of the primary drug.

2. *Potentiation*—When the effects of the primary drug are increased by an interactant, the action is called **potentiation**. The two drugs are not similar and only the primary drug produces measurable effects. The interactant usually potentiates the effect of the primary drug by (a) increasing the amount absorbed; (b) increasing drug concentration at receptor sites; (c) retarding the drug's metabolism into inactive metabolites; or (d) retarding excretion of the drug.

3. *Synergism*—When the combined effect is *greater than* the effect of each drug given alone, it is called **synergism**. The interactant acts by a different mechanism and intensifies the effect of the primary drug.

The following terms are used to indicate a combined effect that is *less than* the expected client response when a drug is given alone.

1. *Antagonism*—The combined effect of two drugs acting against each other and resulting in a *decrease* in the expected client response to either drug is called *antagonism*. The effects of an agonist are decreased by the effects of an antagonist; the resulting effect may be reversible or irreversible. Occasionally, a small quantity of an antagonist is given with an agonist intentionally, either to decrease the side effects or to prolong the duration of the agonist.

2. *Inhibition*—*Any decrease* in the effect of a drug due to an interactant is referred to as **inhibition**. The interactant may have been given prior to, or concurrently with, the administration of the primary drug. The interactant usually inhibits the effects of the primary drug by (a) decreasing the amount absorbed; (b) decreasing drug concentration at receptor sites; (c) increasing the drug's metabolism into inactive metabolites; or (d) increasing excretion of the drug.

[3]Eric Martin, *Hazards of Medication*, 2d ed. (Philadelphia: Lippincott, 1978), p. 356.

[4]Congeners are chemical compounds that are structurally similar to each other and act on the same receptors.

Many client responses to a drug interaction are the result of an alteration in the pharmacokinetics of the primary drug. Knowledge of the sites of potential drug interactions is important in understanding the nature of client responses.

Sites of Drug Interaction

The interactant may alter the absorption, distribution, metabolism, excretion, or action of the primary drug, thereby causing the primary action or therapeutic effect to be increased, decreased, nullified, or rendered completely different.

Absorption

There are several ways in which an interactant can alter the absorption of a primary drug. The interactant may alter any of the following:

1. The motility of the gastrointestinal tract
2. The nature of gastrointestinal contents
3. The characteristics of the primary drug
4. The nature of the primary drug's contact with the absorbing surface

Cathartics, dietary roughage in excessive quantities, and other substances that cause diarrhea will decrease the length of time that orally administered drugs are in contact with the intestinal tract; a high fat content in the diet, on the other hand, will delay gastric emptying. The pH of the gastric contents may be too alkaline or too acidic for optimum absorption of the primary drug. Clients who take sodium bicarbonate preparations, such as Alka-Seltzer, for indigestion, or ascorbic acid (vitamin C), should avoid taking these substances within an hour of taking their medications. Nonabsorbable complexes will form if tetracycline is taken with milk or dairy products. Since mineral oil prevents the absorption of lipid-soluble vitamins, clients should avoid taking mineral oil on a daily basis and take a substitute instead, such as dioctyl sodium sulfosuccinate (Colace).

Distribution

There are four basic ways in which interactants can alter the distribution of a primary drug. The interactant may change any of the following:

1. The rate or amount of circulation to the absorption site, the reception site, or a storage site
2. The chemical characteristics of the circulating primary drug, particularly the degree of ionization
3. The amount of protein binding of the primary drug and thus the amount of free drug available at the site of action
4. The amount of primary drug binding at storage sites and thus the amount available at the action site

Although the intravenous administration of sodium bicarbonate and other pH-altering medications is sometimes required to adjust an abnormal pH, it should be remembered that significant changes in the serum pH can alter the protein binding of a primary drug. Phenobarbital, which is 40 to 60% protein bound, should be administered cautiously to clients who have been taking phenytoin (Dilantin), which is 70 to 95% protein bound, since phenobarbital toxicity may result. Furthermore, clients on long-term phenytoin therapy should be cautioned against taking large quantities of salicylates (aspirin), since they may displace phenytoin from its plasma-binding sites. If the client is already taking a protein-bound drug, the use of another protein-bound drug should be avoided whenever possible; one of the two drugs may be displaced, resulting in toxicity.

Metabolism

An interactant can interfere with primary drug metabolism by promoting either enzyme induction or enzyme inhibition. For example, the regular use of barbiturates will increase microsomal enzyme activity. The primary drug, which is metabolized by the affected microsomal system, will be metabolized at a faster rate than expected and the microsomal enzyme system's ability to metabolize many drugs will be decreased. The primary drug's duration of action and effect are prolonged by MAO inhibitors and other enzyme inhibitors.

Excretion

There are three basic ways in which interactants can alter the excretion of a primary drug.

The interactant may alter the rate or amount of any of the following:

1. Glomerular filtration or renal tubular secretion
2. Tubular reabsorption
3. Biliary excretion

Diuretics are known to cause dramatic alterations in the excretion of sodium, potassium, chloride, and other electrolytes. The excessive loss of certain electrolytes can increase the possibility of primary drug toxicity. Furosemide (Lasix) increases the possibility of drug toxicity from digitalis glycosides and from lithium by promoting the loss of potassium and other electrolytes. But furosemide and other diuretics decrease the excretion of uric acid, thus antagonizing the action of sulfinpyrazone (Anturane), a drug used to treat gout. Although sulfinpyrazone competitively inhibits the tubular reabsorption of uric acid, it also interferes with the excretion of several weak organic acids, including penicillin and the cephalosporins. As a general rule, any drug that alters kidney function will be an interactant with drugs excreted via the kidneys.

Interactants that cause alterations in biliary excretion include some of the antibiotics and antineoplastic agents. Some of the primary drugs that are excreted with the bile into the intestines are ultimately eliminated in the feces. If this method of elimination is blocked, the excess is eliminated via other routes, particularly the urine, so blockage of biliary excretion seldom causes a serious problem.

Drug action

There are five basic mechanisms by which interactants can alter the primary drug at its action site(s). The interactant may do any of the following:

1. Change the affinity of the primary drug for its receptor sites
2. Alter the activity of primary drug inactivating enzymes
3. Compete with the primary drug for receptor sites
4. Change the primary drug's transport mechanism(s)
5. Change the transport mechanisms of an endogenous substance that will alter the primary drug action

Certain drugs have a greater affinity for receptor sites than many other drugs or substances. For example, atropine has a greater affinity than acetylcholine for cholinergic postganglionic receptor sites in smooth muscle, cardiac muscle, and exocrine glands; consequently, it blocks the action of acetylcholine. MAO inhibitors will block the enzyme that destroys amines, including ephedrine and amphetamines, thereby increasing the concentration of sympathomimetic amines at receptor sites. Hypertension and related symptoms can result if the MAO inhibitor is not discontinued at least two weeks prior to the administration of amines. Health team members should have complete knowledge of the range of action and effects of all drugs they administer in order to prevent drug interactions.

TYPES OF INTERACTANTS

An interactant may be a drug, nutrient, or another chemical. More information is available about drug interactants, but other chemicals can be interactants as well, including food additives, drug preservatives, household products, insecticides, herbicides, and other occupational chemicals. These chemicals can gain access to the body by ingestion or injection, through abrasions and lacerations, or through intact skin and mucous membranes.

Many drug interactants are believed to interfere with the pharmacokinetics of the primary drug. It is believed that interactant nutrients and other chemical substances also alter the absorption, distribution, metabolism, and elimination of the primary drug, although some chemicals may interact directly with the primary drug.

Drugs

There are a few commonly used drugs that are known to interact with and alter the absorption of other drugs; they include antacids, antidiarrheal agents, iron preparations, cathartics, sodium bicarbonate, and a few antibiotics, such as neomycin. As a general rule, these medications should not be administered within one hour of other medications. Commonly used interactants that tend to displace drugs from protein-binding sites include oral hypoglycemic agents, barbiturates, salicylates, phenytoin (Dilantin), tranquilizers, and sulfonamides. A drug interaction chart should be consulted before administering another drug to a client who takes any of the above drugs on a regular basis.

Some commonly used drugs that are known to be enzyme inducers include alcohol, barbiturates, several tranquilizers, sedatives, and hypnotics. Enzyme inhibitors include oral anticoagulants, MAO inhibitors, anabolic-type hormones, and oral hypoglycemic agents. Monographs on the above drugs should be reviewed before therapy with another drug is instituted. Urinary excretion of many drugs may be altered by alcohol, diuretics, and sodium bicarbonate.

Alcohol

Caution should be used when administering drugs to a client who has been drinking alcohol; several interactions are known to occur. Alcohol consumption may alter the absorption of drugs. Alcohol is an excellent solvent for many drugs, and even drugs that are not soluble in alcohol can be altered by the presence of alcohol. The entire coating of some drugs may be prematurely dissolved by the alcohol, causing the drug to be released too soon. Even if he or she has not been drinking recently, the client who normally consumes alcohol on a daily basis may have enzyme induction or an alteration in the normal biochemical pathways of the primary drug.

Nutrients

Food may interact directly or indirectly with orally administered drugs. Occasionally the interaction may be beneficial and even prevent irritating side effects; however, drugs taken with food or at mealtime may be subject to altered absorption. The presence of calcium, magnesium, barium, and aluminum can prevent the absorption of tetracycline and other drugs by causing insoluble complexes to be formed. Consequently, these drugs should not be administered one hour before or after the ingestion of milk, cheese, yogurt, or any other foods containing these cations.

Many drugs are lipid-soluble and should not be administered for one hour before or after the ingestion of dietary fats and oils: the absorption of the drug can be hampered by the presence of fats. The opposite effect can also occur. Mineral oil and other oily substances can alter or even prevent the absorption of vitamins A, D, and K present in food.

Substances that alter the pH of the gastric or intestinal contents may adversely affect the absorption of a drug. If a drug has been designed to be absorbed in the normal pH of the stomach or intestines, its absorption will be hampered by the presence of food in the upper GI tract. Highly acidic foods, such as citrus juices and antacids, are common offenders, because they may adversely alter the pH of the gastric contents. Since the ionization of drugs is governed by their pH values, antacids tend to decrease the absorption of weak basic drugs. Consequently, the client will not receive the desired therapeutic effect from the drug.

Chemicals

Chemicals can be accidentally ingested, inhaled, or absorbed through the skin. When toxic levels of carbon tetrachloride, ammonia, insecticides, and other chemicals are absorbed, severe adverse reactions occur. Even small doses of these substances can cause alterations in the pharmacokinetics of primary drugs. Although a cause-and-effect relationship has not been established between many environmental chemicals and drugs, it is known that DDT, many insecticides, and herbicides do alter drug metabolism through enzyme induction or inhibition. When known, drug interactions caused by chemicals are noted in the drug monographs in the classification section of this book.

Laboratory chemicals

Chemicals are used to obtain results in many laboratory tests. The drug a client is taking may cause false results in laboratory tests because of drug/drug metabolite interaction between the therapeutic agent and the laboratory chemicals. Drugs present in the circulation will contaminate urine samples. If the client's clinical picture does not correlate with the laboratory results, the laboratory should be consulted and an alternate test procedure should be used when possible. For example, the metabolites of the antiinflammatory drug tolmetin (Tolectin) can cause a false positive result for proteinuria when acid precipitation test methods are used. However, dye-impregnated reagent strips, such as Uristix, will provide accurate results. When known, these laboratory chemical/drug interactions are noted in the drug monographs in the classification section of this book.

Preventing Interactions with Primary Drug Therapy

I. Establishing a data base
- A. Obtain history of prescribed medications.
  1. Include medications prescribed by *all* physicians.
  2. List the drug or its description, dosage, frequency, and when client takes the drug.
     For example: Valium 5 mg t.i.d.—"after breakfast, midafternoon, and before retiring."
     Waterpill 250 mg b.i.d.—"when my feet swell—usually one in the evening."
  3. Record pharmacy where prescriptions are filled; call pharmacy to verify prescription when necessary.
- B. Obtain history of over-the-counter drugs, all home remedies, and vitamins. List the amount and frequency taken for common ailments, including nausea and vomiting, diarrhea, constipation, sleeplessness, nervousness, cold symptoms, pain and aches, hay fever or other allergies, and any disorders that occur frequently.
- C. Obtain dietary history of foods typically consumed and daily eating schedule.
  1. Ask for a 24-hour recall that includes snacks and liquid breaks.
  2. List the quantity and type of commercially prepared foods.
  3. List the quantity of tea, coffee, cocoa, soda, beer, and so on, consumed daily.
- D. Obtain history of contact with other chemicals.
  1. List environmental pollutants where client lives and works; include method of travel.
  2. List occupational chemicals, specifically if known by client; list type of work and length of employment.
  3. Ask about tobacco and record type and amount smoked or chewed; include amount of smoke created by others at home and at work.
  4. Ask if client uses home-cleaning products and record type of product, frequency of use, and whether gloves are used.
  5. Ask if client uses gardening and pest-control products and record frequency of use, how product is applied, and whether a mask is used.
  6. Ask if client has a wood-burning stove or fireplace at home and record frequency of use, who carries wood, and who builds fire.

II. Assessment
- A. Determine potential interactions between the prescribed drugs.
- B. Determine potential cross-hypersensitivities from known drug allergies.
- C. Determine potential interactions between OTC drugs and prescribed drugs.
- D. Determine potential interactions between nutrients and all drugs, prescribed and OTC.
- E. Determine potential interactions between other chemicals and all drugs, prescribed and OTC.
- F. Determine the presence of microsomal enzyme stimulators and inhibitors and their potential effect on all drugs taken.

III. Management
- A. Notify physician of potential drug interactions and interfering microsomal stimulators and inhibitors; obtain alternative prescriptions when necessary.
- B. Inform client of potential OTC and home remedy interactants and discuss alternatives.
- C. Design a drug therapy schedule with the client that will maximize the therapeutic response and minimize nutrient-drug reactions.
- D. Inform client of potential chemical interactants and how to minimize exposure to the interactants.

REFERENCES

Goldstein, A. 1974. *Principles of drug action: The basis of pharmocology,* 2nd ed. New York: Wiley.

Goodman, L. S. and Gilman, A. 1980. *The pharmacologic basis of therapeutics,* 6th ed. New York: Macmillan.

Levine, R. R. 1978. *Pharmacology: Drug actions and reactions,* 2nd ed. Boston: Little, Brown.

Martin, E. W. 1978. *Hazards of medications,* 2nd ed. Philadelphia: Lippincott.

Wilson, C. O., and others, eds. 1971. *Textbook of organic, medicinal, and pharmaceutical chemistry,* 6th ed. Philadelphia: Lippincott.

PART III

CALCULATING THE DOSAGE OF DRUGS AND SOLUTION CONCENTRATIONS

SINCE THE ACTION of drugs is directly related to the amount of medication administered, the calculation of the appropriate dosage is vital. This part deals with the various arithmetic skills, rules, and methods of determining the dosage of drugs for administration. Chapter 9 is a review of the essential arithmetic skills used when determining drug dosages. The metric, apothecary, and household systems of weights and measures are discussed in Chapter 10 together with the methods for converting from one system to another. Chapter 11 is concerned with the specific rules and methods for determining the appropriate dosage for oral, parenteral, and intravenous medications as well as preparing solutions. The rules for calculating the appropriate dosage for infants and children are also discussed.

Chapters 9 through 11 can be used for self-study. A diagnostic pretest has been included for each chapter to assist the reader to identify areas of weakness. If any of the questions are answered incorrectly, the pretest answer sheet indicates which section of the chapter the reader should review before proceeding. The answers for each of the exercises has been included to assist the reader in determining miscalculations. In order to prevent mistakes, the dosage of all calculated medications should be checked by a second individual before administering the drug.

Chapter 9

Essential Arithmetic Skills

THE NURSE IS often required to use fractions, decimals, percentages, ratios, and proportions when calculating dosages of medications. This chapter reviews the arithmetic skills needed by the nurse when administering medications. Since there are two number systems—the familiar Hindu-Arabic system and Roman numerals—used in the administration of medications, a review of these systems has also been included.

The following is a pretest for this chapter. If all questions are answered correctly, there is no need to read this chapter. However, if any of the questions are answered incorrectly, the answer sheet on page 165 will direct the reader to the section of this chapter that should be reviewed before proceeding to Chapter 10.

PRETEST

Change the following Roman numerals to Hindu-Arabic numbers.

1. XII **2.** XV **3.** IV **4.** III

Change the following Hindu-Arabic numbers to Roman numerals.

5. 2 **6.** 14 **7.** 9 **8.** 8

Change the following mixed numbers to improper fractions.

9. $2\frac{2}{3}$ **10.** $4\frac{5}{6}$

Change the following improper fractions to mixed numbers.

11. $\frac{29}{6}$ **12.** $\frac{51}{5}$

Reduce the following fractions to lowest terms.

13. $\frac{5}{35}$ **14.** $\frac{4}{10}$

Solve the following.

15. $\frac{3}{10} + \frac{2}{10}$ **16.** $\frac{5}{14} + \frac{2}{7}$
17. $\frac{4}{5} - \frac{1}{3}$ **18.** $2\frac{5}{6} - 1\frac{1}{4}$
19. $\frac{1}{2} \times \frac{4}{5}$ **20.** $3 \times 1\frac{1}{3}$
21. $\frac{4}{5} \div \frac{2}{3}$ **22.** $4 \div \frac{3}{4}$

Change the following decimals to common fractions.

23. 0.52 **24.** 0.006

Solve the following.

25. 24.5 + 102.06 **26.** 0.002 + 1.04
27. 20.4 − 1.38 **28.** 0.3 − 0.006
29. 32.04 × 0.3 **30.** 0.09 × 0.1
31. 3.1 ÷ 5 **32.** 2.4 ÷ 0.03

Complete the following table by filling in the blanks with the equivalent percent, fraction, and/or decimal.

	Percent	Fraction	Decimal
33.	30%	______	______
34.	______	$\frac{18}{100}$	______
35.	______	______	0.09

Solve the following.

36. Find 20% of 10 g.
37. Find 0.5% of 25 lb.
38. What percent of 60 g is 15 g?
39. $\frac{4}{6} = \frac{x}{20}$.
40. 1 : 8 :: x : 24.

There are two sets of number symbols used in the administration of medications. These sets of symbols are called **number systems**. A working knowledge of these number systems and the *arithmetic skills* of addition, subtraction, multiplication, and division are essential for the accurate administration of medications. These skills are applied in the form of fractions, decimals, percentages, ratios, and proportions in order to calculate drug dosages.

NUMBER SYSTEMS

When human beings first began to trade, they needed symbols to designate the number of items being traded. Different sets of symbols were created by various tribes to count the items. The number system with which we are most familiar is called the **Hindu-Arabic system**. Symbols used in the Roman Empire are now called **Roman numerals**.

Since the Roman system uses letters as its symbols, the only arithmetic skills that apply are addition and subtraction. The Hindu-Arabic system allows for multiplication and division as well. In addition, people using the Hindu-Arabic system found a way to symbolize a part of a whole number, called a **fraction**.

Hindu-Arabic System

This system uses the following familiar symbols: 0, 1, 2, 3, 4, 5, 6, 7, 8, 9. The arabic numerals are so simple and versatile that they have survived all other systems. The location of each of the symbols within a series of numbers indicates the symbol's value in that location or *digit*.

Example

3284 represents

(3)	+	(2)	+	(8)	+	(4)
thousands		hundreds		tens		units

The Arabic system has the additional advantage of being able to indicate a part of a whole number. The most common way of representing this is by the use of a decimal point.

Roman System

Roman numerals are sometimes seen on sundials, clocks, and as dates—for example, on the cornerstone of buildings. Doctors sometimes write prescriptions for medications in Roman numerals.

The Arabic value of the basic Roman numeral letters are shown in Table 9-1. The symbols I, V, and X are the most frequently used in prescriptions.

TABLE 9-1 Arabic and Roman Numerals

Roman Symbol	Hindu-Arabic Symbol
I (*or* $\dot{\bar{\text{i}}}$)	1
V (*or* $\dot{\bar{\text{v}}}$)	5
X (*or* $\dot{\bar{\text{x}}}$)	10
L	50
C	100
D	500
M	1000

When a Roman symbol is repeated, the symbols are added.

Examples

$$\text{II} = \dot{\bar{\text{i}}} + \dot{\bar{\text{i}}} = 2$$

$$\text{III} = \dot{\bar{\text{i}}} + \dot{\bar{\text{i}}} + \dot{\bar{\text{i}}} = 3$$

A few rules must be followed in order to read and write Roman numerals successfully.

Number of Digits	Meaning	Example
One digit	Symbol represents itself (units)	3
First digit of a two-digit number	Represents tens	23
First digit of a three-digit number	Represents hundreds	623
First digit of a four-digit number	Represents thousands	4623

Rule 1 When the value of the *first* symbol is *larger* than the value of the second symbol, the symbols are *added.*

Examples

VI = 5 + 1 = 6
XV = 10 + 5 = 15
LX = 50 + 10 = 60

Rule 2 When the value of the *first* symbol is *smaller* than the value of the second symbol, the first symbol is *subtracted* from the second symbol.

Examples

IV = 5 − 1 = 4
IX = 10 − 1 = 9
XL = 50 − 10 = 40

Rule 3 Any one symbol can be used only *three* times in the same sequence, and its value is *added.* However, if there is a larger symbol of comparable value, it is used instead.

Examples

III = 3
XV = 15 (instead of VVV)
XXX = 30
CL = 150 (instead of LLL)

Rule 4 When there are three or more *different* symbols and the values of the symbols become progressively smaller, the symbols are *added.*

Examples

XVII = 10 + 5 + 2 = 17
CLX = 100 + 50 + 10 = 160
DCVII = 500 + 100 + 5 + 2 = 607

Rule 5 When there are three or more *different* symbols and the value of *one* of the symbols is *larger* than the value of the symbol preceding it, the value of the smaller symbol is *subtracted* from the larger symbol (Rule 2), and then the *resulting value* is *added* to the value of the other symbols.

Examples

XIV = 10 + (5 − 1) = 10 + 4 = 14
LIX = 50 + (10 − 1) = 50 + 9
= 59
CDX = (500 − 100) + 10 = 400 + 10
= 410
MCMLXXIV = 1000 + (1000 − 100) + 50 + 20 + (5 − 1)
= 1000 + 900 + 50 + 20 + 4
= 1974

EXERCISE A

Change the following Roman numerals to Hindu-Arabic numbers.

1. M	**2.** C	**3.** XIII
4. XC	**5.** CCC	**6.** LXXX
7. LXVI	**8.** MCCXXIII	**9.** XXIV
10. LIV	**11.** XCVII	**12.** MCMXXIV

EXERCISE B

Change the following Hindu-Arabic numbers to Roman numerals.

1. 10	**2.** 50	**3.** 7
4. 23	**5.** 29	**6.** 34
7. 150	**8.** 552	**9.** 68
10. 127	**11.** 19	**12.** 95
13. 415	**14.** 954	

FRACTIONS

A fraction is a method of considering a part of a whole unit. The number on the bottom (or *denominator*) represents the whole unit and the number on the top (or *numerator*) represents the number of parts being considered. For example, the fraction $\frac{3}{4}$ indicates that only 3 sections out of the whole unit 4 are being considered. The denominator is 4 and the numerator is 3.

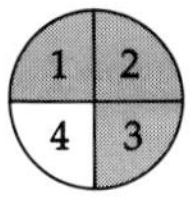

There are several kinds of fractions used when calculating drugs and solutions:

1. *Common fraction*—A fraction in which both the numerator and denominator are whole numbers. There are two types:
   a. *Proper fraction*—A fraction in which the number of sections being considered is *smaller* than the whole unit; that is, the numerator is smaller than the denominator. For example, the fraction $\frac{5}{6}$ is proper because the numerator is smaller than the denominator.

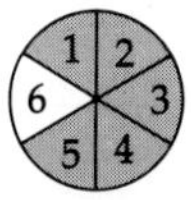

   b. *Improper fraction*—A fraction in which the number of sections being considered is *larger* than the whole unit; that is, the numerator is larger than the denominator. For example, $\frac{9}{6}$ is improper because the numerator is larger than the denominator.

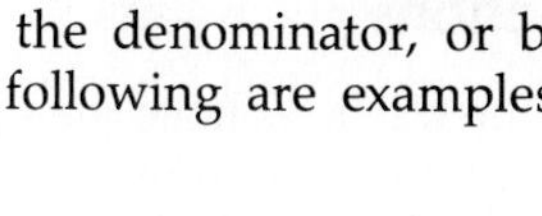

2. *Complex fraction*—A fraction in which either the number of sections being considered, the whole unit, or both are fractions; that is, the numerator, the denominator, or both are fractions. The following are examples of complex fractions:

$\dfrac{3}{\frac{2}{5}}$ Denominator is a fraction

$\dfrac{\frac{2}{3}}{8}$ Numerator is a fraction

$\dfrac{\frac{5}{6}}{\frac{1}{2}}$ Both numerator and denominator are fractions

Note the extended line that separates the numerator from the denominator.

3. *Mixed number*—A combination of a whole number and a fraction, for example, $1\frac{3}{4}$. This number can also be written as $\frac{7}{4}$ since the whole number 1 can also be divided into 4 sections.

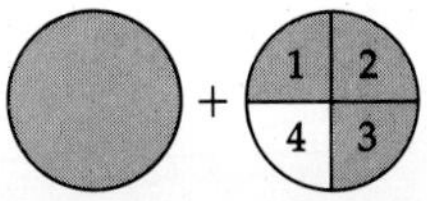

Changing Mixed Numbers to Improper Fractions

A whole number can be divided into equal sections once it is known how many sections are desired.

Example In $2 = \frac{8}{4}$ each whole unit has 4 sections. Therefore 2 whole units would have 8 sections.

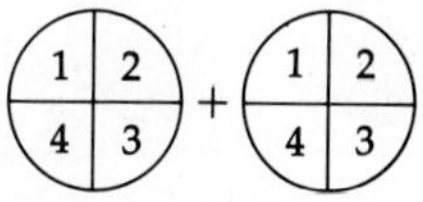

As in the above example, the number of sections in each whole unit can be added. It is, however, faster to multiply the whole number times the number of sections each unit represents.

Example The conversion $3 = \frac{6}{2}$ can therefore be done in the following ways:

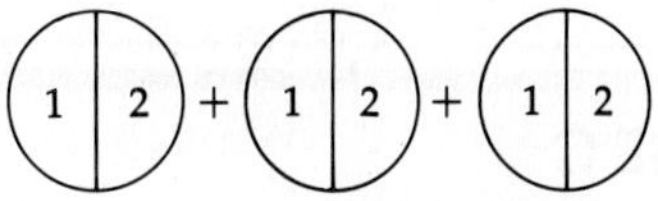

$$2 + 2 + 2 = 6 \quad \therefore \frac{6}{2}$$

or

$$2 \text{ sections} \times 3 \text{ whole units} = 6 \quad \therefore \frac{6}{2}$$

A mixed number gives the number of sections desired in its fraction.

Example $2\frac{3}{4} =$

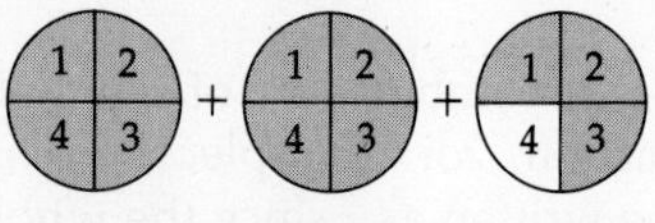

$4 + 4 + 3 = \frac{11 \text{ sections}}{4 \text{ whole units}}$

or

$(4 \text{ sections} \times 2 \text{ units}) + 3 \text{ sections} = \frac{11}{4}$

Changing Improper Fractions to Mixed Numbers

The number of whole numbers in an improper fraction can be obtained by separating out the number of whole units.

Example

$\frac{13}{5} = \frac{5}{5} + \frac{5}{5} + \frac{3}{5}$

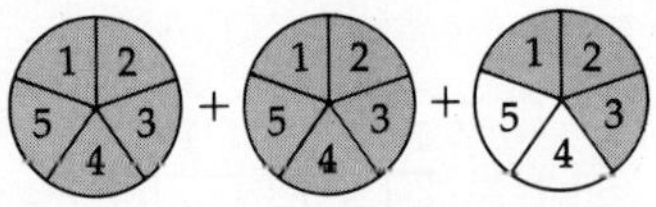

$1 + 1 + \frac{3}{5} = 2\frac{3}{5}$

or

$\frac{13}{5} = \quad 5\overline{)13}$ gives 2, 10, 3 sections left $= 2\frac{3}{5}$

EXERCISE C

Change the following mixed numbers to improper fractions.

1. $5\frac{3}{5}$
2. $2\frac{7}{16}$
3. $8\frac{4}{6}$
4. $7\frac{5}{7}$
5. $12\frac{1}{2}$

EXERCISE D

Change the following improper fractions to mixed numbers.

1. $\frac{11}{8}$
2. $\frac{7}{2}$
3. $\frac{16}{4}$
4. $\frac{11}{5}$
5. $\frac{200}{7}$

Reducing Fractions

Small fractions are often easier to work with than large fractions. Most large fractions can be reduced to a smaller one by *dividing the numerator and denominator by the same number.* Since the resulting fraction is smaller than the original fraction, this is called reducing a fraction to its **simplest** or **lowest term**.

Examples

$$\frac{30}{60} = \frac{30 \div 30}{60 \div 30} = \frac{1}{2}$$

$$\frac{2}{8} = \frac{2 \div 2}{8 \div 2} = \frac{1}{4}$$

Note When the numerator and denominator are divided by the *same number,* the value of the fraction does not change.

EXERCISE E

Reduce the following fractions to lowest terms.

1. $\frac{10}{60}$
2. $\frac{5}{50}$
3. $\frac{7}{21}$
4. $\frac{6}{54}$
5. $\frac{2}{16}$
6. $\frac{6}{15}$
7. $\frac{8}{20}$
8. $\frac{9}{30}$

Adding Fractions

Rule 1 If the fractions have the same *denominator* (whole units), the number of sections *(numerator)* can be *added* together.

Example

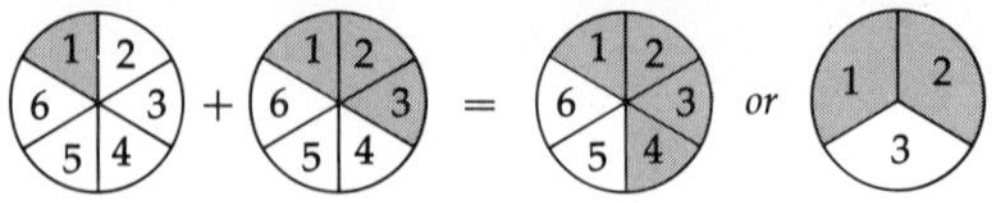

$\frac{1}{6} + \frac{3}{6} = \frac{4}{6}$ or $\frac{2}{3}$

Note When possible, the fraction should be reduced to its simplest term.

Rule 2 If the fractions have *different denominators* (whole units), the lowest number of whole units *(common denominator)* that each denominator can fit into equally is first found and then the *numerators* can be added.

Examples

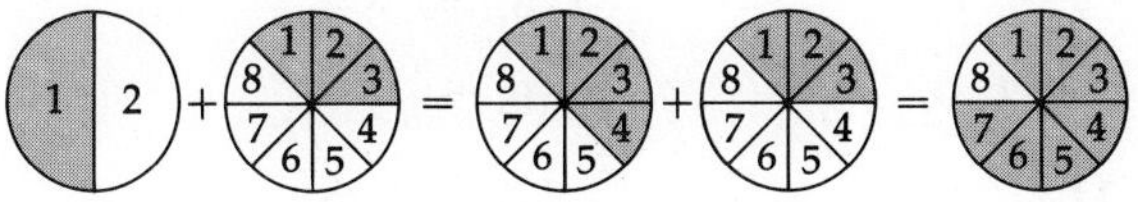

$$\frac{1}{2} + \frac{3}{8} = \frac{4}{8} + \frac{3}{8} = \frac{7}{8}$$

$$\frac{1}{5} + \frac{3}{4} = \frac{4}{20} + \frac{15}{20} = \frac{19}{20}$$

Note When it is difficult to find a *common denominator,* the denominator of the fractions can be multiplied to produce a common denominator. In the example above, the lowest common denominator of $\frac{1}{5} + \frac{3}{4}$ can be found by multiplying the 5 by the 4 to equal 20.

Rule 3 When adding mixed numbers, the fraction is separated from the whole number and then each part is added separately.

Example

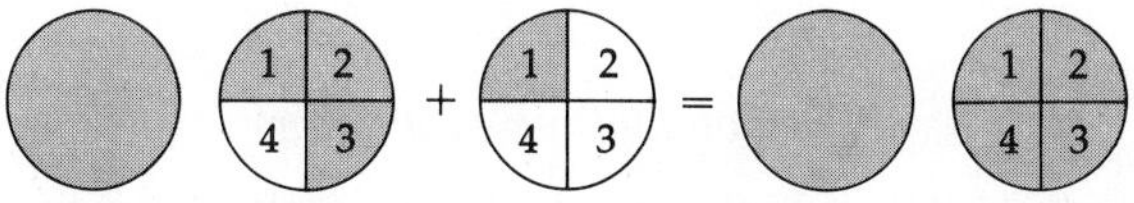

$$1\frac{3}{4} + \frac{1}{4} = 1\frac{4}{4} = 2$$

EXERCISE F

Add the following fractions.

1. $\frac{3}{6} + \frac{2}{6}$ **2.** $\frac{3}{16} + \frac{7}{16}$

3. $\frac{7}{12} + \frac{3}{12}$ **4.** $\frac{4}{14} + \frac{2}{10}$

5. $1\frac{2}{3} + \frac{3}{8}$ **6.** $5\frac{2}{5} + 1\frac{1}{3}$

Subtracting Fractions

Rule 1 If the fractions have the same whole units (or denominators), then the number of sections (numerator) can be subtracted.

Examples

$$\frac{5}{8} - \frac{2}{8} = \frac{3}{8} \qquad \frac{7}{6} - \frac{4}{6} = \frac{3}{6} \quad or \quad \frac{1}{2}$$

Note When possible, the answer should be reduced to its simplest term.

Rule 2 If the fractions have different whole units (denominators), then the lowest common denominator is found first and then the number of sections (numerators) can be subtracted.

Example

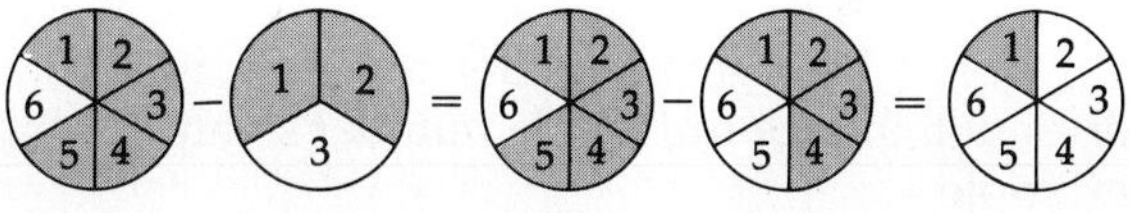

$$\frac{5}{6} - \frac{2}{3} = \frac{5}{6} - \frac{4}{6} = \frac{1}{6}$$

Rule 3 When subtracting mixed numbers, the fractions and then the whole numbers are subtracted.

Examples

$$1\frac{3}{8} - \frac{1}{8} = 1\frac{2}{8} \quad \text{or} \quad 1\frac{1}{4}$$

$$1\frac{3}{6} - \frac{5}{6} = \frac{4}{6} \quad \text{or} \quad \frac{2}{3}$$

Note A whole number can be divided into sections; in the latter case this is 6 sections.

EXERCISE G

Subtract the following fractions.

1. $\frac{5}{3} - \frac{1}{3}$ **2.** $\frac{5}{18} - \frac{3}{18}$

3. $\frac{12}{15} - \frac{3}{5}$ **4.** $\frac{9}{24} - \frac{3}{12}$

5. $\frac{2}{3} - \frac{1}{4}$ **6.** $5\frac{1}{4} - 2\frac{1}{16}$

7. $4\frac{5}{8} - 4\frac{1}{4}$

Multiplying Fractions

When multiplying two fractions, the number of sections (numerator) and then the whole units (denominator) are multiplied. The answer should be in its simplest form.

Example

$$\frac{2}{3} \times \frac{3}{4} = \frac{2 \times 3}{3 \times 4} = \frac{6}{12} \quad or \quad \frac{1}{2}$$

When multiplying a fraction with a whole number, a 1 is placed under the whole number (denominator) before proceeding as above.

Example

$$\frac{3}{4} \times 3 = \frac{3}{4} \times \frac{3}{1} = \frac{3 \times 3}{4 \times 1} = \frac{9}{4} \quad or \quad 2\frac{1}{4}$$

Note Placing a 1 under a whole number does not change the whole number's value. For example,

$$10 = \frac{10}{1} = 1\overline{)10} \;\to\; 10$$

(1 into 10 goes 10 times: 10 − 10 = 0)

When multiplying a fraction by a mixed number, the mixed number is first changed to an improper fraction and then the two resulting fractions are multiplied.

Example

$$2\frac{3}{4} \times \frac{1}{2} = \frac{11}{4} \times \frac{1}{2} = \frac{11 \times 1}{4 \times 2} = \frac{11}{8} \quad or \quad 1\frac{3}{8}$$

Shortcut The process of multiplying fractions can be shortened by first *dividing* the numbers above the line and the numbers below the line by the *same common number.* This is commonly called **cancelling out.**

Example

$$\frac{1}{\cancel{8}_{4}} \times \frac{\cancel{2}^{1}}{6} = \frac{1 \times 1}{4 \times 6} = \frac{1}{24}$$

EXERCISE H

Multiply the following fractions.

1. $\frac{1}{2} \times \frac{3}{5}$
2. $\frac{2}{15} \times \frac{5}{4}$
3. $\frac{2}{4} \times \frac{4}{10}$
4. $\frac{3}{8} \times \frac{2}{3}$
5. $\frac{5}{6} \times 2$
6. $\frac{9}{10} \times 4$
7. $2 \times \frac{3}{4}$
8. $10 \times \frac{4}{5}$
9. $3\frac{5}{7} \times \frac{1}{3}$
10. $5\frac{7}{16} \times \frac{3}{4}$
11. $\frac{1}{6} \times 2\frac{1}{2}$
12. $\frac{12}{15} \times 6\frac{1}{8}$

Dividing Fractions

When dividing two fractions, the second fraction *(divisor)* is first *inverted* and then the resulting fractions are *multiplied.* The answer should be in its simplest form.

Examples

Two fractions

$$\frac{1}{3} \div \frac{1}{8} = \frac{1}{3} \times \frac{8}{1} = \frac{1 \times 8}{3 \times 1} = \frac{8}{3} \quad \text{or} \quad 2\frac{2}{3}$$

Fraction and whole number

$$\frac{2}{5} \div 3 = \frac{2}{5} \div \frac{3}{1} = \frac{2}{5} \times \frac{1}{3} = \frac{2 \times 1}{5 \times 3} = \frac{2}{15}$$

Fraction and mixed number

$$\frac{3}{7} \div 1\frac{1}{2} = \frac{3}{7} \div \frac{3}{2} = \frac{3}{7} \times \frac{2}{3} = \frac{3 \times 2}{7 \times 3} = \frac{6}{21} \quad or \quad \frac{2}{7}$$

Shortcut: cancelling out

$$\frac{7}{9} \div \frac{1}{3} = \frac{7}{9} \times \frac{3}{1} = \frac{7 \times \cancel{3}^{1}}{\cancel{9}_{3} \times 1} = \frac{7 \times 1}{3 \times 1} = \frac{7}{3} \quad or \quad 2\frac{1}{3}$$

EXERCISE I

Divide the following fractions.

1. $\frac{1}{2} \div \frac{1}{3}$
2. $\frac{2}{4} \div \frac{7}{8}$
3. $\frac{1}{3} \div \frac{2}{3}$
4. $\frac{3}{5} \div \frac{1}{4}$
5. $1\frac{3}{4} \div \frac{1}{2}$
6. $2\frac{5}{6} \div \frac{1}{3}$
7. $\frac{4}{5} \div 10$
8. $\frac{8}{9} \div 3$
9. $4 \div \frac{1}{2}$
10. $12 \div \frac{2}{5}$
11. $\frac{4}{7} \div 3\frac{1}{4}$
12. $\frac{7}{10} \div \frac{1}{3}$

DECIMALS

The decimal system is another way of writing fractions. However, in this system the whole unit is either a 10 or a multiple of 10 (100, 1000, 10,000, and so on). The *decimal point* allows one to add, subtract, multiply, and divide these fractions with the same ease as whole numbers.

Remember that the Arabic system of whole numbers uses the location of the number to indicate its value.

Example

3225 tablets = 3 thousand + 2 hundred + 2 tens + 5 units

If a decimal point is placed after the number, it does not change the number of tablets indicated.

Example

3225 tablets = 3225.

If the decimal point is followed by zeros, it still does not change the number of tablets, since the zero indicates that there is nothing occupying that place.

Example

3225 tablets = 3225. = 3225.000

Note As many zeros can be added as necessary without changing the value of the number.

The values of the places located before the decimal point are as follows:

Thousands	Hundreds	Tens	Units .
3	2	2	5 .

Decimal Fractions

Similar values are used to indicate the places on the *right-hand* side of the decimal point *(decimal fraction)* as are used to indicate the whole number places.

.	Tenths	Hundredths	Thousandths
.	2	5	8

A zero can be placed in front of the decimal point without changing the fraction's value, since the zero indicates that nothing occupies that place.

Example

.258 = 0.258

Note One should always place a zero in front of the decimal point when indicating a decimal fraction. When the decimal point is written too lightly, the zero indicates the proper location of the decimal point. This helps reduce medication errors.

A decimal fraction can be written as a common fraction by placing the number of sections indicated *(numerator)* over the value of the last place indicated *(denominator).*

Examples

$$0.1 = \frac{1}{10}$$

$$0.25 = \frac{25}{100}$$

$$0.348 = \frac{348}{1000}$$

Note The *number of zeros* in the denominator is *equal* to the *number of places* on the *right-hand* side of the decimal point.

EXERCISE J

Change the following decimal fractions to common fractions.

1. 0.3
2. 0.9
3. 0.24
4. 0.58
5. 0.289
6. 0.04
7. 0.043
8. 0.209
9. 0.004
10. 0.025

Adding Decimals

When whole numbers are added, the tens, hundreds, thousands, and so on, are placed under each other and then added. (The tens are added to the tens; the hundreds are added to the hundreds . . .). The same procedure is used with decimals. *Line up* the *decimals* and the *places* and then *add*.

Example

	hundreds	tens	units	tenths	hundredths
	5	2	5 .	0	4
+	4	7	5 .	0	6
1	0	0	0 .	1	0

EXERCISE K

Add the following decimals.

1. 285.4 + 32.5 **2.** 782.0 + 3.4
3. 92.01 + 8.72 **4.** 0.48 + 9.72
5. 0.45 + 0.22 **6.** 0.04 + 0.008
7. 0.142 + 0.104

Subtracting Decimals

To subtract decimals, *line up* the *decimal points* and the *places* and then *subtract* the numbers.

Example

	hundreds	tens	units	tenths	hundredths
	4	2	5 .	1	0
−	2	1	5 .	0	8
	2	1	0 .	0	2

Note A zero was added at the end of 425.1 to make the subtraction easier (425.1 = 425.10).

EXERCISE L

Subtract the following decimals.

1. 25.5 − 20.2 **2.** 10.25 − 8.15
3. 1.08 − 0.02 **4.** 0.102 − 0.082
5. 324.56 − 100.48 **6.** 10.3 − 0.045
7. 8.25 − 0.4

Multiplying Decimals

Multiplication of decimals is similar to the multiplication of whole numbers. First, the numbers are multiplied. Then *all* the *decimal places* on the *right-hand* side of the decimal point in both numbers are *counted*. The *decimal point* is *placed* by counting *back* the appropriate number of decimal places from the *right-hand* side of the *answer.*

Example

```
  10.1     1 decimal place
×  0.2     1 decimal place
  2.02     2 decimal places in answer
```

Example

```
  25.0     1 decimal place
× 0.11     2 decimal places
  2 50
 2 5 0
 2. 750    3 decimal places in answer
```

EXERCISE M

Multiply the following decimals.

1. 25.2 × 0.3 **2.** 210. × 0.02
3. 38.3 × 1.2 **4.** 74.01 × 2.501
5. 0.04 × 0.5 **6.** 1.48 × 2.5
7. 48.3 × 0.3 **8.** 0.09 × 1.4

Dividing Decimals

When dividing decimal numbers, the decimal point in the answer *(quotient)* is placed directly above the decimal point in the number being divided *(dividend)* and then division (by the *divisor*) is performed as with whole numbers.

```
        Quotient
Divisor)Dividend
```

Example

$10.2 \div 2 = 2\overline{)10.2}$ Place decimal point in quotient

$= 2\overline{)10.2}$ with quotient 5.1 Divide

If the *divisor* also has a decimal point, it must first be changed into a *whole number* by *moving* the *decimal point* over the same number of places in *both* the *divisor* and the *dividend.* Then the decimal point is placed in the answer (quotient) above the decimal point in the number being divided (dividend) and the division is performed.

Examples

$100.55 \div 0.5 = 0.5\overline{)100.55} = 5.\overline{)1005.50}$

$= 5.\overline{)1005.50}$ with quotient 201.10

$26 \div 0.02 = 0.02\overline{)26.0} = 02.\overline{)2600.0}$

$= 2.\overline{)2600.0}$ with quotient $1300.$

EXERCISE N

Divide the following decimals.

1. 54.5 ÷ 4
2. 2.04 ÷ 6
3. 98.4 ÷ 3
4. 42.3 ÷ 2.4
5. 74.6 ÷ 3.2
6. 5.10 ÷ 0.25
7. 98 ÷ 2.6
8. 0.175 ÷ 0.5

PERCENTAGES

When the term 100% is used, it often means perfect or complete. For example, a grade of 100% in school means that everything is correct. The term *percent* therefore means the number of sections being considered as compared with 100. A percent can be written in three ways:

1. A percent, with the symbol %
2. A fraction
3. A decimal

Examples

$$30\% = \frac{30}{100} = 0.30$$

$$5\% = \frac{5}{100} = 0.05$$

$$\frac{1}{2}\% \text{ or } 0.5\% = \frac{\frac{1}{2}}{100} \text{ or } \frac{1}{200} = 0.005$$

Remember The fraction $\frac{\frac{1}{2}}{100}$ is one-half of 1% and can be simplified as follows:

$$\frac{\frac{1}{2}}{100} = \frac{1}{2} \div 100 = \frac{1}{2} \div \frac{100}{1}$$

$$= \frac{1}{2} \times \frac{1}{100} = \frac{1 \times 1}{2 \times 100} = \frac{1}{200}200$$

Notes

1. When a percent is written with the symbol %, the whole unit of 100 is understood.
2. When a percent is written as a fraction, the number of sections being considered (numerator) are placed over the whole unit 100 (denominator).
3. When a percent is written as a decimal, the hundredth place is used to indicate the number of sections in the whole unit.

units	tenths	hundredths
0	.3	0

EXERCISE O

Complete the following table by filling in the blanks with the equivalent percent, fraction, and/or decimal.

	Percent	Fraction	Decimal
1.	25%	_____	_____
2.	_____	$\frac{2}{100}$	_____

	Percent	Fraction	Decimal
3.	____	____	0.10
4.	____	____	0.03
5.	____	$\frac{85}{100}$	____
6.	64%	____	____
7.	____	$\frac{20}{100}$	____
8.	____	____	0.004
9.	$\frac{1}{3}$%	____	____
10.	____	$\frac{1}{400}$	____

Finding the Percent of a Number

When preparing solutions, it is sometimes necessary to find the percent of a number. First, the *percent* is written as a *decimal* and then the number is *multiplied* by the decimal.

Example Find 20% of 10 g.

Firstly, 20% = 0.20 (converting the percent to a decimal). Then, multiplying

$$\begin{array}{r} 10 \\ \times 0.20 \\ \hline 2.00 \text{ g} \end{array}$$

Example Find $\frac{1}{4}$% of 20 g.

Firstly, $\frac{1}{4}$% or 0.25% = 0.0025. Then, multiplying

$$\begin{array}{r} 20 \\ \times 0.0025 \\ \hline 100 \\ 40 \\ \hline 0.0500 \end{array} \quad \text{or} \quad 0.05 \text{ g}$$

EXERCISE P

Solve the following.

1. Find 10% of 80 lb.
2. Find 3% of 20 g.
3. Find 25% of 10 g.
4. Find $\frac{1}{2}$% of 200 lb.
5. Find 5% of 1 g.

Finding What Percent One Number Is of Another

When finding the percent one number is of another, it is necessary to first form a *fraction* by placing the number to be considered over the *total* number. The fraction is then reduced to its *simplest* form and then to a percent.

Example Johnny weighed 70 lb before he became sick. During his illness he lost 14 lb. What percent of his body weight has Johnny lost?

$$\frac{14 \text{ lb}}{70 \text{ lb}} = \frac{2}{10} = \frac{1}{5}$$

$$\frac{1}{5} = 5\overline{)1.00}^{\,0.20} = 0.20 = 20\%$$

Johnny has lost 20% of his body weight.

EXERCISE Q

Solve the following.

1. What percent is 20 g of 55 g?
2. Harry normally weighs 150 lb. However, he loses 25 lb. What percent of his body weight has Harry lost?
3. What percent of a mixture is water if the mixture contains 300 cc of water and 50 cc of hydrogen peroxide?

RATIOS

Ratio is a term used to express the relationship between two different quantities. The ratio is often written as a fraction. A solution that contains 1 part hydrogen peroxide and 2 parts water is a ratio of 1 to 2. This ratio can be written as $\frac{1}{2}$ or 1:2.

A relationship between two quantities is often written as a ratio with a diagonal line (*x*/*y*) and is read as *per.* For example, the rate at which intravenous fluids run is often called *drops per minute* (gtt/min.).

PROPORTIONS

A **proportion** consists of *two ratios* that are *equal*. A solution that contains 1 part hydrogen peroxide and 2 parts water ($\frac{1}{2}$) and a solution that contains 2 parts hydrogen peroxide and 4 parts water ($\frac{2}{4}$) are two equal ratios and therefore can be written as a proportion.

$$\frac{1}{2} = \frac{2}{4}$$

Instead of being written as a fraction, this proportion can also be written as follows:

1 : 2 : : 2 : 4
(One is to two) as (two is to four)

To find out if two ratios are equal, and therefore a proportion, the terms are *cross multiplied*. If the results are the same, the ratios are equal.

Example Is $\frac{1}{4}$ equal to $\frac{2}{8}$?

$\frac{1}{4} = \frac{2}{8}$ Cross multiply

$4 \times 2 = 1 \times 8$
$8 = 8$ Compare the results

The answer is the same; therefore the ratios are equal.

Example Is $\frac{1}{2}$ equal to $\frac{3}{6}$?

1 : 2 : : 3 : 6 Multiply the two outside numbers (extremes) and the two inside numbers (means)

$1 \times 6 = 2 \times 3$
$6 = 6$ Compare results

The answer is the same; therefore it is a proportion.

SOLVING FOR AN UNKNOWN QUANTITY

Since proportions consist of two equal ratios, they are useful in determining drug dosages when there is an unknown quantity. An x is often used to represent the unknown quantity.

Example How many eighths is $\frac{1}{4}$ equal to?

$\frac{1}{4} = \frac{x}{8}$
$4x = 1 \times 8$
$4x = 8$
$x = 2$

1 : 4 : : x : 8
$4x = 1 \times 8$
$4x = 8$
$x = 2$

EXERCISE R

Solve the following for x.

1. $\frac{5}{8} = \frac{x}{16}$ **2.** $\frac{20}{50} = \frac{x}{25}$
3. 1:3::x:9 **4.** 4:36::x:10
5. $\frac{5}{15} = \frac{x}{30}$ **6.** $\frac{1}{4} = \frac{x}{10}$
7. 2:16::x:9 **8.** 30:64::x:8

ANSWERS TO PRETEST

1. 12 **2.** 15 **3.** 4
4. 3 **5.** II **6.** XIV
7. IX **8.** VIII

If any of the above are answered incorrectly, start with Number Systems (page 154).

9. $\frac{8}{3}$ **10.** $\frac{29}{6}$
11. $4\frac{5}{6}$ **12.** $10\frac{1}{5}$

If any of the above are answered incorrectly, start with Fractions (page 156).

13. $\frac{1}{7}$ **14.** $\frac{2}{5}$

If any of the above are answered incorrectly, start with Reducing Fractions (page 158).

15. $\frac{1}{2}$ **16.** $\frac{9}{14}$

If any of the above are answered incorrectly, start with Adding Fractions (page 158).

17. $\frac{7}{15}$ **18.** $\frac{19}{12}$ *or* $1\frac{7}{12}$

If any of the above are answered incorrectly, start with Subtracting Fractions (page 159).

19. $\frac{2}{5}$ **20.** 4

If any of the above are answered incorrectly, start with Multiplying Fractions (page 160).

21. $\frac{6}{5}$ *or* $1\frac{1}{5}$ **22.** $\frac{16}{3}$ *or* $5\frac{1}{3}$

If any of the above are answered incorrectly, start with Dividing Fractions (page 160).

23. $\frac{52}{100}$ **24.** $\frac{6}{1000}$

If any of the above are answered incorrectly, start with Decimals (page 161).

25. 126.56 **26.** 1.042

If any of the above are answered incorrectly, start with Adding Decimals (page 162).

27. 19.02 **28.** 0.294

If any of the above are answered incorrectly, start with Subtracting Decimals (page 162).

29. 9.612 **30.** 0.009

If any of the above are answered incorrectly, start with Multiplying Decimals (page 162).

31. 0.62 **32.** 80

If any of the above are answered incorrectly, start with Dividing Decimals (page 162).

33. $\frac{30}{100} = 0.3$ **34.** $18\% = 0.18$
35. $9\% = \frac{9}{100}$

If any of the above are answered incorrectly, start with Percentages (page 163).

36. 2 g **37.** 0.125 lb

If any of the above are answered incorrectly, start with Percentages (page 163).

38. 25%

If the above is answered incorrectly, start with Finding What Percent One Number Is of Another (page 164).

39. 13.3 **40.** 3

If any of the above are answered incorrectly, start with Ratios (page 164).

ANSWERS TO EXERCISES

Exercise A

1. 1000 **2.** 100 **3.** 13 **4.** 90 **5.** 300
6. 80 **7.** 66 **8.** 1223 **9.** 24 **10.** 54
11. 97 **12.** 1924

Exercise B

1. X **2.** L **3.** VII **4.** XXIII **5.** XXIX
6. XXXIV **7.** CL **8.** DLII **9.** LXVIII
10. CXXVII **11.** XIX **12.** XCV **13.** CDXV
14. CMLIV

Exercise C

1. $2\frac{8}{5}$ **2.** $3\frac{9}{16}$ **3.** $5\frac{2}{6}$ **4.** $5\frac{4}{7}$ **5.** $2\frac{5}{2}$

Exercise D

1. $1\frac{3}{8}$ **2.** $3\frac{1}{2}$ **3.** 4 **4.** $2\frac{1}{5}$ **5.** $28\frac{4}{7}$

Exercise E

1. $\frac{1}{6}$ **2.** $\frac{1}{10}$ **3.** $\frac{1}{3}$ **4.** $\frac{1}{9}$ **5.** $\frac{1}{8}$ **6.** $\frac{2}{5}$ **7.** $\frac{2}{5}$
8. $\frac{3}{10}$

Exercise F

1. $\frac{5}{6}$ **2.** $\frac{10}{16}$ or $\frac{5}{8}$ **3.** $\frac{10}{12}$ or $\frac{5}{6}$ **4.** $\frac{17}{35}$
5. $\frac{49}{24}$ or $2\frac{1}{24}$ **6.** $10\frac{1}{15}$ or $6\frac{11}{15}$

Exercise G

1. $1\frac{1}{3}$ **2.** $\frac{1}{9}$ **3.** $\frac{1}{5}$ **4.** $\frac{1}{8}$ **5.** $\frac{5}{12}$ **6.** $\frac{51}{16}$ **7.** $\frac{3}{8}$

Exercise H

1. $\frac{3}{10}$ **2.** $\frac{1}{6}$ **3.** $\frac{1}{5}$ **4.** $\frac{1}{4}$ **5.** $1\frac{2}{3}$ **6.** $3\frac{3}{5}$ **7.** $1\frac{1}{2}$
8. 8 **9.** $\frac{26}{21}$ or $1\frac{5}{21}$ **10.** $4\frac{5}{64}$ **11.** $\frac{5}{12}$
12. $\frac{147}{30} = 4\frac{27}{30}$

Exercise I

1. $1\frac{1}{2}$ **2.** $\frac{4}{7}$ **3.** $\frac{1}{2}$ **4.** $\frac{12}{5}$ or $2\frac{2}{5}$ **5.** $\frac{7}{2}$ or $3\frac{1}{2}$
6. $\frac{17}{2}$ or $8\frac{1}{2}$ **7.** $\frac{2}{25}$ **8.** $\frac{8}{27}$ **9.** 8 **10.** 30
11. $\frac{16}{91}$ **12.** $\frac{21}{10}$ or $2\frac{1}{10}$

Exercise J

1. $\frac{3}{10}$ **2.** $\frac{9}{10}$ **3.** $\frac{24}{100}$ **4.** $\frac{58}{100}$ **5.** $\frac{289}{1000}$ **6.** $\frac{4}{100}$
7. $\frac{43}{1000}$ **8.** $\frac{209}{1000}$ **9.** $\frac{4}{1000}$ **10.** $\frac{25}{1000}$

Exercise K

1. 317.9 **2.** 785.4 **3.** 100.73 **4.** 10.2
5. 0.67 **6.** 0.048 **7.** 0.246

Exercise L

1. 5.3 **2.** 2.1 **3.** 1.06 **4.** 0.02 **5.** 224.08
6. 10.255 **7.** 7.85

Exercise M

1. 7.56 **2.** 4.2 **3.** 45.96 **4.** 185.09901
5. 0.02 **6.** 3.7 **7.** 14.49 **8.** 0.126

Exercise N

1. 13.625 or 13.6 **2.** 0.34 **3.** 32.8
4. 17.625 or 17.6 **5.** 23.3125 or 23.3 **6.** 20.4
7. 37.692307 or 37.7 **8.** 0.35

Exercise O

1. $\frac{25}{100} = 0.25$ **2.** $2\% = 0.02$ **3.** $10\% = \frac{10}{100}$
4. $3\% = \frac{3}{100}$ **5.** $85\% = 0.85$ **6.** $\frac{64}{100} = 0.64$
7. $20\% = 0.20$ **8.** $\frac{1}{4}\% = \frac{4}{1000}$ **9.** $\frac{1}{300} = 0.003$
10. $\frac{1}{4}\% = 0.0025$

Exercise P

1. 8 lb **2.** 0.6 g **3.** 2.5 g **4.** 1 lb **5.** 0.05 g

Exercise Q

1. 36% **2.** 17% **3.** 86%

Exercise R

1. 10 **2.** 10 **3.** 3 **4.** 1.1 **5.** 10 **6.** 2.5
7. 1.125 **8.** 3.75

REFERENCES

Anderson, E. M. 1972. *Workbook of solutions and dosage of drugs*. 9th ed. St. Louis: C. V. Mosby.

Eisenbach, R. 1977. *Calculating and administering medications*. Philadelphia: F. A. Davis.

Martin, E. W. 1969. *Techniques of medication: A manual on the administration of drug products*. Philadelphia: Lippincott.

Richardson, L. I., and Richardson, J. K. 1976. *The mathematics of drugs and solutions with clinical applications*. New York: McGraw-Hill.

Sackheim, G. I., and Robins, L. 1974. *Programmed mathematics for nurses*. 3rd ed. New York: Macmillan.

Swartz, C. E. 1973. *Math for the first two years of college science*. Englewood Cliffs, N.J.: Prentice-Hall.

Chapter 10

Metrology

METROLOGY IS THE science of weights and measures and it is therefore essential that nurses who administer medications understand this subject. There are three systems presently used in pharmacology: the metric system, the apothecary system, and the household system. The ability to convert dosages of medications within each system and between different systems is vital. Some medication dosages are prescribed in one system (such as the apothecary system) but the dosage form may be measured in another system (usually the metric system). The nurse must therefore be able to convert the apothecary measurement into the equivalent metric measurement in order to administer the correct dosage. In addition, since many clients take medications at home using ordinary teaspoons and tablespoons, the nurse must be able to convert dosages ordered in the metric or apothecary systems into the equivalent household measurement.

This chapter presents the three systems of weights and measures. It also provides the reader with methods of converting from one system to another. A number of practice exercises have been included.

The following is a pretest for this chapter. If all questions are answered correctly, there is no need to read this chapter. However, if any of the questions are answered incorrectly, the answer sheet on page 180 will direct the reader to the section of this chapter that should be reviewed before proceeding to the Chapter 11.

PRETEST

Fill in the blanks with the correct metric abbreviation or word.

1. 450 ml = 450 ______ (word)
2. 96 kilograms = 96 ______ (abbreviation)
3. 52 centimeters = 52 ______ (abbreviation)
4. 5 g = 5 ______ (word)

Solve the following equivalents.

5. 260 cc = ______ l **6.** 5 l = ______ ml
7. 6 g = ______ mg **8.** 7.2 kg = ______ g

Write out the meaning of each of the following abbreviations.

9. ʒ iss = ______ **10.** f℥ ii = ______
11. ♏ v = ______

Express the following using the appropriate apothecary abbreviations.

12. 5 g = ______ **13.** $\frac{1}{8}$ gr = ______
14. 20 f ʒ = ______

Solve the following equivalents.

15. f℥ vii = fʒ ______
16. pt iii = f℥ ______
17. 240 ♏ = f℥ ______
18. ℥ xviii = lb ______
19. 120 mg = gr ______
20. 72 kg = lb ______
21. 0.6 mg = gr ______
22. 15 cc = ʒ ______
23. 0.5 ml = ♏ ______
24. gr xx = ______ g
25. f℥ viss = ______ ml
26. gr $\frac{1}{150}$ = ______ mg
27. 4 cc = ______ gtt
28. 25 ml = ______ t
29. 30 ♏ = ______ T
30. f℥ iv = ______ glassful

SYSTEMS OF WEIGHTS AND MEASURES

There are several systems used to determine the weight and size of objects. The ancient Egyptians, Romans, and Greeks often measured the length of objects by using hands, fingers, arms, and/or fists as guides. For example, a Roman mile was equal to 1000 paces and one Roman pace was equal to five Roman feet. Since one person's foot was not always the same length as another's foot, there was a lack of uniformity in the measurement.

The Hebrews used the *talent* to measure the weight of objects. A talent was equal to the load an adult could carry comfortably and this weight was subdivided into smaller units called *geraks* and *shekel*. But the weight of the talent varied according to the region in which one lived.

The ancient civilizations often used their agricultural products to determine the capacity of containers. Grain, usually wheat grain, was used for dry measures and wine for wet measures. The Greeks determined capacity by the saucerful, cupful, and wine jar. There were four saucers *(oxybaphon)* in a cup *(kotyle)*, 12 cups in a pitcher *(chous)*, and 12 pitchers in a wine jar *(amphora)*. Here again, the size of one man's cup was not necessarily the same size as another's cup. When nations began trading products with other nations, there was a need for uniformity and greater accuracy in weight and measurement, so the number of metrology systems decreased. The avoirdupois, troy, and apothecary systems survived, but they all used the grain as the basic unit (see Table 10-1). Since the size and weight of a grain varied, Henry III tried to standardize the Imperial grain in 1266 by passing a statute indicating that the English penny should weigh "32 grains of wheat well dried and gathered out of the middle of the ear." Another problem of the surviving systems was that the same measure could have two different values. For example, the British gallon contains 160 oz, whereas the American gallon contains only 128 oz (see Table 10-2).

Because of the lack of precision in the metrology systems, French scientists began, during the late 18th century, to develop a system of weights and measures that relied on permanent natural standards. The basic unit of length, a *meter,* was defined to be $\frac{1}{10,000,000}$ of the distance from the North Pole to the equator, and a platinum bar of this length was placed in the French Archives. The *gram,* the basic unit of weight, was defined to be 1 cc of water at its greatest density (4°C). A platinum model of the kilogram (1000 g) was also placed in the Archives. The *metric standards* were legally adopted by France in 1799.

The *metric system* grew in popularity, particularly among the scientific community. On May 20, 1875, at an international meeting in France, the treaty of the Convention of the Meter was signed. Eighteen countries, including the United States, soon ratified the treaty. Since there was some error in the original measurement, it was decided to accept the metric standards of the Archives, and each country received a copy of the standards for their own Archives. The treaty also led to the establishment of the International Bureau of Weights and Measures, which was given custody of the international standards.

The metric system is accepted by most countries as the official method of determining weights and measures. However people are reluctant to change from their familiar systems of measurement, so it is necessary for health professionals to be able to convert from one system to the other. The metric system is the primary system used in medicine, although prescriptions for older drugs are sometimes written in the apothecary system. Since the household system, an even older method of measurement that uses cooking utensils, is often used in the home, *household measurements* are also presented in this chapter.

TABLE 10-1 Systems of Weights

Avoirdupois Weight								
Pound		Ounces						Grains
1	=	16					=	7000
		1					=	437.5
Troy Weight								
Pound		Ounces				Pennyweights		Grains
1	=	12			=	240	=	5760
		1			=	20	=	480
						1	=	24
Apothecary Weight								
Pound		Ounces		Drams		Scruples		Grains
1	=	12	=	96	=	288	=	5760
		1	=	8	=	24	=	480
				1	=	3	=	60
						1	=	20

TABLE 10-2 Systems of Capacity

Imperial Measure (British)

Gallon		Quarts		Pints		Fluidounces		Fluidrams		Minims
1	=	4	=	8	=	160	=	1,280	=	76,800
				1	=	20	=	160	=	9,600
						1		8	=	480
								1	=	60

Apothecary (U.S.)

Gallon		Quarts		Pints		Fluidounces		Fluidrams		Minims
1	=	4	=	8	=	128	=	1,024	=	61,440
				1	=	16	=	128	=	7,680
						1	=	8	=	480
								1	=	60

METRIC SYSTEM

The metric system is the most exact system of measurement and has therefore replaced older systems in most scientific work, including pharmacology. The metric standards for the United States are preserved by the U.S. Bureau of Standards in Washington, D.C.

The metric units of measurement are shown in Table 10-3.

TABLE 10-3 Metric Units of Measurement

Type Measurement	Name of Unit	Abbreviation
Length—linear distance	meter	M *or* m
Weight (solids)	gram	G *or* g* Gm *or* gm
Capacity—volume of liquids	liter	L *or* l

*The G or g alone is sometimes confused with the abbreviation for grain (gr).

The metric system is based on the decimal scale of numbers. Greek prefixes are used to indicate measurements greater than the standard units and Latin prefixes are used to indicate subdivisions of the standard units (see Table 10-4).

Table 10-4 Prefixes in the Metric System

Quantity	Prefix	Abbreviation
1000	kilo-	k
100	hecto-	h
10	deka-	dk
0.1	deci-	d
0.01	centi-	c
0.001	milli-	m

For example, a length of 1000 meters is written 1 kilometer (1 km) and one-hundredth of a gram is written 1 milligram (1 mg or 1mgm).

EXERCISE A

Fill in the blanks with the correct metric abbreviation or word.

1. 9 meters = 9 ______ (abbreviation)
2. 5 decimeters = 5 ______ (abbreviation)
3. 48 km = 48 ______ (word)
4. 0.08 cm = 0.08 ______ (word)
5. 4 grams = 4 ______ (abbreviation)
6. 84 hg = 84 ______ (word)
7. 0.6 dg = 0.6 ______ (word)
8. 98 milliliters = 98 ______ (abbreviation)
9. 7 l = 7 ______ (word)
10. 0.68 centiliters = 0.68 ______ (abbreviation)

The *meter* was the first standard unit of measurement to be determined. The yard is often compared to the meter (1 m = 39.37 in.) and the mile to the kilometer (1 km = 0.6214 mile). In medicine, the most frequently used linear measures are the centimeter and the millimeter. For example, infants' heads are measured in centimeters and blood pressure is measured in millimeters of mercury.

Units for capacity and weight were derived from the meter. The *liter* is the standard unit of capacity or volume of a liquid. A liter was defined to be the volume of water contained in a cube that has 10 cm on all sides (Figure 10-1). Therefore,

$$1 \text{ liter} = 10 \text{ cm} \times 10 \text{ cm} \times 10 \text{ cm} = 1000 \text{ cc}$$

cc is the common abbreviation for cubic centimeters (cm^3 = cc). Since one-thousandth of a liter can also be called a milliliter (ml), a milliliter is equal to a cubic centimeter (1 ml = 1 cc).

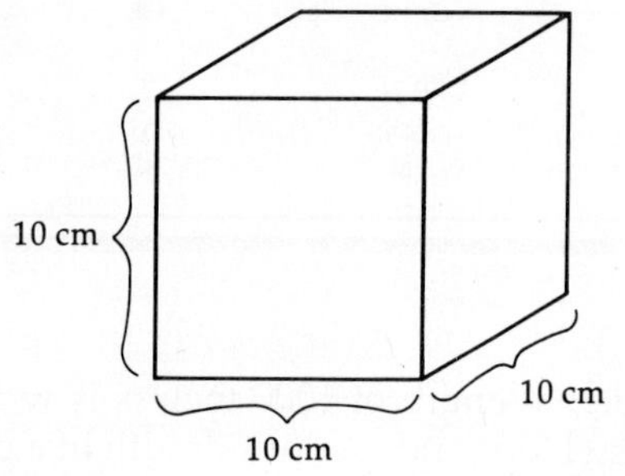

FIGURE 10-1

The *gram* is the most commonly employed unit of weight in pharmacology. It is defined as the weight of 1 cc of water at a temperature of 4° C, the temperature at which water is the most dense. The milligram (mg or mgm) and the kilogram (kg or kgm) are also used frequently in medicine. The milligram and gram are often used for medications whereas the kilogram is usually utilized to measure the weight of clients.

Changing Units

Since the metric system is the most precise method of measurement, it is the system most frequently used when determining drug dosages. It is therefore necessary to know how to change from one unit to another. Because the metric system is based on decimals, it is as easy to change units as it is to count change for a dollar bill, which is also based on 10s. A dollar contains 10 dimes or 100 pennies or 1000 mills (the latter unit, however, is no longer minted since it lost its usefulness). Similarly, a gram contains 10 dg or 100 cg or 1000 mg. Table 10-5 lists some commonly used equivalents.

In order to convert from one unit to the other, it is sometimes helpful to set up a proportion between the units of a *known ratio* and an *unknown ratio* (see Chapter 9). Then the proportion can be solved for the unknown quantity.

Example How many liters are there in 2500 ml?

It is *known* that there are 1000 ml in 1 l. Therefore,

Known ratio	*Unknown ratio*
$\frac{1000 \text{ ml}}{1 \text{ l}}$	$\frac{2500 \text{ ml}}{x \text{ l}}$

Cross multiply:

$$1000x = 2500$$
$$x = 2500 \div 1000$$
$$x = 2.5 \text{ l in } 2500 \text{ ml}$$

Reminder In order for this method of proportions to provide the correct answer, the numerators of both ratios must have the *same units* (ml) as must the denominators (liter).

TABLE 10-5 Commonly Used Equivalents

Weight (Dry Measures)	
1 milligram = 0.001 gram	
1 gram = 1000 milligrams	
1 gram = 0.001 kilograms	
1 kilogram = 1000 grams	
Volume (Liquid Measures)	
1 milliliter = 0.001 liter	
1 liter = 1000 milliliters	
Volume to Weight	
1 milliliter = 1 cubic centimeter	

Note Writing the unit with its quantity can help the solver to be sure that both the numerators and both the denominators have the same units, respectively.

Example How many milligrams are there in 3.6 g?

It is *known* that there are 1000 mg in 1 g. Hence,

Known ratio	*Unknown ratio*
$\frac{1000\text{ mg}}{1\text{ g}}$	$\frac{x\text{ mg}}{3.6\text{ g}}$

Cross multiply:

$$x = 1000 \times 3.6$$
$$x = 3600\text{ mg in } 3.6\text{ g}$$

Example How many milliliters are there in 1.5 liters?

It is *known* that 1 cc = 1 ml and since there are 1000 ml in 1 l there are also 1000 cc in 1 l. Therefore,

Known ratio	*Unknown ratio*
$\frac{1000\text{ ml}}{1\text{ l}}$	$\frac{x\text{ ml}}{1.5\text{ l}}$

Cross multiply:

$$x = 1000 \times 1.5$$
$$x = 1500\text{ cc in } 1.5\text{ l}$$

Another method of finding the unknown quantity is to *move the decimal point*. In the example above involving the number of milligrams in 3.6 g, the answer was 3600.0 mg. Note that both the problem and the answer had a 3 and a 6, but that the decimal point was moved three places to the right (3.6 to 3600.0) when 3.6 was multiplied by 1000. The unknown quantity (mg) is a smaller unit of measure than the known quantity (g), therefore there will be an increase in the number of units.

Rule 1 When the *unknown quantity* is a *smaller* unit than the known quantity, the decimal point is moved to the *right* the same number of spaces as the number of zeros in the known ratio.

Example How many milliliters are there in 1.8 liters? (See Figure 10-2.)

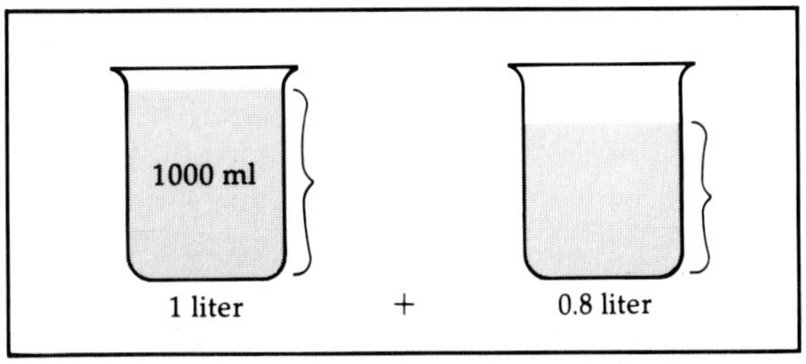

FIGURE 10-2

It is *known* that there are 1000 ml in 1 l. As the problem is going from a larger unit (liters) to an unknown amount of a smaller unit (milliliters), there must be an *increase* in the number of the smaller units. Therefore, the numbers would be multiplied, which would move the decimal point to the *right*.

Since there are 1000 ml in 1 l, and further since there are three zeros in 1000, the decimal point would be moved three places to the right.

1.8 l = 1,800 ml *or* 1800 ml

Example How many grams are there in 32 k?

It is *known* that there are 1000 g in 1 k. Now, grams are a smaller unit than kilograms and as there are three zeros in 1000 g (=1 k), the decimal point is therefore moved three places to the *right*.

32 kgs = 32,000 *or* 32,000 g

When the unit of the unknown quantity is larger than that of the known quantity, the solution requires division and therefore the decimal point would be moved to the left.

Rule 2 When the *unknown quantity* is a *larger* unit of measure than the known quantity, the decimal point is moved to the *left* the same number of spaces as the number of zeros in the known ratio.

Example How many grams are there in 6800 mg?

It is *known* that there are 1000 mg in 1 g. Since grams are a larger unit than milligrams and there are three zeros in 1000 mg (= 1 g), the decimal point is therefore moved three places to the *left*.

6800 mg = 6,800 g *or* 6.8 g

Either setting up a proportion or moving the decimal point will give a correct answer. Moving the decimal point is, of course, faster than solving a proportion. However, when in doubt as to which direction the decimal point should be moved, the proportion method is recommended.

EXERCISE B

Solve the following equivalents.

1. 5g = ______ mg
2. 2.8 kg = ______ g
3. 4824 kg = ______ g
4. 284 mg = ______ g
5. 28,004 g = ______ kg
6. 760 ml = ______ l
7. 4.9 l = ______ ml
8. 28 ml = ______ cc
9. 450 cc = ______ l
10. 1.4 l = ______ ml

APOTHECARY SYSTEM

The word apothecary means a person who prepares and sells drugs—our present-day pharmacist. Several centuries ago, when the preparation and sale of medicinal products became a profession separate from medicine the pharmacist adopted several methods to measure small quantities of drugs. That used for measuring liquids had been used in the wine industry and that for measuring dry or powdered substances was based on standardized quantities for the pound, ounce, dram, scruple, and grain. Since the apothecary used these measures consistently, this method of measurement soon became known as the *apothecary system*.

The more precise method of measurement, the metric system, will no doubt replace the older apothecary system in the near future. However, the apothecary system is still used by some physicians and pharmacists, particularly for drugs that have been used for centuries, such as digitalis. Consequently, it is necessary for all health professionals to know both systems of measurement and how to convert from one system to the other.

Units of Dry Measure

The basic unit of dry weight is the *grain,* which is based on the weight of a single grain of wheat. There are 20 grains in a *scruple,* but the scruple is seldom used now. The *dram* is the next largest unit and it is equal to 60 grains. There are 8 drams in an ounce and 12 oz in a pound. (See Table 10-6.)

Units of Liquid Measure

The *minim* is the amount of water weighing 1 grain and is the basic unit used for measuring fluids. There are 60 minims in a fluid*dram* and 8 fluidrams in a fluid*ounce*. The word fluid (fl) is used as a prefix to indicate a liquid is being measured instead of a dry substance. A *pint* contains 16 fluidounces and there are 2 pints in a *quart*. The next largest unit, a *gallon,* contains 4 quarts. (See Table 10-7.)

Writing Units of Measure

In the apothecary system the symbol of the unit is usually written first and then the quantity is listed using the lowercase Roman numerals.

Examples

2 drams is written ʒi̇i̇
4 ounces is written ʒi̇v
8 grains is written gr ʒvi̇i̇i̇

Note The "one" is dotted so that it will not be confused with an "L" for 50 or in the case of 2 "ones" it will not be confused with a "v" for five.

TABLE 10-6 Units of Dry Measure

Unit	Symbol	Equivalent Units
Grain	gr	
Scruple	℈	20 grains
Dram	ʒ	3 scruples (60 grains)
Ounce	℥ *or* oz	8 drams
Pound	lb	12 ounces

TABLE 10-7 Units of Liquid Measure

Unit	Symbol	Equivalent Units
Minim	♏	1 grain (dry measure)
fluidram	fʒ	60 minims
fluidounce	f℥ *or* fl oz	8 fluidrams
pint	O* *or* pt	16 fluidounces
Quart	qt	2 pints
Gallon	C† *or* gal	4 quarts

*The symbol for pint (O) comes from the Latin word *Octarius;* but since the symbol can be mistaken for a zero, it is seldom used.

†The symbol for gallon (C) comes from the Latin word *Congius* and is sometimes abbreviated as "Cong."

EXERCISE C

Write out the meaning of each of the following abbreviations.

1. gr iii = ______
2. gr xii = ______
3. ♏ x = ______
4. fl ʒ iiss = ______
5. pt vi = ______
6. fl ℥ ss = ______
7. gal xxv = ______
8. gr $\frac{1}{3}$ = ______

Express the following using the appropriate apothecary abbreviations.

9. 10 drams = ______
10. 3 quarts = ______
11. 9 fluidounces = ______
12. 4 grains = ______
13. 35 minims = ______
14. $\frac{1}{8}$ grains = ______
15. 7 ounces = ______
16. $7\frac{1}{2}$ grains = ______

Fractional quantities are usually expressed in Hindu-Arabic numbers. However, the fraction $\frac{1}{2}$ is often written with a separate symbol (ss), from the Latin word *semis* meaning one-half.

Examples

$\frac{1}{4}$ grain is written gr $\frac{1}{4}$
$2\frac{1}{2}$ grains is written gr iiss

Hindu-Arabic numbers are also used when the whole unit is written out in full or when large quantities are being expressed. In such cases, the numbers precede the unit.

Examples

5 ounces
$7\frac{1}{8}$ grains
3 fluidrams
10 minims

Examples

gal LVii is written 57 gal
lb CLX is written 160 lb

Note When it is understood that the substance is a fluid, the term fluid or its abbreviation is often dropped.

Changing Units

It is often necessary to change from one unit to another in the apothecary system. For example, a measuring flask may be calibrated for minims when the dosage required is in drams. The conversion can be performed as described previously by first setting up a proportion between the *known ratio* (minims and drams) and the *unknown ratio* and then solving for the unknown quantity.

Example How many minims are there in ʒ iii?

It is *known* that there are 60 ♏ in 1 dram. Hence,

Known ratio	*Unknown ratio*
$\frac{60\ ♏}{1\ \text{dram}}$	$\frac{x\ ♏}{3\ \text{drams}}$

Cross multiply:

x = 180 ♏ in 3 drams

Reminder In order for this method of proportions to provide the correct answer, the ratios must be set up with the *same units* in the numerators and denominators, respectively. In the above example, minims were in the numerators and drams were in the denominators.

Note Writing the unit with its quantity can help the solver to check that both the numerators and both the denominators have the same units, accordingly.

Example How many fluidrams are there in ℥ i̇vss?

It is *known* that there are 8 fluidrams in 1 fluidounce. Therefore,

Known ratio	*Unknown ratio*
$\frac{8 \text{ fluidrams}}{1 \text{ fluidounce}}$	$\frac{x \text{ fluidrams}}{4.5 \text{ fluidounces}}$

Cross multiply:

$$x = 8 \times 4.5$$
$$x = 36.0$$
$$x = 36 \text{ fluidrams in } 4\tfrac{1}{2} \text{ fluidounces}$$

Note The fraction $4\frac{1}{2}$ was changed to a decimal (4.5) in order to make the multiplication easier. However, the 8 can be multiplied by $4\frac{1}{2}$ as follows:

$$8 \times 4\frac{1}{2} = (8 \times 4) + (8 \times \frac{1}{2})$$
$$= 32 + 4$$
$$= 36$$

Sometimes the known ratio is not the ratio required to solve the problem. In this case, the known ratio can often be converted into the required units by a proportion.

Example How many grains are there in ℥ i̇i̇ ?

It is *known* that there are 60 gr in 1 dram and 8 drams in 1 oz (Figure 10-3). As the number of grains in 1 oz is unknown this must be determined first.

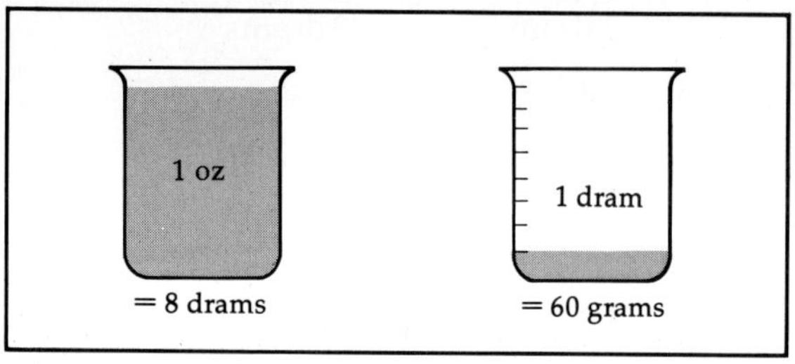

FIGURE 10-3

If 1 oz contains 8 drams and 1 dram contains 60 gr then

$$1 \text{ oz} = 8 \text{ (drams)} \times 60 \text{ (grains)}$$
$$1 \text{ oz} = 480 \text{ gr}$$

Now the numerator (grains) and the denominator (ounces) of each ratio have the same unit of measure and the problem can be solved.

Known ratio	*Unknown ratio*
$\frac{480 \text{ gr}}{1 \text{ oz}}$	$\frac{x \text{ gr}}{2 \text{ oz}}$

Cross multiply:

$$x = 480 \times 2$$
$$x = 960 \text{ gr in } 2 \text{ oz}$$

Note When the unknown quantity (x) is *smaller than* the desired quantity, *multiplication* is required to solve the problem. However, when the unknown quantity is *larger than* the desired quantity, *division* is required.

Example How many pounds are there in 18 oz?

It is *known* that there are 12 oz in 1 lb. Since the unknown quantity (pounds) is larger than the desired unit (ounces), division is required in the solution.

Known ratio	*Unknown ratio*
$\frac{12 \text{ oz}}{1 \text{ lb}}$	$\frac{18 \text{ oz}}{x \text{ lb}}$

Cross multiply:

$$12x = 18$$
$$x = 18 \div 12$$
$$x = 1\tfrac{1}{2} \text{ lb in } 18 \text{ oz}$$

EXERCISE D

Solve the following equivalents.

1. fʒ i̇i̇i̇ = gr ______	**2.** f℥ xi̇ = fʒ ______
3. lb xxx = oz ______	**4.** fʒ xi̇i̇ ♏ ______
5. f℥ i̇x = fʒ ______	**6.** gal i̇i̇ = pt ______
7. lb vss = oz ______	**8.** ʒ$\frac{1}{4}$ = gr ______

9. qt i̇ss = f℥ _____ **10.** 144 oz = lb _____
11. 480 gr = oz _____ **12.** fʒ xii̇ = f℥ _____
13. pt xxi̇v = gal _____ **14.** 450 ♏ = ʒ _____

CHANGING UNITS BETWEEN SYSTEMS

Sometimes it is necessary to change a dosage written in the apothecary system to a metric unit and vice versa. Some of the more useful equivalents are listed in Table 10-8.

TABLE 10-8 Useful Approximate Equivalents

Metric System	Apothecary System
Weight	
1 mg	1/60 grain
60 mg	1 grain
1 g	15 grains (or 16 gr)*
454 g	1 pound
1 kg	2.2 pounds
Volume	
1 ml	16 minims (or 15♏)†
4 ml (*or* 5 ml)	1 fluidram
30 ml	1 fluidounce
1000 ml *or* 1 l	1 quart

*Either equivalent can be used for conversion (1 g = 15.432 gr).
†Either equivalent can be used for conversion (1 ml = 16.23 ♏).

As indicated in Table 10-8, there are no exact equivalents between the apothecary and the metric systems of measurement. Consequently, the solver can select either of the approximate equivalents when converting between the systems. It is recommended that the equivalent that will convert the desired quantity evenly should be used in order to make the computation easier and/or the dosage more accurate to measure. The conversion is performed as described previously using the method of proportions.

Example How many minims are there in 0.5 ml?

The *known* approximate equivalent is 1 ml = 15 or 16 ♏. Therefore,

$$\frac{0.5\text{ ml}}{x\ ♏} = \frac{1\text{ ml}}{15♏} \qquad \frac{0.5\text{ ml}}{x\ ♏} = \frac{1\text{ ml}}{16\ ♏}$$

$$x = 7.5\ ♏ \qquad x = 8\ ♏$$

Note As a syringe is calibrated in whole minims only, the equivalent 1 ml = 16 ♏ should be used since 8 ♏ and not 7.5 ♏ can be measured on a syringe.

Example How many grams are there in 75 gr?

The *known* approximate equivalent is 1 g = 15 or 16 gr. Hence,

$$\frac{75\text{ gr}}{x\text{ g}} = \frac{15\text{ gr}}{1\text{ g}} \qquad \frac{75\text{ gr}}{x\text{ g}} = \frac{16\text{ gr}}{1\text{ g}}$$

$$15x = 75 \qquad 16x = 75$$

$$x = 5\text{ g} \qquad x = 4.6875\text{ g}$$

Note Since the systems are not always directly interchangeable, the use of the equivalent 1 g = 15 gr not only makes the computation easier, it also yields the even answer of 5 g. If a medication was packaged in 1-g tablets, the exact dosage of five tablets would be administered.

Example How many grams (drug's measurement) are there in gr xxiv (dosage ordered)?

It is *known* that there are 15 or 16 gr in 1 g. Therefore,

Known ratio *Unknown ratio*

$$\frac{16\text{ gr}}{1\text{ g}} \qquad \frac{24\text{ gr}}{x\text{ g}}$$

Cross multiply:

$$16x = 24$$

$$x = 1.5\text{ g}$$

Example How many grains (drug's measurement) are in 0.3 mg (dosage ordered)?

It is *known* that there are 60 mg in 1 gr. Hence,

Known ratio *Unknown ratio*

$$\frac{1\text{ gr}}{60\text{ mg}} \qquad \frac{x\text{ gr}}{0.3\text{ mg}}$$

Cross multiply:

$$60x = 0.3 \qquad 60x = \frac{3}{10}$$

$$x = \frac{0.3}{60} \qquad x = \frac{\frac{3}{10}}{\frac{60}{1}}$$

$$x = 0.005 \text{ gr} \qquad x = \frac{3}{10} \times \frac{1}{60}$$

$$x = \frac{3}{600} = \frac{1}{200}$$

$$x = \frac{1}{200} \text{ gr}$$

Remember The apothecary system uses fractions instead of decimals. However, the measurements can be converted to the metric system.

EXERCISE E

Convert the following metric units to apothecary units.

1. 45 mg = gr ______
2. 90 mg = gr ______
3. 7.5 g = gr ______
4. 0.25 g = gr ______
5. 96 kg = lb ______
6. 0.4 mg = gr ______
7. 10 mg = gr ______
8. 30 ml = ʒ ______
9. 0.2 ml = ♏ ______
10. 750 ml = pt ______

Convert the following apothecary units to metric units.

11. fʒ viiss = ______ ml
12. gr xxx = ______ g
13. gr $\frac{1}{600}$ = ______ mg
14. gr $\frac{1}{40}$ = ______ mg
15. gr iss = ______ g
16. fʒ iss = ______ ml
17. ♏ ix = ______ ml
18. pt v = ______ l
19. f℥ iiiss = ______ ml
20. ♏ iv = ______ ml

HOUSEHOLD MEASUREMENTS

When measuring medications in the home, clients use articles that are familiar and commonplace; for example, cups, water glasses, tablespoons, teaspoons, and droppers. (See Table 10-9.) Since clients seldom have metric or apothecary calibrated containers in the home, health professionals need to know how to convert metric and apothecary dosages into their appropriate household measurements. The commonly accepted equivalents are listed in Table 10-10 and Table 10-11. Also see Figure 10-4.

TABLE 10-9 Household Units

Unit	Symbol	Equivalent Units
Drop	gtt*	—
Teaspoon	t *or* tsp	60 drops
Tablespoon	T *or* tbsp	3 teaspoons
Ounce	oz	2 tablespoons
Cupful	c *or* cup	6 ounces
Glassful	—	8 ounces

*The symbol gtt comes from the Latin word *gutta* meaning drop.

TABLE 10-10 Useful Approximate Equivalents

Metric System	Household System
1 ml	15 drops (*or* 16 drops)
4 ml (*or* 5 ml)*	1 teaspoon
15 ml (*or* 16 ml)	1 tablespoon
30 ml	1 ounce
180 ml	1 cupful
240 ml	1 glassful

*Either equivalent can be used for conversion purposes.

TABLE 10-11 Useful Approximate Equivalents

Apothecary System	Household System
1 minim	1 drop
1 fluidram	1 teaspoon (15 or 16 drops)
4 fluidrams	1 tablespoon
1 fluidounce	1 ounce (2 tablespoons)
6 fluidounces	1 cupful
8 fluidounces	1 glassful

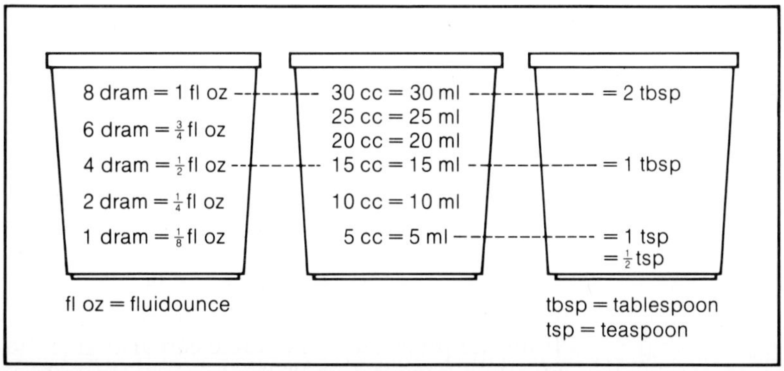

FIGURE 10-4

To convert a measurement from the metric or apothecary systems to a household unit, the method of proportions previously described is used.

Example How many drops are there in 2 ml?

It is *known* that there are 15 drops in 1 ml. Therefore,

Known ratio	*Unknown ratio*
$\frac{15\text{ gtt}}{1\text{ ml}}$	$\frac{x\text{ gtt}}{2\text{ ml}}$

Cross multiply:

$$x = 15 \times 2$$
$$x = 30 \text{ gtt in } 2 \text{ ml}$$

Remember The numerators of both ratios must have the same unit (gtt) as must the denominators (ml).

Example How many teaspoons are there in 10 ml?

It is *known* that there are 5 ml in 1 t. Hence,

Known ratio	*Unknown ratio*
$\frac{5\text{ ml}}{1\text{ t}}$	$\frac{10\text{ ml}}{x\text{ t}}$

Cross multiply:

$$5x = 10$$
$$x = 10 \div 5$$
$$x = 2 \text{ t in } 10 \text{ ml}$$

Note Either equivalent can be used for conversion; here, the conversion unit of 5 ml rather than 4 ml was used.

Example How many tablespoons are there in 10 drams?

It is *known* that there are 4 drams in 1 T. Thus,

Known ratio	*Unknown ratio*
$\frac{4\text{ drams}}{1\text{ T}}$	$\frac{10\text{ drams}}{x\text{ T}}$

Cross multiply:

$$4x = 10$$
$$x = 10 \div 4$$
$$x = 2.5 \text{ T in } 10 \text{ drams}$$

EXERCISE F

Convert the following metric dosages into household measurements.

1. 3 ml = ______ gtt
2. 480 ml = ______ glassful
3. 45 ml = ______ T
4. 12 ml = ______ t
5. 450 ml = ______ cupful
6. 1.6 ml = ______ gtt

7. 840 ml = ______ glassfuls
8. 15 ml = ______ t
9. 10 ml = ______ t
10. 40 ml = ______ T

Convert the following apothecary dosages into household measurements.

11. 13♏ = ______ gtt
12. fʒiii = ______ t
13. fʒxvi = ______ T
14. f℥ xxxvi = ______ cupful
15. fʒiiss = ______ t
16. f℥iss = ______ T
17. fʒii = ______ gtt
18. fʒss = ______ gtt
19. 20 f℥ = ______ glassfuls
20. ℥ss = ______ t

Accuracy of Dosage

The metric system is the most precise method of measuring and the older apothecary system is relatively precise, but household measurements tend to be inaccurate for several reasons. Firstly, tableware teaspoons and tablespoons can hold variable amounts of liquids, depending on the style. The capacity of teaspoons has been shown to vary from 3.5 to 6.5 ml of water whereas tablespoons can hold more than 16 ml of water. In fact, the ordinary tablespoons can hold from 20 to 28 ml of water. However, it has been noted that cooking teaspoons and tablespoons do generally hold between 4 and 5 ml and 15 and 16 ml, respectively.

Secondly, the capacity of spoons will vary depending on whether the spoon is heaped with medication or leveled. Even with liquid drugs this can be a problem since the thicker, or more viscous, the fluid the more the spoon will hold without running over. For example, more milliliters of Maalox (a thick suspension) can be put in a spoon than can Coca-Cola syrup (a thinner solution). Many liquid antibiotics are thick syrups and can therefore create an overdose hazard.

Another difficulty with tableware spoons is that when the spoon is held slightly tilted and not in a horizontal position, the capacity of the spoon decreases. Cooking spoons are more accurate measures because the design usually requires that they are held in the horizontal position, so there is little variation in the capacity. However, since the use of cooking spoons could be a sanitary hazard if they are not disinfected properly, their use for administering medications is not advocated.

Since many medications are poisonous in large quantities, accuracy of dosage is critical, particularly for small children. Some over-the-counter drugs now come with calibrated containers for measuring the dosage. Clients should be encouraged to save these measuring containers or to buy a calibrated "medicine glass" from the pharmacy. The nurse can also give the client an accurately calibrated container, such as the disposable ones used in many hospitals.

Clients who measure their own medications should also be shown how to read the bottom of the meniscus. If the client reads the dosage from the top of the meniscus, he or she will be taking less than the desired dose. Undermedication of drugs that require specific drug levels in the blood, such as some antibiotics, can cause problems for clients, so they should always be taught to read the bottom of the meniscus with the measuring container on a level surface. See Figure 10-5.

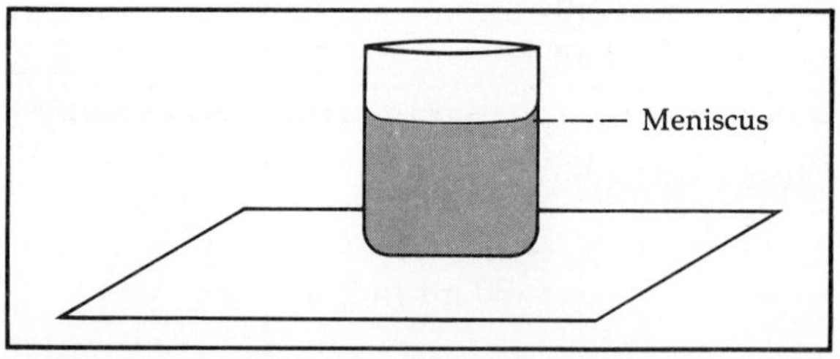

FIGURE 10-5

ANSWERS TO PRETEST

1. milliliters
2. kg
3. cm
4. grams

If any of the above are answered incorrectly, start with Metric System (page 171).

5. 0.260
6. 5000
7. 6000
8. 7200

If any of the above are answered incorrectly, start with Changing Units (page 172).

9. $1\frac{1}{2}$ drams
10. 2 fluidounces
11. 5 minims
12. gr v
13. gr $\frac{1}{8}$
14. 20 fʒ (*or* fʒ xx)

If any of the above are answered incorrectly, start with Apothecary System (page 174).

15. 56
16. 48
17. 0.5
18. 1.5

If any of the above are answered incorrectly, start with Changing Units (page 175).

19. 2
20. 158.4
21. $\frac{1}{100}$
22. 3 (*or* 3.75)
23. 8 (*or* 7.5)
24. 1.25 (*or* 1.3)
25. 195
26. 0.4

If any of the above are answered incorrectly, start with Changing Units Between Systems (page 177).

27. 60
28. 5 (*or* 6.25)
29. 0.5
30. 0.5

If any of the above are answered incorrectly, start with Household Measurements (page 178).

After successfully completing the above pretest, pages 183–205 should be read.

ANSWERS TO EXERCISES

Exercise A

1. m **2.** dm **3.** kilometer **4.** centimeter **5.** g **6.** hectogram **7.** decigram **8.** ml **9.** liters **10.** cl

Exercise B

1. 5000 **2.** 2800 **3.** 4,824,000 **4.** 0.284 **5.** 28.004 **6.** 0.76 **7.** 4900 **8.** 28 **9.** 0.450 **10.** 1400

Exercise C

1. 3 grains **2.** 12 grains **3.** 10 minims **4.** $2\frac{1}{2}$ fluidrams **5.** 6 pints **6.** $\frac{1}{2}$ fluidounces **7.** 25 gallons **8.** $\frac{1}{3}$ grain **9.** 3^x ℥ **10.** qt iii **11.** ℥ ix **12.** gr iv **13.** 35 ♏ **14.** gr $\frac{1}{8}$ **15.** ℥ vii **16.** gr viiss

Exercise D

1. 180 **2.** 120 **3.** 360 **4.** 720 **5.** 72 **6.** 16 **7.** 66 **8.** 15 **9.** 48 **10.** 12 **11.** 1 **12.** $1\frac{1}{2}$ **13.** 3 **14.** $7\frac{1}{2}$

Exercise E

1. $\frac{3}{4}$ **2.** $1\frac{1}{2}$ **3.** 120 (*or* 112.5) **4.** 4 (*or* 3.75) **5.** 211.2 **6.** $\frac{1}{150}$ **7.** $\frac{1}{6}$ **8.** 6 (*or* 7.5) **9.** 3 (*or* 3.2) **10.** 1.5 **11.** 30 (*or* 37.5) **12.** 2 (*or* 1.875) **13.** $\frac{1}{10}$ **14.** $1\frac{1}{2}$ **15.** 0.1 **16.** 6 (*or* 7.5) **17.** 0.6 (*or* 0.5625) **18.** 2.5 **19.** 105 **20.** 0.25 (*or* 0.267)

Exercise F

1. 45 **2.** 2 **3.** 3 (*or* 2.8) **4.** 3 (*or* 2.4) **5.** 2.5 **6.** 24 **7.** 3.5 **8.** 3 (*or* 3.75) **9.** 2 (*or* 2.5) **10.** 2.5 (*or* 2.67) **11.** 13 **12.** 3 **13.** 4 **14.** 6 **15.** 2.5 **16.** 3 **17.** 30 **18.** 7.5 **19.** 2.5 **20.** 4

REFERENCES

Anderson, E. M. 1972. *Workbook of solutions and dosage of drugs*. 9th ed. St. Louis: C. V. Mosby.

Richardson, L. I., and Richardson, J. K. 1976. *The mathematics of drugs and solutions with clinical applications*. New York: McGraw-Hill.

Sackheim, G. I., and Robins, L. 1974. *Programmed mathematics for nurses*. 3rd ed. New York: Macmillan.

Whisler, B. L. *Mathematics for Health Professionals*. Monterey, CA: Duxbury Press, 1979.

Chapter 11

Posology

POSOLOGY IS THE branch of medical science that deals with the dosage of medications. Since the action of a drug is directly related to the quantity given, the correct dosage is vital. This chapter includes the calculations required to administer the correct dosages of oral, parenteral, and intravenous medications as well as the preparation of solutions. The rules for determining the appropriate dosages for infants and children are also presented.

The following is a pretest for this chapter. If all questions are answered correctly, there is no need to read this chapter. However, if any of the questions are answered incorrectly, the answer sheet on page 205 will direct the reader to the section of this chapter that should be reviewed before proceeding to Chapter 12.

PRETEST

Solve the following dosage problems.

1. *Desired:* Phenobarbital, 45 mg po. *Available:* Phenobarbital, 15-mg tablets. How many tablets should be given?
2. *Desired:* Ampicillin, 750 mg po. *Available:* Ampicillin oral suspension, 250 mg/5 ml. How many milliliters should be administered?
3. *Desired:* Terpin hydrate with codeine, gr $\frac{1}{5}$ po. *Available:* Elixir of terpin hydrate with codeine, 2 mg/ml. How many milliliters should be administered?
4. *Desired:* Morphine, gr $\frac{1}{8}$ IM. *Available:* Morphine sulfate, 10 mg/ml. How many milliliters should be administered?
5. *Desired:* Regular insulin, 30 U (H). *Available:* Regular insulin, 40 U/ml. Shade the correct dosage on each syringe.
   (a) Administer with an insulin syringe calibrated for U-40 insulin.

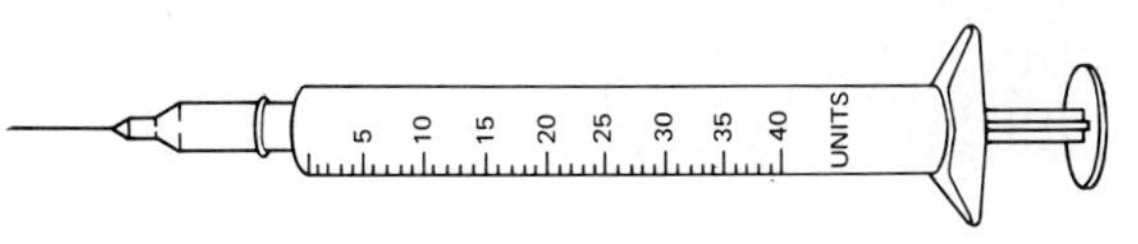

   (b) Administer with a disposable TB syringe.

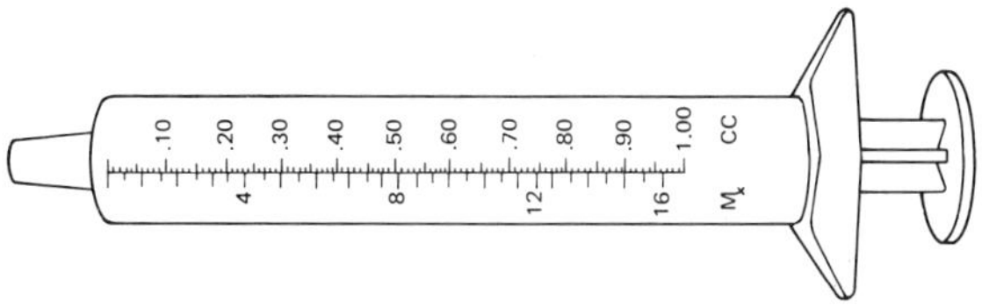

   (c) Administer with a 2.5-ml syringe.

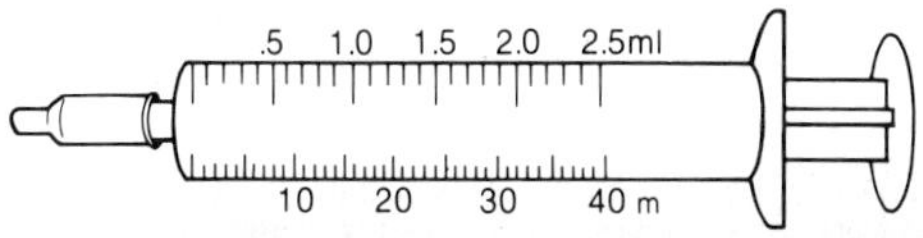

6. *Desired:* Dilantin, 100 mg IM. *Available:* Sodium phenytoin (Dilantin), 250 mg in an ampule. *Directions:* Add sterile water in accompanying ampule to yield 5 ml of solution.
   (a) What is the strength of the resulting solution?
   (b) How many milliliters should be given?
7. *Give:* 2500 ml of 5% D/W IV in 24 hours. *IV administration set:* 15 gtt/ml.
   (a) How many gtt/min. should the IV run?
   (b) How many ml/hr will the client receive?
8. *Give:* Erythromycin 750 mg q8h IV via Soluset. *Available:* Erythromycin powder, 250 mg in a 10-ml vial. *Directions:* Add 10 ml of sterile water to yield 100 mg/1.1 ml. Should be given for 30 minutes. Prepared solution may be added to 5% D/W or NS IV's. *IV administration set:* 60 gtt/ml.
   (a) How many milliliters of reconstituted erythromycin should be added to the Soluset?
   (b) If the Soluset is filled to the 100-ml mark, how many gtt/min. should the medicated solution run?
9. Using Fried's Rule, find the appropriate pediatric dose. A 5-month-old infant weighs 14.6 lb and is to receive phenobarbital. The adult dosage is 0.1 g.
10. Using Clark's rule, find the appropriate pediatric dose.
    (a) A 10-year-old child weighs 88 lb and is to receive aspirin. The adult dosage is 10 gr.
    (b) A 14-year-old child weighs 50 kg and is to receive digoxin. The adult maintenance dosage is 0.5 mg.
11. A 6-year-old child who weighs 58 lb is to receive neomycin q6h po. Neomycin 50 mg/

kg/24 hr is the recommended dose. What is the dosage of each divided dose?

12. Prepare 100 fluid ounces of 1 : 10,000 potassium permanganate solution from potassium permanganate crystals. How much solute should be used?
13. Prepare 750 ml of 10% lysol solution from 50% lysol solution.
    (a) How much solute should be used?
    (b) How much solvent should be used?

FACTORS AFFECTING DRUG DOSAGE

The average *therapeutic dose* is the quantity of a drug that will cause the desired action without producing toxic or lethal effects. It is based on a 150-lb adult and is determined by animal experimentation and experience with clients.

There are several basic factors that influence the dosage of a drug. Two of the primary factors are the age and weight of a client. Infants and children require smaller dosages, not only because of their smaller size, but also because they cannot absorb, metabolize, and excrete many drugs as well as an adult. Elderly clients often require less than the average adult dose because of alterations in their physiologic functioning. Variations among average adults must also be considered because every adult does not weigh 150 lb. Women, for example, who tend to weigh less, often require a smaller dose. Obese individuals require less medication than their weight would indicate, because adipose tissue does not absorb most medications and therefore should be discounted in obese clients when determining dosages.

The absorption, metabolism, and excretion of drugs also affect the dosage of medications. Drugs that are absorbed and excreted rapidly need to be given at frequent intervals in order to provide the desired effect. However, drugs that are excreted slowly should be given at longer intervals in order to prevent them accumulating. As many drugs are metabolized by the liver and excreted by the kidneys, clients with liver or kidney diseases will often metabolize and excrete drugs too slowly. Consequently, these clients tend to accumulate the drug in their bodies.

The route of administration can also affect the dosage. The action of most drugs occurs after the drug enters the bloodstream. Therefore, medications given intravenously usually require smaller dosages than those given intramuscularly or subcutaneously. Furthermore, because food in the GI tract can interfere with the absorption of drugs, orally and rectally administered drugs tend to be absorbed the slowest and often require higher dosages.

ORAL DOSAGES

Almost 90% of all prescribed medications are administered orally. Tablets and capsules are the most commonly prescribed oral drugs, but some medications are administered orally in the form of liquids, lozenges, and powders or granules. Determination of the drug dosage of an oral medication varies according to its dosage form.

Whole Tablets and Capsules

The drug forms shown in Figure 11-1 must be administered in their entirety. Since the quantity of these drug forms is fixed, the dosage amount must be one or more tablets or capsules. If a smaller dosage is required, the drug must either be obtained from a pharmacist as a tablet with a smaller dose or in a different dosage form, such as a liquid or a scored tablet.

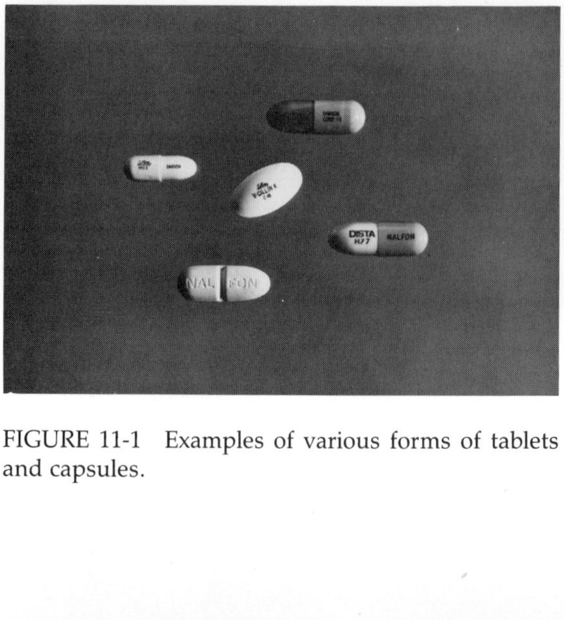

FIGURE 11-1 Examples of various forms of tablets and capsules.

Example A prescription asks for Compazine, 5 mg po.

Only 10-mg tablets of this antiemetic are immediately available, but 5 mg tablets can be obtained from a pharmacist. Therefore, the correct dosage can be procured and then administered.

Example A prescription asks for phenobarbital, 7.5 mg po. This barbiturate comes in 15-, 30-, 60-, and 100-mg tablets. However, the drug is also available in an elixir containing 4 mg/ml. The medication therefore can be given as a liquid but not as a tablet.

Many adults can only swallow a tablet smaller than 1.5 c in diameter. The "OOO" capsule, which is 3 cm long and 1 cm wide, is now seldom used. (See Figure 11-2.) A client should not be required to swallow more tablets than necessary, although sometimes large amounts of a drug are necessary in order to achieve the desired effect. To determine the number of tablets or capsules required, a proportion (see Chapter 9) is set up between the *available ratio* (available dose) and the *desired ratio* (desired dose) and then solved for the required number of tablets or capsules.

Example

- *Desired*—Aspirin, 15 gr po
- *Available*—Aspirin tablets containing 5 gr each

Available ratio	*Desired ratio*
$\frac{5\text{ gr}}{1\text{ tablet}}$	$\frac{15\text{ gr}}{x\text{ tablets}}$

Cross multiply:

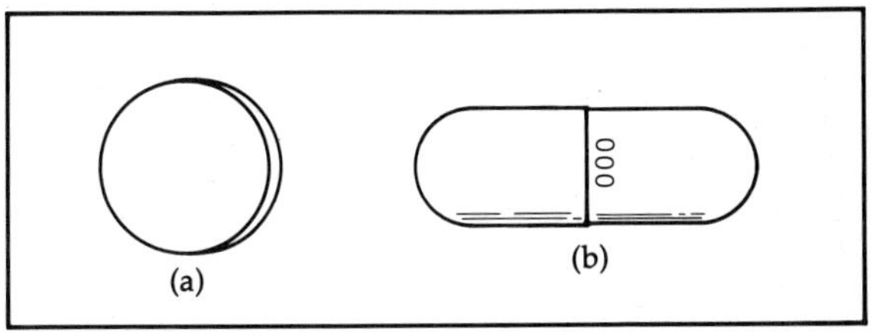

FIGURE 11-2 (*a*) 1.5-mm tablets (actual size). (*b*) OOO capsule.

$$5x = 15$$
$$x = 15 \div 5$$
$$x = 3 \text{ tablets of aspirin}$$

Remember The numerators of both ratios must have the same unit (gr) as must the denominators (tablets).

Shortcut When *more than one* tablet is required, the dosage can be calculated faster by simply *dividing* the *desired* dose by the *available* dose.

Example

- *Desired*—Gantrisin, 2000 mg po
- *Available*—Gantrisin tablets containing 500 mg each

Proportion method

$$\frac{500\text{ mg}}{1\text{ tablet}} = \frac{2000\text{ mg}}{x\text{ tablets}}$$
$$500x = 2000$$
$$x = 2000 \div 500$$
$$x = 4 \text{ tablets of 500 mg each}$$

Shortcut Method

$$\frac{\text{Desired dose}}{\text{Available dose}} = \frac{2000\text{ mg}}{500\text{-mg tablet}}$$
$$= 4 \text{ tablets of Gantrisin}$$

Notes The above prescription for Gantrisin could have been written as 2 g instead of 2000 mg.

Both methods require that the *available dose* and the *desired dose* have the *same unit of measure.* (See Chapter 11, if you need assistance in converting from one unit of measure to another.)

EXERCISE A

How many tablets are required for the following dosages?

1. *Desired:* Seconal, 100 mg po. *Available:* 50-mg capsules.
2. *Desired:* Aspirin, gr viiss po. *Available:* gr iiss tablets.

3. *Desired:* Atropine sulfate, gr $\frac{1}{150}$ po. *Available:* gr $\frac{1}{300}$ tablets.
4. *Desired:* Digitoxin, 0.2 mg po. *Available:* 0.05-mg tablets.
5. *Desired:* Codeine sulfate, gr ss po. *Available:* 15-mg tablets.

Liquids and Scored Tablets

The proportion method can be used to determine *divided doses* of liquids and scored tablets for oral administration. Scored tablets are compressed drug forms that have indented lines through the center and can be safely broken along the line to yield half of the tablet's dosage. For example, a 10-mg tablet can be broken in half to yield 5 mg in each half (see Figure 11-3). One of the half tablets can then be given for a desired dose of 5 mg.

When the dosage of a liquid medication is ordered by volume no calculation is necessary.

Examples

Milk of magnesia, ʒ iss po
Maalox, 30 ml po
Donnatol, 5 ml po
Tincture of opium, gtt v in 30 ml water po

The volume can be measured with a medicine glass, a syringe, or a dropper. For dosages smaller than 5 ml a syringe or a dropper should be used, but for 5 ml (1 dram) or more a medicine glass can be utilized (see Figure 11-4). When using a medicine glass the following rules should be observed in order to ensure an accurate measurement:

1. The medicine glass should be placed on a *level surface,* such as a counter top, to prevent any tilting of the glass.

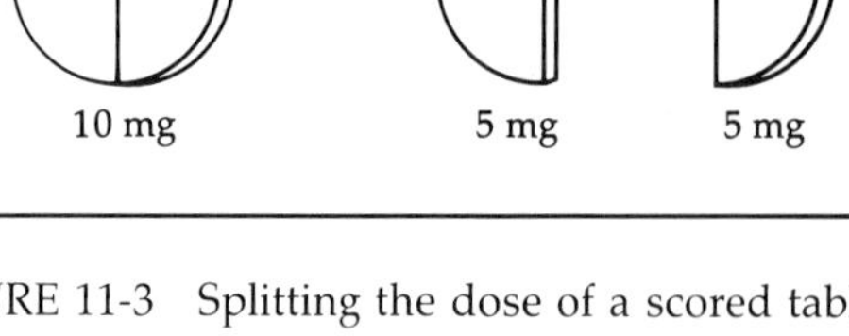

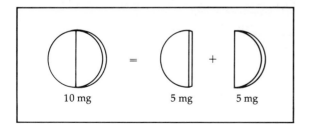

FIGURE 11-3 Splitting the dose of a scored tablet.

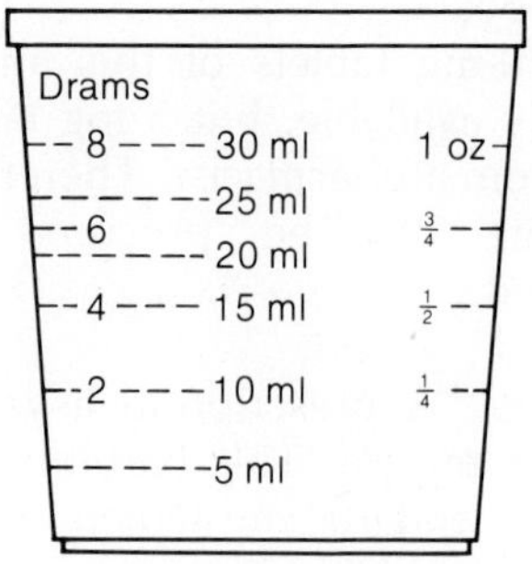

FIGURE 11-4 A medicine glass.

2. The observer should be positioned directly *in front of* and *at eye level* with the medicine glass to avoid any parallax.
3. The dosage should be read at the *bottom* of the *meniscus* to prevent errors due to adhesion or cohesion of the liquid with the glass.

(The instructions for the use of a syringe are presented later in this chapter.)

The number of drops in 1 ml can vary greatly depending on the size of the opening (lumen) and the viscosity and temperature of the liquid. Medications that have a higher viscosity and are refrigerated create a larger drop. Consequently, drug companies frequently include a specially calibrated dropper with drugs that require this form of measurement. The medication should always be measured with its accompanying dropper. If for some reason the dropper is unusable, the pharmacist should be informed of the drug's name and dosage form and the pharmacist will provide a new dropper.

When liquid medications are ordered by dosage instead of volume, a calculation is required. The drug label will indicate the amount of drug in a specific volume—for example, 10 mg/ml or 5 mg/4 ml. This represents the *available ratio* and the proportion method can be used to determine the volume of the desired dose.

Example

- *Desired*—Sudafed, 60 mg po

- *Available*—Pseudoephedrine hydrochloride (Sudafed) syrup, 6 mg/ml

Available ratio $\frac{6\text{ mg}}{1\text{ ml}}$ *Desired ratio* $\frac{60\text{ mg}}{x\text{ ml}}$

Cross multiply:

$$6x = 60$$
$$x = 60 \div 6$$
$$x = 10 \text{ ml of pseudoephedrine hydrochloride}$$

Shortcut The dosage can be calculated faster by simply *dividing* the *desired* dose *by* the *available dose* and then *multiplying by* the *volume* of the available dose.

$$\frac{\text{Desired dose}}{\text{Available dose}} \times \text{Volume (of available dose)} = \text{Amount to administer}$$

$$\frac{60\text{ mg}}{6\text{ mg}} \times 1\text{ ml} = 10\text{ ml of pseudoephedrine hydrochloride}$$

Example

- *Desired*—Erythromycin, 200 mg po
- *Available*—Erythromycin suspension, 25 mg/ml

Proportion method

$$\frac{25\text{ mg}}{1\text{ ml}} = \frac{200\text{ mg}}{x\text{ ml}}$$
$$25x = 200$$
$$x = 200 \div 25$$
$$x = 8 \text{ ml of erythromycin suspension}$$

Shortcut method

$$\frac{200\text{ mg}}{25\text{ mg}} \times 1\text{ ml} = 8\text{ ml of erythromycin suspension}$$

Remember Both methods of determining the number of milliliters to administer require that the *ratios* have the *same unit of measure* (mg/ml).

Measuring in Units and Milliequivalents

Although the metric and apothecary systems of measuring medications by weight and/or volume are accurate enough for most drugs, some medications require more precision than these systems can provide. Therefore some drugs, such as penicillin, are measured in *units* (U) of activity. Even other drugs require such minute quantities to create the desired effect that they must be measured by the chemical-combining power of the drug. Therefore, medications, such as potassium chloride, are measured in *milliequivalents* (mEq).

Whether a medication is ordered in units or milliequivalents, the proportion and/or the shortcut methods can be used to determine the desired dosage.

Example

- *Desired*—Penicillin G, 200,000 U po
- *Available*—Penicillin G, 50,000 U/tablet

Proportion method

$$\frac{50{,}000\text{ U}}{1\text{ tablet}} = \frac{200{,}000\text{ U}}{x\text{ tablets}}$$
$$50{,}000x = 200{,}000$$
$$x = 200{,}000 \div 50{,}000$$
$$x = 4 \text{ tablets of penicillin G}$$

Shortcut method

$$\frac{200{,}000\text{U}}{50{,}000\text{U}} \times 1\text{ tablet} = 4\text{ tablets of penicillin G}$$

Example

- *Desired*—Potassium triplex, 30 mEq po
- *Available*—Potassium triplex, 15 mEq/5 ml

Proportion method

$$\frac{15\text{ mEq}}{5\text{ ml}} = \frac{30\text{ mEq}}{x\text{ ml}}$$
$$15x = 150$$
$$x = 150 \div 15$$
$$x = 10 \text{ ml of potassium triplex/18}$$

Shortcut method

$$\frac{30\text{ mEq}}{15\text{ mEq}} \times 5\text{ ml} = 10\text{ ml of potassium triplex}$$

Exercise B

Solve the following dosage problems.

1. *Desired:* Sudafed, 30 mg po. *Available:* Pseudoephedrine hydrochloride (Sudafed) syrup, 6 mg/ml.
2. *Desired:* Ampicillin, 500 mg po. *Available:* Ampicillin suspension, 250 mg/5 ml.
3. *Desired:* Phenobarbital, 30 mg po. *Available:* Phenobarbital elixir, 4 mg/ml.
4. *Desired:* Erythromycin, 600 mg po. *Available:* Erythromycin suspension, 0.2 g/5 ml.
5. *Desired:* Potassium chloride, 20 mEq po. *Available:* Kaon (potassium chloride) elixir, 40 mEq/30 ml.
6. *Desired:* Penicillin G, 1,000,000 U po. *Available:* Penicillin G, 500,000 U/tablet.
7. *Desired:* Mycostatin, 400,000 U po. *Available:* Nystatin (Mycostatin) oral suspension, 100,000 U/ml.
8. *Desired:* Terpin hydrate with codeine, gr $\frac{1}{6}$ po. *Available:* Elixir of terpin hydrate with codeine, 2 mg/ml.

INJECTABLES

Although oral drugs are the most frequently prescribed, injectable medications are often required for clinic and hospitalized clients. Whether the site of injection is just under the skin (intradermal), in subcutaneous tissue (subc), or into a muscle mass (IM), the method of calculating the dosage is similar to determining liquid oral dosages.

Since injectable medications are administered into tissues they are prepared under sterile conditions. Years ago, injectable medications were prepared from tablets in a very time-consuming process. Now, they can be obtained in four forms. Most injectables are available as solutions packaged in single-dose sterile ampules or sterile multidose vials (see Figure 11-5). However, since some drugs deteriorate quickly in solution, these drugs arrive as dry powders in sterile ampules or vials. (See Chapter 12 for information on dosage forms.) A number of frequently used medications, such as penicillin, are available in prefilled disposable syringes.

Prepared Injectable Solutions

Either the proportion or shortcut method can be used to determine the amount of injectable to be administered. There are, however, some variations, depending on the dosage and its form. Determining the dosage of *prepared injectable solutions* is the same as calculating the dosage of liquid oral medications. The label on the ampule or vial will indicate the quantity per volume.

Example

- *Desired*—Demerol, 35 mg. 1 IM
- *Available*—Demerol, 25 mg/ml

Proportion method

$$\frac{25\text{ mg}}{1\text{ ml}} = \frac{35\text{ mg}}{x\text{ ml}}$$
$$25x = 35$$
$$x = 35 \div 25$$
$$x = 1.4\text{ ml of Demerol 25 mg/ml}$$

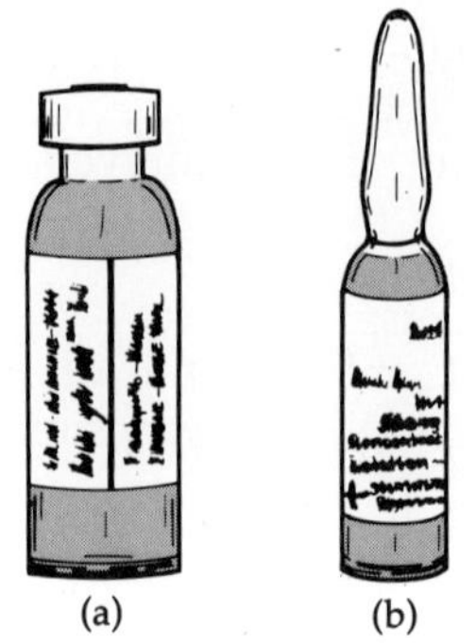

FIGURE 11-5 (*a*) Ampule. (*b*) Vial.

Shortcut method

$$\frac{35 \text{ mg}}{25 \text{ mg}} \times 1 \text{ ml} = 1.4 \text{ ml of Demerol}$$

Once the dosage has been calculated the next step is to prepare the syringe. A 2.5-ml syringe is calibrated for each 0.1 ml, as well as minims, and most 5 ml-syringes are calibrated for each 0.2 ml. However, larger capacity syringes, such as 10, 20, and 50 ml, are generally only calibrated for each 0.5 ml. Consequently, the selection of the syringe size is important in determining the correct dosage. In the above example, a 2.5-ml or 5-ml syringe could have been used. Figure 11-6 shows a 2.5-ml syringe filled to the 1.4-ml mark.

Example

- *Desired*—Lasix, 10 mg. 1 IM
- *Available*—Lasix, 20 mg/2 ml

Proportion method

$$\frac{20 \text{ mg}}{2 \text{ ml}} = \frac{10 \text{ mg}}{x \text{ ml}}$$
$$20x = 20$$
$$x = 1 \text{ ml of Lasix 20 mg/2 ml}$$

Short-cut method

$$\frac{10 \text{ mg}}{20 \text{ mg}} \times 2 \text{ ml} = 1 \text{ ml of Lasix}$$

Example

- *Desired*—Procaine penicillin, 400,000 U IM
- *Available*—Procaine penicillin, 300,000 U/ml

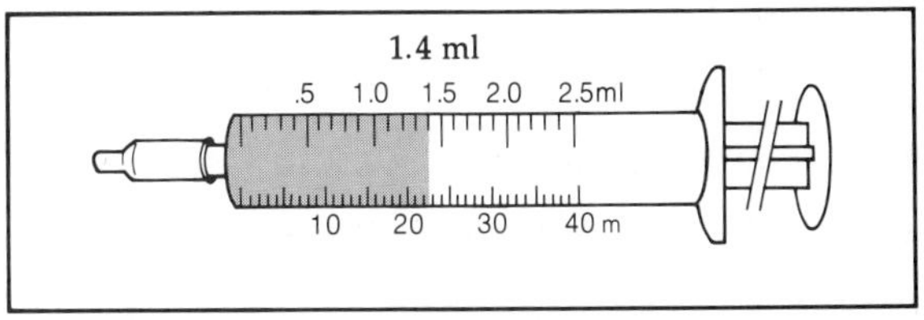

FIGURE 11-6 A 2.5-ml syringe filled to the 1.4-ml mark.

Proportion method

$$\frac{300{,}000 \text{ U}}{1 \text{ ml}} = \frac{400{,}000 \text{ U}}{x \text{ ml}}$$
$$300{,}000x = 400{,}000$$
$$x = 400{,}000 \div 300{,}000$$
$$x = 1.33 \quad or \quad 1.3 \text{ ml of procaine penicillin}$$

Shortcut method

$$\frac{400{,}000 \text{ U}}{300{,}000 \text{ U}} \times 1 \text{ ml} = 1.3 \text{ ml of procaine penicillin}$$

Note In this case a syringe calibrated for each 0.1 ml must be used.

Since most small syringes are only calibrated in tenths of a milliliter, the dosage must be rounded off to the nearest tenth. If the hundredth number is *between* 0 and 4, the number is rounded off to the *next lowest* tenth, as in the preceding example. If, however, the hundredth number is *between* 5 and 9, the answer is rounded off to the *next highest* tenth.

Examples

If the answer is 1.33 ml, it is rounded to 1.3 ml.
If the answer is 0.78 ml, it is rounded to 0.8 ml.
If the answer is 2.06 ml, it is rounded to 2.1 ml.
If the answer is 1.42 ml, it is rounded to 1.4 ml.

EXERCISE C

1. *Desired:* Demerol, 30 mg IM.
   Available: Meperidine hydrochloride (Demerol), 50 mg/ml.
2. *Desired:* Gentamycin, 70 mg IM.
   Available: Gentamycin sulfate, 40 mg/ml.
3. *Desired:* Procaine penicillin, 750,000 U IM.
   Available: Procaine penicillin, 300,000 U/ml.
4. *Desired:* Lanoxin, 0.05 mg IM.
   Available: Digoxin ((Lanoxin), 0.2 mg/2 ml.
5. *Desired:* Morphine, gr $\frac{1}{4}$ IM.
   Available: Morphine sulfate, 10 mg/ml.

Solutions of Less Than One Milliliter

Medications that require small, exact dosages are measured with special syringes. The total capacity of *insulin* and *TB* syringes is 1 ml. An insulin syringe is calibrated in 100 or 40 subdivisions (see Figure 11-7) and is so called because insulin is available in 40 U/ml and 100 U/ml. It is therefore important to select a syringe with the correct scale.

Example

- *Desired*—NPH insulin, 25 U (H)
- *Available*—NPH insulin, 40 U/ml

If the U-40 scale on an insulin syringe is used, it is not necessary to calculate the dosage, only to fill the syringe to the correct marking (see Figure 11-8).

Example

- *Desired*—PZI insulin, 55 U
- *Available*—PZI insulin, 100 U/ml

In this case, a U-100 syringe is required and is filled to the 55 mark.

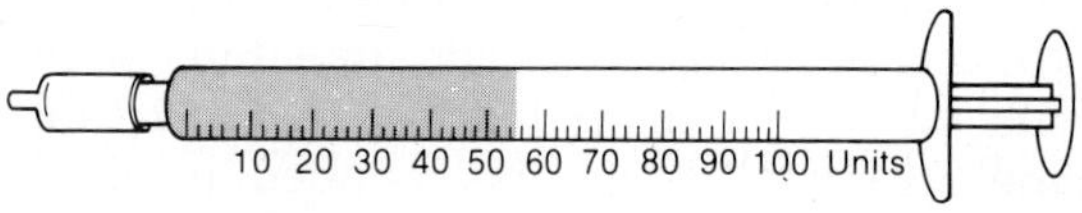

Although it is preferable to use an insulin syringe, situations may arise when only 2.5-ml syringes are available. If this is the case the insulin dosage must be determined in either milliliters or minims. As the millimeter scale has 10 subdivisions and the minim scale 16, the minim scale is preferred.

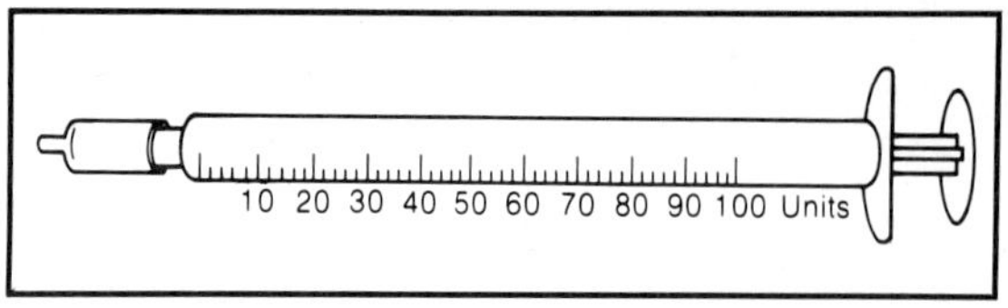

FIGURE 11-7 A U-100 insulin syringe.

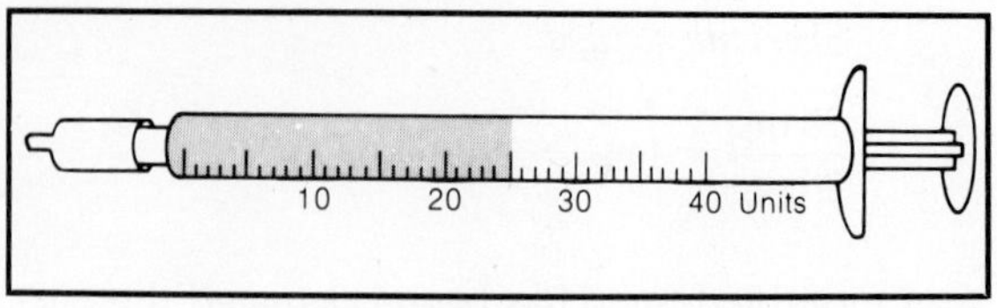

FIGURE 11-8 A U-40 insulin syringe filled to the 25-U mark.

Example

- *Desired*—Regular insulin, 15 U (H)
- *Available*—Regular insulin, 40 U/ml

Proportion method

$$\frac{40\ \text{U}}{16\ \text{♏}} = \frac{15\ \text{U}}{x\ \text{♏}}$$

$$40x = 240$$

$$x = 240 \div 40$$

$$x = 6\ \text{♏ of insulin}$$

Note 16 minim/ml should be used when calculating injectable dosages of less than 1 ml, such as insulin.

The *TB* syringe was originally designed for skin tests to detect tuberculin reactivity and was made of glass. Since the tuberculin bacillus cannot be destroyed by autoclaving the glass syringes, the title *TB syringes* was allocated so that they would not be used for anything else. *Glass TB syringes should not be used for anything except TB skin testing.* TB syringes, which have 100 subdivisions in 1 ml, are now available in a disposable form and are useful for measuring small dosages, since they have never been used for the tuberculin bacillus. When insulin syringes are not available, but disposable TB syringes are, the latter can be used if the needle is changed to an appropriate size.

Example

- *Desired*—Regular insulin, 30 U (H)
- *Available*—Regular insulin, 40 U/ml

Since 1 ml (= 100 subdivisions on disposable TB syringe) contains 40 U of insulin, the *available ratio* consists of dividing 40 U by 100.

Proportion method

$$\frac{40\text{ U}}{100\text{ subs}} = \frac{30\text{ U}}{x\text{ sub}}$$
$$40x = 3000$$
$$x = 3000 \div 40$$
$$x = 75\text{ subdivisions of insulin}$$

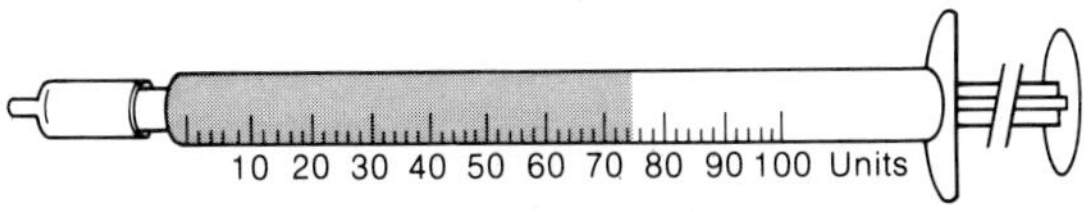

EXERCISE D

Solve the following problems and shade the correct dosage on each syringe.

1. *Desired:* Regular insulin, 25 U (H). *Available:* Regular insulin, 40 U/ml.
   (a) Administer with an insulin syringe calibrated for U-40 insulin.

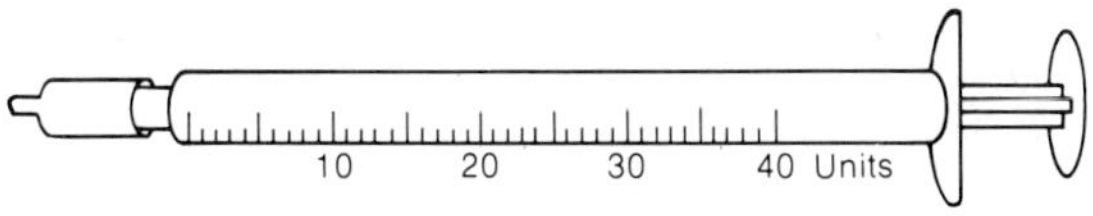

   (b) Administer with a disposable TB syringe.

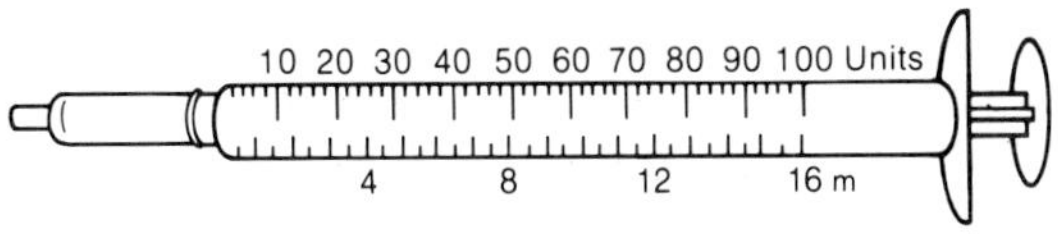

   (c) Administer with a 2.5-ml syringe.

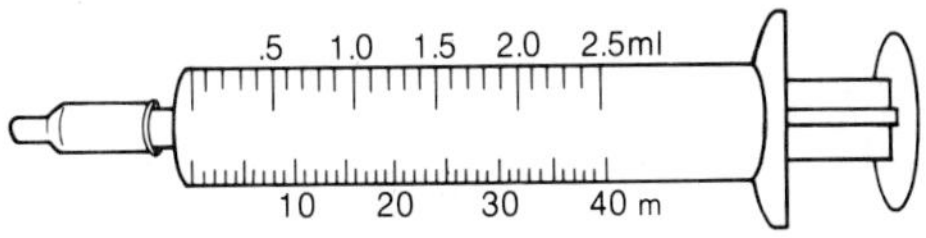

2. *Desired:* PZI insulin, 37 U (H). *Available:* PZI insulin, 100 U/ml.
   (a) Administer with a U-100 insulin syringe.

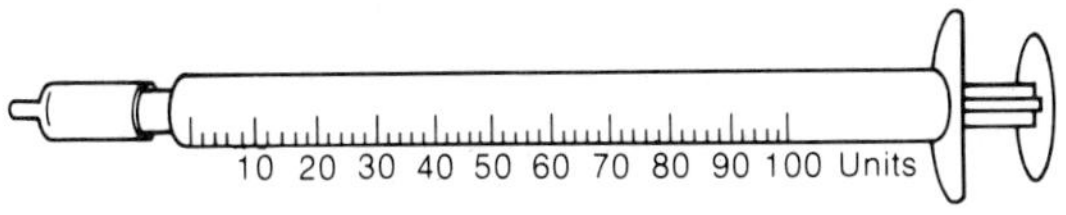

   (b) Administer with a 2.5-ml syringe.

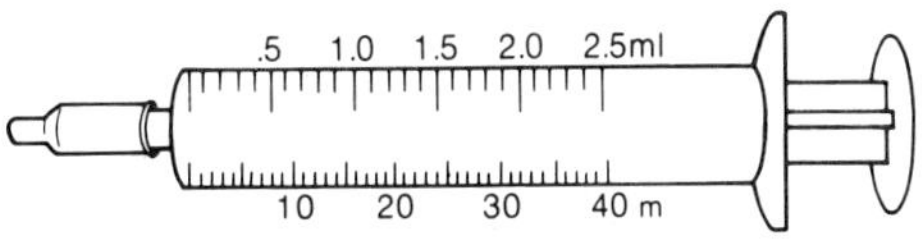

3. *Desired:* NPH insulin, 60 U (H). *Available:* NPH insulin, 100 U/ml.
   (a) Administer with an insulin syringe calibrated for U-100 insulin.

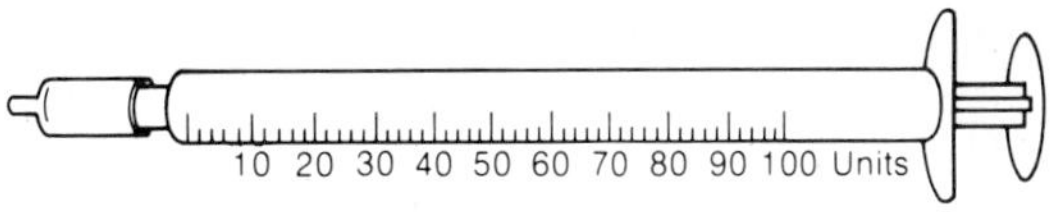

   (b) Administer with a 2.5-ml syringe.

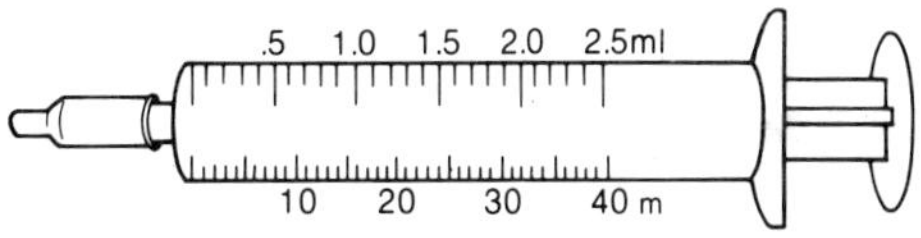

Dosages of Dry Injectables

Some injectable medications are packaged as powders or crystals in sterile containers because they tend to deteriorate rapidly in solution. The dry drug is made into a sterile solution just prior to administration in a process called **reconstitution**. Most of these drugs are dissolved in either sterile saline or sterile water; however, some require a special diluent which comes packaged with the drug. The type of diluent is specified on the directions that accompany the drug.

The volume of fluid used in reconstituting the drug varies according to the site of injection and the characteristics of the drug. Full details of the amounts of fluid that injection sites can safely accept are presented in Chapter 14—note, however, that *intramuscular* injections should be 1 ml or less whenever possible. When the drug is very irritating to body tissues, the medication should be prepared in as much solution as the injection site can safely tolerate. Pharmaceutical companies often include directions that state the recommended amount of fluid for each route of administration.

The quantity of fluid that is added to a powdered medication does not always create the same quantity of solution. In some cases, the resulting solution is greater than the amount of diluent added because the dry medication also occupies space. This is called the **displacement factor**. For example, when 1 g of carbenicillin (Geopen) 1 is diluted with 3.6 ml of sterile water, the reconstituted solution is equal to 4.0 ml—the dissolved drug expanded the solution by 0.4 ml. (See Figure 11-9.) Pharmaceutical companies often specify the strength of the reconstituted solution when the recommended amount of diluent is added.

In summary, the following information is required when reconstituting a dry injectable:

1. Type of diluent
2. Amount of diluent
3. Strength of reconstituted solution

The recommended reconstitution directions from the pharmaceutical company may be on the drug monograph inserted in the drug package. If the dry medication is not accompanied by pharmaceutical directions, a pharmacist can supply the information.

Example

- *Desired*—Geopen, 500 mg IM
- *Available*—Carbenicillin (Geopen), 1 g in a 5-ml vial
- *Directions*—Add 3.6 ml of sterile water, which yields 4.0 ml of solution. The strength of the resulting solution is 1 g/4.0 ml.

Proportion method

$$\frac{1000\text{ mg}}{4.0\text{ ml}} = \frac{500\text{ mg}}{x\text{ ml}}$$

$$1000x = 2000$$

$$x = 2000 \div 1000$$

$$x = 2.0\text{ ml of Geopen}$$

Note Since both numerators must have the same unit of measure, the available dosages' units (grams) was changed to the desired dosages' units (milligrams).

Example

- *Desired*—Penicillin G, 600,000 U IM
- *Available*—Potassium penicillin G, 1,000,000 U in a 10-ml vial
- *Directions*—Add 1.6 ml of sterile water, which yields 2 ml of solution. The strength of the resulting solution is 1,000,000 U/2 ml.

Proportion method

$$\frac{1{,}000{,}000\text{ U}}{2\text{ ml}} = \frac{600{,}000\text{ U}}{x\text{ ml}}$$

$$1{,}000{,}000\,x = 1{,}200{,}000$$

$$x = 1{,}200{,}000 \div 1{,}000{,}000$$

$$x = 1.2\text{ ml of penicillin G}$$

Occasionally, the dry medication will not dissolve readily in the recommended amount of diluent, therefore a few more minims should be added. The volume of the resulting solution can then be measured in a syringe.

In both of the preceding examples the drugs were in multidose vials. The medication that is not used (500 mg Geopen and 400,000 U penicillin G, respectively) can be stored in a refrigerator and used at a later date. However, because these drugs tend to deteriorate after reconstitution, the vials should be labeled with the time and date the drug was reconstituted. For example, Geopen deteriorates in 72 hours and should not be administered if more than 72 hours have elapsed after reconstitution. The strength of the reconstituted solution should also be marked on the vial (that is, Geopen 500 mg/ml). If a reconstituted vial is *not labeled* with the time, date, and strength of the solution, it should *not be used.*

EXERCISE E

In the following problems determine (a) the strength of the resulting solution and (b) the dosage.

1. *Desired:* Geopen, 250 mg IM. *Available:* Carbenicillin (Geopen), 1 g in a 5-ml vial. *Directions:* Add 3.6 ml of sterile water, which yields 4.0 ml of solution.
2. *Desired:* Penicillin, 300,000 U IM. *Available:* Penicillin G, 1,000,000 U in a 10-ml vial. *Directions:* Add 4.5 ml of sterile water, which yields 5 ml of solution.
3. *Desired:* Ampicillin, 250 mg IM. *Available:* Sodium ampicillin, 1 g in a 5-ml vial. *Directions:* Add 3.4 ml of sterile water, which yields 4 ml of solution.

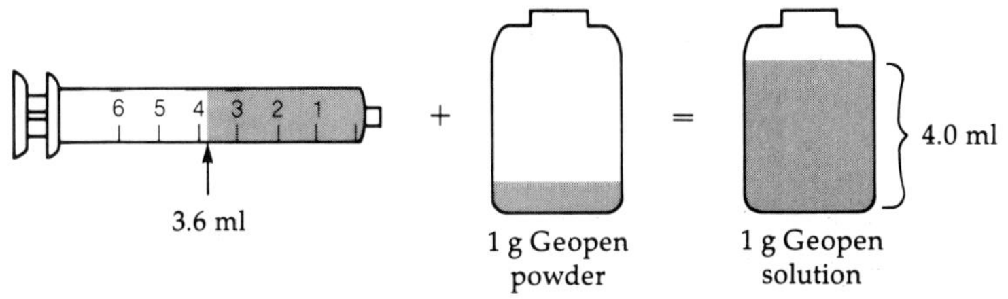

FIGURE 11-9 Reconstitution of 1 g of Geopen.

4. *Desired:* Ancef, 500 mg IM. *Available:* Cefazolin sodium (Ancef), 1 gm in a multidose vial. *Directions:* Add 3.0 ml of sterile water, which yields 3.0 ml of solution.
5. *Desired:* Ritalin, 5 mg IM. *Available:* Methylphenidate hydrochloride (Ritalin), 100 mg in a 10-ml vial. *Directions:* Add 10 ml of sterile aqueous solvent, which yields 10 ml of solution.

INTRAVENOUS FLUIDS AND MEDICATIONS

Intravenous (IV) medications are most commonly given to correct electrolyte imbalances, to combat systemic infections, or to treat disorders. The drug can be administered in the following ways:

1. *IV bolus or IV push*—Injected directly into a vein
2. *Continuous drip*—Added to the bottle of IV fluids being administered
3. *Volume control set*—Added periodically to a separate IV fluid chamber
4. *Piggyback setup*—Added to a separate fluid container that is then intermittently attached to a continuous IV set

See Chapter 14 for detailed information on IV equipment. All of these methods require some variation in the preparation of medication dosage and in the regulation of the IV fluid being given. Irritating drugs can cause damage to the vein, so they are prepared in more dilute strengths than injectable medications. IV drugs also cause stronger and more immediate effects than drugs given by other routes.

IV Bolus

The preparation of a drug bolus is similar to that of injectable medications except that it is usually more dilute and is administered over a period of time. For example, Ancef is often given as 225 mg/1.0 ml IM, but the recommended IV strength is only 50 mg/1.0 ml injected into the vein over a period of at least 3 to 5 minutes. (The preferred method is to give the Ancef in 100 ml of fluid over a period of 30 minutes. This strength is 5 mg/ml.) The recommended strength can be found on the drug container or in the drug insert. Many adverse reactions can occur if the drug is too strong.

The rate at which an IV bolus is given is just as important as the drug's strength. Since the effects of the drug occur within seconds, toxic and other adverse reactions may result if the drug is administered too quickly. For example, phenytoin (Dilantin) may be given via an IV bolus to a convulsing client, but the rate should not exceed 50 mg/min. If this rate is exceeded, the client may experience severe bradycardia, hypotension, or both.

Drugs that are highly protein-bound must be given rapidly to ensure an immediate effect. The antihypertensive drug diazoxide (Hyperstat) must be administered via an IV bolus in 30 seconds or less because the drug is more than 90% bound to the blood's circulating protein.

Only physicians and certified IV nurses should administer an IV bolus. The nurses caring for the client are responsible for preparing the appropriate drug strength and monitoring the client's response to the drug. The intended and untoward responses to IV bolus drugs can be found in the drug insert or in the drug monograph.

Calculating Continuous IV Drip Rates

Because of the numerous problems involved in giving an IV drug bolus, most IV medications are administered in an even more dilute form over a longer period of time. For example, electrolytes and vitamins are often added to the client's continuous IV container. The regulation of IV fluids, as well as IV fluids with drug additives, is calculated on the basis of the number of drops per minute (gtt/min). Since the size of a drop will vary according to the size of the opening, the IV administration set must be checked to determine the number of drops in each milliliter. The drops per milliliter (gtt/ml) varies between different IV administration sets and can range from 10 to 60 gtt/ml.

Once the number of drops per minute has been calculated, the next step is to determine the volume of fluid and the time period over which it is to be administered. The physician's prescription will often state the desired time period over which the volume of fluid is to be given.

Examples of typical IV orders are as follows:

1. Give 1000 ml of 5% D/W with Berocca C q8h IV.
2. Give 500 ml of 5% D/W with 20 mEq potassium chloride (KCL) q12h IV.
3. IV orders—1000 ml q12h, 1000 ml Ringer's lactate, 1000 ml 5% D/W with MVI
4. Give 50 ml/hr. Alternate 500 ml 5% D/W with 500 ml NS.
5. Daily IV's—1000 ml 5% D/W with 10 ml MVI and 40 mEq KCL, 2000 ml 5% D in 0.45 NS.
6. IV of 5% D/W to KVO.

The first four examples specify the time period. In the fifth example it is assumed that the fluid will be given over a 24-hour period. Since continuous IV fluids should be given at a constant rate, the nurse should administer 1000 ml q8h until the physician clarifies the order. In the sixth example *KVO* means *keep the vein open*. It is used when clients require only intermittent IV medication and instructs the administrator not to puncture the vein each time the medication is administered. Each agency has its own protocol for the KVO drip rate, but the drip rate must be sufficiently rapid to keep the vein open. Five minidrops per minute (5 ml/hr) is usually adequate. The vein of an infant can usually be kept open with as little as 2 ml/hr.

In summary, the following information is needed before the drip rate of a continuous IV can be determined:

1. Calibration size of the IV administration set (gtt/ml)
2. Type of fluid in which to administer the medication
3. Volume of fluid to be administered
4. Time period over which the fluid is to be administered

The volume of fluid is then converted to drops and the hours converted to minutes.

Example Give 1000 ml 5% D/W q8h. The IV administration set is calibrated for 15 gtt/ml.

First, 1000 ml must be converted to drops (gtt).

Proportion method

$$\frac{15\text{ gtt}}{1\text{ ml}} = \frac{x\text{ gtt}}{1000\text{ ml}}$$
$$x = 1000 \times 15$$
$$x = 15{,}000\text{ gtt}$$

Shortcut

$$\frac{15\text{ gtt}}{1\text{ ml}} \times 1000\text{ ml} = 15{,}000\text{ gtt}$$

Next, hours (q8h) must be converted to minutes. Since there are 60 minutes in 1 hour, there are 480 minutes in 8 hours.

$$60\text{ minutes} \times 8\text{ hours} = 480\text{ minutes}$$

Finally, the number of drops are divided by the number of minutes to give the number of drops per minute.

$$15{,}000\text{ gtt} \div 480\text{ minutes} = 31\text{ gtt/min.}$$

The answer of 31.25 was rounded off to 31.

Therefore the number of drops per minute can be calculated as follows:

$$\frac{\text{Desired ml} \times \text{gtt/ml of IV set}}{\text{Desired hr} \times 60\text{ min.}} = \frac{\text{Total gtt}}{\text{Total min.}} = \text{gtt/min.}$$

This method requires the use of large numbers and it not only takes longer to divide large numbers, but there is also a chance of error in computation. Another way of obtaining the drip rate without using large numbers is the following:

1. Find the number of milliliters to be given in each hour.

$$\frac{1000\text{ ml}}{8\text{ hr}} = 125\text{ ml/hr}$$

2. Convert the number of milliliters (per hour) to drops by multiplying the milliliters by the drop calibration of the IV set.

$$125\text{ ml} \times 15\text{ gtt} = 1875\text{ gtt}$$

3. Divide the number of milliliters (per hour) by 60 minutes (1 hour).

$$\frac{1875\text{ gtt}}{60\text{ min.}} = 31.25 \quad or \quad 31\text{ gtt/min.}$$

This alternative method of determining the number of drops per minute can be calculated as follows:

$$\frac{\text{Desired ml/hr}}{60\text{ min.}} \times \text{gtt/ml of IV set} = \text{gtt/min.}$$

Minidrip sets

Drip rate calculations are simplified when a minidrip set is used. This set is calibrated for 60 gtt/ml, and since there are 60 minutes in an hour, the two factors cancel each other out. Therefore, the number of desired milliliters per hour is the same as the number of drops per minute. Thus,

$$\text{ml/hr} = \text{gtt/min.}$$

only if a 60 gtt/min IV administration set is used.

Example Give 100 ml of 5% D/W each hour. The IV administration set is calibrated for 60 gtt/ml.

Proportion method

$$\frac{100\text{ ml} \times 60\text{ gtt/ml}}{1\text{ hr} \times 60\text{ min./hr}} = \frac{6000\text{ gtt}}{60\text{ min.}} = 100\text{ gtt/min.}$$

Alternative method

$$\frac{100\text{ ml}}{{}_1\cancel{60}\text{ min.}} \times \cancel{60}^1\text{ gtt/ml} = 100\text{ gtt/min.}$$

Therefore 100 ml/hr = 100 gtt/min.

Volume control sets

Volume control sets (see Figure 11-10) contain a small fluid chamber within the IV tubing. This setup is useful for neonates, infants, and other clients who require small volumes of IV fluids. When the small fluid chamber is filled with the required volume of fluid, the upper clamp is closed. The small fluid chamber will hold 100 ml or more and is calibrated in 1.0 ml. The most commonly used sets (Buretrol and Soluset) have drip chambers calibrated for 60 gtt/ml. If the desired number of milliliters per hour is not stated in the IV order, the nurse must first determine this volume and then calculate the drops per minute.

Example Give 750 ml of Ringer's lactate daily via Buretrol.

The desired number of milliliters per hour are:

$$\frac{750\text{ ml}}{24\text{ hr}} = 31\text{ ml/hr}$$

Since the set is calibrated for 60 gtt/ml, the drip rate is 31 gtt/min. The small fluid chamber is therefore filled to the 31 mark, care being taken to read the bottom of the meniscus.

IV pumps

The flow rates of all the IV administration sets presented thus far are adjusted by clamps and this procedure takes valuable nursing time. When IV pumps are used to regulate flow rates, the nurse simply sets the rate selector and the pump controls the rate automatically. Peristaltic and gravity pumps operate on a drops per minute basis but piston pumps control IV flow rates on the basis of milliliters per hour. The nurse should become familiar with the IV pump before using it for a client because the pump is a machine and can malfunction. Flow rates should be checked at least once every 8 hours to be sure that the pump is functioning properly and is delivering the desired rate.

Intermittent Infusions

Many IV drugs that do not require continuous infusion, are too dangerous to administer via an IV bolus. These drugs are administered inter-

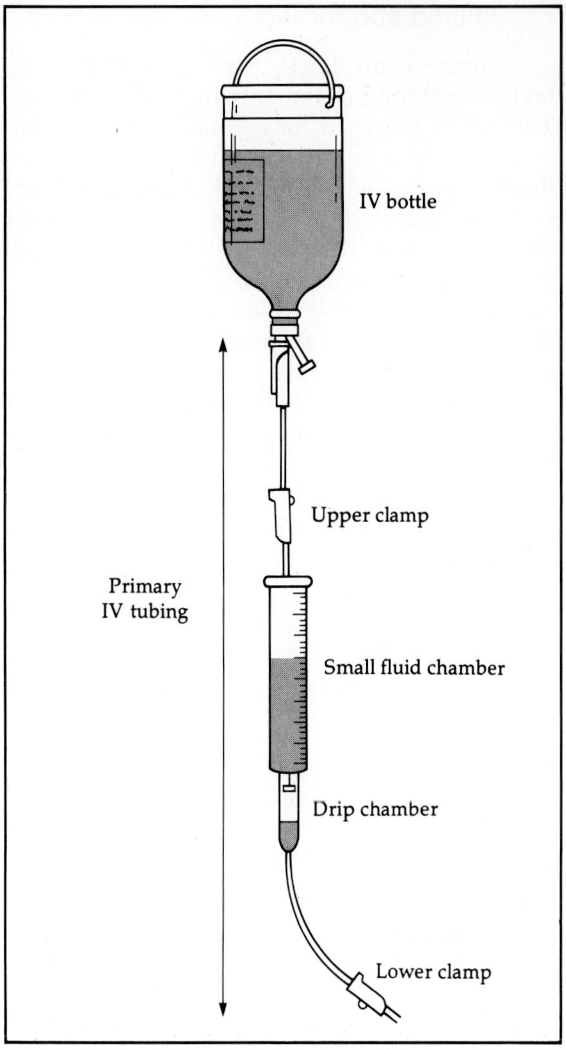

FIGURE 11-10 Volume control set.

mittently through a volume control set in the primary line, or via a secondary line, commonly called a **piggyback**. As with continuous infusions, certain information must be known before the drip rate can be determined:

1. Calibration size of the IV administration set (gtt/ml)
2. Type of fluid in which to administer the medication
3. Volume of fluid to be administered
4. Time period over which the fluid is to be administered

Intermittent IV orders, like all medication orders, indicate the drug name, route, and frequency of administration. In addition, the physician should specify the type of IV fluid, the volume of fluid, and the time interval over which the medication is to be administered. If any of this information is omitted or questionable, the nurse should consult the physician or pharmacist, follow the recommendations indicated on the drug insert, or follow agency protocol.

Some IV medications can be added to any type of IV fluid, but many drugs are either physically or chemically incompatible with certain solutions. For example, although most drugs can be administered in 5% D/W, diazepam (Valium) forms a precipitate when mixed with IV dextrose solutions. All known drug incompatibilities will be listed on the drug insert.

Most intermittent IV drugs are administered in 50 or 100 ml of IV fluid over a 30-minute time period, or longer, depending on the drug's irritating qualities and potential adverse reactions. Neonates, infants, and clients on a restricted fluid intake often receive 50 ml, whereas adults usually receive 100 ml. The volume of IV fluid should be equal to or greater than the recommended amount.

Although some IV drugs come already prepared as solutions, many antibiotics and other drugs must first be reconstituted before they can be added to the IV fluid for administration. It is important to follow the manufacturer's directions carefully for reconstituting the drug. Examples of recommended pharmaceutical directions are:

1. A reconstituted solution of 1 g cefazolin sodium (Ancef) should be administered in 100 ml or more of sodium chloride, 5% or 10% D/W, or lactated Ringer's solution.
2. A 2-ml solution of 300 g cimetidine hydrochloride (Tagamet) should be administered in 100 ml of 5% or 10% D/W, sodium chloride, or lactated Ringer's solution.
3. A reconstituted solution of 2 g carbenicillin should be further diluted in at least 20 ml of 5% D/W, sodium chloride, 5% D in 0.45 NS, or lactated Ringer's solution before administering.

The method of administration of intermittent IV medications varies according to the type of administration set used.

Piggyback or secondary lines

The piggyback is prepared by drawing the desired amount of drug into a sterile syringe and injecting it into a 50- or 100-ml container of IV fluid, using strict aseptic techniques. The container should be labeled with the time and date of administration and the type and quantity of drug. The line from this secondary container is injected into the client's primary line and the flow rate is adjusted accordingly.

Example Give clindamycin (Cleocin) 600 mg q6h IV in 100 ml 5% D/W over 30 minutes.

The secondary line is calibrated for 10 gtt/min.

Proportion method

$$\frac{100\text{ ml} \times 10\text{ gtt/min.}}{30\text{ min.}} = \frac{1000}{30}$$
$$= 33.3 \quad \textit{or} \quad 33\text{ gtt/min.}$$

Alternative method

$$\frac{100\text{ ml}}{30\text{ min.}} \times 10\text{ gtt/min.} = 3.3 \times 10$$
$$= 33.3 \quad \textit{or} \quad 33\text{ gtt/min.}$$

Example Give 250 mg of Geopen q6h IV in 100 ml 5% D/W. Carbenicillin (Geopen), 1 g of dry powder, is available and the IV administration set is calibrated for 10 gtt/ml.

Reconstitution of Geopen, yields a solution strength of 1000 mg/4.0 ml. Therefore,

$$\frac{1000\text{ mg}}{4.0\text{ ml}} = \frac{250\text{ mg}}{x\text{ ml}}$$
$$1000x = 1000$$
$$x = 1000 \div 1000$$
$$x = 1.0\text{ ml of Geopen}$$

The next step is to prepare a sterile syringe containing 1.0 ml Geopen and inject the medication into a 100-ml container of 5% D/W. Now, milliliters must be converted to drops:

$$\frac{10\text{ gtt}}{1\text{ ml}} = \frac{x\text{ gtt}}{100\text{ ml}}$$
$$x = 10 \times 100$$
$$x = 1000\text{ gtt of IV fluid}$$

Since the minutes are not indicated, 100 ml of medicated solution will be administered to the adult client over a 30-minute time period. Thus, the number of drops per minute is:

$$\frac{1000\text{ gtt}}{30\text{ min.}} = 33\text{ gtt/min.}$$

Volume control sets

Volume control sets are prepared by first drawing the required amount of drug into a syringe. Then both volume control clamps are then *closed* and the medication is injected through the port into the small fluid chamber. The upper clamp is *opened* and the drug is diluted with the desired amount of IV fluid. Then the upper clamp is *closed*. The bottom clamp can now be *opened* and the flow rate regulated. Because the client's continuous IV fluid is being used to dilute the intermittent drug, the nurse must be certain that the intermittent drug is not only compatible with the IV solution but also with any drugs that might have been previously added to the solution. The flow rate for volume control sets is not calculated in milliliters per hour since the medication is usually given over a shorter time period. In order to minimize errors, the alternative method of determining the drip rate is recommended.

Example Give cimetidine hydrochloride (Tagamet) 300 mg q6h IV via Soluset with 100 ml of solution. The continuous IV solution is 5% D/W and a Soluset is calibrated for 60 gtt/ml.

Assuming a 30-minute time period, minutes are first convested to hours because ml/hr = gtt/min. Hence,

$$\frac{60\text{ min.}}{1\text{ hr}} = \frac{30\text{ min.}}{x\text{ hr}}$$
$$60x = 30$$
$$x = 0.5\text{ hr}$$

Substituting in the formula:

$$\frac{100\text{ ml}}{0.5\text{ hr}} = 200\text{ gtt/min.}$$

The same answer is obtained by the alternative method:

Alternative method

$$\frac{100\text{ ml}}{30\text{ min}} \times 60\text{ gtt/ml} = 200\text{ gtt/min.}$$

Example Give Ancef 500 mg q6h IV via Buretrol in 50 ml IV fluid. Cefazolin sodium (Ancef), 500 mg dry powder in 10-ml vial, is available and a Buretrol is calibrated for 60 gtt/ml.

The first step is to reconstitute the Ancef with 2 ml diluent, which yields a solution strength of 500 mg/2.2 ml. Next, 2.2 ml of this solution is drawn into a sterile syringe and injected into the Buretrol chamber, which is filled to the 50-ml mark. The flow rate can then be determined as follows, assuming a 30-minute time period.

$$\frac{50\text{ ml}}{30\text{ min.}} \times 60\text{ gtt/ml} = 100\text{ gtt/min.}$$

EXERCISE F

Solve the following problems.

1. *Give:* 3500 ml of 5% D/W IV in 24 hours. *IV administration set:* 15 gtt/ml. How many gtt/min. should the IV run?
2. *Give:* 1500 ml of NS IV in 10 hours. *IV administration set:* 60 gtt/ml. How many gtt/min. should the IV run?
3. *Give:* 2000 ml of 5% D/W IV in 12 hours. *IV administration set:* 20 gtt/ml. How many gtt/min. should the IV run?
4. *Give:* 1000 ml of 5% D/W, 1000 ml of Ringer's lactate IV in 24 hours. *IV administration set:* 15 gtt/ml. How many gtt/min. should the IV run?
5. *Give:* 1000 ml of 5% D/W with 30 mEq KCl IV in 6 hours. *Available:* Potassium chloride (KCL), 40 mEq in 20 ml. *IV administration set:* 20 gtt/ml.
   (a) How many milliliters of KCL should be added to the IV bottle?
   (b) How many gtt/min. should the IV run?
6. *Give:* 500 ml of 5% D/W with 15 mg folic acid IV in 4 hours. *Available:* Folvite (folic acid), 5 mg/ml in 10-ml vial. *IV administration set:* 15 gtt/ml.
   (a) How many milliliters of folic acid should be added to the IV bottle?
   (b) How many gtt/min. should the IV run?
7. *Give:* Vancocin 250 mg q6h via Soluset. *Available:* Vancomycin (Vancocin), 500 mg in a 10-ml vial. *Directions:* Add 10 ml of sterile water to yield 500 mg/10.8 ml. Should be given over a period of 20 to 30 minutes. Prepared solution may be added to 5% D/W or NS IVs. *IV administration set:* 60 gtt/ml.
   (a) How many milliliters of reconstituted Vancocin should be added to the Soluset?
   (b) If the Soluset is filled to the 100-ml mark, how many gtt/min. should the medicated solution run?
8. *Give:* Erythromycin 500 mg q6h IV via Soluset. *Available:* Erythromycin powder, 250 mg in a 10-ml vial. *Directions:* Add 10 ml of sterile water to yield 100 mg/4.1 ml. Should be given for 30 minutes. Prepared solution may be added to 5% D/W or NS IVs. *IV administration set:* 60 gtt/ml.
   (a) How many milliliters of reconstituted erythromycin should be added to the Soluset?
   (b) If the Soluset is filled to the 75-ml mark, how many gtt/min. should the medicated solution run?
9. *Give:* 1000 ml 5% D/W IV in 12 hours, 1000 ml NS IV in 12 hours. Add 7,500,000 U of penicillin G to each 1000 ml of IV fluid. *Available:* Potassium penicillin G, 5,000,000 U in a 50-ml vial. *Directions:* Add 22.5 ml of sterile water to yield 200,000 U/ml. *IV administration set:* 15 gtt/ml.
   (a) How many milliliters of reconstituted penicillin G should be added to each IV?
   (b) How many gtt/min. should the IV run?
10. *Give:* 500 ml 5% D/W with 200 mg of Aramine added to IV to maintain B.P. above 100 systolic. *Available:* Metaraminol tartrate (Aramine) 10 mg/ml. How many milliliters of Aramine should be added to the IV?
11. *Give:* 2000 ml of Ringer's lactate IV in 24 hours. *IV administration set:* 10 gtt/ml.
    (a) What should be the gtt/min. on the rate selector of a gravity pump?
    (b) What should be the ml/hr on the delivery rate of a piston pump?

PEDIATRIC DOSAGES

Clinical trials conducted by pharmaceutical companies to examine the effects of drug dosage generally engage adults, so consequently very few medications indicate the recommended drug dosage for infants and children. There are several rules for determining the dosage for infants and children, but these rules are based on the child's age, weight, or surface area and do not consider the child's physiologic development. For example, a rule-computed dosage of narcotics is often too great a dosage for children because their tolerance to narcotics is less than that of an adult. Consequently, the rules can only serve as guidelines in determining the proper dosage for infants and children.

Rules Based on Age, Weight, and Surface Area

Age

The following three rules use the age of the infant or child to determine the dosage. These rules only indirectly consider the child's size, weight, and physiologic development.

Fried's rule This rule is useful for infants and children up to the age of two years old. Fried's rule calculates the child's dose by dividing the age of the infant in months by 150 and multiplying the answer by the adult dose. Thus,

$$\frac{\text{Age in months}}{150} \times \text{Adult's dose} = \text{Child's dose}$$

Young's rule This rule is useful for children between the ages of 1 and 12. The dose is obtained by dividing the age of the child in years by the sum of the child's age plus 12 and dividing the answer by the adult dose. Hence,

$$\frac{\text{Age in years}}{\text{Age} + 12} \times \text{Adult's dose} = \text{Child's dose}$$

Cowling's rule This rule determines the dose for a child by dividing the age of the child on his next birthday by 24 and multiplying the answer by the adult dose. Therefore,

$$\frac{\text{Age at next birthday}}{24} \times \text{Adult's dose} = \text{Child's dose}$$

Young's and Cowling's rules assume that the child would be 24 years old before the adult dosage can be tolerated.

Weight

Clark's rule Clark's rule determines dosage by the weight of the child or infant and assumes that the average adult weight is 150 lb (or 68 kg). Since the desired action of drugs is often affected by a client's weight, Clark's rule usually provides a more accurate dosage than the age rules. However, this rule does not consider the child's physiologic development or his ability to metabolize and excrete a drug. Clark's rule calculates the child's dose by dividing the child's weight in pounds (or kilograms) by 150 (or 68) and multiplying the answer by the adult dose. Thus,

$$\frac{\text{Weight in pounds}}{150} \times \text{Adult's dose} = \text{Child's dose}$$

$$\frac{\text{Weight in kilograms}}{68} \times \text{Adult's dose} = \text{Child's dose}$$

Surface area

Rules based on body surface area have been developed in an attempt to overcome the difficulties encountered with age and weight rules. However, the surface area of a child is seldom known and a normogram chart of body surface area must be consulted. Here again, the charts do not account for all the individual differences in infants and children.

Surface area rule This rule assumes that the average adult has a surface area of 1.7 m^2. However, some charts assume a value of 1.73 m^2. The average body weight of an individual with a surface area of 1.7m^2 is approximately 150 lb. Since it is easier to determine a client's body weight, Clark's rule is often preferred when determining a child's dose. The surface area rule determines the dose for a child by dividing the child's surface area by 1.7 and multiplying the answer by the adult dose. Hence,

$$\frac{\text{Surface area in square meters}}{1.7} \times \text{Adult's dose} = \text{Child's dose}$$

Example How many grains of aspirin should be given to a 6-month-old infant who weighs 7.0 kg (15.4 lb) and has a surface area of 0.37 m^2. The adult dose of aspirin is 10 gr.

Fried's rule

$$\frac{6\text{ months}}{150} \times 10\text{ gr} = x\text{ gr}$$
$$0.04 \times 10 = x$$
$$0.4\text{ gr} = x$$

Clark's rule

$$\frac{15.4\text{ lb}}{150} \times 10\text{ gr} = x\text{ gr}$$
$$0.10 \times 10 = x$$
$$1.0\text{ gr} = x$$

Surface area rule

$$\frac{0.37\text{ m}^2}{1.7} \times 10\text{ gr} = x\text{ gr}$$
$$0.22 \times 10 = x$$
$$2.2\text{ gr} = x$$

Note The surface area rule can lead to overmedication in infants, and Fried's rule can result in undermedication. The most reliable, and therefore most frequently used rule, is Clark's rule, which is based on body weight.

Example How many milligrams of Garamycin should be given to a petite 5-year-old who weighs only 15.5 kg (34 lb) and has a surface area of 0.65 m^2. The adult dose of gentamicin (Garamycin) is 80 mg.

Young's rule

$$\frac{5\text{ years}}{5 + 12} \times 80\text{ mg} = x\text{ mg}$$
$$0.29 \times 80 = x$$
$$23.2\text{ mg} = x$$

Cowling's rule

$$\frac{6\text{ years}}{24} \times 80\text{ mg} = x\text{ mg}$$
$$0.25 \times 80 = x$$
$$20\text{ mg} = x$$

Clark's rule

$$\frac{34\text{ lb}}{150} \times 80\text{ mg} = x\text{ mg}$$
$$0.23 \times 80 = x$$
$$18.4\text{ mg} = x$$

Surface area rule

$$\frac{0.65}{1.7} \times 80\text{ mg} = x\text{ mg}$$
$$0.38 \times 80 = x$$
$$30.4\text{ mg} = x$$

Note The surface area rule can result in overmedication; Cowling's & Clark's rules are preferred.

Example How many milligrams of Dilantin should be given to a stocky 12-year-old who weighs 50 kg (110 lb) and has a surface area of 1.51 m^2. The adult dose of phenytoin (Dilantin) is 100 mg tid.

Young's rule

$$\frac{12\text{ years}}{12 + 12} \times 100\text{ mg} = x\text{ mg}$$
$$.5 \times 100 = x$$
$$50\text{ mg} = x$$

Cowling's rule

$$\frac{13\text{ years}}{24} \times 100\text{ mg} = x\text{ mg}$$
$$0.54 \times 100 = x$$
$$54\text{ mg} = x$$

Clark's rule

$$\frac{110\text{ lb}}{150} \times 100\text{ mg} = x\text{ mg}$$
$$0.73 \times 100 = x$$
$$73\text{ mg} = x$$

Surface area rule

$$\frac{1.51}{1.7} \times 100\text{ mg} = x\text{ mg}$$
$$0.89 \times 100 = x$$
$$89\text{ mg} = x$$

Note Both age rules can lead to undermedication in the older child whereas Clark's rule and the surface area rule provide a more reasonable dosage. These are therefore preferred.

Commonly Used Rules

Fried's and Clark's rules are the most frequently used methods of determining dosages for infants and children because they are less likely to result in overmedication. Fried's rule is usually used for infants up to the age of 2 years and Clark's rule is generally used for children older than 2 years although it is sometimes used for infants too.

Since the metric system will eventually replace the apothecary system, the metric conversion for Clark's rule has been included. It is becoming more common for pediatric dosages to be ordered according to kilograms of body weight rather than pounds. The dosages of some medications, particularly antibiotics, are sometimes given per kilogram of body weight per 24 hours. Some examples are as follows:

1. Amoxicillin oral suspension, 20 mg/kg/24 hr
2. Phenytoin (Dilantin), 5 mg/kg/24 hr
3. Neomycin sulfate tablets, 50 mg/kg/24 hr

When medications are ordered in this manner, there is no need to use Fried's or Clark's rules, since the amount of medication can be directly computed. After determining the total amount of medication the child should receive in 24 hours, the amount is divided by the frequency of administration. Thus,

$$\text{Child's weight} \times \text{24-hour dosage} = \frac{\text{Frequency of administration}}{\text{Each divided dose}}$$

Example An 8-year-old weighs 29.5 kg and is to receive gentamicin q8h IV. Gentamicin IV: 6 mg/kg/24 hr

$$\frac{29.5\,\text{kg} \times 6\,\text{mg}}{3} = x$$

$$\frac{177}{3} = x$$

$$59\,\text{mg} = x$$

Therefore, 59 mg of gentamycin is given every eight hours.

Since none of the rules makes provision for all the physiologic differences between children, all clients should be closely observed for signs of over- or undermedication.

EXERCISE G

1. Use Fried's rule to find the appropriate pediatric dose.
   (a) A 3-month-old infant is to receive tetracycline. The adult dosage is 500 mg.
   (b) A 14-month-old infant is to receive phenobarbital (Luminal). The adult dosage is 60 mg.
   (c) A 9-month-old infant is to receive aspirin. The adult dosage is 10 gr.
2. Use Young's rule to find the appropriate pediatric dose.
   (a) A 3-year-old child is to receive phenytoin (Dilantin). The adult dosage is 100 mg tid.
   (b) A 9-year-old child is to receive meperidine (Demerol). The adult dosage is 75 mg.
   (c) A 7-year-old child is to receive gentamicin (Garamycin). The adult dosage is 80 mg.
3. Use Cowling's rule to find the appropriate pediatric dose.
   (a) A 2-year-old child is to receive tetracycline. The adult dosage is 500 mg.
   (b) A 6-year-old child is to receive streptomycin. The adult dosage is 500 mg.
   (c) A 10-year-old child is to receive morphine sulfate. The adult dosage is 12 mg.
4. Use Clark's rule to find the appropriate pediatric dosage.
   (a) A 3-month-old infant weighs 12 lb and is to receive phenytoin (Dilantin). The adult dosage is 100 mg tid.
   (b) An 18-month-old infant weighs 10.5 kg and is to receive phenobarbital (Luminal). The adult dosage is 0.1 gm.
   (c) A 4-year-old child weighs 36 lb and is to receive ampicillin. The adult dosage is 500 mg.
   (d) An 8-year-old child weighs 30 kg and is to receive nafcillin (Nafcil). The adult dosage is 250 mg.
   (e) An 11-year-old child weighs 41.8 kg and is to receive digoxin (Lanoxin). The adult maintenance dosage is 0.5 mg.
5. Use the surface area rule to find the appropriate pediatric dosage.
   (a) A 10-month-old infant has a surface area of 0.40 m^2 and is to receive streptomycin. The adult dosage is 500 mg.
   (b) A 15-month-old infant has a surface area of 0.48 m^2 and is to receive atropine. The adult dosage is gr $\frac{1}{150}$.
   (c) A 7-year-old child has a surface area of

0.95 m^2 and is to receive meperidine (Demerol). The adult dosage is 75 mg.

6. Use the manufacturer's recommended dosage per kilogram of body weight and find the dosage of each divided dose.
   (a) A 12-year-old child who weighs 43.2 kg is to receive neomycin tablets q6h × 3 days. Neomycin 50 mg/kg/24 hr is the recommended dose.
   (b) A 3-year-old child who weighs 30 lb is to receive tobramycin q8h IM. Tobramycin 3 mg/kg/24 hr is the recommended dose.

SOLUTIONS

Dosage calculations for oral and most injectable medications involve administering given quantities of *pure* or full strength (100%) drugs. When dealing with solutions, however, the drugs have to be diluted, often with large volumes of water, to desired strengths. The pure drug being dissolved is called the **solute** and the diluting fluid is called the **solvent**.

The solute can be a gas, liquid, or solid. Most of the gaseous solutions, such as hydrogen peroxide and carbonated magnesium citrate, are prepared by the manufacturer. In order to prevent a change in the gas solution's strength, the pharmaceutical directions must be carefully observed. For example, hydrogen peroxide must be kept in an airtight container away from sunlight or heat otherwise the molecular oxygen will be released leaving only water. Solutions made from solid or liquid solutes often require further preparation before they can be administered. All drugs for solutions that come packaged as crystals, powders, tablets, and liquids are considered *pure* or *full strength drugs* unless the label indicates otherwise. The strength of liquids that are available in diluted forms will be indicated on the label—for example, 95% alcohol solution or a 1:10,000 potassium permanganate solution.

The strength of a solution can be written either as a percent or as a ratio of pure drug to diluting fluid. When a solution's strength is expressed as a *percent,* it indicates the quantity of pure drug in 100 parts of diluent. Therefore, a 10% boric acid solution contains 10 g of boric acid in 100 ml of solution. Although the strength of most solutions is expressed as a percent, potent drugs are often written as ratios. When a solution's strength is given as a ratio it specifies the quantity of drug, usually in grams, that is in the solution. For example, a 1:10,000 potassium permanganate solution has 1 g of potassium permanganate in 10,000 ml of solution. (Note that a 1:5000 strength of this solution can be irritating to body tissues.)

When a physician orders a solution strength not commercially available, the volume of liquid that must be added to the available drug to make the desired strength must be calculated. A proportion can be used to determine this quantity as follows:

$$\frac{\text{Desired strength}}{\text{Available strength}} = \frac{\text{Amount of solute}}{\text{Volume of solution}}$$

This formula can be rearranged by multiplying each side of the proportion by the volume of solution so that only the amount of solute to be used is on the right-hand side. Thus,

$$\frac{\text{Desired strength}}{\text{Available strength}} \times \begin{array}{c}\text{Volume of}\\ \text{desired solution}\end{array} = \begin{array}{c}\text{Amount}\\ \text{of solute}\end{array}$$

If a liter of solution is required, liters must first be changed to milliliters (1 l = 1000 ml).

Solutions from Pure Solute

Example Prepare 1000 ml of 5% boric acid solution from boric acid crystals. (Note that crystals are pure drugs.)

Proportion method

$$\frac{5\%}{100\%} = \frac{x\,\text{g}}{1000\,\text{ml}}$$
$$100x = 5000$$
$$x = 5000 \div 100$$
$$x = 50\,\text{g}$$

Alternative method

$$\frac{5\%}{100\%} \times 1000\,\text{ml} = x\,\text{g}$$
$$0.05 \times 1000 = x$$
$$50\,\text{g} = x$$

Therefore, 50 g of boric acid crystals are added to 100 ml of water to make a 5% solution.

Example Prepare 500 ml of 10% sodium chloride solution from sodium chloride 0.5-g tablets.

Proportion method

$$\frac{10\%}{100\%} = \frac{x\,\text{g}}{500\,\text{ml}}$$
$$100x = 5000$$
$$x = 5000 \div 100$$
$$x = 50\,\text{g}$$

Alternative method

$$\frac{10\%}{100\%} \times 500\,\text{ml} = x\,\text{g}$$
$$0.1 \times 500 = x$$
$$50\,\text{g} = x$$

Using the information that one tablet contains 0.5 g, the number of tablets necessary for 50 g can be determined as follows:

$$\frac{0.5\,\text{g}}{1\text{ tablet}} = \frac{50\,\text{g}}{x\text{ tablets}}$$
$$0.5x = 50$$
$$x = 50 \div 0.5$$
$$x = 100\text{ tablets}$$

Thus, 100 tablets of sodium chloride are added to 500 ml of water to make a 10% solution.

When the drug required for a solution comes prepared as a liquid, the volume that the drug occupies should be subtracted from the total solution in order to determine the quantity of diluting fluid.

Example Prepare 2000 ml of 20% lysol solution from full strength liquid Lysol.

Proportion method

$$\frac{20\%}{100\%} = \frac{x\,\text{ml}}{2000\,\text{ml}}$$
$$100x = 2000 \times 20$$
$$100x = 40{,}000$$
$$x = 40{,}000 \div 100$$
$$x = 400\,\text{ml}$$

Alternative method

$$\frac{20\%}{100\%} \times 2000\,\text{ml} = x\,\text{ml}$$
$$0.2 \times 2000 = x$$
$$400\,\text{ml} = x$$

Since a solution of 2000 ml is desired, the volume (400 ml) of the Lysol solute is subtracted from the total volume.

$$2000\text{ ml} - 400\text{ ml} = 1600\text{ ml}$$

Therefore, 1600 ml of water are added to 400 ml of full strength liquid Lysol to make 2000 ml of a 20% Lysol solution.

Solutions from Concentrated Solute

Liquid solutes are sometimes available in concentrations that are less than full strength. Here again, the proportion method can be used to determine the quantities of solute and liquid needed to make the desired solution.

Example Prepare 1 l of 2% Lysol solution from 10% Lysol solution.

Proportion method

$$\frac{2\%}{10\%} = \frac{x\,\text{ml}}{1000\,\text{ml}}$$
$$10x = 1000 \times 2$$
$$10x = 2000$$
$$x = 2000 \div 10$$
$$x = 200\,\text{ml}$$

Alternative method

$$\frac{2\%}{10\%} \times 1000\,\text{ml} = x\,\text{ml}$$
$$0.2 \times 1000 = x$$
$$200\,\text{ml} = x$$

Since a solution of 1000 ml is required, the volume of diluent is:

$$1000\text{ ml} - 200\text{ ml} = 800\text{ ml}$$

Thus, 800 ml of water are added to 200 ml of 10% Lysol solution to make 1000 ml of 2% Lysol solution.

Apothecary Measurement of Solutions

Sometimes an order for a solution or a drug may be in the apothecary system rather than the metric system. This is particularly true for solutions that have been used for many decades. In such cases, the apothecary measurements can be converted to metric measurements or the required dosage can be determined using the apothecary system. The metric system uses grams per milliliter whereas the apothecary system uses grains per minim and fractions are often used instead of percents. The arithmetic is generally easier when the metric system is used.

Example Prepare 32 fluid ounces of 1:10,000 potassium permanganate from potassium permanganate crystals.

The first step is to convert fluid ounces to minims. Using the conversion 480 minims = 1 fluid ounce, 32 fluid ounces = 15,360 minims.

Next, the quantity of solute is determined. Note here that a ratio can also be written as a fraction (that is, 1:10,000 = $\frac{1}{10{,}000}$) and that the whole unit 1 indicates a 100% solute in the apothecary system. If the solute is a diluted solution, its fraction is inserted.

Proportion method

$$\frac{1}{10{,}000} = \frac{x\ \text{gr}}{15{,}360\ \text{♏}}$$
$$1x = \frac{1}{10{,}000} \times 15{,}360$$
$$x = 1.5\ \text{g}$$

Alternative method

$$\frac{1}{10{,}000} \times 15{,}360\ \text{♏} = x\ \text{gr}$$
$$\frac{1}{10{,}000} \times \frac{1}{1} \times 15{,}360 = x$$
$$\frac{1}{10{,}000} \times 15{,}360 = x$$
$$1.5\ \text{gr} = x$$

This problem can also be solved by first converting to the approximate metric equivalents and then using the proportion or alternative method. Thus, 32 fluid ounces = 1000 ml and 1:10,000 = 1/10,000 = 0.01%.

Proportion method

$$\frac{0.01\%}{100\%} = \frac{x\ \text{g}}{1000\ \text{ml}}$$
$$100x = 1000 \times 0.01$$
$$100x = 10$$
$$x = 10 \div 100$$
$$x = 0.1$$

Alternative method

$$\frac{0.01\%}{100\%} \times 1000\ \text{ml} = x\ \text{g}$$
$$0.0001 \times 1000 = x$$
$$0.1\ \text{g} = x$$

Therefore, 1.5 gr or 0.1 g of crystals are added to 32 fluid ounces to make a 1:10,000 potassium permanganate solution.

Solution Strength in Ratio Form

When a solution's strength is written in ratio form, the ratio can be converted to a percent (see Chapter 9) and then the proportion or alternative method can be used to solve the problem.

Example Prepare 500 ml of 1:4 hydrogen peroxide solution from full strength hydrogen peroxide solution.

The ratio 1:4 ($\frac{1}{4}$) is equivalent to 25%. Now, the problem can be solved.

Proportion method

$$\frac{25\%}{100\%} = \frac{x\ \text{ml}}{500\ \text{ml}}$$
$$100x = 500 \times 25$$
$$100x = 12{,}500$$
$$x = 12{,}500 \div 100$$
$$x = 125\ \text{ml}$$

Alternative method

$$\frac{25\%}{100\%} \times 500\ \text{ml} = x\ \text{ml}$$
$$0.25 \times 500 = x$$
$$125\ \text{ml} = x$$

Since a solution of 500 ml is desired, the volume of diluent is:

$$500\ \text{ml} - 125\ \text{ml} = 375\ \text{ml}$$

Therefore, 375 ml of water are added to 125 ml of hydrogen peroxide to make 500 ml of 1:4 hydrogen peroxide solution.

EXERCISE H

1. Prepare 1000 ml of 50% sodium chloride solution from sodium chloride 0.5-g tablets.

2. Prepare 500 ml of 3% boric acid solution from boric acid crystals.
3. Prepare 500 ml of 1:2000 mercuric chloride solution from mercuric chloride 500 mg tablets.
4. Prepare 400 ml of 5% Lysol solution from 50% Lysol solution.
5. Prepare 1 l of 1:8000 potassium permanganate solution from potassium permanganate 0.5-g tablets.
6. Prepare 250 ml of 40% glycerin solution from full strength liquid glycerin.
7. Prepare 16 fluid ounces of 1:500 sodium chloride solution from sodium chloride 15-gr tablets.
8. Prepare 250 ml of 1:10,000 epinephrine solution from 1:1000 epinephrine solution.
9. Prepare 750 ml of NS (0.9% solution) from sodium chloride crystals.
10. Prepare 1 l of 5% vinegar solution from full strength vinegar solution.

ANSWERS TO PRETEST

1. 3 tablets

If the above is answered incorrectly, start with Whole Tablets and Capsules (page 184).

2. 15 ml
3. 6 ml

If any of the above are answered incorrectly, start with Liquids and Scored Tablets (page 186).

4. 0.75 ml *or* 12 ♏

If the above is answered incorrectly, start with Injectables (page 188).

5. a. 30 units on the U-40 scale

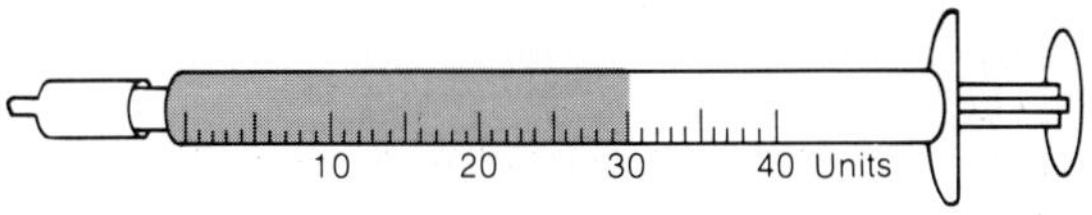

b. 75 units

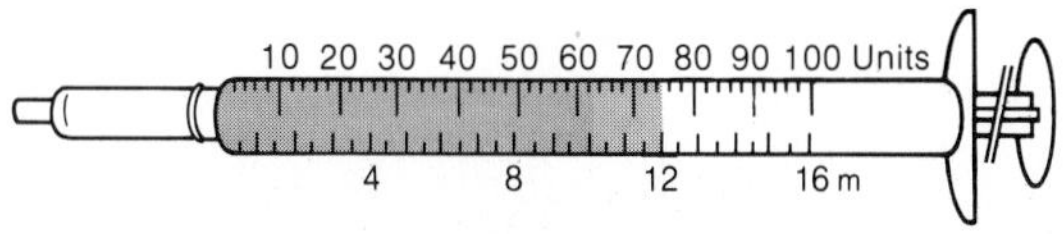

c. 12 ♏

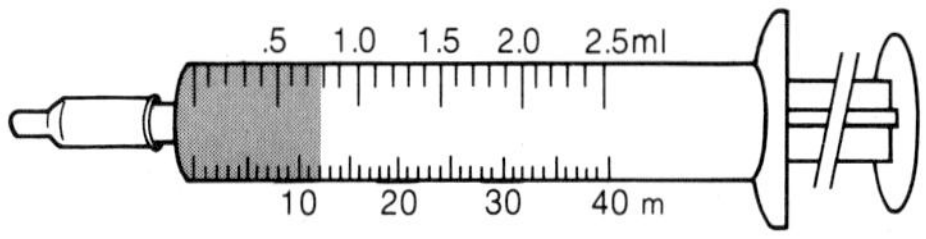

If any of the above are answered incorrectly, start with Solutions of Less Than One Milliliter (page 190).

6. a. 50 mg/ml
   b. 2 ml

If any of the above are answered incorrectly, start with Dosages of Dry Injectables (page 191).

7. a. 26 gtt/min
   b. 104.17 *or* 104 ml/hr
8. a. 8.25 ml
   b. 200 gtt/min

If any of the above are answered incorrectly, start with Intravenous Fluids and Medications (page 193).

9. 3.3 mg (*or* 0.0033 g)
10. a. 5.9 gr
    b. 0.37 mg
11. 330 mg

If any of the above are answered incorrectly, start with Pediatric Dosages (page 198).

12. Add 4.8 gr (*or* 0.003 g) to 100 fluid ounces of water.
13. a. 150 ml of 50% Lysol solution
    b. 600 ml of water

If any of the above are answered incorrectly, start with Solutions (page 202).

ANSWERS TO EXERCISES

Exercise A

1. 2 capsules 2. 3 tablets 3. 2 tablets
4. 4 tablets 5. 2 tablets

Exercise B

1. 5 ml 2. 10 ml 3. 7.5 ml 4. 15 ml
5. 15 ml 6. 2 tablets 7. 4 ml 8. 5 ml

Exercise C

1. 0.6 ml 2. 1.75 ml 3. 2.5 ml 4. 0.5 ml
5. 1.5 ml

Exercise D

1. a. 25 units on U-40 scale

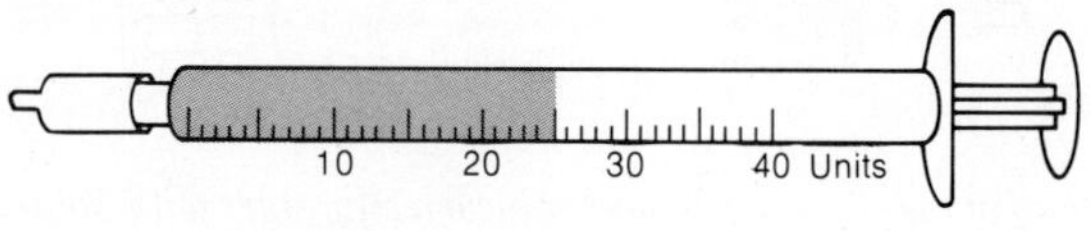

b. 62.5 units

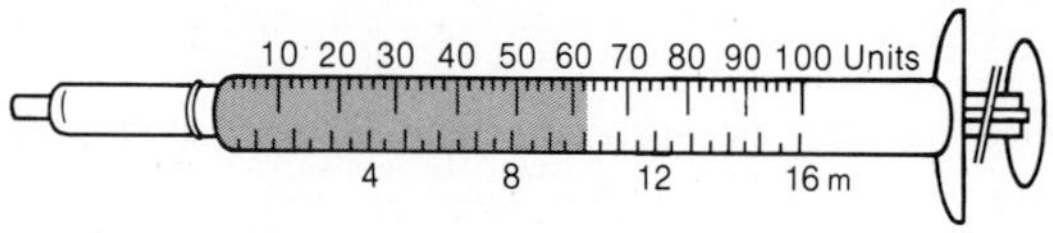

c. 10 ♏

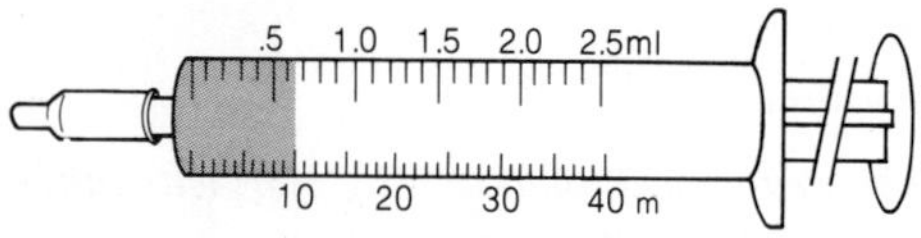

2. a. 37 units

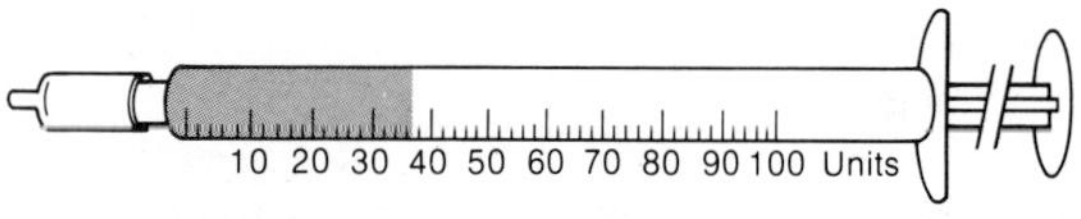

b. 5.9 or 6 ♏

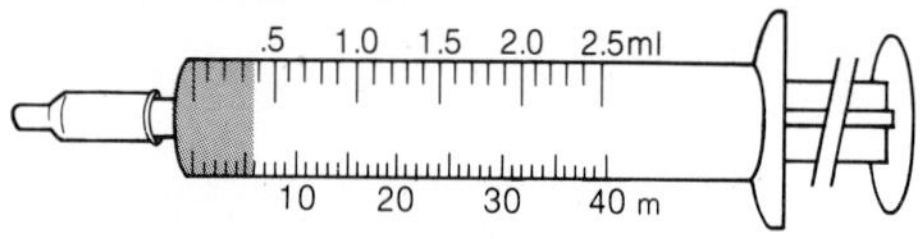

3. a. 60 units on U-100 scale

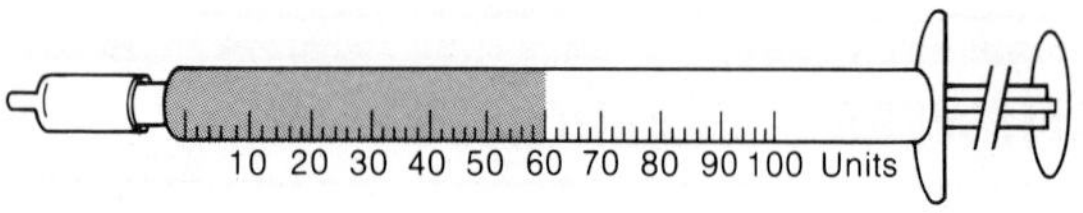

b. 9.6 or 10 ♏

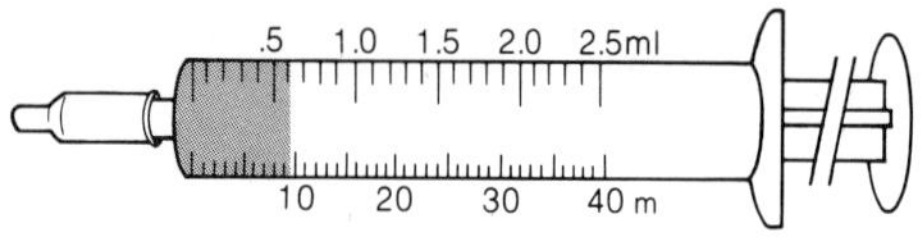

Exercise E

1. a. 250 mg/ml **b.** 1 ml **2. a.** 200,000 U/ml **b.** 1.5 ml **3. a.** 250 mg/ml **b.** 1 ml **4. a.** 333 mg/ml **b.** 1.5 ml **5. a.** 10 mg/ml **b.** 0.5 ml

Exercise F

1. 36 gtt/min. **2.** 150 gtt/min. **3.** 56 gtt/min. **4.** 21 gtt/min **5. a.** 15 ml **b.** 56 gtt/min. **6. a.** 3 ml **b.** 31 gtt/min. **7. a.** 5.4 ml **b.** 200 gtt/min. **8. a.** 20.5 ml **b.** 150 gtt/min. **9. a.** 37.5 ml (1 vial + 12.5 ml from a second vial) **b.** 21 gtt/min. **10.** 20 ml **11. a.** 13.8 *or* 14 gtt/min. **b.** 83 ml/hr

Exercise G

1. a. 10 mg **b.** 5.6 mg **c.** 0.6 gr **2. a.** 20 mg **b.** 32 mg **c.** 29 mg **3. a.** 62.5 mg **b.** 146 mg **c.** 5.5 mg **4. a.** 8 mg **b.** 15 mg (*or* 0.015 g) **c.** 120 mg **d.** 110 mg **e.** 0.31 mg **5. a.** 118 mg **b.** 0.0019 gr (*or* 0.11 mg) **c.** 42 mg **6. a.** 540 mg **b.** 13.6 mg

Exercise H

1. Add 1000 tablets (500 g) to 1000 ml of water. **2.** Add 15 g to 500 ml of water. **3.** Add $\frac{1}{2}$ tablet (250 mg) to 500 of water. **4.** Add 360 ml of water to 40 ml of 50% Lysol solution. **5.** Add $\frac{1}{4}$ tablet (125 mg) to 1000 ml of water. **6.** Add 150 ml of water to 100 ml of full strength glycerin. **7.** Add 1 tablet (15 gr) to 16 fluid ounces of water. **8.** Add 225 ml of water to 25 ml of 1:1000 epinephrine solution. **9.** Add 6.75 g to 750 ml of water. **10.** Add 950 ml of water to 50 ml of full strength vinegar.

REFERENCES

Anderson, E. M. 1972. *Workbook of solutions and dosages of drugs.* 9th ed. St. Louis: C. V. Mosby.

Blume, D. M. 1974. *Dosage and solutions.* 2nd ed. Philadelphia: F. A. Davis.

Campbell, J. 1978. The BSA method of calculating pediatric drug dosages. *Maternal-Child Nursing.* 3:357.

Eisenbach, R. 1977. *Calculating and administering medications.* Philadelphia: F. A. Davis.

Engram, B. 1981. Computing IV flow rates. *Nursing 81.* 11:89.

Fleischman, M. R. 1975. *Dosage calculation: Method and workbook.* Publication 10-1560. New York: National League for Nursing.

Keane, C. B., and Fletcher, S. M. 1980. *Drugs and solutions.* 4th ed. Philadelphia: W. B. Saunders.

Richardson, L. I., & Richardson, J. K. 1976. *The mathematics of drugs and solutions with clinical applications.* New York: McGraw-Hill.

Sackheim, G. I., and Robins, L. 1974. *Programmed mathematics for nurses.* 3rd ed. New York: Macmillan.

Sager, D. P., and Kovarovic, S. B. 1980. *Intravenous medications.* Philadelphia: J. B. Lippincott.

PART IV

THE ADMINISTRATION OF MEDICATIONS

Drug preparation and administration Medications are administered to create a systemic action, a local action, or both. To produce its intended systemic effect, a medication must first be absorbed. The absorption of a drug is affected by many factors, including (1) the concentration of the drug; (2) the circulation at the site of drug contact; (3) the characteristics of the absorbing surface; (4) the route of administration; and (5) the drug form used.

Since the amount and rate of circulation and the characteristics of the absorbing surface are dependent on the route of administration, the latter is the primary factor in determining the rate and uniformity of a drug's absorption. Some drugs, like insulin, are inactivated by digestive juices when given orally; others, such as magnesium sulfate, act locally as a cathartic when given orally but cause depression of the central nervous system when injected intramuscularly. In fact, some drugs are dangerous if given by the wrong route. For example, norepinephrine (Levophed) can only be given intravenously, since it will cause destruction of the surrounding tissue if given intramuscularly. Consequently, the route of administration is as important as the dosage of a drug in producing the intended therapeutic effect.

The routes of administration can be classified according to the nature of their absorbing surfaces. The mucous membrane of the *alimentary tract* is the most frequently prescribed route, used when systemic action is desired. Many medications, also given for their systemic effects, are injected into body tissues or directly into the circulation. This method is called the *parenteral* route. Still others are applied *topically* to the skin, usually for their local action. Occasionally, medications are applied to *mucous membranes,* such as the urethra, generally to provide a local effect. If the absorbing surface is sterile, the medication must be sterile. If the surface normally contains microorganisms, on the other hand, the medication does not have to be sterile but should be as free of microorganisms as possible. Table IV-1 summarizes the characteristics of the common routes.

Procedures for ordering, distributing, and administering drugs are changing rapidly; but the nurse continues to have the responsibility for actual preparation and administration of individual drug doses for the client. Whatever the particular agency's medication procedure may be, there can be no substitute for the nurse's technical skill, knowledge, and judgment; particularly in those situations where routine agency procedures may not apply. In some agencies, nurses are still calculating dosages, preparing dilutions, and converting from apothecary to metric systems or vice versa. However, in the past few years many health agencies have instituted the unit-dose medication system.

Unit-dose distribution system This system provides single premeasured and packaged doses for clients, thereby eliminating the time-consuming tasks of calculating and measuring dosages. Hospitals using the unit-dose system provide mobile medication carts with individual compartments containing each client's medications, stored separately from the medications of all other clients (see Figure IV-1). Medications to be administered during a specific time period—for example, 12 to 24 hours—are placed in the client's compartment. The medications are prepared and delivered to the client care area by the pharmacy department. This method provides a double-check system that significantly decreases the risk of medication errors. In addition, there must be provision on the medication cart for a locked cabinet or drawer in which to store controlled drugs and an area for other stock supplies and emergency drugs (see Figure IV-2).

The unit-dose system frees the nurse from much of the time-consuming work of calculat-

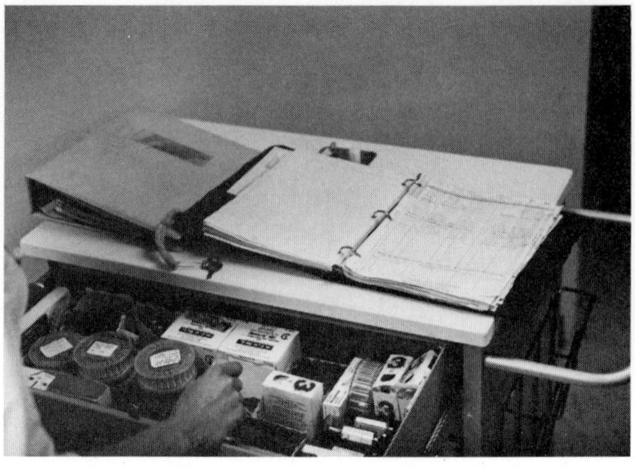

FIGURE IV-1 A unit-dose medication cart showing stock supplies in top lockable drawer.

TABLE IV-1 Characteristics of Common Routes of Drug Administration

Route	Absorbing Surface	Usual Abbreviation	Commonly Used Action	Sterile or Clean Preparation	Usual Dosage Form
Alimentary Tract					
Oral	Mucous membrane of stomach and/or intestines	po	Systemic	Clean	Tablets Capsules Suspensions Solutions
Sublingual	Mucous membrane under the tongue	SL	Systemic	Clean	Tablets
Buccal	Mucous membrane of mouth	—	Systemic	Clean	Lozenges
Rectal	Mucous membrane of rectum and/or colon	PR, or per rectum	Local	Clean	Suppositories Solutions Ointments
Parenteral					
Intramuscular	Muscle	IM	Systemic	Sterile	Solution or suspension
Hypodermic or subcutaneous	Subcutaneous tissue	(H), SQ, SC, or subcu	Systemic	Sterile	Solution or suspension
Intradermal	Dermis layer of skin	ID or intraderm	Local	Sterile	Solution
Intravenous	—	IV	Systemic	Sterile	Solution
Intraarterial	—	—	Systemic	Sterile	Solution
Intracardiac	Endocardium and/or tunica intima	—	Local and systemic	Sterile	Solution
Intraperitoneal	Peritoneal cavity	—	Systemic	Sterile	Solution
Intrasynovial	Synovial sac of a joint	—	Local	Sterile	Solution or suspension
Topical					
Unbroken skin	Epidermis	—	Local	Clean	Lotions Ointments Creams
Open skin area	Dermis	—	Local	Sterile	Aqueous solutions
Other Mucous Membranes					
Eye	Conjunctiva	OD or Rt. eye, os or L eye, or OU, both eyes	Local	Sterile	Ophthalmic solution Ophthalmic ointment

TABLE IV-1 ***Continued***

Route	Absorbing Surface	Usual Abbreviation	Commonly Used Action	Sterile or Clean Preparation	Usual Dosage Form
Urethra	Urethral mucosa	Ureth	Local	Sterile	Bougie (suppository)
Vagina	Vaginal mucosa	Vag	Local	Clean	Solution Ointment Foams Suppository
Nose	Nasal mucosa	—	Local	Clean	Aqueous solution
Respiratory tract	Bronchial tree mucosa	inhal	Local and systemic	Sterile	Vaporized aqueous solution

ing, measuring, and pouring, and is decidedly more accurate and safer than older methods. In no way, however, does it allow nurses to forfeit their responsibilities concerning medications. *Safe* administration, close *observation* and *assessment*, client *teaching*, relevant *communications*, and accurate *recording* are vital nursing functions. Because the unit-dose system is quick and efficient, the nurse actually has more time to spend in direct client care, thereby facilitating the fulfillment of these vital responsibilities.

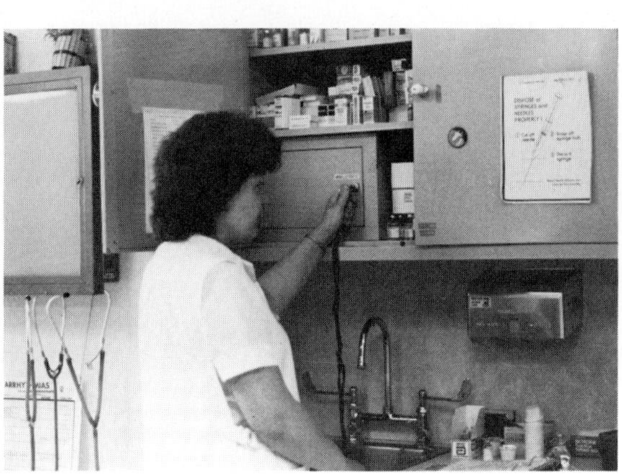

FIGURE IV-2 A nurse preparing to remove a narcotic from the double-locked narcotic cabinet.

Medication orders These orders are written on the client's chart or permanent record, on a specific order form designed only for this purpose, or in a special "physicians' order" book. In some situations, the doctor may give a verbal order or a telephone order to the nurse, in which case the nurse writes the order on the client's record as soon as possible, and the doctor signs his or her name under the order.

The medication order must be clearly written and must include the following information:

1. Client's name
2. Date and time the order is written
3. Name of medication
4. Dosage and schedule of administration
5. Route of administration

Only standard abbreviations should be used and the medication order must be signed by the physician. If any of the above information is missing from the order, or if any part is illegible or questionable, it is the nurse's responsibility to contact the physician for clarification before transcribing the order or administering the drug. (See Chapter 2 for abbreviations and further explanation.)

Agency controls Every health agency has its own specific procedures for controlling, preparing, and administering medications. There are, however, certain measures that are basic to the nurse's role and responsibility:

1. All drugs should be stored in locked cabinets or closets. When the unit-dose system is used, the medication carts should be equipped with locks.

2. Narcotics and other drugs under legal restriction must be double-locked in an area that is not accessible to the public. In the unit-dose system, narcotics are either stored in a separate locked drawer in the medication cart or in a double-locked area in the nurse's station. Each dose is recorded in a special record book. (See Figure IV-2)

3. All drug container labels must be complete and legible. If the label becomes stained or loosened, the container must be returned to the pharmacy. Under no circumstances should the nurse take the responsibility for relabeling a drug container.

4. Drugs for internal administration should be stored separately from topical medicines. In the unit-dose system, topical drugs are usually stored in a separate compartment in the medicine cart.

5. Drugs that are out-dated, changed in color, or of questionable purity must be returned to the pharmacy. In the unit-dose system, any drugs left over after discontinuance of the medication or the client's discharge from the agency must be returned to the pharmacy.

The nurse who is preparing medications for administration should be free from distractions. Ideally, preparation should take place in the medicine closet or another quiet area. In the unit-dose system, the medicine cart can be wheeled away from the nurses' stations or brought directly to the client's unit. In any case, preparation for administering drugs requires the nurse's *total* concentration.

Critical elements in drug preparation There are five key safety factors that the nurse must consider for every drug dose prepared and administered. The *right drug* must be given to the *right client* at the *right time* in the *right dose* by the *right route*. Table IV-2 summarizes the critical elements involved in ensuring that drugs are prepared and administered accurately.

Critical elements in drug administration The administration of medications is a professional responsibility requiring both cognitive and technical expertise. Every clinical agency has its own standard procedure for administering drugs, and equipment and techniques will vary from agency to agency. However, the following basic guidelines and safety measures for drug administration are pertinent to all clinical settings:

1. Never administer a drug that has been prepared by someone else (unless that person is a pharmacist).

2. Never administer a drug without being thoroughly familiar with its action, recommended dosage, route of administration, and side effects or toxic effects or both.

3. Always identify the client by reading his or her identification band and calling him or her by name, or by having client recite his or her name to the nurse.

4. Always have client swallow oral medications in the nurse's presence. *Never* leave medicines at the client's bedside, unless specifically ordered by the physician.

5. Always explain the administration procedure to the client, including information about the drug in the explanation when appropriate.

6. *Always* wash your hands before administering medications by any route.

The administration of medications has great psychological and physical significance for the client. It follows that the nurse's attitude toward drug administration is of great importance to the client. The nurse's skill in the technical aspects of administration, along with a supportive approach, can do much to enhance the desired effect of the drug.

Variations in agency procedures Every health agency has its own well-defined procedures for preparing and administering medications. In addition to the foregoing, generally accepted precautions, it is the nurse's responsibility to become thoroughly familiar with his/her agency's specific procedure. Some agencies have developed self-study programs or in-service courses that newly employed nurses must take

TABLE IV-2 Critical Elements in Drug Preparation

Key Safety Factor	Critical Elements: From Stock Supply	Critical Elements: Unit-Dose System
The right drug	Check container label with order and/or medicine card *three times:* when removing drug from shelf; when pouring drug into container for administration; when returning container to shelf or drawer.	Check prepackaged unit label with order when removing from client's storage compartment.
The right client	Check name on medication order and/or medication Kardex. Proceed to pour, checking three times, as described above.	Check drugs in client's compartment against order on physician's order sheet or medication Kardex.
The right time sequence	Check medication order with medication container label. Be sure agency time schedule correlates with desired effect of drug.*	Be sure agency time schedule correlates with desired effect of drug.*
The right dose	Check medication order with label on container *three times,* as described above. If calculation is required, verify dosage by having someone else check your calculations.	Check unit-dose label with order when removing drug from client's compartment.
The right route	Check medication order with label on container *three times,* as described above. Be sure stock dosage form conforms to route ordered by physician.	Check unit-dose drug form with order.

*With certain drugs, maintenance of an adequate blood level of the drug is critical, which means that the prescribed time schedule must be strictly observed. Furthermore, some drugs are more effectively absorbed on an empty stomach, so they are given before meals. Others are more effectively absorbed in the presence of food in the stomach and must be given with meals or immediately after a meal.

before they are permitted to prepare and administer medications.

In some agencies using the unit-dose system, medications are dispensed from the client's compartment with only the medication Kardex or the client's medication order sheet as the source of information about administration. Agencies may require individual medication cards for each medication. These cards must contain all the elements of the physician's order and are often color-coded according to route of administration, time of day, or type of drug. The cards are placed in or under the medication dose when it is taken to the client's unit. No matter what system is used, the critical elements involved in preparing and administering medications are applicable in all situations.

Chapter 12

Drug Dosage Forms and Packaging

DRUG FORMS AND RELATED NURSING MANAGEMENT

Drugs are available in a variety of forms that are designed for several different routes of administration. Many drugs are prepared in more than one form and dosage, so that the prescribing professional, and the client, have a choice of route. For example, some antibiotics are available in tablet, capsule, suspension, or liquid form for oral administration, and in parenteral form for IM or IV administration.

Drug forms are generally prepared by pharmaceutical companies or by a licensed pharmacist, but the nurse sometimes needs to change a drug form before administering it to a client. For example, certain drugs are very unstable in suspension, so the powdered drug must be mixed with a suitable liquid just prior to administration.

The following list describes the drug forms that are available, along with related implications for nursing management. Figure 12-1 (see pp. 222–223) illustrates the more common drug forms and packaging.

Drug form	*Nursing management*
Tablet—Powdered drug that has been compressed into a disc. Tablets vary greatly in size and weight, depending on actual dosage of the active drug, as well as on the coating, filler, or binder used to prepare them. Some tablets are scored (indented in the middle), so that they can be broken in half easily.	Uncoated tablets may be broken or crushed for the client who has difficulty in swallowing.
Coated tablet—Compressed drug covered with sugar or another flavored coating to make it more palatable or more attractive.	Coated tablets should be administered in whole form, since the coating disguises the unpleasant taste of the drug.
Enteric coated tablet—Tablet coated with a substance that will not dissolve until it reaches the small intestine. Drugs that are irritating to the gastric lining and would therefore cause gastric distress are prepared this way.	Enteric coated tablets should never be broken or crushed, since the coating is present to prevent irritation to the stomach lining. Check to be sure tablet is not passed undigested—occasionally the coating fails to dissolve in the intestine.
Sublingual tablet—Small disc that is placed under the tongue and that dissolves quickly, thereby releasing the active substance for direct absorption into the bloodstream.	Sublingual tablets must be dissolved under the tongue, which is highly vascular. This method facilitates rapid absorption into the bloodstream, causing the drug to take effect within one to five minutes. They should not be chewed or swallowed.
Tablet triturate—Disc made by moistening the powdered drug with a liquid that is quickly evaporated, such as alcohol, or with powdered sugar. The discs are then molded and dried; they disintegrate quickly in water.	Because of rapid disintegration of disc in water, tablet should be swallowed quickly to prevent unpleasant taste from drug.
Capsule—Small, hollow container, usually made of gelatin and glycerin, used to enclose a drug. Capsules may be used to conceal a bitter taste. They range in length from	Uncoated capsules may be opened and contents swallowed for more rapid disintegration and absorption of drug, or for client who has difficulty swallowing capsules. The

Drug form	*Nursing management*
12 to 28 mm and are produced in a variety of colors. The drug contained in the capsule may be in powder, granule, or liquid form.	unpleasant taste of the capsule contents may be disguised by administering with a palatable liquid, provided one has determined that the liquid will not change the desired action of the drug.
Enteric coated capsule—Capsule coated with a substance that will not dissolve in gastric secretions. Disintegration takes place in the alkaline secretions of the small intestine.	Enteric coated capsules must be swallowed in whole form, since coating is designed to prevent irritation to the stomach.
Sustained-release capsule or prolonged-action capsule—Tiny drug particles (granules) contained in the capsule are coated with a variety of substances that are designed to dissolve at different times. This drug form provides for continuous release of small doses of the drug over an extended time period, which can range from 2 to 12 hours, depending on the coatings used.	These capsules must never be opened or broken apart before ingestion. Changing the form could result in rapid absorption and overdose.
Troche—Drug mixed with sugar and a mucilage, then molded into a flat, round or square shape. It is designed to dissolve in the mouth, thereby releasing large doses of the drug for local effect. Troches are also called *lozenges.*	Troches should be permitted to dissolve in the mouth and should never be swallowed whole or chewed, since they are designed for local effect in the mouth and/or throat.
Pill—Drug mixed with a sticky substance (excipient) that facilitates its being molded into a shape convenient for swallowing. Pills are usually oval or round in shape, and seldom contain more than 5 gr of the drug. The word *pill* is often mistakenly used to refer to tablets and capsules.	Pills may be broken or crushed to make swallowing easier.
Powder—Very fine particles of one or more drugs for internal or external use.	Powders must be mixed with a suitable liquid (indicated on package label) before oral ingestion. (External powders may not require dilution before use.)
Effervescent powder—Powdered drugs mixed with sodium bicarbonate or citric acid. When mixed with a liquid, these powders release carbon dioxide, causing the effervescence (bubbling). They are also available in tablet form.	With effervescent powders (and tablets), the client should be made aware that he or she will be swallowing a bubbling liquid (like a carbonated beverage). Drink should be swallowed while effervescing, since the bubbling sensation masks the taste of the medication.
Aqueous solution—One or more drugs dissolved in water or normal saline.	*Waters, liquors, mucilages,* and *infusions* may have a pungent or

Drug form	Nursing management
	unpleasant taste. The nurse should be prepared to offer fruit juice, milk, or other suitable liquid to the client immediately after ingestion of the drug.
Water (aqua)—Solution of a volatile or aromatic substance (drug) in distilled water.	
Liquor—Solution of a nonvolatile substance in distilled water	
Mucilage—Thick, gummy substance (usually a vegetable preparation) used to suspend insoluble drugs in water	
Infusion—Solution made by steeping a substance (usually a plant part) in hot or cold water in order to release the active ingredient.	
Syrup—Aqueous solution saturated with sugar. It usually contains a flavoring agent that assists in disguising the taste of the drug mixed in the syrup.	*Syrups* are sweetened and usually flavored, but there may be a lingering aftertaste from the dissolved drug.
Alcoholic solution—One or more drugs dissolved in alcohol.	Alcoholic solutions should not be administered to the alcoholic client.
Spirit or essence—Volatile drug dissolved in alcohol.	Spirits are potent preparations, seldom given in doses of more than 4 ml. They have a strong alcoholic taste; offer juice, milk, or water after ingestion. They are never injected—administer orally only.
Elixir—Spirit that has been sweetened and/or flavored.	Elixirs have a strong but sweet taste. Be prepared to offer a suitable liquid after ingestion, unless preparation is for cough. They are never injected; administer orally only.
Tincture—Solution made by extracting from the crude source those constituents of a drug that are soluble in alcohol.	Potent preparations, tinctures are given in small (4 ml or less) doses. They are never injected. Offer a suitable liquid after ingestion.
Fluid extract—Alcoholic solution of drugs prepared so that 1 ml of the solution contains 1 g of the active drug. Fluid extracts are, therefore, 100% in strength.	These are the most concentrated of the fluid preparations and may precipitate (come out of solution) when exposed to light. They are packaged in dark brown or green bottles, and should never be used if precipitate has formed. They are never injected. Administer orally in small (4 ml or less) doses.
Extract—Drug dissolved in alcohol (a fluid extract), with the	Extracts are usually used as the active ingredient in other

Drug form	*Nursing management*
solvent then evaporated. The extract is up to four times stronger than the fluid extract. The preparation may be semisolid or solid in consistency, or, sometimes, semiliquid with a syrupy consistency.	dosage forms, such as tablets. Dry, powdered extracts, such as liver extract, should be mixed in a suitable liquid for oral administration.
Aqueous suspension—Finely divided particles (powders) of a drug in a fluid. They are not dissolved in the fluid.	Aqueous suspensions for *intramuscular or subcutaneous injection* are prepared with sterile water or physiological saline; they cannot be administered intravenously or intra-arterially. Aqueous suspensions for *ophthalmic* use are also sterile and may contain an added bacteriostatic agent. *Oral* suspensions are not sterile and must never be administered by any other route. All suspensions must be thoroughly agitated before administration, since the particles settle to the bottom of the fluid upon standing. Avoid freezing since resuspending particles again may be difficult or impossible.
Mixture—Powdered solid suspended in a liquid medium. A mixture contains more than one drug.	
Emulsion—Fats or oils suspended in water, supplemented by an agent that coats the small oily drops, thereby helping to stabilize the suspension.	
Magma—Large particles of insoluble drugs suspended in water.	
Gel—Drug in crystalline form (chemically combined with water to form tiny crystals), suspended in water. The suspended particles are smaller than those in a magma.	
Topical drug forms—Drugs designed to be applied to a definite local area, usually to an external surface.	
Ointment—Drug or mixture of drugs added to a semisolid base, such as petroleum jelly or lanolin. Some ointments contain a base that is water soluble. Ointments may be designed to produce local effects on the skin	The fatty base used to prepare ointments is designed to keep the active ingredients in prolonged contact with the tissue. In order to prevent the ointment from being rubbed off by clothing or bed covers, the nurse may need to cover the affected area with a dry, sterile dressing

Drug form	*Nursing management*
or to be absorbed through the skin, or as specially prepared ophthalmic medications.	*Ophthalmic ointments* are sterile and prepared with a base that is not irritating to the eye. All ointments in jars should be removed with a sterile tongue blade to avoid contaminating the remaining contents.
Liniment—Liquid suspension containing a drug or mixture of drugs in oil, alcohol, or water.	Liniments are applied by rubbing, which provides a counterirritant effect and improves circulation to the affected area.
Lotion—Liquid medicinal suspension applied externally. Various lotions are designed for protection, lubrication, cleansing, cooling, or antipruritic effects.	Lotions are applied by gently but firmly patting onto the skin, in order to avoid further irritation, inflammation, or itching of the affected part.
Paste—Preparation similar to an ointment in consistency, but with a base composed of nonfatty ingredients that do not soften or melt at body temperature. Pastes are designed to absorb secretions or to provide a protective barrier on the skin surface.	These thick, stiff preparations are patted onto the skin, in order to avoid further irritation, inflammation, or itching of the affected part.
Plaster—Combination of substances formed into a thick, sticky mass, spread onto cloth or paper, and then applied to the skin.	Body heat causes plasters to soften and adhere to the skin. They are seldom used today. They have a counterirritant effect—that is, the superficial inflammatory reaction has a beneficial effect on the underlying or adjacent body part.
Poultice—Hot, moist pack composed of wet linseed or flaxseed in a cotton covering, designed to supply moist heat to an area.	If left on the skin too long, poultices can cause maceration (softening and breakdown) of the skin. Considered a home remedy, they are rarely used today.
Suppository—Drug mixed with a fatty base and molded into shapes suitable for insertion into the rectum, vagina, or urethra. They melt at body temperature, releasing the active ingredients for a local or systemic effect. They are shaped into cylinders or cones; the base substance is soap, glycerinated gelatin, or cocoa butter. A urethral suppository is called a *bougie*.	*Rectal* suppositories may be designed for *local* effect (such as relief of hemorrhoidal pain and itching), or for *systemic* effect, by absorption of the active ingredient through the rectal mucosa (as in aminophylline suppositories). *Vaginal* suppositories are designed for local effect on the vaginal mucosa or the cervix. *Urethral* suppositories are designed for local effect and must be administered using aseptic technique. *All* suppositories must be inserted fully into the appropriate body cavity to prevent expulsion and loss of the drug. In hot weather or very warm environments, suppositories must be refrigerated to prevent melting.

PACKAGING AND LABELING OF DRUGS

The federal Food, Drug and Cosmetic Act includes many features pertaining to accuracy in medication container labels, in information inserts accompanying drug packages, and in advertising. See Chapter 4 for more information on legislation controlling labeling and packaging of drugs.

A variety of packaging is used for the different drug forms but, according to federal legislation, every package label must include (1) an accurate statement of the contents, including quantity, kind, and proportion of ingredients; (2) directions for use and warnings against unsafe use; and (3) the name of the manufacturer.

In clinical agencies where staff pharmacists dispense drugs, the containers delivered to the client's unit may not contain all this information, but just the name of the drug, the dosage per unit, and, sometimes, the client's name. If the nursing staff needs more information, the pharmacist can supply it.

Packaging for Drugs for the Alimentary Tract

Multidose containers These containers are available in a variety of sizes and shapes and can contain a few or many units. They are made of clear or colored glass or plastic and may be transparent or opaque. The container lids may screw on and off, snap on and off, or open only when in one designated position ("child-proof" caps). Multidose containers are used for tablets, capsules, troches, pills, powders, aqueous solutions, alcoholic solutions, extracts, and aqueous suspensions.

Unit-dose packaging This type of packaging consists of single-unit packages prepared by the pharmacist for a particular client. Each individual dose is sealed in paper, cellophane, plastic, or a small bottle, and appropriately labeled. Unit-dose packaging can be used for all drug forms for which multidose containers are appropriate.

In *strip-packaging* individual units of a drug are separated on a paper or plastic strip and held in place with a tightly sealed, clear plastic covering. Each drug unit can be ejected for administration without dislodging the others. Strip-packaging can be used for tablets, capsules, troches, and pills.

In *blister-packaging* individual units of a drug are sealed in plastic bubbles similar to unit-dose packaging but prepared by the manufacturer rather than the pharmacist. Figure 12-2 illustrates one type of blister-strip packaging and one type of ampule.

Suppositories This drug form can be packaged in any of three ways:

1. *Multidose boxes*—Individual suppositories are usually foil-wrapped and packed in boxes of five or more. In hot weather or very warm environments, the box should be refrigerated to prevent melting of contents.

2. *Blister-packaging*—Individual suppositories are sealed in plastic bubbles or foil; they should be refrigerated as necessary.

3. *Jars*—Some suppositories, such as glycerin, are bulk-packaged in glass jars with screw-on lids; they should be refrigerated as necessary.

Packaging for Parenteral Drugs

The term *parenteral* literally refers to any route other than the gastrointestinal one. In practice, the parenteral designation is usually used only for those drugs given by injection; therefore, parenteral packaging must be sterile.

Vials Vials are small glass containers with nonremovable rubber tops through which a needle is inserted to withdraw the solution. They are usually multidose—that is, they contain enough solution for a number of doses of medication. If the vial contains a powdered form of the drug, the appropriate amount and type of sterile diluent must be used to dissolve it before injection.

Ampules Small, sealed glass containers holding a single dose of a drug are called ampules. The narrow top of the ampule must be broken off according to the manufacturer's directions before the drug can be withdrawn.

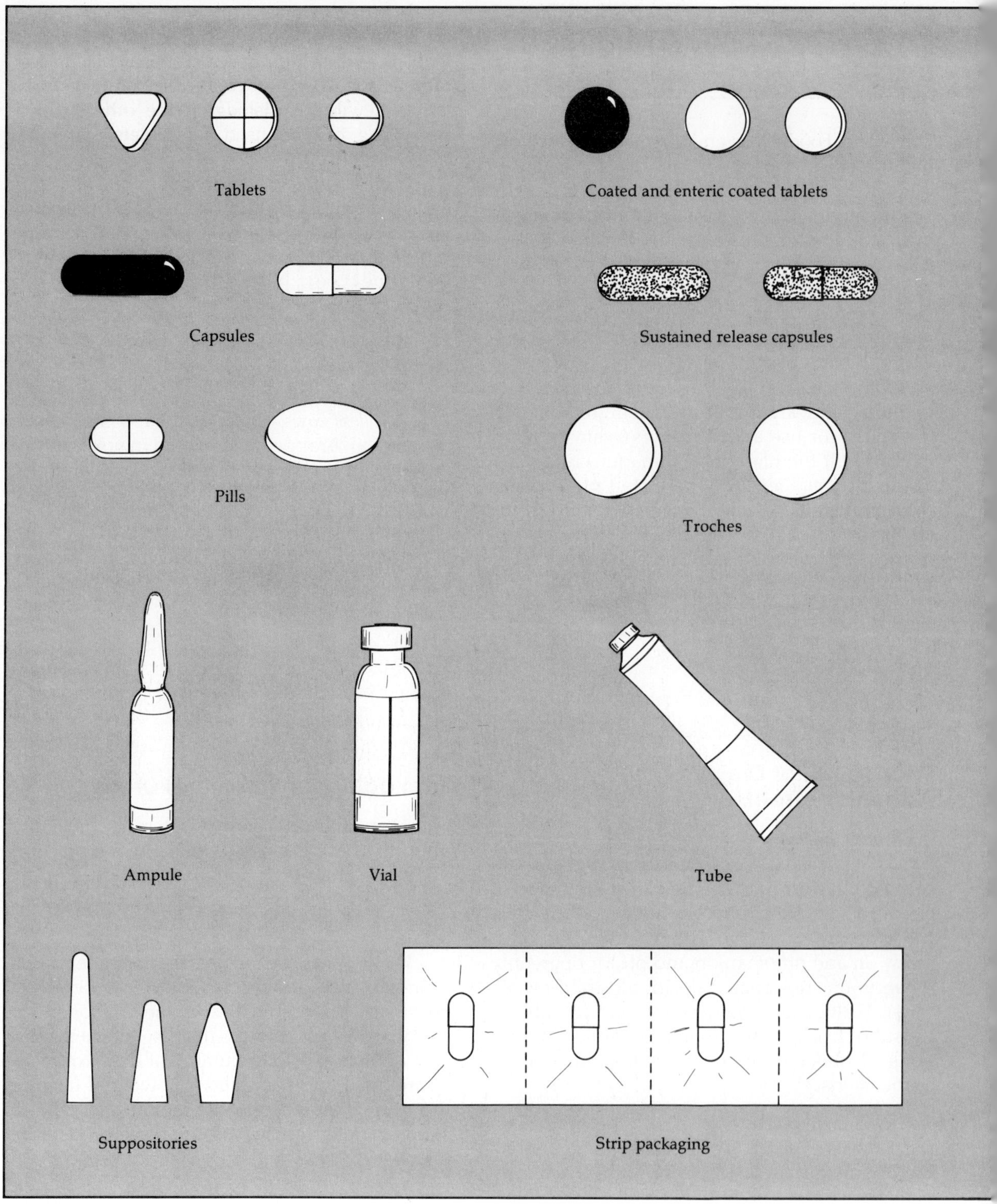
Tablets
Coated and enteric coated tablets
Capsules
Sustained release capsules
Pills
Troches
Ampule
Vial
Tube
Suppositories
Strip packaging

FIGURE 12-1

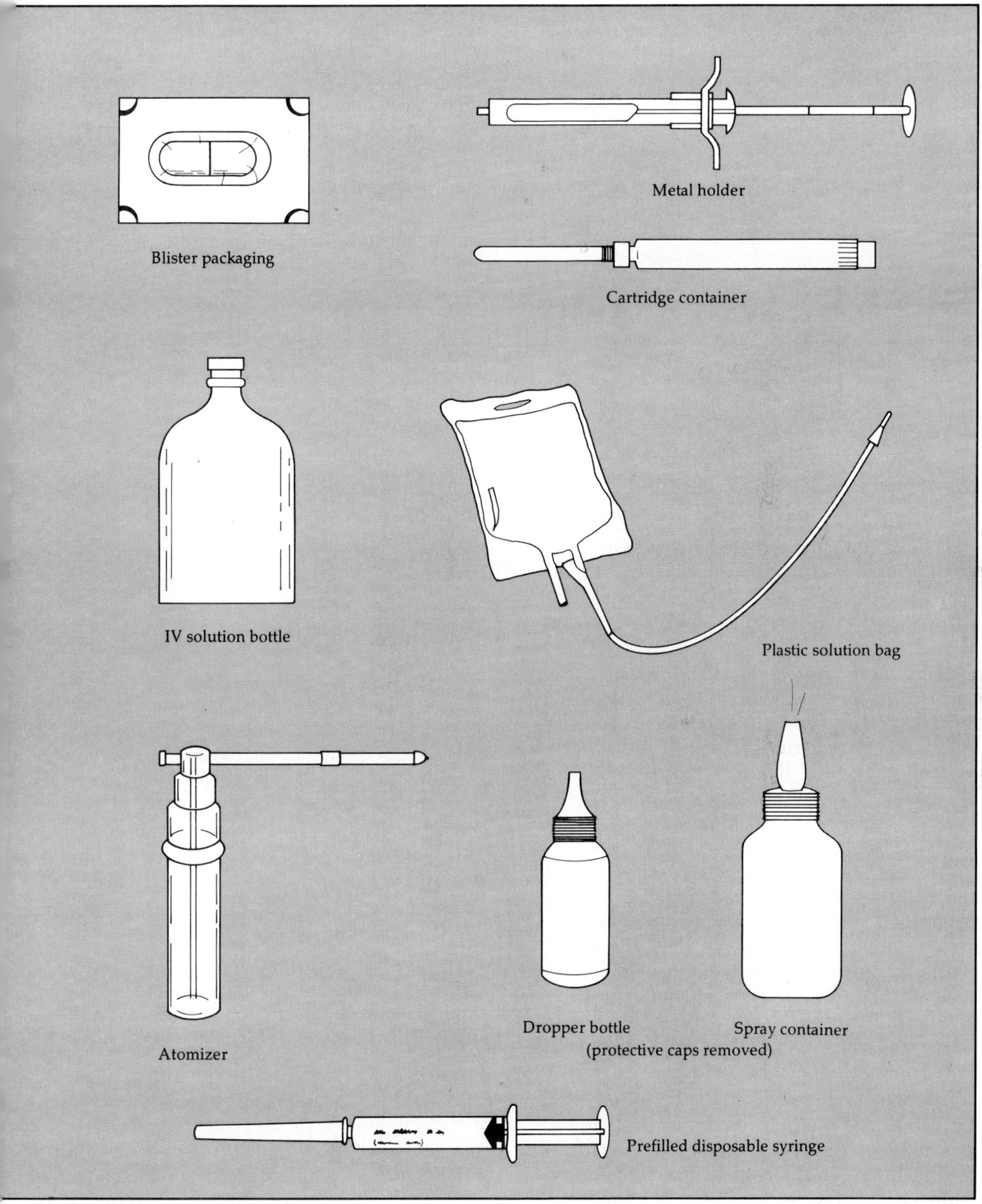

FIGURE 12-1 *(Continued)*

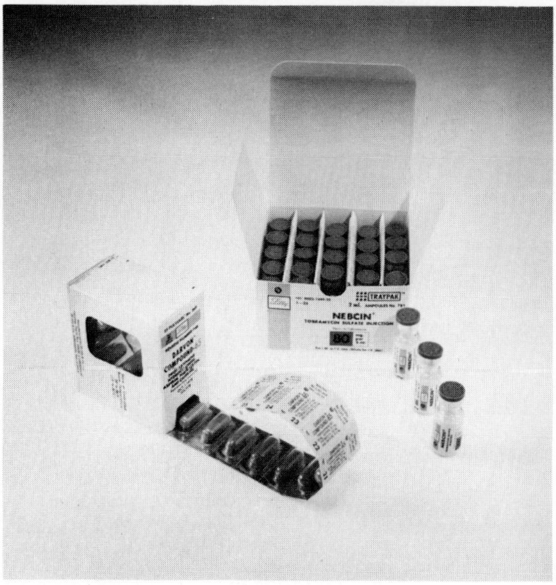

FIGURE 12-2

Prefilled disposable syringes These packaged units contain a syringe filled with the drug preparation and an attached needle. Some commonly used drugs, such as furosemide, haloperidol, and diazepam, are available in this form.

Cartridge container A single dose of a drug is sealed in a glass cartridge with a needle attached and the cartridge unit is placed in a holder with a plunger for injection. The cartridge and needle are disposable, and the metal or plastic holder is reusable. Cartridges may come in blister packages.

Bottles Solutions prepared for administration by intravenous drip are packaged in glass bottles of 250 to 1000 ml capacity, with volume designations imprinted in the glass. The top is usually a nonremovable rubber plug with a metal covering and thin rubber seal. Both the metal covering and the pliable rubber seal are removed before use, allowing the IV administration set to be inserted into the rubber plug.

Plastic bags Whole blood, plasma, packed cells, and some intravenous solutions are packaged in heavy plastic bags with volume designations printed on the bags. The IV administration set is either packaged with the bag or attached at the time of administration.

Packaging for Topical Drugs

Jars These cylindrical containers, made of glass or plastic, with a screw-on or snap-on lid, come in a variety of sizes. They may be transparent or opaque and are used for ointments, pastes, and creams.

Bottles These glass or plastic containers come in a variety of shapes, sizes, and colors. The top is usually narrower than the base of the container and has a screw-on lid. Bottles are used for liniments and lotions.

Tubes These soft, metal or plastic containers usually contain several ounces of a medication. The top is narrower than the body of the tube and has a screw-on cap. Tubes are used for ointments and lotions.

Sprays These soft, plastic containers come in varying sizes and release a fine mist of the medicated solution. Some topical antiseptic solutions are packaged as sprays.

Packaging of Drugs for Other Routes of Administration

Inhalation drugs

It is important to remember that some inhaled drugs are not limited in their systemic effects to the respiratory tract; they are also absorbed into the circulation through the pulmonary alveoli. Therefore, it is important not to exceed the prescribed dosage.

Sprays or atomizers These devices change medicated liquid in the container into a vapor for inhalation. Sprays are packaged as small, flexible plastic containers. Many nasal decongestants are packaged as sprays. Atomizers are packaged as push-button cans or in glass bottles to be used with screw-on atomizer tops.

Metered-dose nebulizers These devices are small glass or plastic containers filled with medicated solutions. The stem protruding from the container attaches to a mouthpiece. When the container and mouthpiece are pushed together, a measured amount of medicated vapor is released. Many bronchodilators are packaged as metered-dose nebulizers.

Drugs for the eye, ear, and nose

Dropper bottles These soft plastic containers have tops designed to release one drop of liquid medication when squeezed. They are used primarily for sterile ophthalmic solutions and for nasal and optic solutions.

Containers with screw-on medicine droppers The required dosage is drawn into the calibrated dropper and released by squeezing the bulb. They are used for the same purposes as dropper bottles.

Tubes These soft, metal or plastic containers usually contain 1 oz or less of the medication. The top is narrower than the body of the tube and has a screw-on cap. Tubes are used for ointments and lotions. Ophthalmic drugs packaged in tubes must be labeled "For ophthalmic use only." The medication is sterile.

Drugs for vaginal and urethral application

Blister-packaging Individual suppositories are sealed in plastic bubbles. They are refrigerated as necessary. Urethral suppositories come in sterile packages and must be administered using aseptic techniques.

Applicators Applicators may be prefilled by the pharmaceutical company or filled from stock supply just before use. A cartridge and plunger are calibrated to deliver a specified amount of the desired preparation. They are used for vaginal applications.

Foil-wrapped suppositories Individual suppositories are foil-wrapped and packed in boxes of five or more. In hot weather or very warm environments, the box should be refrigerated to prevent the contents melting.

SUMMARY

It is evident that there is a great variety in both dosage forms and drug packaging. Drug forms that are packaged similarly may be prepared for very different uses and must never be interchanged. For example, several bacteriostatic ointments are packaged in small tubes; some of them are prepared for application to the skin and others for ophthalmic use. *Only* the ophthalmic preparations may be used in the eye.

Finally, anyone administering medications must be familiar with the nursing implications of each dosage form and mode of packaging. Even the most potent drug will be ineffective if it is expelled in an undissolved state. Any medication could be dangerous if absorbed in a way that was not intended.

REFERENCES

Ansel, H. 1979. *Introduction to pharmaceutical dosage forms.* Philadelphia: Lea and Febiger.

Palmer, H. A., and Fraser, G. L. 1978. Crushing tablets, opening capsules: When is it safe? *RN* 41:53.

Swarbrick, J., ed. 1973. *Dosage form design and bioavailability.* Philadelphia: Lea and Febiger.

Chapter 13

Alimentary Tract Administration

MEDICATIONS THAT ARE administered into the gastrointestinal tract can be introduced for absorption in the oral cavity, swallowed for absorption in the stomach or intestines or both, or administered rectally. The oral route is the most convenient, as well as the most economical, way of providing a systemic action, but it is not without disadvantages. Irritating drugs can cause gastrointestinal complications, such as nausea, vomiting, and diarrhea, and the rate of drug absorption is slower for the oral route than for the parenteral one.

Irregular absorption of drugs can also occur due to such factors as (1) the inactivation of some medications by either the stomach acids or the intestinal enzymes; (2) the formation of unabsorbable complexes due to the drug's interaction with food or other drugs; and (3) the anatomical and physiological variations of some clients. Then, too, the client's cooperation in swallowing the prescribed medication is necessary. The oral route cannot be used for an unconscious client, nor for a client who has difficulty swallowing. Such an individual may need an alternative route, particularly if the medication cannot be crushed or given in a liquid form.

THE ORAL CAVITY

The mucous membrane of the mouth and pharynx is composed of thick, stratified, squamous epithelium and is therefore less sensitive to irritating drugs than other mucous membranes of the body. However, the thickness of the epithelium can cause slower absorption in this area than through other mucous membranes. Since the taste buds are located on the tongue, orally administered drugs should have an agreeable taste if the client's cooperation is to be gained.

Drug solutions that are applied for their local effect in the oral cavity are called **mouthwashes.** Solutions that are intended for the pharynx are called **gargles.** The primary purpose of these solutions is to cleanse or disinfect the structures or both, but they also have some aesthetic value. Since saliva is secreted most of the time and then swallowed, drugs administered for their local effect need to be repeated approximately every hour; the client should not be given water after taking the drug.

Drugs that are given orally to provide a systemic action must be held in the oral cavity until dissolved. When the medication is held against the mucous membrane of the cheek, it is called **buccal** administration. When the drug is held beneath the tongue, near the sublingual vein, it is termed **sublingual** administration. In both cases, the medication must be held, without swallowing, until the drug has dissolved. The tablets dissolve more quickly if the mucous membranes are moist; therefore, the client's mouth should be rinsed before administering the drug. When a rapid systemic action is required, these methods are better than swallowing because the drug is not destroyed by the digestive enzymes nor is it rapidly metabolized by the liver, since the portal circulation is initially by-passed. Nitroglycerin, a coronary vasodilator, can produce its therapeutic effects in one to two minutes when given sublingually; if it were swallowed it would be rapidly destroyed by the liver.

THE STOMACH AND SMALL INTESTINES

Even though clients often prefer to swallow their medications, it usually takes at least one hour for drugs administered this way to start to produce their therapeutic effects. This route is therefore inappropriate when an immediate action is required, such as in emergency situations. Drug solutions are usually absorbed faster than drugs in solid form, since drugs must be dissolved before they can be absorbed. Therefore, many drugs given for their local effect, such as antacids, should be given with little or no water. When a systemic effect is desired, the drug should be given with at least 100 ml of water to increase the rate of dissolution.

Factors That Alter Oral Drug Absorption

In general, the higher up in the alimentary tract a drug is absorbed, the sooner the therapeutic effects will occur. The gastric mucosa, however, will only absorb a few drugs, so the primary absorbing surface of the oral route is the intestinal tract. The absorption of drugs through the mucosa into the bloodstream is dependent on several factors, including the area's pH, the rate of gastric emptying, intestinal motility, the solubility of the drug in gastrointestinal fluids, the drug concentration or dosage and the presence of food in the intestines.

The *pH of the upper gastrointestinal tract* is very acid (approximately 1), and then becomes progressively more alkaline until it reaches approximately 8 in the lower intestine. An acid pH, such as that of the stomach, ionizes weak bases, whereas a more alkaline environment, such as that of the intestines, ionizes weak acids. Consequently, weak bases, such as morphine and ephedrine, are poorly absorbed in the stomach and more readily absorbed in the intestines, and weak acids, such as alcohol and aspirin, are more readily absorbed in the stomach.

The more ionized a substance is, the greater difficulty it will have passing through lipid membranes, such as the gastric and intestinal mucosae. Strong acids and bases are quickly ionized and are therefore poorly absorbed through the gastrointestinal tract. Drugs that are completely ionized and lipid insoluble, such as the antibiotic streptomycin, are absorbed very slowly.

The stomach can be artificially alkalinized by the administration of poorly absorbed bases, such as antacids. This technique decreases the gastric absorption of weak acids, such as aspirin, and increases the absorption of weak bases. When this alteration is intended, it is important to give the antacid simultaneously with the drug.

Some medications are destroyed by the acidity of the stomach, but many of them can be protected from the stomach's environment by an enteric coating, which should never be broken. If a smaller dose is required or the client is unable to swallow the drug in its coated form, the drug should be reordered in a different form or for a different route of administration.

The *motility of the gastrointestinal tract* also affects the absorption of drugs. The slower the stomach empties and the slower the rate of intestinal peristalsis, the longer a drug is in contact with the absorbing membranes. The absorption of many drugs is therefore increased as the motility of the tract decreases. However, if the emptying of the stomach is delayed, drugs that are absorbed in the small intestine will have delayed therapeutic effects. Medications that are unstable in gastrointestinal fluids, as well as drugs that tend to interact with food to form complexes, will undergo decreased or delayed absorption. Such medications should be given at least two hours before or after meals.

When the *circulation to the gastrointestinal tract* is impaired, the absorption of a swallowed medication is impaired as well. Shock, hemorrhage, and cardiovascular collapse decrease the circulation to the intestines and therefore alter drug absorption from the gastrointestinal tract (see Figure 13-1). These conditions, as well as extreme pain and delirium also delay the emptying of the stomach. Consequently, there is danger of drug toxicity when the client's circulation is normalized.

The absorption of drugs is also influenced by the *concentration of drug* in the gastrointestinal tract. In most cases, the greater the drug's concentration gradient, the more of it will be absorbed. Consequently, when the drug dosage is increased, there is a corresponding increase in the amount of drug absorption.

The *presence of food* in the stomach can delay the emptying of the stomach contents into the small intestine. If a drug is absorbed in the intestines and is taken after meals, the drug will have delayed absorption. Drugs can also interact with food, drugs, or other chemicals, forming unabsorbable complexes, so the *presence of other substances in the stomach also affects drug absorption.* Oral iron preparations react with the calcium phosphate in milk and become unavailable for absorption. On the other hand, the absorption of some drugs is enhanced by the presence of certain foods, drugs, or other chemicals in the stomach. Vitamin C enhances the absorption of iron, so oral iron preparations should be given with orange juice rather than with milk.

Preparation and Administration of Oral Medications

Critical elements in the preparation and administration of oral medications are presented in Tables 13-1 and 13-2, respectively.

Narcotics and other drugs requiring legal control and recording are sometimes packaged in controlled dispensers. Each dosage compartment is numbered. The dose can be ejected directly into the medicine cup by moving the opening on the container to the next number.

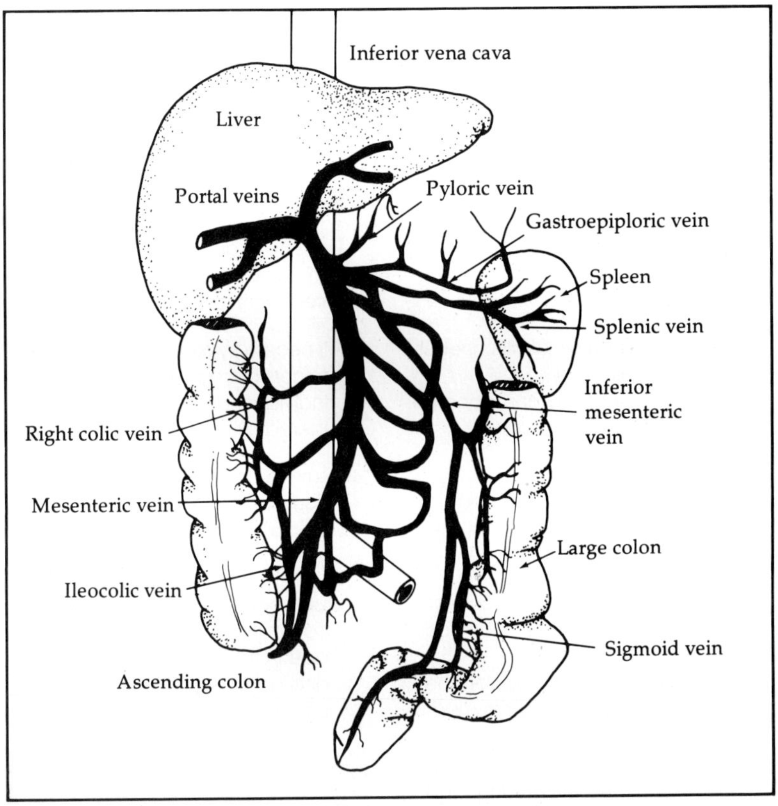

FIGURE 13-1 Venous circulation from the gastrointestinal tract.

The actual procedure and critical elements are otherwise the same as those listed for stock supply preparation.

THE RECTUM

Most rectal medications are given for their local action on either the contents of the colon or the tissues of the rectum, but the rectal route can also be used for systemic therapeutic effects. The rectal mucosa is similar to the intestinal mucosa and is therefore capable of absorbing drugs. As with the upper GI tract, weak acids and bases are absorbed readily and stronger acids and bases are more ionized and therefore poorly absorbed. However, the absorption of drugs by this route tends to be irregular and incomplete.

The superior hemorrhoidal vein drains into the mesenteric vein and then into the portal circulation, but the middle and inferior hemorrhoidal veins drain into the hypogastric vein and then directly into the inferior vena cava. Consequently, drugs absorbed in the lower two-thirds of the rectum do not pass through the liver and escape potential destruction by that organ (see Figure 13-2).

Although the normal function of the rectum is to expel its contents rather than retain them, there is a wide variation in the ability of different individuals to expel and retain rectal contents. Clients who frequently have fecal matter in the rectum without the impulse to defecate are better able to retain medications administered by this route. Clients who have exceptionally sensitive rectums tend to expel medications before sufficient time for absorption has elapsed. Since fecal matter will retard the absorption of rectal medications administered for their systemic effects, these drugs should be administered after the client has defecated.

The rectal route of administration is more

TABLE 13-1 Preparation Procedure for Oral Medications

	Critical Elements	
Procedure	**Stock Supply**	**Unit-Dose System**
Verify medication order according to agency policy.		
Wash hands.	Use sink nearest medicine cupboard.	Use sink nearest medicine cart—may be in client's room or treatment room.
Assemble equipment.	Clear working area of all unnecessary supplies. Gather together tray and appropriate containers for drugs.	All necessary supplies and containers are on medicine cart. Individual doses can be administered directly from package.
Select medication.	Take container from shelf. Hold at eye level and compare label with *every* element of medication order (first check).	Remove package from compartment. Compare label with ***every*** element of medication order.
Remove lid and pour medication.	*Solids:* Shake required amount into *lid* of medicine bottle, then transfer to medicine cup. Once the medication has left the bottle or lid, it is *never* returned to the stock container. Fingers should touch only *outside* surfaces of lid, bottle, and medicine cup, to prevent contamination of contents.	Open package and drop medication into cup *or* open package in the client's presence and administer directly from package.
	Liquids: Place lid *upside down* on working surface to prevent contamination of inside of lid. Holding bottle with label against palm of hand (to prevent soiling the label), pour required amount into calibrated medicine cup. Hold cup at *eye level* and read dose from bottom of meniscus.	Open package in presence of client and administer directly from package. *Caution:* If the unit-dose package is *different* than the prescribed dose, follow the procedure listed under *Stock Supply.* Double-check dose with order before administering drug to client.
Check dose with order.	Hold container at eye level and compare label with order (second check). Place stock container and lid on working surface with lid upside down.	
Place client's medication on tray.	Follow agency procedure, but always keep medicine card together with poured medicine.	
Check dose with order. Return bottle to shelf.	Replace lid; hold container at eye level and compare label with order (third check). Return bottle to shelf.	

TABLE 13-2 Procedure for Administration of Oral Medications

Procedure	Critical Elements
Bring medication to client. Identify client and explain procedure as necessary.	*Tablets and Capsules:* Instruct client to place as far back on tongue as possible, for ease in swallowing. *Liquids:* Cough syrups are *not* followed by water; antacids may be followed by no more than 10 ml of water. *Sublingual tablets:* Explain to client that medication must be placed under the tongue and remain there until dissolved. *Buccal tablets:* Explain to client that medication must be retained against the mucosa of the cheek until dissolved. *Troches:* Explain to client that medication must dissolve in the mouth and should not be swallowed whole or chewed.
Administer medication.	Hand medication to client. Pour water into cup and hand to client. Remain with client until drug is swallowed or dissolved. If client is incapacitated or restrained, the nurse places medication in client's mouth, under tongue or cheek, and holds water cup to client's lips while he or she drinks it.
Discard medicine container appropriately.	If client is unable to take the medication for any reason, the medication is discarded, if it was poured from stock supply,* or returned to client's medication compartment, if it is an unopened unit-dose.
Record medication.	Follow agency procedure for recording administration of medication immediately after leaving client.

*If it is necessary to discard a controlled substance, the record in the narcotic control book must be signed by *two* licensed nurses. However, unopened, individually packaged doses of controlled substances may be returned to the locked storage compartment.

inconvenient than the oral route. If a client has inflamed hemorrhoids or an anal fistula, the rectal insertion of drugs may be too painful. However, the rectal route is useful when (1) the client cannot take the drug orally, due to vomiting, unconsciousness, or inability to swallow; (2) the drug would be destroyed or inactivated by the gastric or intestinal environments; or (3) the client, such as a child or a psychotic adult, refuses to swallow.

Common practice in the past has been to determine rectal dosages by doubling the oral dose, based on the fact that the rectal mucosa absorbs drugs irregularly. However, more recent studies have indicated that the proper rectal dose must be determined for each drug. For example, the rectal dose of aminophylline, aspirin, and digitalis is greater than the oral dose, whereas the rectal dose of atropine and morphine is more toxic than the oral route and must be administered rectally in smaller doses. Drugs given as rectal suppositories and ointments take longer to be absorbed, than do drugs given as rectal solutions via retention enemas. The average adult rectum can comfortably retain about 120 ml of solution, so medicated retention enemas should be less than 120 ml. The client should lie quietly for 20 minutes following a suppository or 30 minutes following a retention enema so the medication will not be prematurely evacuated.

Preparation and Administration of Suppositories

Since most suppositories are prepared by the pharmaceutical manufacturers, no preparation is required in mixing or drawing up the medication. The only preparation required is the assembling of all necessary equipment. After washing the hands, the nurse verifies the medication order

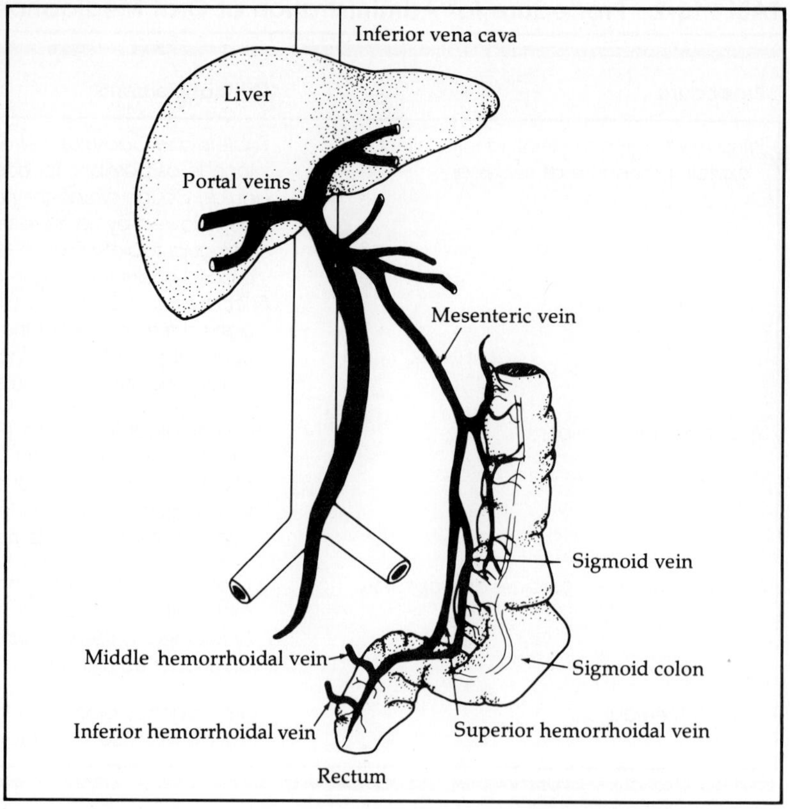

FIGURE 13-2 Venous circulation from the rectum and sigmoid colon.

as in all other routes of administration. On the medication tray are assembled the following items:

1. Suppository package
2. Appropriate antiseptic sponges for cleansing external area of insertion—check agency procedure manual for cleansing solutions used
3. Clean gloves or finger cot
4. Sterile water-soluble lubricant

Once the equipment needed for suppository insertion is assembled, the client is positioned on his or her side with the upper leg flexed. The nurse opens the suppository wrapper, squeezes a small amount of lubricant onto the inside of the wrapper and puts on the glove. The anal area is exposed, and the lubricated suppository is gently inserted at least 2 in. beyond the internal anal sphincter. The suppository must be in direct contact with the rectal mucosa. Then inserting the suppository, the finger should follow the wall of the rectum. If the suppository is inserted into a stool mass, it will be ineffective.

REFERENCES

Aman, R. A. 1980. Treating the patient, not the constipation. *American Journal of Nursing.* 80:1634.

Bauwens, E., and Clemmons, C. 1978. Foods that foil drugs. *RN* 41:79.

Black, C. D., Popovich, N. G., and Black, G. 1977. Drug interactions in the GI tract. *American Journal of Nursing.* 77:1426.

Hill, R. B., and Kern, F. 1977. *The gastrointestinal tract: Structure and function in disease.* Baltimore: Williams and Wilkins.

Chapter 14

Parenteral Administration

METHODS AND ROUTES OF PARENTERAL ADMINISTRATION

The term *parenteral* is derived from the Greek words *para* and *enteron,* and means *not through the intestinal tract;* the term has come to refer more narrowly to the administration of medication by injection through one or more layers of skin tissue. The methods of administering sterile solutions are by means of either a syringe and a needle, a hypodermic injector, or other less painful devices that have recently been invented.

The parenteral routes have many advantages over the oral route. Drugs that are destroyed or inactivated by the gastrointestinal environment, as well as medications that are poorly absorbed orally, can be administered parenterally. This route is often preferred when rapid absorption of a drug is required, particularly in emergency situations. The therapeutic response is often seen within minutes of an intravenous injection of a medication. Parenteral administration is especially useful for clients who are unconscious, uncooperative, or unable to retain oral drugs. The parenteral routes are also used for drugs that are irritating to the gastrointestinal tract.

However, the parenteral routes have several disadvantages. Because medications are absorbed rapidly and completely, there is little or no time to counteract any adverse effects. If a client is allergic to a drug, parenteral administration could be fatal. It is particularly important to note any known drug allergies in the client's history so that those potentially dangerous substances will not be administered.

With drugs that are known to sometimes produce severe allergic reactions, it is advisable to do a *skin test* on the client before the substance is administered. If clients have a documented allergy to the substance, however, they should be given neither drug nor skin test. A skin test consists of an intradermal injection of a small amount of the diluted drug. If the injected site becomes red and inflamed after a specified amount of time has passed, the client is probably allergic to the medication and it should be used with caution, if at all. Note that some clients have a histamine reaction to all injections.

Drugs that are to be injected must be sterile; they are therefore generally more expensive than oral medications. Many drugs are painful when injected and can cause considerable local tissue damage. If an irritating drug is absorbed poorly for any reason, it may cause a sterile abscess to form. Factors that reduce absorption include lack of circulation to the site, injection into edematous tissue, and too small an absorbing surface area; therefore, the injection site must be selected carefully. If microorganisms are accidentally injected with the medication, an infection will develop, so parenteral medications must be administered with great care and skill.

Types of Needles for Parenteral Use

Needles are available in a variety of lengths and gauges (thickness or size of lumen). The *higher* the gauge number, the *smaller* the size of the lumen, and vice versa. For example, a 25-gauge needle is smaller in diameter than an 18-gauge needle. Furthermore, more viscous solutions require a lower-gauge needle than do thin, watery solutions.

Needle lengths vary from 0.25 to 6 in., with the shorter needles generally being of higher gauge (smaller lumen) and the longer needles being of lower gauge (larger lumen). The size of the needle selected for parenteral injection depends upon the following factors:

1. The consistency of the medication being administered
2. The route of administration (intradermal, subcutaneous, intramuscular, and so on)
3. The client's general condition and tissue structure

Figure 14-1 shows a needle designed for parenteral use.

There are no hard-and-fast rules governing needle length and gauge for the different routes of injection. However, the nurse must be thoroughly familiar with the anatomical structure of the skin and underlying tissues to select the appropriate needle. The nurse must also be aware of the client's age and condition when selecting the needle. For example, slender, elderly clients generally have thinner subcutaneous tissue than younger people; therefore, the nurse may choose to use a 1-in. needle for an intramuscular injection rather than the usual 1.5-in. needle. Table 14-1 provides a general guide to needle selection for the *average* adult client; it must be modified as necessary.

Types of Syringes for Parenteral Use

Syringes are available in a variety of styles and capacities. They are usually made of glass or plastic and range in capacity from 1 to 50 ml. Most syringes in use today are of the disposable type; however, glass syringes are used on sterilized trays prepared by institutions, such as lumbar-puncture trays, and when the suction created by large glass syringes is required for irrigation.

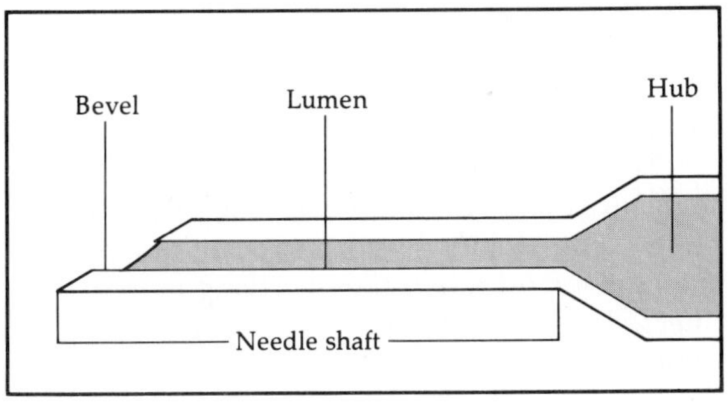

FIGURE 14-1 Diagram of a hollow, metal needle for parenteral use.

Insulin syringe Most insulin syringes are used *only* for administering insulin because they have a total capacity of 1 ml and are calibrated for 40 or 80 *units* rather than milliliters. However, the newer disposable insulin syringes are calibrated for 100 units and can be used for measuring minute doses of drugs. (See Figure 14-2.)

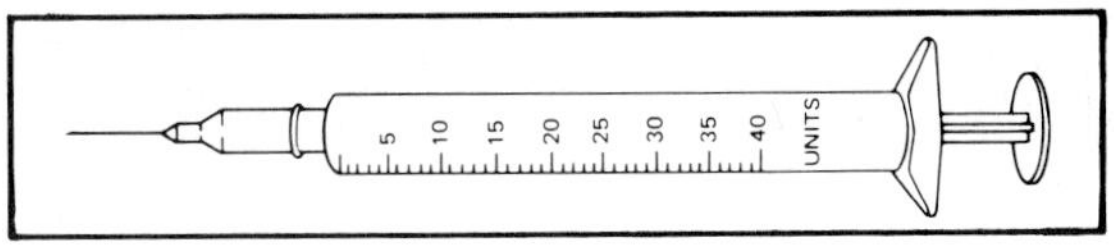

FIGURE 14-2 Insulin syringes.

Tuberculin syringe TB syringes are used primarily for tuberculin skin tests and, if in a disposable form, for very small doses of drugs. These syringes are calibrated for each 0.01 ml (hundredths of a milliliter) and have a total capacity of 1 ml. (See Figure 14.3.)

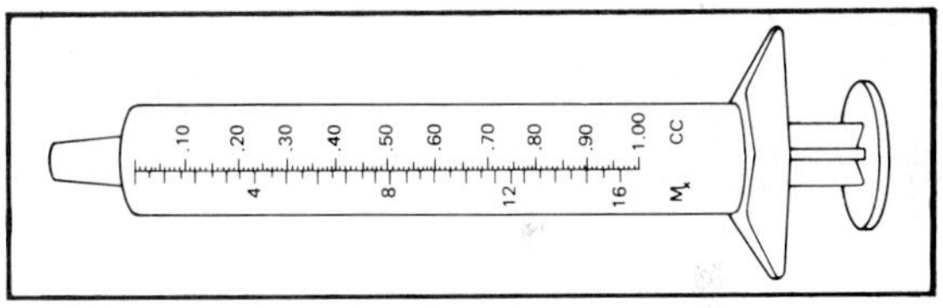

FIGURE 14-3 Tuberculin syringe.

Regular disposable syringe These syringes come prepackaged in paper or plastic with or without a needle already attached. They range in capacity from 3 to 50 ml. A syringe packaged in paper or thin plastic can be removed by pulling the layers apart at one end. A syringe packaged in rigid plastic containers is opened by twisting the plastic cap at the plunger end to break the seal. (See Figure 14-4.)

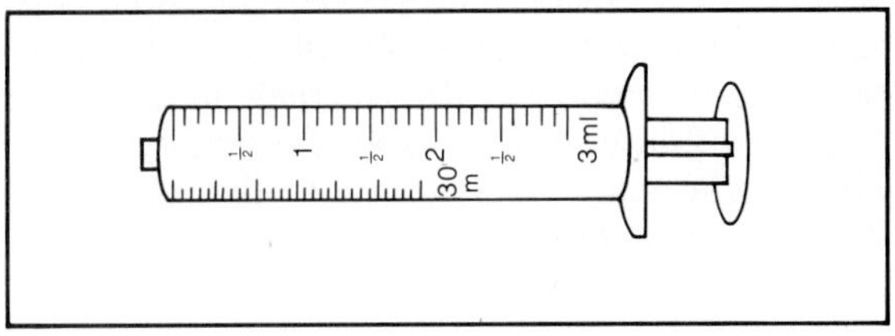

FIGURE 14-4 Regular disposable syringe.

TABLE 14-1 Guide to Needle Selection for Parenteral Use

Route of Administration	Needle Length	Needle Gauge
Intradermal	$\frac{3}{8}$ in.	25–27
Subcutaneous	$\frac{5}{8}$ in.	25–27
Intramuscular	1–2 in.	16–23
Intravenous	1–3 in.*	18–23
Intraperitoneal[†]	$\geq\frac{1}{2}$–3 in.	20–25
Intraarticular[†]	$\geq\frac{1}{2}$–3 in.	20–25
Intracardiac[†]	$\geq\frac{1}{2}$–3 in.	20–25
Intracathecal[†]	$\geq\frac{1}{2}$–3 in.	20–25

*The needle length depends on the client's particular anatomy.
[†]Usually administered by a physician.

Disposable unit-dose syringe The syringe and needle are packaged as a unit and the syringe can be used only for the matching unit-dose medication. The medication may come prepackaged in the syringe or in a separate *medication vial* that simply screws into place at the plunger end of the syringe cylinder. The needle end inside the syringe then punctures the medication vial and the unit is ready for use. (See Figure 14-5.)

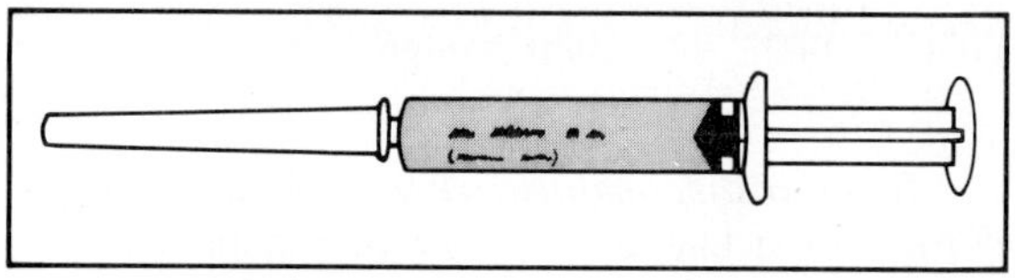

FIGURE 14-5 Prefilled unit-dose syringe.

Cartridge units These units can be used only with appropriate reusable plastic or metal cartridge holders. The medication is sealed in a glass tube with a needle attached and protected by a rubber sheath (see Figure 14-6). The *metal* cartridge holder is hinged at the plunger end and provides an opening for the needle and cartridge to be inserted into the holder (see Figure 14-7). The needle end is screwed into the matching threads at the bottom of the holder and then the plunger is swung back up into place and screwed to the matching threads at the top of the medication cartridge. The rubber sheath protecting the needle should not be removed during this preparation; it remains in place until the medication is administered.

The *plastic* cartridge holder is similar in design to the metal one, but the plunger end is not hinged. The plunger is pulled straight back to permit insertion of the medication cartridge in the side opening of the holder. The needle end of the cartridge and the plunger are then screwed into place, as with the metal holder.

INTRAMUSCULAR ADMINISTRATION

The injection of a drug deep into the body of a striated muscle is called an *intramuscular (IM) injection*. Medications given via IM injection are generally absorbed faster than those injected subcutaneously. Muscle tissue will also accommodate many irritating substances that would cause necrosis of subcutaneous tissues.

There are, however, several disadvantages to the use of the intramuscular route. Many major blood vessels and nerve tracts run adjacent to the bones, and when the overlying muscles are injected, the risk of damaging a nerve tract, penetrating a bone, or entering a blood vessel is higher than it is with subcutaneous injections. Severe pain or permanent nerve damage, possibly resulting in paralysis, can be caused not

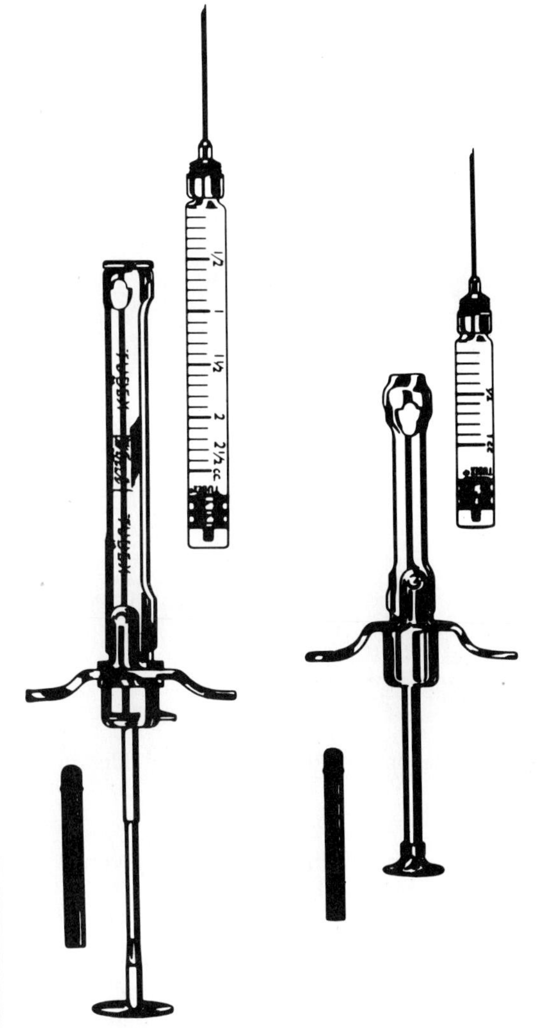

FIGURE 14-6 Metal cartridge holder with prefilled cartridge.

only by puncturing a nerve tract, but also by injecting the fluid too close to a nerve tract and causing compression of the nerve. Local tissue injury or necrosis can occur if the injected muscle is unable to accommodate the irritating characteristics of a drug or the quantity of fluid given.

In order for a muscle to be injected safely, the needle must be long enough to penetrate the skin, subcutaneous tissue, and part of the muscle mass. The depth of subcutaneous tissue varies greatly in different parts of the body and among individuals. For example, some obese clients may have large quantities of adipose tissue in their legs or abdomen, but relatively little in their arms; elderly clients may only have a thin layer because people tend to lose some of their subcutaneous tissue as they get older; emaciated clients also tend to have thin subcutaneous layers. In general, the abdomen and thighs have thicker subcutaneous layers than other parts of the body.

The distance the needle is inserted should be determined according to the client and the selected site. A quick method of estimating the required needle length is to grasp a 2- to 3-in. (5 to 7 cm) lateral expansion of the tissue over the potential site while the underlying muscle is in a relaxed state, and move it back and forth gently. The freely movable tissue is subcutaneous tissue; the more stationary tissue is muscle.

The skin and subcutaneous tissue can become irritated by some medications given intramuscularly if the drug is allowed to come in contact with them. Irritating IM drugs can be displaced away from the needle before the needle is withdrawn by including a small air bubble (0.1 to 0.3 ml) in the syringe before administering it. However, this technique may be inadequate with highly irritating drugs. To prevent subcutaneous tissue injuries, a special technique called the *Z-track* technique (described later in this chapter) is used to displace each tissue layer before the medication is administered; the drug is thereby locked in when the layers return to their normal positions. All irritating drugs should be given in large muscle masses only.

The absorption of a medication is determined primarily by its solubility in the muscle fluid. If the drug is water soluble in the muscle fluid, it will cause little or no local tissue damage and will be absorbed rapidly. Medications that tend to be insoluble in the muscle fluid will sometimes cause local tissue damage and pain. Some of the low solubility drugs are packaged with an anesthetic to decrease the pain.

Occasionally, it is desirable to prolong the action of a drug by slowing the absorption rate. This can be achieved by preparing drugs in suspension (rather than solution) or in oil. For example, benzathine penicillin G in suspension can act for several days. In addition, several hormones prepared for injection are available in oil,

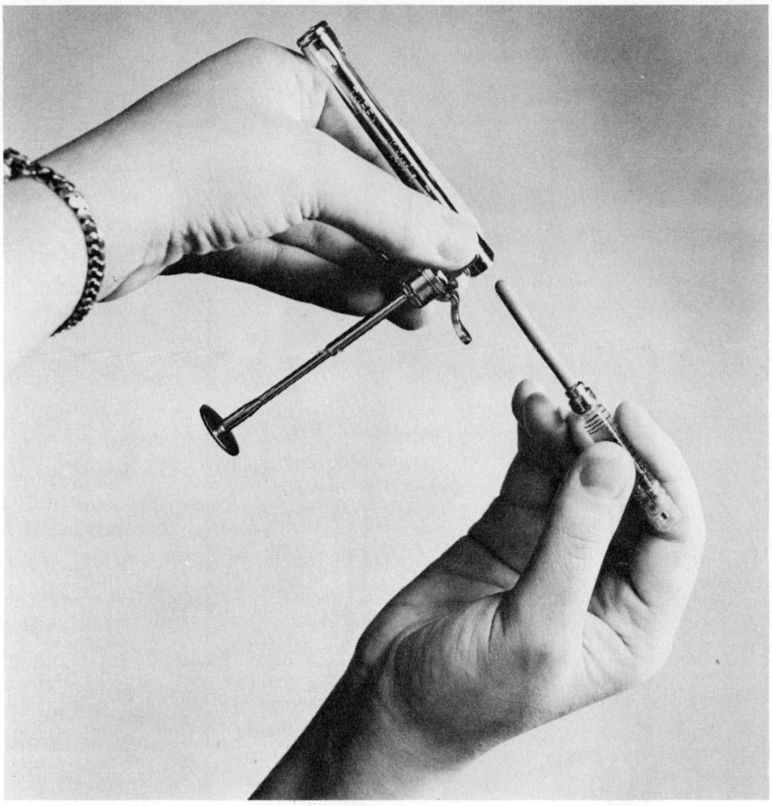

FIGURE 14-7 Inserting medication cartridge into metal holder.

such as desoxycorticosterone acetate, a hormone of the adrenal cortex used in the treatment of Addison's disease.

In fact, it is possible to sustain the action of a drug for several weeks by artificially slowing the absorption to a minimum. Preparations used for this purpose are termed *depot* (storehouse) or *repository* (replacement) injections. A depot of a compressed tablet or pellet is usually administered subcutaneously and a repository fluid is generally given intramuscularly. For example, the female hormone estrogen is sometimes given for replacement therapy in menopausal clients. The absorption of estradiol cypionate (estrogen) is so slow that the effects can last four weeks or more.

Sites for Intramuscular Injections

Injection sites must be selected carefully to accommodate the medication and to prevent injury to the client. The guidelines for selecting a site are as follows:

1. Irritating medications should be given in large muscle masses only.
2. The muscle mass selected must be able to accommodate the quantity of fluid injected.
3. Unused muscles should not be used for injections, since they may have atrophied.
4. Undeveloped muscles often have too small a muscle mass to accommodate an injection (a child's buttock should not be injected unless the child can walk).
5. Muscle masses located near nerve tracts or major blood vessels should be avoided.
6. A second injection should not be given into a site that still contains fluid or medication from a previous injection.
7. The selected muscle mass must have adequate circulation to absorb the fluid and medication injected.

There are several appropriate muscle sites for IM injections in the upper arm, the buttock, and the thigh.

The deltoid

The triangular deltoid muscle, which extends from the clavicle and scapula over the shoulder to insert in the middle of the humerus, can accommodate up to 2 ml of fluid and is convenient to use. However, since this area contains many pain nerve endings, injection can be rather painful. The deltoid muscle contains two main nerve routes: the radial nerve runs beneath the humerus in the axillary area and then runs laterally over the middle of the humerus, with a major branch of the brachial artery (see Figure 14-8).

However, the main nerve and blood vessel routes are avoided when the body of the deltoid is injected. The recommended injection site is the midlateral aspect of the upper arm between the acromion process and the axillary fold. This area of the upper arm should be completely exposed when administering an IM injection to ensure proper identification of the injection site.

Muscles are easier to inject when relaxed and there is often less pain if the muscle is in this state. Therefore, since the main action of the deltoid muscle is abduction of the arm, the arm should be placed against the trunk before injection, with the client standing, sitting, or lying.

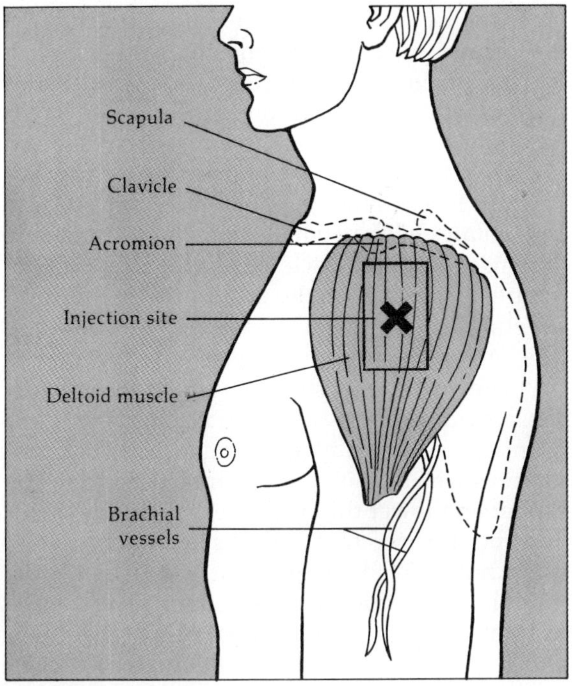

FIGURE 14-8 Deltoid injection site.

Gluteal region

Potential injection sites in the gluteal region include the gluteus maximus, the gluteus medius, and the gluteus minimus, an area extending from the iliac crest to the lower surface of the buttocks. However, only the *upper outer quadrant* of the buttocks can be injected safely because the major blood vessels and nerve tracts that supply the legs run from the spinal area down through the middle and lower parts of the gluteal region. (See Figure 14-9.) Paralysis of the legs can result if the sciatic nerve is injected.

The sciatic nerve is a large nerve tract composed of nerves from the fourth and fifth lumbar region and the first, second, and third sacral segments of the spinal cord. Branches of the sciatic nerve include the tibial nerve, the common peroneal nerve, and the nerve to the hamstrings. Damage to the tibial branch can cause footdrop and sensory disturbances; damage to the common peroneal or hamstring branch can also cause sensory disturbances as well as paralysis. Great care must be taken to avoid the sciatic nerve and its branches when administering injections into the gluteal region.

Furthermore, aspirating for blood is essential when giving an IM injection as there is a danger of puncturing a blood vessel. The inferior gluteal artery supplies blood to the gluteus maximus and piriformis, as well as to the sciatic nerve

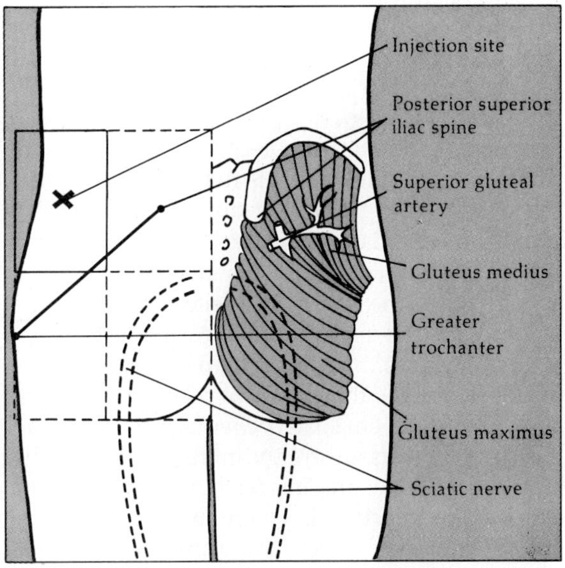

FIGURE 14-9 Dorsogluteal site.

and the skin over the buttocks. The superior gluteal artery supplies the gluteus medius, gluteus minimus, and the skin over the sacrum. These main arteries are embedded deep within the muscles, but some of their branches are more superficial, as are the veins, that drain the region.

Because of the massive size of the muscles in the gluteal region, this area is suitable for the injection of irritating drugs, even in the emaciated client. In fact, the gluteal region is the only recommended site for injecting colloidal iron preparation, iron dextran (Imferon). The gluteal region is also capable of accommodating 6 to 8 ml of injected fluid in the normal-sized adult. However, it is recommended that only 5 ml be injected in each buttock to prevent irritation of the muscle. Caution should be taken in the obese client; the bony landmarks may be difficult to identify due to the thick layer of subcutaneous tissue. If the iliac crest cannot be located, another site should be used.

The gluteal muscles are not fully developed in children until they are able to walk. Consequently, the gluteal region should be avoided until the child can walk independently, usually between the ages of 12 and 18 months.

The *gluteus maximus* is one of the largest muscle masses in the body. It helps the body to attain an upright position by extending and laterally rotating the thigh. It also braces the knee when the thigh is fully extended. To relax this muscle for an injection the client should lie on the abdomen with toes pointed inward. The nurse then elevates the client's lower legs with a pillow or rolled blanket. The injection is administered in the *upper outer quadrant,* which is located by dividing the buttock into four equal sections. This area is sometimes called the *dorsogluteal site,* indicating that the needle is to be inserted in the lower portion of the upper outer quadrant. The gluteus medius is a desirable site, because it can be used for all patients. This area is sometimes referred to as the *ventrogluteal* site. The minimus, underlying the medius, is the smallest of the gluteal muscles, but since the overlying medius is a thick muscle, the muscle mass is thick enough to use even in emaciated clients. The skin and subcutaneous tissue are thinner here than in the dorsogluteal site, and it is farther from the sciatic nerve. The injection is given about 1 in. (3 cm) below the iliac crest in normal-sized adults (between the sides of a V formed by the palm of the hand positioned over the greater trochanter, with the first finger on the anterior superior spine of the iliac crest and the second finger opened in a V on the iliac crest). (See Figure 14-9.)

If these landmarks cannot be identified, as in obese clients, another site should be selected.

The gluteus medius and gluteus minimus abduct and rotate the thigh medially. Relaxation of these muscles can be achieved by having the client lie either on the abdomen or on the side with both legs together. The gluteal region should be avoided in children and adults who are incontinent since such a condition creates a greater chance of infection in these injection sites.

The thigh

The large muscle group in the anterior and lateral aspect of the thigh is called the *quadriceps femoralis* and is composed of four muscles: the rectus femoralis, the vastus lateralis, the vastus medialis, and the vastus intermedius. These muscles are thick and contain few major blood vessels and nerves. The skin surface over the quadriceps also has few sensory nerve endings. Therefore, the anterior and lateral aspects of the thigh are satisfactory injection sites.

The *vastus lateralis* is the largest of the quadriceps muscles. It is so large that as much as 15 ml can be injected into the thickest part in a normal-sized adult. However, no more than 5 ml should be injected at one time because larger quantities can cause muscle irritation, pain, and muscle spasms. Because of its massive size, the lateralis is recommended for injections in infants and young children; but no more than 2 ml should be injected. The muscle begins as a broad aponeurosis, attached to the greater trochanter, and extends down to a flat tendon that is inserted in the lateral aspect of the patella.

The long, rather slender vastus lateralis muscle provides several appropriate injection sites. Damage to the muscle's aponeurosis and tendon, as well as injury to other structures in the upper and lower thigh, can be avoided by dividing the distance from the greater trochanter to the knee into four equal parts and using the middle two sections for injections. The muscle is located in the anterior lateral part of the thigh.

In the midthigh area, the layer of subcutaneous tissue over the muscle posterior border is thicker than that over the muscle itself. Consequently, the muscle's posterior border can be palpated by identifying the thickened subcutaneous area. To avoid the major blood vessles and nerve tracts located on the posterior side of the femur, the needle is injected into the thigh's anterior lateral area, at least 1 in. (2.5 cm) from the vastus lateralis' posterior border. (See Figure 14-10.)

The anterior thigh contains the *rectus femoralis* muscle, which is bordered medially by the *vastus medialis.* The *vastus intermedius* lies beneath the rectus femoralis, so there is a large area of muscle mass in the anterior thigh. These muscles are relatively free of major blood vessels and nerve tracts. The anterior thigh contains more sensory nerve endings than the lateral thigh, so the rectus femoralis is *only used when other sites are unavailable for injection.*

The rectus femoralis begins as two tendons originating in the iliac spine and the acetabulum of the hip. The muscle extends down over the anterior surface of the thigh and ends in a long flat tendon that is inserted in the lower surface of the patella. To avoid damage to the muscle's tendons, only the anterior midthigh area should be injected. The recommended site can be identified by dividing the distance from the greater trochanter into two sections and drawing an imaginary line. The injection should be given at the level of the line or just above the line. (See Figure 14-11.)

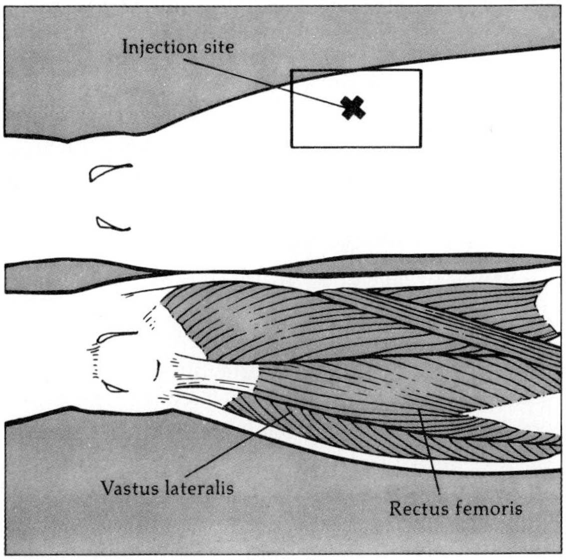

FIGURE 14-10 Vastus lateralis site.

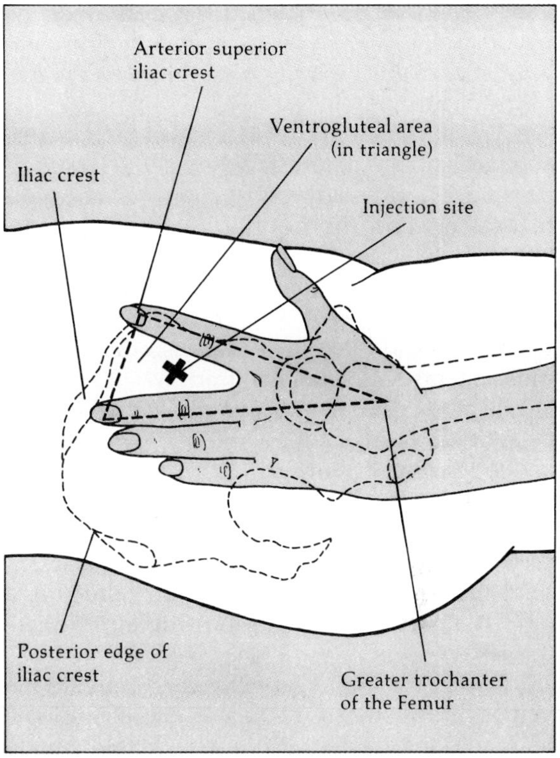

FIGURE 14-11 Ventrogluteal injection site.

The quadriceps femoralis group of muscles extends the whole length of the leg. The muscles are in a relaxed state when the clients are lying down with their knees flexed. Since infants' knees are normally flexed, their legs should be kept in this position while sites in the quadriceps femoralis are being injected. However, the comfort of an adult client is increased when lying on the side with the knees flexed.

Pediatric Intramuscular Injections

Special precautions should be taken when administering an intramuscular injection to an infant or a small child. Whenever possible, needles with a smaller diameter and a shorter length should be used. Narrow needles cause less local injury to tissues than thicker ones. A needle becomes narrower as the needle gauge number increases. For example, a 21-gauge needle (often used for adult IMs) is considerably larger than a 25-gauge needle (often used for IMs in children). However, some medications are so thick that they cannot be expelled through a narrow needle, so needle selection depends on the characteristics of the medication as well as on the size of the client.

The thickness of the skin, subcutaneous tissue, and muscle determine the needle length to be used. The tissue thickness should be assessed before selecting the needle length so that the appropriate tissue layer is injected. Although intramuscular injections are usually given to adults with a 1.5-in. (3.5 cm) to a 2-in. (5 cm) needle, a 1-in. (2.5 cm) needle is adequate for most infants and small children.

To avoid pain, infants and small children pull away from an injection, sometimes resulting in dislodgement or contamination of the needle. Consequently, children must be restrained either with special equipment designed for this purpose or by another individual. The body part is held firmly with one hand as the other hand quickly injects the needle into the appropriate tissue layer.

Injections should generally be given into the ventrogluteal site or the vastus lateralis muscle in infants and small children. The deltoid muscle is too small and the minimus muscle (dorsogluteal site) is not fully developed in children until they can walk independently (see Figure 14-12).

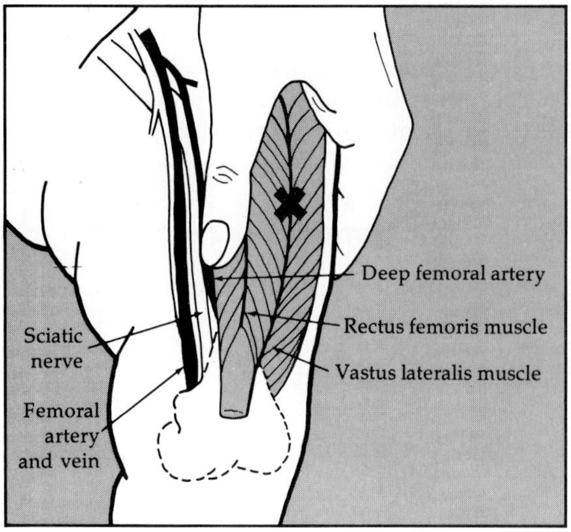

FIGURE 14-12 Rectus femoralis injection site in the left leg.

Intramuscular Self-Administration

Sometimes it is necessary to teach a client how to self-administer a medication intramuscularly. For example, many clients with myasthenia gravis must have an intramuscular injection of neostigmine daily. Since these clients must be able to see what they are doing and have both hands free to manipulate the syringe, the sites must be selected carefully. The vastus lateralis and rectus femoralis muscles of both thighs are accessable to self-administered intramuscular injections.

The client should be taught to rotate the sites of injection so that the injected tissue has a chance to recover. Some medications are absorbed very slowly, so the characteristics of the medication must be considered as well. Since each injection site should be used as infrequently as possible, a schedule of rotating sites should be kept on a calendar by the client.

Preparation and Administration of Intramuscular Injections

Table 14-2 presents the critical elements involved in the preparation of IM injections and Table 14-3 presents the critical elements involved in the administration of IM injections.

Intramuscular medication can also be administered by the *Z-track technique.* This method of administration is used for drugs that are very irritating to the skin and subcutaneous tissue or that would discolor the skin if they leaked from the injection site. When this technique is used, the path of the needle is sealed off after the skin is released, thereby preventing leakage of the drug into the subcutaneous tissue. The upper outer quadrant of the buttock is the preferred site for Z-track injections. (See Figure 14-13.)

The procedure is the same as that shown in Table 14-3, with the following exceptions:

1. An *air bubble is left in the syringe* before injection.
2. The skin is pulled to *one side* before injection and *held there during* the injection and the *withdrawal* of the needle.
3. After the drug has been injected, 10 seconds are allowed to pass before the needle is withdrawn.
4. After the needle is withdrawn, the skin is released.
5. The site is *not massaged.*

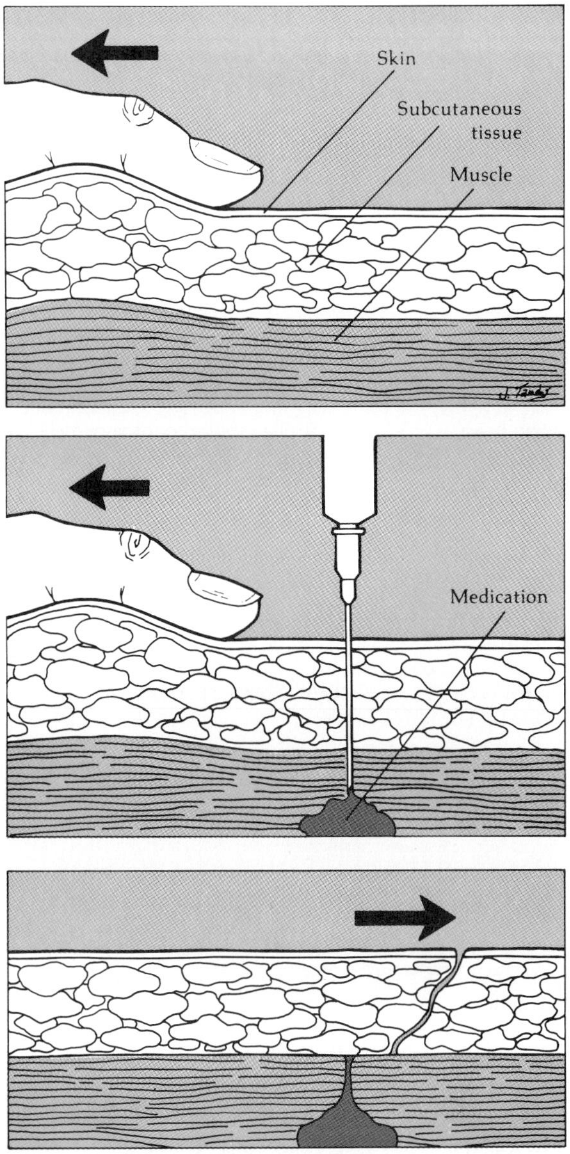

FIGURE 14-13 Z-track tissue displacement.

SUBCUTANEOUS ADMINISTRATION

The injection of substances into the loose tissue beneath the skin is called a *subcutaneous* or *hypodermic injection*. The term *hypodermic*, which literally means *under the derma* or skin, and the term *subcutaneous*, meaning *under the cutis* or skin, are used interchangeably. Subcutaneous tissue is a layer of fibrous proteins widely interspaced with collections of fat cells. Since the cells of this tissue are primarily fat cells, the tissue is sometimes called *adipose tissue*. Subcutaneous tissue contains blood vessels, nerves, and lymphatic vessels.

Sites for Subcutaneous Injections

The thickness and fat content of the subcutaneous layer varies in different parts of the body and is influenced by heredity, sex hormones, eating habits, and age. In most areas of the body it is thicker than the dermis, but it is absent in some locations, such as the anterior surface of the tibia and the eyelids.

Hypodermic injections are given in areas where there are relatively large quantities of subcutaneous tissue well supplied with blood and lymphatic vessels, such as the outer surfaces of the upper arms, the thighs, the abdomen, the gluteal region of the buttocks, and the lateral aspects of the chest (axillary line area). The use of the latter side is suitable in men and infants, but there may be too little subcutaneous tissue in women for this site to be used. The upper arm is often the most accessible and therefore the most frequently used site. However, the thighs and especially the abdomen contain fewer pain nerve endings than the arms, so they are often the preferred sites for subcutaneous injections. (See Figure 14-14.)

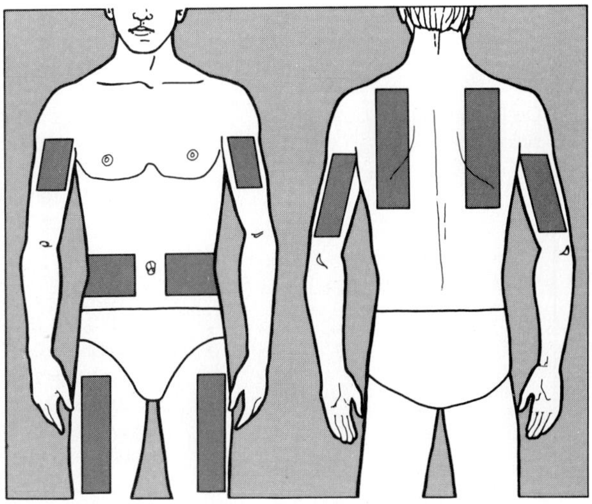

FIGURE 14-14 Sites for subcutaneous injection.

TABLE 14-2 Preparation Procedure for Intramuscular Injection

	Critical Elements	
Procedure	**Stock Supply**	**Unit-Dose System***
Verify medication order according to agency policy.		
Wash hands.	Use sink nearest medication area.	
Assemble equipment.	Clear working area. Gather together tray, correct size syringe, needle, and antiseptic sponges.	Gather together tray, correct size syringe, needle, and antiseptic sponges.
Select medication.	Take container from storage area. Hold at eye level and compare label with *every* element of medication order (first check).	Individually labeled container may be in client's compartment, in refrigerator, or in locked cabinet.
Cleanse the medication container.	*Vial:* Using antiseptic sponge briskly scrub the rubber top of vial. Discard sponge. Place another sponge over vial's rubber top and place vial on tray. *Ampule:* Snap top of ampule until all liquid is in bottom section of ampule. Using antiseptic sponge, clean neck of ampule. Break off top, using sponge to protect fingers. Discard top and sponge. Place ampule on tray.	*Vial:* Same as stock supply. *Ampule:* Same as stock supply.
Assemble needle and syringe. (See page 235 for types of syringes.)	Open sterile package containing syringe and needle according to packaging directions. Attach needle to syringe if necessary, keeping protective sheath on needle to prevent contamination.	Assembly: Same as stock supply.
Remove protective sheath from needle.	Pull rubber or plastic sheath straight off and place sheath on tray.	Same as stock supply.
Draw up required dose into syringe.	*Vial:* Draw up air in syringe equal to amount of medication required. Remove sponge from top of vial and insert needle into cleansed rubber stopper of vial, with bevel up. Inject air into air in vial. Withdraw required dose by pulling plunger up to correct calibration. If there is an air bubble in syringe, pull plunger back slightly beyond required dose. Remove needle from vial. *Ampule:* Insert needle into opening of ampule, being careful not to touch sides of ampule.	*Vial:* Same as stock supply. *Ampule:* Same as stock supply.

TABLE 14-2 ***Continued***

Procedure	Critical Elements: Stock Supply	Critical Elements: Unit-Dose System*
	Withdraw required dose by pulling back on the plunger. If there is an air bubble in syringe, pull plunger back slightly beyond required dose. Remove needle from ampule.	
Expel air and read dosage.	Hold syringe with needle straight up, and *gently* push on plunger to expel air from syringe. With calibrations on syringe at *eye level,* check dose with medication order card (second check).	Same as stock supply.
Replace protective sheath on needle.	Be careful not to contaminate needle by touching it to outside of sheath. Place syringe on tray with medicine card.	Be careful not to contaminate needle by touching it to outside of sheath.
Return medicine container to appropriate place.	*Vial:* Compare label with medicine order (third check). Return multidose vial to storage area. *Ampule:* Compare label with medicine order (third check). Discard ampule.	*Vial:* Compare label with medicine order again (third check). Discard remaining contents in single-dose vial. *Ampule:* Compare label with medicine order (third check). Discard ampule.

*A *true* unit-dose injection is already prepared and ready for immediate administration.

The injection site should be carefully selected, particularly in elderly and debilitated clients. The skin of the aged becomes thinner and loses some of its subcutaneous tissue, which accounts for the wrinkled appearance of the elderly. If hypodermic injections are necessary, they should be given in areas that still retain a thick subcutaneous layer, such as the abdomen and thighs. These sites are also recommended in the very thin or emaciated client.

Areas that have poor circulation should also be avoided, since the injected medication will be absorbed slowly and irregularly. Such areas include scar tissue. In clients who have arteriovenous shunts—for example, individuals in renal failure undergoing hemodialysis—the shunt extremity should not be injected. In fact, hypodermic injections should not be administered in all clients who are undergoing a generalized decrease in circulation, such as individuals in shock.

The absorption of drugs administered subcutaneously depends on the following factors:

1. The drug's ability to penetrate a lipid membrane
2. The molecular size of the medication
3. The quantity of blood capillaries in the area
4. The concentration of the drug

The capillary walls behave like a lipid membrane in that they are penetrated by diffusion or filtration. Most lipid-soluble drugs diffuse the capillary membranes rapidly, so the drug's effect is often seen within minutes. On the other hand, the rate at which water-soluble drugs penetrate the capillary wall is dependent on their molecular size. The smaller the molecules, the faster the drug will enter the bloodstream. Insoluble and nondiffused substances are carried away by the lymphatic system, which moves much more slowly than the blood, so the action of these substances is delayed.

TABLE 14-3 Procedure for Administration of Intramuscular Injection

Procedure	Critical Elements
Bring prepared medication and equipment to client. Identify client and explain procedure.	Bring the following equipment to bedside: syringe with medication; antiseptic sponges; and medicine card, if used by agency.
Select injection site.	Expose site to be used, making sure it is different from location of previous injection.
Cleanse injection site.	Using an antiseptic sponge, cleanse injection site with a circular motion from the center outward.
Prepare syringe for injection.	Holding syringe in one hand, grasp needle guard with other hand and pull it straight off, being careful not to contaminate needle by touching it to outside of needle guard. Hold syringe with needle pointing straight up.
Inject medication.	Stretch cleansed skin between thumb and index finger or pinch skin gently (depending on site, condition, and age of client). Insert needle at a 90-degree angle with *pointed end of bevel first.* Release skin. Pull back on plunger to be sure needle is not in a blood vessel. If blood is aspirated, withdraw the needle, discard needle and syringe, and repeat procedure using new equipment and medication. If no blood enters the syringe, inject medication by pushing plunger slowly.
Remove needle.	Press down on site of injection with antiseptic sponge while quickly withdrawing needle. Gently massage site in circular motion *if indicated.* Cover needle with guard.
Discard syringe and needle in designated containers.	Agencies have special containers for breaking and disposing of needles and syringes, so they cannot be used again.
Record medication.	Follow agency procedure for recording medication immediately after leaving client.

The more capillaries there are in the injection site, the greater is the surface area available for absorption, and the faster the drug will be absorbed. Absorption from edematous tissue is poor, so injections into this tissue should be avoided.

Occasionally it is desirable to have a drug absorbed slowly. It is possible to slow the rate of absorption by decreasing the blood flow to the area—for example, by applying an ice bag over the injection site. The blood flow can also be reduced by adding a small amount of a vasoconstrictor, such as epinephrine, to the medication being injected. Some local anesthetics come prepared with epinephrine for injection so that the effect of the anesthetic will be prolonged. If a vasoconstrictor is used, the injected area should be observed frequently for a marked decrease in the circulation, a development that could lead to tissue necrosis.

If desired, the absorption rate can be increased by applying a hot water bottle to the site, which will increase the blood flow. Since diffusable drugs are absorbed rapidly anyway, there is little value in rubbing or massaging the injection site. However, the absorption of nondiffusable or poorly diffusable substances can be increased by movement of the body part involved, since these substances must be transported through the lymphatic system before reaching the bloodstream.

For example, if the upper arm is injected, the client can be instructed to move the arm frequently.

Most injected drugs are either in solution or suspension. Remember that a solution is a liquid containing the dissolved drug and a suspension is a mixture of liquid and drug. Since drugs must be in solution before they can be absorbed, solutions produce faster action than suspensions. When it is desirable to have a drug absorbed slowly in order to prolong its action, a suspension of the drug may be ordered. For example, the effects of an injection of regular insulin, a solution, last 6 to 8 hours, whereas the effects of protamine zinc insulin, a suspension, last 24 to 28 hours. Medications in an oleaginous liquid (in oil) also often take longer to act than the same drug in sterile water. For example, the effects of an injection of epinephrine *solution* will only last a few hours, but an injection of epinephrine in oil will last 12 hours or more.

The volume of medication that can be comfortably absorbed from the subcutaneous tissue is generally 2.0 ml. However, larger volumes can be absorbed if the injection site is infiltrated with the enzyme *hyaluronidase*. The subcutaneous infusion of large quantities of fluid (800 to 1000 ml) is called *hypodermoclysis*. Hyaluronidase decomposes (hydrolyzes) mucopolysaccharides such as hyaluronic acid, which is a viscous component of the interstitial fluid of many tissues and acts like a cement to the tissues. When this acid is broken down and liquefied by hyaluronidase, the tissues become more permeable and the absorption of injected fluids increases considerably. Only very soluble nonirritating fluids are administered by this method; however, the client may still complain of soreness in the injected tissue. Sterile normal saline or half normal saline is the solution infused in most cases, but 5% dextrose solutions can also be used. Dextrose solutions tend to irritate the tissue sooner than saline solutions.

The solution must be infused slowly to prevent the tissues from becoming distended. Distention of the tissue will decrease the solution's absorption rate by collapsing the adjacent blood and lymph vessels. The infusions must be given in areas that have a thick layer of subcutaneous tissue; therefore, the thigh is the most frequently used site.

Hypodermoclysis injections can be used to infiltrate infected eschar tissues of burn clients. Using sterile technique, the appropriate antibiotic is mixed with 25 ml of normal saline and administered at a rate slow enough to prevent swelling of the eschar site (approximately 30 minutes). Each injection covers and therefore treats a diameter of about 13 cm (6 in.) of eschar. The entire eschar can be treated at the same time by the use of multiple hypodermoclysis injections positioned at 13-cm intervals.

Although subcutaneous tissues can absorb irritating substances more comfortably than the oral route, the skin can become irritated if these drugs are allowed to come in contact with the skin during injection. Consequently, it is recommended that an air bubble of 0.1 to 0.3 ml be injected so that the irritating drug is displayed away from the needle tip before the needle is removed. It is also recommended that irritating medications be given in the abdominal subcutaneous tissue, since it has fewer nerve endings than the other sites.

As with other parenteral routes, hypodermic injections are used when the oral route is unsuitable and when the effects of a drug are needed quickly. However, infections can be introduced by this route if sterile technique is not strictly observed and there is also the danger of injecting directly into a vein. This risk can be eliminated if, after inserting the needle, the syringe's plunger is pulled back to see if blood is aspirated. If blood is aspirated, a blood vessel has been punctured, and the medication should not be given into that site.

Subcutaneous injections are frequently given with a $\frac{5}{8}$ in. (1.5 cm) length needle in infants, children, and adults, whereas a $\frac{3}{8}$ in. (1 cm) length needle may be needed for premature infants and emaciated children.

Subcutaneous Self-Administration

Many diabetic clients must give themselves daily subcutaneous injections of insulin. Subcutaneous injections can be self-administered in the upper thigh and the abdomen (see Figure 14-14). To avoid injecting the same site twice, the client should keep a calendar and mark off the sites used daily.

Preparation and Administration of Subcutaneous Injections

The preparation procedure for subcutaneous administration is the same as for intramuscular injection, using an appropriately sized needle (see Table 14-2). Table 14-4 presents the critical elements involved in the administration of subcutaneous injections, and Figure 14-15 shows needle angles for subcutaneous injections.

INTRADERMAL ADMINISTRATION

The injection of substances into the skin's dermis (corium layer) is called *intradermal administration*. The terms *intracutaneous* and *endermic* are also sometimes used to indicate this route. The epidermis consists of a stratified epithelium with an outer tough, horny mass of cells that must rely on the capillaries just beneath them for nutrients. The dermis, on the other hand, consists of tough connective tissue, elastic fibers, lymphatics, and a rich supply of capillaries and nerve endings.

With the exception of the cells lining the sebaceous glands, normal, healthy skin is resistant to the absorption of any substance, so only small volumes of nonirritating solution can be used, usually 0.1 to 0.2 ml. Consequently, intradermal injections are only useful for local effects, such as skin testing for allergies or diagnostic testing for such diseases as tuberculosis. When the skin requires puncturing or incising for certain procedures, the nerve endings of the dermis layer can be locally anesthetized by injecting small quantities of an anesthetic, such as procaine.

A 25- or 27-gauge needle, $\frac{3}{8}$ in. (1 cm) long, is used for intradermal injections for infants, children, and adults.

Preparation and Administration of Intradermal Injections

The preparation procedure for intradermal injection is the same as for intramuscular injection (see Table 14-2) except that a disposable tuberculin (TB) syringe is usually used to draw up the medication. This is because very small amounts are administered (less then 0.4 ml) and the TB syringe is calibrated in hundredths of a milliliter.

Intradermal injections are usually administered in the flexor surface of the forearm, which has a relatively thin epidermis and is therefore useful for this type of injection. The area between the scapulae is also used. During administration, the skin is held taut to prevent it from moving while the thin, short needle is inserted.

Figure 14-16 shows the position of the needle for intradermal injection. The needle is inserted almost parallel to the skin surface at an angle of 10 or 15 degrees. The expected reaction time to the injected solution, which causes a temporary stinging sensation and raises a wheal in the skin (Figure 14-17), varies with the drug and the client's sensitivity to the solution. With the exception of

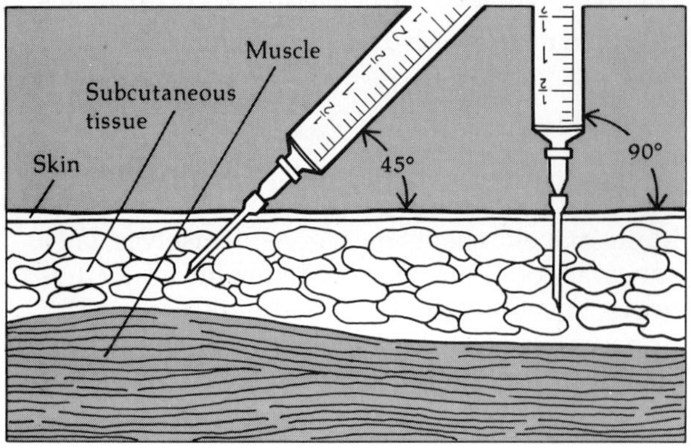

FIGURE 14-15 Angle for subcutaneous injection.

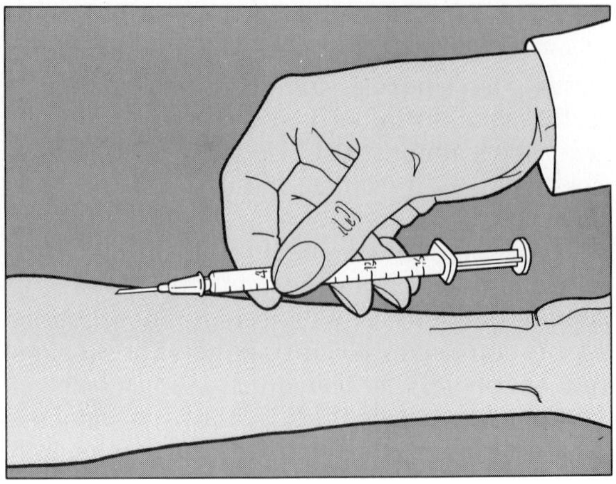
FIGURE 14-16 Intradermal injection syringe position.

TABLE 14-4 Procedure for Administration of Subcutaneous Injection

Procedure	Critical Elements
Bring prepared medication and equipment to client. Identify client and explain procedure.	Bring the following equipment to bedside: syringe with medication; antiseptic sponges; and medicine card, if used by agency.
Select injection site.	Expose site to be used, making sure it is different from location of previous injection.
Cleanse injection site.	Using an antiseptic sponge, cleanse injection site with a circular motion, from the center outward.
Prepare syringe for injection.	Holding syringe in one hand, grasp needle guard with other hand and pull it straight off, being careful not to contaminate needle by touching it to outside of needle guard. Hold syringe with needle pointing straight up. Expel air bubble by pushing *gently* on plunger. (For irritating drugs, do not expel air bubble.)
Inject medication.	Pinch cleansed skin gently between thumb and index finger. Insert needle at a 45-degree angle with *pointed end of bevel first.* Release skin. Pull back on plunger to be sure needle is not in a blood vessel. If blood is aspirated, withdraw needle, discard needle and syringe, and repeat procedure using new equipment and medication. If no blood appears, inject medication by pushing plunger slowly.
Remove needle.	Press down on site of injection with antiseptic sponge while quickly withdrawing needle. Massage site *gently* in a circular motion.* Cover needle with guard.
Discard syringe and needle in designated containers.	Agencies have special containers for breaking and disposing of needles and syringes, so they cannot be used again.
Record medication.	Follow agency procedure for recording medication immediately after leaving client.

*Heparin injection should *not* be massaged.

aspiration, which is not necessary, the administration procedure is the same as that for intramuscular injection.

INTRAVENOUS ADMINISTRATION

Medicated solutions that are administered directly into the venous circulation are called *intravenous (IV) injections* or *infusions*. An *IV injection* means that the solution is forced into the vein with a syringe, whereas an IV *infusion* means that the solution enters the vein by force of gravity. While only small quantities of fluid can be injected, large quantities can be infused intravenously. The terms *IV push* or *IV bolus* are used to indicate the injection of small quantities of medicated solution into a vein. The German word *phleboclysis* (literaly means to cleanse a vein) and the term *venoclysis* and *continuous IV* are sometimes used to indicate the slow infusion of large quantities of solutions into a vein to (1) replace fluids; (2) provide nutrients; and (3) introduce medications. Some drugs need to be administrated

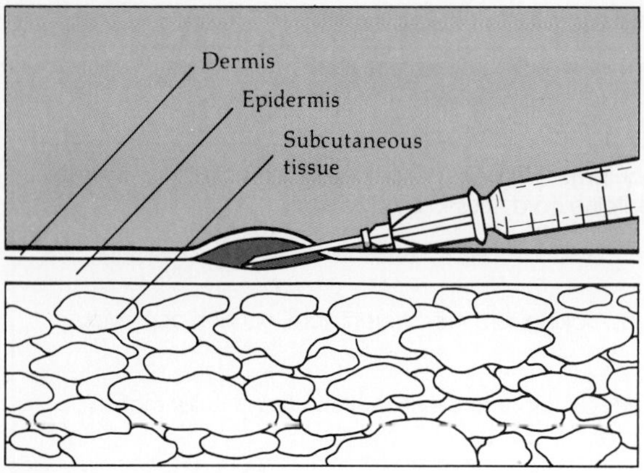

FIGURE 14-17 Formation of a small wheal after intradermal injection.

periodically but are too irritating or dangerous to give via IV bolus. The term *intermittent infusion* is used to denote the administration of diluted medications over 20 to 60 minutes. Intermittent infusions may be given through specialized IV administration tubing called *volume control sets* or via a secondary line added to the continuous IV administration sets. Since infusions are regulated by how fast the solution is allowed to drip into a drip chamber, the term *IV drip* is also used to indicate the infusion of medicated solutions.

The action of drugs given intravenously is immediate, often within 30 seconds or less, because the medication does not have to be absorbed through a membrane before it enters the circulation. Consequently, this route is preferred in emergency situations or when the drug dosage must be adjusted to the clients response. For example, when a client is in shock and blood pressure has fallen dangerously low, certain drugs can be diluted with sterile fluid and given IV to keep the blood pressure in a safe range. The faster the IV drips, the more drug is administered to the client. If the client's blood pressure then becomes too high, the IV drip can be slowed. The term *titrating* is sometimes used to indicate that the dosage of a drug is being controlled by the speed or rate of the IV infusion. When an individual's response to a drug is controlled by titration, the expression *"monitoring the clients response,"* is often used. Drugs that are titrated according to the client's response include dopamine, lidocaine, and Isuprel. Titrating enables the rate of drug administration to be controlled as accurately as possible. An *infusion pump* set for the desired rate of administration or a minidrop chamber (60 gtt/ml) are recommended for this procedure.

Methods of Entering Veins

A vein can be entered externally by puncturing it with a sterile needle called a *venipuncture* or by surgically cutting a small incision into the vein called a *venous cutdown.* A sterile 21- or 22-gauge needle attached to a syringe is commonly used to give a single dose of a medication intravenously. However, if the client has an IV infusion running, the discomfort of a puncture can be avoided by administering the drug through the tubing. When the client requires several doses of a drug over a period of time, such as antibiotics, a continuous infusion is usually set up to keep the vein open, called a *KVO,* and the medication is given through a secondary line connected to the KVO administration set.

The needle gauge must be smaller than the diameter of the inside of the vein. When intravenous injections were first given to infants a cutdown was often necessary since the 25-gauge hypodermic needles were either too large or too awkard to use in the small superficial scalp veins of infants. Consequently, a small gauge needle that would lie flat against the infant's head was designed. These needles are called *scalp veins, winged tips,* or *butterflies* because the needle area is in the shape of a butterfly. (See Figure 14-18.) Butterflies are now available in 21- to 28-gauge needles and are not only useful for infants but also small children, the small veins of the hand, individuals with low venous pressure, and clients who have veins that rupture easily.

Since injection needles have a sharp point and are inflexible, they tend to puncture clear through a vessel when the client moves. Consequently, injection needles are more useful when administering anesthetics or when the client needs the vein punctured for short periods (for example, a 4-hour chemotherapy treatment). When a venipuncture is reqired for longer periods of time, a flexible piece of tubing, called a *catheter* or *cannula,* is often inserted either through the lumen of a needle (intracath) or as a sheath covering the needle (angiocath). The needle is then withdrawn. Angiocaths are short (usually $1\frac{1}{2}$ to

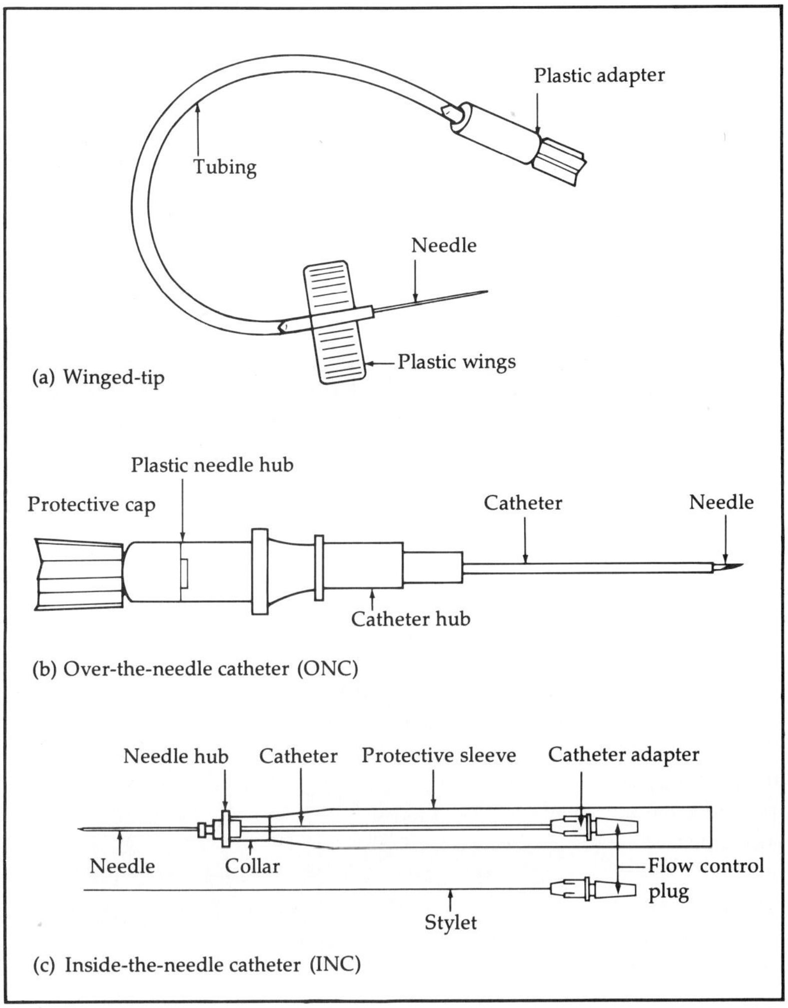

FIGURE 14-18 Types of catheters and needles used for venipuncture.

3 in. long) and are used in peripheral vessels whereas intracaths are long (up to 36 in.) and are used for insertion into large vessels, such as the superior vena cava for the purpose of hyperalimentation or central venous pressure monitoring. (See Figure 14-18.)

The risk of infection is much less with a small puncture wound through the skin, but, when it is impossible to administer an IV by an external venipuncture, a venous cutdown is often performed by the physician. The skin over the vein is surgically incised and sterile tubing (catheter) is inserted into one of the larger surface veins through a small cut. The catheter is then sutured into place and the skin is sutured shut. Consequently, *an IV cutdown that stops running should not be removed and the physician should be notified immediately.*

Sites for Venipuncture

The large superficial veins with little or no subcutaneous tissue covering them, such as are found in the antecubital space, the wrist, and the dorsal surface of the hand, are easily punctured, and so are suitable for IV injection. However, the dorsal metacarpal veins of the hand have a smaller lumen than most of the veins in the wrist and forearm. In the elderly, the dorsal metacarpal veins often stand out and appear large because of atherosclerotic changes in the vessels, but the vessel lumen is often smaller and less pliable than veins in the normal adult. Because of the small lumen size and the mobility of the hand, a small gauge scalp vein is recommended for injection into these vessels.

The accessory cephalic vein, which curves over the radial surface on the thumb side of the wrist, is often prominent in adults and is large enough to accommodate a large gauge needle. However, it is often difficult to enter because there are no adjacent structures to hold it in place during venipuncture. The flexible angiocaths and intracaths are usually used for this vessel since rotation and flexion of the wrist could cause a needle to dislodge. Great care should be taken to keep the wrist in a comfortable but stationary position.

In the antecubital space, the medial cephalic vein is often reserved for punctures of short duration, such as obtaining blood for analysis and for administering medications via IV push. This vessel has a large lumen and is easily punctured, even in children. The basilic vein is also frequently used, but it is surrounded by a great deal of subcutaneous tissue in many individuals and is therefore more difficult to puncture. (See Figure 14-19, top.)

The numerous veins on the anterior surface of the lower arm, which include the medial antibrachial vein, the accessory cephalic vein, and other vessels that lead into the cephalic and basilic vein, can also be used, but these vessels have large quantities of subcutaneous tissue surrounding them and are therefore difficult to puncture except by individuals experienced in IV injection. (See Figure 14-19, bottom.)

The veins on the dorsal surface of the foot and the medial surface of the ankle are sometimes used, but IV injection in the lower extremities poses more risks than does injection in the arms. There is a great danger of clot (thrombus) formation if a varicose vein is injected. Even in a client with normal veins, ambulation is impossible with an infusion in the foot or ankle. This immobility in turn results in decreased venous circulation in the legs and stasis of blood can cause thrombus formation. When a thrombus breaks loose, it is called an *embolus,* and it will travel with the blood until it lodges in a vessel that is smaller than the clot. Emboli from the legs can lodge in the pulmonary circulation and cause serious impairment of respiration or brain function.

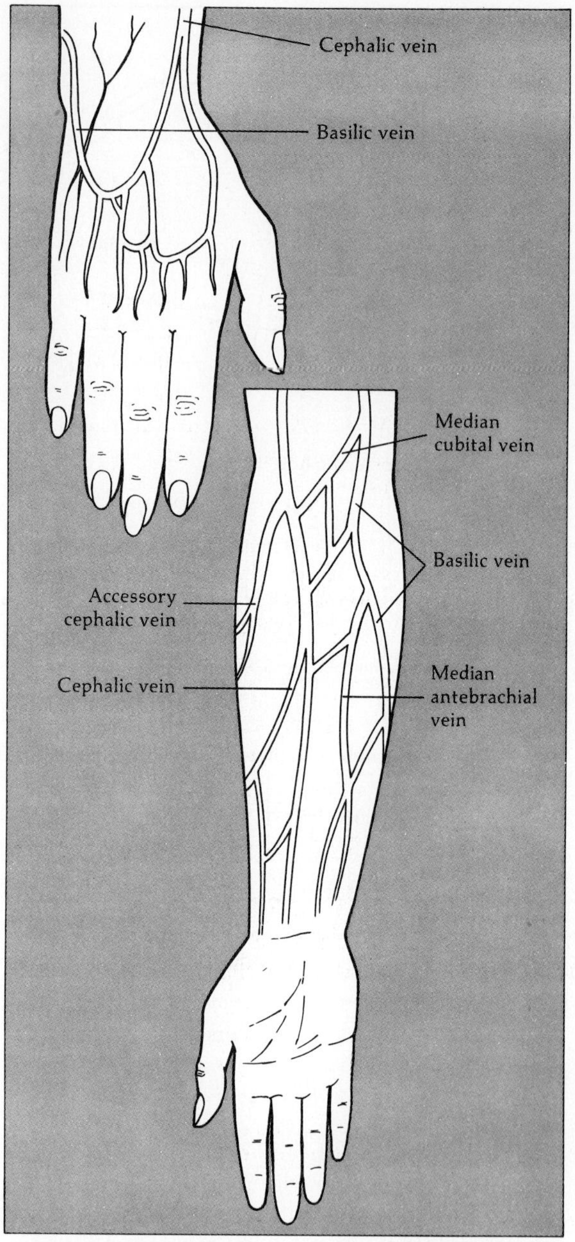

FIGURE 14-19 Dorsal and ventral views of the veins of the hand and forearm.

The risks of leg venipuncture often outweigh the advantages. If a client must have an intravenous infusion in the leg, the client should be observed frequently for thrombus or embolus formation and venous circulation should be enhanced by (1) using a bed cradle to keep the weight of the bed linen from compressing the veins; (2) elevating the entire leg about 20 degrees, with the trunk no higher than 45 degrees; and (3) teaching the client isometric leg exercises.

In infants and small children, the arm veins are often too small for IV injections. Instead, the external jugular vein can be used in children and the superior longitudinal sinus in infants. An angiocath is often used in the jugular vein and a scalp vein needle in the sinus. Precautions must be taken to prevent the child from touching the IV site; covering the hands of an infant is usually sufficient, but elbow restraints are often needed for small children.

When none of the above sites for intravenous infusion is available, a cutdown is performed by the physician. The deeper but larger upper basilic or brachial vein is often used.

Intravenous Solutions

Medications and infusions given intravenously must be *clear, sterile,* and *isotonic solutions.* Suspensions and oily solutions (with the exception of fat emulsions) can cause vessel blockage and pulmonary embolisms if inadvertently given IV. Medications that are packaged in powdered form must be *completely dissolved* before they are administered IV.

As the blood is slightly alkaline and has a normal pH of 7.4, all IV solutions should have a pH as close to 7.4 as possible. If the solution is markedly hypotonic, it can cause the client's red blood cells to burst or hemolyze; if it is markedly hypertonic, it can destroy the red blood cells by shrinking them. However, there are situations in which a hypertonic solution is necessary, such as extreme fluid imbalance. In these cases, the client must be watched closely for blood cell destruction, signaled by fever, diaphoresis and chills, and the IV rate carefully monitored.

Certain irritating solutions that can cause destruction of muscle and subcutaneous tissue can be given safely IV without damaging the relatively insensitive lining of the veins. These drugs must be diluted adequately and injected slowly. Precautions are taken to prevent the irritating medication from coming in contact with other tissues by (1) changing to a new sterile needle for injection after filling the syringe to the required dose; (2) administering an isotonic solution after the drug is given IV; and (3) withdrawing 1 to 2 ml of blood into the syringe before removing the needle. If the irritating drug does escape into the surrounding tissue, called an *infiltration* or *extravasation,* the IV should be stopped immediately and the physician notified. For example, the potent cardiovascular agent, norepinephrine (Levophed), will cause necrosis and sloughing upon infiltration and the affected area must be injected with phentolamine (Regitine) by the physician as soon as possible to minimize the destruction of tissue.

Great care must also be taken to prevent the injection of microorganisms. The medication and solutions used must be sterile and the drug must be prepared under sterile conditions. When diluting a powdered drug with a solution from a multidose vial, a previously unopened vial should be used. In addition, the IV tubing should be changed at least every 24 hours. If the solution is inadvertently contaminated with pathogens, symptoms will often appear with 30 minutes. These symptoms may include fever, chills, nausea, vomiting, and even shock in severe cases. In such cases, the IV should be stopped or the IV bottle changed immediately and vital signs taken every 15 minutes until the physician arrives. The contaminated IV bottle should be saved so that the organism can be identified by culture and the appropriate antibiotic administered.

The intravenous route has several advantages: (1) absorption barriers are avoided; (2) large volumes of fluid can be accommodated; (3) irritating, acidic, and alkaline solutions can be given; and (4) continuous monitoring of a drug's action can be maintained. However, this route is considered the most dangerous method of giving medications. Because drug action is virtually immediate, often occurring within 30 seconds or less, allergic reactions can arise within minutes and can result in serious harm or even death. Once the medication is administered IV, there is no way to retard its effect. Also, there is the danger of giving too much of a drug, particularly to emaciated and drug-sensitive clients.

Since the individual who administers a drug is held legally responsible for the results, IV medications should be given only by those health professionals who understand both the drug and the risks involved. Many IV medications are administered by a physician. However, a great number of nurses have been certified to give some IV drugs, particularly in emergency settings. Other health professionals—for example, some paramedics—are also able to administer IV medications when necessary.

Drug Incompatibilities

A *drug incompatibility* occurs when the combination of two or more substances results in an undesired physical or chemical reaction. Chemical incompatibilities occur when two substances react to produce new compounds or when the reaction leaves one or both substances inactive therapeutically. Such incompatibilities may be invisible and are therefore difficult to detect. Nurses should consult a pharmacist and become acquainted with drugs in order to prevent a chemical reaction. Physical incompatibilities, on the other hand, are often visible since the solution may form a precipitate, become hazy or cloudy, form bubbles due to the creation of gas, or change the color of the solution.

There are three main factors affecting compatibility: (1) length of exposure; (2) ionic instability; and (3) the pH of the resulting solution. For example, potassium penicillin will remain stable for 24 hours in sterile water, but only 6 hours in 5% D/W solution; erythromycin remains stable for 24 hours in sterile normal saline, but only 6 hours in 5% D/W. Most barbiturates, phenytoin (Dilantin), and a number of other drugs should be given via IV bolus in order to avoid precipitation. Since many drugs, particularly antibiotics, remain stable and soluble in a solution with a relatively neutral pH, these drugs will form a precipitate if combined with a drug that makes the resulting solution highly acidic or highly alkaline. Therefore, antibiotics should be well diluted and administered through a secondary line or piggyback. The drug manufacturer's recommendations should be carefully followed.

When a client must receive incompatible drugs, the solutions can be given (1) at different time periods; (2) through different IV administration sites; or (3) by different routes. As in hyperalimentation, there are occasions in which several drugs must be added to the same IV container. In such cases, the solution should be prepared by a pharmacist.

Known drug incompatibilities are listed in the drug's packaged brochure or can be obtained from a drug incompatibility chart (see Table 14-5). In fact, any solution that becomes cloudy, changes its color, or forms a precipitate should not be given since the solution has undergone a change. In addition to drug incompatibilities, other factors, such as the age of the solution and its reaction with the container, can cause changes. IV solutions should never be given after the expiration date on the label.

With the exception of a few substances, 5% dextrose and water are compatible with most drugs. Medications should never be added to whole blood, blood products, plasma expanders (for example, dextran), or protein hydrolysates (Amigen) since numerous incompatibilities can occur.

Preparation and Administration of Intravenous Injections

Although IV medications used to be given by the physician, it is now fairly common for clinical agencies to allow licensed professional nurses to give IV medications after they have been trained and supervised appropriately. Direct administration of a drug by venipuncture is referred to as IV push or IV bolus, to distinguish it from adding medications to large amounts of intravenous infusion solutions.

Any accessible vein may be used for IV injection, but the veins of the forearm are preferred because they are close to the surface and are large enough to be penetrated easily. An 18- to 22-gauge needle, 1 to 2 in. long, is used for IV injection.

The preparation procedure for IV injection is the same as that for intramuscular injection (see Table 14-2). The procedure for administration of IV injection is shown in Table 14-6.

IV Bolus Through a Y Port

When a client already has an IV, the discomfort of a second venipuncture can be avoided by administering the drug through the Y port in an existing IV tubing. The procedure for giving a drug in this way is shown in Figure 14-20 and summarized in Table 14-7.

TABLE 14-5 Commonly Used Drugs Known to Have Several Incompatibilities

Aminophylline	Meperidine (Demerol)
Amobarbital (Amytal)	Morphine sulfate
Ampicillin	Penicillin G
Ascorbic acid (vitamin C)	Pentobarbital (Nembutal)
Cephalothin (Keflin)	Phenytoin (Dilantin)
Chloramphenicol	Phenobarbital (Luminal)
Diazepam (Valium)	Procainamide (Pronestyl)
Digoxin	Sodium bicarbonate
Ephedrine sulfate	Tetracycline
Epinephrine (Adrenalin)	Thiopental sodium (Pentothal)
Erythromycin	Vancomycin
Furosemide (Lasix)	Vitamin B
Heparin	Warfarin sodium (Coumadin)

Continuous Intravenous Infusion

An intravenous infusion is administered when the amount of solution required is 250 ml or more. Infusions may be ordered for short periods of time in order to administer specific medications, or for several days in succession to keep the client adequately hydrated and in electrolyte balance. Infusions are also used for the administration of certain drugs, such as antibiotics, and to keep a vein open for emergency drug administration.

There are several types of intravenous solution containers and administration sets available, and it is wise to study the package directions before beginning to assemble the unit.

It is important to be aware that intravenous infusions are administered by the gravity method rather than by injection under manual pressure. Therefore, the solution container must be hung on a device high enough above the level of the client to overcome the client's venous pressure.

All intravenous administration sets consist of long lengths of plastic tubing to which a glass or plastic drip chamber is attached. The chamber permits the nurse to determine the rate (drops per minute) at which the solution is entering the client's circulation. Since administration sets made by different manufacturers deliver drops of *different volume*, the nurse *must read* the packaging information to ascertain how many drops will equal 1 ml of solution. The range for different sets is from 10 to 20 drops per milliliter; that for minidrop sets is 50 to 60 drops per milliliter. This information is essential to the nurse in determining the proper flow rate required for carrying out the physician's order. (See Chapter 11 for calculating drops per minute.)

There is a variety of setups commonly in use for intravenous infusions. The simplest consists of a bottle or bag of sterile solution; a length of sterile plastic tubing with a drip chamber at one end; a movable clamping device somewhere along the tubing; and a narrower tip for attaching to a needle or catheter at the other end of the tubing

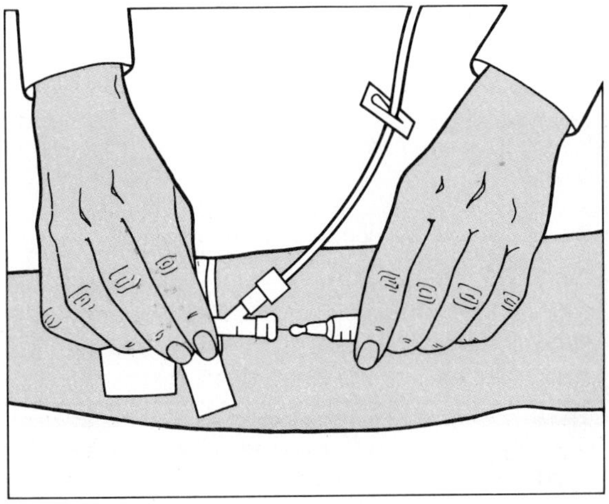

FIGURE 14-20 Administering intravenous medication through an intravenous line.

TABLE 14-6 Procedure for Administration of Intravenous Injection (IV Push or IV Bolus)

Procedure	Critical Elements
Bring prepared medication and equipment to client. Identify client and explain procedure.	Bring the following equipment to bedside: syringe with medication; antiseptic sponges; tourniquet; and medicine card, if used by agency.
Select vein for venipuncture.	In many clients, the veins of the forearm are visible beneath the skin.
Apply tourniquet.	Wrap tourniquet around extremity about 3 in. above venipuncture site. Amount of tension should be sufficient to distend veins below the tourniquet so they are palpable and visible. Have client open and close fist if the forearm is used.
Palpate the selected vein.	Tap the vein lightly 2 in. in either direction, to ascertain its size and direction.
Cleanse injection site.	Using an antiseptic sponge, briskly wipe the injection site. Do not touch cleansed site again with fingers.
Prepare syringe for injection.	Remove needle guard. Expel *all* air from syringe.
Stretch skin at injection site.	Place thumb just below injection site and pull skin downward so it is taut.
Pierce skin and vein with needle.	Insert needle at a 45-degree angle with the *pointed end of bevel first.* Continue moving tip of needle toward and into the vein. While holding the syringe barrel stationary, gently pull back on the plunger. Blood will flow into the syringe when the vein has been entered.
Release the tourniquet.	Holding syringe in one hand, release the tourniquet with the other hand.
Inject medication.	Push plunger evenly, injecting drug into vein. Observe the recommended rate of IV administration for the particular drug.* Observe client for any untoward reactions.
Withdraw needle.	With one hand, place antiseptic sponge over injection site. Withdraw needle quickly and apply *firm* pressure with sponge for *about one minute.*
Discard syringe and needle in designated containers.	Agencies have special containers for breaking and disposing of needles and syringes, so that they cannot be used again.
Record medication.	Follow agency procedure for recording medication immediately after leaving client.

*Each drug monograph indicates the recommended rate of IV drug administration. Although most drugs are given slowly, about five minutes or more, some must be given quickly, about 30 seconds, because of protein binding.

TABLE 14-7 Procedure for Administration of IV Bolus Through a Y Port

Procedure	Critical Elements
Identify type of IV solution client is receiving.	If any incompatibilities exist between IV bolus and clients present IV solution, the bolus cannot be given at this site.
Prepare medication.	Be certain that the drug is adequately diluted in the appropriate solution for IV administration.
Bring prepared medication to client. Identify client and explain procedure.	Bring the following equipment to bedside: syringe with medication; antiseptic sponges; and medication card, if used by agency.
Check present IV site for infiltration and patency.	Do not administer drug if site is infiltrated, restart the IV.
Locate Y port closest to client in IV tubing. Cleanse Y port.	Using an antiseptic sponge, briskly wipe the injection site in Y port. Do not touch cleansed site again with fingers.
Inject medication.	While holding lower part of Y port firmly, insert needle about 1 in. into injection site. Fold and pinch IV tubing just *above* the Y port so that the medication does not flow back into the client's IV container. Push plunger at the recommended rate for the drug, injecting drug down tubing into client. Observe client for any untoward reactions. Stop giving the drug if a reaction occurs.
Withdraw needle.	Hold lower part of Y port firmly and withdraw needle. Check that IV solution returns to appropriate rate.
Discard equipment.	Agencies have special containers for breaking and disposing of needles and syringes, so that they cannot be used again.
Record medication.	Follow agency procedure for recording medication immediately after leaving client.

(see Figure 14-21). The glass solution container (or the cap that covers the container opening) must have an air vent so that when fluid leaves the container it is replaced with an equal volume of air. Otherwise the IV will not run. Different manufacturers have varying methods of venting the bottles. Plastic bags do not require air vents since the flexible walls of these containers collapse to equalize the pressure as fluid leaves the bag.

It is possible to set up two containers of solution by using Y tubing. In this setup, the appropriate clamps can be regulated to allow solution to leave either of the two containers.

The Y setup is sometimes used for blood transfusions—one of the two containers contains the blood and the other contains normal saline (0.9%). Although the drop chamber contains a special filter to prevent large particles from entering the client's circulation, the container of blood should have an additional filter. Dextrose solutions cause clumping of erthrocytes, therefore the IV line is flushed with normal saline before and after the blood transfusion is given.

When blood must be transfused rapidly, either an in-line or an external *blood pump* (Figure 14-22) can be used. A "Blood Pump Administration

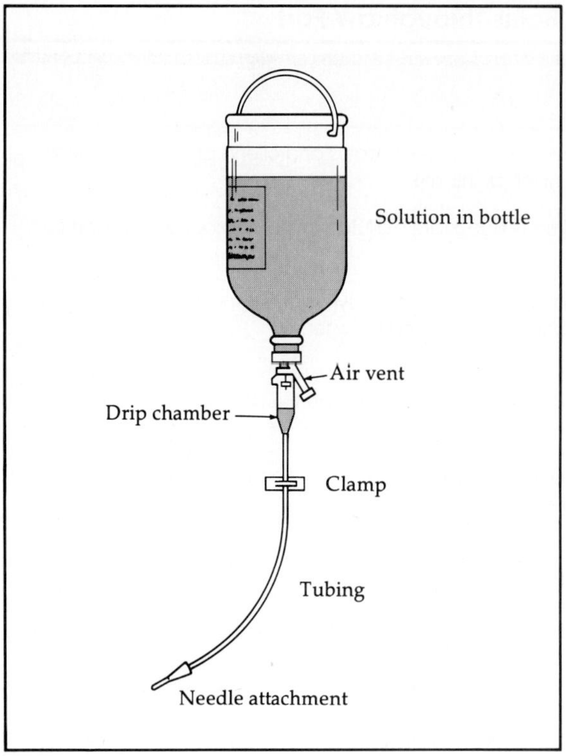

FIGURE 14-21 Basic setup for intravenous infusion.

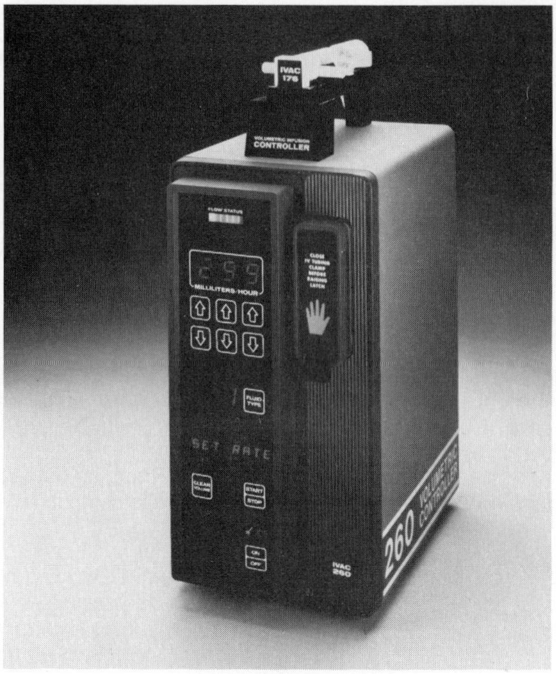

FIGURE 14-22 Blood pump.

Set" contains a pump chamber that can be squeezed manually and filled by inverting the tubing. The external blood pump is often called a *blood cuff,* since it consists of an aneroid cuff that slips over the blood bag. The desired flow rate is obtained by inflating the cuff. As the bag empties, the cuff loses pressure and must be reinflated.

Drip rates

There are three basic methods used to control IV drip rates:

1. An *infusion pump* is a device that accurately controls the rate of IV administration. When the drip rate is preset, it will be consistently maintained by the machine.

2. When specialized equipment is unavailable, the flow rate can be controlled more accurately with a *minidrip IV set* (60 gtt/min.) than with a standard IV administration set (10 to 20 gtt/min.). When small adjustments are required, it is often easier to raise or lower the IV pole, to increase or decrease the rate, respectively, than it is to alter the IV drip regulator.

3. A specialized type of IV tubing, called *memory tubing,* has been designed to maintain a preset drip rate. Research in the use of this tubing indicates that the drip rate will not vary more than a small percentage in 12 hours. Information about this tubing can be obtained from the manufacturer.

When a medication must be administered at a specific rate over a prolonged period of time, an *IV pump* is recommended. These machines can be set up for the desired rate of delivery. There are several types on the market (see Figure 14-23) and each pump has its own set of operating instructions. The pump's manual should be read before attempting to operate it and should be kept with the machine at all times.

The *syringe pump* was designed to deliver an IV bolus at a controlled rate. It can be used to give diluted IV medications or to keep the vein of neonates open since it can be set to deliver less than 1 ml per hour.

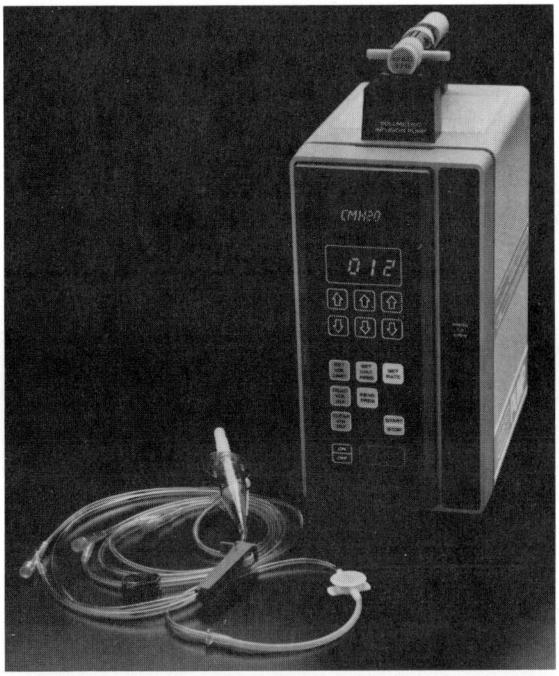

FIGURE 14-23 Infusion pump.

Both the peristaltic and gravity pumps have a dial that can be set for the desired drops per minute and a drop sensor which is attached to the drip chamber of the IV set. The *peristaltic pump* operates by exerting pressure against the IV tubing; the *gravity pump* operates through the use of gravity. Many of these pumps can be run on batteries as well as electricity.

The most sophisticated pump is the *piston pump*. Special tubing containing a pump chamber is required and must be carefully filled before the pump will operate properly. A drop sensor is attached to the IV drip chamber and the pump is inserted into the machine. The desired delivery rate is measured in milliliters per hour, not drops per minute.

It should be remembered that all machines can malfunction. The rate of IV fluid delivery should be checked manually during each shift.

Preparation

Critical elements in the preparation of IV infusions are shown in Table 14-8.

Administration

Large volumes of fluids may be given by intravenous infusion, using gravity to permit the fluid to enter the vein. The solution for infusion is ordered by the physician, as is the total volume to be administered in a specific time period.

The techniques for venipuncture are exactly the same as those for intravenous injection. When the needle or catheter is in place, it is attached to the tubing from the prepared infusion setup. The hub of the needle and a short section of the attached tubing must be securely taped to the client's extremity to prevent the needle being dislodged (see Figures 14-24 and 14-25). Table 14-9 presents the critical elements in this procedure.

Additives

Drugs can be (1) added directly to a client's infusion bag or bottle; (2) given as a bolus in the infusion line; or (3) administered mixed in a separate infusion setup that is then added to the client's existing infusion line.

When additives to the basic intravenous solution are ordered by the physician, they may be injected directly into the container. Common additives include vitamins and minerals, such as potassium chloride. The medication is prepared in a syringe using the same procedure for intramuscular injections (see Table 14-2). The added medication is injected into the IV container through the cleansed rubber stopper of the solution bottle or the injection port on solution bags. The bag or bottle is then rotated gently to ensure thorough mixing of the contents.

If two or more additives are ordered, the nurse must be certain that they are compatible in solution. The literature packaged with the medication is a good source for this information. If there is any question about mixing two or more drugs together, the agency pharmacist should be consulted.

After the solution is prepared, the container must be labeled with the following information:

1. Name of medication added
2. Dosage of each additive
3. The date they were added
4. The time they were added

TABLE 14-8 Preparation Procedure for Intravenous Infusions

Procedure	Critical Elements
Wash hands.	Use sink nearest IV supply cabinet.
Assemble equipment.	Gather together container of required solution, appropriate IV tubing, two correct size needles, several antiseptic sponges, tourniquet, and tape. An IV pole should be at the client's bedside. In addition, a syringe and arm restraint may be needed.
Check IV order.	Read container label and compare with *every* element of physician's order (first check).
Remove protective shields from container caps.	For bottles, remove metal shield according to directions. For plastic bags, expose insert area as directed on package.
Cleanse caps.	Using an antiseptic sponge, briskly cleanse insert areas on bottles or plastic bags.
Insert sterile tubing into solution container.	Open tubing package, noting directions on package. Remove protective shield from pointed end of drip chamber, being careful not to contaminate tip. Insert tip of drip chamber into cleansed rubber stopper of bottle or into cleansed seal on plastic bag. Hold container *firmly* in one hand, while pushing tip into seal with other hand.
Close clamp on tubing.	*Metal clamp:* Slide so that the narrowest part of slit is over tubing. *Screw clamp:* Turn clockwise to tightest position.
Attach needle to end of tubing.	Remove protective cap from end of tubing. Insert hub of needle onto end of tubing by pushing firmly. Leave protective sheath on needle until administration time.
Recheck label on container with physician's order.	Compare label with all elements of order (second check).
Take assembled setup and additional supplies to client's unit.	IV pole is placed on appropriate side of bed (side of extremity to be used for infusion). Other equipment is placed on bedside table or cart.
Hang container on pole and expel air from tubing.	Remove protective sheath on needle. Open clamp. Fill drip chamber one-quarter to one-half full, let solution run through tubing until drops flow from needle. All air should now be expelled from tubing. Close clamp. Replace protective sheath on needle.

Most agencies use preprinted, self-adherent labels for this purpose (see Figure 14-26). After the container has been labeled, the basic procedure for preparation of continuous IV infusion is followed (see Table 14-8).

Intermittent Intravenous Drug Administration

Many medications for intravenous therapy are sometimes ordered as intermittent doses, such as every six or eight hours. There are several

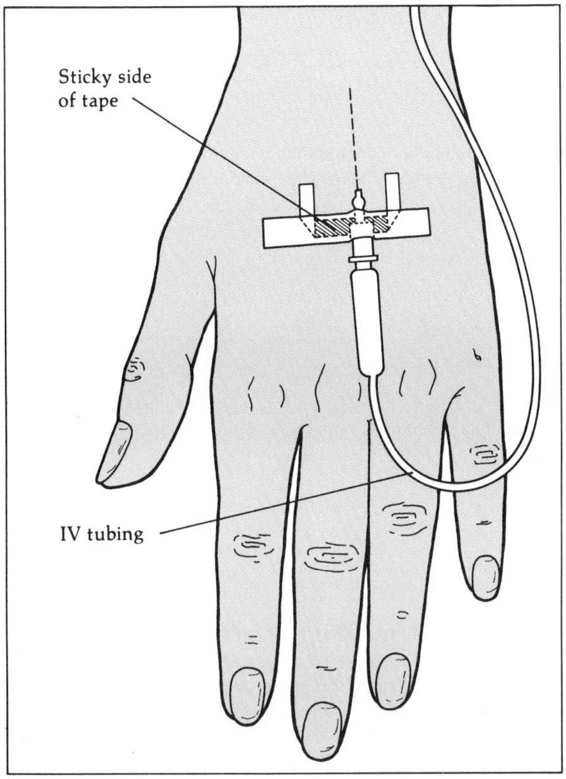

FIGURE 14-24 Tape the plastic catheter securely.

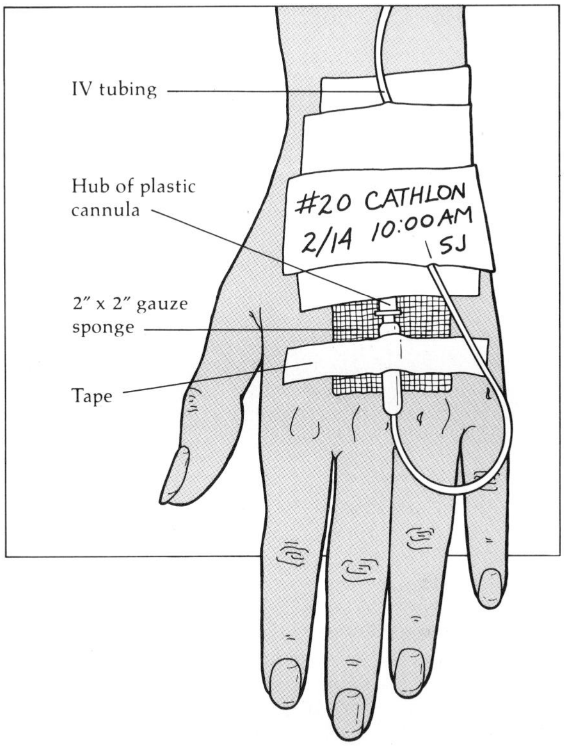

FIGURE 14-25 IV site dressing.

methods used for this type of administration: (a) volume control setup; (b) piggyback setup, and (c) heparin lock setup. In each of these methods, the medication is prepared exactly as for intramuscular injection.

Volume control set

Some IV administration sets, such as Buretrol and Soluset, contain a small fluid chamber within the IV tubing and are termed *volume control sets.* The small fluid chamber will hold 100 ml or more and there is a line for each millimeter. The drip chamber is calibrated at 60 gtt/min. When the lower clamp is opened, fluid from the IV container fills the small fluid chamber at least halfway up the desired fluid level. The upper clamp is then closed and the medication is gently injected into the cleansed rubber-covered port on top of the fluid chamber. (The formation of an unwanted air bubble in the fluid can be prevented by touching the side of the small fluid container with the syringe needle while injecting the medication.) When the upper clamp is opened, the fluid fills the small fluid chamber to the desired level (60 ml). Before this clamp is closed, the bottom of the meniscus should be read. The IV rate is regulated at the desired speed by opening the lower clamp. Irritating drugs should be diluted in 100 ml of solution and infused slowly. The small fluid chamber must be labeled with the drug name, dose, date, and time started. Most medications are infused over a 30- or 60-minute time period.

When clients are on severe fluid restriction, the volume control set may be attached directly to the client's continuous IV solution container. However, before the medication is added to the small fluid chamber the compatibility of the continuous IV solution and the drug should be checked. Alternatively, the volume control set can be attached to a second IV solution container, which is then run into the client's continuous IV tubing. This is the preferred method because it prevents potential incompatibilities.

TABLE 14-9 Procedure for Administration of Intravenous Infusion

Procedure	Critical Elements
Bring prepared infusion setup to bedside. Identify client and explain procedure.	Bring the following equipment to bedside: prepared infusion setup; antiseptic sponges; tourniquet; padded restraining board, if necessary; tape; sterile 2 × 2 gauze; bacteriostatic ointment, if used by agency; IV pole, and extra syringe and needle or catheter.
Hang solution on IV pole.	Container should be at least 18 in. above client. Be sure pole is on same side of bed as venipuncture site selected.
Open clamp on tubing.	Be sure tubing is filled with solution. Let several drops run from needle (or end of tubing) to be sure *all air is expelled from system.*
Close clamp on tubing. Select vein for venipuncture and continue as described in Table 14-6, up to and including releasing the tourniquet.	
Remove syringe from needle and attach tubing.	Grasp hub of needle firmly with one hand and gently twist off syringe; place syringe on tray or bedside table. Attach end of tubing to hub of needle without contaminating the connecting end of tubing.
Open clamp or tubing.	Open clamp until solution drips slowly into drip chamber.
Secure needle and tubing to extremity.	Place *one* dry 2 × 2 gauze under hub to prevent pressure on skin. Tape hub of needle securely to extremity. Cover taped needle with sterile gauze square. Form a small loop with tubing, close to needle, and tape securely to extremity. Attach padded restraint board if necessary.*
Adjust clamp to provide proper flow rate.	Flow rate depends on physician's order and type of administration set used by agency.
Remove unnecessary equipment from bedside.	Dispose of syringe and needles according to agency procedure.
Record infusion.	Follow agency procedure for recording continuous infusions immediately after leaving client.

*If the venipuncture site is in the antecubital fossa, it will be necessary to restrain the joint to prevent the needle being dislodged from the vein.

Piggyback or secondary line

In the *piggyback setup,* a small bag of IV solution (50 or 100 ml) is attached to a standard IV administration set or a shorter set of tubing with a drip chamber called a *secondary line* administration set (see Figure 14-27). This tubing is filled with the solution so that no air enters the client's vein. The medication is added into a small bag of IV solution, after which the bag is labeled with the drug's name, dose, date, and time. A sterile needle is attached to the end of this secondary tubing and then the needle is completely inserted through the cleansed Y extension in the client's continuous or *primary* IV administration set. The primary tubing may be

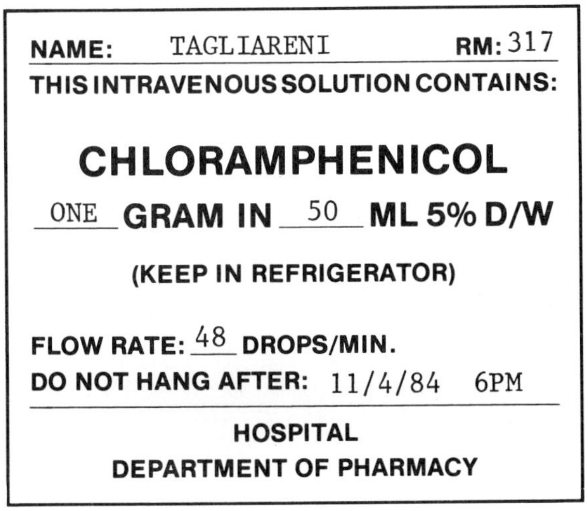
NAME: TAGLIARENI RM: 317
THIS INTRAVENOUS SOLUTION CONTAINS:

CHLORAMPHENICOL

ONE GRAM IN 50 ML 5% D/W

(KEEP IN REFRIGERATOR)

FLOW RATE: 48 DROPS/MIN.
DO NOT HANG AFTER: 11/4/84 6PM

HOSPITAL
DEPARTMENT OF PHARMACY

FIGURE 14-26 Examples of preprinted labels.

clamped or the primary container may be hung about one foot lower than the medicated secondary container (Figure 14-27a). The IV flow rate is regulated to the desired speed for the medicated solution. The primary solution will begin to run after the medication has entered the vein if the primary container was lowered instead of clamped at the outset. For simultaneous administration of medicated solution and primary solution, the secondary set is connected to the lower (or secondary) port, and the containers are hung at equal levels (Figure 14-27b). If intermittent administration is desired, the primary tubing is clamped during medication administration.

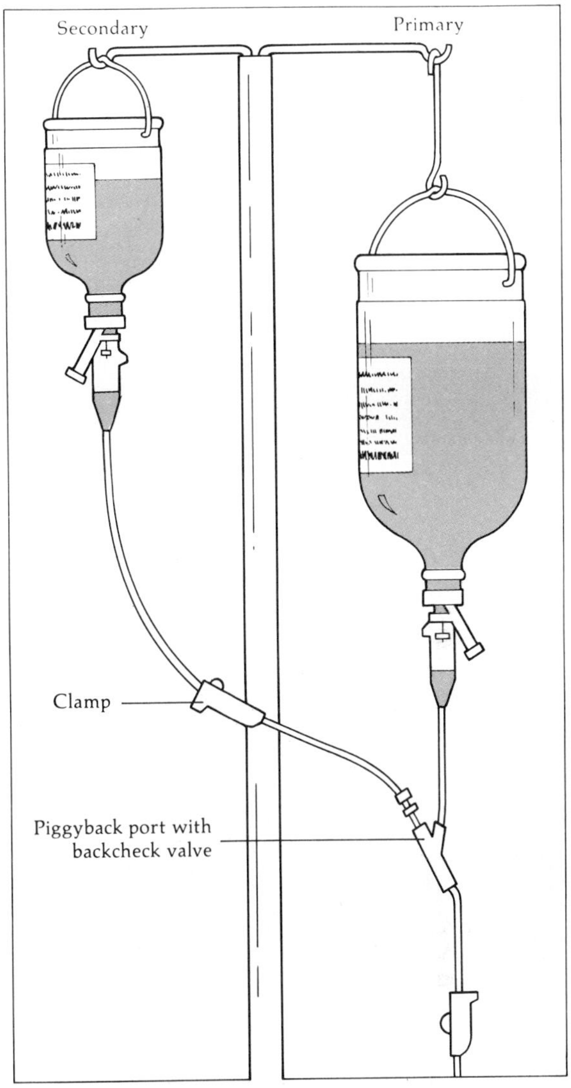

FIGURE 14-27(a) A piggyback intravenous setup.

Heparin lock

The *heparin lock* or *heparin well* setup is used when a client requires intermittent doses of IV medication, but does not need a continuous infusion. A small needle attached to a thin plastic tubing is left in the vein. The distal end of the short tubing is covered with a rubber seal, through which the medication is injected at the designated times. The medication is prepared exactly as for intramuscular injections. In addition, a syringe containing 3 ml of sterile isotonic saline is prepared and another syringe containing heparin is prepared. (See Figure 14-28.)

Each clinical agency has its own protocol to follow when using a heparin lock. One procedure for administering medications via the heparin lock setup is as follows:

1. Cleanse rubber cap on heparin lock with antiseptic sponge.
2. Inject 1 to 1.5 ml of sterile isotonic saline.
3. Administer medication (needle at end of tubing is inserted into rubber cap).
4. When medication has been infused, remove tubing with needle from heparin lock. Cleanse rubber cap with antiseptic sponge.
5. Inject 1 to 1.5 ml of sterile isotonic saline.
6. Inject 100 U of heparin for flush.

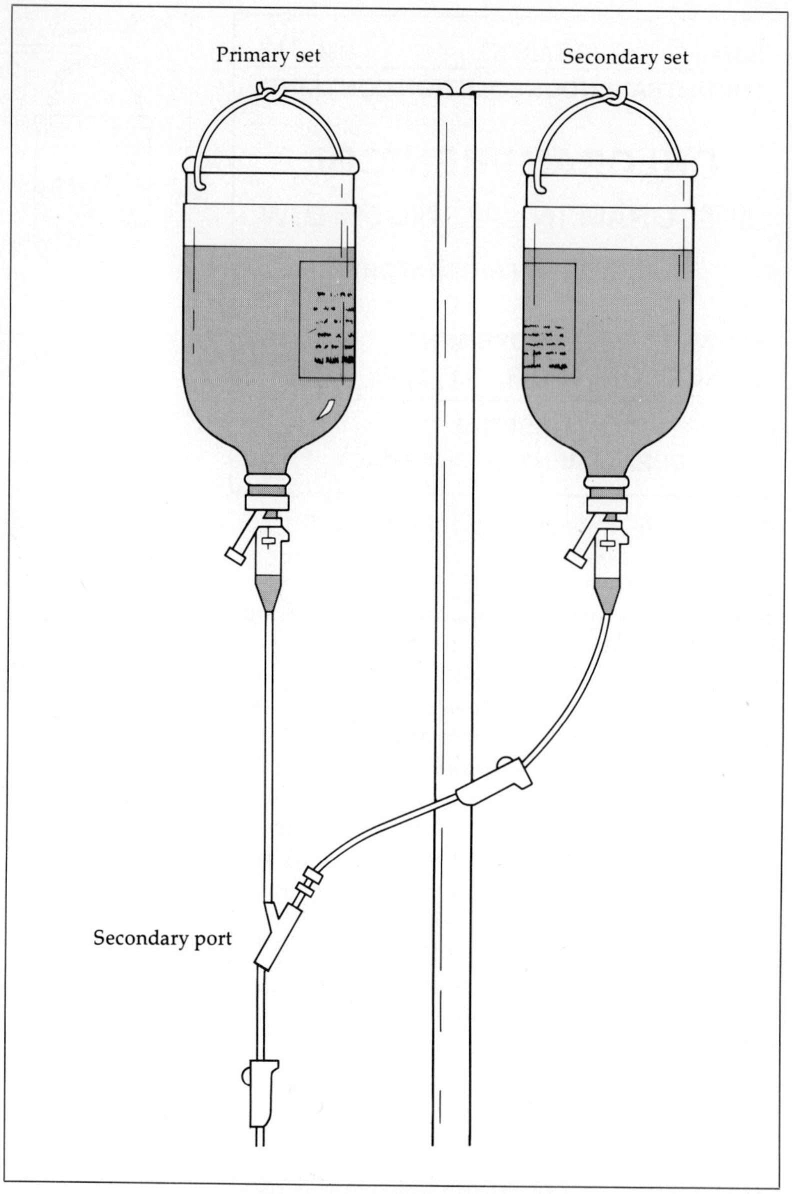

FIGURE 14-27(b) Primary and secondary sets for simultaneous administration.

The heparin remains in the tubing and serves to keep the needle and tubing patent until the next dose of medication.

Summary

The importance of the nurse's knowledge, skill, and judgment in administering intravenous medications and infusions cannot be overemphasized. The desired effect of the drug is instantaneous and any untoward or toxic effects may occur with equal rapidity. The client's condition and reaction to the medication must be assessed frequently and any untoward reaction is an indication for *immediate* discontinuance of the intravenous therapy and prompt notification to the physician. Swelling and/or constant discomfort at the venipuncture site is an indication of infiltration and also calls for discontinuance of the intravenous therapy at that venipuncture site. Many solutions, safely administered by the

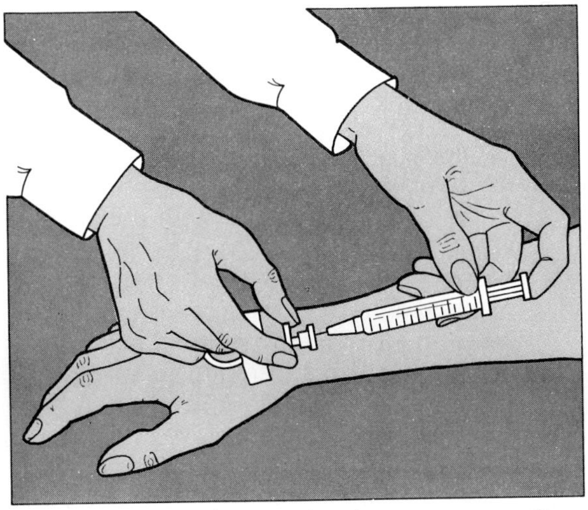

FIGURE 14-28 Administering intravenous medication through a heparin lock.

intravenous route, are very irritating to other tissues and can cause tissue breakdown and necrosis.

Total Parenteral Nutrition (Hyperalimentation)

Total parenteral nutrition (TPN) is used for clients who are unable to digest and absorb nutrients from the alimentary tract. When it is necessary to infuse large quantities of hypertonic solutions for the purpose of providing nutrition, especially proteins, the usual peripheral intravenous sites are too small. Consequently, TPN is provided by placing a catheter in the vena cava where the large blood volume rapidly dilutes the hypertonic solution.

Baseline laboratory studies are done prior to initiating TPN to determine the need for specific additives. Daily laboratory studies are continued until the client is stabilized and are then obtained on a weekly basis. Specific amounts of additives will vary from day to day depending on the client's changing needs.

Solutions used for TPN are high in calories and protein in order to provide sufficient energy for metabolism and nitrogen for protein synthesis. Basic TPN solutions, therefore, always contain hypertonic dextrose (50%), protein hydrolysates or amino acids, and other electrolytes and vitamins needed to correct particular deficiencies in clients. In most agencies, the pharmacist will add the prescribed electrolytes and other substances to the commercially prepared hyperalimentation solutions under strict aseptic conditions, preferably under a laminar flow hood. The usual additives include potassium, sodium, chloride, calcium, phosphate, vitamins C, D, and K, folic acid, magnesium, and trace elements, such as zinc and manganese. If regular insulin is to be used in the hyperalimentation solution, it must be added just prior to administration so that the insulin will retain its effectiveness. Again, strict aseptic technique must be followed in order to prevent contamination of the solution.

Clients placed on TPN usually receive three bottles of solution per 24-hour period. The quantity of the basic solution plus the quantity of the additives must be considered when calculating the milliliters per hour to be infused. For example, 1000 ml of basic solution plus 140 ml of additives equals 1140 ml total fluid to be given over an 8-hour period. This indicates an infusion rate of 175 ml/hr. The use of an infusion pump is recommended since it is vital that the flow rate is maintained as accurately as possible. If the infusion drips too slowly, the client will be deprived of sufficient caloric intake. If it is infused too rapidly, the hypertonicity of the solution will cause massive diuresis and lead to dehydration and electrolyte imbalances.

Catheter insertion

The TPN catheter is inserted by the physician into the superior vena cava by way of the right or left subclavian vein. This insertion site allows for freedom of movement and can be easily maintained with sterile occlusive dressings. Alternative catheter insertion sites include the external jugular vein and a peripheral vein, usually the brachial vein. However, these alternative sites are less desirable because they limit the client's movement or, in the case of the brachial vein, predispose to phlebitis. (See Figure 14-29.)

The following is a list of equipment needed for catheter insertion:

- Sterile gloves and drapes
- Sterile gown and mask, if agency policy
- Acetone
- An antiseptic solution, such as iodine solution

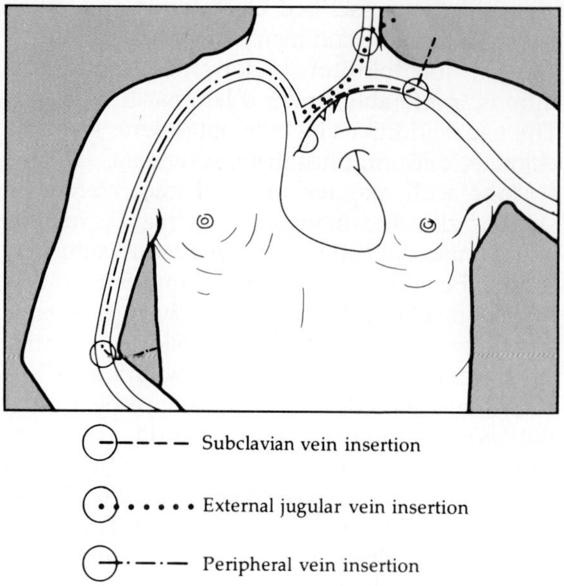

FIGURE 14-29 Catheter placement for hyperalimentation (CVP line).

- Sterile 4 × 4 gauze pads
- Sterile hemostat and scissors
- Alcohol swabs
- Xylocaine, or other local anesthetic
- Two 5 to 10 ml syringes
- Isotonic saline solution
- A 2-in., 14-gauge needle
- Hyperalimentation catheter
- Suture materials
- 5% D/W IV solution (500 ml)
- Antimicrobial ointment
- Tincture of benzoin
- Occlusive tape

The procedure for catheter insertion is as follows:

1. The isotonic dextrose IV solution and tubing are prepared according to the procedure on page 260. A microfilter is added to the distal end of the tubing in order to prevent air and particulate matter from entering the bloodstream inadvertently.
2. To facilitate venous distention, the client is placed in the Trendelenburg position while lying on a rolled towel positioned between the shoulders. The client's head should be turned to the side opposite the insertion site.
3. The area of catheter insertion is cleansed and painted with an antiseptic solution and surrounded with sterile drapes.
4. The physician injects a local anesthetic, inserts the catheter, and sutures the catheter in place. During catheter insertion, the client is asked to perform the Valsalva maneuver in order to prevent air embolism.
5. After the catheter has filled with blood or is cleared with sterile normal saline the IV tubing is connected to the catheter.
6. Antimicrobial ointment is applied and the site is covered with a sterile dressing.
7. An x-ray is taken with the client in high Fowler's position, to affirm correct catheter placement.
8. If catheter placement is correct, hyperalimentation solution can be substituted for the isotonic IV solution. An infusion pump should be used to maintain the prescribed drip rate.
9. The final dressing is applied, using sterile gloves. The insertion site is covered with a sterile dressing. The surrounding area is swabbed with tincture of benzoin and occlusive tape is applied. The catheter-tubing connection should be accessible.
10. The tubing connections should be taped to avoid accidental separation.
11. The tubing is taped to the dressing and the dressing is labeled with the date of application (Figure 14-30).

Nursing care

To reduce the possibility of infection, the tubing and filter should be changed every 24 to 48 hours, with the client in the supine position. While detaching the used tubing from the catheter and replacing it with new tubing, the client should be instructed to perform the Valsalva

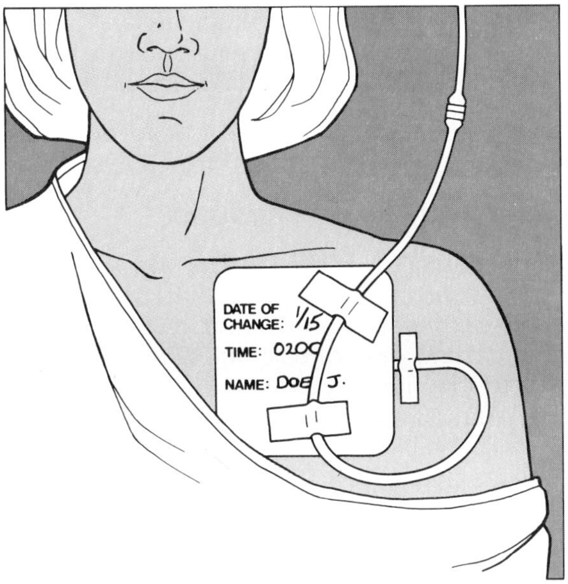

FIGURE 14-30 Hyperalimentation dressing.

maneuver to prevent air embolism. The dressing should be changed every 48 to 72 hours using strict aseptic technique. The use of a face mask by the nurse is highly recommended and the client's face should be turned away from the dressing site.

The client beginning TPN is vulnerable to a number of untoward effects. Because of the potential development of hyperglycemia, the client's urine should be tested for sugar and ketones every six hours. The urinary sugar content may be as great as twice the normal level and there may be a small amount of acetone. Higher amounts usually indicate severe hyperglycemia, which could progress to metabolic acidosis. As there is great individual variation in renal thresholds for glucose, daily serum glucose measurements should be done during the stabilization phase of TPN therapy. A sudden rise in urinary sugar content may be the first sign of infection. In any case, urinary sugar content should not be the sole determinant of insulin administration.

The client's vital signs should be monitored every four hours initially and weight should be checked daily. Accurate intake and output monitoring is essential. An elevated blood pressure, moist respirations, and neck vein distention may indicate fluid overload with impending pulmonary edema and congestive heart failure.

Daily serum electrolytes, osmolarity, BUN, and creatinine levels should also be monitored, especially during the first week (stabilization phase) of TPN. Common electrolyte imbalances include hypo- or hypernatremia, hypokalemia, and hypophosphatemia. Imbalances are corrected by adding the appropriate electrolyte to the hyperalimentation solution. Another serious imbalance, called the *HHNK state* (hyperglycemic, hyperosmolar, nonketotic state), can also occur. This life-threatening hyperglycemic condition can only be diagnosed by laboratory data. Unlike the hyperglycemia of diabetes mellitus, this condition occurs in the absence of ketoacidosis. The key factors to check include an elevated glucose level, often over 600 mg%, an elevated serum osmolality, often over 300 mOsm/kg, the absence of ketonuria, and a normal or low serum potassium level. The client with HHNK is treated with hypotonic IV solutions and potassium supplements as indicated.

Following are several additional precautions to help avoid complications of TPN:

1. Never administer blood, take blood samples, measure CVP, or add any medications or other solutions to the TPN line. The deposits and precipitates that may form are a source of infection and thrombosis.
2. Never use hyperalimentation solution that is cloudy or is left over from a previous administration.
3. Always keep hyperalimentation solution refrigerated until an hour prior to use. The solution should be close to room temperature when administered.
4. Observe client for signs and symptoms of local or systemic infection, phlebitis, or thrombosis, for which TPN clients are at increased risk.
5. For clients on long-term TPN, it is important to be especially vigilant in observing for insidious changes that may indicate deficiencies in trace elements and/or fatty acids. For example, the development of dermatitis with nose and mouth lesions, brittle nails, hair loss, mental changes, fever, diarrhea, may be signs of zinc deficiency and can occur from 2 to 20 weeks following initiation of TPN. Similarly, fatty acid deficiency can result in hair loss, dry skin with poor skin turgor, and poor wound healing.

Fatty acid deficiency is treated with intravenous fat emulsions. These fat emulsions can be administered in a peripheral vein since they are isotonic. They can also be administered through the secondary port of the hyperalimentation tubing if the filter beyond this port is removed. (The fatty acid molecules will not pass through the filter.) In either case, the drip rate should be 1 ml/min. for the first 30 minutes while observing for dyspnea, chest pain, rise in temperature, sweating, vomiting, or allergic reactions. If no reactions occur, the rate can be increased to no more than 125 ml/hr. For many clients on long-term TPN, the physician routinely prescribes 1000 to 1500 ml of fat emulsion each week.

Discontinuation

TPN should never be discontinued abruptly since rebound hypoglycemia could occur. Administration can be tapered off gradually by reducing the drip rate at a rate of 30 to 60 ml each hour. For clients who are eating 1500 calories or more each day and receive insulin in the hyperalimentation solution, a dextrose solution is substituted for the hyperalimentation solution and the drip rate is gradually decreased over a 4- to 8-hour period.

When the TPN is discontinued, the sutures holding the catheter are removed, and the catheter is slowly withdrawn while maintaining manual pressure over the insertion site. Sterile gloves and other supplies are a necessity. Antimicrobial ointment is applied and a pressure bandage is left in place for one hour, after which a Band-Aid or 2 × 2 gauze pad may be used to cover the site.

It is important to inspect the catheter for damage after it is removed, and the catheter tip should be sent to the laboratory for culture. If there is any damage to the catheter, the client should be observed for possible embolism.

OTHER PARENTERAL ROUTES

Administration of medication via the other parenteral routes requires special training and is generally done only by physicians; therefore, the actual procedures will not be delineated here. However, the general indications and special considerations will be presented for the following routes: intracardiac, intraarticular, intraperitoneal, and intrathecal.

Intracardiac Administration

Epinephrine or related drugs are sometimes injected directly into the heart after cardiac arrest in an effort to stimulate the heart muscle to resume functioning. Intracardiac injection is also associated with other resuscitation measures, including artificial respiration, closed cardiac massage, and defibrillation if the arrest is caused by ventricular fibrillation.

Intracardiac injection is performed by inserting the needle to the left of the sternum between the fourth and fifth rib, and the drug is injected during the expiratory phase of respiration. The resulting stimulus to the myocardium often causes resumption of normal sinus rhythm. As it is possible for the stimulus to cause ventricular fibrillation, the intracardiac injection procedure is used only when a defibrillator (and other supportive equipment) is available.

Intraarticular Administration

Corticosteroids and antibiotics are sometimes injected directly into the synovial sacs of joints to relieve pain, stiffness, swelling, inflammation, infection, or a combination of these symptoms. Intraarticular administration provides for a high, local concentration of the drug along with the potential for a prolonged effect, without causing the undesirable side effects of systemic therapy. This technique is practical when only one or two joints are affected; in clients with generalized joint disease, such as rheumatoid arthritis, the appropriate drugs must be given systemically.

Joints must be injected under strict aseptic conditions to avoid the introduction of pathogens. The involved joint should be x-rayed and studied carefully before the procedure is carried out, so that trauma to surrounding nerves and blood vessels is avoided.

Corticosteroids should not be administered intraarticularly when the joint is infected. Steroids reduce resistance to infection and their prolonged use in infected joints can lead to necrosis and joint destruction. The client should be told that discomfort in the injected joint usually intensifies for several hours before relief of pain and stiffness begins.

Intraperitoneal Administration

The vascular peritoneum is a large, semipermeable membrane that permits water and various solutes to move in either direction by osmosis and diffusion. The intraperitoneal route of drug administration, directly into the peritoneal cavity, is usually used for *dialysis* to remove excess body wastes or fluid, or both, excessive electrolytes, or toxic substances resulting from the ingestion of drugs or poisons. In acute, potentially reversible renal failure caused by drug toxicity, transfusion reaction, or other trauma, peritoneal dialysis is an important and often lifesaving procedure.

The electrolyte composition of the dialyzing solution is usually the same as that of *normal* plasma, so that abnormal concentrations in the client's plasma will be corrected through both osmosis and diffusion. The percentage of dextrose in the dialyzing solution controls the tonicity of the solution. A *slightly hypertonic* solution is used for removing excess *quantities* or undesirable *kinds* of solutes from the plasma. A *more hypertonic* solution is used for removing excess *fluid* from the body.

The peritoneal catheter is inserted by the physician using strict aseptic technique. The client should be weighed before the first dialysis and daily thereafter. Accurate recording of intake and output is essential. Frequent monitoring of vital signs is necessary, especially during the first treatment. The peritoneal cavity of the adult client is injected with 2 liters of dialyzing solution, warmed to body temperature. A smaller amount is instilled in infants and children. In either case, the fluid is allowed to enter as rapidly as possible without causing respiratory distress from sudden pressure on the diaphragm. This instillation can usually be accomplished in 10 to 15 minutes.

When the bottles have emptied but the tubing still contains fluid, the clamp is closed. The dialyzing fluid is left in the abdomen for a length of time ranging from 30 minutes to 2 hours to allow for maximum exchange of solutes, fluid, or both across the peritoneal membrane. At the end of the prescribed exchange period, the fluid is allowed to drain from the abdomen by gravity into a drainage container on the floor. The procedure may be repeated immediately or the peritoneal catheter may be left in place for the next prescribed dialyzing treatment. If the difference between the volume of the instilled fluid and that of the drained fluid is more than 500 ml either way, the physician should be notified immediately.

Drugs most often added to dialyzing solutions include antibiotics for prevention of peritonitis, heparin to keep the catheter patent, potassium, and sodium bicarbonate. Antineoplastic drugs can also be administered by intraperitoneal injection for local effect. Drugs administered by this route are absorbed more quickly than if given intramuscularly, but the action is not as rapid as occurs with intravenous administration. Peritoneal dialysis is contraindicated when there is abdominal pathology, including adhesions, and immediately after abdominal surgery.

Intrathecal Administration

The term *intrathecal injection* refers to the introduction of a needle into the subarachnoid space, the space occupied by the cerebrospinal fluid. This procedure, which is sometimes referred to as *subdural* or *intraspinal puncture*, is generally performed either to withdraw a small amount of cerebrospinal fluid for diagnostic purposes or to administer an anesthetic agent directly into the subarachnoid space. It is also used to instill medication directly into the cerebrospinal fluid and, more rarely, to remove some fluid when the cerebrospinal pressure is dangerously high.

Removal of even a small volume of cerebrospinal fluid must be done very slowly and with careful monitoring of the patient during the procedure. The normal pressure in this fluid is 40 to 130 mm of water; if the pressure is altered too quickly, the patient will complain of headache, dizziness, and nausea. A 20-mm change in the patient's blood pressure during the procedure is another indication that a pressure change is occurring too rapidly. In the patient who has recently had a cerebrovascular accident, a sudden lowering of cerebrospinal pressure can precipitate renewed bleeding.

Intrathecal injection is performed by inserting a needle and stylus into the space between the fourth and fifth lumbar vertebrae. In the average adult, the subarachnoid space is reached when the needle is advanced 2.5 to 3 in. (6.3 to 7.5 cm) beyond the skin; in a small child, the depth is 0.5 to 1 in. (1.3 to 2.5 cm). The syringe attached to the needle usually contains a small amount of lidocaine, which is slowly released as the needle is advanced. When the involved tissues are anesthetized in this manner, the procedure is almost painless.

When this procedure is to be performed, the patient is usually positioned on his or her side, with the back close to the edge of the bed. The knees should be drawn up close to the chest with the head forward as much as possible. This position permits maximum widening of the intervertebral spaces and clear visualization of the vertebrae.

The patient must remain motionless while the needle is in the subdural space to prevent tearing of the meninges or breakage of the needle. Any medication introduced into the cerebrospinal fluid should be warmed to body temperature before instillation. Antiinfective agents are sometimes administered directly into the subarachnoid space in clients with meningitis.

Strict aseptic technique is mandatory for intrathecal injection. The skin must be disinfected as for surgery and the physician performing the procedure must observe sterile technique. When the procedure is completed, the puncture site is covered with a small sterile dressing.

The most frequent complaint of the patient after intracathecal injection is headache. Since headache is one of the symptoms resulting from a drop in cerebrospinal pressure, it is thought that this "spinal headache" is due to slow, temporary leakage of the fluid through the hole in the meninges. The patient should be kept in bed for 24 to 48 hours after the procedure to lessen the possibility of headache. *Any* exercise will aggravate all symptoms associated with a drop in cerebrospinal pressure.

REFERENCES

Anderson, M. A., Aker, S. N., and Hickman, R. O. 1982. The double-lumen Hickman catheter. *American Journal of Nursing*. 82:272.

Borgen, L. 1978. Total parenteral nutrition in adults. *American Journal of Nursing*. 78:224.

Geolot, D. H., and McKinney, N. P. 1975. Administering parenteral drugs. *American Journal of Nursing*. 75:788.

Greenblatt, D. J., and Kock-Weser, J. 1976. Intramuscular injection of drugs. *New England Journal of Medicine*. 295:542.

Hays, D. 1974. Do it yourself the Z-track way. *American Journal of Nursing*. 74:1070.

Huey, F. L. 1983. What's on the market? A nurse's guide. *American Journal of Nursing*. 83:902.

Hutchison, M. M. 1982. Administration of fat emulsions. *American Journal of Nursing*. 82:275.

Medication errors: A case study. 1979. *Hospitals*. 53:61.

Millam, D. A. 1979. How to insert an IV. *American Journal of Nursing*. 79:1268.

Morris, M. E. 1979. Intravenous drug incompatibilities. *American Journal of Nursing*. 79:1288.

Newton, E. 1979. Route, site, & technique: Three key decisions in giving parenteral medication. *Nursing 79*. 9:18.

Nursing Photobook. 1980. *Giving medications*. Horsham, PA: Intermed Communications.

Nursing Photobook. 1980. *Managing IV therapy*. Horsham, PA: Intermed Communications.

Rollins, W. 1980. What nurses should know about administering new drugs. *Nursing Law and Ethics*. 1:1.

Steel, J. 1983. Too fast or too slow—the erratic IV. *American Journal of Nursing*. 83:898.

Chapter 15

Dermal Administration

MOST MEDICATIONS THAT are applied topically to the skin are intended to provide a local rather than a systemic action. The skin is the body's barrier against hazards, but some medications can penetrate its protective mechanisms. The absorption of drugs through the intact skin is called **percutaneous absorption.** However, this form of absorption is very slow and irregular, so it is seldom relied on when systemic effects are desired.

THE SKIN

The skin is the largest body organ and can account for as much as 15% of the body weight. The skin of an average adult ranges in thickness from 0.5 mm (0.02 in.) on the eyelids to 6.25 mm (0.25 in.) on the soles of the feet and the upper back. The outer surface of the skin, called the *epidermis*, is the primary protector of the body, whereas the *dermis* layer (*corium*) provides the nutrition, acts like a cushion, and supports most of the skin's appendages, such as hair, nails, and various glands. (See Figure 15-1.)

The epidermis is avascular, paper thin, and equally thick over most of the body. It is subdivided into several *strata* or sublayers. Most of the epidermis consists of the same type of cells, called *keratinocytes*, but their appearance changes as they are forced to the surface by the production of new cells from the innermost layer. Each stratum obtains its name from the appearance of its cells. The innermost layer, called the *stratum germinatum*, is where the well-defined, columnar-shaped keratinocytes originate. A few *melanocytes*, which produce dark-brown pigmented granules containing the complex protein called *melanin*, also originate in this stratum. Melanin shields the dermis from destructive ultraviolet rays and is one of the chief determinants of skin color. Therefore, individuals with genetically dark skin coloring have more protection from the sun's ultraviolet rays than those with fair coloring.

Of the three ultraviolet wavelengths emitted from the sun, the shortest wavelength (UVC) does not penetrate the earth's upper atmosphere, but the middle wavelength (UVB) can penetrate the epidermis and cause a sunburn. Certain medications, such as the tetracyclines, sulfonamides, and phenothiazines, can cause the skin to be sensitive to UVA, the longest wavelength; the areas of skin exposed to light will become reddened or even blister. This *photosensitivity* reaction to drugs is discussed more fully in Chapter 8. Clients taking drugs that are reported to cause photosensitivity reactions should be cautioned against overexposure to sunlight.

Other medications can cause either a diffuse or a patchy darkening of the skin by stimulating the production of melanin or by leaving deposits of the drug, or its metabolites, in the skin. These drugs include silver products (for example, silver nitrate), iron (ferrous sulfate), and some oral contraceptives. Clients taking these drugs should also be warned of a possible change in skin color.

As the keratinocytes move up through the *stratum granulosum* and the *stratum lucidum* of the epidermis, they become dehydrated, less defined in shape, and less active metabolically. Their protein content changes as well. By the time they reach the outer layer, called the *stratum corneum*, they are completely flat, tightly packed, and essentially dead. Their protein becomes a hard scleroprotein, called *keratin*. Keratin is so tough that it is even insoluble in gastric juices. Consequently, the stratum corneum is often referred to as the hard, horny layer.

This outer layer is so compactly filled with dehydrated cells that it (1) prevents the body from losing fluids and electrolytes from the dermis; (2) resists microorganisms; (3) provides protection against chemicals; and (4) resists mild electrical currents. Gradually the outer dead cells rub off. In normal, healthy skin, the progression of keratinocytes from their origin in the stratum germinatum to their sloughing off at the surface takes approximately four weeks.

The epidermis protects the fluid-filled dermis layer below it. The junction between the two skin layers contains projections of dermis, called papillae, and corresponding depressions of epidermis called epidermal pegs. The dermal papillae contain numerous capillaries, from which the epidermis receives its nutrients and oxygen, as well as lymphatics and nerves.

The dermis is considerably thicker than the epidermis in most parts of the body. The dermis of an average adult can range from almost 4 mm (0.16 in.) over the back to just over 1 mm (0.04 in.) on the palm of the hand.

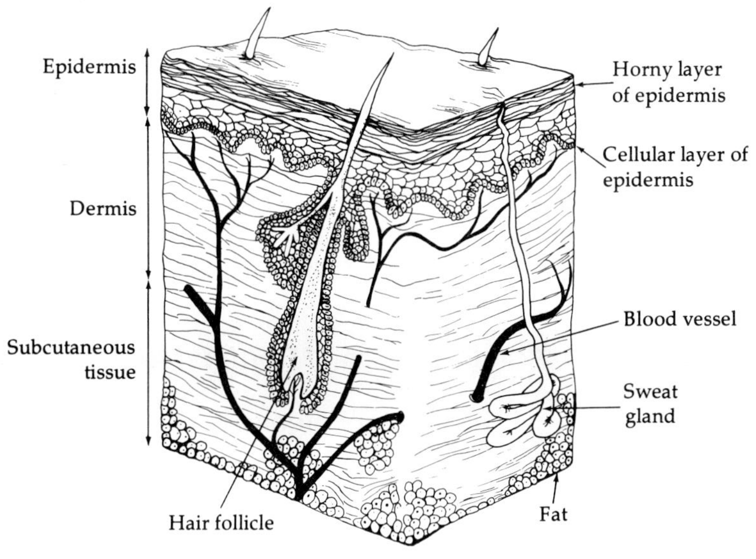

FIGURE 15-1 Cross section of skin.

The dermal layer is composed primarily of connective tissue containing many small blood vessels, lymphatics, glands, and hair shafts. Although the hair has little if any protective function, disturbances in hair growth can be a side effect of some medications. Some drugs, such as phenytoin (Dilantin), can increase the quantity of hair, called **hypertrichosis,** and others can cause a loss of hair, called **alopecia.** Medications that may cause alopecia include anticoagulants, particularly heparin, antineoplastics, some oral contraceptives, and vitamin A in excessive quantities.

Factors Affecting Absorption Through the Skin

The glands of the skin appear to be located in the dermis, but they are actually specialized cells of the epidermis located in the epidermal pegs. The sweat glands (eccrine and apocrine) provide little protection to the skin, but the sebaceous glands secrete a concentrated lipid called *sebum.* Sebum lubricates the skin and helps to prevent water from penetrating the skin's surface. It is thought that sebum may even have antibacterial and antifungal properties.

Drugs are absorbed better through the skin if the sebum is washed off before the medication is applied. If the medication is applied in the form of wet dressings, or applied after a shower or tub bath, it will be absorbed more easily, since the skin's surface sebum and outer stratum corneum cells have been washed away. Sometimes drugs that are intended to penetrate the skin's surface are packaged with a wetting agent that will decrease the skin's surface tension. On the other hand, when the intent is to apply the drug to the skin's surface only, the medication should be administered to intact, dry skin.

Topical absorption is also affected by the condition of the skin. Drug absorption is faster when the medication is applied to thin or broken skin, or skin with little sebum. For example, when an antiperspirant or deodorant is applied immediately after bathing and shaving, the harsh chemicals can penetrate the skin's surface and cause pain by stimulating the nerve endings in the dermal layer.

The functioning of sebaceous glands is stimulated by the sex hormone androgen. Since androgen is produced primarily between puberty and menopause, that is the time when sebum provides the most protection; young children and older people have relatively little sebum. Infants, however, are born with a protective coating called *vernix caseosa,* which contains large quantities of sebum produced under the influence of the mother's androgen in utero.

When the vernix of infants and the sebum of adolescents and adults is washed off, the skin absorbs medications more readily. Drugs that are intended for topical use only must therefore be applied with caution to infants and children since their skin tends to absorb medications more rapidly. The use of soaps containing hexachlorophene was discontinued in newborn nurseries when it was discovered that hexachlorophene could cause neurological damage to infants, particularly premature infants. Soaps containing hexachlorophene should not be used on clients who have little sebum or who have large open areas on their skin, since the drug could be absorbed into the bloodstream.

The absorption of topically applied medications can be hastened by the following procedures:

1. Washing the skin surface well, using friction to remove the sebum and surface cells
2. Soaking the body part in water or a medicated solution for at least 15 minutes
3. Applying wet dressings or compresses containing a solution of the medication and wrapping the body part in plastic
4. Applying medications that are in a fatty or oily base (ointments) and then applying an occlusive barrier such as plastic wrap.

Conversely, medications penetrate more slowly when they are applied to dry, nonwashed, intact skin. When medication is applied to the skin, the skin should be evaluated periodically for signs of irritation from the drug, and the client should be observed for possible toxic signs and symptoms from systemic effects.

Preparation Procedure for Dermal Medications

The critical elements involved in the preparation procedure for dermal medications are shown in Table 15-1.

Administration of Dermal Medications

Ointments or creams

Since ointments are usually fatty preparations, they soften and melt at body temperature, thereby releasing the active ingredients. It is usually necessary to cover the affected area with a dry, sterile dressing after application of an ointment to protect clothing and keep the medication from being rubbed off. When an ointment is to be administered, the following supplies are needed: (1) ointment, (2) sterile tongue blades, and (3) sterile dressings and tape. If the area to be treated is extensive, a sterile glove may be used to apply the ointment.

After explaining the procedure to the client and exposing the area to be treated, the nurse removes the "old" ointment either by scraping with a sterile tongue blade or by wiping with a

TABLE 15-1 PREPARATION PROCEDURE FOR DERMAL MEDICATIONS

	Critical Elements	
Procedure	**Liquids (Liniments, Lotions)**	**Solids (Ointments, Pastes)**
Wash hands.		
Gather together equipment.	Assemble tray, sterile gauze or cotton, sterile glove.	Assemble tray, sterile tongue blade, sterile gauze, and dressing supplies, if needed.
Select medication.	Remove container from storage area.	Same as liquids.
	Hold at eye level and compare label with *every* element of medication order.	Same as liquids.
	Place on tray with other equipment.	Same as liquids.

sterile dressing. (For burn patients, a daily bed bath, shower, or hydrotherapy treatment may be prescribed to aid in removing topical medications.) The ointment jar or tube is opened and the cover placed on the tray or bedside table with the inner surface facing upward. The ointment is removed from the jar with a sterile tongue blade and applied to the skin. If necessary, the nurse may put on a sterile glove at this time and use the gloved hand to spread the ointment. If more ointment is needed, a new sterile tongue blade can be used to remove the medication from the jar. The treated area is then covered with a dry, sterile dressing, as necessary.

Lotions

Lotions are gently patted onto the affected skin surface. A dressing is usually not required, since lotions dry rather quickly. The following supplies are needed: (1) lotion, (2) sterile gauze or cotton balls, (3) sterile glove. After exposing the area to be treated, the nurse opens the lotion container, placing the cap face up on the tray, opens the gauze package, and puts on a sterile glove. The lotion is poured onto the gauze held in the gloved hand and gently patted onto the affected skin.

Liniments

The active ingredients in liniments are mixed into a lubricant base, which facilitates application by rubbing. The nurse exposes the area to be treated and puts on sterile gloves. The liniment is poured onto a gauze square, as with lotions. It is applied by gently rubbing into the skin until the skin reddens, indicating circulation to the area has improved. A dressing is not necessary.

Pastes

Pastes are used very infrequently. They are applied exactly like ointments, but they are much thicker in consistency and do not readily melt at body temperature.

THE EAR

Although the external ear is a body cavity, it is lined with epidermal tissue and is therefore subject to the same considerations as other dermal surfaces. The exception to this is when there is suspected or definite perforation of the tym-

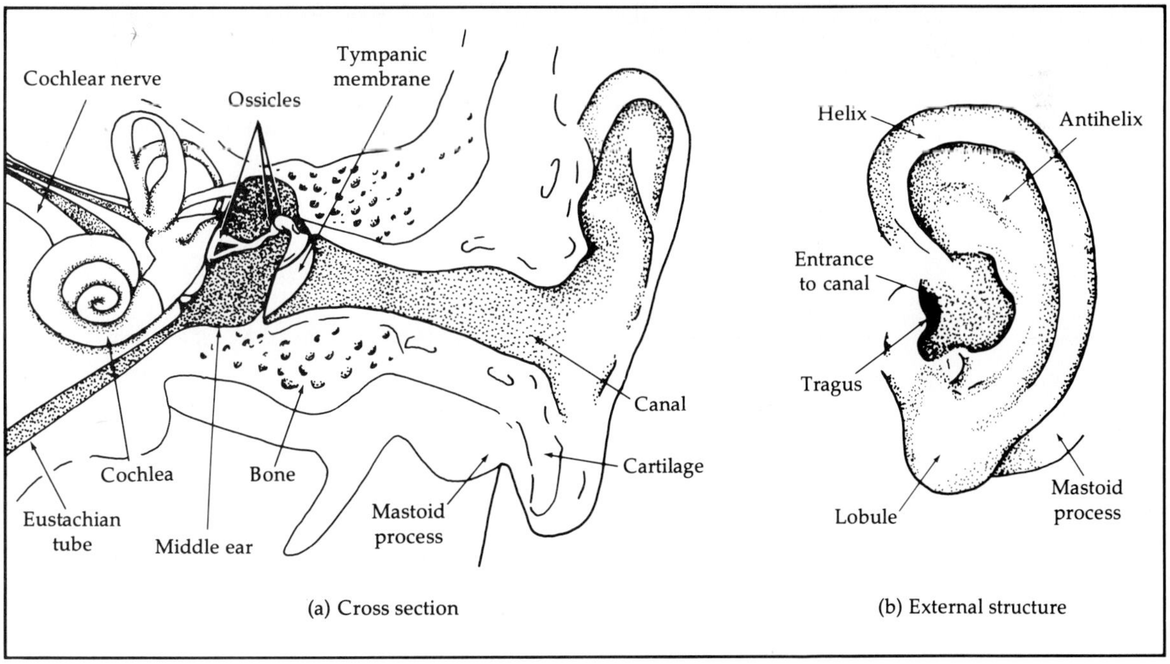

FIGURE 15-2 Internal cross section and external structures of the ear.

panic membrane, in which case, the aural cavity is treated as a mucous membrane. (See Figure 15-2.)

Medications administered to the external ear are for treatment of local conditions, and they are usually instilled as drops. The solution should be warmed to body temperature so the client does not become dizzy from thermal stimulation of the semicircular canals. If the tympanic membrane is intact, the administration of ear drops is a clean, rather than a sterile, procedure.

Administration of Drugs to the Ear

For instillation of ear drops, the client should be positioned so that the ear to be treated faces upward. In the adult, the upper part of the external ear is pulled upward and backward to straighten the canal. For a child under three, the external ear is pulled downward and backward. The prescribed amount of medication is dropped into the external auditory meatus without touching the opening. The tragus can be gently pressed over the meatus for one or two seconds to assist the movement of the drug into the canal.

The client must remain in this position for at least 15 minutes to prevent the medication from leaking out of the ear. If, for any reason, the client cannot keep the affected ear uppermost, a small cotton or gauze pledget can be placed *loosely* in the opening to keep the medication in contact with the canal. To prevent the pledget from absorbing the instilled medication, a few drops of the medication can be applied to it. The pledget will usually fall out on its own accord.

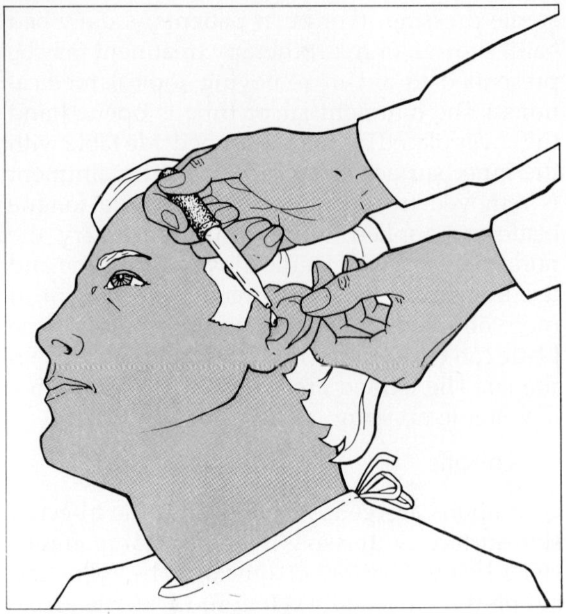

FIGURE 15-3 Administering ear drops.

REFERENCES

Hawkins, K. 1978. Wet dressings: Putting the damper on dermatitis. *Nursing 78.* 8:64.

Matus, N. R. 1977. Topical therapy: Choosing & using the proper vehicle. *Nursing 77.* 7:8.

Chapter 16

Administration via Other Routes

MUCOUS MEMBRANES LINE the body cavities and passages that communicate with the air; they are usually composed of cells or glands that secrete a watery fluid (mucus). When water-soluble medications in aqueous solution are applied to mucous membranes, they are quickly absorbed into the bloodstream. The effect of drugs applied to these membranes can be local or systemic, or both; consequently, the recommended dosage must be carefully observed to prevent systemic toxicity.

The secretions of the mucous membranes have several important characteristics that should be kept in mind when medications are applied. The colloid particles in the mucus retain moisture, thereby keeping the membrane soft. The mucus also contains the enzyme *muramidase* (lysozyme), which is a bacteriolytic agent. These natural barriers to invading pathogenic organisms should not be continuously washed away, so the careless use of irrigating solutions on mucous membranes should be avoided.

As a general rule, solutions applied to mucous membranes should be isotonic so they do not change the normal fluid and electrolyte balance in the cells. Plain water is *hypotonic* and will diffuse into the cells, causing edema. Because edematous tissue has decreased resistance to infection and trauma, plain water is not used on injured mucous membranes. Slightly *hypertonic* solutions may be used on injured mucous membranes to reduce edema of the tissue.

The mucous membranes, aside from those in the alimentary tract, are located in the nose, eye, urethra, vagina, and respiratory tract.

THE NOSE AND SINUSES

The nasal passages contain turbinates that protrude into the nasal cavity and increase the internal surface area of the nose (see Figure 16-1). Gaseous and liquid medications both penetrate well, but liquids require positional assistance in order to spread across the convoluted nasal surfaces. The client is placed in a supine position without a pillow and the liquid medication is instilled into the vestibule. The client's neck is then gently extended backward so the drug will spread under the turbinates and into the posterior nasal passageways. Aerosols are often preferred to liquid medications when the drug is instilled to assist sinus drainage.

Since the nasal mucosa is sensitive and highly vascular, it tends to be easily irritated, often resulting in spontaneous sneezing, and becomes edematous rapidly. Consequently, nasal medications should be nonirritating and should be instilled without touching the sensitive vestibule.

Although the nasal mucosa has been treated locally for years, it is now being used for the administration of a few systemic medications. The nasal route has two advantages over the oral route:

1. Circulation from the nose does not pass through the liver before entering the general circulation, so nasal administration is more effective for drugs that are rapidly metabolized by the liver, provided the drugs can be produced in a nonirritating form.
2. Drugs administered nasally cannot interact with food and other oral medications.

For these two reasons, the nasal route is under investigation as a means of administering more systemic drugs.

The most commonly used drug forms for nasal administration are sprays and drops, although ointments, jellies, and lotions are also available. Since the nasal surfaces are very convoluted, only aerosols with very finely divided particles will be dispersed over a large proportion of the nasal mucosa. Nose drops are generally used for temporary relief of congestion from upper respiratory infection or for local anesthetic action. Many of the spray or drop preparations are available without a prescription and are widely used for the relief of cold symptoms. When these vasoconstrictor drops or sprays are used too frequently, or for more than three consecutive days, the nasal mucosa will become irritated and edematous. This irritation is referred to as the *rebound effect,* since its symptoms are the opposite of the desired effects of the medication.

Nose drops are prepared either as aqueous solutions or as emulsions that adhere to the mucous membrane and have more prolonged contact with the tissues. Ointments and jellies also adhere to the mucous membrane and are used for their prolonged emollient action. Oily liquids are not used in the nose because of the danger of aspiration into the lungs.

Tampons are usually used in the nose for the

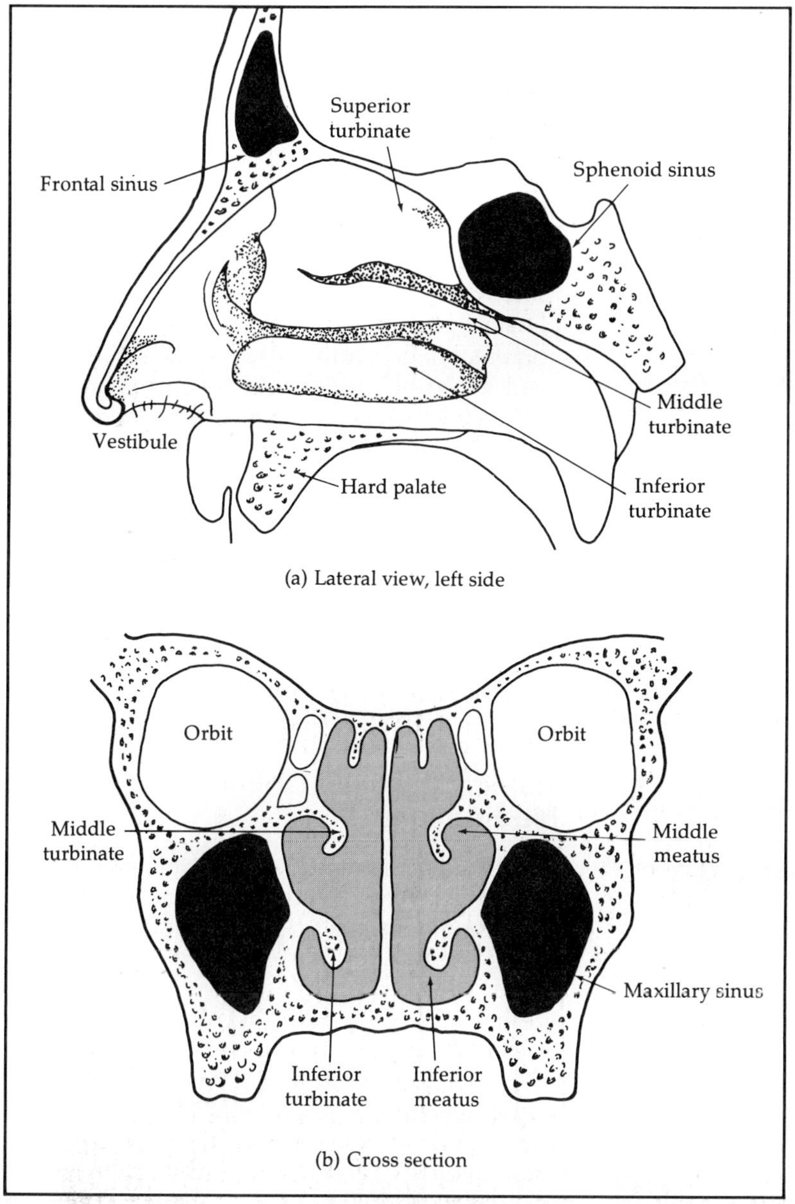

FIGURE 16-1 Lateral and cross-sectional views of the nasal cavity.

control of bleeding. Occasionally they may be used for the continuous delivery of medication to the mucous membrane—for example, in cases of severe nasal or sinus infection. The tampon used for nasal bleeding is usually oxidized cellulose, which absorbs the blood and swells, thereby stopping the bleeding by direct pressure. The material changes to a gelatinous mass and can be removed after about 24 hours. Tampons in the nose should be used judiciously because they are irritating to the sensitive mucosa, and their interference with normal secretory and ciliary activities of the nose can lead to paranasal sinus infection.

Administration of Drugs into the Nose

Sprays Directions on the drug container for administration should be followed. The client should blow his or her nose before the spray is instilled. One or two sprays is the usual dosage, with the client's head kept upright. The client should inhale through the nose after the spray is instilled.

Drops The following procedure should be followed when nose drops are administered:

1. The client should clear the nose before drops are instilled.
2. Place client in dorsal recumbent position, with neck hyperextended. (The head is either tilted backwards over the edge of the bed or a pillow is placed under the shoulders; see Figure 16-2.)
3. Place tip of dropper no more than 0.5 in. into the nostril, without touching the tip of the nose.
4. Instruct client to breathe through his or her mouth, and instill required number of drops into each nostril.
5. Instruct client to remain in this position for about five minutes, so the medication can be dispersed and absorbed.
6. Offer the client tissues to expectorate solution from the mouth.

Jellies and Ointments The following procedure should be followed when jellies and ointments are administered:

1. The client should clear the nose before medication is instilled.
2. Squeeze required amount of medication into opening of nostril.
3. Instruct client to close the mouth, close the other nostril with finger pressure, and inhale deeply.

THE EYE

The eyes contain many delicate structures that must be carefully maintained to ensure unimpaired vision. The cornea and anterior aspect of the sclera are covered by a thin serous membrane called the *conjunctiva,* which lines the inner aspect of the eyelids and forms a natural sac between the eyelids and the eyes (see Figure 16-3). The conjunctiva is extremely sensitive and only very mild medications are used. Since the eye structures are essentially free of microorganisms, only sterile solutions can be used, and caution must be taken to prevent contamination of the tip of the drug container.

Medications for administration to the conjunctiva are prepared in solutions, lotions, suspensions, or ointments. The various liquid preparations can be administered as drops, or can be used to bathe or irrigate the eye. Although ophthalmic drugs are applied for local effect, it should be noted that the conjunctiva is an absorbing surface and the rate of absorption is increased when inflammation is present. Since liquid medications are quickly washed away by normal eye secretions, ointments are often used at night because of their prolonged retention in the eye. When ointments are instilled, the client should be aware that vision in the medicated eye will be blurred for some time after administration.

Administration of Ophthalmic Medications

Eye medication, whether ointment or liquid, must be sterile, labeled "for ophthalmic use only," and be at room temperature. The nurse should take the medication, sterile gauze squares or clean cotton balls, and sterile physiological saline to the bedside. Any visible secretions around the eye should be carefully wiped away with a cotton ball soaked in saline before the eye medication is administered. After explaining the procedure, the client is instructed to look upward. The nurse then places a cotton ball or gauze square under the lower lid and presses gently downward with the thumb over the bony rim of the orbit, exposing the conjunctival sac. Pressure must never be applied to the eyeball itself. See Figure 16-4.

The solution or ointment is then placed into the conjunctival sac from a point below the client's field of vision. The tip of the applicator should be about 1 in. away from the eye and should never come in direct contact with any part of the eye. Under *no* circumstances should the medication ever be dropped on the sensitive cornea.

When the lower lid is released following instillation of the medication, the client should

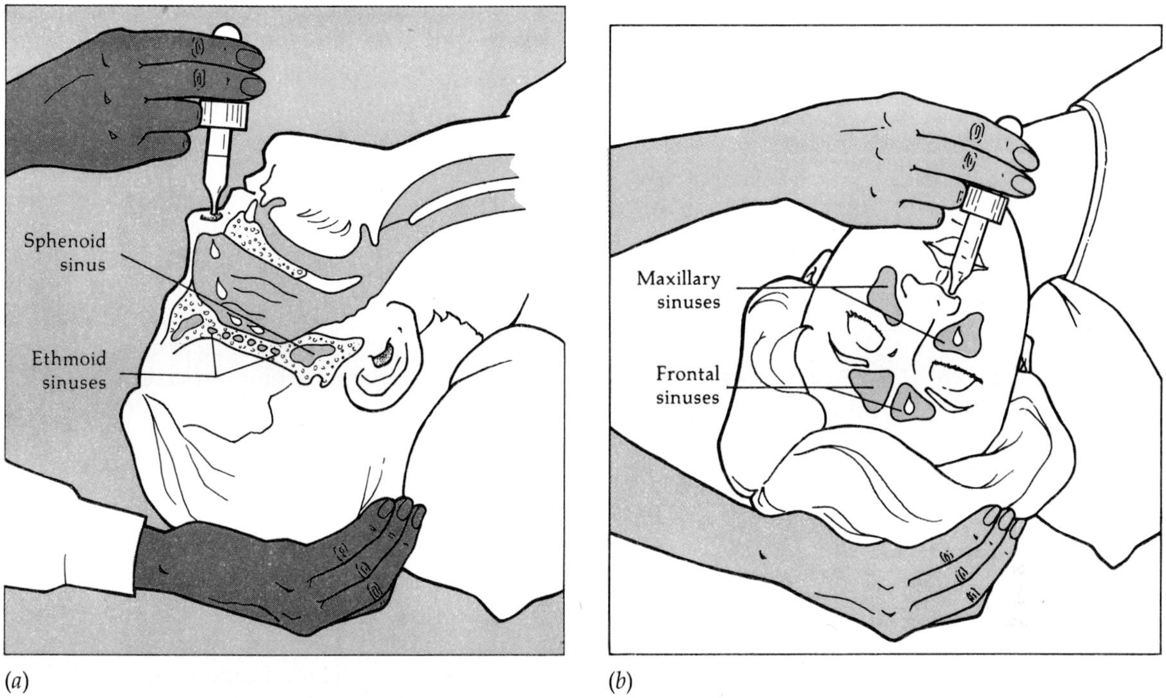

FIGURE 16-2 (*a*) Proetz position for ethmoid or sphenoid sinus medications, (*b*) Parkinson position for maxillary and frontal sinus medications.

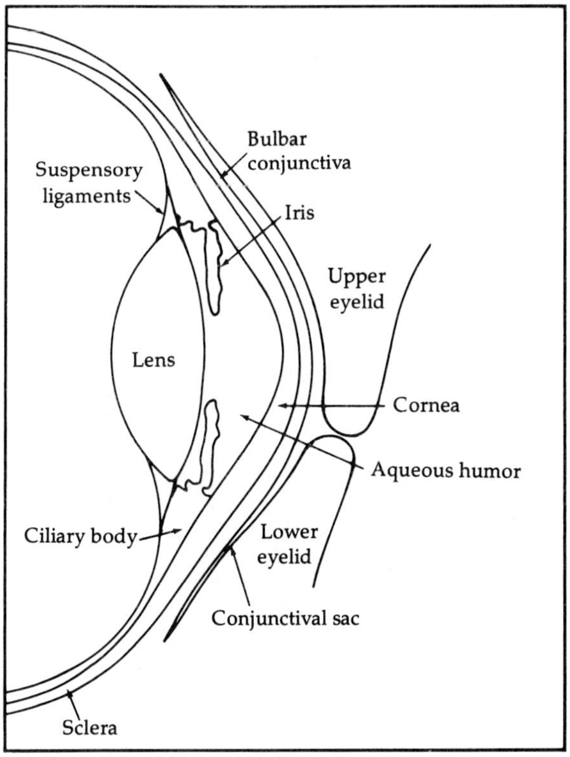

FIGURE 16-3 Structures of the eye.

close the eye for a few seconds and rotate the eyeball to facilitate dispersion of the medication. If the medication is capable of causing a systemic effect, the nurse should apply gentle pressure to the lacrimal duct at the inner corner of the eye for about two minutes. This pressure will prevent the medication from being absorbed into the circulation through the nasal mucosa.

THE URETHRA

The urethral mucosa is highly sensitive and tends to absorb medications into the circulation; therefore, it should be treated only with nonirritating drugs. Genitourinary infections are usually treated with systemic drugs, but occasionally a drug may be instilled for its local effect.

Administration of Drugs into the Urethra

Urethral medication is usually prepared in suppository form. Insertion of a urethral supposi-

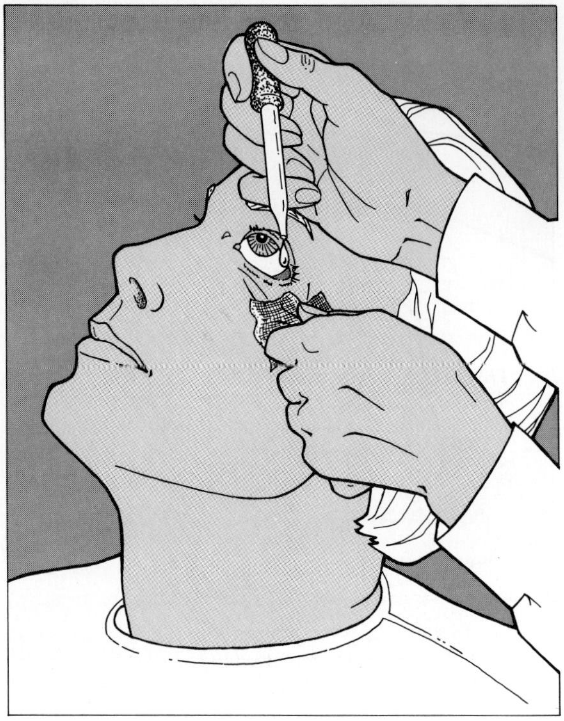

FIGURE 16-4 Administering eye drops.

tory, called a *bougie,* demands strict aseptic technique. The procedure is exactly the same as for urinary catheterization, with the urethral suppository taking the place of the catheter. (A nursing fundamentals book should be consulted for a description of the catheterization procedure.) The client should void before insertion of the urethral suppository and should be instructed *not* to void for at least 30 minutes after the medication is inserted. It will probably be more comfortable for the client to remain in a recumbent position for 30 minutes after the urethral instillation.

THE VAGINA

The vagina is one of the least sensitive mucosae, but it tends to absorb drugs readily because of its vascularity. Therefore, possible systemic effects of a drug must be considered before it is administered vaginally.

Although the normal vaginal secretions tend to be resistant to pathogens, infections do occur. Consequently, systemic medications are often preferred to locally applied drugs for the treatment of vaginal infections.

Regular vaginal douching is not advisable for the healthy individual because the beneficial action of the normal vaginal secretion is lost. However, when chronic infection or inflammation occurs, regular douching with a prescribed medicated solution may be ordered. (A nursing fundamentals book should be consulted for a description of the douching procedure.)

Administration of Drugs into the Vagina

The various drugs for the treatment of vaginal infections and inflammations are available as suppositories, creams, jellies, ointments, and powders that are dissolved before use. The supplies needed are the medication (suppository or medication in an applicator), cotton balls or gauze soaked with appropriate antiseptic solution, and sterile gloves.

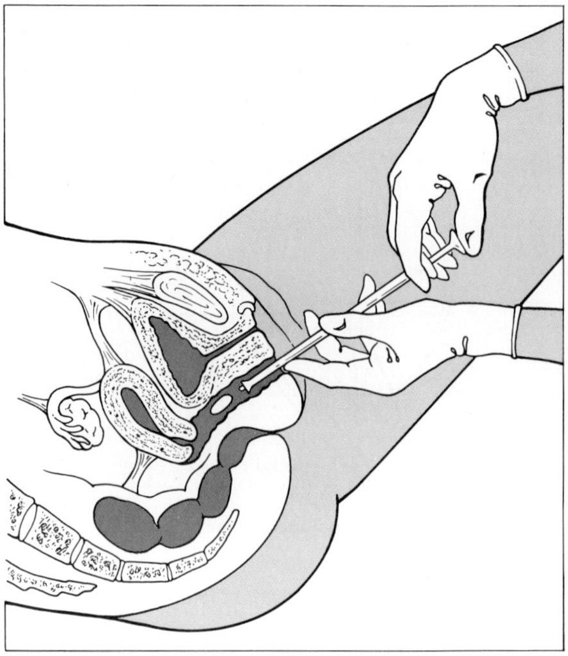

FIGURE 16-5 Correct insertion of vaginal medication.

The client should void before the medication is instilled. The nurse unwraps the medication and cotton balls and puts on gloves. With one hand the nurse exposes the vaginal orifice and cleanses the labia from front to back with the cotton balls. Using a gloved index finger, the nurse advances the suppository, pointed end first, into the vagina. Resistance will be felt when the fornix or cervix is reached.

An applicator is inserted to a depth of 2 in. and is slowly withdrawn while the plunger is pushed to release the medication. The client should be instructed to remain in a recumbent position for at least 30 minutes after instillation of the medication. (See Figure 16-5.)

THE RESPIRATORY TRACT

The lungs provide a highly vascular surface with an area of approximately 60 m^2 in the average adult. Therefore, the systemic effects of an inhaled drug occur almost as rapidly as if the drug were administered intravenously.

The rate of a drug's diffusion across the pulmonary membrane is affected by (1) the solubility of the drug in body fluids; (2) the drug's diffusion gradient; (3) the thickness of the membrane through which the drug passes; (4) the temperature of the body; and (5) the molecular weight of gaseous drugs and the particle size of liquid and solid drugs. The various laws of physics that pertain to the movement of gases, liquids, and solids should be reviewed.

Inhaled medications must be vaporized or nebulized and *must* be water-soluble in order to prevent damage to the client's lung tissue. The commercially prepared solutions for inhalation are packaged with explicit directions for their use. These include nasal sprays and hand-operated nebulizers for oral inhalation. Also available are empty containers with screw-on atomizer tops and nebulizer containers that can be attached to oxygen delivery equipment.

Administration of Drugs into the Respiratory Tract

A drug is *vaporized* when it is converted from its solid or liquid state into a gaseous state. A drug is *nebulized* when it is reduced to small particles from its liquid state. The size of these particles depends upon the type of nebulizing apparatus used. The hand-operated nebulizers usually produce larger particles, whereas those connected to an electrically operated or oxygen source produce very tiny particles, and are therefore more effective in reaching the more remote lung tissues. Nebulization is achieved by passing air under pressure through the liquid or by vibrating the liquid very rapidly.

Inhalation drugs given by *vapor* are volatile drugs; that is, they quickly evaporate when exposed to air. These drugs are packaged in very small ampules.

Nonvolatile drugs can be administered by simple steam inhalation or by nebulization. For steam inhalation, the drug is dissolved in water and the solution is heated to about 100°F or until it produces steam. The heating can be done on an ordinary kitchen stove or with electrically operated heaters, called *bubble humidifiers* or *molecular humidifiers*. The client inhales the steam, inspiring deeply. The warmth and moisture have a local soothing effect. The client should inhale the steam through the mouth, because contact with the membranes in the nose will cause swelling and further respiratory obstruction. The other respiratory membranes are also sensitized by the moist heat, so the client should not be exposed to marked changes in temperature and humidity for at *least* one hour after the steam inhalation. The water reservoir should be emptied and refilled with fresh water every 4 to 6 hours.

For nebulization, the medicated solution is contained either in a hand-operated device that releases the mist when a bulb is compressed with the hand; or is part of a pressure system using oxygen or air passed through the solution.

Hand-operated nebulizers Hand-operated devices include mininebulizers and metered-dose nebulizers. The mininebulizer, although attached to a pressure source, is controlled by the client's own inspiratory and expiratory efforts. When instructing clients in their use, the nurse should stress the following:

1. The client should sit as straight as possible (high Fowler's position) to facilitate maximum chest expansion.
2. The client should close lips tightly around mouthpiece, inhale deeply, and wait 5 sec-

onds before exhaling so the medication can permeate lung tissues.

3. Unless disposable, the mouthpiece should be rinsed after each use to prevent clogging.

It is most important for the client to be observed for potential side effects of inhaled medications. Drugs such as epinephrine and isoproterenol can cause marked blood pressure and cardiac changes. Clients inhaling these drugs should have vital signs monitored closely, particularly during the first few administrations. Clients should be instructed never to exceed the prescribed dosages, without their physicians' approval.

Nebulizers attached to pressure sources When a nebulizer is attached to a pressure source, the tube conducting the gas under pressure must always be below the level of the solution. The oxygen pressure provided by wall units is generally set at 50 lb/in^2. The flow rate is set high enough (usually at 10 to 12 L/min.) so that the steam is visible at the distal end of the tubing. The tubing from the nebulizer may be connected to a basal catheter, a nasal cannula, a face mask, or a tent. Nebulizers can also be attached to IPPB (intermittent positive pressure breathing) machines connected to the air or oxygen source. The IPPB machine causes forced dilatation of the bronchi and alveoli in clients whose tidal volume is compromised by acute or chronic respiratory disease. In either case, it is important to keep pressure and flow rates at recommended levels, and to maintain correct water levels in the nebulizer reservoirs. Dry air, particularly heated dry air, can cause irritation to respiratory mucous membranes.

In preparing solutions for inhalation, sterile water or saline is used. When the nebulized solution is administered via an endotracheal or tracheostomy tube, the solution is prepared using sterile technique, and the container and tubing must also be sterile.

For administration by nebulizer, vaporizer, or atomizer, only *one drug* should be given at a time, even if several are prescribed. Mixing drugs can cause undesirable reactions or one drug may be inactivated when combined with another.

Volatile drugs When administering volatile drugs, the ampule or capsule is taken to the bedside along with some gauze squares. The ampule is broken open and the contents are poured onto the gauze. The client then inhales the vapor *only* two or three times, since these drugs are potent and often irritating, and they take effect very rapidly. The client's eyes should be kept closed or covered to prevent irritation to the cornea from the vapor.

It is important to remember that the effects of many inhalation drugs are not limited to the respiratory tract; that is, the drug is absorbed into the circulation through the pulmonary alveoli. Therefore, the prescribed dosages should never be exceeded.

REFERENCES

Chrow, L. 1978. On the use of selected bronchodilators in the asthmatic and non-asthmatic patient. *American Association of Nurse Anesthetists Journal.* 46:389.

Lehnert, B., and Schachter, E. 1980. *The pharmacology of respiratory care.* St. Louis: C. V. Mosby.

Nursing Photobook. 1980. *Providing respiratory care.* Horsham, PA: Intermed Communications.

Saunders, W., and Gardier, R. 1976. *Pharmacotherapy in otolaryngology.* St. Louis: C. V. Mosby.

Waddleton, C. 1978. Drugs in eye infections. *Nurses Drug Alert.* 2:100.

Webber-Jones, J., and Bryant, M. 1980. Over-the-counter bronchodilators. *Nursing 80.* 34.

Ziment, I. 1978. *Respiratory pharmacology and therapeutics.* Philadelphia: W. B. Saunders.

Chapter 17

Introduction to the Drug Monographs

A DRUG MONOGRAPH is a systematic summary of the pertinent facts about a single drug. Since several companies may manufacture the same generic drug and sell it under different names, drug monographs are usually written about generic drugs.

The style in which a drug monograph is written varies according to the audience to which it is directed. Monographs written for chemists emphasize the drugs' chemical structure and only briefly mention therapeutic uses and dosages. On the other hand, monographs intended for pharmacists emphasize the drugs' chemical structure, primary therapeutic uses, related dosages, and biotransformation processes. Brief statements on precautions, warnings, and adverse reactions are also given. In addition to this information, pharmacists need to know how the drug is supplied and by which companies.

Drug monographs written for physicians and nurses are similar to those designed for pharmacists. These monographs briefly describe the drugs' chemical and physical characteristics, but their emphasis is on the therapeutic indications, contraindications, precautions, warnings, adverse and toxic effects, and specific client assessment factors. Monographs for nurses also include specific information related to the administration of drugs, precautions for storage and administration, and nursing management factors. This chapter indicates the type of information included in drug monographs intended for health team members.

DRUG NAMES

The names of most drugs have evolved during the process of researching new substances for their medicinal value. Some drugs, however, have several names. In order to prevent unnecessary confusion in the naming of drugs, the United States and several other countries have formulated guidelines, but there is a lack of consistency on the international level. Thus, a name used for a drug in one country may be used for an entirely different substance in another.

A drug's *chemical name* indicates the nature of the constituent atoms and their arrangement and is used by chemists to reproduce the substance in the laboratory. The United States has specific rules for writing the chemical structure of a drug. For example, the chemical name of an antiinflammatory drug similar to aspirin is 1 - (*p*-chorobenzoyl) - 5-methoxy-2-methylindole-3-acetic acid (Indomethacin). The structure-activity relationship between two similar substances can be recognized from the chemical names or from a comparison of the abbreviated sketches of the drugs' chemical structures. (See Figure 17-1.)

If a substance is thought to have a medicinal value, its chemical name is shortened to one that will be understood more readily by non-chemists. The *generic name* usually reflects some of the drug's chemical features; sometimes an abbreviation of the chemical name is used. Some commonly used drugs have more than one generic name. To avoid confusion, the council for each drug compendium selects one *official name* for each drug for use in its manual. As these councils have not always agreed on the same official names, the official name is followed by the initials of the compendium in which it is listed. For example, epinephrine solution, U.S.P., is the same as adrenaline solution, B.P. When two compendia accept the same official name, the drug may be written with both sets of initials. Much of the confusion about drug nomenclature has been eliminated in the United States through the joint efforts of the American Pharmaceutical Association, the American Medical Association, the Federal Food and Drug Administration, and members of the official compendia councils. Members of each of these groups formed the U.S. Adopted Names Council and established guidelines for the acceptance of proposed and official names.

When the same drug is manufactured by more than one company, each company selects a *trade name* or *brand name* for that drug for advertising purposes which is registered with the U.S. Patent Office so that no other manufacturer can use the same trade name. The trademark will not be accepted by the U.S. Patent Office if the name is misleading. The symbol ® is written after a registered trade name, as in Amytal® sodium, Achromycin®, and Aquamephyton® injectable. The symbol™ appears after some drugs and indicates a trademark name, as in Codalan™, Disonate™, and Rid™.

When a generic name is used on a prescrip-

Generic name:	
Epinephrine	Ephedrine
Sketch of chemical structure:	

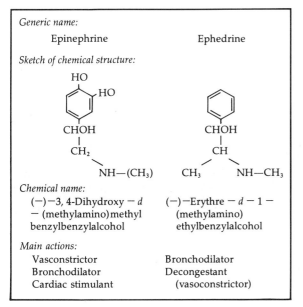

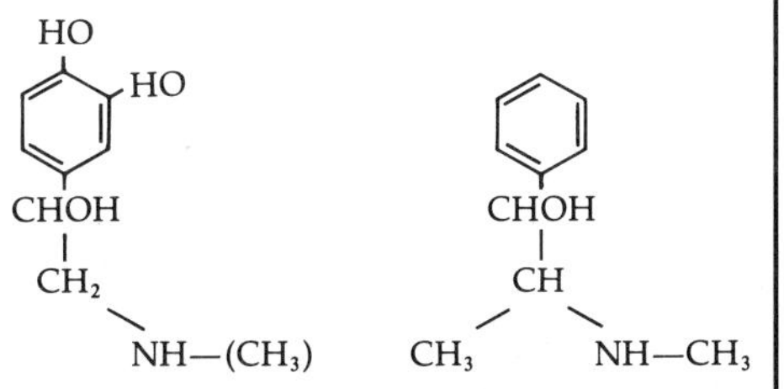

Chemical name:	
(−)−3, 4-Dihydroxy − *d* − (methylamino)methyl benzylbenzylalcohol	(−)−Erythre − *d* − 1 − (methylamino) ethylbenzylalcohol
Main actions:	
Vasconstrictor Bronchodilator Cardiac stimulant	Bronchodilator Decongestant (vasoconstrictor)

FIGURE 17-1 Structure-activity relationship: Abbreviated chemical structure sketch of two related drugs.

tion, the pharmacist is not restricted to a particular brand, so the least expensive generic drug can be dispensed. In most cases, there is little difference between the products manufactured by different companies. For example, the tricyclic antidepressant amitriptyline hydrochloride, U.S.P., produced by Merck, Sharp, and Dohme under the trade name Elavil is the same as Endep produced by Roche Laboratories. However, minor differences in bioavailability, buffer additives, and other characteristics do sometimes occur. For example, a company may add flavoring (fruit flavor) to make its product more acceptable to young children or use a dye in preparing the drug. If a client is hypersensitive to the dye but not to the generic drug, the physician will prescribe a brand that is prepared without the dye.

TYPE OF DRUG REGULATION

Drugs can be divided into four groups according to the regulations and controls to which they are subjected.

Over-the-counter (OTC) drugs are medicinal agents that can be purchased without a prescription; they include cold remedies, vitamins, and antidiarrhea, antiemetic, analgesic, and antiseptic agents. Many of these products are available in supermarkets, discount houses, and other stores. Although some poisons can also be obtained from these kinds of stores, poisons considered highly hazardous must be purchased from a licensed pharmacist who keeps detailed records of poison sales. As described in Chapter 5, an OTC drug package must contain information on the product's uses.

Prescription (R_x) drugs must be prescribed by a licensed physician and dispensed by a licensed pharmacist. They are considered too hazardous to be taken without medical supervision and include antibiotics, potent antiallergenics, bronchodilators, diuretics, cardiotonics, and antiinflammatory agents. Depending on state laws, physicians may dispense sample prescription drugs or larger quantities in rural areas.

Most *controlled substances* require a prescription from a licensed physician that must also include the physician's DEA number. There are five subcategories or schedules for controlled substances, as described in Chapter 6, and each schedule specifies the type of regulations to which the drug is subjected. In most cases, only limited supplies of these drugs can be prescribed and dispensed. Pharmacists must keep detailed records of all controlled drugs dispensed.

Experimental (Exp) drugs can be prescribed only by selected physician-investigators. These drugs are first tested on animals and then released by the FDA for clinical study on a small sample of clients. If the FDA permits the drug to be released for further clinical trials, a physician must submit an application for use of the drug on selected clients, as described in Chapter 5. Since experimental drugs are seldom mass produced, they are usually expensive and difficult to obtain.

CLASSIFICATION OF DRUGS

In drug monographs, the classification of drugs may be based on (1) the body system affected; (2) the drug's intended purpose; (3) the drug's primary action in the body; (4) the drug's chemical nature; or (5) a combination of these groupings. Classifying drugs assists health team members in identifying important characteristics of groups of drugs. However, many drugs affect more than one body system, act on several sites, and produce more than one effect. For example, epinephrine, U.S.P., has been classified as a bronchodilator, a cardiac stimulant, a vasopressor, an adrenergic agent, a sympathomimetic amine, and a catecholamine—each of these groupings identifies a different characteristic of the drug. Drug classifications that use chemical groupings are more specific in describing drug action and effects but require a more complete understanding of chemistry and physiology. In pharmacotherapeutics, grouping drugs according to primary action or intended purpose of administration is distinctly advantageous because it communicates the pertinent information to health team members.

The drug monographs in this text use more than one classification method. In most chapters, drugs are classified according to intended purpose or primary action, but some chapters classify the drugs according to chemical structure because it indicates the nature of drugs more explicitly. The chapters based on chemical classifications list the drugs in particular groupings and monographs on each drug can also be found in the chapter dealing with the particular drug's purpose or primary action. Health team members should be familiar with the different types of drug classifications since a variety of methods for grouping the same drugs are used in pharmacological literature.

CONTENTS OF A DRUG MONOGRAPH

Action

The first major section of a drug monograph describes the known action of the drug in the body, including the receptors that are stimulated or inhibited, and the resulting effects. For newly released drugs, data from animal studies are often presented, although animal research can only give general guidelines about drug action and effects in human beings.

Indications For Use

Included under this heading are diseases, illnesses, and other health problems for which the drug may be therapeutically useful. In some cases, the limitations of the drug's usefulness are included. For example, when antibiotics are effective against certain microorganisms but not against others, both categories of pathogens are mentioned. Furthermore, if an antibiotic has limited effectiveness against severe infections in certain parts of the body, such as bacteremia and meningitis, these limitations are often listed. When a drug has been thoroughly reviewed, the FDA includes it in published evaluations of drugs' effectiveness against particular illnesses. The FDA categories include "effective," "probably effective," "less-than-effective," and "ineffective;" most ineffective drugs have been recalled from the market.

Contraindications; Warnings and Precautions

The conditions under which a particular drug should never be used, or used with great caution, are presented in this section of the drug monograph. *Contraindication* is the absolute category, indicating that the drug will definitely cause harm and probably cause a life-threatening situation in the client for whom it is contraindicated. In some cases, a hypersensitivity to one drug may cause a hypersensitivity to another drug, an effect particularly common with chemically related drugs (congeners and isomers). When known, cross-hypersensitivities will be indicated in statements such as the following: "Drug X should not be given when the client has a known hypersensitivity to drug Y." Occasionally, a client is hypersensitive to a whole class of drugs, such as penicillins. Note here that although the generic names include *-cillin,* the trade names may not have this identifying suffix; for example, Geopen and Pyopen are trade names for carbenicillin. Great care must be taken to prevent these drugs from being administered to clients who are allergic or hypersensitive to penicillin.

Other contraindications may embrace specific pathologies. For example, drug monographs of estrogens and estrogen-containing drugs include the following statement: "Do not give if the client has (1) a known or suspected estrogen-dependent neoplasm; (2) a known or suspected pregnancy; (3) abnormal uterine bleeding; or (4) active thrombophlebitis or thrombolism." The presence of a systemic fungal infection is a contraindication for certain steroids. Sometimes a particular drug may be indicated for a certain disease, but it may be contraindicated in a specific form of the disease. For example, the antidiabetic agent tolazamide, U.S.P., is contraindicated in juvenile or labile (brittle) diabetes.

When the safe therapeutic use of a drug is unknown but the drug is thought to have a high potential for producing severe adverse reactions in clients with certain conditions, the conditions may be listed as contraindications in statements such as the following; "May cause harmful teratogenic effect—do not use during pregnancy;" or "Effect in a child is unknown—do not use in children under 12 years."

Since knowledge about drug interactions has expanded, interactions between drugs are usually listed separately. However, when a particular drug-drug interaction is known to cause severe toxic or other life-threatening adverse reactions, it may appear as a contraindication. For example, certain sympathomimetics and other drugs that interact with monoamine oxidase (MAO) are metabolized at significantly reduced rates (about one-tenth the normal rate) in clients who have had recent therapy with MAO inhibitors, producing severe toxic effects when the normal dosage is administered. Depending on the potential severity of drug-drug interactions, drug monographs may list them as warnings or precautions rather than interactions.

Warnings are given when a drug is potentially capable of causing a serious adverse reaction. A warning differs from contraindication in that the latter states the possibility of a severe adverse reaction in *all* clients with the indicated condition whereas the former is a statement of a potentially severe adverse reaction in *some* clients with the indicated condition. Information about (1) hypersensitivities or idiosyncracies; (2) potential effects of prolonged therapy, such as tolerance or dependence; (3) illnesses that may potentiate toxic or adverse effects; and (4) the drug's association with an altered state of health, such as risk of carcinogenesis, may be stated as warnings. Indications of the drug's safety record in pregnant women and in children are frequently listed as warnings. For example, many sulfonamides include a warning statement such as the following; "Although sulfonamides have not been completely tested in animals or humans, the incidence of cleft palate was significantly greater in the offspring of rats and mice who were treated with high doses of sulfonamides during pregnancy".

Precautions list some of the dangers that may occur when a drug is administered to some clients. Potential drug tolerance, drug abuse, and illnesses in which the drug may cause a toxic effect are usually presented as precautions rather than warnings. A warning is a stronger statement than a precaution. As long as a drug is used carefully in clients with an illness listed under precautions, the incidence of adverse reactions is low. Suggestions or specific tests for monitoring potential adverse effects are indicated. For example, most potassium supplements state the following as a precaution: "Hyperkalemia may result: obtain frequent serum potassium levels and periodic EKGs, and assess client's clinical status. Tingling of the extremities, listlessness, mental confusion, and other symptoms are associated with hyperkalemia."

Information about drug degradation may be listed as precautions. For example, the monograph for epinephrine injection, U.S.P., cautions the drug handler not to remove the ampules from the package until they are to be used because epinephrine is degraded by light.

Drug interactions can also be included under precautions. For example, the diuretic chlorothiazide, U.S.P., may cause hypokalemia when given concurrently with adrenocorticotrophic hormone (ACTH). Alterations in the client's laboratory results may also be indicated as precautions. For example, thiazides may cause a decrease in serum protein-bound iodine (PBI) levels. It is the responsibility of the entire health team to prevent adverse reactions, and a knowledge of a drug's contraindications, warnings, and precautions helps to prevent them.

Parameters of Use

Although seldom grouped under one heading, characteristics, such as absorption qualities, methods of metabolism, amount of protein binding, and methods of excretion, that limit a drug's therapeutic usefulness are included in drug monographs. Since biotransformation characteristics are often altered by the client's state of health, many of these characteristics will be found under the headings *Action, Toxic Effects,* and *Untoward Reactions.* For example, a number of toxic and other adverse reactions occur due to the inability of the client's body systems, such as the liver or kidneys, to process the drug normally. Most drug biotransformation data are based on studies of healthy adults with normal liver, kidney, and other body functions, but in reality, many clients on drug therapy have pathologic conditions that alter their ability to metabolize drugs. Another limitation of research data arises from the fact that research subjects only receive the drug being tested whereas in clinical practice clients often receive two or more drugs. Even if the drugs do not interact directly, either drug may alter the body's ability to process the other, resulting in an adverse or toxic reaction.

Research data concerning a drug's ability to cross the placenta or the blood-brain barrier, or to pass into a dialyzing fluid, are available for some drugs. Most drugs taken by pregnant clients will cross into the fetal circulation. Teratogenic studies are now required for all new drugs released in the United States and the results are listed separately in most drug monographs. Identical studies are also being conducted on many drugs that have been used clinically for decades, but progress is slow and the results may not be available for several years. It is important to remember that teratogenic studies are conducted on *animals* and that human physiology is different from animal physiology.

Although research conditions limit the availability of information on drug characteristics, the data does provide guidelines for treatment. In the drug monographs in this text, the known parameters of drug use are grouped with related precautions to assist in the recognition of pertinent data related to potential untoward reactions.

Untoward Reactions

All medications can cause effects unrelated to the purpose for which they are given. These untoward effects can be beneficial, nonhazardous, or adverse. Most drug monographs list only the toxic drug effects, adverse reactions, and hypersensitivity reactions, both allergic and idiosyncratic. With many drugs, it is difficult to distinguish between the secondary and primary effects, so the secondary effects are seldom listed in a separate category.

Many drug monographs list *adverse reactions* according to the body system involved, even though there may be more than one. This method assists health team members in identifying adverse drug reactions. *Toxic drug reactions* frequently disappear as soon as the drug is discontinued. When the drug is essential to the client's regime, the drug dosage may be reduced rather than abruptly discontinued. Occasionally, an antidote is required for a toxic reaction; the appropriate antidote for each drug can be found in the monograph under the headings *Drug Interactions* or *Toxic Effects.*

The presence of an adverse drug reaction or a *hypersensitivity reaction* is an indication for discontinuing the drug immediately. Although the appropriate measures used to treat these reactions are seldom listed in a drug monograph, it is the responsibility of the health team members to be familiar with them. Most pharmacology textbooks describe the treatment of severe reactions such as anaphylaxis, serum sickness, and blood dyscrasia. A comprehensive list of adverse drug reactions and their treatment is given in Chapter 8.

Secondary drug effects seldom require treatment. Color changes in the urine or feces, for example, need to be explained to the client to avoid unnecessary alarm. Annoying secondary effects, such as the dizziness experienced by some clients taking antihypertensive or diuretic agents, will usually subside when the dosage is reduced. In such cases, the physician may change the drug or prescribe a small dose of a drug that counteracts the annoying symptom, if the secondary effect becomes hazardous to the client. Some medications cause annoying secondary effects in all clients and are compounded with a counteracting drug. For example, aminophylline is used as a bronchodilator but can cause nervousness, insomnia, tachycardia, and extrasystole. These secondary effects are minimized by giving small quantities of a barbiturate.

Drug Interactions

Since drugs are chemicals, they can interact directly or indirectly with other chemical substances. Unwanted interactions can cause abnormal alterations in the results of laboratory tests. The absorption of orally administered drugs can be drastically altered by the ingestion of certain foods. Cigarette smoking, the consumption of alcohol, and the absorption of many other chemical substances can also affect a client's ability to metabolize certain drugs. Some drug monographs include this information, but some require the reader to use other sources of information on drug interactions. When possible, this text lists all known interactions under the heading *Drug Interactions.* A brief explanation about the effects of the interactions is also given.

Administration

Most drug monographs contain information on the normal range and the acceptable routes of administration. The dosage is usually based on the needs of the *average adult,* who weighs 150 lb or 68 kg. Thin clients usually require smaller doses and obese clients sometimes require larger doses for the desired therapeutic response to occur. The upper limit of a dosage range should not be exceeded because toxic effects can occur. When studies have been conducted to determine the safe therapeutic range in children, information on the dosage per kilogram of body weight is given. Since the physiology of a child is somewhat different from that of an adult, some drugs are not recommended for use in children.

Drugs that rely on normal functioning kidneys for excretion may be retained in clients with impaired kidney function and induce toxic reactions. The creatinine clearance test is often used to determine the ability of the kidneys to adequately excrete a drug. When the research data is available, drug monographs include administration recommendations for clients with a specific creatinine clearance level. For example, the antiinfective agent cephradine is usually administered every 6 to 12 hours; clients with a creatinine clearance test of 15 to 19 ml/min. receive the drug every 12 to 24 hours; if the test is 10 to 14 ml/min., the drug administration is every 24 to 40 hours, and so forth.

The purposes for which a drug is administered sometimes require different dosages in order to induce the desired therapeutic effect. For example, propranolol, a beta-adrenergic blocker, is used to treat cardiac arrhythmias, hypertension, and angina pectoris. Although as much as 640 mg daily may be required to control hypertension, angina may be controlled with only 160 mg daily. Information concerning these and other pertinent aspects of drug dosage appear under the heading *Administration.*

Available Drug Forms

Information on drug forms and packaging is outlined under this heading. (See Chapter 12 for a detailed explanation of drug forms and packaging.) This information assists the health team members in identifying the drug, since several drug companies may manufacture the same generic drug. All known drug forms are listed when necessary.

Nursing Management

Specific information related to the administration of a drug to ensure proper management is included in this section of drug monographs. In this text, the information is divided into four subsections for easy retrieval; planning factors, administration factors, evaluation factors, and client teaching factors.

Planning factors include items that should be considered before drug therapy is instituted: baseline data that should be obtained; equipment or antidotes that should be available in the event of adverse reactions; and other precautions that should be considered.

Administration factors include those factors pertaining to recommended techniques of administration—for example, appropriate diluents, IV titration tables, and other related factors for the Z-track method of intramuscular injection. Other considerations are whether a drug should be given between meals, before meals, after meals, or with meals.

Evaluation factors include a listing of the data that should be collected to determine the onset of untoward reactions and factors that should be evaluated when clients are on prolonged drug therapy.

Client teaching factors include items that clients should understand when they are taking a drug. Clients taking *any* drug should be informed of (1) the type of drug they are taking; (2) the drug's action; (3) untoward reactions; and (4) drug administration precautions. Beyond these general considerations, each drug has specific factors about which the client and/or his or her family should be informed. For example, clients on thiazide diuretics need to be informed that because potassium is lost from the body, they need to eat adequate quantities of potassium-rich foods to prevent serious electrolyte disturbances. Good oral hygiene needs to be emphasized to clients on the anticonvulsant phenytoin. Clients taking propranolol must be warned against abrupt withdrawal of the drug since angina or a myocardial infarction may be precipitated.

PART V

FOOD SUPPLEMENTS

AN ADEQUATE, WELL-BALANCED diet supplies all the proteins, carbohydrates, fats, vitamins, and minerals normal clients need to remain healthy. Food supplements are useful when clients are very young or old, have a stressful situation or an illness that prevents adequate nutrition, or are debilitated. When there is a specific nutrient deficiency, it should be evaluated and treated.

Infants and children grow rapidly and may require calcium, phosphorus, and vitamin B supplements in their diet. Young adult woman tend to eat inadequate amounts of iron-rich foods and often require iron supplements. Insufficient intake of ascorbic acid (vitamin C) occurs in all adults who reside in cold climates during the winter months. Certain nutrients, such as calcium and the B vitamins, tend to be poorly absorbed in elderly clients; consequently, supplemental vitamins may be required to prevent illness. Restoration of health and the prevention of further deterioration in debilitated clients and clients under stress can also be checked by the proper supplements. It should be remembered that most vitamin and mineral preparations are formulated for specific types of clients and that the selection of an over-the-counter preparation should be chosen with care.

Millions of clients buy multivitamin and mineral preparations in the United States. Production of these agents is one of the fastest growing industries today. However, because most clients do not have sufficient knowledge to select the appropriate formulation, the same over-the-counter preparation is often given to every member of the household without realizing that excessive ingestion of certain vitamins and minerals can actually cause an imbalance in some family members. For example, teenagers who drink large quantities of milk may ingest excessive quantities of calcium and vitamin D when given certain formulations. Hypervitaminosis A and D can develop in young children who are given adult preparations. The use of fluoride-containing preparations can cause darkening of the teeth in adults. It should be remembered that many food manufacturers add certain vitamins and minerals during processing. Careful assessment of the client's nutritional intake should be done before determining whether a preparation should be administered and if so, which one.

When *total parenteral nutrition,* or hyperalimentation, is needed by a client, specific formulations are prescribed by the physician to meet the nutritional needs of the client. These formulations are usually prepared by a pharmacist since admixtures are included. During hyperalimentation, the client's serum electrolyte and glucose levels, total protein, and other tests should be evaluated frequently and correlated with the clinical picture. Prolonged hyperalimentation may result in a deficit of trace elements, such as zinc, and these deficiencies should be assessed periodically. (See Chapter 14 for the details concerning the administration of total parenteral nutrition.)

Even minor alterations in certain minerals can cause illness—for example, potassium has a relatively narrow serum safety level. Clients on potassium—depleting diuretics often require supplemental potassium. However, excessive potassium intake (hyperkalemia) through ingestion of supplements or IV therapy can result in cardiac conduction disturbances whereas a deficit of potassium (hypokalemia) can lead to arrhythmias and hypotension. Frequent assessment of a client on mineral supplements is essential for detecting excessive and inadequate levels early.

Although vitamin and mineral preparations are often regarded as just replacements for inadequate intake, many of these substances can be used therapeutically. For example, several vitamin B compounds are used as hematopoietic agents; magnesium substances can be used as an antacid, a cathartic, or an anticonvulsant; and some iron preparations are used as diagnostic agents.

Chapter 18

Vitamins

PEOPLE HAVE KNOWN for centuries that certain foods are essential to prevent certain diseases. Scurvy was the first disease to be associated with a specific food deficiency. In 1804, the British Navy eradicated scurvy in sailors by issuing a daily ration of lemon or lime juice. But it was not until the 20th century that scientists discovered that certain foods contained a small quantity of a substance that was not synthesized in the body, namely *vitamins*. Funk coined the term *vitamine* to describe the substance in rice polishings that cured polyneuritis in pigeons and beriberi in man. Since this substance, later to be revealed as thiamine, was thought to be a nitrogenous compound, or *amine*, essential for life, or *vita* (Latin for life), the substance became known as *vitamine*. The *e* was dropped when other organic, nonnitrogenous compounds in this class were discovered.

CHARACTERISTICS OF VITAMINS

Vitamins are a group of organic substances that are not proteins, carbohydrates, fats, minerals, or organic salts but are essential for normal growth and development. These substances must be obtained from plant or animal sources as they cannot be synthesized by the body. Only small quantities are required by the body and the well-balanced diet contains adequate amounts.

Situations in which adequate amounts of one or more vitamins are lacking in the body may be due to inadequate intake of vitamin-containing food, inadequate absorption from the gastrointestinal tract, or increased need for the vitamin. Children who refuse to eat vegetables may lack one or more vitamins; adults who lack intrinsic factor are unable to absorb their ingested vitamin B_{12} and develop pernicious anemia; chronic illnesses and other forms of physiological stress may deplete the body's stores of certain vitamins and pregnancy increases the requirements for certain vitamins and minerals. Therefore, specific vitamin and multivitamin preparations are sometimes required as drugs to prevent illness or to treat a disorder. See Table 18-1 for a summary of disorders caused by vitamin deficiency.

Vitamins are complex chemical substances that are divided into two broad categories: fat-soluble vitamins (A, D, E, and K) and water-soluble vitamins (B and C). These categories are further divided into vitamins with similar properties, the largest of which is the B complex vitamins. Since any one vitamin, such as vitamin D, can exist in nature in more than one form, vitamins are usually referred to by their chemical name or vitamin letter with a subscript number. For example, vitamin D_2 is called *ergocalciferol* and vitamin D_3 *cholecalciferol*. The various forms of a vitamin often vary in their potency, sources in nature, and tolerance in humans, but their actions in human biochemical and physiologic processes are similar.

RECOMMENDED DAILY ALLOWANCES

Vitamins have attained much attention and misunderstanding by the public. Some groups advocate the massive ingestion of vitamin preparations for the purpose of curing hyperactivity, depression, and almost every disorder known to medicine. This type of quackery can be dangerous since the excessive ingestion of vitamins, particularly the fat-soluble vitamins, can cause hypervitaminosis. Consequently, committees have been formed in many countries to establish minimum daily requirements. In the United States, a Food and Nutrition Board was established under the auspices of the National Research Council. This board evaluates research on vitamins and releases research information to the public, including recommended daily allowances (RDA).

Vitamin doses exceeding the RDA can be administered without untoward effects. Excessive quantities of the water-soluble vitamins are excreted by the body via the kidneys. Therefore, the ingestion of excessive amounts of water-soluble vitamins is not only often unnecessary, but it can also be a waste of money. The fat-soluble vitamins, on the other hand, are stored in the liver and other body tissues and are not eliminated as readily by the body. Although the body is able to store and therefore tolerate relatively large quantities of ingested fat-soluble vitamins, acute or chronic vitamin toxicity can occur and should be avoided.

TABLE 18-1 Summary of the Major Actions and Deficiency States of Vitamins

VITAMIN	Major Action in Body	Deficiency State
A (retinol)	Formation of rhodopsin (visual purple); formation and maintenance of epithelial cells	Night blindness; xerophthalmia; various disorders of the skin and mucous membranes
D (calciferol)	Assists in the absorption and excretion of calcium and phosphorus; development and maintenance of bone	Rickets in children; osteomalacia in adults
E (tocopherol)	Antioxidant that protects erythrocytes from hemolysis; assists in the prevention of selenium deficiency	Hemolytic and other anemias; selenium deficiency (depigmentation of teeth, liver necrosis, muscle atrophy)
K	Biosynthesis of certain blood coagulation factors including prothrombin	Hypoprothrombinemia; hemorrhagic disease of newborns
C (ascorbic acid)	Formation and maintenance of intercellular ground substance; antioxidant that protects enzyme activity; assists in the absorption of iron and the conversion of folic acid to folinic acid; assists the immune system	Scurvy; slowed healing process (burns, surgery, trauma); certain hemorrhagic disorders
B_1 (thiamine)	Coenzyme factor in carbohydrate metabolism	Beriberi; neuritis
B_2 (riboflavin)	Coenzyme factor essential in cellular respiration and metabolism	Ariboflavinosis
B_3 (niacin)	Coenzyme factor essential in cellular respiration and carbohydrate metabolism; vasodilation	Pellagra; certain psychoses
B_5 (pantothenic acid)	Essential constituent of coenzyme A; involved in carbohydrate, fat, and protein metabolism	No specific deficiency state; slowed healing process (burns, surgery, trauma)
B_6 (pyridoxine)	Coenzyme factor in protein metabolism	Certain types of anemia; neuritis and convulsions have occurred
B_{12} (cyano-cobalamin)	Coenzyme factor in protein metabolism; hematopoiesis; maintenance of nerves' myelin coating	Pernicious anemia
Folic acid	Coenzyme factor in several metabolic processes; hematopoiesis	Megaloblastic anemia; anemia of pregnancy

FAT-SOLUBLE VITAMINS

GENERIC NAMES Vitamin A, retinol (retinoic acid, retinal, retinyl ester, neovitamin A, hepaxanthin A, alpha-, beta-, or gamma-carotenes, oleovitamin A)

TRADE NAMES Acon, Alphalin, Anatola, Aquasol A, A-Vita

(OTC) (RX)

CLASSIFICATION Fat-soluble vitamin, antiexophthalmic

Source Vitamin A exists in many forms including an alcohol (retinol), an aldehyde (retinal), an acid (retinoic acid), an ester (retinyl ester), or an epoxide (hepaxanthin A). Carotenes are synthesized by deep yellow and green plants, ingested by humans, and subsequently metabolized to vitamin A. The carotenes can be produced synthetically or concentrated from plant sources. Concentrates of vitamin A may be produced synthetically or obtained from fish oil (cod-liver oil).

Action Vitamin A is essential to humans and is required for the following biochemical and physiologic processes;

1. The formation of rhodopsin (visual purple) in the rods of the retina; rhodopsin is necessary for visual adaptation to dim light.
2. The formation of photosensitive pigments in the cones of the retina.
3. Essential to the formation and maintenance of epithelial cells throughout the body, including the skin and mucous membranes. A deficiency of vitamin A causes mucous membranes to become dry and prone to infection; the cornea hardens (xerophthalmia), and keratinization of the skin occurs.
4. Essential for normal growth and development; the exact mechanisms are unknown. A deficiency of vitamin A causes teeth and bone malformations and affects fetal development.

Indications for Use Vitamin A deficiency: xerophthalmia and follicular hyperkeratosis, kwashiorkor. Conditions causing malabsorption and poor storage of vitamin A: celiac disease, steatorrhea (sprue), colitis (chronic diarrhea), extensive bowel surgery, biliary obstruction, hepatitis, cirrhosis of the liver, infancy (due to poor storage), advanced age, clients who have a low intake of protein. States of increased requirements: pregnancy, lactation, infancy, persistent fever, infectious diseases (pneumonia).

Contraindications Hypervitaminosis A.

Warnings and Precautions Excessive ingestion can cause hypervitaminosis A. Water-miscible formulations are required in clients who have disorders of fat absorption. There is a greater tendency for acute toxicity when water-miscible formulations are ingested in large amounts. Should never be given via IV push since anaphylaxis may occur.

Untoward Reactions Hypervitaminosis A: blood plasma levels greater than 1000 IU/dl. Acute poisoning is characterized by increased intracranial pressure (headache, irritability, drowsiness), vomiting, and peeling of skin. Chronic ingestion is characterized by irritability, anorexia, formation of tender nodules on the head and extremities, abnormal bone growth, joint pain, hepatosplenomegaly with jaundice, loss of body hair, pruritis, and dry, hyperpigmented skin. Hypercarotenemia is characterized by a yellow discoloration of the skin of the palms, ear lobes, and soles of the feet. The sclera is not affected.

Parameters of Use

Absorption Actively transported through the GI tract except in disorders of fat absorption. Beta-carotene is the primary source of dietary vitamin A. Water-miscible formulations (retinol and its esters) are absorbed faster and more completely than oily formulations. Plasma levels peak in about 4 hours.

Small amounts cross the placenta. No more than 6000 IU should be taken daily during pregnancy. Large amounts can enter breast milk. Nursing infants have developed toxicity.

Storage About 90% is stored in the liver; small amounts are stored in the kidneys, eyes, lungs, and body fat. Liver storage is able to maintain plasma levels for 3 to 12 months.

Excretion The metabolite glucuronide is secreted in bile (some is reabsorbed); water-soluble metabolites are excreted in urine and feces. Nephritis and other disorders may cause the excretion of unchanged vitamin A.

Drug Characteristics Easily oxidized and is unstable in the presence of light; acetate and palmitate preparations are more stable than other formulations. Store in airtight containers that are resistant to light; store container in a dark area.

Drug Interactions Mineral oil absorbs carotene and prevents its absorption by the body. Vitamin A alcohols, whether synthetically produced or obtained from dietary animal sources, are not affected. Cholestyramine resin may antagonize the absorption of vitamin A. Deoxycholic acid increases the rate of fat-soluble vitamin absorption.

Administration The dosage varies according to the needs of the client. One IU is equal to 0.6 mcg of beta-carotene, 0.3 mcg of retinol, 0.34 mcg of retinol acetate, or 0.54 mcg of retinol palmitate.

- *Commonly used oral dosages in mild deficiency states:* Adults: 15,000 IU daily; Infants and children: 5,000 to 10,000 IU daily.
- *Commonly used IM or oral dosages in severe deficiency states:* Adults: 50,000 to 100,000 IU daily for 2 weeks; Children: 17,500 to 35,000 IU daily for 10 days; Infants: 7,500 to 15,000 IU daily for 10 days.

Available Drug Forms Capsules, tablets, oral liquids with dropper; ampules and multidose vials.

Nursing Management

Planning factors When possible, complete a dietary history to determine the client's daily intake of carotene and vitamin A from dietary sources, including fortified foods and self-administered vitamin supplements. Consult a dietitian as needed.

Administration factors The recommended daily allowances of vitamin A: Infants: 1500 IU; Ages 1 to 3 years: 2000 IU; Ages 3 to 9 years: 2500 to 3500 IU; Ages 9 to 12 years: 4500 IU; Ages 12 to 18 years: 5000 IU; Adults: 5000 IU; Pregnancy: 6000 IU; Lactation: 8000 IU.

Evaluation factors

1. Improvement in the client's clinical status should be assessed weekly. If nyctalopia (night blindness) does not improve within 2 weeks, other causes should be investigated. Examine skin and mucous membranes.
2. Examine clients for chronic toxicity monthly.

Client teaching factors

1. Warn clients who have an adequate intake of vitamin A against taking self-administered supplements of the vitamin.

2. Instruct client to store drug in a cool dry place away from light. Discuss potential sites for drug storage.

GENERIC NAMES Vitamin D_2, ergocalciferol; vitamin D_3, cholecalciferol (OTC) (RX)

TRADE NAMES Activated Ergosterol, Calciferol, Deltalin, Drisdol, Geltabs, Radiostol, Viosterol; Activated 7-Dehydrocholesterol

Source The term vitamin D is used to indicate a group of sterol compounds with antirachitic properties. Vitamin D_2 is formed when ergosterol, a precursor found in plants and yeast, is exposed to ultraviolet light (irradiation). Some breads are fortified with vitamin D_2. When 7-dehydrocholesterol is irradiated, it forms vitamin D_3. Fish liver oils and fortified milk are sources of vitamin D_3. When a client's skin is exposed to sunlight (ultraviolet rays), vitamin D_3 is formed. Since vitamin D does not occur naturally in many foods, several common food stuffs, including milk, bread, and cereal, are fortified with vitamin D.

Action Vitamin D is essential to humans and is required for the following biochemical and physiologic processes:

1. Increases the intestinal absorption of calcium, probably by stimulating the synthesis of a new protein and thereby increasing mucosal permeability to calcium.
2. The intestinal absorption of phosphorus accompanies the absorption of calcium, and vitamin D may activate a mechanism for phosphate absorption that is independent of calcium absorption.
3. Renal excretion of calcium and phosphates is altered by the plasma levels of these ions. If the plasma concentration of these ions is below their renal threshold level, they will not be excreted. Vitamin D increases the tubular reabsorption of phosphates. (Parathyroid hormone influences the renal excretion of these ions, particularly calcium.)
4. Stimulates the development of osteoclasts and prolongs their life span.
5. Increases the rate of mineral accretion and promotes mineral resorption by bone.
6. Is distributed into many tissues and functions in the movement of various cations, including magnesium. Is also thought to affect citrate metabolism.
7. Plays a role in the maintenance of normal parathyroid hormone activity.

Indications for Use Rickets in children (massive doses are required for refractory rickets); osteomalacia (adult rickets) due to poor absorption of vitamin D or A; infantile tetany due to a low level of plasma calcium; hypoparathyroidism; states of increased requirements: infancy, pregnancy, lactation.

Contraindications Hypervitaminosis D or A, hypercalcemia, hyperphosphatemia, severe impairment of renal function, including osteodystrophy.

Warnings and Precautions Excessive ingestion can cause hypervitaminosis D. Bile salts may be required in clients with hepatic or biliary dysfunction. Malabsorption of vitamin D may occur in clients with celiac syndrome, sprue, and colitis. Individuals vary in their sensitivity to vitamin D. Use with caution in clients with cardiovascular disorders.

Untoward Reactions Hypervitaminosis D or vitamin D toxicity: serum levels greater than 135 IU/dl. Initial symptoms include anorexia, nausea, vomiting, diarrhea, or constipation. Prolonged ingestion causes calcification of soft tissues, including the kidneys, lungs, and heart. Altered glomerular filtration occurs and results in polyuria, albuminuria, hematuria, and eventually renal failure. Hypercalcemia and hyperphosphatemia may occur and result in a number of symptoms. (See Calcium and Phosphorus for further details.)

Parameters of Use

Absorption Readily absorbed from the GI tract. Poorly absorbed when inadequate quantities of bile salts are present in the GI tract. Normal serum levels: 50 to 135 IU/dl.

Crosses the placenta. Can cause toxicity in the fetus if excessive quantities are ingested. No more than 400 IU should be taken daily during pregnancy. Enters breast milk. Assess nursing baby for excessive intake.

Storage High concentrations are found in the liver initially; some is bound to blood proteins (globulin); redistributed to tissues for storage in spleen, bones, brain, skin, and other tissues. Although stored in smaller quantities than vitamin A, a cumulative effect (toxicity) can result.

Excretion Large quantities are excreted in bile (some is reabsorbed); nearly 50% of orally ingested vitamin D is eliminated in feces; some vitamin D and its metabolites are excreted by the kidneys.

Drug Characteristics Easily oxidized and is unstable in the presence of light. Store in airtight containers that are resistant to light; store container in a dark area.

Drug Interactions Mineral oil absorbs vitamin D and therefore inhibits its absorption. Mineral oil should be taken at least 4 hours prior to or after vitamin D. Deoxycholic acid increases the rate of fat-soluble vitamin absorption. Barbiturates accelerate and change the metabolism of vitamin D through enzyme induction. Supplemental doses of vitamin D are required with prolonged barbiturate consumption. Anticonvulsants, including phenytoin, primidone, ethotoin, and mephenytoin, inactivate vitamin D by enzyme induction. Clients on anticonvulsant therapy require daily supplemental doses of vitamin D. Oral contraceptives potentiate the action of cholecalciferol by inhibiting the vitamin's metabolism. Clients on oral contraceptives should receive few or no supplemental doses of vitamin D.

Administration The dosage varies widely according to the needs of the client. One IU is equal to 0.025 mcg of vitamin D_3.

- *Rickets, osteomalacia, infantile tetany:* 1000 to 4000 IU daily.
- *Refractory rickets:* 50,000 top 500,000 IU daily.
- *Hypoparathyroidism:* 50,000 to 250,000 IU daily. (Dosage is based on serum calcium levels.)

- *Commonly used oral dosage in severe deficiency states:* 400 IU daily.

Available Drug Forms Capsules, tablets, oral liquids with dropper; ampules and multidose vials.

Nursing Management

Planning factors

1. When possible, complete a dietary history to determine the client's daily intake of vitamin D from dietary sources, including fortified foods and self-administered vitamin supplements. Consult a dietitian as needed. (A quart of fortified milk usually contains 400 IU of vitamin D.)
2. Baseline serum calcium, urinary calcium, potassium, and urea should be taken.
3. Notify the physician if the client has inadequate hepatic and renal function.

Administration factors

1. Oral bile salt supplements should be given simultaneously with vitamin D in clients with bile salt deficiency.
2. The recommended daily allowance of vitamin D for infants, children, and adults if 400 IU daily.
3. Only water-miscible solutions can be used for the IV route of administration.

Evaluation factors

1. Serum calcium levels should be taken weekly or monthly, particularly in clients being treated for hypoparathyroidism.
2. Vitamin D toxicity should be assessed at least monthly. If it occurs, treat with a low-calcium diet that is deficient in vitamin D; force fluids and treat symptomatically. Occasionally, urinary acidifiers may be prescribed to increase the renal excretion of calcium. Phenobarbital may be used to accelerate the metabolism of vitamin D. Because vitamin D is cumulative, several weeks of treatment are usually required to normalize serum calcium levels.
3. Clients with hyperphosphatemia will require dietary restriction of phosphates in order to avoid calculi in the kidneys and other soft tissues.

Client teaching factors

1. Warn clients who have an adequate intake of vitamin D against taking self-administered supplements of the vitamin.
2. Instruct client to store drug in a cool, dry place away from direct light. Discuss potential sites for drug storage.

GENERIC NAMES Vitamin E, alpha-tocopherol

TRADE NAMES Aquasol E, E-Ferol Succinate, Eprolin, Ecofrol, Econ, Tocopherex

CLASSIFICATION Fat-soluble vitamin (OTC) (RX)

Source Alpha-, beta-, gamma-, and delta-tocopherol are substances that have a similar biological function and are collectively called vitamin E. The most potent and the most significant tocopherol is alpha-tocopherol. Vegetable oils, particularly wheat germ oil, are the richest source of vitamin E. Smaller quantities are found in green leafy vegetables, egg yolks, cereals, and muscle meats.

Action Although vitamin E is essential to rat reproduction, there is no evidence of an antisterility function in humans. Little is known about the action of vitamin E in humans. Some authorities believe that its function is yet to be discovered; whereas others believe that it acts as an antioxidant agent. Some of the effects of vitamin E deficiency have been attributed to a lack of selenium (depigmentation of teeth, liver necrosis, muscle dystrophy). Animal research has demonstrated the following physiologic functions of vitamin E:

1. Necessary for the structure and function of smooth, skeletal, and cardiac muscle as well as the vessel walls.
2. Maintenance of liver tissue integrity; prevents liver necrosis.
3. An antioxidant that protects the integrity of erythrocytes from oxidizing agents; protects cells from hemolysis.
4. Related to the metabolism of unsaturated fatty acids; may protect the lipid matrix of body cells.
5. Assists in the body's utilization of vitamin A.

Indications for Use Macrocytic, megaloblastic anemia that accompanies protein-caloric malnutrition; hemolytic anemia that can occur in premature infants and in malabsorption syndromes; acanthocytosis syndrome; minor skin disorders; used as a preservative in some vitamin A formulations.

Contraindications None known.

Warnings and Precautions High dosages may cause hemorrhage in vitamin K-deficient clients. Has little or no therapeutic value in the following disorders: sterility, habitual abortion, muscular dystrophy, schizophrenia.

Untoward Reactions Prolonged excessive doses may cause muscle weakness, fatigue, and creatinuria. Thrombophlebitis has been reported in clients who used megadoses of vitamin E.

Parameters of Use

Absorption Believed to be absorbed completely from the GI tract, except in disorders of fat absorption. Probably requires the presence of bile salts for complete absorption. Associated with beta-lipoproteins in the plasma.

Crosses the placental barrier; the amount transferred is apparently limited to the immediate needs of the fetus. Large amounts can enter breast milk. Breast-fed babies receive approximately twice the amount of vitamin E as bottle-fed babies.

Storage Found in all tissue cells. Prolonged deprivation (months) is required for signs for vitamin E deficiency to occur.

Excretion Large quantities are excreted slowly by the liver in bile and eliminated with feces. Small quantities are excreted as metabolites by the kidneys.

Drug Characteristics Stable in heat, strong acids, and visible light but will deteriorate slowly when exposed to air or ultraviolet light. Acts as an antioxidant; store in airtight containers.

Drug Interactions Mineral oil may decrease the absorption of orally administered vitamin E; do not give concurrently. Cholestyramine resin may inhibit the absorption of orally administered vitamin E; do not give concurrently. Deoxycholic acid increases the rate of fat-soluble vitamin absorption. Iron salts should not be given concurrently with supplemental vitamin E preparations; vitamin E decreases the therapeutic value of iron salts. Warfarin preparations should not be administered concurrently with vitamin E; vitamin E may reduce the level of vitamin K-dependent coagulation factors, and hemorrhage may occur.

Administration Dosage varies according to the needs of the client. One IU is equal to 1 mg of pure alpha-tocopherol acetate. Usual dosage: 30 to 200 IU po or IM daily.

Available Drug Forms Tablets containing 30, 50, 100, or 200 mg; capsules containing 30, 50, 100, or 200 mg; intramuscular preparations containing 30, 100, or 200 mg/ml; topical ointments, creams, lotions, and oils containing variable quantities of vitamin E; multivitamin tablets, capsules, and liquids containing small quantities of vitamin E.

Nursing Management

Planning factors

1. When possible, complete a dietary history to determine the client's daily intake of vitamin E from dietary sources, including fortified foods and self-administered vitamin supplements. Consult a dietitian as needed.
2. Diets high in unsaturated fatty acids increase the client's requirements for vitamin E.

Administration factors

1. Water-miscible vitamin E preparations are absorbed more completely than other drug forms.
2. The recommended daily allowances of vitamin E are: Infants: 5 IU; Preschool children: 10 IU; Ages 6 to 10 years: 15 IU; Ages 10 to 14 years: 20 IU; Ages 14 to 18 years: 25 IU; Adult males: 30 IU; Adult females: 25 IU; Pregnancy and lactation: 30 IU.

Client teaching factors

1. Warn client against taking more than 300 IU daily.
2. Instruct client to store drug in an airtight container.

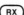

GENERIC NAMES Vitamin K_1, phytonadione (RX)

TRADE NAME Aquamephyton, Konakion, Mephyton, Mono-Kay, Phytomenadione

CLASSIFICATION Fat-soluble vitamin, prothrombogenic

Source There are three main groups of substances that have a similar biological activity and are collectively called vitamin K, namely, phytonadione or phylloquinone (K_1), the menaquione compounds (K_2), and menadione (K_3). Green leafy vegetables and many vegetable oils are a dietary source of vitamin K_1. Since K_2 is synthesized by the normal intestinal flora (gram-positive bacteria), most healthy individuals have a constant, adequate supply of vitamin K. (Newborns have a sterile intestine at birth and may require supplemental vitamin K.) Vitamin K_2 may be prepared from putrefied fish meal. Vitamin K_3 is produced synthetically.

Action Although the specific mechanism by which it acts is unknown, vitamin K is essential for the biosynthesis of certain coagulation factors. It is believed that vitamin K acts as a catalytic enzyme or coenzyme for the synthesis of prothrombin, factor VII (proconvertin), the Christmas factor IX, and the Stuart factor X.

Indications for Use Hypoprothrombinemia that may result in bleeding or hemorrhage due to vitamin K deficiency. Conditions that cause hypoprothrombinemia due to inadequate dietary intake or intestinal synthesis of vitamin K, including hemorrhagic disease of the newborn, extensive bowel resection, or prolonged antibiotic therapy. Conditions that cause malabsorption of vitamin K, including malabsorption syndrome (celiac disease and sprue), colitis and chronic diarrhea, excessive use of laxatives, or biliary diseases. Drug-induced hypoprothrombinemia caused by anticoagulant therapy (particularly with warfarin derivatives), prolonged therapy with salicylates, certain venoms, or excessive vitamin A intake. Mild liver disease and injury.

Contraindications Elevated serum prothrombin levels, severe liver disease (hepatitis, cirrhosis).

Warnings and Precautions Not effective as an antidote against the anticoagulant heparin. Whole blood may be required during the first 2 to 3 hours to control severe bleeding. Excessive correction of drug-induced hypoprothrombinemia will increase the hazard presented by the preexisting thromboembolic phenomenon.

Untoward Reactions Anaphylaxis and other severe reactions have occurred after IV administration. Transient reactions, including "odd sensations of taste and flushing", dizziness, rapid and weak pulse, diaphoresis, dyspnea, and hypotension, may occur. Large doses may cause hyperbilirubinemia in newborns.

Parameters of Use

Absorption Vitamin K_1 and K_2 require the presence of bile salts for GI absorption. If inadequate, bile salts must be given concurrently for adequate absorption. Enters the bloodstream via the lymphatics. Readily absorbed from IM sites. Effect occurs in: 15 minutes (IV); 1 to 2 hours (IM); 6 to 12 hours (oral). Effect lasts 12 to 14 hours after parenteral administration. Whole blood may be required during the interim. Bleeding can usually be controlled in 3 to 8 hours after parenteral administration.

Crosses placenta. Although not recommended currently, vitamin K can be given to mothers 12 to 24 hours before delivery to prevent hemorrhagic disease of the newborn.

Storage Little storage in body tissues.

Metabolism Not completely understood; some glucuronide is formed.

Excretion Metabolites excreted in bile and urine. Most of the unchanged fecal vitamin K is formed by intestinal flora.

Drug Characteristics Degraded rapidly by sunlight but stable when exposed to air. Must be protected from light at all times.

Drug Interactions Mineral oil will decrease the GI absorption of orally administered vitamin K; do not give concurrently. Cholestyramine resin decreases the GI absorption of vitamin K; do not give concurrently. Deoxycholic acid increases the rate of fat soluble vitamin absorption. Antibiotics (tetracyclines, sulfonamides) decrease the ability of the intestinal flora to produce vitamin K. They can induce a vitamin K deficiency. Anticoagulants (oral) are inhibited by vitamin K. Vitamin K is used as an antidote for excessive drug-induced anticoagulation activity.

Administration

- *Single recommended dosage for prophylaxis in newborns:* 0.5 to 2 mg IM (or subc) immediately after birth.
  Therapeutic dosages vary according to the client's prothrombin time—the longer the prothrombin time, the higher the dosage required.
- *Inadequate intake or malabsorption:* 5 to 10 mg po daily; 2 to 20 mg IM daily.
- *Drug-induced, mild to moderate hemorrhage:* Single dose of 1 to 20 mg subc or IM, repeated if necessary.
- *Drug-induced, severe hemorrhage:* Single does of up to 50 mg subc or IM, repeated if necessary. Occasionally, the IV route may be necessary.

Available Drug Forms Tablets containing 5 mg; 0.5-ml ampules containing 1 mg; 1-ml ampule containing 10 mg/ml; 2.5-ml ampule containing 10 mg/ml; 2.5-ml multidose vials containing 10 mg/ml; 5-ml multidose vials containing 10 mg/ml. Konakion can be given only intravenously (aqueous dispersion); Mephyton tablets are yellow compressed tablets scored on one side; Aquamephyton can be given intravenously; however, it is recommended that it be given IM or subc whenever possible (aqueous colloidal solution).

Nursing Management

Planning factors

1. Baseline complete blood cell count (CBC), serum prothrombin time (PT), and partial prothrombin time (PTT) should be obtained.
2. A serum bilirubin should be obtained on infants before the drug is administered.
3. Daily minimum requirements are met by the average diet and by intestinal flora production.
4. The offending drug (anticoagulant) must be discontinued until hypoprothrombinemia has been corrected.
5. Store in dark area. Do not remove protective packaging until ready to use.

Administration factors

1. The recommended daily allowances of vitamin K are: Infants: 1 to 5 mcg/kg of body weight; Children and adults: 0.03 mcg/kg of body weight.
2. When administering IM:
   (a) Inject into a large muscle mass and use an appropriate length needle to ensure a deep injection.
   (b) Since it can be irritating to skin and other tissues, the Z-track method can be used to ensure the medication's entrapment in muscle tissue.
3. When administering IV:
   (a) Double-check to ensure that the phytonadione available can be administered IV.
   (b) Only normal saline, 5% D/W, or 5% D/S can be used as diluent. Dilute 1 ml of vitamin K with at least 9 ml diluent; diluting 1 ml with 19 ml of diluent is recommended.
   (c) Have epinephrine available for immediate use in the event of an anapholactoid response.
   (d) Administer medication at the rate of 0.5 mg/min. or slower and observe client continuously for adverse reactions.
   (e) Monitor vital signs every 5 minutes for 30 minutes following administration. If any adverse reactions occur, notify physician immediately. Then monitor vital signs periodically.

Evaluation factors

1. Obtain PT and PTT as indicated by physician (about q6h). Monitor vital signs frequently until hypoprothrombinemia is corrected and bleeding ceases. Notify physician if bleeding and hypotension persists, since the client's condition may be unresponsive to vitamin K therapy.
2. When indicated, observe client for reoccurrence of preexisting thromboembolic phenomenon.

GENERIC NAMES Vitamin K_3, menadione (RX)

TRADE NAME Hykinone (Menadione Sodium Bisulfate), Hescor K

CLASSIFICATION Fat-soluble vitamin, prothrombogenic

Source Synthetic substitute for vitamin K that is very soluble in water.

Action Menadione can be given parenterally. Naturally occurring vitamin K supplements are preferred for prophylactic and therapeutic use because this synthetic formulation can cause severe adverse reactions. Hescor K is a combination of menadione, hesperidin, and ascorbic acid. (See phytonadione for further details.)

Indications for Use Hypoprothrombinemia due to vitamin K deficiency induced by antibiotics, salicylates, obstructive jaundice, or biliary fistulas.

Contraindications Elevated serum prothrombin levels, severe liver disease, in neonates.

Warnings and Precautions Clients with glucose-6-phosphate dehydrogenase defect may develop hemolysis. Whole blood may be required within the first 2 to 3 hours to control bleeding. Use with caution in clients with hepatic dysfunction. Not given during last trimester of pregnancy. Can cause hyperbilirubinemia, brain damage, and even death of the neonate, particularly the premature neonate.

Untoward Reactions Anemia due to hemolysis of erythrocytes, polycythemia, and splenomegaly have been reported. Renal and hepatic damage can occur. May induce hyperbilirubinemia or hemolysis of erythrocytes in neonates.

Parameters of Use

Absorption Vitamin K_3 and its water-soluble derivatives do not require the presence of bile salts for GI absorption; readily absorbed from IM site. Effect occurs in: 1 to 2 hours (IM); and 6 to 10 hours (oral). Effect lasts 12 to 14 hours.

Crosses placenta freely.

Storage Little storage in body tissues.

Metabolism Completely metabolized by the body. Glucuronide and sulfate conjugates are formed; glucuronide competes with bilirubin for detoxification. May induce hyperbilirubinemia or hemolysis of erythrocytes.

Excretion Metabolites excreted in urine.

Drug Characteristics Causes irritation to skin and mucous membranes, particularly when in powder form. Avoid contact with skin or mucous membranes. Give oral dosages with food or after meals in order to avoid irritation to gastric mucosa.

Drug Interactions See phytonadione for further details.

Administration Dosages vary according to the client's prothrombin time; the longer the prothrombin time, the higher the dosage required.

- *Inadequate synthesis due to antibiotic therapy:* 5 mg po daily.
- *Hypoprothrombinemia due to malabsorption:* Adults: 5 to 15 mg IM daily; Children: 5 to 10 mg po or IM daily.

Available Drug Forms Tablets containing 5 mg; ampules containing 10 mg/ml; ampules containing 75 mg/2 ml (for liver function test).

Nursing Management

Planning factors

1. Baseline complete blood cell count (CBC), serum prothrombin time (PT), and partial prothrombin time (PTT) should be obtained.
2. The offending drug (antibiotic) should be discontinued.
3. Protect drug solution from light. Store in dark area.

Administration factors

1. Daily minimum requirements are met by the average diet and by intestinal flora production.
2. Official daily needs must be established.
3. Deep IM route is preferred.

Evaluation factors See phytonadione for further details.

GENERIC NAMES Vitamin K_3, menadiol sodium diphosphate

TRADE NAMES Kappadione, Synkayvite (RX)

CLASSIFICATION Fat-soluble vitamin, prothrombogenic

Source A water-soluble analog of vitamin K that is derived from menadione.

Action It is converted to menadione in the body. Has been used to treat hypoprothrombinemia due to vitamin K deficiency and as a test to distinguish between obstructive jaundice and other liver diseases (75 mg administered IV). Has also been used experimentally to increase the selectivity of radiotherapy against certain types of tumor cells.

See Menadione for indications for use, contraindications, warnings and precautions, untoward reactions, parameters of use, and drug interactions.

Administration Adults: 5 to 15 mg daily or bid; Children: 5 to 10 mg daily or bid. May be given orally, subc, IM, or IV.

Available Drug Forms Tablets containing 5 mg; ampules containing 5 or 10 mg/ml; ampules containing 75 mg/2 ml.

Nursing Management (See phytonadione for further details.)

1. Store at room temperature (59 to 86 F).
2. Controls bleeding in 1 to 2 hours.
3. Effect is rapid after IV but has a longer duration when given subc, IM, or orally (8 to 24 hours).

WATER-SOLUBLE VITAMINS

GENERIC NAMES Vitamin C, ascorbic acid; calcium ascorbate; sodium ascorbate (OTC) (RX)

TRADE NAMES Ascor, Ascorbicap, Best C, C-Long, Cebid, Cecon, Cemill, Cetane, Cevalen, Cevi-bid, Ce-vi-sol, Cevitamic Acid, Lemascorb, Solucap C, Saro-C; Cal-scorbate; Cenolate, Cetane, Cevita, C-ject, Liqui-cee

CLASSIFICATION Water-soluble vitamin, antiscorbutic

Source Although vitamin C is synthesized from glucose by most animals, humans lack an essential enzyme for the conversion of 1-glucuronic acid to ascorbic acid. Consequently, we must rely on naturally occurring sources, such as citrus fruits, tomatoes, cabbage, potatoes, berries, peppers, pineapple, broccoli, asparagus, and other green vegetables. Numerous drinks and several cereals are fortified with vitamin C and it is used to prevent the oxidation and rancidity of some foods.

Action Ascorbic acid is essential to humans and is required for the following physiologic processes:

1. Formation and maintenance of the intercellular "cement," namely, ground substance and collagen. It therefore prevents scurvy and maintains the integrity of bone cartilage, the dentin of teeth, and the vascular walls.
2. Powerful antioxidant that protects several enzyme activities and may prevent the oxidation of epinephrine.
3. Enhances the intestinal absorption of iron and assists in the removal of iron from ferritin (iron's storage complex).
4. Assists in the conversion of folic acid (folacin) to folinic acid (leucovorin) in the liver.
5. Associated with the formation of the vasoconstrictor substance serotonin (hydroxytryptamine). Serotonin aids in the maintenance of vascular tone.
6. Assists in the metabolism of two naturally occurring amino acids, tyrosine and phenylalanine. Phenylanine is involved in the synthesis of epinephrine and thyroxine.
7. High doses of vitamin C may increase the hepatic microsomal enzyme system to metabolize various poisons faster.
8. Related to the formation of interferon, prostaglandins, T-lymphocytes, immunoglobulins, and other body defense mechanisms.

Indications for Use Treatment and prevention of scurvy; methemoglobinema; enhancement of the intestinal absorption of iron; stress conditions, including wound healing, surgery, burns, tuberculosis, and other infections; malnutrition; certain hemorrhagic disorders.

Contraindications None known.

Untoward Reactions Large doses taken orally may cause gastric irritation and diarrhea. Has the potential for causing kidney stones in high-risk individuals. May cause hemolytic anemia in clients who have a glucose-6-phosphate dehydrogenase deficiency.

Parameters of Use

Absorption Readily absorbed from GI tract and from most parenteral sites. Since it is poorly absorbed from fat tissue, the drug should be given deep into muscle.

Present in human milk but lacking in cows' milk. Bottle-fed infants must receive supplemental vitamin C.

Distribution Generalized; highest quantities found in glandular tissues (adrenal), liver, white blood cells, and the brain.

Storage Limited (about 1500 mg); tissue stores are depleted within days during stress situations.

Excretion Excreted by the kidneys when the renal threshold is exceeded (plasma levels in excess of 1.4mg% for most individuals). No toxicity has been reported but high dosages taken daily may cause kidney stones in high-risk clients. Excessive excretion can cause acidification of urine. Give cautiously to clients who are prone to gout and crystalluria. Large doses increase the excretion of weak bases and inhibit the excretion of weak acids.

Drug Characteristics Less stable than other vitamins; easily oxidized when exposed to air, heat, and light. Store in airtight containers away from light and heat. Dry preparations are somewhat stable in air but aqueous solutions decompose rapidly when exposed to air. Liquid preparations and juices must be stored in tightly sealed containers.

Drug Interactions Salicylates will increase the renal excretion of vitamin C. But since vitamin C is an acidifying agent, this acid will increase the absorption of orally administered salicylates and decrease the excretion of weak acids such as salicylates. Consequently, salicylates and other weak acids are potentiated by vitamin C. Do not administer oral salicylates. Observe client for salicylate toxicity when drugs are taken concurrently. Sulfonamides must be given cautiously with vitamin C, if at all. The vitamin decreases the renal excretion of sulfonamides while the excretion of vitamin C is enhanced. The urine becomes excessively acid and crystalluria and the precipitation of cystine, oxalate, and urate stones may result. Smoking may increase the metabolism and excretion of vitamin C and result in a subclinical or mild deficiency state. Barbiturate excretion is decreased by vitamin C while the vitamin's excretion is enhanced. Therefore, the sedative effect of barbiturates is potentiated and toxicity may occur. Some weak bases, such as antipyrine, atropine, meperidine, and guanidine, are excreted faster. Consequently, the vitamin causes inhibition of these drugs. Warfarin preparations are inhibited by vitamin C. This results in a shortening of the prothrombin time. The mechanism is unknown. Mineral oil may inhibit the absorption of vitamin C; do not give concurrently. Iron preparations (ferrous) are potentiated by large doses of vitamin C. Vitamin B_{12} is destroyed by vitamin C; do not give concurrently.

Laboratory Interactions False-positive results for urine glucose tests (Benedict's solution, Clinitest, Tes-Tape); false increase in serum uric acid (nonenzymatic method); false-positive results for occult blood in stool.

Administration Dosage varies according to the needs of the client. Usual dietary supplemental dosages: Adults: 250 to 1000 mg daily; Teenagers: 250 to 500 mg daily; Children: 250 mg daily; Infants: 100 to 250 mg daily. Up to 4000 mg daily have been prescribed. Dosage can be given orally, IM, or IV.

Available Drug Forms *Oral use (OTC):* Tablets containing 50, 100, 250, 500, 1000, or 1500 mg; chewable tablets containing 250 or 500 mg; capsules containing 250 or 500 mg; sustained release capsules containing 500 or 1000 mg; liquid containing 300 mg/ml. Parenteral use (Rx): 1-ml and 2-ml ampules containing 250 or 500 mg/ml; 30-ml vials containing 250 or 500 mg/ml.

Nursing Management

Planning factors

1. When possible, complete a dietary history to determine the client's daily intake of vitamin C from die-

tary sources, including fortified foods and self-administered vitamin supplements. Consult a dietician as needed.

2. Smokers, geriatrics, alcoholics, and clients with hyperthyroidism, fever or infection may develop a mild or subclinical deficiency of vitamin C—petechiae, sensitive gums that bleed when teeth are brushed, easy bruising, limb and joint pain, pallor, and anorexia.
3. Subclinical deficiencies are more prevalent in cold climates when fresh fruits and vegetables are not readily available.
4. Bottle-fed infants who are not on supplemental vitamin C should be given 1 to 2 bottles of a juice rich in vitamin C daily (orange juice).

Administration factors

1. The total daily requirements for various age groups and stress situations have not been determined. The recommended daily allowances of vitamin C are: Infants: 35 mg; Children: 40 mg; Teenage boys: 45 to 55 mg; Teenage girls: 45 to 50 mg; Adults: 60 mg; Pregnancy: 80 mg; Lactation: 100 mg.
2. When administering orally:
   (a) Give with a full glass of water after meals.
   (b) Large daily dosages are given in divided doses to prevent gastric irritation.
3. When administering IM:
   (a) Give deep into large muscle mass.
   (b) Rotate sites to avoid undue local irritation.
4. When administering IV:
   (a) Known to be incompatable with aminophylline, chloramphenicol, sodium succinate, chlordiazepoxide (Librium), conjugated estrogens (Premarin), dextran, phytonadione (Aquamephyton), penicillin, and vitamin B_{12}.
   (b) A second IV site should be used for all incompatible drugs.
   (c) Administer slowly in dilute form. If given too rapidly, the drug may cause dizziness and lightheadedness.

Client teaching factors

1. Instruct client to store drug in tightly sealed containers away from light.
2. Advise client to take no more than 250 mg at any one time. Divided doses should be used.
3. Caution client not to take vitamin C with other medications, including multivitamins containing B vitamins.

GENERIC NAMES Vitamin B_1, thiamine hydrochloride

(OTC) (RX)

TRADE NAMES Aperrine HCL, Betalin S, Betaxin, Bewon, THIA, Thiamine Chloride, Vitamin D_1, Vitamin F

CLASSIFICATION Water-soluble vitamin (enzyme cofactor), antiberiberi, antineuritic

Source Thiamine is a naturally occurring vitamin of the B-complex group. It is found in wheat germ, lean pork, dried beans, whole wheat, and other enriched grains. Eggs, fish, and some vegetables contain smaller quantities of thiamine. It occurs as free thiamine, as thiamine pyrophosphate, or as a cocarboxylase protein complex. Preparations of the vitamin are obtained from yeast, liver concentrates, or produced synthetically.

Action Thiamine is essential for the functioning of many, if not all, of the body organs and tissues. Its physiologically active form, thiamine pyrophosphate, acts as a coenzyme during the intermediate stages of carbohydrate metabolism. Thiamine assists in the decarboxylation of pyruvic acid and other alpha-ketoacids. Consequently, the body's need for thiamine is directly related to the number of calories, particularly carbohydrate calories, used for energy production.

Indications for Use Treatment and prevention of thiamine deficiency, including beriberi and subclinical states (anorexia, muscular weakness, paresthesia, restlessness, pallor, weight loss, hypotension, lowered body temperature). Alcoholic neuritis due to inadequate intake. Conditions that may cause malabsorption of thiamine, including prolonged diarrhea, ulcerative colitis, upper intestinal resections, and advanced age. States of increased requirement: pregnancy (neuritis), lactation. States of increased metabolism: hyperthyroidism, fever, infections, infancy, adolescence.

Contraindications None reported for orally administered thiamine. Toxic reactions have occurred after the rapid IV administration of large dosages.

Warnings and Precautions Parenteral route of drug administration is used only in severe cases or when oral administration is not feasible. When beriberi occurs in breast-fed infants, the mother should be treated as well.

Untoward Reactions Toxic reactions after IV administration include muscular weakness and labored breathing followed by death due to respiratory failure. Anaphylactic reactions have been reported after IV administration, but rarely.

Parameters of Use

Absorption Only about one-quarter of oral thiamine is absorbed through the duodenum and small intestine; the rest is eliminated via the feces. Clients should consume food and oral supplements approximately four times the recommended daily intake. Complete and rapid absorption from IM sites; IM is the preferred method for correcting severe deficiency.

Crosses placenta. Enters breast milk freely. Breast-fed infants will receive adequate quantities of thiamine only if the mother has consumed adequate amounts.

Storage Occurs in all body tissues, particularly the brain, liver, heart, and kidneys. Tissue stores are depleted rapidly when there is little or no intake of thiamine. Subclinical symptoms may appear within days or a few weeks after the onset of chronic diarrhea.

Metabolism Approximately 1 mg is used each day, but approximately 4 mg should be consumed daily by healthy adults.

Excretion Excessive intake of pyrimidine causes unchanged thiamine to be eliminated in urine.

Drug Characteristics Dry form stable to heat and light. Aqueous solutions are less stable to heat than dry formations. Prolonged cooking (boiling) causes some loss of potency.

Drug Interactions Thiamine may enhance the therapeutic effects of muscle relaxants.

Administration The dosage varies according to the carbohydrate metabolism and energy requirements of the client. (Adults: 0.23 to 0.5 mg/1000 calories.)

- *Commonly used dosages in mild deficiency states:* 5 to 10 mg po daily.
- *Commonly used dosages in severe deficiency states:* 30 to 100 mg po, IM, or IV daily.

Available Drug Forms Tablets containing 5 to 250 mg; oral liquids containing various amounts; ampules or multidose vials of sterile solution for injection containing 100 mg/ml.

Nursing Management

Planning factors

1. When possible, complete a dietary history to determine the client's daily intake of thiamine from dietary sources, including fortified foods and self-administered vitamin supplements. Consult a dietitian as needed.
2. Although beriberi (both dry and wet) is endemic in Asia, it seldom occurs in the United States. However, subclinical cases of thiamine deficiency are thought to be prevalent in the United States, particularly among infants, adolescents, geriatrics, fad dieters, pregnant women, alcoholics, and the clinically ill clients.

Administration factors

1. The recommended daily allowances of thiamine (assuming an average caloric intake) are: Infants: 0.2 to 0.5 mg; Children: 0.6 to 1.0 mg; Teenage boys: 1.3 to 1.5 mg; Teenage girls: 1.1 to 1.2 mg; Adult males: 1.2 to 1.4 mg; Adult females: 1.0 mg; Pregnancy: 1.2 mg; Lactation: 1.5 mg.
2. Large amounts are given in divided doses in order to maximize tissue storage.
3. When administering IM:
   (a) Used only when vomiting or other GI disturbances are present.
   (b) Administer deep into muscle and rotate sites since tissue irritation can occur.
4. When administering IV:
   (a) Used only in severe deficiency states until symptoms begin to subside (2 to 3 days).
   (b) A skin test should be done prior to administration.
   (c) Can be administered in 100 ml of IV fluid over 1 hour or more.

Evaluation factors

1. Rapid IV administration can cause severe untoward reactions; a mild transitory drop in blood pressure can occur. Keep patient in bed during administration and monitor blood pressure frequently.
2. Assess the therapeutic effectiveness daily by determining the improvement in the client's clinical status. Serum pyruvic acid levels will decline to normal levels, the legs become stronger, and paresthesia decreases. Cardiac symptoms will gradually disappear (bounding radial pulses, tachycardia, palpitations, flattened or inverted T waves, shortened Q-T interval). Irritability, insomnia, depression, and anorexia subsides.

Client teaching factors

1. Explain to clients that raw vegetables are higher in Vitamin B_1 content than boiled vegetables.
2. Caution clients to store liquid preparation in a cool area.

GENERIC NAMES Vitamin B_1, thiamine mononitrate

TRADE NAMES Thiamine Nitrate, Vitamin B_1 Mononitrate

(OTC) (RX)

CLASSIFICATION Water-soluble vitamin, antiberiberi, antineuritic (enzyme cofactor)

Source Synthetically produced salt of thiamine.

Action This compound is more stable than thiamine hydrochloride in the dry state and is therefore the preferred compound for many multivitamin preparations. (See Thiamine Hydrochloride for further details.)

See Thiamine Hydrochloride for indications for use, contraindications, warnings and precautions, untoward reactions, parameters of use, drug interactions, administration, available drug forms, and nursing management.

GENERIC NAMES Vitamin B_2 riboflavin

TRADE NAMES Hyrye, Lactoflavin, Vitamin G

CLASSIFICATION Water-soluble vitamin (enzyme cofactor)

(OTC) (RX)

Source Riboflavin is a naturally occurring vitamin of the B-complex group. It is found in milk (2 mg/quart), milk products, some organ meats (liver, heart), yeast, and some green vegetables. It occurs in the free form as well as combined with phosphorus and certain proteins. Preparations are obtained from yeast, liver concentrates, milk, or produced synthetically.

Action Riboflavin is essential for the functioning of many, if not all, of the body organs and tissues. It is known to form at least two coenzymes, flavin mononucleotide (FMN) and flavin adenine dinucleotide (FAD), which are essential to cellular metabolism. FMN assists in deamination (removal of the amino group from certain proteins) and FAD assists in several aspects of cellular respiration. Much of riboflavin's metabolism and physiologic activity is still unknown.

Indications for Use Treatment and prevention of riboflavin deficiency, ariboflavinosis. Adjunct in the treatment of other vitamin B deficiencies, including beriberi and pellagra. The bone marrow depression and optic neuritis induced by chloramphenicol and other antibiotics may be reduced by riboflavin.

Contraindications None known.

Warnings and Precautions Riboflavin deficiency rarely occurs alone. The disorder accompanies other vitamin B deficiencies.

Untoward Reactions Toxicity has not been reported. Large doses may cause clients' urine to turn bright yellow.

Parameters of Use

Absorption Readily absorbed from the upper GI tract; readily absorbed when given parenterally. Deficiency may occur when there is a disturbance of the upper GI tract, such as a segmental resection.

Distribution To all organs and tissues. Bound to plasma proteins and has the potential of being displaced from plasma binding sites by some drugs and vice versa.

Storage Little storage in tissues; small quantities found in liver, kidneys, and heart. Deficiencies may occur if tissue needs are not supplied daily.

Metabolism Little is known; combines with phosphoric acid and proteins.

Excretion Only about 9% is eliminated normally in urine; when large doses are absorbed, large quantities are eliminated unchanged in urine; some fecal excretion. Vitamin B_2 has low toxicity since excess is excreted freely.

Drug Characteristics Stable to dry heat but is easily destroyed by light; less stable when exposed to moisture; unstable in alkaline solutions. Store in tightly sealed containers placed in a dark place.

Administration Dosage varies according to the needs of the client.

- *Commonly used dosages in mild deficiency states:* 2 to 5 mg po daily.
- *Commonly used dosages in severe deficiency states:* 5 to 10 mg po daily. Up to 50 mg given in divided doses has been used. Dosages may be given IM, subc, or IV when GI absorption is not feasible.

Available Drug Forms Tablets containing 2, 5, or 10 mg; vials containing 5 mg/ml. Found in several multivitamin preparations, including Albafort, Alba-Lybe, Al-Vite, B-C-Bid, Besta, Eldercaps, Eldertonic, Glutofac, Hemo-Vite, Mega-B, Megadose, Obron-6, Rovite, Therabid, and Vicon-C.

Nursing Management

Planning factors

1. When possible, complete a dietary history to determine the client's daily intake of riboflavin from dietary sources, including fortified foods and self-administered vitamin supplements. Consult a dietitian as needed.
2. Riboflavin deficiency is usually related to a deficiency of B vitamins. Vitamin B complex therapy is usually required.

Administration factors

1. The recommended daily allowances of riboflavin vary according to total caloric and protein intake, body size, metabolic rate, and rate of growth. Intakes for healthy individuals are: Infants: 0.4 to 0.6 mg; Young children: 0.6 to 1.2 mg; Teenagers: 1.3 to 1.5 mg; Adult men: 1.7 mg; Adult women: 1.5 mg; Pregnancy: 1.8 mg; Lactation: 2.0 mg.
2. Large amounts should be given in divided doses to maximize tissue levels.

Evaluation factors Evaluate therapeutic effectiveness by assessing for cheilosis, glossitis, seborrheic dermatitis, corneal vascularization (redness), burning sensation in hands and feet, and other signs of vitamin B deficiency.

Client teaching factors

1. Instruct client to protect drug from light.
2. Emphasize the necessity for a well-balanced diet to prevent deficiencies.
3. Inform client of possible discoloration of urine.

GENERIC NAMES Vitamin B_3, niacin, nicotinic acid; niacinamide, nicotinic acid amide (OTC) (RX)

TRADE NAMES Diacin, Niac, Niacels, Nicobid, Nico-400, Nicocap, Nicolar, Nico-Span, Nicotinex, SK-Niacin, Tega-Span, Tinic, Vasotherm, Vastran Forte, Wampocap; Nicotinamide

CLASSIFICATION Water-soluble vitamin (enzyme cofactor), antipellagra

---

Source Niacin is a naturally occurring vitamin of the B-complex group. Niacin is easily converted to niacinamide. Niacin and its amide are produced by animals and a few plants. Meats, liver, peanuts, beans, peas, and some grains are rich in niacin. The precursor of niacin is tryptophan, but it takes approximately 60 mg of tryptophan to produce 1 mg of niacin. Therefore, a niacin equivalent is about 60 mg of tryptophan. White rice, corn, oats, and most fruits and vegetables contain little or no niacin. Milk and eggs are low in niacin but high in tryptophan.

Action Niacin and its amide, along with riboflavin, are essential to tissue respiration and carbohydrate metabolism. They are enzyme cofactors that assist in the conversion of proteins and fats to glucose. They also assist in the oxidation of glucose to release energy. Niacin, but not its amide, causes vasodilation, particularly in the peripheral vascular system, but little if any vasodilation of the cerebral and coronary arteries. Large doses of niacin, but not its amide, can inhibit lipolysis by interfering with cholesterol synthesis, and therefore, lowers the plasma levels of cholesterol, triglycerides, and free fatty acids. The term *niacin* is preferred to *nicotinic acid* in order to avoid confusing the vitamin with the poison nicotine.

Indications for Use Treatment and prevention of niacin deficiency: pellagra, psychoses due to dietary deficiency, alcoholic encephalopathy due to dietary deficiency, malabsorption caused by certain cancerous growths in the GI tract. Hartnup's disease (genetic disorder of tryptophan transport). Niacin (but not the amide) may be of some benefit in certain peripheral vascular disorders and hyperlipidemia. States of increased requirements: infancy, adolescence, pregnancy, lactation. Used to differentiate niacin deficiency psychosis from other psychoses. Confusion and delirium disappear within 24 hours in clients with niacin deficiency.

Contraindications Hypersensitivity to niacin or its amide, active peptic ulcer, gastritis, hemorrhage, hypotension, severe liver disorders.

Warnings and Precautions Should be used cautiously in clients with a history of allergies, diabetes, peptic ulcer, gout, and liver or gallbladder disease.

Untoward Reactions Large doses may irritate the GI tract and cause vomiting, diarrhea, and flatulence. Large doses may alter liver function tests and induce hyperglycemia; diabetic clients may require additional insulin. Hyperuricemia and gout may be aggravated by large doses. Circulatory collapse has occurred after rapid IV administration. Transient side effects from niacin preparations include flushing with onset in 1 hour, headache, and hypotension.

Parameters of Use

Absorption Readily absorbed from all sites; give with a full glass of water after meals.

Storage Distributed to all tissues but little stored for any period of time; a deficiency state can occur within weeks.

Metabolism Several conversions occur through enzyme systems; some metabolites are biologically active (NAD, NADP); the liver is the primary site for conversion to metabolites. Hepatic dysfunction can delay the conversion to inactive metabolites.

Excretion Metabolites are eliminated primarily in the urine; large doses may cause it to be excreted unchanged in urine. May cause glucosuria.

Drug Characteristics Niacin is stable to heat in dry form as well as solution. Prolonged exposure to light may cause deterioration. Store in a dark area; discard if a discoloration occurs. Niacinamide is more stable in solution and more compatible with thiamine chloride than niacin.

Drug Interactions Hypoglycemic agents may be antagonized by niacin and niacinamide since larger doses of the vitamin may increase serum glucose levels. Postural hypotension and excessive vasodilation may occur when used concurrently with adrenergic blocking agents (agents used to treat hypertension).

Administration Dosage varies according to the needs of the client and the intended purpose of the drug.

- *Commonly used dosages in mild deficiency states:* 25 to 50 mg po daily, bid, or tid.
- *Commonly used dosages in severe deficiency states:* Tablet: 25 to 50 mg po 4 to 10 times daily; Timed-release capsule: 125 to 250 mg po bid; Parenterally: 25 to 50 mg bid or tid.
- *Commonly used dosages of niacin for vasodilation:* 50 mg po bid or tid.
- *Commonly used dosages of niacin for hyperlipidemia:* 500 to 3000 mg po daily in divided doses.

Available Drug Forms *Niacin:* Tablets containing 50, 100, or 250 mg; timed-release capsules containing 125, 250, 400, or 500 mg; elixir containing 50 mg/tsp; ampules and multidose vials containing 1 or 10 mg/ml; present in numerous multivitamin tablets, capsules, and elixirs. *Niacinamide:* Tablets containing 500 mg; ampules and multidose vials containing 50 or 100 mg/ml; present in numerous multivitamin tablets, capsules, and elixirs.

Nursing Management

Planning factors

1. When possible, complete a dietary history to determine the client's daily intake of niacin from dietary sources, including fortified foods and self-administered vitamin supplements. Consult a dietitian as needed.
2. Small doses given frequently will maximize the desired therapeutic effect.

Administration factors

1. The recommended daily allowances of niacin or trypotophan are: Infants: 5 to 8 mg; Teenage boys: 17 to 20 mg; Teenage girls: 15 to 16 mg; Adult males: 18 mg; Adult females: 13 mg; Pregnancy: 15 mg; Lactation: 20 mg; Senior citizens: 13 to 14 mg.
2. When administering orally, give with a full glass of water to maximize absorption.
3. When administering IM, administer deep into large muscle mass.
4. When administering IV:
   a. A skin test should be done prior to administering niacin or its amide since anaphylactic reactions may occur. The amide is usually tolerated better than niacin.
   b. Administer slowly. Can be administered in 50 to 100 ml of IV fluid over 1 hour.
   c. Have client remain in bed during drug administration.

Evaluation factors

1. If GI disturbances occur with niacin, niacinamide may be better tolerated.
2. Blood sugar and liver function tests should be taken weekly.
3. Diabetics should be followed daily to determine niacin's effect on their insulin requirements.
4. Assess the presence of side effects every 15 minutes following IV administration. If hypotension or dizziness occur, have the client rest in bed until the side effects subside (approximately 60 to 90 minutes). Notify physician.
5. Assess the therapeutic effectiveness daily by deter-

mining the improvement in the client's clinical status. Dramatic improvement in the skin and mucous membrane lesions may occur in severe deficiencies; tongue swelling eases; the presence of excessive oils on the skin decreases; burning sensation of skin subsides; nausea and vomiting disappear.

Client teaching factors

1. Instruct client to store drug in a dark area and to discard drug if discoloration occurs.
2. Instruct client to take drug after meals.

GENERIC NAMES Vitamin B_5, pantothenic acid; calcium pantothenate, racemic calcium pantothenate; panthenol

(OTC) (RX)

TRADE NAMES Pantothenic acid; Calpanate, Dextro-Calcium Pantothenate

CLASSIFICATION Water-soluble vitamin, chick antidermatitis factor

Source Although pantothenic acid is widely distributed throughout living tissue, the quantity is so minute that the calcium malts of pantothenic acid have been found to be a more economical source. Panthenol is the alcohol analog of pantothenic acid. Pantothenic acid is synthesized by intestinal bacteria and can be found in yeast, liver, kidney, egg yolks, and skimmed milk. Beef, dairy products, and numerous green or yellow vegetables are also good sources of the acid.

Action Pantothenic acid is an essential constituent of coenzyme A (Co A or acetyl Co A) and Co A is an important activating agent in many metabolic processes, particularly those involving acetylation. It is involved in the processes of carbohydrate, fat, and protein metabolism, the formation of steroid hormones and the heme for hemoglobin synthesis. It may also be involved in the elimination of some drugs (sulfonamides). Specific deficiency states have not been identified but are related to deficiencies of other B vitamins.

Indications for Use There are no established therapeutic uses for pantothenic acid. May be useful in situations of extreme metabolic stress, such as severe burns, extensive injuries, and severe infections. Often used in conjunction with other B vitamins in clients with a general vitamin B deficiency. Has not been proven effective in the treatment of alopecia, the prevention of gray hair, or retardation of the aging process.

Warnings and Precautions Daily requirements not established. A well-balanced diet provides 10 to 20 mg daily. The body excretes about 6 mg daily.

Administration Usual dosage: 10 mg po daily. Range: 10 to 50 mg daily.

Available Drug Forms Found in several multivitamin preparations, including Al-Vita, B-C-Bid, Besta, Eldercaps, Hemo-Vite, Megadose, Obron-b, Rovite, and Therabid.

Nursing Management

1. It is considered to be a nontoxic vitamin.
2. Since it is found widely in nature, a deficiency of pantothenic acid is unlikely.
3. There is no scientific evidence to indicate that pantothenic acid supplements will retard the aging process.

GENERIC NAMES Vitamin B_6, pyridoxine hydrochloride

(OTC) (RX)

TRADE NAMES Beesix, Hexa-Betalin, Hexavibex, Hydoxin

CLASSIFICATION Water-soluble vitamin (enzyme cofactor)

Source Pyridoxine is a naturally occurring vitamin of the B-complex group. It exists in nature as pyridoxol (pyridoxine), pyridoxal and pyridoxamine. All three forms are biologically active. Liver, kidney, other meats, seafood, legumes, yeast, and cereals of wheat or corn are good sources of pyridoxine. Milk, eggs, and most vegetables contain limited amounts.

Action Pyridoxine is an essential coenzyme in metabolism. In the body the natural pyridoxine substances are converted to pyridoxal phosphate. Although it is not completely understood, pyridoxal serves several key roles in metabolism including the following:

1. Assists in energy transformation in brain and nerve cells.
2. Decarboxylation of amino acids.
3. Assists in transamination reactions (transfer of amino group in amino acids).
4. Involved in the formation of niacin from its precursor tryptophan and assists in the conversion of tryptophan to serotonin, a potent vasoconstrictor that stimulates cerebral activity.
5. Assists in the transfer of sulfur from sulfur-containing amino acids.
6. Is probably involved with the incorporation of certain glucose metabolites into the heme of red blood cells.
7. May be involved in the active transport of amino acids from the intestinal tract and the transport of amino acids into cells.
8. Assists in the conversion of linoleic acid, an essential fatty acid, to its metabolites.

Although no specific deficiency state has been identified, certain anemias, convulsions, neuritis, and irritability have been related to vitamin B_6 deficiency. Other vitamin B deficiencies are probably involved.

Indications for Use Prevention of pyridoxine deficiency; treatment of a B-complex deficiency; hypersensitivity to pyridoxine; hypochromic microcytic anemia; peripheral neuritis due to isoniazid; convulsions and anemias due to a deficiency of vitamin B_6 (inborn error of metabolism); states of increased requirement: pregnancy, lactation; may be of some benefit in alcoholic polyneuritis, controlling nausea and vomiting due to pregnancy and radiation therapy, drug-induced optic neuritis, and other neurological disorders; isoniazid poisoning.

Contraindications Hypersensitivity to pyridoxine.

Warnings and Precautions Clients taking levodopa should not ingest more than 5 mg of pyridoxine daily. Excessive intake of protein will increase the requirements for pyridoxine. Although humans can tolerate up to 25 mg/kg daily, 3 to 4 g/kg has induced convulsions in animals.

Untoward Reactions Paresthesia and somnolence have been reported.

Parameters of Use

Absorption Absorbed readily from the upper portion of small intestine.

Distribution In all body tissues.

Half-life About 20 days; deficiency states are usually corrected in 3 weeks.

Metabolism Poorly understood but it is converted to pyridoxal phosphate. Degraded in liver to 4-pyridoxic acid.

Excretion 4-Pyridoxic acid is excreted by the kidneys; large doses may cause excessive pyridoxal excretion.

Drug Characteristics Pyridoxine is stable to heat, acid, and alkali, but it is sensitive to light. Store in dark area away from direct light.

Drug Interactions Pyridoxine has been useful in counteracting some of the neurologic side effects of anticholinergic agents. Pyridoxine is of some value in preventing chloramphenicol-induced optic neuritis. Isoniazid inhibits the action of pyridoxine; clients taking isoniazid should have supplemental pyridoxine. Levodopa action is reduced by pyridoxine; supplemental pyridoxine should not be given when levodopa is required. Supplemental dosages of pyridoxine are of some value in decreasing the drug-induced urinary retention, dry mouth, and other side effects of tricyclic antidepressants.

Administration Dosage varies according to the needs of the client and the amount of protein in the diet.

- *Commonly used dosages to prevent deficiency:* 2 to 5 mg po daily.
- *Commonly used dosages for vitamin B_6 errors in metabolism:* Initial dose of 600 mg po or IM daily; Maintenance dose of 30 mg po or IM daily.
- *Commonly used dosages in drug-induced deficiency states:* Initial dose of 100 mg po daily for 3 weeks; Maintenance dose of 30 to 50 mg po daily.
- *Commonly used dosages for isoniazid poisoning (10 g or more):* Initial dosage of 4 g IV then 1 g IM q30min, until an equal amount of pyridoxine has been given.

Available Drug Forms Tablets containing 10, 25, or 50 mg; vials and ampules containing 50 or 100 mg/ml; multidose vials containing 50 or 100 mg/ml; present in many multivitamin tablets, capsules, and elixirs.

Nursing Management

Planning factors

1. When possible, complete a dietary history to determine the client's daily intake of pyridoxine from dietary sources, including fortified foods and self-administered vitamin supplements. Consult a dietitian as needed.
2. Pyridoxine deficiency is seldom seen without simultaneous deficiencies of other B vitamins.
3. Women taking oral contraceptives may develop a pyridoxine deficiency.

Administration factors

1. Daily requirement is unknown. Adults require at least 1.2 mg daily (100 g of dietary protein).
2. The recommended daily allowances are: Adults: 2 mg; Pregnancy: 2.5 mg; Lactation: 2.5 mg.
3. Large dosages should be given in divided doses, such as 50 mg bid.
4. Drug can be administered IV in 50 ml of IV fluid over 30 minutes.

Evaluation factors Assess the therapeutic effectiveness daily by determining the improvement in the client's clinical status: improvement in seborrhealike skin lesions around eyes, nose, and mouth, glossitis, stomatitis, convulsions and other CNS disturbances, and anemia.

Client teaching factors

1. Explain the necessity of life-long maintenance dosages to clients with vitamin B_6 inborn errors in metabolism.
2. Instruct clients taking levodopa to check the quantity of pyridoxine in OTC multivitamin preparations before using them.
3. Instruct client to store drug in a dark area.

GENERIC NAMES Vitamin B_{12}, cyanocobalamin, cobalamin

OTC RX

TRADE NAME Berubigen, Betalin 12, B-Twelve, Bevidox, Cobavite, Cobin, Crystimin, Dodex, Kaybovite, Redisol, Rubesol, Rubramin PC, Sytobex, Vi-Twel

CLASSIFICATION Water-soluble vitamin (extrinsic factor), hematopoietic

---

Source This vitamin does not occur in plants but exists as vitamers (cobalamins B_{12a}, B_{12b}, B_{12c}, B_{12d}) in animal proteins. Foods rich in vitamin B_{12} include the organ meats (liver, kidney), clams, oysters, crabs, salmon, sardines, tuna, flounder, haddock, eggs, and lean muscle meats. Milk and some cheeses contain small quantities. Cyanocobalamin is produced by certain microorganisms, such as *Streptomyces griseus*. The vitamin is mass produced from these microorganisms and from animal livers.

Action Vitamin B_{12} is the only vitamin that contains cobalt, which gives the vitamin its red color. The vitamin is essential for normal growth of cells, hematopoiesis, development of epithelial tissue, and maintenance of the myelin coating of nerves. It is involved in several metabolic interactions with other nutrients, particularly folic acid, thymine, and choline. The primary actions of the vitamin include the following:

1. The maturation of normal RBCs. Folic acid can temporarily substitute for vitamin B_{12} in this process. Both folic acid and vitamin B_{12} are required for DNA and RNA synthesis.
2. Methylation of certain substances. Probably acts as a coenzyme in reactions involving amino acids and other substances essential for cell reproduction, myelin synthesis, and normal growth.

A deficiency of vitamin B_{12} causes pernicious anemia (macrocytic and megaloblastic), demyelination of certain large spinal nerve fibers (particularly of the posterior columns), a loss of peripheral sensation, and sometimes paralysis.

Indications for Use Pernicious anemia; inadequate absorption due to lack of intrinsic factor caused by destructive lesions of the gastric mucosa (ingestion of corrosives), gastric atrophy, or gastrectomy; inadequate absorption due to sprue, regional ileitis, ileal resection, ileal neoplasia, or pancreatic disease (low bowel pH); inadequate absorption due to intestinal parasites, such as the fish tapeworm, or bacteria competing for the vitamin.

Contraindications History of sensitivity to vitamin B_{12} or cobalt; Hereditary optic nerve atrophy (Leber's disease).

Warnings and Precautions Rapid IV administration may cause anaphylaxis. Use with caution in clients with cardiac disorders, pulmonary disorders, hypertension, or a history of congestive heart failure, since hypokalemia and fluid overload may occur. Use with caution in clients with gout since hyperuricemia may occur. Correction of deficiency may reveal the presence of polycythemia vera.

Untoward Reactions Intense therapy has caused anaphylaxis, hypokalemia, congestive heart failure, pulmonary edema, and peripheral vascular thrombosis. Mild transient diarrhea, feeling of generalized swelling, and flushing are common. Rash with or without pruritis has occurred. Irritation and pain at injection site is common.

Parameters of Use

Absorption Ingested vitamin B_{12} is readily absorbed from the ileum when intrinsic factor, a mucoprotein secreted by the stomach is present. Intrinsic factor also protects the vitamin's binding to specific beta- and alpha-globulins (normal range 200 to 900 pg). When necessary, intrinsic factor is given simultaneously with the vitamin. Calcium must be present in the ileum for B_{12} to be absorbed. Some free vitamin diffuses through the intestinal mucosa (approximately 1%). Diffusion is enhanced when large dosages are ingested. Levels peak 8 to 12 hours after ingestion. Vitamin B_{12} is not absorbed when intestinal pH is below 5.5. When necessary, intestinal pH can be corrected with sodium bicarbonate or other alkalis. The vitamin is absorbed from IM and subc sites. Plasma levels peak approximately 1 hour after parenteral injection.

Crosses placenta freely. Infant blood levels are higher than mothers'.

Storage Primarily in liver, 1 to 10 mg in normal individuals. Smaller quantities are found in the kidneys, heart, muscle, pancreas, spleen, bone marrow, and other tissues. Clinical deficiency states may take as long as 6 years to appear. Liver disease, such as hepatitis, may cause release of liver stores and mask symptoms of B_{12} deficiency.

Metabolism Converted to the active coenzymes methylcobalamin and deoxyadenosylcobalamin in the tissues.

Excretion In bile, approximately 3 to 7 mcg daily. Small quantities are secreted in pancreatic and gastric juices. Most is reabsorbed from GI tract; only about 1 mcg is eliminated via feces. Only the free B_{12} is eliminated via urine (less than 0.25 mcg daily); the administration of large doses will increase the free B_{12} levels in the blood and therefore cause the rapid urinary excretion of the vitamin.

Drug Interactions Vitamin C destroys vitamin B_{12}; do not administer concurrently. Do not administer vitamin B_{12} with juices high in vitamin C. Alcohol causes a malabsorption of vitamin B_{12}. Colchicine inhibits the absorption of ingested vitamin B_{12}. *p*-Aminosalicylic acid inhibits the absorption of ingested vitamin B_{12} and decreases the urinary excretion of the vitamin. Potassium chloride inhibits the absorption of ingested vitamin B_{12} by decreasing the intestinal pH. Prednisone increases the absorption of ingested vitamin B_{12}. Chloramphenicol may cause a poor therapeutic hematopoietic response to vitamin B_{12}, since it interferes with the normal maturation of erythrocytes. Supplemental vitamin B_{12} may help prevent chloramphenicol-induced optic neuritis.

Administration Dosage varies according to the needs of the client.

- *Initial therapy for severe deficiency:* Adults: 30 mcg IM or subc daily for 5 to 10 days, up to 250 mcg have been used; Children: 30 to 100 mcg IM or subc for 5 to 10 days.
- *Maintenance therapy in pernicious anemia:* 100 to 250 mcg IM or subc once per month for life.
- *Most other forms of deficiency states:* Maintained on 1 to 60 mcg po daily for life or until the underlying condition is corrected.
- *Nutritional supplement for debilitated clients:* 1 to 25 mcg daily.

Available Drug Forms Multidose vials containing 30, 50, 60, 100, 120, or 1000 mcg/ml; ampules containing 50 or 1000 mcg/ml; tablets and capsules containing various dosages.

Nursing Management

Planning factors

1. A history of previous untoward effects to drugs should be obtained.
2. An intradermal test with 0.1 mcg should be administered before parenteral therapy is initiated.
3. A complete blood count as well as vitamin B_{12} and folic acid blood levels should be determined prior to initiating therapy.
4. Although dietary deficiency is seldom seen in normal individuals, it has occurred in clients who are strict vegetarians. The deficiency symptoms may be acute in breast-fed infants of strict vegetarians.
5. Obtain baseline serum electrolyte levels.

Administration factors

1. The recommended daily allowances of vitamin B_{12} are: Infants: 0.3 mcg; Teenagers: 3 mcg; Adults: 2 to 25 mcg. Minimum daily intake: 0.1 mcg. These doses are easily supplied by a well-balanced diet, since two glasses of milk, 2 eggs, and 8 oz of meat yield 4.8 mcg.
2. Administering vitamin B_{12} with meals may enhance absorption, provided the meal is devoid of vitamin C. Food and juices rich in vitamin C can be given either 1 hour before or 2 hours after meals.
3. Administer IM solution deep into subcutaneous tissue or inject into a large muscle mass to prevent local irritation.
4. When administering IV:
   a. Reserved for severe cases in which other routes of administration are not feasible.
   b. Incompatible with dextrose and alkaline solutions. Administer in normal saline devoid of other substances.

Evaluation factors

1. Obtain serum electrolyte levels daily for the first 5 days.
2. Evaluate the client's clinical status at least three times a day during the first 5 days of therapy. As resumption of normal erythropoiesis may increase the potassium requirements dramatically, severe hypokalemia may occur. Pulmonary edema and congestive heart failure have been known to occur during initial therapy.
3. The clinical symptoms (paresthesia, palpitations, external dyspnea, incoordination, GI disturbances, fatigue) and blood count should improve within 48 hours. Complete disappearance in irreversible neurologic symptoms can take as long as 18 months. Concurrent physical therapy has been of some benefit. (If the deficiency is of long standing, permanent damage may have occurred to the spinal column.)

Client teaching factors

1. Clients with pernicious anemia must be educated about their disorder: the need for life-threatening parenteral therapy and the consequence of avoiding their monthly injections.
2. Instruct client to store drug in a dark area.

GENERIC NAMES Folic acid, pteroylglutamic acid

TRADE NAME Folacin, Folvite (RX)

CLASSIFICATION Water-soluble vitamin, hematopoietic

Source Folic acid is a B-complex vitamin that consists of three acids, including glutamic acid, the only amino acid metabolized by the brain. The vitamin occurs naturally in many plants and animals. Foods rich in folic acid include organ meats (liver, kidneys), fresh green leafy vegetables, asparagus, and yeast. Canning and prolonged cooking of vegetables destroys their folic acid content.

Action Folic acid is essential for normal growth of cells and hematopoiesis. It is involved in several metabolic reactions with other nutrients, including vitamin B_{12}. Although folic acid itself is not active physiologically in humans, it is rapidly converted by the body to an active metabolite, tetrahydrofolic acid (THFA). THFA acts as a coenzyme that will accept and transfer single carbon units in several metabolic processes, including the synthesis of purines, thymine and other pyrimidine compounds, and some amino acids. The primary actions of the vitamin include the following:

1. Maturation of normal erythrocytes. Folic acid is required for DNA synthesis and can substitute for vitamin B_{12} in this maturation process.
2. Promotes normal growth by participating in the intermediate metabolism of DNA and certain amino acids.

A deficiency of folic acid causes a megaloblastic anemia similar in hematologic characteristics to pernicious anemia (deficiency of vitamin B_{12}). Although folic acid will improve the blood picture in pernicious anemia by acting as a substitute for vitamin B_{12} in erythropoiesis, the neurological damage caused by a deficiency of vitamin B_{12} will continue since folic acid cannot substitute for vitamin B_{12} in RNA synthesis. (RNA is required for the normal maintenance of the central nervous system.) Other signs and symptoms of folic acid deficiency include glossitis, diarrhea, malaise, and insomnia.

Indications for Use Folic acid deficiency or megaloblastic anemia. Conditions that cause malabsorption, including sprue, celiac disease, regional jejunitis, and jejunal diverticulosis. Conditions related to an inadequate intake, including malnutrition, infancy and childhood (often associated with infection and/or diarrhea), alcoholism (alcohol can block folic acid metabolism), advanced age, food fads, excessive dieting, prolonged cooking of food. States of increased requirements: pregnancy (particularly the third trimester), lactation, liver disease, rheumatic arthritis, malignant diseases, alcoholism, chronic infections. Deficiency states associated with certain medications, including anticonvulsants, antimalarial agents, and prolonged use of salicylates or oral contraceptives. As an adjunct in the treatment of pernicious, aplastic, and hemolytic anemia.

Contraindications Aplastic, normocytic, or other anemias in which the causative factor is unknown since folic acid may mask the symptoms of the underlying disease process.

Warnings and Precautions Folic acid in doses above 0.1 mg daily may obscure pernicious anemia (deficiency of vitamin B_{12}) by causing a remission in the blood picture while neurologic damage continues to progress. Orotic aciduria, pyridoxine-deficient megaloblastic anemia, and vitamin E-deficient megaloblastic anemia do not respond to therapy with folic acid.

Untoward Reactions Reported to be nontoxic to humans. Hypersensitivity reactions, including rash, malaise, and bronchospasm, have been reported, but rarely. A generalized feeling of warmth and flushing have been reported after IV administration.

Parameters of Use

Absorption Rapidly absorbed from the proximal section of the small intestines; structural or functional disorders of the upper GI tract may cause malabsorption. Present in blood 30 minutes following oral dose.

Freely crosses placenta and appears in milk. Lactating mothers need increased quantities of folic acid, since breast milk removes relatively large amounts of folic acid, thus causing megaloblastic anemia in the mother.

Storage About 50% stored in liver; total body storage is about 5 to 10 mg. Inadequate intake will cause body storage to be depleted in 2 to 3 months.

Metabolism Rapidly converted to active metabolites including THFA. The metabolites, not folic acid, are active in humans.

Excretion Within 24 hours by sweat glands and kidneys as metabolites and small quantities of unchanged drug. A minimal amount of tubular reabsorption occurs.

Drug Characteristics Destroyed by light. Store in a dark place.

Drug Interactions Oral Contraceptives interfere with the absorption of folic acid. Anticonvulsants, particularly phenytoin, may cause a deficiency of folic acid. If folic acid supplements are given concurrently with anticonvulsants, there may be a reduction in seizure control. The antineoplastic activity of folic acid antagonists, particularly pyrimethamine, will be blocked if folic acid is administered concurrently. Chronic consumption of alcohol results in poor liver storage of folic acid and inhibition of certain enzyme systems required for folic acid metabolism and function.

Administration

- *Initial therapeutic dose for adults and children:* 1.0 mg daily.
- *Usual maintenance doses:* Adults: 0.4 mg; Children under 4 years: 0.4 mg; Infants: 0.1 mg daily; Pregnancy and lactation: 0.8 mg. May be administered orally, IM, or IV.

Available Drug Forms Tablets containing 1 mg; multidose vials containing 10 ml with 5 mg/ml; added to some parenteral multivitamin preparations (MVI-12) and numerous prescription multivitamin preparations.

Nursing Management

Planning factors

1. When possible, complete a dietary history to determine the client's daily intake of folic acid from dietary sources, including prescription and self-administered vitamin supplements. It should be remembered that prolonged cooking will destroy most of the food's folic acid content. Consult a dietitian as needed.
2. Obtain a drug history of all medications taken in the last year to determine whether the folic acid deficiency is due to drug interaction. If a potential drug interaction is uncovered, withdrawal of the offending agent may be necessary.
3. The presence of pernicious anemia must be ruled out before initiating therapy with folic acid. Injectable vitamin B_{12} is necessary to treat pernicious anemia.
4. Oral folic acid is preferred to parenteral preparations. Parenteral administration may be necessary initially for severe deficiencies, nausea, vomiting, and malabsorption disorders.
5. Clients with alcoholism, hemolytic anemia, and chronic infections may require a large maintenance dose.

Administration factors

1. The recommended daily allowances of folic acid are: Infants and children under 4 years: 0.15 mg; Children over 4 years: 0.4 mg; Adults: 0.4 mg; Pregnancy: 0.8 mg; Lactation: 0.5 mg.
2. Administer IM solution deep into a large muscle mass. Subcutaneous injections have been used but are not recommended.
3. When administering IV:
   (a) Dilute in at least 100 ml of IV solution and infuse over 1 hour.
   (b) It can be added to 500 to 1000 ml of the client's daily infusions.
   (c) Protect the IV solution from direct sunlight.

Evaluation factors

1. The client's blood picture should begin to improve within 2 to 5 days. Improvement of other symptoms may take 1 week or more. Therapeutic doses are often necessary for the first 2 weeks before the client can be started on a daily maintenance dose. The client's response to therapy should be observed and charted daily.
2. Clients receiving anticonvulsant drugs must be closely followed since seizure activity may reoccur.

Client teaching factors

1. Instruct client to store drug in a dark area.
2. Emphasize the need for regular hematologic tests and medical checkups until the anemia has subsided.
3. Diet education is usually necessary to prevent the reoccurrence of deficiency.

GENERIC NAMES Calcium leucovorin, folinic acid

TRADE NAME Calcium Folinate, Leucovoria (RX)

CLASSIFICATION Water-soluble vitamin, hematopoietic

Source Calcium leucovorin is the formyl derivative and active form of folic acid, namely 5-formyl tetrahydrofolic acid (THFA). Calcium leucovorin is not only useful as a source of folic acid for megaloblastic anemias, but can also be used as an antidote against folic acid antagonists, since it is already in the active form and does not require the action of folate reductase.

Action See Folic Acid.

Indications for Use Antidote for folic acid antagonists; megaloblastic anemias due to sprue, nutritional deficiency, pregnancy, and infancy; when oral therapy is not possible.

Contraindications See Folic Acid.

Warnings and Precautions Should not be used alone for pernicious anemia (vitamin B_{12} deficiency). Should be administered within 1 hour. Follow the administration for an overdose of folic acid antagonist. Little or no antidote effect will occur if calcium leucovorin is given 4 or more hours after the folic acid antagonist.

Untoward Reactions Hypersensitivity reactions including bronchospasm, rash, and malaise have occurred, but rarely.

Parameters of Use See Folic Acid.

Drug Interactions See Folic Acid.

Administration

- *Megaloblastic anemia:* No more than 1 mg IM daily.
- *Antidote against folic acid antagonists:* Amounts equal to the weight of the antagonist; Usual dosage: 6 mg IM; Range: 250 mcg to 15 mg.

Available Drug Forms Ampules containing 3 mg in 1 ml of solution; vials containing 50 mg of dry powder, which is reconstituted with 5 ml of diluent to yield 10 mg/ml.

Nursing Management

Planning factors

1. Calcium leucovorin and appropriate diluent should be kept at all locations where folic acid antagonists are administered.
2. Baseline complete blood cell count (CBC) and other blood work should be obtained.

Administration factors

1. Reconstitute dry powder with bacteriostatic water for injection, U.S.P., which contains benzyl alcohol. Reconstituted solution must be used within 7 days.
2. If the diluent is not available, dilute with water for injection, U.S.P., only and administer immediately. Discard remaining drug since a precipitate will begin to form.
3. No additional therapeutic results occur if more than 1 mg is given.
4. When administering IM:
   (a) Administer deep into large muscle mass.
   (b) If a large dosage is required, administer two equal doses at two different sites.
5. Administer within 1 hour of the folic acid antagonist for best effect.

Evaluation factors Monitor the client's vital signs frequently. Notify physician immediately if respiratory distress occurs and treat appropriately. (See folic acid for further details.)

Client Teaching Factors See Folic Acid.

OTHER VITAMIN SUBSTANCES

GENERIC NAMES *p*-aminobenzoic acid; potassium *p*-aminobenzoate

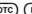

TRADE NAME PABA; Potaba (OTC) (RX)

CLASSIFICATION Water-soluble factor, structural component of folic acid

Source Small amounts occur naturally in cereal, eggs, milk, and meats.

Action Although PABA does not fit all the criteria of a true vitamin, it has vitaminlike characteristics and some individuals consider PABA to be a member of the vitamin B-complex since it has been found to be essential to the growth of several microorganisms. Unlike lower organisms, humans and other mammals are unable to convert PABA to folic acid. Therapeutic doses have been found to be rickettsiostatic but not in individuals infected with typhus, Rocky Mountain spotted Fever, and tsutsugamushi disease. When combined with salicylates, PABA increases the blood level of salicylates by interfering with their analgesic effect. PABA's antifibrotic activity may be required to increase oxygen uptake at the tissue level; however, PABA's therapeutic effectiveness as an antifibrotic agent has not been established. Since PABA does play a role in melanin formation it is sometimes added to sun-screening lotions.

Indications for Use Use as an antirickettsial agent has been replaced by other more effective agents. Therapeutic effectiveness of potassium *p*-aminobenzgoate (Potaba) for scleroderma, dermatomyositis, morphea, linear scleroderma, pemphigus, and Peyronie's disease is under investigation. Combined with salicylate for use as an analgesic for rheumatic fever and other disorders.

Contraindications Concurrent therapy with sulfonamides.

Warnings and Precautions Nutritional achromotrichia (graying of hair) cannot be treated effectively with PABA in humans.

Untoward Reactions Anorexia and nausea may occur infrequently and require discontinuation of drug until symptoms subside; then a lower dosage can be restarted; if a rash or fever develops, discontinue the drug.

Parameters of Use

Absorption Rapid from GI tract. Some systemic absorption may occur from topical preparations.

Distribution Is widely found in serum, spinal fluid, urine, and sweat.

Metabolism Rapidly conjugated with glycine to form *p*-aminohippuric acid in the liver. Metabolism is slowed in clients with hepatic dysfunction.

Excretion By kidneys as metabolites.

Drug Interactions Potentiates the action of salicylates, such as aspirin. Decreases the antiinfective action of sulfonamides and pyrimethamine. Since these agents inhibit the growth of microorganisms by preventing the formation of folic acid, concurrent therapy with PABA causes competitive inhibition. Displaces folic acid antagonists (methotrexate) and penicillin from plasma protein binding sites and therefore may cause toxicity. Decreases the action of *p*-aminosalicylic acid. Probenecid inhibits the urinary excretion of PABA and thereby elevates serum PABA levels.

Administration

- *Commonly used dosages of Potaba for antifibrosis:* Adults: 12 g po daily in 4, 5, or 6 divided doses; Children: 1 g/kg of body weight po daily in divided doses.
- *Commonly used dosages of analgesic preparations:* 300 mg added to 300 mg of aspirin per tablet.

Available Drug Forms *Potaba:* Tablets containing 0.5 g; capsules containing 2.0 g; Envules containing 0.5 g; containers holding 100 g or 1 lb of powder. Found in some multivitamins (Mega-B), some analgesics (Pabirin), and some sun-screening lotions (Presun).

Nursing Management

Planning factors

1. Determine whether client has nausea before administering drug.
2. Check drug incompatibilities before initiating drug therapy.
3. Dissolve 100 g of powder in 1 quart of water to yield a 10% Potaba solution.
4. Prepared Potaba solution may be kept for 7 days under refrigeration.

Administration factors

1. Determine whether client has nausea before administering drug.
2. Dissolve Potaba tablets in 3 to 4 fl oz of water before administering
3. Administer with meals or with a snack, such as milk and crackers.

Evaluation factors

1. If client develops nausea, do not administer drug and notify physician.
2. Watch clients who are receiving PABA and salicylates for acute salicylate toxicity (headaches, dizziness, ringing in the ears, confusion, thirst, nausea and vomiting, diarrhea, hyperventilation).
3. Measure and record the size and shape of fibrotic patches every 2 or 3 days.
4. Observe clients using topical preparations for systemic PABA toxicity (anorexia, nausea).

Client teaching factors

1. Advise client to avoid taking drug on an empty stomach.
2. Instruct client to notify physician if nausea persists.
3. Instruct client to avoid salicylates; advise client to check the contents of OTC sedative analgesics and cold remedies for the presence of salicylates.

GENERIC NAME Biotin (OTC) (RX)

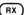

TRADE NAMES Factor, Vitamin H

CLASSIFICATION Water-soluble vitamin, skin factor

Source Both the free and combined forms of biotin occur naturally and can be used by humans. Sources high in biotin include peaches, raspberries, egg yolks, liver, kidney, yeast, nuts, and grains.

Action Biotin is considered to be part of the B-complex group. Because it was found to correct a syndrome characterized by dermatitis, hair loss, and paralysis in rats who were fed large quantities of egg whites, it has been called the "anti–egg white injury factor." The injurious component in egg white is a protein called avidin. Biotin corrects the syndrome by combining with avidin in the intestines to produce a nonabsorbable complex. Although biotin is produced by intestinal bacteria, the avidin-induced injury can occur in individuals who eat large quantities of egg whites, but rarely. Biotin is a necessary coenzyme for carboxylation (carbon dioxide fixation or addition) and for deamination. Therefore, biotin is involved in numerous metabolic processes, including the synthesis of some fatty acids and amino acids, the formation of purines, and the deamination of amino acids.

Indications for Use There are no established uses for biotin. Avidin syndrome, characterized by dermatitis on the extremities, an ashen, pallid appearance, anemia, muscular aches and pains, hyperesthesia, and depression. May be used in conjunction with other B vitamins in clients with a B-complex deficiency. May be of some benefit as an adjunct in the treatment of severe seborrhea and psoriasis.

Administration Minute quantities given orally in certain multivitamin preparations.

Available Drug Forms Found in some multivitamin preparations (Berocca Plus, Mega-B, Megadose).

Nursing Management

1. It is considered to be a nontoxic vitamin.
2. Since it is found widely in nature, a deficiency of biotin is unlikely.
3. Daily requirement has not been established.

GENERIC NAMES Choline, choline bitartrate (RX)

CLASSIFICATION Water-soluble vitamin factor

Source Often found in protein foods. Good food sources include egg yolks, meats, legumes, and some cereals.

Action Choline is involved in many biological processes. It is the precursor of acetylcholine, a methyl donor in intermediate metabolism (transmethylation), and acts as a lipotropic agent for fatty livers. Choline is a constituent of the phospholipid lecithin, which is essential for the normal transport of fat. A deficiency of choline causes hemorrhagic kidney degeneration in animals.

Indications for Use No longer used as a lipotropic agent for clients with hepatitis, cirrhosis, and other disorders that cause fatty liver deposits. Ilopan-Choline may help relieve the gas retention associated with gastritis, gastric hyperacidity, irritable colon, regional ileitis, cholecystitis, splenic flexure syndrome, and postoperative gas retention.

Contraindications None known.

Warnings and Precautions Do not administer Ilopan-Choline within 1 hour of succinylcholine. Use caution when administering large doses to nursing mothers and pregnant women. The safety and effectiveness of large dosages in children has not been established.

Untoward Reactions A generalized rash, urticaria, and a dull headache have been reported, but rarely. No causal relationship has been found to date.

Parameters of Use

Absorption Fairly readily absorbed from GI tract. Before absorption, some choline is converted to trimethylamine and its oxide by intestinal bacteria.

Excretion By kidneys primarily as trimethylamine.

Drug Interactions Allergic reactions of unknown causes have been reported when Ilopan-Choline is given concurrently with antibiotics, narcotics, and barbiturates, but rarely.

Administration Small quantities are added to some multivitamin preparations (80 mg in Megadose). Ilopan-Choline contains 25 mg of choline per tablet and 2 or 3 tablets are given tid.

Available Drug Forms Found in some multivitamin preparations (Ilopan-Choline, Mega-B, Megadose). *Ilopan-Choline:* Tablets containing 50 mg dexpanthenol (pantothenic acid) and 25 mg choline. Its derivatives are used as cholinergic agents (carbachol, Urecholine) and as short-acting muscle relaxants (choline chloride succinate).

Nursing Management

Administration factors

1. Administer drug between meals.
2. Give drug with a full glass of water.
3. Drug remains stable at room temperature.

Evaluation factors

1. Measure abdominal girth and auscultate bowel sounds before initiating drug therapy with Ilopan-Choline.
2. Auscultate bowel sounds before each administration of Ilopan-Choline and compare results.
3. Measure abdominal girth before morning dose of Ilopan-Choline.

GENERIC NAME Inositol (OTC) (RX)

CLASSIFICATION Water-soluble vitamin

Source Inositol is found in most plants and animals. Good food sources include fruits, cereals, eggs, milk, liver, and other meats.

Action Inositol is an isomer of glucose and is readily converted to glucose by the body and vice versa and has been called a "muscle sugar." It does have some lipotropic effect, but has been found to have little or no therapeutic value in diseases that cause fatty liver deposits. There is some evidence to indicate that it may be useful in reducing elevated serum cholesterol levels. It has been found that a deficiency of inositol causes stunted growth, alopecia, and severe dermatitis in mice. Inositol has been used to promote epithelialization in humans but without any convincing results.

Indications for Use No known therapeutic use.

Parameters of Use

Absorption Easily absorbed from the GI tract. Normal blood levels: 0.5 mg/100 ml.

Storage Widely distributed; large quantities stored in heart and skeletal muscle. Also found in the brain and red blood cells. Either stored or converted to glucose and used by body.

Excretion Small quantities excreted by kidneys.

Administration Small quantities are added to some multivitamin preparations (80 mg in Megadose).

Available Drug Forms Inositol is no longer an official drug, but it is found in some multivitamin (Mega-B, Megadose) and topical preparations (Amino-Cerv).

Nursing Management

1. Daily requirement has not been established.
2. A well-balanced diet provides about 1000 mg daily.

Chapter 19

Minerals

CHARACTERISTICS OF MINERALS

The major minerals in the body include sodium, potassium, calcium, phosphorus, magnesium, sulfur, and chlorine. Sodium is the primary cation in extracellular fluid and potassium is the primary intracellular cation. Calcium, which is often combined with phosphorus, is present in greater quantities than any other mineral in the body; most of the calcium is found deposited in bones and teeth. Nearly 70% of the magnesium in the body is found in bones combined with calcium and phosphorus.

The essential mineral sulfur is found complexed with proteins, fats, and as sulfates of sodium, potassium, and magnesium. The normal serum sulfur level is 0.7 to 1.5 mEq/l. Proteins contain adequate quantities of dietary sulfur, thus preventing a deficiency.

Chlorine occurs in the body as the chloride ion and accounts for almost 3% of the total mineral content. The normal serum level of chloride is 95 to 105 mEq/l, but even greater quantities occur in cerebrospinal fluid (125 mEq/l). When the serum pH becomes acidic, the kidneys reabsorb large quantities of bicarbonate ion and the reabsorption of chloride ions is decreased. The opposite occurs when the blood becomes alkaline. This chloride shift also assists in the maintenance of blood pH: the chloride ion replaces the bicarbonate ion in red blood cells, thus maintaining the polarity of the red blood cells, and the bicarbonate ion adjusts the blood pH.

The trace minerals include iron, copper, cobalt, iodine, manganese, zinc, and molybdenum. Iron, copper, and cobalt are important factors in the hemopoietic process: iron and copper are both required for the formation of hemoglobin and cobalt is an essential constituent of vitamin B_{12}, which is required for red blood cell formation. Monographs of these trace minerals are included with the hemopoietic agents.

Iodine is an important trace element required for the synthesis of thyroid hormones. It is found in nature primarily as iodides. A deficiency of iodine causes simple or nontoxic goiter. The "Goiter Belt" in the United States has little or no iodine in the soil and therefore in the food grown. Iodized salt has helped to prevent iodine deficiencies in these goiter areas of the midwest.

Although relatively large quantities of zinc are required by the body, little manganese and molybdenum are needed. Manganese activates several biological processes, including aspects of protein, carbohydrate, and fat metabolism, as well as urea formation. Molybdenum is a component of several body enzymes, including xanthine oxidase and aldehyde oxidase. Zinc is an essential constituent of carbonic anhydrase, carboxypeptidase, and the tissue enzyme lactic dehydrogenase. Since zinc readily combines with insulin, the pancreas uses zinc to store insulin. Interest in zinc has been increasing over the last two decades because it may be involved in the function of the liver and the nervous system.

The body cannot tolerate large deviations in most serum electrolytes. Although only relatively small shifts in potassium and calcium levels can occur before symptoms appear, comparatively large alterations in serum magnesium levels and moderate changes in sodium levels can be endured. Dramatic changes in any of these electrolytes can cause death. See Table 19-1 on electrolyte disturbances for more details.

MINERAL SUPPLEMENTS

Calcium is used in several gastric antacids since it readily reacts with hydrochloric acid to form salts. Sodium is used to prepare numerous medications that can be tolerated by the body. These compounds must be used judiciously in clients with restricted sodium intake. Sodium, phosphate, calcium, and magnesium are all used in laxative preparations. (See Chapter 77 for further details.) Iodine, in the form of iodide, has been used as an expectorant. When these mineral-containing medications are used, clients must be observed for excessive intake and treated accordingly.

MAJOR MINERALS AND ELECTROLYTES

Sodium

GENERIC NAMES Sodium chloride (OTC) (RX)

TRADE NAMES Salt Tablets, Sodium Chloride Injection, Normal Saline

CLASSIFICATION Electrolyte supplement

Table 19-1 Summary of Electrolyte Disturbances

Electrolyte	Alteration	Laboratory Findings	Clinical Signs and Symptoms	Causes
Sodium	Whole body deficit (isotonic dehydration)	Little change in serum electrolytes; elevated serum proteins; elevated hematocrit	Lowered body temperature and blood pressure; elevated heart rate and respiration; oliguria progressing to anuria	Fluid and sodium lost in equal quantities; surgical procedures
	Hypernatremic dehydration	Normal serum sodium level (occasionally elevated above 150 mEq/l); elevated hematocrit and serum proteins	Elevated temperature; lowered blood pressure; apprehension and weakness progressing to confusion and convulsions; oliguria progressing to anuria; dry mucous membranes and tongue	Loss of water in excess of sodium lost; severe vomiting; excessive sweating; excessive diuresis; excessive intake of sodium
	Hyponatremia	Low serum sodium level (occasionally below 120 mEq/l)	Absence of thirst; polyuria (oliguria in renal insufficiency); nausea, vomiting, diarrhea, abdominal cramps; muscle twitching; irritability, disorientation, confusion, convulsions, coma	Loss of sodium in excess of water lost; excessive fluid intake; excessive tap water enemas; low-sodium diet with excessive water intake; excessive IV intake of dextrose in water solutions
Potassium	Hyperkalemia	Elevated serum potassium level (above 5 mEq/l)	Peaked T waves, flattening and widening P waves, A-V dissociation and ventricular fibrillation; intestinal cramps and diarrhea; weakness progressing to flaccid paralysis; oliguria progressing to anuria; inability to speak	Decreased urinary output or excessive intake of potassium; massive trauma or tissue injury (burns); wasting diseases; impaired renal function

Table 19-1 *Continued*

Electrolyte	Alteration	Laboratory Findings	Clinical Signs and Symptoms	Causes
	Hypokalemia	Lowered serum potassium level (below 3 mEq/l)	Weak pulse and lowered blood pressure; flattening T waves, A-V conduction abnormalities; cardiac arrest; intestinal muscular weakness, distention, paralytic ileus; weakness, lethargy, confusion	Diabetic ketoacidosis; hyperaldosteronism; excessive diuresis; diarrhea; intestinal fistulas; severe vomiting
Calcium	Hypercalcemia	Elevated serum calcium level (above 5.8 mEq/l); lowered serum phosphate level; Sulkowitch urine test indicates calcium precipitation	Nausea, vomiting, diarrhea or constipation; shortened Q-T interval, peaked T waves close to QRS, arrhythmias, ventricular fibrillation; lethargy, confusion, apathy; kidney stones; infection and flank pain around bones	Hyperparathyroidism; renal impairment of calcium excretion; excessive intake of calcium and vitamin D; excessive mobilization of calcium from bones
	Hypocalcemia (tetany)	Lowered serum calcium level (below 4.5 mEq/l); elevated serum phosphate level; hypokalemia masks the symptoms of tetany	Tingling and paresthesia due to vascular spasms, prolongation of Q-T interval, 2:1 heart block; painful tonic muscle spasms, facial spasms (tics) progressing to convulsions; positive Chvostek's sign and Trousseau's sign	Acute pancreatitis; accidental removal of parathyroid during thyroidectomy; inadequate intake during pregnancy and lactation; inadequate intake of vitamin D; multiple blood transfusions with citrated blood

Table 19-1 *Continued*

Electrolyte	Alteration	Laboratory Findings	Clinical Signs and Symptoms	Causes
Magnesium	Hypermagnesemia	Elevated serum magnesium level (above 10 mEq/l)	Depresses A-V and intraventricular conduction; vasodilation causing lowered blood pressure; lowered cardiac output and elevated temperature of skin; absence of knee jerk (above 10 mEq/l); S-A and A-V block (above 15 mEq/l); respiratory depression (above 17 mEq/l); cardiac arrest (above 20 mEq/l)	Renal impairment of magnesium excretion; excessive intake of magnesium sulfate (laxatives, antacids, IV)
	Hypomagnesemia	Lowered serum magnesium level (below 1.5 mEq/l); elevated serum cholesterol; elevated alpha- and beta-lipoproteins	Hyperactive reflexes progressing to tetany; short P-Q interval and flat or inverted T waves; positive Chvostek's sign; twitching and jerking movements progressing to convulsions; hallucinations, delusions, confusion, combative behavior	Prolonged hyperalimentation without magnesium supplements.

Source Foods high in sodium include whole milk, meat, eggs, and certain vegetables. Canned foods, processed cheese, and frozen peas contain large quantities of sodium.

Action Sodium is the most abundant cation of extracellular fluid and is the primary determinant of osmotic water balance. Cellular permeability, and therefore the normal functioning of body cells, is affected by sodium-glucose metabolism, sodium-potassium pump, and the transmission of neuromuscular impulses. There is a direct relationship between serum sodium levels and blood pressure, urinary output, and cardiac contractions (upstroke velocity and the amplitude of myocardial action potential).

Indications for Use Hyponatremia due to inadequate sodium intake (sodium-restricted diets) or excessive loss of sodium (diarrhea); as an adjunct in the treatment of heat stroke with hyponatremia; dehydration when there is a concurrent loss of sodium; GI disturbances associated with hyponatremia.

Contraindications Hypernatremia, acute pulmonary edema, severe sodium restriction.

Warnings and Precautions Use with caution in clients with cardiac disorders and renal impairment; in the elderly and clients with hypertension.

Untoward Reactions Hypernatremia can occur. The signs and symptoms include apprehension, weakness, abdominal cramps, thirst, fever, oliguria with a high specific gravity, and lowered blood pressure. If untreated, agitation, confusion, and convulsions may follow. Electrolyte disturbances including hypokalemia may occur. Large doses or rapid administration may precipitate pulmonary edema or aggravate congestive heart failure.

Parameters of Use

Absorption Readily absorbed from GI tract; about 5% lost in feces. Diarrhea increases the loss of sodium. Normal serum levels of sodium: 136 to 145 mEq/l or 310 to 340 mg/100 ml. Normal serum levels of chloride: 95 to 106 mEq/l.

Excretion Primarily via the kidneys; sweat glands may excrete more water than sodium. Excretion is regulated by aldosterone.

Drug Interactions Many medications contain sodium salts (sodium bicarbonate).

Administration

- *Prevention of heat stroke:* 250 to 500 mg po prn followed by 8 fl oz of water.
- *Heat stroke with hyponatremia:* 1000 ml of 0.9% or 0.45% sodium chloride solution IV as needed. (Often alternated with 5% D/W.)
- *Hyponatremia:* 1000 ml of 0.89% sodium chloride solution is usually adequate.

Available Drug Forms Tablets containing 250 or 500 mg; sterile multidose vials for reconstituting powdered medications; sterile IV solutions containing 0.9% sodium chloride (normal saline) or 0.45% sodium chloride (0.5 normal saline); also available as 5% dextrose solution.

Nursing Management

Planning factors

1. Baseline serum electrolytes must be obtained.
2. The average American diet contains 4 to 6 g of sodium daily.
3. The normal adult body can function well on 2 g of sodium daily.
4. Other supportive measures are essential for clients with heat stroke (see a medical surgical textbook). IV dextrose solution may be required to prevent acidosis (ketosis).

Administration factors

1. A relatively wide range of serum levels are tolerated in normal adults. However, even slightly excessive infusion rates may precipitate pulmonary edema in the elderly and clients with cardiac or renal dysfunction.
2. IV sodium chloride should be administered at a constant rate unless otherwise ordered by the physician.
3. Never inject normal saline solution for irrigation.

Evaluation factors

1. Assess clients for fluid overload and alterations in sodium levels frequently.
2. Monitor vital signs, blood pressure, and urinary output.
3. Serum electrolytes should be obtained frequently. The frequency depends on the severity of the condition.

Client teaching factors

1. Inform clients that heat stroke can best be prevented by avoiding excessive exposure to heat.
2. Salt tablets should not be used by the elderly or clients with cardiac or renal dysfunction unless under the supervision of a physician.

Potassium

GENERIC NAME Potassium chloride (oral) (RX)

TRADE NAMES K-Lor, K-Lyte, K-Lyte/CL, K-Tab, Kaochlor, Kaochlor S-F 10%, Kaon-CL, Kaon-CL-10, Kaon-CL 20%, Kato, Kay Ciel Elixir 20%, Klorvess 10%, Klotrix, Micro-K, Rum-K, SK Potassium 10% and 20%, Slow-K

CLASSIFICATION Electrolyte supplement

Source Foods rich in potassium include bananas, dried figs and peaches, orange juice, nuts, legumes, and meat.

Action Potassium is the primary intracellular cation and it is involved in several physiological processes. Potassium is required for the maintenance of normal intracellular tonicity and the contraction of cardiac, skeletal, and smooth muscles and the transmission of nerve impulses. It is also required for other processes, including the storage of glycogen and nitrogen. Even relatively slight deviations in normal serum potassium levels (3.8 to 4.5 mEq/l) can cause serious consequences, particularly in the elderly, neonates, infants, and debilitated clients. The symptoms of hypokalemia include a decrease in smooth muscle excitability (anorexia, vomiting, abdominal distention, paralytic ileus) and skeletal muscle excitability (flaccid muscles, weakness), cardiac arrhythmias (bradycardia, first degree heart block), EKG changes (prolonged Q-T interval, S-T depression, depression or inversion of T waves, development of U waves), and hypotension with a weak pulse. Several drugs, including the thiazide diuretics and the corticosteroids, can cause hypokalemia.

Indications for Use Prevention and treatment of potassium deficiency; states of inadequate potassium intake, including malnutrition and excessive dieting; states of excessive potassium loss, including the use of thiazide diuretics and corticosteroid therapy; states of massive trauma or excessive stress, including burns, crushing injuries, and extensive surgery.

Contraindications Hyperkalemia; severe renal impairment (oliguria, anuria, azotemia); when potassium-sparing diuretics (spironolactone, triamterene) are being given; severe hemolytic anemia.

Warnings and Precautions Use with caution in clients with chronic renal failure. Acute alkalosis can cause low serum potassium levels in the absence of a total body deficit of potassium.

Untoward Reactions Hyperkalemia may occur in clients who have renal impairment (geriatrics, neonates, clients with kidney disorders). The signs and symptoms include EKG changes (peaked T waves, loss of P waves, S-T depression, prolonged Q-T interval), oliguria that progresses to anuria, and GI disturbances (colic, diarrhea). Severe hyperkalemia (serum level of 9 to 10 mEq/l) causes muscle paralysis, speech difficulties, and conduction arrhythmias that lead to cardiac arrest. Hemodialysis may be required. GI disturbances are common following the administration of oral supplements. The mucosa may be irritated to the point of bleeding. The early signs and symptoms include nausea, vomiting, diarrhea, abdominal distention, and discomfort. GI hemorrhage can result, particularly in geriatric clients and clients with a preexisting alteration of the intestinal mucosa (history of peptic ulcer, ulcerative colitis).

Parameters of Use

Absorption Rapidly absorbed from GI tract; high potassium concentration in any one area will cause GI irritation. Continuously recycled in GI tract as a component of digestive juices. Little is excreted in the feces normally. Vomiting and diarrhea may cause severe hyperkalemia. Normal serum levels: 3.5 to 5.0 mEq/l or 14 to 20 mg/100 ml. EKG changes usually appear when serum potassium reaches 7 to 8 mEq/l. Crosses placenta and is found in breast milk. Lactating mothers should bottle-feed their babies.

Excretion Primarily via the kidneys. Aldosterone conserves sodium ions and causes the loss of potassium ions.

Drug Interactions Concomitant therapy with potassium and potassium-sparing diuretics or potassium salt substitutes may result in hyperkalemia. Adequate dosages of potassium salts will prevent digitalis toxicity that can occur when digitalis and thiazide diuretics are administered concurrently.

Administration Dosage is highly individualized according to the client's actual and expected potassium loss.

- *Mild potassium loss daily:* Adults: 20 to 30 mEq po daily given in divided doses; Children: 10 to 15 mEq po daily given in divided doses.
- *Moderate potassium loss daily (concurrent use of digitalis and thiazide diuretics):* Adults: 25 to 100 mEq po daily given in divided doses; Maximum daily dose: 200 mEq.

Available Drug Forms See tables for available drug forms.

TABLETS

Trade Name	Potassium Content	Remarks
K-Tab	10 mEq	Slow release, film-coated tablet
Kaon-CL	6.7 mEq	Controlled release, sugar-coated tablet (wax matrix); contains FD&C yellow No. 5
Kaon-CL-10	10 mEq	Controlled release, sugar-coated tablet (wax matrix)
Klotrix	10 mEq	Slow release, film-coated tablet (wax matrix)
Micro-K	8 mEq	Controlled release over 8 to 10 hours

PACKETS OF DRUG POWDER

Trade Name	Potassium Content	Remarks
Kato	20 mEq	Tomato-flavored
Kay Ciel	20 mEq	Packets of powder
KCL	20 mEq 20 mEq	Unflavored
Klor-Con	20 mEq	Fruit-flavored, contains saccharin
Klor-Con-25	25 mEq	
K-Lor	15 mEq 20 mEq	Fruit-flavored
K-Lyte/CL	25 mEq	Effervescent tablets and powders

Nursing Management

Planning factors

1. Serum electrolytes must be obtained before initiating therapy.
2. Renal function tests (serum creatinine, creatinine clearance test) should be done prior to initiating drug therapy, particularly in the elderly and clients with known or suspected renal impairment. Determine client's intake and output.
3. Assess client's daily intake of potassium from dietary sources, including salt substitutes such as Co-Salt. Consult a nutritionist and physician as needed. The use of Diasal should be included.
4. A well-balanced diet contains 2 to 4 g of potassium daily.
5. Store in a dry area. Check powder packets for perforation before using.

LIQUIDS

Trade Name	Potassium Content	Remarks
Kaon-Cl 20%	40 mEq/15 ml	Contains saccharin, flavoring, and 5% alcohol
Kaochlor	20 mEq/15 ml	Contains sugar, saccharin, flavoring, 5% alcohol, FD&C yellow No. 5
Kaochlor S-F 10%	20 mEq/15 ml	Contains sugar
Kay Ciel Elixir 20%	20 mEq/15 ml	Contains 4% alcohol, no sugar
KCL		
5%	20 mEq/30 ml	
10%	15 mEq/11.25 ml	
10%	20 mEq/15 ml	
10%	30 mEq/22.5 ml	
10%	40 mEq/30 ml	
KCL Elixir		Sugar-free
10%	20 mEq/15 ml	
20%	40 mEq/15 ml	
Klor 10%	20 mEq/15 ml	
Klor-Con 20%	40 mEq/15 ml	
Klorvess 10%	20 mEq/15 ml	Cherry-flavored, contains 1% alcohol
Rum-K	20 mEq/10 ml	Contains butter rum synthetic flavor, 4 to 6 fl oz alcohol, sugar-free
SK Potassium 10%	40 mEq/30 ml	
20%	80 mEq/30 ml	

Administration factors

1. Follow manufacturer's directions for dilution of liquids and powders to prevent GI irritation. When diluting:
   a. Dissolve powders completely in diluent (cold water, juice) before administering.
   b. Liquids must be further diluted in water or juice (3 to 4 fl oz for 10 mEq, 6 to 8 fl oz for 15 to 20 mEq).
   c. Extra fluids are recommended.
2. Give with meals or immediately following a meal. (K-Lyte should be sipped over a 5 to 10-minute period.)
3. Follow tablets with a full glass of water.

Evaluation factors

1. Monitor intake and output. If oliguria occurs, notify physician.
2. Observe for signs and symptoms of hyperkalemia.
3. Serum electrolytes should be obtained daily until dosage is stabilized, then periodically (weekly, monthly).

Client teaching factors

1. Instruct client to follow manufacturer's directions for diluting powders and liquids.
2. Warn client to avoid taking medication on an empty stomach.
3. Instruct client to drink at least one glass of fluid following drug administration.
4. Instruct client to store drug in a dry area, not in kitchen or bathroom, and to inspect powder packets before using. If packet is perforated, it should not be used.
5. Instruct client to seek medical advice if nausea, vomiting, diarrhea, or oliguria occur.
6. The client and family should be made aware of the initial signs and symptoms of hyperkalemia. The drug should be discontinued and the physician notified if symptoms occur.

GENERIC NAME Potassium chloride (injection)

CLASSIFICATION Electrolyte supplement (RX)

See potassium chloride (oral) for Source.

Action Potassium is the primary intracellular cation. It is required for the maintenance of normal intracellular tonicity and the contraction of cardiac, skeletal, and smooth muscles and the transmission of nerve impulses. Parenteral potassium chloride is preferred when treating severe hypokalemia, postoperative clients, and clients who are unable to tolerate oral potassium salts. See potassium chloride (oral) for further details.

Indications for Use Prevention and treatment of potassium deficiency; states of inadequate potassium intake, including hyperalimentation, comatose clients, and severe malnutrition; states of excessive potassium loss, including vomiting, diarrhea, intestinal surgery (ileostomy, bowel resections), continuous intestinal drainage, and prolonged diuresis; recovery period after massive trauma or excessive stress, including burns, crushing injuries, and extensive surgery.

Contraindications Hyperkalemia, severe renal impairment or dehydration, when potassium-sparing diuretics are being given, hemolytic anemias, uncontrolled adrenal disorders (Addison's disease), heat stroke.

Warnings and Precautions Use with caution in the initial treatment of diabetes acidosis, crushing injuries, severe trauma, and burns since hyperkalemia may occur. Use with caution in clients with renal impairment. Acute alkalosis can cause low serum potassium levels in the absence of a total body deficit of potassium.

Untoward Reactions Hyperkalemia; phlebitis and irritation to the vein used for drug therapy (client may complain of a burning or stinging sensation if the infusion is administered too fast).

Parameters of Use

Absorption Rapidly absorbed from GI tract. Continuously recycled in GI tract as a component of digestive juices. Nasogastric suctioning, vomiting, and diarrhea can deplete body potassium rapidly. Normal serum levels: 3.5 to 5.0 mEq/l. Hyperkalemia: moderate: 7 to 8 mEq/l; severe: 9 to 10 mEq/l.

Crosses placenta and is found in breast milk. May cause hyperkalemia in fetus. Lactating mothers should bottle-feed their babies.

Excretion Primarily via the kidneys. Aldosterone conserves sodium ions and causes the loss of potassium ions.

Drug Interactions Concomitant therapy with potassium and potassium-sparing diuretics can cause hyperkalemia. Adequate dosages of potassium salts will prevent digitalis toxicity that can occur when digitalis and thiazide diuretics are administered concurrently. Intravenous potassium may augment the effects of the antidiabetic agent acetohexamide by facilitating the metabolism of glucose and increasing the secretion of insulin.

Administration Dosage is highly individualized according to the client's actual and expected potassium loss. Range: 20 to 30 mEq added to IV infusions daily. Must be well diluted in IV solutions and administered over several hours. Do not exceed 200 mEq in 24 hours. Should not be given via IV bolus.

Available Drug Forms Vials containing 20 mEq in 10 ml and 40 mEq in 20 ml (2 mEq in each ml); multidose vials containing 60 mEq in 30 ml (2 mEq in each ml).

Nursing Management

Planning factors

1. Serum electrolytes must be obtained before initiating therapy.
2. Renal function tests (serum creatinine, creatinine clearance) should be done prior to initiating drug therapy, particularly in the elderly and clients with known or suspected renal impairment.
3. Determine client's intake and output. If oliguria or anuria is present, notify physician.

Administration factors

1. Be careful to avoid getting drug on hands when withdrawing the required dosage. The solution is hypertonic and can cause irritation of the skin and a burning sensation in open cuts.
2. Rotate the container of IV solution after injecting potassium. Usually added to 1000 ml of the client's daily IV fluids.
3. Check the patency of the IV before starting drug. If in doubt, restart the IV, since potassium chloride can be very irritating to the vein. Rotate IV sites frequently.

Evaluation factors

1. Check for signs of hyperkalemia frequently, particularly when large dosages (40 mEq or more) are being administered.
2. Serum electrolytes should be obtained frequently (daily).
3. Monitor intake and output. If oliguria occurs, notify physician.
4. When possible, the client should have cardiac monitoring to detect the early signs of hypokalemia (prolonged Q-T interval, S-T depression, depression or inversion of T waves, development of U waves) and hyperkalemia (peaked T waves, loss of P waves, S-T depression, prolonged Q-T interval).
5. Treatment of hyperkalemia may require one liter of 10% D/W with 30 to 40 units of regular insulin to promote the transfer of potassium from the serum to the intracellular fluid. If the client is also acidotic, 150 to 300 mEq of sodium bicarbonate IV may be required. Hemodialysis is an effective measure for removing potassium from the body.

GENERIC NAME Potassium acetate (RX)

CLASSIFICATION Potassium supplement

See potassium chloride (oral) for Indications for use, Contraindications, Warnings and precautions. Untoward reactions, Parameters of use, Drug interactions, Administration, and Nursing management.

Source Salt of potassium that is produced synthetically.

Action Potassium acetate is very soluble in water and is used as a potassium supplement. Potassium is the primary intracellular cation. It is required for the maintenance of normal intracellular tonicity and the contraction of cardiac, skeletal, and smooth muscles and the transmission of nerve impulses. The acetate salt of potassium tends to be less irritating to the GI tract than potassium chloride.

Available Drug Forms An ingredient of Trikates.

GENERIC NAME Potassium acid phosphate (RX)

TRADE NAME K-Phos

CLASSIFICATION Urinary Acidifier

See potassium chloride (oral) for Indications of use, Contraindications, Warnings and precautions, Untoward reactions, Parameters of use, Drug interactions, and Nursing management.

Action Assists in keeping calcium from precipitating in the urinary tract. See potassium chloride (oral) for further details.

Administration Two tablets po qid with a full glass of water.

Available Drug Forms Tablets containing 250 mg phosphorus, 298 mg sodium, and 45 mg potassium.

GENERIC NAME Potassium bicarbonate (RX)

CLASSIFICATION Potassium supplement

See potassium chloride (oral) for Contraindications, Warnings and precautions, Untoward reactions, Parameters of use, Drug interactions, and Administration.

Source Synthetically produced.

Action Used in effervescent potassium supplements. Freely soluble in water but almost insoluble in alcohol. The bicarbonate salt may be less irritating to the GI tract than other oral potassium salts. (See potassium chloride (oral) for further details.)

Available Drug Forms An ingredient of K-Lyte, KEFF, Klorvess, and Trikates.

Nursing Management Dissolve tablet in 4 fl oz or more of water before administering. (See potassium chloride (oral) for further details.)

GENERIC NAME Potassium carbonate (RX)

CLASSIFICATION Potassium supplement

See potassium chloride (oral) for Contraindications, Warnings and precautions, Untoward reactions, Parameters of use, Drug interactions, and Administration.

Source Synthetically produced.

Action Used in effervescent potassium supplements. May be less irritating to GI tract than other oral potassium salts. (See potassium chloride (oral) for further details.)

Available Drug Forms An ingredient of KEFF.

Nursing Management Dissolve tablet in 4 fl oz or more of water before administering. (See potassium chloride (oral) for further details.)

GENERIC NAME Potassium citrate (RX)

CLASSIFICATION Potassium supplement

See potassium chloride (oral) for Indications for use, Contraindications, Warnings and precautions, Untoward reactions, Drug interactions, Administration, and Nursing management.

Action Used in oral potassium supplements (also systemic alkalizers). Freely soluble in water but almost insoluble in alcohol. (See potassium chloride (oral) for further details.)

Parameters of Use

Absorption Absorbed and metabolized to potassium bicarbonate.

Excretion Less than 5% excreted unchanged. See potassium chloride (oral) for further details.

Available Drug Forms An ingredient of Bi-K, K-Lyte, Polycitra, Trikates, and Twin-K.

GENERIC NAME Potassium gluconate (RX)

TRADE NAME Kaon

CLASSIFICATION Potassium supplement

See potassium chloride (oral) for Indications for use, Contraindications, Warnings and precautions, Parameters of use, and Drug interactions.

Action Ammonium chloride can be used concurrently to supply chloride ion; but ammonium chloride is not used if liver impairment is present. (See potassium chloride (oral) for further details.)

Untoward Reactions Hypersensitivity reactions to FD&C yellow No. 5 coloring. Hypochloremic alkalosis may occur in clients with a salt-free diet. Ammonium chloride can be used as a source of the chloride ion. (See potassium chloride (oral) for further details.)

Administration 40 mEq po daily; 2 tablets po qid after meals and at bedtime; 15 ml of elixir po in 1 fl oz or more of water bid.

Available Drug Forms Tablets containing 5 mEq of elemental potassium; sugar-free elixir containing 20 mEq/15 ml, saccharin, aromatics, and 5% alcohol; available in grape or lemon-lime flavor (lemon-lime flavor contains FD&C yellow No. 5 coloring). An ingredient of Bi-K and Kolyum.

Nursing Management The elixir must be further diluted before administering. Add elixir to 4 fl oz or more of water or orange juice. (See potassium chloride (oral) for further details.)

Combination Potassium Supplement Preparations

See potassium chloride (oral) for Action, Indications for use, Contraindications, Warnings and precautions, Untoward reactions, Parameters of use, Drug interactions, and Nursing management.

TRADE NAME Bi-K (RX)

CLASSIFICATION Oral potassium supplement

Administration Dissolve 15 ml of liquid in 6 to 8 fl oz of water or fruit juice bid, tid, or qid with meals or a snack.

Available Drug Forms Generic contents in 15 ml of liquid. Total potassium content: 20 mEq as potassium citrate and potassium gluconate. Sorbitol and saccharin as additives.

TRADE NAME Kaochlor-Eff (RX)

CLASSIFICATION Oral potassium supplement

Administration Dissolve 1 tablet in 3 fl oz or more of water or other liquid bid.

Available Drug Forms Generic contents in each tablet: potassium chloride: 0.6 g; potassium bicarbonate: 1 g; potassium citrate: 0.22 g. Total potassium content: 20 mEq. Betaine hydrochloride, saccharin, artificial citrus fruit flavor, and FD&C yellow No. 5 as additives.

TRADE NAME KEFF (RX)

CLASSIFICATION Oral potassium supplement

Administration Dissolve 1 tablet in 4 fl oz or more bid, tid, or qid after meals.

Available Drug Forms Generic contents in each tablet: potassium chloride: 1.118 g; potassium bicarbonate: 0.401 g; potassium carbonate: 0.069 g. Total potassium content: 20 mEq. Betaine hydrochloride, saccharin, artificial flavorings, and colors as additives.

TRADE NAME Klorvess (RX)

CLASSIFICATION Oral potassium supplement

Administration Dissolve one tablet or packet in 3 to 4 fl oz of cold water or fruit juice.

Available Drug Forms Generic contents in each granule or tablet: potassium chloride: 1.125 g; potassium bicarbonate: 0.5 g. Total potassium content: 20 mEq. 0.913 g L-lysine monohydrochloride as an additive.

TRADE NAME K-Lyte D.S. (RX)

CLASSIFICATION Oral potassium supplement

Administration Dissolve one tablet in 6 to 8 fl oz of cold or ice water daily or bid. Taken with meals and sipped over a 5 to 10-minute period.

Available Drug Forms Generic contents in each effervescent tablet: potassium bicarbonate: 2.5 g; potassium citrate: 2.7 g. Total potassium content: 50 mEq. 2.1 g citric acid, saccharin, natural and artificial flavorings, and color as additives.

TRADE NAME K-Lyte/CL (RX)

CLASSIFICATION Oral potassium supplement

Administration Dissolve 1 tablet in 6 to 8 fl oz of cold or ice water daily or bid. Taken with meals and sipped over a 5 to 10-minute period.

Available Drug Forms Generic contents in each effervescent tablet and measured scoop of powder: potassium chloride: 1.5 g; potassium bicarbonate: 0.5 g. Total potassium content: 25 mEq. 0.91 g L-lysine monohydrochloride, 0.55 g citric acid, saccharin, natural and artificial flavorings, and color as additives.

TRADE NAME K-Lyte/CL 50 (RX)

CLASSIFICATION Oral potassium supplement

Administration Dissolve 1 tablet in 6 to 8 fl oz of cold or ice water daily or bid. Taken with meals and sipped over a 5 to 10-minute period.

Available Drug Forms Generic contents in each effervescent tablet: potassium chloride: 2.24 g; potassium bicarbonate: 2 g. Total potassium content: 50

mEq. 3.65 g L-lysine monohydrochloride, 1 g citric acid, saccharin, natural and artificial flavorings, and color as additives.

TRADE NAME Kolyum (RX)

CLASSIFICATION Oral potassium supplement

Administration Dissolve 15 ml of liquid in at least 30 ml of water bid for adults. Dissolve 5-g packet of powder in 3 to 4 fl oz of cool water for adults. Both can be used for children.

Available Drug Forms Generic contents in 15 ml of liquid or 5-g packet of powder: potassium chloride: 0.25 g; potassium gluconate: 3.9 g. Total potassium content: 20 mEq. Sorbitol as an additive.

TRADE NAME Trikates (RX)

CLASSIFICATION Oral potassium supplement

Administration Dissolve 5 ml of liquid in 3 to 4 fl oz of tomato or orange juice tid or qid after meals.

Available Drug Forms Generic contents in 5 ml of liquid: potassium bicarbonate: 0.5 g; potassium citrate: 0.5 g; potassium acetate: 0.5 g. Total potassium content: 15 mEq. Glycerin, saccharin, water, and aromatics as additives.

TRADE NAME Twin-K (RX)

CLASSIFICATION Oral potassium supplement

Administration Dissolve 15 ml of liquid in 16 fl oz of water or fruit juice bid, tid, or qid with meals or a snack.

Available Drug Forms Generic contents in 15 ml of liquid: Total potassium content: 20 mEq as potassium citrate and potassium gluconate. Sorbitol and saccharin as additives.

Other Electrolyte Replacement Preparations

TRADE NAME Bicitra (RX)

CLASSIFICATION Systemic alkalizer

Action Sodium citrate is metabolized to sodium bicarbonate. This supplement is used to replace sodium bicarbonate in the body. Only 5% sodium citrate is excreted unchanged by the kidneys. Sodium salts may have a laxative effect.

Indications for Use Used for chronic metabolic acidosis (renal disorders) and alkalization of urine.

Contraindications Severe kidney failure, clients on sodium restriction.

Administration Adults: 10 to 30 ml diluted in 1 to 3 fl oz of water po after meals and at bedtime; Children: 5 to 15 ml diluted in 1 to 3 fl oz of water po after meals and at bedtime.

Available Drug Forms Generic contents: sodium citrate, citric acid. Sugar-free.

Nursing Management

1. More palatable if liquid is chilled before administering.
2. Follow each drug administration with a full glass of water.

TRADE NAME Hydra-Lyte (RX)

CLASSIFICATION Oral electrolyte replacement preparation

Indications for Use Replaces electrolytes and water lost during mild or moderate diarrhea; useful in children as well as adults.

Administration Ingested po freely to quench thirst. Offer to children every 1 to 2 hours.

Available Drug Forms Foil-lined packets. Generic contents in each packet: water, dextrose, sucrose, sodium chloride, sodium citrate, sodium bicarbonate, artificial flavorings, coloring. Each packet contains: sodium: 84 mEq; chloride: 50 mEq; bicarbonate: 10 mEq; potassium: 10 mEq; glucose: 27 mM; sucrose: 1 mM.

Nursing Management

1. Discontinue all other food intake.
2. Unflavored gelatin can be added to make a gelatin dessert.

TRADE NAME Pedialyte (RX)

CLASSIFICATION Oral electrolyte replacement preparation

Action Glucose content prevents ketosis; particularly useful for the replacement of electrolytes in infants and young children.

Indications for Use Replaces electrolytes and water lost during mild and moderate diarrhea.

Administration Children over 5 years: 2 liters or more daily; Infants and very young children: Determined by body weight (a 17-lb toddler requires 1 liter daily).

Available Drug Forms Ready-to-use bottles containing 8 fl oz. Generic contents in each liter: water, dextrose, potassium citrate, sodium chloride, sodium citrate, citric acid, magnesium chloride, calcium chloride. Each liter contains: sodium: 30 mEq; potassium: 20 mEq; calcium: 4 mEq; magnesium: 4 mEq; chloride: 30 mEq; citrate: 28 mEq; dextrose: 50 g; calories: 200.

Nursing Management

1. Discontinue all other food intake.
2. May be used at home for moderate diarrhea in small children.
3. After opening, store in refrigerator.

TRADE NAME Polycitra (RX)

CLASSIFICATION Systemic alkalizer

Action Citrates are metabolized to potassium and sodium bicarbonate. Also used for alkalinization of urine.

Indications for Use Excessive loss of sodium and bicarbonate ions; chronic metabolic acidosis (urinary uric acid and cystine calculi); adjunct in the treatment of gout with uricosuric agents.

Contraindications Severe renal failure, untreated Addison's disease, severe myocardial damage.

Administration Adults: 15 to 30 ml diluted in water given after meals; Children: 5 to 15 ml diluted in water given after meals.

Available Drug Forms Syrup containing glucose; Polycitra LC, which is a sugar-free liquid. Generic contents in 5 ml of liquid: potassium citrate: 500 mg; sodium citrate: 500 mg; citric acid: 334 mg. Each 5 ml contains: potassium: 5 mEq; sodium: 5 mEq. Total bicarbonate: 10 mEq.

Nursing Management

1. The liquid is more palatable if chilled before administering.
2. Follow each drug administration with a full glass of water.

Cation-Exchange Resin

GENERIC NAME Sodium polystyrene sulfonate

TRADE NAME Kayexalate (RX)

CLASSIFICATION Cation-exchange resin

Action This drug is a sulfonic-type resin prepared in sodium form. It is able (in vitro) to exchange approximately 3.1 mEq of potassium per gram of drug; however, it actually removes (in vivo) about 1 mEq of potassium per gram. The sodium ions are released from the drug in the GI tract and exchanged for potassium ions in the client's serum, particularly in the large intestines. The efficiency of the exchange process is limited, unpredictable, and depends on the concentration of the ions and the duration of contact. The drug will also exchange small quantities of other cations, particularly calcium and magnesium.

Indications for Use Hyperkalemia (chronic renal failure). Frequently used to control serum potassium levels until the client can be prepared for hemodialysis (transferred to a dialysis unit and an A-V shunt inserted). Rapidly developing hyperkalemia is associated with states of rapid tissue breakdown (burns, severe trauma, motor vehicle accident victims).

Contraindications Hypokalemia, congestive heart failure (sodium overload).

Warnings and Precautions Hypocalcemia should be corrected before instituting therapy. Should be administered rectally if nausea and vomiting are present. Elevated potassium levels can occur in the absence of a total potassium excess. Fecal impaction should be treated before instituting therapy. Use with caution in digitalized clients; in clients who have an intolerance to sodium (severe hypertension, marked edema).

Untoward Reactions GI disturbances, including nausea, vomiting, and constipation, are common, particularly when high dosages are administered orally. Fecal impaction can occur, particularly in the elderly. When these reactions occur, rectal drug administration should be used. Hypokalemia can occur. Early signs include agitation, confusion, and delayed thought processes; EKG changes and cardiac arrhythmias (premature atrial, nodal, or ventricular contractions, tachycardia). Marked muscular weakness will progress to flank paralysis and cardiac arrest in severe hypokalemia. Digitalis toxicity may occur in digitalized clients as serum potassium levels decrease. Hypocalcemia can occur, particularly after prolonged drug therapy. Symptoms include tingling of the fingers and facial muscle spasms that progress to tetany. Positive Chvostek's and Trousseau's signs will be present. Convulsions will occur in marked hypocalcemia.

Parameters of Use Water-soluble golden brown powder that is odorless and tasteless. Solution may be flavored with syrup (1 to 2 ml) to make it more palatable orally.

Absorption Nonabsorbable, but the sodium in the drug is exchanged for potassium. Hypernatremia can occur in susceptible clients.

Exchange Primarily in large intestines; small amount in stomach and small intestines; moderate amount in rectum. If tolerated, oral administration is more effective. Instill enema into sigmoid colon when possible. Forms a suspension with sorbitol; sorbitol draws water into GI tract and prevents constipation. Aqueous vehicle (sorbitol or water) can be warmed before adding Kayexalate.

Do not warm Kayexalate; heating changes its exchange properties.

Drug Interactions Systemic alkalosis can occur when cation-exchange resins are administered orally with cation-donating antacids and laxatives (magnesium hydroxide, aluminum carbonate) and the resin's potassium exchange capability is impaired; do not use concurrently. Digitalis toxicity can occur as the serum potassium exchange capability is impaired; do not use concurrently.

Administration Dosage depends on the serum potassium level and estimated total potassium excess. Adults: 15 to 60 g po daily, bid, tid, or qid or 25 to 60 g by retention enema q6h retained for 2 to 6 hours; Infants and young children: Dosage based on the exchange rate of 1 mEq of potassium per gram of resin.

Available Drug Forms Jars containing 1 lb of powder (453.6 g). One gram of Kayexalate contains 4.1 mEq of sodium.

Nursing Management

Planning factors

1. Serum electrolytes and calcium and magnesium levels should be taken before initiating therapy. Hypocalcemia should be corrected before starting resin.
2. An EKG is recommended and the client should be on continuous cardiac monitoring (telemetry) during drug therapy.
3. An intake and output record should be kept.
4. Oral resin suspension can be prepared and stored at room temperature for a 24-hour period. Label the suspension with date and time of preparation and discard after 24 hours.
5. If the client is receiving food, the suspension (or powder) can be mixed with the food and taken at mealtime. Sorbitol can be given separately.
6. Obtain the following equipment when a retention enema is prescribed:

   A. *Adults and older children*

   i. 30 cc 3-way Foley catheter, size 28 or 30.
   ii. Enema bag or large funnel with 2 ft of tubing and an adaptor.
   iii. 200-ml container for stirring or agitating suspension.
   iv. Water-filled syringe to inflate catheter balloon.
   v. An enema drainage system (adaptor, tubing, bucket) capable of holding 3000 ml.

   B. *Infants and small children*

   i. 5 to 10 cc 3-way Foley catheter, size 16, 18, or 20.
   ii. Enema bag, funnel, or "open" bulb syringe with 2 ft of tubing and an adaptor.
   iii. 100-ml container for stirring or agitating suspension.
   iv. Water-filled syringe to inflate catheter balloon.
   v. A well-vented urinary drainage system is usually adequate.
7. A tap-water enema should be given as a retention enema before instituting drug therapy.

Administration factors

1. Use level teaspoons when measuring dosage. Four level teaspoons equals 15 g (about 3.5 g in each level teaspoon). A sterile tongue blade can be used to remove powdered drug from the jar.
2. When administering drug orally:
   a. Oral suspension is made with the prescribed quantity of water, sorbitol, or both.
   b. There should be at least 3 to 4 ml of fluid per gram of drug (at least 25 to 30 ml of fluid for 15 g of drug).
   c. A little cherry or other flavoring can be added to make the solution more palatable.
   d. Typical example of oral suspension:

Drug powder	15 g
Sorbitol	30 ml
Water	19 ml
Flavoring	1 ml
Total	15 g in 50 ml

   e. The solution can be stirred or agitated gently in a small jar (baby food jar). Allow the suspension to stand and gently stir or agitate every 5 or 10 minutes until a caramellike suspension forms (about 30 minutes).
   f. If too little fluid is used, a thick paste will form. The paste should not be administered since it has a greatly reduced exchange surface and may cause a fecal impaction. Notify physician.
3. When administering drug through a nasogastric tube:
   a. Prepare oral suspension.
   b. Check location of nasogastric tube before instilling drug. Accidental administration into the lungs will cause pneumonia.
   c. Instill medicated solution.
   d. Flush tube with 20 to 30 ml of water.
   e. Clamp tube for at least 2 hours.
4. When administering drug as a retention enema:
   a. Enema suspension is made with the prescribed quantity of water, sorbitol, or both.
   b. There should be at least 3 to 4 ml of fluid per gram of drug (at least 120 to 160 ml of fluid for 40 g of drug).
   c. Typical example of retention enema suspension:

Drug powder	40 g
Sorbitol	100 ml
Water	50 ml
Total	40 g in 150 ml

   d. The fluid should be at room temperature or warmer. The fluid can be heated before adding the drug. Be sure the suspension is cooled to body temperature before administering the enema.
   e. Insert lubricated tip of 3-way Foley catheter into sigmoid colon (about 20 cm or 8 in. for an adult) and inflate balloon until resistance is felt. Tape catheter in place.
   f. Clamp outlet opening (with a rubber band).
   g. Instill medicated suspension via gravity while continuously stirring the fluid to keep the drug particles in suspension.

h. Flush the tubing with 50 ml of water and clamp the tube (with a rubber band).
i. If fluid begins to leak out of the rectum, the hips can be elevated on a small pillow or the client can assume a side-lying, knee-chest position if possible. A slightly thicker solution can be used at the next administration.
j. The enema is retained for several hours and then the outlet opening is attached to a drainage system and the enema fluid drained.
k. A tap-water cleansing irrigation enema is given at body temperature to remove the resin. About 2000 ml is administered through the 3-way intake and continually drained out the outlet tubing.

5. When administering an enema as a retention enema to infants and small children:
   a. Follow the same procedure for adults.
   b. 25 to 50 ml is usually adequate to flush the suspension.
   c. A 500-ml cleansing enema is usually adequate.
   d. Consult the pediatrician about the quantities of fluid to use.

Evaluation factors

1. Serum electrolytes and calcium and magnesium levels should be determined at least once every 24 hours.
2. Observe client frequently (every 2 to 4 hours) for signs of hypokalemia.
3. Continuous cardiac monitoring with readings every 2 hours should be done.
4. If signs of hypokalemia or hypocalcemia occur, obtain serum electrolyte levels and notify physician.
5. If nausea and vomiting occur, notify physician and obtain an order for an alternative route of drug administration.
6. Monitor intake and output.
7. When retention enemas are used, maintain a flow sheet.

Calcium

GENERIC NAME Calcium gluconate (RX)

CLASSIFICATION Electrolyte supplement

Source Foods rich in calcium include milk, cheese, and other dairy products. Foods with less calcium content include leafy vegetables, legumes, and nuts. Drug is prepared from food concentrates or synthetically.

Action Calcium gluconate is used to replace calcium ions when there is a deficit. Although calcium gluconate contains one-third the amount of calcium contained in calcium chloride, the gluconate is less irritating and therefore better tolerated than calcium chloride. Nearly all of the calcium in the body is found as skeletal phosphate and carbonate in bone and teeth. Serum calcium must be maintained within a narrow range (9 to 10.5 mg/100 ml) since it plays a dramatic role in numerous physiologic processes including:

1. Several steps of the normal blood clotting process including the formation of prothrombin and stable fibrin.
2. Initiation of muscle contraction in skeletal, cardiac, and smooth muscles.
3. Increases myocardial contractility and ventricular excitability; but prolongs systole.
4. Normal transmission of nerve impulses (the release of acetylcholine).
5. Activation of certain enzymes, including adenosinetriphosphatase (ATPase).
6. Affects the permeability of cell walls and thereby assists in the control of intracellular fluid.

As calcium forms numerous insoluble complexes with food acids (oxalic acid, phytic acid), nearly 70% of dietary calcium is not absorbed. Vitamin D is required for calcium absorption from the GI tract. Protein and carbohydrate, particularly lactose, intake enhance calcium absorption, but excessive fat and fatty acids decrease it due to the formation of insoluble calcium soaps. An appropriate relationship between calcium and phosphorus intake is also required.

Indications for Use Prevention and treatment of hypocalcemia during states of increased need: pregnancy, lactation, infancy, growth spurts in children. Tetany due to hypocalcemia. Treatment of hypocalcemic states associated with malnutrition, rickets, vitamin D deficiency, malabsorption disorders, hypoparathyroidism, parathyroid surgery, neonatal tetany, and advanced renal failure. Prevention and treatment of hypocalcemia caused by multiple blood transfusions containing citrate (exchange transfusions, multiple transfusions for the treatment of GI bleeding, aortic aneurysm). As an adjunct in the treatment of cardiac arrest and profound cardiovascular collapse. (It enhances electrical defibrillation and can increase contractility when peripheral pulses are absent but QRS complexes are present.) May be used as an adjunct in the treatment of magnesium sulfate overdose and lead colic. (Acts as an antidote.) May be used to decrease the pain and muscle spasms caused by the venom of the black widow spider.

Contraindications Hypercalcemia, milk-alkali syndrome.

Warnings and Precautions Use with caution in digitalized clients; in clients with renal impairment and clients known to have a history of kidney stones; in clients with Addison's disease and other states of adrenocortical deficiency; in clients with hyperthyroidism or hyperparathyroidism as they may develop hypercalcemia rapidly due to an increased rate of calcium resorption from bones.

Untoward Reactions Acute hypercalcemia can occur, producing a variety of symptoms, including muscle and joint pain; decreased excitability of muscles and nerves that progresses to tetany; EKG changes (shortening of the Q-T interval, bradycardia, and other arrhythmias); flank pain, polyuria, azotemia, and calcium precipitating in the urine; lethargy, confusion, irritability, nausea, vomiting, and paralytic ileus. Serum calcium levels must be obtained to confirm hypercalcemia. GI disturbances can occur after ingestion of calcium and may cause nausea, vomiting, abdominal pain, irritation of a previous peptic ulcer, and constipation.

Vein irritation and phlebitis can occur when solutions of calcium salts are administered IV. Too rapid an IV injection can cause local burning sensations, tingling sensations, hypotension, a feeling of extreme warmth, a chalky taste in the mouth, and cardiac arrest. Local irritation at IM sites can occur.

Parameters of Use

Absorption Mostly from the upper GI tract, particularly the duodenum. About one-third is absorbed when serum levels are normal. An acidic pH and hypocalcemia increase the absorption of calcium. Vitamin D enhances the active transport of calcium from the GI tract; an adequate intake of vitamin D is required. Parathyroid hormone is released when serum calcium levels drop and increases calcium absorption, mobilization from bone, and renal excretion of phosphate. Normal serum levels: 9 to 10 mg/100 ml or 5 mEq/l.

Distribution Widely; some remains as ionized calcium. It is the ionized calcium that is used in physiologic processes such as blood clotting. About one-half of the calcium in body fluids is bound to plasma proteins. Myocardial response may last as long as 2 hours. The duration of the cardiac response depends on the severity of the hypocalcemic state.

Excretion Excreted by kidneys. Unabsorbed calcium is excreted in feces; some calcium enters the digestive juices and is excreted in the feces. Large quantities are reabsorbed in hypocalcemia; but in hypercalcemia little calcium is reabsorbed.

Drug Interactions Calcium salt solutions enhance the effects of digitalis glycosides, thus increasing the chance of arrhythmias and digitalis toxicity. Calcium salts form insoluble complexes with tetracycline and other antibiotics; do not administer concurrently. Vitamin D increases the intestinal absorption of calcium. IV injections of calcium salt solutions are incompatible with numerous drugs, including sodium bicarbonate, digoxin, digitoxin, diazepam, and phenytoin. Administer calcium salts alone and flush the IV tubing before giving another drug.

Administration The dosage and rate of administration varies widely according to the severity of hypocalcemia. Usual adult dosage: 1 g po tid; Range: 3 to 15 g po daily; Children: 500 mg/kg/day in divided doses.

Available Drug Forms Tablets containing 500 mg or 1 g (4.5 mEq); ampules containing 10 ml of a 10% solution (4 mEq).

Nursing Management

Planning factors

1. Serum electrolytes and calcium and phosphorus levels should be taken before initiating drug therapy.
2. Obtain a history to determine the past or present occurrence of a peptic ulcer and kidney stones and the use of oral calcium salts. Notify physician if client has a history of either disorder.
3. A well-balanced diet containing dairy products provides ample quantities of calcium.
4. Determine the amount of dietary calcium ingested daily. Consult physician and dietitian as needed.
5. Schedule drug administration at least 2 hours after meals.
6. Seizure precautions (padded rails, padded tongue blades) should be instituted in clients with severe hypocalcemia.

Administration factors

1. The recommended daily allowances of calcium are: Infants: 400 to 600 mg; Children: 700 to 1400 mg; Adults: 800 mg; Pregnancy and lactation: 1300 mg.
2. Administer drug with water, not milk, as an interaction may occur.
3. Instruct client to drink several extra glasses of water to avoid calcium precipitation in the genitourinary system.
4. When administering IV:
   a. Check patency of IV before giving. If in doubt, restart IV in a large vein since vein irritation may occur.
   *b. IV bolus is not recommended because cardiac arrest and other untoward reactions may occur. When necessary, such as during cardiac resuscitation, a syringe pump is recommended.
   c. Physician should prescribe rate of drug administration. Administer slowly; do not exceed 0.5 ml/min. of a 10% solution.
   d. May be added to 50 ml of 5% D/W and infused over 20 to 30 minutes.

Evaluation factors

1. Serum calcium levels should be taken frequently, depending on the severity of hypocalcemia. Serum electrolytes and phosphate levels should be determined periodically.
2. Record intake and output.
3. Check urine for signs of precipitation, particularly the early morning specimen. If noticeably cloudy, obtain serum calcium levels and notify physician.
4. Cardiac monitoring is recommended when administering calcium salt solutions IV.

Client teaching factors

1. Instruct client to take calcium salts at least 2 hours after meals and to avoid taking other medications at the same time.
2. Instruct clients to drink at least 1 quart of extra fluid daily.
3. Instruct client or client's family to inspect morning urine for marked cloudiness. If it occurs, they should notify physician.
4. Instruct client to notify physician if nausea, vomiting, or abdominal pain occurs.
5. Instruct client to consult physician before using a home remedy for constipation.

GENERIC NAME Calcium chloride (RX)

CLASSIFICATION Electrolyte supplement

See calcium gluconate for Source, Parameters of use, and Drug interactions.

Action Calcium chloride is used to replace calcium ions when there is a severe deficit or tetany is present. Although it contains approximately three times the amount of calcium as calcium gluconate, calcium chloride is more irritating to tissues. Since calcium chloride provides additional chloride to the serum, the drug also causes acidosis with a resulting diuresis that may persist up to 48 hours. (See calcium gluconate for further details.)

Indications for Use Tetany due to hypocalcemia. Treatment of hypocalcemia caused by multiple blood transfusions containing citrate. As an adjunct in the treatment of cardiac arrest and profound cardiovascular collapse. (It enhances electrical defibrillation and can increase contractility when peripheral pulses are absent but QRS complexes are present.)

Contraindications Hypercalcemia, severe renal impairment.

Warnings and Precautions Use with caution in digitalized clients; in clients with renal insufficiency and clients known to have a history of kidney stones.

Untoward Reactions Acute hypercalcemia can occur, producing a variety of symptoms, including muscle and joint pains; decreased excitability of muscles and nerves that progresses to tetany; EKG changes (shortening of the Q-T interval, bradycardia, and other arrhythmias); flank pain, polyuria, azotemia, and calcium precipitating in the urine; lethargy, confusion, irritability, nausea, vomiting, and paralytic ileus. Serum calcium levels must be obtained to confirm hypercalcemia. Local vein irritation will occur if drug is injected frequently or too rapidly. Peripheral vasodilation and a cutaneous burning sensation may occur. A moderate drop in blood pressure is relatively common. Accidental injection into subcutaneous tissue may cause tissue necrosis.

Administration The dosage and rate of administration varies widely according to the severity of hypocalcemia. Intravenously: 250 to 1000 mg IV by bolus or infusion; Intracardiac: 200 to 400 mg injected into ventricular chamber and into heart muscle.

Available Drug Forms Ampules containing 5 or 10 ml of a 5% solution (5 ml contains 14 mEq); ampules containing 10 ml of a 10% solution (14 mEq).

Nursing Management

Planning factors

1. Serum electrolytes and calcium and phosphorus levels should be taken before initiating drug therapy.
2. Obtain a history to determine the past or present occurrence of a peptic ulcer and kidney stones and the use of oral calcium salts. Notify physician if client has a history of either disorder.
3. Determine the amount of dietary calcium ingested daily. Consult physician and dietitian as needed.
4. Oral drug administration is no longer recommended due to untoward reactions from GI irritation.

Administration factors

1. Check patency of IV before giving. If in doubt, restart IV in a large vein since vein irritation may occur.
2. Physician should prescribe rate of drug administration. Inject slowly; do not exceed 0.5 ml/min. of a 5% solution or 1.0 ml/min. of a 10% solution. A syringe pump is recommended.
3. May be added to 50 ml of 5% D/W and infused over 20 to 30 minutes.
4. Flush IV line before and after administering drug.

Evaluation factors

1. Serum calcium levels should be taken frequently, depending on the severity of hypocalcemia. Serum electrolytes and phosphate levels should be determined periodically.
2. Record intake and output.
3. Check urine for signs of precipitation, particularly the early morning specimen. If noticeably cloudy, obtain serum calcium levels and notify physician.
4. Cardiac monitoring is recommended when administering calcium salt solutions IV.

GENERIC NAME Calcium carbonate (OTC)

TRADE NAMES Equilet, Precipitated Chalk, Dicarbosil, Titralac, Tums

CLASSIFICATION Antacid, calcium supplement

Indications for Use Gastric irritation, mild calcium deficiency.

Warnings and Precautions Do not exceed 8 g daily. Frequently causes constipation. Prolonged use may cause hypercalcemia, alkalosis, hypomagnesemia, hypophosphatemia, or renal calculi.

Administration Supplement: 1 to 2 g po tid; Antacid: 500 to 1000 mg po between meals and at bedtime.

GENERIC NAME Calcium lactate (OTC)

CLASSIFICATION Calcium supplement

Action Lactate assists in the absorption of calcium. (See calcium gluconate for further details.)

Indications for Use Mild calcium deficiency.

Administration 1 to 5 g po tid with meals. Each gram contains 6.5 mEq of calcium.

Available Drug Forms An ingredient of several prenatal and multivitamin preparations.

GENERIC NAME Calcium glubionate (OTC)

TRADE NAME Neo-Calglucon

CLASSIFICATION Calcium supplement

Indications for Use A dietary supplement, hypoparathyroidism, osteoporosis, rickets.

Administration Adults: 1 to 2 tbsp of syrup daily, bid or tid; Children under 4 years: 2 tsp of syrup daily; Infants: 50 to 150 mg/kg daily given in 3 doses. Each teaspoon (5 ml) of syrup provides 115 mg of calcium.

Nursing Management

1. 5.0 mg of benzoic acid added as a preservative.
2. Often given with vitamin D.

GENERIC NAME Calcium glycerophosphate (RX)

CLASSIFICATION Calcium supplement

Action Similar to calcium gluconate but can be injected IM with little or no irritation.

Indications for Use Tetany, hypoparathyroidism.

Warnings and Precautions Not recommended for infants and young children.

Available Drug Forms Ampules of 10 ml; multidose vials of 60 ml. An ingredient of Calphosan.

Administration 1 to 2 IM injections of 10 ml weekly.

Combination Calcium Supplement Preparations

See calcium gluconate for Action, Indications for use, Contraindications, Warnings and precautions, Untoward reactions, Parameters of use, Drug interactions, and Nursing management.

TRADE NAME Calcet (OTC)

CLASSIFICATION Calcium supplement

Indications for Use Used as a general or prenatal dietary supplement and for treatment of nocturnal leg cramps.

Administration

- *Prevention of deficiency:* 2 tablets po at bedtime.
- *Deficiency:* 1 tablet midmorning, 1 tablet midafternoon, and 2 tablets bedtime.

Available Drug Forms Generic contents in each yellow-coated tablet: calcium carbonate: 240 mg; calcium lactate: 240 mg; calcium gluconate: 240 mg; vitamin D_2: 100 IU. Total calcium content: 152.8 mg.

TRADE NAME Ca-Plus (OTC)

CLASSIFICATION Calcium supplement

Warnings and Precautions Use with caution in clients with a diet high in oxalic acid; concurrent administration produces insoluble calcium oxalate.

Administration 1 tablet qid.

Available Drug Forms Generic contents in each tablet: calcium-protein complex: 280 mg.

TRADE NAME Calphosan (RX)

CLASSIFICATION Calcium supplement

Warnings and Precautions Not recommended for small children.

Administration 1 or 2 injections of 10 ml weekly for 4 to 5 weeks, then as needed.

Available Drug Forms Generic contents in 10 ml ampule: calcium lactate: 50 mg; calcium glycerophosphate: 50 mg. 0.25% phenol added as a preservative.

TRADE NAME Calphosan B-12 (RX)

CLASSIFICATION Calcium supplement

Warnings and Precautions Not recommended for small children.

Administration 1 or 2 injections of 10 ml weekly for 4 to 5 weeks, then as needed.

Available Drug Forms Generic contents in 10-ml ampule: calcium lactate: 50 mg; calcium glycerophosphate: 50 mg; vitamin B_{12}: 300 mcg.

TRADE NAME Dical-D (OTC)

CLASSIFICATION Calcium supplement

Indications for Use When dairy product intake is restricted.

Administration 1 capsule tid with meals. Chew 1 wafer bid with meals.

Available Drug Forms Generic contents in each gelatin capsule: dibasic calcium phosphate: 500 mg; vitamin D_2: 133 IU; phosphorus: 90 mg. Calcium to phosphorus ratio: 1.3 to 1. Also contains cornstarch as an additive. Generic contents in each wafer: dibasic calcium phosphate: 1 g; vitamin D_2: 200 IU; phosphorus: 180 mg. Calcium to phosphorus ratio: 1.29 to 1. Total calcium content: 232mg. Also contains dextrose, sucrose, talc, stearic acid, mineral oil, salt, natural and artificial flavorings as additives.

TRADE NAME Os-Cal (OTC)

CLASSIFICATION Calcium supplement

Indications for Use When low dietary intake exists.

Administration 1 tablet po tid at mealtime.

Available Drug Forms Generic contents in each tablet: calcium carbonate: 625 mg; vitamin D_2: 125 USP units. Total calcium content: 250 mg.

TRADE NAME Os-Cal-Gesic (OTC)

CLASSIFICATION Antiarthritic

Indications for Use For the temporary relief of symptoms associated with arthritis.

Administration Initially 2 tablets po qlh times 3 or 4 doses; then 1 to 2 tablets po qid.

Available Drug Forms Generic contents: calcium carbonate: 250 mg; vitamin D_2: 50 USP units; salicylamide: 400 mg. Total calcium content: 100 mg.

Phosphorus

GENERIC NAMES Sodium phosphate; potassium phosphate

TRADE NAMES Neutra-Phos; Neutra-Phos K (OTC)

CLASSIFICATION Electrolyte supplement (RX)

Source Milk, dairy products, and lean meats are good sources of phosphorus and calcium. Can be prepared from food concentrates or produced synthetically.

Action The sodium and potassium phosphate salts are used to supplement the dietary intake of phosphorus. Like calcium, phosphorus is metabolically regulated by the parathyroid hormone and the two minerals have a definite serum ratio. More than 80% of body phosphorus is found combined with calcium in bones and teeth. The remaining phosphorus is widely distributed throughout the tissues and is involved in various aspects of carbohydrate, protein, and fat metabolism. The mineral is found in phospholipids, phosphatides, enzymes, and in high-energy phosphate compounds such as ATP. The dietary intake of calcium and phosphorus does not change with age, with the exception of infants who require a slightly lower phosphorus intake.

Indications for Use Seldom required therapeutically. Hypophosphatemia due to (1) inadequate absorption, such as sprue and celiac disease; (2) imbalance of calcium-phosphorus ratio, such as that which can occur in rickets and other bone disorders; and (3) hyperparathyroidism. The primary symptom of hypophosphatemia is muscular weakness. Also used in laxative preparations (see Chapter 77) and in urinary acidifiers.

Contraindications Hypoparathyroidism, severe renal impairment, hypervitaminosis D.

Untoward Reactions Symptoms of phosphorus toxicity are: GI disturbances (nausea, vomiting, diarrhea, particularly at large dosages); liver dysfunction (hypertrophy with tenderness, hypoglycemia, hypoprothrombinemia); oliguria. Chronic ingestion of excessive dosages may cause cirrhosis of the liver and renal insufficiency.

Parameters of Use

Absorption Readily absorbed from upper GI tract; about 75% of ingested phosphorus is absorbed. Vitamin D enhances absorption of calcium and phosphorus. Excessive calcium intake may result in the formation of insoluble calcium-phosphorus compounds. Normal serum levels: Inorganic phosphorus: 2.6 to 4.8 mg/100 ml; Phospholipids: 150 to 350 mg/100 ml. Serum must be tested promptly for accurate results.

Distribution Bone, teeth, extracellular fluid, cell membranes, collagen, and intracellular fluid. Primarily found as inorganic phosphate.

Excretion By kidneys; active reabsorption by tubules is regulated by parathyroid hormone; low serum phosphorus causes increased reabsorption. Renal impairment causes an increase in serum phosphorus, which in turn depresses serum calcium levels. Normal urine phosphorus: 0.9 to 1.3 g/24 hours. High urinary concentrations in the distal tubule convert sodium basic phosphate to sodium acid phosphate, thus causing the excretion of hydrogen ions.

Drug Interactions Large dosages or the chronic ingestion of antacid, including aluminum hydroxide, may decrease the absorption of phosphorus due to the formation of unabsorbable compounds. Vitamin D increases the absorption of phosphorus. Excessive intake of calcium salts will decrease the absorption of phosphorus because of the formation of unabsorbable compounds.

Administration Dosage and duration of administration varies with the client's age and severity of hypophosphatemia. Usual dosage for adults and children over 4 years: 250 mg to 2 g po daily in divided doses after meals and at bedtime; Infants and children under 4 years: 200 to 800 mg po daily in divided doses.

Available Drug Forms Capsules containing 250 mg phosphorus (14.25 mEq); unit-dose powders for reconstitution to 75 ml containing 250 mg phosphorus. Multidose powders for reconstitution to 1 gallon of solution. Neutra-Phos also contains 164 mg (7.125 mEq) of sodium and 278 mg (7.125 mEq) of potassium per dose. (Do not use for clients on sodium restriction.) Neutra-Phos K also contains 556 mg (14.25 mEq) of potassium and is sodium-free.

Nursing Management

Planning Factors

1. Serum phosphorus and calcium levels should be taken before instituting drug therapy. Twenty-four hour urine specimens for phosphate content should also be done.
2. Determine dietary intake of phosphorus and calcium. Consult dietitian and physician as needed.
3. Determine intake and output. If oliguria exists consult physician before administering drug.
4. Schedule drug administration for after meals and at bedtime.
5. Reconstituted solution may be kept in refrigerator to increase palatability.
6. Potassium drug salts should be used in clients on low-sodium diets.

Administration factors

1. Drug is always given in solution.
2. Reconstitute solution as directed by manufacturer. Capsules are to be reconstituted in one-third of a glass of water. Do not take whole.
3. Reconstituted solution does not require further dilution but may be followed with a small quantity of water.
4. Excessive intake of drug may cause laxative effect.
5. Fluid should be encouraged during meals.

Evaluation factors

1. Serum phosphorus and calcium levels should be taken periodically (weekly, monthly).
2. Monitor intake and output. If oliguria occurs, notify physician.

Client teaching factors

1. Warn client against taking capsules whole.
2. Teach client how to reconstitute powders and capsules.
3. Instruct client to notify physician if urinary output decreases or if diarrhea occurs.
4. Caution client to limit fluid intake at time of drug administration but to take adequate quantities of fluid at other times.

Combination Phosphorus Preparations

TRADE NAME K-Phos (RX)

CLASSIFICATION Electrolyte supplement, urinary acidifier

Indications for Use Urinary acidifier that aids in the prevention of calcium deposits in the urinary tract, the control of genitourinary infections by acidifying urine, the control of odor and turbidity of ammoniacal urine, and increases the effectiveness of certain antibiotics.

Contraindications Renal insufficiency, severe liver impairment, Addison's disease, hyperkalemia.

Warnings and Precautions Use with caution in clients on sodium-restricted diets. May cause a laxative effect, nausea, and hyperacidity.

Administration 2 tablets po qid with a full glass of water.

Available Drug Forms Generic contents in each tablet: potassium acid phosphate: 155 mg; sodium acid phosphate: 350 mg; potassium: 44.5 mg; sodium: 67 mg. Total elemental phosphorus: 125.6 mg.

TRADE NAME K-Phos No. 2 (RX)

CLASSIFICATION Electrolyte supplement, urinary acidifier

See K-Phos for Indications for use and Contraindications.

Warnings and Precautions Do not exceed 8 tablets in 24 hours. Acid-ash diet is recommended.

Administration 1 tablet po daily with a full glass of water.

Available Drug Forms Generic contents in each tablet: potassium acid phosphate: 305 mg; sodium acid phosphate: 700 mg; potassium: 88 mg (2.25 mEq); sodium: 134 mg (5.83 mEq). Total elemental phosphorus: 250 mg.

TRADE NAME K-Phos Neutral (RX)

CLASSIFICATION Electrolyte supplement, urinary acidifier

See K-Phos for Indications for use and Contraindications.

Warnings and Precautions Use with caution in clients on sodium-restricted diets. Excessive dosages may cause a laxative effect. Keep container tightly closed.

Administration 1 to 2 tablets po with a full glass of water.

Available Drug Forms Generic contents in each tablet: dibasic sodium phosphate: 852 mg; potassium acid phosphate: 155 mg; sodium acid phosphate: 130 mg; sodium: 298 mg; potassium: 45 mg; Total elemental phosphorus: 250 mg.

TRADE NAME K-Phos Original (RX)

CLASSIFICATION Electrolyte supplement, urinary acidifier

See K-Phos for Contraindications.

Indications for Use May be used in clients on sodium-restricted diets. (See K-Phos for further details.)

Warnings and Precautions Excessive dosages may cause a laxative effect. The high potassium content may cause gastrointestinal ulcerations; use with caution in clients with a history of hyperacidity or peptic ulcer. Administer with caution to clients taking digitalis.

Administration Before stirring and administering, soak tablet 2 to 5 minutes.

Available Drug Forms Generic contents in each tablet: potassium acid phosphate: 500 mg; potassium: 144 mg (3.67 mEq). Total elemental phosphorus: 14 mg.

TRADE NAME Uroqid-Acid (RX)

CLASSIFICATION Electrolyte supplement, urinary acidifier

Action Methenamine releases formaldehyde, a germicidal agent, in the urinary system if the urinary pH is 5.0 or less. Phosphate acidifies the urine to enhance the formation of formaldehyde.

Indications for Use Management of chronic urinary tract infection.

Contraindications Moderate or severe renal insufficiency, severe hepatic impairment.

Warnings and Precautions May cause dysuria. Use with caution in clients on sodium-restricted diets.

Administration Initially: 3 tablets po qid; Maintenance: 1 to 2 tablets po qid.

Available Drug Forms Generic contents in each tablet: sodium acid phosphate: 200 mg; methenamine mandelate: 350 mg.

TRADE NAME Uroqid-Acid No. 2 (RX)

CLASSIFICATION Electrolyte supplement, urinary acidifier

See Uroquid-Acid for Action, Indications for use, and Contraindications.

Warnings and Precautions Use with caution in clients on sodium-restricted diets.

Administration Initially: 2 tablets po qid; Maintenance: 2 to 4 tablets po daily in divided doses.

Available Drug Forms Generic contents in each tablet: sodium acid phosphate: 500 mg; methenamine mandelate: 500 mg.

TRADE NAME Uro-KP-Neutral (OTC)

CLASSIFICATION Electrolyte supplement, urinary acidifier

See K-Phos for Contraindications and Warnings and precautions.

Indications for Use Urinary acidifier, phosphate supplement.

Administration 6 capsules po daily in divided doses.

Available Drug Forms Generic contents in each capsule: sodium as dibasic sodium phosphate: 226.8 mg; potassium as dibasic potassium phosphate: 49.8 mg. Total elemental phosphorus: 172.8 mg.

TRADE NAME Thiacide (RX)

CLASSIFICATION Electrolyte supplement, urinary acidifier

Indications for Use Urinary antiinfective agent and acidifier. Since it is sodium-free, the drug can be used for clients on sodium-restricted diets.

Contraindications Renal failure, hyperkalemia.

Warnings and Precautions Use with caution in digitalized clients.

Administration Maintenance: 2 to 4 tablets po daily in divided doses.

Available Drug Forms Generic contents in each tablet: potassium acid phosphate: 250 mg; methenamine: 500 mg.

Magnesium

GENERIC NAME Magnesium sulfate (injection)

CLASSIFICATION Electrolyte supplement, anticonvulsant

RX

Source Magnesium is widely distributed in nature. Rich food sources are nuts, seafood, dried beans, and soybeans. It is usually prepared synthetically.

Action Next to potassium, magnesium is the second most abundant cation in intracellular fluid. Nearly 70% of the body's magnesium is found combined with calcium and phosphorus in bone. Body muscles contain more magnesium than calcium; but unlike calcium, there is normally very little magnesium in serum (1.4 to 2.5 mg/100 ml or 1.5 to 3 mEq/l). The body can tolerate relatively wide variations in this range. Magnesium is necessary for several intracellular enzyme reactions and it serves as a catalyst or coenzyme factor in carbohydrate and protein metabolism. It is useful as a central nervous system depressant because it blocks the release of acetylcholine and may even desensitize muscles to neurologic impulses. Most individuals can tolerate a serum magnesium level as high as 12 mEq/l or greater before heart block, respiratory paralysis, and cardiac arrest occur. It prolongs cardiac conduction time and depresses impulse formation at the sinoatrial node (cardiac pacemakers).

Indications for Use Anticonvulsant, treatment of eclampsia, cardiac depressant (calcium antagonist). (See magnesium sulfate (oral) for use as a laxative (Chapter 77) and other indications.)

Contraindications Severe renal insufficiency, congestive heart failure, heart block.

Warnings and Precautions Use with caution just prior to delivery as it will cause CNS depression in the neonate and augment the effect of certain anesthetics. Use with caution in clients with renal insufficiency since renal excretion of magnesium is impaired. Clients with hypertension or congestive heart failure may develop sodium overload.

Untoward Reactions Hypermagnesemia can occur, particularly in clients with impaired renal function. The early symptoms include depression of deep tendon reflexes and finally the absence of the patellar reflex. As the serum magnesium level increases heart block, respiratory paralysis, hypotension, flaccid paralysis, and cardiac arrest occur. Other electrolyte imbalances including hypernatremia can occur. Complete heart block may occur in digitalized clients.

Parameters of Use

Absorption Effects occur: in minutes (IV); about 1 hour (IM). Effects last: 30 to 60 minutes (IV); 3 to 4 hours (IM). Normal serum levels: 1.4 to 2.5 mg/100 ml or 1.5 to 3 mEq/l.

Crosses placenta; may cause fetal distress.

Distribution Widely distributed throughout the body fluids. Some protein binding occurs.

Excretion Rapidly by the kidneys. Duration of effect is prolonged in renal impairment. Reabsorption of magnesium ions occurs in hypomagnesemia.

Drug Interactions Heart block may occur in clients receiving digitalis glycosides. Profound CNS depression can occur if magnesium sulfate is administered concurrently with other anticonvulsant and CNS depressants, such as anesthetics, barbiturates, and narcotics. Calcium gluconate can be used to counteract hypermagnesemia (antidote).

Administration Dosage depends on the effect desired and the client's serum magnesium level. Impairment of urinary clearance of magnesium should be considered.

- *Anticonvulsant loading dose:* 10 g of a 50% solution IM; 4 g of a 10% solution slow IV injection or infusion.
- *Maintenance dose:* 3 to 4 g IM q4-6h as needed; 500 to 1000 mg/hour IV as needed.
- *Prophylaxis and mild deficiency:* 35 to 400 mg po daily; 500 to 1000 mg IM or IV daily as needed.

Available Drug Forms Ampules of 10% solution containing 1 g in 10 ml for IV use; ampules of 50% solution containing 5 g in 10 ml for IM use.

Nursing Management

Planning factors

1. Serum electrolytes and calcium and magnesium levels should be taken before instituting drug therapy.
2. When appropriate, determine the quantity of dietary magnesium ingested daily. Consult dietitian and physician as needed.
3. Seizure precautions should be instituted in clients with convulsive disorders.
4. Vital signs, blood pressure, and deep tendon reflexes, including knee jerk, should be recorded before administering drug.
5. Calcium gluconate and a 20-ml syringe and needle should be kept at the bedside when parenteral injections are given.

Administration factors

1. Deficiency states in man are unlikely but may occur in chronic malnutrition. May be required in clients on prolonged hyperalimentation.
2. The recommended daily allowances are: Adult men: 350 mg; Adult women: 300 mg; Pregnancy and lactation: 450 mg.
3. When administering IM:
   a. IM injections are frequently avoided because of the volume of injectable fluid required and the discomfort that occurs at the injection site. Use a 50% magnesium solution.
   b. Avoid IM injections in children.
   c. Assess IM sites for potential fluid accommodation. Do not give more than 5 ml in one site.
   d. Prepare required number of syringes for the total dosage required. Two syringes and needle sites may be required to administer a loading dose. Change needles before administering.
   e. Administer each injection deep into the muscle mass. Both gluteal areas may be required to administer the total loading dose. The Z-track method of administration is recommended.
   f. Rotate injection sites.
   g. Examine injection sites frequently for irritation.
   h. Monitor vital signs and blood pressure every 30 minutes.
4. When administering IV:
   a. Loading dose can be given via IV bolus but slowly. Do not exceed 150 mg per minute (1.5 ml/min. of a 10% solution or 0.3 ml of a 50% solution).
   b. Check patency of IV before administering drug.
   c. The loading dose can be added to 50 or 100 ml of 5% D/W and infused over 30 minutes.
   d. The maintenance dose can be added to 5% D/W or another compatible infusion solution. The drug dose, infusion volume, and rate of drug administration should be prescribed by the physician. An infusion pump is highly recommended but a carefully observed microdrip IV administration set can be used.
   e. When 5 g magnesium sulfate (10 ml of 50% solution) are added to 500 ml of 5% D/W, the following infusion rates are used:

MAGNESIUM SULFATE

Drug Order		Infusion Rate		
mg/hr	mg/min.	ml/h (pump)	macro-gtt/min.* (15 gtt/ml)	micro-gtt/min. (60 gtt/ml)
500	8.3	50	12.5	50
600	10	60	15	60
700	11.6	70	17.5	70
800	13.3	80	20	80
900	15	90	22.5	90
1000	16.6	100	25	100

*Not recommended.

   f. When 5 g of magnesium sulfate (50 ml of 10% solution) are added to 500 ml of 5% D/W to yield a total infusion volume of 550 ml, the following infusion rates are used:

MAGNESIUM SULFATE

Drug Order		Infusion Rate		
mg/hr	mg/min.	ml/h (pump)	macro-gtt/min.* (15 gtt/ml)	micro-gtt/min. (60 gtt/ml)
500	8.3	55	13.75	55
600	10	66	16.5	66
700	11.6	77	19.25	77
800	13.3	88	22	88
900	15	99	24.75	99
1000	16.6	110	27.5	110

*Not recommended.

   g. Vital signs and blood pressure should be monitored constantly when IV loading dose is administered and every 10 to 15 minutes when infusion is running.
   h. Cardiac monitoring is highly recommended.
   i. The knee jerk reflex should be checked every 10 minutes when IV loading is administered and every 30 minutes when infusion is running.
   j. Monitor fetal heart rate frequently in pregnant women.

Evaluation factors

1. Serum magnesium levels should be obtained about 15 to 30 minutes after the IV loading dose is absorbed and about 2 to 3 hours after the IM loading dose.
2. Serum electrolytes and calcium levels should be obtained frequently (q4-12h).
3. The following changes frequently occur at the indicated serum magnesium level:

MAGNESIUM SULFATE

Common Effects	Magnesium Level (mEq/l)
Depression of reflexes (therapeutic level)	4–7
QRS complex widens, P-Q interval is prolonged	5–10
Knee jerk reflex absent	> 10
Respiratory depression	10–15
S-A and A-V heart block, hypotension	12–16
Respiratory arrest	> 15
Cardiac arrest	> 25

4. The absence of the knee jerk reflex is an indication of excessive drug levels. Slow the rate of administration to KVO and notify physician. (Withhold additional IM injections.)
5. Bradycardia, hypotension, and a respiratory rate below 12/min. are also indications of excessive toxicity.
6. Oliguria (less than 30 ml of urine/h) may precipitate excessive drug levels. Notify physician if this occurs.
7. Fetal distress may occur in pregnant women; notify physician immediately.
8. The newborn may have a weak cry, depressed heart rate, and flaccid muscles. Treat accordingly.

GENERIC NAME Magnesium carbonate (OTC)

CLASSIFICATION Antacid

Administration 1 to 2 tablets or 15 to 30 ml po qid between meals and at bedtime.

Available Drug Forms An ingredient of Escort and Gaviscon.

Nursing Management Suspension should be shaken well before measuring dosage. (See Chapter 75 on antacids for further details.)

GENERIC NAME Magnesium gluconate (OTC)

CLASSIFICATION Magnesium supplement

Indications for Use Dysmenorrhea states (decreases uterine contractions and pain), hypomagnesemia.

Administration 500 to 1000 mg po with a full glass of water bid or tid 30 minutes before meals. 500 mg provides about 29 mg of magnesium.

Available Drug Forms Found in some multivitamin preparations.

GENERIC NAME Magnesium hydroxide (OTC)

CLASSIFICATION Antacid

Indications for Use Gastric irritation, used to buffer aspirin tablets.

Administration As directed po qid between meals and at bedtime.

Available Drug Forms An ingredient of several antacids, including Aludrox, Camalox, Gelusil-M, Kudrox, and Maalox. Found together with aspirin in some analgesics, such as Cama Inlay tablets.

Nursing Management Suspensions should be shaken well before measuring dosage. (See Chapter 75 on antacids for further details.)

GENERIC NAME Magnesium oxide (OTC)

CLASSIFICATION Magnesium supplement

Indications for Use Hypomagnesemia, used to buffer salicylate analgesics.

Administration As directed.

Available Drug Forms An ingredient of several multivitamin preparations, including Beeleth, Berocca-Plus, Hyalex, and Optilets.

GENERIC NAME Magnesium-protein complex

TRADE NAME Mg-Plus (OTC)

CLASSIFICATION Dietary supplement

Indications for Use Malnutrition, hypomagnesemia.

Warnings and Precautions Excessive doses may have a laxative effect.

Administration 1 tablet po daily, bid, or tid. Each tablet contains 133 mg of magnesium from soy protein and yeast.

TRACE MINERALS

Iodine

GENERIC NAMES Potassium iodide; potassium iodide solution

TRADE NAMES Kisol, Pima; SSKI (RX)

CLASSIFICATION Iodine supplement, expectorant

Action Iodine is necessary for the synthesis of the thyroid hormones thyroxine and triiodothyronine. Thyroxine regulates cell metabolism. A dietary deficit in iodine causes enlargement of the thyroid gland which is commonly called simple or nontoxic goiter. Although little iodine is required by the body, individuals who seldom eat seafood and who mainly ingest foods grown in iodine-deficient soil are prone to developing iodine-deficiency goiters. Small doses of potassium iodide can be used to treat these goiters and to prevent deficiency states during growth and development periods, particularly pregnancy and lactation. The iodine salts are often preferred to iodine as they are less toxic. Iodine salts act as an expectorant by liquefying tenacious bronchial secretions; they are often used as an ingredient of bronchodilators and cough syrups. Although excessive dosages of iodine salts cause little or no change in the normal thyroid, the thyroid of clients with hyperthyroidism will respond by decreasing its size and vascularity and by increasing firmness of the gland. The quantity of thyroid hormones secreted is decreased temporarily. Therefore, the drug is useful in preparing a client for thyroidectomy and in treating hyperthyroidism. But as the body adjusts to the increase in iodide, the symptoms of hyperthyroidism will return after prolonged drug therapy.

Indications for Use Prevention of iodine deficiency, iodine-deficiency goiter (simple goiter), preoperative preparation for thyroidectomy, hyperthyroidism (myxedema), expectorant when bronchial secretions are scant but thick (chronic bronchitis, asthma, bronchiectasis, emphysema).

Contraindications Hypersensitivity to iodine and iodides, tuberculosis, acute bronchitis, severe renal impairment.

Warnings and Precautions Use with caution during pregnancy since high dosages or prolonged drug use may cause untoward reactions in the fetus. Prolonged use of high dosages may cause hypothyroidism. Use with caution in clients with a history of peptic ulcer or other disorders associated with upper GI irritation.

Untoward Reactions GI disturbances, including nausea, vomiting, diarrhea, epigastric discomfort, and a slight metallic taste, are common. Small bowel lesions, including stenosis and ulceration, have been associated with potassium salts. Discontinue drug if abdominal pain, distention, nausea, vomiting, or GI bleeding occur. Hypersensitivity reactions, including angioedema, laryngeal edema and hemorrhages in skin or mucous membranes, can occur within hours. Generalized skin eruption, fever, arthralgia, enlarged lymph nodes, and eosinophilia may also occur. Iodism (chronic iodine poisoning) may occur with prolonged drug therapy. The symptoms include metallic taste, stomatitis, increased salivation, coryza, sneezing, periorbital edema, pulmonary edema, and circulatory collapse.

Parameters of Use

Absorption From small intestines as iodide; little free iodine is absorbed from the GI tract. Normal serum levels of potassium iodide: 4 to 8 mcg/100 ml.

Crosses placenta and enters breast milk; use with caution in pregnancy. Lactating mothers should bottle-feed their babies.

Distribution Widely; about 30% in thyroid gland. Enters saliva and gastric juices; may cause metallic taste, oral lesions, and other GI disturbances. It is bound to plasma proteins as iodide and thyroxine.

Metabolism Thyroxine is metabolized by the liver and iodine is excreted in bile.

Excretion Primarily via the kidneys in 2 to 3 days.

Drug Characteristics Unstable in moist air. Store in airtight container and keep in dry area.

Drug Interactions The concurrent use of oral thiazide diuretics may predispose the client to GI ulcerations. The concurrent use of lithium may predispose the client to hypothyroidism If essential, lower dosages of iodine salts may be necessary. The concurrent use of antithyroid agents is not recommended.

Laboratory Interactions Alterations in thyroid function tests, including elevation of serum protein-bound iodine (PBI) can occur; alteration in urinary 17-hydroxycorticosteroid can occur.

Administration

- *Prophylaxis:* 200 mg po daily for 10 days twice a year; 150 to 300 mcg in a multivitamin preparation daily or iodized salt (approximately 75 mcg/g of salt).
- *Thyroidectomy:* 300 mg po tid or qid for 10 to 14 days before surgery; Range: 300 mg to 1800 mg daily.
- *Expectorant:* Adults: 300 to 600 mg po tid or qid; Children: 150 to 300 mg po qid.

Available Drug Forms Enteric release tablets containing 120 or 300 mg; syrup containing 300 mg in 5 ml; saturated oral solution (SSKI) containing 300 mg in 0.3 ml provided with calibrated dropper marked at the 0.3 ml and 0.6 ml level; oral solution containing 500 mg in 15 ml. An ingredient in some multivitamin preparations, including Calinate-FA, En Cebrin, Filibon, Stuart Prenatal, Eldec, Megadose, and Os-Cal.

Nursing Management

Planning factors

1. Thyroid function tests (PBI, T_3, T_4) should be done before drug therapy is instituted.
2. A dietary history to assess the total daily intake of iodine and iodine compounds should be obtained. (Remember to include iodized salt, cough syrups, and bronchodilators.)
3. Many radiopaque substances (Telepaque) contain iodine and may disrupt PBI tests for months.
4. Adequate hydration of the client may prevent the need for expectorants. When appropriate, encourage fluids in clients with respiratory disorders.
5. Determine if there is an allergy to iodine or iodine compounds. Notify physician.

Administration factors

1. The recommended daily allowances are: Adult males: 130 mcg; Adult females: 100 mcg; Pregnancy and lactation: 150 mcg.
2. Iodine solutions are added to 3 to 4 fl oz of water before administering and followed by a full glass of water. The salty taste of potassium iodide can be disguised in milk or fruit juice.
3. Tablets and syrup should be taken with a full glass of water, milk, or fruit juice.
4. Iodine compounds should be given after meals to prevent GI irritation.

5. The client should be observed frequently for hypersensitivity reactions after the first dose (first 3 to 4 hours).
6. Store drug in airtight containers away from light.

Evaluation factors

1. If lacrimal or nasal secretions increase and frequent sneezing occurs, notify physician.
2. Assess client daily for clinical signs of iodism since results of thyroid function tests are inaccurate during drug therapy.
3. If signs and symptoms of GI disturbances occur, give drug with milk or food. If symptoms persist, notify physician as a small bowel lesion may be developing.

Client teaching factors

1. Inform client that vomitus may have a purple color.
2. Instruct client to notify nurse or physician if symptoms of iodism occur.
3. Instruct client to drink adequate quantities of fluid.
4. Inform client to take drug after meals or with milk or food to prevent GI disturbances. If disturbances persist, instruct the client to notify physician.

GENERIC NAME Sodium iodide (RX)

CLASSIFICATION Iodine supplement

Action Sodium iodide is similar to potassium iodide but is less prone to cause GI ulcerations. It is used to replace body iodine in deficiency states such as goiter. The sodium salt is preferred in the treatment of thyroid toxicosis because hyperkalemia could occur with potassium iodide. (See potassium chloride for further details.)

Indications for Use Prevention of iodine deficiency, iodine-deficiency goiter, as an adjunct in the treatment of thyroid toxicosis.

Contraindications Hypersensitivity to iodine or iodides, tuberculosis, acute bronchitis, severe renal impairment.

Warnings and Precautions Use with caution during pregnancy since high dosages or prolonged drug use may cause goiter formation or other untoward reactions in the fetus. Prolonged use of high dosages may cause hyperthyroidism.

Untoward Reactions GI disturbances, including nausea, vomiting, diarrhea, epigastric discomfort, and a slight metallic taste are common. Hypersensitivity reactions, including angioedema, laryngeal edema and hemorrhages in skin or mucous membranes, can occur within hours. Generalized skin eruptions, fever, arthralgia, enlarged lymph nodes, and eosinophilia may also occur. Iodism (chronic iodine poisoning) may occur with prolonged drug therapy. The symptoms include metallic taste, stomatitis, increased salivation, coryza, sneezing, periorbital edema, pulmonary edema, and circulatory collapse.

Parameters of Use

Absorption From small intestines as iodide; little free iodine is absorbed from the GI tract.

Crosses placenta and enters breast milk. Use with caution during pregnancy. Lactating mothers should bottle-feed their babies.

Distribution Widely, about 30% in thyroid gland. Enters saliva and gastric juices; may cause metallic taste, oral lesions, and other GI disturbances. It is bound to plasma proteins as iodine and thyroxine.

Metabolism Thyroxine is metabolized by the liver and the iodine is excreted in bile.

Excretion Primarily via kidney in 2 to 3 days.

Drug Interactions The concurrent use of oral thiazide diuretics may predispose the client to GI ulcerations. The concurrent use of lithium may predispose the client to hyperthyroidism. If essential, lower dosages of iodine salts may be necessary. The concurrent use of antithyroid agents is not recommended.

Laboratory Interactions Alterations in thyroid function tests, including elevation of serum protein-bound iodine (PBI) may occur; alteration in urinary 17-hydroxycorticosteroid can occur.

Administration

- *Prophylaxis:* 200 mg po daily for 10 days twice a year. Use of iodized salt yields approximately 75 mcg/g of salt.
- *Iodine deficiency:* 300 mg po tid or qid.
- *Thyroid toxicosis:* 1000 to 2000 mg IV by continuous drip for 24 hours; then 600 mg po tid, qid, or q6h.

Available Drug Forms Tablets containing 200 or 300 mg; ampules containing 1000 or 2000 mg/20 ml.

Nursing Management

Planning factors

1. Thyroid function tests (PBI, T_3, T_4) should be done before drug therapy is instituted.
2. A dietary history to assess the total dietary intake of iodine and iodide compounds should be obtained. (Remember to include iodized salt, cough syrups, and bronchodilators.)
3. Many radiopaque substances (Telepaque) contain iodine and may disrupt PBI for months.
4. Adequate hydration of the client may prevent the need for expectorants. When appropriate, encourage fluids in respiratory clients.
5. Obtain vital signs before instituting drug.
6. Store drug in airtight containers away from light.

Administration factors

1. The recommended daily allowances are: Adult males, 130 mcg; Adult females: 100 mcg; Pregnancy and lactation: 150 mcg.
2. Tablets and syrup should be taken with a full glass of water, milk, or fruit juice.

3. Iodine compounds should be given after meals to prevent GI irritation.
4. Oral potassium or sodium iodide is administered as soon as the crisis is over; usually in 24 hours.
5. When administering IV:
   a. Check the patency of IV before starting drug; if site is questionable, restart IV before adding drug. Infiltrated drug solutions are irritating to tissues.
   b. An infusion pump is recommended.
   c. Keep IV bottle away from direct sunlight.

Evaluation factors

1. If lacrimal or nasal secretions increase and frequent sneezing occurs, notify physician.
2. Assess client daily for clinical signs of iodism since results of thyroid function tests are inaccurate during drug therapy.
3. If signs and symptoms of GI disturbances occur, give oral drug preparations with milk or food. If symptoms persist, notify physician.
4. When administering IV:
   a. Monitor vital signs and check for signs of toxicity frequently (q1-2h).
   b. Record intake and output. If oliguria occurs, notify physician.

Client teaching factors

1. Instruct client to notify nurse or physician if symptoms of iodism occur.
2. Instruct client to drink at least 1 extra quart of fluid each day.
3. Inform client to take drug after meals to prevent GI disturbances.

GENERIC NAME Iodized sodium chloride (OTC)

TRADE NAME Iodized Salt

CLASSIFICATION Iodine supplement

Indications for Use Prevention of iodine deficiency.

Administration Contains approximately 75 mcg of sodium or potassium iodide per gram of sodium chloride.

GENERIC NAME Strong Iodine Solution (RX)

TRADE NAME Lugol's Solution, Compound Iodine Solution

Classification Iodine supplement

Source Contains 5% iodine and 10% potassium iodide in distilled water.

Indications for Use Often used for 10 to 14 days prior to surgery to prepare clients for thyroidectomy; iodine deficiency.

Warnings and Precautions May be irritating to the GI tract.

Administration 0.3 ml po in a full glass of water tid or qid. See potassium iodide for further details.

GENERIC NAME Ammonium iodide (RX)

CLASSIFICATION Expectorant

Indications for Use As an adjunct in the treatment of bronchitis, bronchial asthma, emphysema, and cystic fibrosis; used after surgery to prevent chronic sinusitis atelectasis.

Administration 200-mg capsule tid after meals. See potassium iodide for further details.

GENERIC NAME Riodine (OTC)

CLASSIFICATION Iodine supplement

Source Organic compound containing iodine and castor oil.

Indications for Use Iodine deficiency.

Administration 200-mg capsule tid after meals.

GENERIC NAME Iodinated glycerol (RX)

TRADE NAME Organidin

CLASSIFICATION Expectorant

Source Isomeric mixture produced from the interaction of iodine and glycerol. Viscous, amber liquid; contains about 50% organically bound iodine and no free iodine or inorganic iodide.

Indications for Use As an adjunct in the treatment of bronchitis, bronchial asthma, emphysema, and cystic fibrosis; used after surgery to prevent chronic sinusitis atelectasis.

Warnings and Precautions May cause acne in adolescents.

Administration Adults: 60 mg (20 gtt or 2 tablets) qid with 6 to 8 fl oz of fluid or 1 tsp elixir po qid. Children: Depends on body weight.

Available Drug Forms A 5% solution containing 50 mg/ml (1 drop equals about 3 mg); tablets containing 30 mg; 12% elixir containing 60 mg/5 ml. See potassium iodide for further details.

Iodine-Containing Antiseptic Preparations

GENERIC NAME Iodine tincture (RX)

TRADE NAME Tr of Iodine

CLASSIFICATION Iodine-containing topical antiseptic

Source 2% iodine and 2.4% iodine in alcohol.

Indications for Use Traditionally used as an antiinfective agent for lacerations and abrasions.

Warnings and Precautions Causes burning sensation when applied due to irritation of tissues. Erythema and vesicles will form if applied to moist skin.

GENERIC NAME Phenolated iodine solution (RX)

TRADE NAME Carbolized Iodine Solution

CLASSIFICATION Iodine-containing topical antiseptic

Source 5% compounded aqueous solution and 6% phenol in glycerin and water.

Indications for Use Traditionally used as an antiinfective agent for lacerations and abrasions. Less irritating than tincture of iodine.

GENERIC NAME Iodine ointment (RX)

TRADE NAMES Regular Iodized Ointment, Stainless Iodized Ointment

CLASSIFICATION Iodine-containing topical antiseptic

Source Regular: Contains 4% iodine and 4% potassium iodine in glycerin; Stainless: Contains 5% iodine in paraffin, oleic acid, and petroleum.

Indications for Use Traditionally used as an antiinfective agent for lacerations and abrasions. Less irritating than tincture of iodine.

GENERIC NAME Thymol iodine (RX)

TRADE NAME Thymol Powder Aristol

CLASSIFICATION Iodinc containing topical antiseptic

Source Thymol is a phenol prepared from thymol oil. The addition of iodine is said to increase the effectiveness of this antiinfective agent.

Indications for Use Used as an antiinfective agent in open skin lesions such as decubitus ulcers.

Nursing Management

1. Applied like a dusting powder.
2. Residue should be completely removed before reapplying powder.

GENERIC NAME Iodine solution (RX)

TRADE NAME Roma-Nol

CLASSIFICATION Iodine-containing topical antiseptic

Indications for Use Used as an antiinfective agent for skin and mucous membrane injuries and lesions.

Nursing Management

1. Lacks the toxic and irritating qualities of tincture of iodine.
2. May require 3 to 4 applications before full effect occurs.

GENERIC NAME Iodoform (RX)

TRADE NAMES Iodoform Powder, Iodoform Gauze, Iodoform Ointment, Triiodomethane

CLASSIFICATION Iodine-containing topical antiseptic

Action Iodoform is insoluble in water, has a persistent, offensive odor, and is a somewhat effective germicidal preparation. When the powder is sprinkled into the laceration or wound, iodine is slowly liberated. The gauze and ointment have a less offensive odor and the gauze may be used to pack open wounds. Other antiseptics have replaced the use of iodoform in many areas.

Available Drug Forms Jars of powder; gauze impregnated with iodoform and available in various widths; 10% ointment.

Nursing Management

1. When necessary, treated area should be cleansed with normal saline using aseptic technique. Gently dry area with sterile, absorbent gauze before reapplying drug.
2. Wound usually cleansed and treated 2 or 3 times a day.
3. Iodoform packing should not be removed unless specifically ordered by the physician.

GENERIC NAME Povidone-iodine (OTC)

TRADE NAMES Aerodine, Betadine, Femidine, Isodine

CLASSIFICATION Iodine-containing topical antiseptic

Action Povidone-iodine is a nontoxic, water-soluble iodine complex that contains 10% iodine. The iodine is slowly released and provides a germicidal effect against numerous microorganisms, including viruses, fungi, gram-positive and gram-negative organisms, yeasts, and protozoa. This iodine compound is relatively nonirritating to tissues and causes little or no burning sensation when applied to open lesions.

Indications for Use Preparation of the skin for surgery, venipuncture, and other invasive procedures; infections of the skin and mucous membranes, including monilial and trichomonas forms of vaginitis; disinfection of hands prior to using surgical or antiseptic technique.

Contraindications Hypersensitivity to iodine or iodine compounds.

Untoward Reactions Skin irritation may occur and result in erythema and swelling; discontinue drug if these symptoms occur and notify physician.

Administration

- *Skin preparation:* Apply directly to skin; scrub should be lathered at least 5 minutes before rinsing.
- *Laceration and wounds:* Apply directly to wound or apply to sterile gauze bandage before covering area.
- *Vaginal douche:* 1 to 2 tbsp in 1000 ml of lukewarm water daily.
- *Vaginal gel:* Insert one applicatorful (50 ml) at bedtime.

Available Drug Forms Solution, surgical scrub, skin cleanser, Helafoam solution with broad spectrum microbicidal activity (used to prevent infection in burns and wounds); ointment, aerosol spray, vaginal douche solution, vaginal gel (requires a prescription).

Nursing Management

1. May be irritating to the conjunctiva. Avoid contact with the eyes.
2. Starched linens and clothing will stain a purple-brown color. The stain will fade or disappear when natural fabrics are washed, but tends to remain in synthetic fabrics. Use disposable covers and avoid contact with fabrics.

Radiographic Iodine Compounds

GENERIC NAME Iodoalphionic acid (RX)

CLASSIFICATION Radiographic iodine compound

Action Radiographic substance that concentrates in gallbladder. Occasionally, x-rays are repeated the next day after a double drug dose.

Indications for Use Cholecystography.

Contraindications Acute or chronic renal failure, active GI disorders.

Untoward Reactions Dysuria, vomiting, diarrhea, burning sensation upon swallowing, pruritus, flatulence.

Parameters of Use

Excretion Primarily via the kidneys.

Administration 3 g po with several glasses of water following a fat-free late afternoon meal.

Nursing Management NPO until x-rays are taken the next morning.

GENERIC NAME Iopanoic acid (RX)

TRADE NAME Telepaque

CLASSIFICATION Radiographic iodine compound

Action A contrast media that is readily absorbed. It is eliminated in bile and concentrated in the gallbladder. The drug has a relatively low toxicity. Occasionally, x-rays are repeated the next day after a double drug dose.

Indications for Use Cholecystography.

Contraindications Acute or chronic renal failure, active GI disorders.

Administration 3 g po with several glasses of water following a fat-free supper (given 10 hours before x-rays).

GENERIC NAME Iophendylate (injection) (RX)

TRADE NAME Pantopaque

CLASSIFICATION Radiographic iodine compound

Indications for Use Myelography.

Contraindications Within 10 days of a lumbar puncture or when lumbar puncture is contraindicated.

Administration Dosage varies. Injected by physician at time of testing.

Nursing Management Must be removed after x-rays; what little drug remains takes several months to absorb.

GENERIC NAME Sodium diatrizoate (injection)

TRADE NAME Hypaque (RX)

CLASSIFICATION Radiographic iodine compound

Action A contrast media that is rapidly excreted unchanged via the kidneys.

Indications for Use Urography.

Administration 30 ml of a 50% solution injected IV over 3 to 5 minutes. Onset: 5 minutes by normal kidney; up to 30 minutes in renal insufficiency.

Nursing Management If crystals form in drug solution, heat in warm water until crystals disappear. It can then be safely used.

GENERIC NAME Meglumine diatrizoate (injection)

TRADE NAMES Cardiografin, Gastrografin, Renografin (RX)

CLASSIFICATION Radiographic iodine compound

Indications for Use Angiography, urography, occasionally used as a contrast media for the GI tract.

Administration Dosage varies according to the type of x-ray procedure ordered. Can be administered by several routes, including IV, oral, IM, and enema.

GENERIC NAME Meglumine iodipamide (injection)

TRADE NAMES Cholografin, Meglumine (RX)

CLASSIFICATION Radiographic iodine compound

Indications for Use Cholangiography, cholecystography.

Administration 20 ml of a 52% solution over 10 minutes.

GENERIC NAME Sodium iodipamide (injection)

TRADE NAME Cholografin Sodium (RX)

CLASSIFICATION Radiographic iodine compound

Indications for Use Cholangiography, cholecystography.

Administration 40 ml of a 20% solution IV.

GENERIC NAME Meglumine iothalamate (injection)

TRADE NAME Conray (RX)

CLASSIFICATION Radiographic iodine compound

Action A water-soluble isomer of meglumine diatrizoate that is used for vascular studies. Since it is excreted rapidly in the kidneys, it can also be used for urography.

Indications for Use Cerebral angiography, peripheral angiography, venography, urography, cholangiography, cholecystography.

Administration Dosage varies according to procedure.

GENERIC NAME Sodium iothalamate (injection)

TRADE NAMES Angio-Conray, Conray-400 (RX)

CLASSIFICATION Radiographic iodine compound

Indications for Use Intravascular angiocardiography, aortography, urography.

Contraindications Cerebral angiography.

Administration Dosage varies according to body weight and purpose of procedure.

UNESSENTIAL MINERALS

Fluoride

GENERIC NAME Sodium fluoride (RX)

TRADE NAME Fluoritab, Luride, Pediaflor, Thera-Flur-N

CLASSIFICATION Dental caries prophylactic

Action Fluorine combines with calcium to form the apatite molecule of teeth and the fluorapatite crystals in bone. The inclusion of fluoride ions in teeth causes the enamel to be harder, thus resulting in resistance to tooth decay. Fluoride must be ingested on a daily basis throughout the development of teeth in order to be effective. However, some benefit occurs when children receive fluoride treatments and use fluoride rinses.

Indications for Use Useful to growing children for the prevention of dental caries.

Contraindications Water supply containing 0.7 parts per million (ppm) or more of fluoride.

Warnings and Precautions Use with caution in clients on sodium-restricted diets (renal failure, cardiac disorders); use in adults may cause discoloration of teeth; fluoride content of water should be known in order to prevent excessive intake of fluoride.

Untoward Reactions Mottling of teeth (fluorosis) and osteosclerosis due to prolonged intake or ingestion in adult clients. Toxicity can occur from accidental ingestion of more than 250 mg of sodium fluoride. Signs and symptoms include GI disturbances (nausea, vomiting, diarrhea, epigastric discomfort, excessive salivation), a decrease in serum protein-bound iodine, paralysis, hypotension, convulsions, and respiratory depression. Ingestion of over 500 mg can be fatal. Skin reactions, including urticaria, eczema, and dermatitis, have been reported, but rarely.

Parameters of Use

Absorption Readily absorbed from GI tract and through skin and lungs. The highly soluble compounds, such as sodium fluoride, are absorbed more completely.
Enters breast milk.

Distribution Widely; but mainly concentrated in bone, teeth, and kidneys.

Excretion Primarily via the kidneys; some excreted in sweat and feces.

Administration Dosage depends on age (tooth formation) and amount of fluoride in water ingested.

- *When the water supply is 0.2 ppm or less:* Children from birth to 2 years: 0.25 mg po daily; Ages 2 to 3 years: 0.5 mg po daily; Ages 3 to 12 years: 1.0 mg po daily.
- *When the water supply is 0.2 to 0.7 ppm:* Children from birth to 2 years: 0.125 mg po daily; Ages 2 to 3 years: 0.25 mg po daily; Ages 3 to 12 years: 0.5 mg po daily.
- *When the water supply is over 0.7 ppm:* No supplement required.

Available Drug Forms *Fluoritab:* Scored tablets containing 1 mg fluorine. *Fluorliquid:* Liquid containing 0.25 mg/gtt in polyethylene squeeze-type dropper bottles. *Luride drops:* Squeeze bottles of 30 ml peach-flavored solution containing 0.125 mg fluoride ion. *Luride Lozi-Tabs:* Tablets containing 0.25, 0.5, or 1.0 mg. *Luride-SF:* Tablets containing 1.0 mg without artificial flavoring or coloring. *Pediaflor drops:* 1 dropperful (1.0 ml) contains 0.5 mg. *Thera-Flur-N:* Gel-drops for topical application. An ingredient in several pediatric multivitamin preparations, including Poly-Vi-Flor and Tri-Vi-Flor.

Nursing Management

Planning factors

1. Determine the quantity of fluoride in the client's drinking water. Notify physician if greater than 0.7 ppm.
2. The recommended daily allowances are: Birth to 3 years: 0.5 mg; Over 3 years: 1 mg.
3. Topical gel and rinses should be applied at bedtime after teeth have been brushed.

Administration factors

1. Tablets can be swallowed and should be followed with a full glass of water.
2. Chewable tablets can be dissolved in mouth or chewed and may provide additional benefit from local contact with teeth.
3. Gel-drops are applied to the inner surface of the mouth-piece applicator and administered as follows:
   a. Spread gel-drops evenly over the inner surface of applicator.
   b. Place applicator over upper and lower teeth at the same time.
   c. Instruct the client to bite down lightly for 6 minutes.
   d. Remove the applicator and rinse mouth.
   e. Clean the applicator with cold water.
4. Liquid can be added to infant's formula or water.

Evaluation factors Excessive ingestion can cause mottling of teeth. Check teeth monthly. Notify physician or dentist if mottling is observed.

Client teaching factors

1. Instruct client to consult physician when relocating so that fluoride water content can be determined before continuing medication.
2. Warn client about excessive ingestion.

GENERIC NAME Acidulated phosphate fluoride solution

TRADE NAME Phos-Flur Oral Rinse (RX)

CLASSIFICATION Fluoride preparation

Indications for Use
Prevention of dental caries.

Administration

- *Daily rinse for children over 6 years:* Rinse vigorously with 5 to 10 ml for 1 minute, then expectorate.
- *Daily supplement for children over 3 years:* Rinse with 5 ml and swallow. (If water contains less than 0.3 ppm.)

Available Drug Forms
Each 5 ml contains 1.0 mg fluoride from sodium fluoride in a 0.1 m phosphate solution. Cherry, lime, and orange flavors are saccharin- and sugar-free; cinnamon flavor contains saccharin.

Nursing Management

1. Teeth should be brushed thoroughly before using rinse.
2. Rinse should not be swallowed if client lives in an area where water has 0.7 ppm fluoride content.
3. Can be used as a dietary supplement if water contains 0.3 to 0.7 ppm.
4. Lime-flavored solution contains FD&C yellow No. 5 (tartrazine). When first using drug, watch client for allergic reactions (bronchial asthma).

GENERIC NAME Sodium fluoride—0.2% neutral solution

TRADE NAME Point-Two Dental Rinse (RX)

CLASSIFICATION Fluoride preparation

Indications for Use
Prevention of dental caries.

Administration

- *Weekly rinse for children 6 to 12 years:* Rinse vigorously with 5 ml for 1 minute, then expectorate. Do not eat or drink for 30 minutes.
- *Weekly rinse for children over 12 years:* Rinse vigorously with 10 ml for 1 minute, then expectorate. Do not eat or drink for 30 minutes.

Available Drug Forms
Each 5 ml contains 5 mg fluoride from sodium fluoride in a mint-flavored aqueous solution containing 6% alcohol.

Nursing Management

1. Do not swallow.
2. Not for use in children under 6 years.
3. If accidentally swallowed, treat with milk or antacids to prevent GI disturbances.

GENERIC NAME Acidulated sodium fluoride gel-drops

TRADE NAME Thera-Flur (RX)

CLASSIFICATION Fluoride preparation

Indications for Use
Prevention of dental caries.

Administration
Daily topical application for children over 3 years: 4 to 8 gtt on applicator and held in mouth for 6 minutes at bedtime.

Available Drug Forms
Contains 0.5% fluoride as sodium fluoride in a lime-flavored aqueous solution containing 0.1 M phosphate.

Nursing Management
Teeth should be brushed well before using. (See sodium fluoride for further details.)

Chapter 20

Multivitamin Preparations

REQUIREMENTS FOR MULTIVITAMIN PREPARATIONS

Millions of dollars are spent on multivitamin preparations in the United States yearly. The use of vitamin supplements far in excess of the recommended daily allowance (RDA) is neither necessary or financially prudent for healthy individuals who ingest a well-balanced diet. Since the body's requirements can change daily according to the amount of exercise, pathogens encountered, and other situations in which certain vitamin requirements are increased, taking a multivitamin preparation containing near or slightly in excess of the RDA can be beneficial as a prophylactic agent. However, multivitamin preparations containing highly excessive quantities of vitamins should be avoided unless there is a therapeutic need and research has proven the therapeutic efficacy of the preparation for that disorder.

Situations in which supplemental multivitamin preparations are required include vitamin deficiencies resulting from (1) inadequate intake; (2) increased body requirements; (3) inadequate absorption; and (4) physiologic stress. Minerals are sometimes added to the preparations; but again, there should be a demonstrated need for the mineral. Inadequate intake is usually due to the type of life style and poor dietary habits. For example, many individuals who dislike vitamin-containing vegetables, omit them from the diet; busy individuals often eat at the neighborhood hamburger stand and may not eat a well-balanced diet regularly. Although a well-chosen multivitamin preparation can assist in preventing deficiencies it cannot totally compensate for bad nutrition.

Normal body requirements increase dramatically during children's growth periods, pregnancy, and lactation. Consequently, specific multivitamin and mineral preparations have been developed to meet the increased needs of these normal body changes. Small quantities of fluoride have been shown to assist in the prevention of dental caries in children and are therefore added to some pediatric multivitamin preparations. However, because excessive ingestion of fluoride can cause discoloration of the teeth, fluoride-containing preparations require a prescription.

Inadequate absorption of vitamins can occur in several gastrointestinal disturbances, including chronic diarrhea, alcoholism, pernicious anemia, and sprue. Geriatric clients may have inadequate absorption of several vitamins and therefore may require a well-chosen supplemental multivitamin preparation. Whenever possible, the deficiency should be treated with the deficient substance.

In general, prolonged physiologic stress increases the need for water-soluble vitamins. Physiologic stress may be caused by chronic febrile infections, prolonged wasting diseases, hyperthyroidism, extensive surgery or trauma, severe burns, and hemorrhaging. A number of parenteral and orally administered multivitamin preparations are available to treat the deficiencies.

PROBLEMS CAUSED BY MULTIVITAMIN PREPARATIONS

Hypervitaminosis can occur from the chronic ingestion of fat-soluble vitamins, mainly vitamin A and D. Acute toxicity can also occur. Children's preparations are often chewable and contain sweeteners and flavorings. Although the additions increase the palatability of the preparations, children sometimes consider them candy and may ingest the entire contents of the container. All multivitamin preparations should be kept out of the reach of children.

Vitamins are chemicals that can interfere with the action of certain drugs. For example, clients with Parkinson's disease who are taking levodopa should not take multivitamin preparations containing pyridoxine. The vitamin decreases the activity of levodopa.

Multivitamin preparations may obscure a disease that continues to produce harmful effects. For example, preparations containing 0.1 mg of folic acid may correct the anemic blood picture of a client with pernicious anemia while the neurologic manifestations progress.

The selection of an appropriate multivitamin preparation for a client requires a careful assessment of daily intake, daily requirements, and special needs. Collaboration between the nurse, physician, and pharmacist is recommended.

PEDIATRIC

Multivitamin Preparations

TRADE NAME Cari-Tab Softab (RX)

CLASSIFICATION Pediatric multivitamin preparation

Administration Infants: ½ tablet crushed and mixed in food or formula; Ages 2 to 3 years: 1 tablet po daily after meals; Ages 3 to 16 years: 2 tablets po daily after meals.

Available Drug Forms Generic contents in each chewable tablet: *Vitamins:* A (palmitate): 2000 U.S.P. units; D: 200 U.S.P. units; C (ascorbic acid and sodium ascorbate): 75 mg. *Mineral:* fluoride: 0.5 mg.

TRADE NAME Mulvidren-F Softab (RX)

CLASSIFICATION Pediatric multivitamin preparation

Administration Ages 2 to 3 years: ½ tablet po daily; Ages 3 to 16 years: 1 tablet po daily.

Available Drug Forms Generic contents in each chewable tablet: *Vitamins:* A: 4000 U.S.P. units; D: 400 U.S.P. units; C (ascorbic acid and sodium ascorbate): 75 mg; thiamine mononitrate (B_1): 2 mg; riboflavin (B_2): 2 mg; niacinamide (B_3): 10 mg; calcium pantothenate (B_5): 3 mg; pyridoxine (B_6): 1.2 mg; cyanocobalamin (B_{12}): 3 mcg. *Mineral:* fluoride: 1 mg.

TRADE NAME Poly-Vi-Flor (RX)

CLASSIFICATION Pediatric multivitamin preparation

Administration Usual dosage: 1.0 ml of liquid po daily for infants and children under 3 years; 1 tablet po daily for children 2 to 3 years or more.

Available Drug Forms Chewable tablets or liquid. Generic contents in each chewable tablet: *Vitamins:* A: 2500 IU; D: 400 IU; E: 15 IU; C: 60 mg; thiamine (B_1): 1.05 mg; riboflavin (B_2): 1.2 mg; niacin (B_3): 13.5 mg; pyridoxine (B_6): 1.05 mg; cyanocobalamin (B_{12}): 4.5 mcg; folic acid: 0.3 mg. *Mineral:* fluoride: 1 mg. Generic contents in 1 ml of liquid: *Vitamins:* A: 1500 IU; D: 400 IU; E: 5 IU; C: 35 mg; thiamine (B_1): 0.5 mg; riboflavin (B_2): 0.6 mg; niacin (B_3): 8 mg; pyridoxine (B_6): 0.4 mg; cyanocobalamin (B_{12}): 2 mcg. *Mineral:* fluoride: 0.5 mg.

TRADE NAME Poly-Vi-Flor 0.25 mg (RX)

CLASSIFICATION Pediatric multivitamin preparation

Administration Usual dosage: 1.0 ml of liquid po daily for infants and children under 2 years.

Available Drug Forms Generic contents in 1 ml of liquid: *Vitamins:* A: 1500 IU; D: 400 IU; E: 5 IU; C: 35 mg; thiamine (B_1): 0.5 mg; riboflavin (B_2): 0.6 mg; niacin (B_3): 8 mg; pyridoxine (B_6): 0.4 mg; cyanocobalamin (B_{12}): 2 mcg. *Mineral:* fluoride: 0.25 mg.

TRADE NAME Poly-Vi-Flor 0.5 mg (RX)

CLASSIFICATION Pediatric multivitamin preparation

Administration Usual dosage: ½ tablet po daily for children 2 to 3 years or more.

Available Drug Forms Generic contents in each chewable tablet: *Vitamins:* A: 2500 IU; D: 400 IU; E: 15 IU; C: 60 mg; thiamine (B_1): 1.05 mg; riboflavin (B_2): 1.2 mg; niacin (B_3): 13.5 mg; pyridoxine (B_6): 1.05 mg; cyanocobalamin (B_{12}): 4.5 mcg; folacin: 0.3 mg. *Mineral:* fluoride: 0.5 mg.

TRADE NAME Poly-Vi-Flor with Iron (RX)

CLASSIFICATION Pediatric multivitamin preparation

Administration Usual dosage: 1 tablet po daily for children over 3 years; 1.0 ml of liquid po daily for children 2 to 3 years or more.

Available Drug Forms Chewable tablets or liquid. Generic contents in each chewable tablet: *Vitamins:* A: 2500 IU; D: 400 IU; E: 15 IU; C: 60 mg; thiamine (B_1): 1.05 mg; riboflavin (B_2): 1.2 mg; niacin (B_3): 13.5 mg; pyridoxine (B_6): 1.05 mg; cyanocobalamin (B_{12}): 4.5 mcg; folic acid: 0.3 mg. *Minerals:* fluoride: 1 mg; iron: 12 mg. Generic contents in 1 ml of liquid: *Vitamins:* A: 1500 IU; D: 400 IU;

E: 5 IU; C: 35 mg; thiamine (B_1): 0.5 mg; riboflavin (B_2): 0.6 mg; niacin (B_3): 8 mg; pyridoxine (B_6): 0.4 mg. *Minerals:* fluoride: 0.5 mg; iron: 10 mg.

TRADE NAME Poly-Vi-Sol (OTC)

CLASSIFICATION Pediatric multivitamin preparation

Administration Usual dosage: 1.0 ml of liquid po daily for children 2 years of age, 1 tablet po daily for children 4 years of age.

Available Drug Forms Chewable tablets or liquid. Generic contents in each chewable tablet: *Vitamins:* A: 2500 IU; D: 400 IU; E: 35 IU; C: 60 mg; thiamine (B_1): 1.2 mg; riboflavin (B_2): 1.2 mg; niacin (B_3): 13.5 mg; pyridoxine (B_6): 1.05 mg; cyanocobalamin (B_{12}): 4.5 mcg. Generic contents in 1 ml of liquid: *Vitamins:* A: 1500 IU; D: 400 IU; E: 5 IU; C: 35 mg; thiamine (B_1): 0.5 mg; riboflavin (B_2): 0.6 mg; niacin (B_3): 8 mg; pyridoxine (B_6): 0.4 mg; cyanocobalamin (B_{12}): 2 mcg.

TRADE NAME Poly-Vi-Sol with Iron (OTC)

CLASSIFICATION Pediatric multivitamin preparation

Administration Usual dosage: 1 tablet po daily for children over 2 years; 1.0 ml of liquid po daily for infants and children under 4 years.

Available Drug Forms Chewable tablets or liquid. Generic contents in each chewable tablet: *Vitamins:* A: 2500 IU; D: 400 IU; E: 35 IU; C: 60 mg; thiamine (B_1): 1.05 mg; riboflavin (B_2): 1.2 mg; niacin (B_3): 13.5 mg; pyridoxine (B_6): 1.05 mg. *Mineral:* iron: 12 mg. Generic contents in 1 ml of liquid: *Vitamins:* A: 1500 IU; D: 400 IU; E: 5 IU; C: 35 mg; thiamine (B_1): 0.5 mg; riboflavin (B_2): 0.6 mg; niacin (B_3): 8 mg; pyridoxine (B_6): 0.4 mg. *Mineral:* iron: 10 mg.

TRADE NAME Tri-Vi-Flor (RX)

CLASSIFICATION Pediatric multivitamin preparation

Administration Usual dosage: 1.0 ml of liquid po daily for children 2 to 3 years or more; 1 tablet po daily for children over 3 years.

Available Drug Forms Chewable tablets or liquid. Generic contents in 1 ml of liquid: *Vitamins:* A: 1500 IU; D: 400 IU; C: 35 mg. *Mineral:* fluoride: 0.5 mg. Generic contents in each chewable tablet: *Vitamins:* A: 2500 IU; D: 400 IU; C: 60 mg. *Mineral:* fluoride: 1 mg.

TRADE NAME Tri-Vi-Flor 0.25 mg (RX)

CLASSIFICATION Pediatric multivitamin preparation

Administration Usual dosage: 1.0 ml of liquid po daily for infants and children under 2 years.

Available Drug Forms Generic contents in 1 ml of liquid: *Vitamins:* A: 1500 IU; D: 400 IU; C: 35 mg. *Mineral:* fluoride: 0.25 mg.

TRADE NAME Tri-Vi-Flor with Iron (RX)

CLASSIFICATION Pediatric multivitamin preparation

Administration Usual dosage: 1.0 ml of liquid po daily for infants and children under 2 years.

Available Drug Forms Generic contents in 1 ml of liquid: *Vitamins:* A: 1500 IU; D: 400 IU; C: 35 mg. *Minerals:* fluoride: 0.25 mg; iron: 10 mg.

TRADE NAME Tri-Vi-Sol (OTC)

CLASSIFICATION Pediatric multivitamin preparation

Administration Usual dosage: 1 tablet po daily for children over 2 years; 1.0 ml of liquid po daily for infants and children under 4 years.

Available Drug Forms Chewable tablets or liquid. Generic contents in each chewable tablet: *Vitamins:* A: 2500 IU; D: 400 IU; C: 60 mg. Generic contents in 1 ml of liquid: *Vitamins:* A: 1500 IU; D: 400 IU; C: 35 mg.

TRADE NAME Tri-Vi-Sol with Iron (OTC)

CLASSIFICATION Pediatric multivitamin preparation

Administration Usual dosage: 1.0 ml of liquid po daily for infants and children under 4 years.

Available Drug Forms Generic contents in 1 ml of liquid: *Vitamins:* A: 1500 IU; D: 400 IU; C: 35 mg. *Mineral:* iron: 10 mg.

TRADE NAME Vi-Daylin ADC Drops (OTC)

CLASSIFICATION Pediatric multivitamin preparation

Administration Usual dosage: 1.0 ml of liquid po daily for infants and children under 4 years.

Available Drug Forms Generic contents in 1 ml of liquid: *Vitamins:* A: 1500 IU; D: 400 IU; C: 35 mg.

TRADE NAME Vi-Daylin Drops (OTC)

CLASSIFICATION Pediatric multivitamin preparation

Administration Usual dosage: 1.0 ml of liquid po daily for infants and children under 4 years.

Available Drug Forms Generic contents in 1 ml of liquid: *Vitamins:* A: 1500 IU; D: 400 IU; E: 5 IU; C: 35 mg; thiamine (B_1): 0.5 mg; riboflavin (B_2): 0.6 mg; niacin (B_3): 8 mg; pyridoxine (B_6): 0.4 mg; cyanocobalamin (B_{12}): 1.5 mcg.

TRADE NAME Vi-Daylin/F ADC Drops (RX)

CLASSIFICATION Pediatric multivitamin preparation

Administration Usual dosage: 1.0 ml of liquid po daily for infants and children under 4 years.

Available Drug Forms Generic contents in 1 ml of liquid: *Vitamins:* A: 1500 IU; D: 400 IU; C: 35 mg. *Mineral:* fluoride: 0.25 mg.

TRADE NAME Vi-Daylin/F ADC + Iron Drops (RX)

CLASSIFICATION Pediatric multivitamin preparation

Administration Usual dosage: 1.0 ml of liquid po daily for infants and children under 4 years.

Available Drug Forms Generic contents in 1 ml of liquid: *Vitamins:* A: 1500 IU; D: 400 IU; C: 35 mg. *Minerals:* fluoride: 0.25 mg; iron: 10 mg.

TRADE NAME Vi-Daylin/F Drops (RX)

CLASSIFICATION Pediatric multivitamin preparation

Administration Usual dosage: 1.0 ml of liquid po daily for infants and children under 4 years.

Available Drug Forms Generic contents in 1 ml of liquid: *Vitamins:* A: 1500 IU; D: 400 IU; E: 5 IU; C: 35 mg; thiamine (B_1): 0.5 mg; riboflavin (B_2): 0.6 mg; niacin (B_3): 8 mg; pyridoxine (B_6): 0.4 mg. *Mineral:* fluoride: 0.25 mg.

TRADE NAME Vi-Daylin/F + Iron (RX)

CLASSIFICATION Pediatric multivitamin preparation

Administration Ages 2 to 3 years: $\frac{1}{2}$ tablet po daily; Ages 3 or more years: 1 tablet po daily.

Available Drug Forms Generic contents in each chewable tablet: *Vitamins:* A: 2500 IU; D: 400 IU; E: 15 IU; C (ascorbic acid and sodium ascorbate): 60 mg; thiamine (B_1): 1.05 mg; riboflavin (B_2): 1.2 mg; niacin (B_3): 13.5 mg; pyridoxine (B_6): 1.05 mg; cyanocobalamin (B_{12}): 4.5 mcg; folic acid: 0.3 mg. *Minerals:* fluoride: 1 mg; iron: 12 mg.

TRADE NAME Vi-Daylin/F + Iron Drops (RX)

CLASSIFICATION Pediatric multivitamin preparation

Administration Usual dosage: 1.0 ml of liquid po daily for infants and children under 4 years.

Available Drug Forms Generic contents in 1 ml of liquid: *Vitamins:* A: 1500 IU; D: 400 IU; E: 5 IU; C: 35 mg; thiamine (B_1): 0.5 mg; riboflavin (B_2): 0.6 mg; niacin (B_3): 8 mg; pyridoxine (B_6): 0.4 mg. *Minerals:* fluoride: 0.25 mg; iron: 10 mg.

TRADE NAME Vi-Daylin Plus Iron Drops (OTC)

CLASSIFICATION Pediatric multivitamin preparation

Administration Usual dosage: 1.0 ml of liquid po daily for infants and children under 4 years.

Available Drug Forms Generic contents in 1 ml of liquid: *Vitamins:* A: 1500 IU; D: 400 IU; E: 5 IU; C: 35 mg; thiamine (B_1): 0.5 mg; riboflavin (B_2): 0.6 mg; niacin (B_3): 8 mg; pyridoxine (B_6): 0.4 mg; cyanocobalamin (B_{12}): 1.5 mcg. *Mineral:* iron: 10 mg.

TRADE NAME Vi-Daylin Plus Iron ADC Drops (OTC)

CLASSIFICATION Pediatric multivitamin preparation

Administration Usual dosage: 1.0 ml of liquid po daily for infants and children under 4 years.

Available Drug Forms Generic contents in 1 ml of liquid: *Vitamins:* A: 1500 IU; D: 400 IU; C: 35 mg. *Mineral:* iron: 10 mg.

TRADE NAME Vi-Daylin (OTC)

CLASSIFICATION Pediatric multivitamin preparation

Administration Usual dosage: 1 tablet po daily for children and adults.

Available Drug Forms Generic contents in each chewable tablet: *Vitamins:* A: 2500 IU; D: 400 IU; E: 15 IU; C: 60 mg; thiamine (B_1): 1.05 mg; riboflavin (B_2): 1.2 mg; niacin (B_3): 13.5 mg; pyridoxine (B_6): 1.05 mg; cyanocobalamin (B_{12}): 4.5 mcg; folic acid: 0.3 mg.

TRADE NAME Vi-Daylin/F (RX)

CLASSIFICATION Pediatric multivitamin preparation

Administration Ages 2 to 3 years: $\frac{1}{2}$ tablet po daily; Ages 3 years or more: 1 tablet po daily.

Available Drug Forms Generic contents in each chewable tablet: *Vitamins:* A: 2500 IU; D: 400 IU; E: 15 IU; C (ascorbic acid and sodium ascorbate): 60 mg; thiamine mononitrate (B_1): 1.05 mg; riboflavin (B_2): 1.2 mg; niacin (B_3): 13.5 mg; pyridoxine (B_6): 1.05 mg; cyanocobalamin (B_{12}): 4.5 mcg; folic acid: 0.3 mg. *Mineral:* fluoride: 1 mg.

TRADE NAME Vi-Daylin + Iron (OTC)

CLASSIFICATION Pediatric multivitamin preparation

Administration Usual dosage: 1 tablet po daily for children and adults.

Available Drug Forms Generic contents in each chewable tablet: *Vitamins:* A: 2500 IU; D: 400 IU; E: 15 IU; C: 60 mg; thiamine (B_1): 1.05 mg; riboflavin (B_2): 1.2 mg; niacin (B_3): 13.5 mg; pyridoxine (B_6): 1.05 mg; cyanocobalamin (B_{12}): 4.5 mcg; folic acid: 0.3 mg. *Mineral:* iron: 12 mg.

TRADE NAME Vi-Daylin Liquid (OTC)

CLASSIFICATION Pediatric multivitamin preparation

Administration Usual dosage: 1 tsp (5 ml) of liquid po daily for children and adults.

Available Drug Forms Generic contents in 5 ml of liquid: *Vitamins:* A: 2500 IU; D: 400 IU; E: 15 IU; C: 60 mg; thiamine (B_1): 1.05 mg; riboflavin (B_2): 1.2 mg; niacin (B_3): 13.5 mg; pyridoxine (B_6): 1.05 mg; cyanocobalamin (B_{12}): 4.5 mcg.

TRADE NAME Vi-Daylin Plus Iron Liquid (OTC)

CLASSIFICATION Pediatric multivitamin preparation

Administration Usual dosage: 1 tsp (5 ml) of liquid po daily for children and adults.

Available Drug Forms Generic contents in 5 ml of liquid: *Vitamins:* A: 2500 IU; D: 400 IU; E: 15 IU; C: 60 mg; thiamine (B_1): 1.05 mg; riboflavin (B_2): 1.2 mg; niacin (B_3): 13.5 mg; pyridoxine (B_6): 1.05 mg; cyanocobalamin (B_{12}): 4.5 mcg. *Mineral:* iron: 10 mg.

PREGNANCY AND LACTATION

Multivitamin and Mineral Preparations

TRADE NAME Calinate-FA (RX)

CLASSIFICATION Multivitamin and mineral preparation for pregnancy and lactation

Warnings and Precautions Folic acid content may mask the progressive neurologic damage in clients with pernicious anemia.

Administration Usual dosage: 1 tablet po daily before a meal.

Available Drug Forms Generic contents in each tablet: *Vitamins:* A (palmitate): 4000 U.S.P. units; D_2:

400 U.S.P. units; C (sodium ascorbate): 50 mg; thiamine mononitrate (B_1): 3 mg; riboflavin (B_2): 3 mg; niacinamide (B_3): 20 mg; pyridoxine (B_6): 5 mg; *d*-panthenol (B_5): 1 mg; cyanocobalamin (B_{12}): 1 mcg; folic acid: 1 mg. *Minerals:* calcium (carbonate): 250 mg; iodine (potassium iodide): 0.02 mg; iron (fumarate): 60 mg; magnesium (oxide): 0.2 mg; manganese (oxide): 0.2 mg; zinc (oxide): 0.1 mg; copper (oxide): 0.15 mg.

TRADE NAME En-Cebrin (OTC)

CLASSIFICATION Multivitamin and mineral preparation for pregnancy and lactation

Administration Usual dosage: 1 Pulvule po daily.

Available Drug Forms Generic contents in each Pulvule: *Vitamins:* A: 4000 IU; D: 400 IU; C: 50 mg; thiamine mononitrate (B_1): 3 mg; riboflavin (B_2): 2 mg; niacinamide (B_3): 10 mg; pantothenic acid (B_5): 5 mg; pyridoxine (B_6): 1.7 mg; cyanocobalamin (B_{12}): 5 mcg. *Minerals:* calcium (carbonate): 250 mg; copper (sulfate): 1 mg; iodine (potassium iodide): 0.15 mg; iron (fumarate): 30 mg; magnesium (hydroxide): 5 mg; manganese (glycerophosphate): 1 mg; zinc (chloride): 1.5 mg.

TRADE NAME En-Cebrin F (RX)

CLASSIFICATION Multivitamin and mineral preparation for pregnancy and lactation

Warnings and Precautions Folic acid content may mask the progressive neurologic damage in clients with pernicious anemia.

Administration Usual dosage: 1 Pulvule daily.

Available Drug Forms Generic contents in each Pulvule: *Vitamins:* A: 4000 IU; D: 400 IU; C: 50 mg; thiamine mononitrate (B_1): 3 mg; riboflavin (B_2): 2 mg; niacinamide (B_3): 10 mg; calcium pantothenate (B_5): 5 mg; pyridoxine (B_6): 2 mg; cyanocobalamin (B_{12}): 5 mcg; folic acid: 1 mg. *Minerals:* calcium (carbonate): 250 mg; copper (sulfate): 1 mg; iodine (potassium iodide): 0.15 mg; iron (fumarate): 30 mg; magnesium (hydroxide): 5 mg; manganese (glycerophosphate): 1 mg; zinc (chloride): 1.5 mg.

TRADE NAME Engran-HP (OTC)

CLASSIFICATION Multivitamin and mineral preparation for pregnancy and lactation

Administration Usual dosage: 1 tablet po bid.

Available Drug Forms Generic contents in each tablet: *Vitamins:* A: 4000 IU; D: 200 IU; E: 15 IU; C: 30 mg; thiamine (B_1): 0.85 mg; riboflavin (B_2): 1 mg; niacin (B_3): 10 mg; pyridoxine (B_6): 1.25 mg; cyanocobalamin (B_{12}): 4 mcg; folic acid: 0.4 mg. *Minerals:* calcium: 325 mg; iodine: 75 mcg; iron: 9 mg; magnesium: 50 mg.

Nursing Management Store at room temperature away from excessive heat.

TRADE NAME Filibon (OTC)

CLASSIFICATION Multivitamin and mineral preparation for pregnancy and lactation

Administration Usual dosage: 1 tablet po daily.

Available Drug Forms Generic contents in each tablet: *Vitamins:* A (acetate): 5000 IU; D_2: 400 IU; E: 30 IU; C: 60 mg; thiamine mononitrate (B_1): 1.5 mg; riboflavin (B_2): 1.7 mg; niacinamide (B_3): 20 mg; pyridoxine (B_6): 2 mg; cyanocobalamin (B_{12}): 6 mcg; folic acid: 0.4 mg. *Minerals:* calcium (carbonate): 125 mg; iodine (potassium iodide): 150 mcg; iron (fumarate): 18 mg; magnesium (oxide): 100 mg.

TRADE NAME Filibon F.A. (RX)

CLASSIFICATION Multivitamin and mineral preparation for pregnancy and lactation

Warnings and Precautions Folic acid content may mask the progressive neurologic damage in clients with pernicious anemia.

Administration Usual dosage: 1 tablet po daily.

Available Drug Forms Generic contents in each tablet: *Vitamins:* A (acetate): 8000 IU; D_2: 400 IU; E: 30 IU; C: 60 mg; thiamine mononitrate (B_1): 1.7 mg; riboflavin (B_2): 2 mg; niacinamide (B_3): 20 mg; pyridoxine (B_6): 4 mg; cyanocobalamin (B_{12}): 8 mcg; folacin: 1 mg. *Minerals:* calcium (carbonate): 250 mg; iodine (potassium iodide): 150 mcg; iron (fumarate): 45 mg; magnesium (oxide): 100 mg.

TRADE NAME Filibon Forte (RX)

CLASSIFICATION Multivitamin and mineral preparation for pregnancy and lactation

Warnings and Precautions: Folic acid content may mask the progressive neurologic damage in clients with pernicious anemia.

Administration Usual dosage: 1 tablet daily.

Available Drug Forms Generic contents in each tablet: *Vitamins:* A (acetate): 8000 IU; D_2: 400 IU; E:

45 IU; C: 90 mg; thiamine mononitrate (B_1): 2 mg; riboflavin (B_2): 2.5 mg; niacinamide (B_3): 30 mg; pyridoxine (B_6): 3 mg; cyanocobalamin (B_{12}): 12 mcg; folacin: 1 mg. *Minerals:* calcium (carbonate): 300 mg; iodine (potassium iodide): 200 mcg; iron (fumarate): 45 mg; magnesium (oxide): 100 mg.

TRADE NAME Filibon OT (RX)

CLASSIFICATION Multivitamin and mineral preparation for pregnancy and lactation

Indications for Use Particularly useful for pregnant women with hemorrhoids.

Warnings and Precautions Folic acid content may mask the progressive neurologic damage in clients with pernicious anemia. Contains the stool softener, docusate.

Administration Usual dosage: 1 tablet po daily.

Available Drug Forms Generic contents in each film-coated tablet: *Vitamins:* A (acetate): 4000 U.S.P. units; D_2: 400 U.S.P. units; E: 30 IU; C: 60 mg; thiamine mononitrate (B_1): 1.7 mg; riboflavin (B_2): 2 mg; niacinamide (B_3): 20 mg; pyridoxine (B_6): 2.5 mg; cyanocobalamin (B_{12}): 8 mcg; folacin: 1 mg. *Minerals:* calcium (carbonate): 250 mg; iodine (potassium iodide): 150 mcg; iron (fumarate): 30 mg; magnesium (oxide): 100 mg. *Other substances:* docusate sodium: 100 mg.

TRADE NAME Iromin-G (OTC)

CLASSIFICATION Multivitamin and mineral preparation, hematinic supplement

Indications for Use Secondary anemia, anemia during pregnancy and lactation.

Warnings and Precautions Folic acid content may mask the progressive neurologic damage in clients with pernicious anemia.

Administration Usual dosage: 1 tablet po bid or tid with meals.

Available Drug Forms Generic contents in each tablet: *Vitamins:* A (acetate): 4000 U.S.P. units; D_2: 400 U.S.P. units; C: 100 mg; thiamine mononitrate (B_1): 5 mg; riboflavin (B_2): 2 mg; niacinamide (B_3): 10 mg; *d*-calcium pantothenate (B_5): 1 mg; pyridoxine (B_6): 25 mg; cyanocobalamin (B_{12}): 2 mcg; folic acid: 0.8 mg. *Minerals:* calcium (carbonate, gluconate, lactate): 50 mg; iron (gluconate): 38.6 mg.

TRADE NAME Materna 1•60 (RX)

CLASSIFICATION Multivitamin and mineral preparation for pregnancy and lactation

Warnings and Precautions Folic acid content may mask the progressive neurologic damage in clients with pernicious anemia. Contains the stool softener, docusate.

Administration Usual dosage: 1 tablet po daily.

Available Drug Forms Generic contents in each film-coated tablet: *Vitamins:* A (acetate): 8000 IU; D: 400 IU; E: 30 IU; C: 120 mg; thiamine mononitrate (B_1): 3 mg; riboflavin (B_2): 3.4 mg; niacinamide (B_3): 20 mg; pyridoxine (B_6): 4 mg; cyanocobalamin (B_{12}): 12 mcg; folacin: 1 mg. *Minerals:* calcium (carbonate): 250 mg; copper (oxide): 2 mg; iodine (potassium iodide): 0.3 mg; iron (fumarate): 60 mg; magnesium (oxide): 100 mg; zinc (oxide): 15 mg. *Other substances:* docusate sodium: 50 mg.

TRADE NAME Mission Prenatal (OTC)

CLASSIFICATION Multivitamin and mineral preparation for pregnancy and lactation

Warnings and Precautions Folic acid content may mask the progressive neurologic damage in clients with pernicious anemia.

Administration Usual dosage: 1 tablet po daily at bedtime.

Available Drug Forms Generic contents in each tablet: *Vitamins:* A (acetate): 4000 U.S.P. units; D_2: 400 U.S.P. units; C: 100 mg; thiamine mononitrate (B_1): 5 mg; riboflavin (B_2): 2 mg; niacinamide (B_3): 10 mg; *d*-calcium pantothenate (B_5): 1 mg; pyridoxine (B_6): 3 mg; cyanocobalamin (B_{12}): 2 mcg; folic acid: 0.4 mg. *Minerals:* calcium (carbonate, gluconate, lactate): 50 mg; iron (gluconate): 38.6 mg.

TRADE NAME Mission Prenatal F.A. (OTC)

CLASSIFICATION Multivitamin and mineral preparation for pregnancy and lactation

Warnings and Precautions Folic acid content may mask the progressive neurologic damage in clients with pernicious anemia.

Administration Usual dosage: 1 tablet po daily at bedtime.

Available Drug Forms Generic contents in each tablet: *Vitamins:* A: 4000 U.S.P. units; D_2: 400 U.S.P. units; C: 100 mg; thiamine mononitrate (B_1): 5 mg; riboflavin (B_2): 2 mg; niacinamide (B_3): 10 mg; *d*-calcium pantothenate (B_5): 1 mg; pyridoxine (B_6): 10 mg; cyanocobalamin (B_{12}): 2 mcg; folic acid: 0.8 mg. *Minerals:* calcium (carbonate, gluconate, lactate): 50 mg; iron (gluconate): 38.6 mg; zinc (sulfate): 15 mg.

TRADE NAME Mission Prenatal H.P. (RX)

CLASSIFICATION Multivitamin and mineral preparation for pregnancy and lactation

Warnings and Precautions Folic acid content may mask the progressive neurologic damage in clients with pernicious anemia.

Administration Usual dosage: 1 tablet po daily at bedtime.

Available Drug Forms Generic contents in each tablet: *Vitamins:* A: 4000 U.S.P. units; D_2: 400 U.S.P. units; C: 100 mg; thiamine mononitrate (B_1): 5 mg; riboflavin (B_2): 2 mg; niacinamide (B_3): 10 mg; *d*-calcium pantothenate (B_5): 1 mg; pyridoxine (B_6): 25 mg; cyanocobalamin (B_{12}): 2 mcg; folic acid: 1 mg. *Minerals:* calcium (carbonate, gluconate, lactate): 50 mg; iron (gluconate): 38.6 mg.

TRADE NAME Natabec Kapseals (OTC)

CLASSIFICATION Multivitamin and mineral preparation for pregnancy and lactation

Administration Usual dosage: 1 Kapseal po daily.

Available Drug Forms Generic contents in each Kapseal: *Vitamins:* A: 4000 IU; D: 400 IU; C: 50 mg; thiamine (B_1): 3 mg; riboflavin (B_2): 2 mg; niacinamide (B_3): 10 mg; pyridoxine (B_6): 3 mg; cyanocobalamin (B_{12}): 5 mcg. *Minerals:* calcium (carbonate): 600 mg; iron (sulfate): 30 mg.

TRADE NAME Natabec Rx Kapseals (RX)

CLASSIFICATION Multivitamin and mineral preparation for pregnancy and lactation

Warnings and Precautions Folic acid content may mask the progressive neurologic damage in clients with pernicious anemia.

Administration Usual dosage: 1 Kapseal po daily.

Available Drug Forms Generic contents in each Kapseal: *Vitamins:* A: 4000 IU; D: 400 IU; C: 50 mg; thiamine (B_1): 3 mg; riboflavin (B_2): 2 mg; niacinamide (B_3): 10 mg; pyridoxine (B_6): 3 mg; cyanocobalamin (B_{12}): 5 mcg; folic acid: 1 mg. *Minerals:* calcium carbonate: 600 mg; ferrous sulfate: 30 mg.

TRADE NAME Natafort Filmseal (RX)

CLASSIFICATION Multivitamin and mineral preparation for pregnancy and lactation

Warnings and Precautions Folic acid content may mask the progressive neurologic damage in clients with pernicious anemia. Contains the stool softener, docusate.

Administration Usual dosage: 1 tablet po daily.

Available Drug Forms Generic contents in each tablet: *Vitamins:* A: 6000 IU: D: 400 IU; E: 30 IU; C: 120 mg; thiamine (B_1): 3 mg; riboflavin (B_2): 2 mg; niacinamide (B_3): 20 mg; pyridoxine (B_6): 15 mg; cyanocobalamin (B_{12}): 6 mcg; folic acid: 1 mg. *Minerals:* calcium (carbonate): 350 mg; iron (fumarate): 65 mg; magnesium (oxide): 100 mg; zinc (oxide): 25 mg; iodine (potassium iodide): 0.15 mg; *Other substances:* docusate sodium: 50 mg.

TRADE NAME Natalins (OTC)

CLASSIFICATION Multivitamin and mineral preparation for pregnancy and lactation

Administration Usual dosage: 1 tablet po daily.

Available Drug Forms Generic contents in each tablet: *Vitamins:* A (acetate): 8000 IU; D: 400 IU; E: 30 IU; C: (sodium ascorbate): 90 mg; thiamine mononitrate (B_1): 1.7 mg; riboflavin (B_2): 2 mg; niacinamide (B_3): 20 mg; pyridoxine (B_6): 4 mg; cyanocobalamin (B_{12}): 8 mcg; folacin: 0.8 mg. *Minerals:* calcium (carbonate): 200 mg; iron (fumarate): 45 mg; magnesium (hydroxide): 100 mg; iodine (calcium iodate): 150 mcg.

TRADE NAME Natalins RX (RX)

CLASSIFICATION Multivitamin and mineral preparation for pregnancy and lactation

Warnings and Precautions Folic acid content may mask the progressive neurologic damage in clients with pernicious anemia.

Administration Usual dosage: 1 tablet po daily.

Available Drug Forms Generic contents in each tablet: *Vitamins:* A (acetate): 8000 IU; D: 400 IU; E: 30 IU; C: (sodium ascorbate): 90 mg; thiamine mononitrate (B_1): 2.55 mg; riboflavin (B_2): 3 mg; niacinamide (B_3): 20 mg; pantothenic acid (B_5): 15 mg; pyridoxine (B_6): 10 mg; cyanocobalamin (B_{12}): 8 mcg; folacin: 1 mg; biotin: 0.05 mg. *Minerals:* calcium (carbonate): 200 mg; iron (fumarate): 60 mg; magnesium (hydroxide): 100 mg; copper (oxide): 2 mg; zinc (oxide): 15 mg; iodine (calcium iodate): 150 mcg.

TRADE NAME Niferex-PN RX

CLASSIFICATION Multivitamin and mineral preparation for pregnancy and lactation

Warnings and Precautions Folic acid content may mask the progressive neurologic damage in clients with pernicious anemia.

Administration Usual dosage: 1 tablet po daily.

Available Drug Forms Generic contents in each film-coated tablet: *Vitamins:* A: 4000 IU; D_2: 400 IU; C (sodium ascorbate): 50 mg; thiamine mononitrate (B_1): 3 mg; riboflavin (B_2): 3 mg; niacinamide (B_3): 10 mg; pyridoxine (B_6): 2 mg; cyanocobalamin (B_{12}): 3 mcg; folic acid: 1 mg. *Minerals:* calcium carbonate: 312 mg; iron (polysaccharide-iron complex): 60 mg; zinc sulfate: 80 mg.

TRADE NAME Nu-Iron-V RX

CLASSIFICATION Multivitamin and mineral preparation for pregnancy and lactation

Warnings and Precautions Folic acid content may mask the progressive neurologic damage in clients with pernicious anemia.

Administration Usual dosage: 1 tablet po daily.

Available Drug Forms Generic contents in each film-coated tablet: *Vitamins:* A: 4000 IU; D_2: 400 IU; C (sodium ascorbate): 50 mg; thiamine mononitrate (B_1): 3 mg; riboflavin (B_2): 3 mg; niacinamide (B_3): 10 mg; pyridoxine (B_6): 2 mg; cyanocobalamin (B_{12}): 3 mcg; folic acid: 1 mg. *Minerals:* calcium carbonate: 312 mg; iron (polysaccharide-iron complex): 60 mg.

TRADE NAME Pramet F.A. RX

CLASSIFICATION Multivitamin and mineral preparation for pregnancy and lactation

Warnings and Precautions Folic acid content may mask the progressive neurologic damage in clients with pernicious anemia.

Administration Usual dosage: 1 tablet po daily.

Available Drug Forms Generic contents in each film-coated tablet: *Vitamins:* A (acetate and palmitate): 4000 IU; D: 400 IU; C: 100 mg; thiamine mononitrate (B_1): 3 mg; riboflavin (B_2): 2 mg; niacinamide (B_3): 10 mg; calcium pantothenate (B_5): 0.92 mg; pyridoxine (B_6): 5 mg; cyanocobalamin (B_{12}): 3 mcg; folic acid: 1 mg. *Minerals:* calcium (carbonate); 250 mg; iron (sulfate): 60 mg; copper (chloride): 0.15 mg; iodine (calcium iodate): 100 mcg.

TRADE NAME Pramilet F.A. RX

CLASSIFICATION Multivitamin and mineral preparation for pregnancy and lactation

Administration Usual dosage: 1 tablet po daily.

Available Drug Forms Generic contents in each film-coated tablet: *Vitamins:* A (acetate and palmitate): 4000 IU; D: 400 IU; C (sodium ascorbate): 60 mg; thiamine mononitrate (B_1): 3 mg; riboflavin (B_2): 2 mg; niacinamide (B_3): 10 mg; calcium pantothenate (B_5): 1 mg; pyridoxine (B_6): 3 mg; cyanocobalamin (B_{12}): 3 mcg; folic acid: 1 mg. *Minerals:* calcium (carbonate): 250 mg; iron (fumarate): 40 mg; magnesium (oxide): 10 mg; copper (chloride): 0.15 mg; zinc (oxide): 0.085 mg; iodine (calcium iodate): 100 mcg.

TRADE NAME Stuart Prenatal OTC

CLASSIFICATION Multivitamin and mineral preparation for pregnancy and lactation

Administration Usual dosage: 1 tablet po daily after a meal.

Available Drug Forms Generic contents in each tablet: *Vitamins:* A (acetate): 8000 IU; D: 400 IU; E: 30 IU; C: 60 mg; thiamine mononitrate (B_1): 1.7 mg; riboflavin (B_2): 2 mg; niacinamide (B_3): 20 mg; pyridoxine (B_6): 4 mg; cyanocobalamin (B_{12}): 8 mcg; folic acid: 0.8 mg. *Minerals:* calcium (sulfate): 200 mg; iron (fumarate): 60 mg; magnesium (oxide): 100 mg; iodine (potassium iodide): 150 mcg.

TRADE NAME Stuart Prenatal with Folic Acid RX

CLASSIFICATION Multivitamin and mineral preparation for pregnancy and lactation

Warnings and Precautions Contains FD&C yellow No. 5 (tartrazine) and may cause hypersensitivity reactions, particularly in individuals who are allergic to aspirin. Folic acid content may mask the progressive neurologic damage in clients with pernicious anemia.

Administration Usual dosage: 1 tablet po daily after a meal.

Available Drug Forms Generic contents in each tablet: *Vitamins:* A (acetate): 6000 U.S.P. units; D: 400 U.S.P. units; C: 100 mg; thiamine mononitrate (B_1): 3 mg; riboflavin (B_2): 3 mg; niacinamide (B_3): 20 mg; calcium pantothenate (B_5): 5.44 mg; pyridoxine (B_6): 10 mg; cyanocobalamin (B_{12}): 5 mcg; folic acid: 0.3 mg. *Minerals:* calcium (sulfate): 350 mg; iron (fumarate): 65 mg.

TRADE NAME Stuartnatal 1 + 1 (RX)

CLASSIFICATION Multivitamin and mineral preparation for pregnancy and lactation

Warnings and Precautions Contains FD&C yellow No. 5 (tartrazine) and may cause hypersensitivity reactions, particularly in individuals who are allergic to aspirin. Folic acid content may mask the progressive neurologic damage in clients with pernicious anemia.

Administration Usual dosage: 1 tablet po daily after a meal.

Available Drug Forms Generic contents in each tablet: *Vitamins:* A (acetate): 8000 IU; D: 400 IU; E: 30 IU; C: 90 mg; thiamine mononitrate (B_1): 2.55 mg; riboflavin (B_2): 3 mg; niacinamide (B_3): 20 mg; pyridoxine (B_6): 10 mg; cyanocobalamin (B_{12}): 12 mcg; folic acid: 1 mg. *Minerals:* calcium (sulfate): 200 mg; iron (fumarate): 65 mg; magnesium (oxide): 100 mg; iodine (potassium iodide): 150 mcg.

GERIATRIC

Multivitamin Preparations

TRADE NAME Al-Vite (OTC)

CLASSIFICATION Geriatric Multivitamin preparation

Indications for Use Multiple vitamin deficiencies.

Warnings and Precautions Not a reliable substitute for vitamin B_{12} in the management of pernicious anemia.

Drug Interactions Pyridoxine content may decrease the efficacy of levodopa.

Administration Usual dosage: 1 or 2 tablets po daily.

Available Drug Forms Generic contents in each tablet: *Vitamins:* A (palmitate): 10,000 U.S.P. units; D_3: 400 U.S.P. units; E: 25 IU; C: 200 mg; thiamine mononitrate (B_1): 20 mg; riboflavin (B_2): 10 mg; niacinamide (B_3): 100 mg; calcium pantothenate (B_5): 20 mg; pyridoxine (B_6): 6 mg; cyanocobalamin (B_{12}) with intrinsic factor: $\frac{1}{2}$ N.F. units.

TRADE NAME B-C-Bid (RX)

CLASSIFICATION Geriatric multivitamin preparation

Indications for Use Stress conditions, debilitated clients.

Administration Usual dosage: 1 sustained release capsule po bid.

Available Drug Forms Generic contents in each tablet: *Vitamins:* C: 300 mg; thiamine (B_1): 15 mg; riboflavin (B_2): 10 mg; niacinamide (B_3): 50 mg; calcium pantothenate (B_5): 10 mg; pyridoxine (B_6): 5 mg; cyanocobalamin (B_{12}): 5 mcg.

Nursing Management No regurgitation or aftertaste occurs.

TRADE NAME Berocca (RX)

CLASSIFICATION Geriatric multivitamin preparation

Indications for Use Vitamin B-complex and C deficiencies: GI disorders, alcoholism, febrile diseases, prolonged disease, hyperthyroidism, severe burns, recovery from surgery.

Warnings and Precautions Not intended for the treatment of pernicious anemia; folic acid content may mask the progressive neurologic damage.

Administration Usual dosage: 1 tablet po daily.

Available Drug Forms Generic contents in each tablet: *Vitamins:* C: 500 mg; thiamine mononitrate (B_1): 15 mg; riboflavin (B_2): 15 mg; niacinamide (B_3): 100 mg; calcium pantothenate (B_5): 18 mg; pyridoxine (B_6): 4 mg; cyanocobalamin (B_{12}): 5 mcg; folic acid: 0.5 mg.

TRADE NAME Mega-B (RX)

CLASSIFICATION Geriatric multivitamin preparation

Indications for Use Vitamin B-complex deficiencies, stress conditions, debilitated clients who have depletion of B-complex vitamins.

Drug Interactions Pyridoxine content may decrease the efficacy of levodopa.

Administration Usual dosage: 1 tablet po daily.

Warnings and Precautions Not intended for the treatment of pernicious anemia or other primary and secondary anemias.

Available Drug Forms Sugar-, starch-free tablet, contained in a yeast base. Generic contents in each tablet: *Vitamins:* thiamine mononitrate (B_1): 100 mg; riboflavin (B_2): 100 mg; niacinamide (B_3): 100 mg; pantothenic acid (B_5): 100 mg; pyridoxine (B_6): 100 mg; cyanocobalamin (B_{12}): 100 mcg; folic acid: 100 mcg; choline bitartrate: 100 mg; inositol: 100 mg; *d*-biotin: 100 mcg; *p*-aminobenzoic acid: 100 mg.

TRADE NAME Orexin Softab (OTC)

CLASSIFICATION Geriatric multivitamin preparation

Indications for Use A high-potency vitamin supplement for deficiencies of vitamins B_1, B_6, or B_{12}.

Administration Usual dosage: 1 tablet po daily. May be chewed or dissolved in water or fruit juice.

Available Drug Forms Generic contents in each tablet: *Vitamins:* thiamine mononitrate (B_1): 10 mg; pyridoxine (B_6): 5 mg; cyanocobalamin (B_{12}): 25 mcg.

Multivitamin and Mineral Preparations

TRADE NAME Berocca Plus (RX)

CLASSIFICATION Geriatric multivitamin and mineral preparation

Indications for Use Stress conditions, alcoholism, hepatic dysfunction from toxic drugs or poisons, infertility due to hepatic dysfunction.

Warnings and Precautions Not recommended for children. Contains inadequate vitamin D and calcium for pregnancy and lactation. Not intended for the treatment of pernicious anemia or other megaloblastic anemias where vitamin B_{12} is deficient; folic acid content may mask the progressive neurologic damage.

Drug Interactions Pyridoxine content may decrease efficacy of levodopa.

Administration Usual dosage: 1 capsule po daily.

Available Drug Forms Generic contents in each tablet: *Vitamins:* A (acetate): 5000 IU; E: 30 IU; C: 500 mg; thiamine (B_1): 20 mg; riboflavin (B_2): 20 mg; niacinamide (B_3): 100 mg; calcium pantothenate (B_5): 25 mg; pyridoxine (B_6): 25 mg; cyanocobalamin (B_{12}): 50 mcg; folic acid: 0.8 mg; biotin: 0.15 mg; *Minerals:* iron (fumarate): 27 mg; chromium (nitrate): 0.1 mg; magnesium (oxide): 50 mg; manganese (dioxide): 5 mg; copper (oxide): 3 mg; zinc (oxide): 22.5 mg.

TRADE NAME Eldec Kapseals (RX)

CLASSIFICATION Geriatric multivitamin and mineral preparation

Administration Usual dosage: 1 capsule po tid.

Available Drug Forms Generic contents in each capsule: *Vitamins:* A (acetate): 1667 IU; E: 10 IU; C: 66.7 mg; thiamine mononitrate (B_1): 10 mg; riboflavin (B_2): 0.87 mg; niacinamide (B_3): 16.7 mg; *dl*-panthenol (B_5): 10 mg; pyridoxine (B_6): 0.67 mg; cyanocobalamin (B_{12}): 2 mcg; folic acid: 0.33 mg. *Minerals:* calcium carbonate: 66.7 mg; iron (sulfate): 16.7 mg; iodine (potassium iodide): 0.05 mg.

TRADE NAME Eldercaps (RX)

CLASSIFICATION Geriatric multivitamin and mineral preparation

Indications for Use Stressful conditions (surgery), restricted diets, malnutrition, chronic illnesses, infection.

Warnings and Precautions Folic acid content may mask the progressive neurologic damage in clients with pernicious anemia.

Administration Usual dosage: 1 capsule po daily.

Available Drug Forms Generic contents in each capsule: *Vitamins:* A: 4000 IU; D_2: 400 IU; E: 25 IU; C: 200 mg; thiamine mononitrate (B_1): 10 mg; riboflavin (B_2): 5 mg; niacinamide (B_3): 25 mg; *d*-calcium pantothenate (B_5): 10 mg; pyridoxine (B_6): 2 mg; folic acid: 1 mg. *Minerals:* magnesium sulfate: 70 mg; manganese sulfate: 5 mg; zinc sulfate: 110 mg.

TRADE NAME Fosfree (OTC)

CLASSIFICATION Geriatric multivitamin and mineral preparation, calcium supplement

Indications for Use Hypocalcemic tetany (nocturnal leg cramps).

Administration Usual dosage: 1 to 2 tablets po daily at bedtime. Range: 1 tablet daily bid, tid, or qid.

Available Drug Forms Generic contents in each tablet: *Vitamins:* A (acetate): 1500 U.S.P. units; D_2: 150 U.S.P. units; C: 50 mg; thiamine mononitrate (B_1): 5 mg; riboflavin (B_2): 2 mg; niacinamide (B_3): 10 mg; *d*-calcium pantothenate (B_5): 1 mg; pyridoxine (B_6): 3 mg; cyanocobalamin (B_{12}): 2 mcg. *Minerals:* calcium (carbonate, gluconate, lactate): 175.7 mg; iron (gluconate): 14.5 mg.

TRADE NAME Geriplex Kapseals (OTC)

CLASSIFICATION Geriatric multivitamin and mineral preparation

Administration Usual dosage: 1 Kapseal po daily with breakfast.

Available Drug Forms Generic contents in each Kapseal: *Vitamins:* A (acetate): 5000 IU; E: 5 IU; C (sodium ascorbate): 50 mg; thiamine mononitrate (B_1): 5 mg; riboflavin (B_2): 5 mg; niacinamide (B_3): 15 mg; cyanocobalamin (B_{12}): 2 mcg; choline: 20 mg. *Minerals:* calcium phosphate: 200 mg; ferrous sulfate: 30 mg; magnesium sulfate: 4 mg; copper sulfate: 4 mg; zinc sulfate: 2 mg. *Other substances:* aspergillus oryzae enzymes: 2.5 gr.

TRADE NAME Geriplex-FS Kapseals (OTC)

CLASSIFICATION Geriatric multivitamin and mineral preparation

Administration Usual dosage: 1 Kapseal po daily with breakfast.

Available Drug Forms Generic contents in each Kapseal: *Vitamins:* A (acetate): 5000 IU; E: 5 IU; C (sodium ascorbate): 50 mg; thiamine mononitrate (B_1): 5 mg; riboflavin (B_2): 5 mg; niacinamide (B_3): 15 mg; cyanocobalamin (B_{12}): 2 mcg; choline: 20 mg. *Minerals:* calcium phosphate: 200 mg; ferrous sulfate: 6 mg; manganese sulfate: 4 mg; copper sulfate: 4 mg; zinc sulfate: 2 mg. *Other substances:* aspergillus oryzae enzymes: 2.5 gr; docusate sodium: 100 mg.

TRADE NAME Geriplex-FS liquid (OTC)

CLASSIFICATION Geriatric multivitamin and mineral preparation

Administration Usual dosage: 30 ml of liquid po daily (2 tbsp).

Available Drug Forms Generic contents in 30 ml of liquid: *Vitamins:* thiamine (B_1): 1.2 mg; riboflavin (B_2): 1.7 mg; niacinamide (B_3): 15 mg; pyridoxine (B_6): 1 mg; cyanocobalamin (B_{12}): 5 mcg. *Minerals:* iron (ferric ammonium citrate): 15 mg; *Other substances:* alcohol: 18%; polymers of ethylene oxide and propylene oxide: 200 mg.

TRADE NAME Megadose (OTC)

CLASSIFICATION Geriatric multivitamin and mineral preparation

Indications for Use Nutritional supplement for physiologic stress.

Warnings and Precautions Prolonged use may cause vitamin A and D toxicity. Folic acid content may mask the progressive neurologic damage in clients with pernicious anemia.

Drug Interactions Pyridoxine content may decrease the efficacy of levodopa.

Administration Usual dosage: 1 tablet po daily.

Available Drug Forms Generic contents in each tablet: *Vitamins:* A: 25,000 U.S.P. units; D: 1,000 U.S.P. units; E: 100 IU; C (with rose hips): 250 mg; thiamine (B_1): 80 mg; riboflavin (B_2): 80 mg; niacinamide (B_3): 80 mg; pantothenic acid (B_5): 80 mg; pyridoxine (B_6): 80 mg; cyanocobalamin (B_{12}): 80 mcg; folic acid: 400 mcg; choline bitartrate: 80 mg; inositol: 80 mg; biotin: 80 mcg; *p*-aminobenzoic acid: 80 mg; rutin: 30 mg; citrus bioflavonoids: 30 mg; betaine hydrochloride: 30 mg; glutamic acid: 30 mg; hesperidin complex: 5 mg. *Minerals:* calcium gluconate: 50 mg; ferrous gluconate: 10 mg; potassium gluconate: 10 mg; magnesium gluconate: 7 mg; manganese gluconate: 6 mg; copper gluconate: 0.5 mg; zinc gluconate: 25 mg; iodine (from kelp): 0.15 mg.

TRADE NAME Vicon-C (OTC)

CLASSIFICATION Geriatric multivitamin and mineral preparation

Indications for Use Stress conditions (surgery, burns, trauma, febrile illnesses, alcoholism, poor nutrition). Can be used for pregnancy and lactation if diet is adequate in vitamin B_{12}, calcium, folic acid, and iron.

Drug Interactions Pyridoxine content may decrease the efficacy of levodopa.

Administration Usual dosage: 1 capsule po bid or tid.

Available Drug Forms Generic contents in each capsule: *Vitamins:* C: 300 mg; thiamine mononitrate (B_1): 20 mg; riboflavin (B_2): 10 mg; niacinamide (B_3): 100 mg; *d*-calcium pantothenate (B_5): 20 mg; pyridoxine (B_6): 5 mg. *Minerals:* magnesium sulfate: 70 mg; zinc sulfate: 80 mg.

TRADE NAME Vicon-Plus (OTC)

CLASSIFICATION Geriatric multivitamin and mineral preparation

Indications for Use Stress conditions.

Drug Interactions Pyridoxine content may decrease the efficacy of levodopa.

Administration Usual dosage: 1 capsule po bid. Dosage should not exceed 8 capsules daily (vitamin A toxicity).

Available Drug Forms Generic contents in each capsule: *Vitamins:* A: 4000 IU; E: 50 IU; C: 150 mg; thiamine mononitrate (B_1): 10 mg; riboflavin (B_2): 5 mg; niacinamide (B_3): 25 mg; *d*-calcium pantothenate (B_5): 10 mg; pyridoxine (B_6): 2 mg. *Minerals:* magnesium sulfate: 70 mg; manganese chloride: 4 mg; zinc sulfate: 80 mg.

TRADE NAME Vicon Forte (OTC)

CLASSIFICATION Geriatric multivitamin and mineral preparation

Indications for Use Prevention of deficiencies associated with restricted diets, improper food intake, and alcoholism. Increased requirements that occur during chronic illnesses, infection, burns, and stress of surgery.

Warnings and Precautions Not intended for the treatment of pernicious anemia; folic acid content may mask the progressive neurologic damage.

Administration Usual dosage: 1 capsule po daily.

Available Drug Forms Generic contents in each capsule: *Vitamins:* A: 8000 IU; E: 50 IU; C: 150 mg; thiamine mononitrate (B_1): 10 mg; riboflavin (B_2): 5 mg; niacinamide (B_3): 25 mg; *d*-calcium pantothenate (B_5): 10 mg; pyridoxine (B_6): 2 mg; cyanocobalamin (B_{12}): 10 mcg; folic acid: 1 mg. *Minerals:* magnesium sulfate: 70 mg; manganese chloride: 4 mg; zinc sulfate: 80 mg.

TRADE NAME Vicon with Iron (OTC)

CLASSIFICATION Geriatric multivitamin and mineral preparation

Indications for Use Prevention of vitamin deficiencies in women of childbearing age; prevention of zinc deficiencies accompanying acute and chronic infections, surgery, alcoholism, and drug therapy.

Drug Interactions Pyridoxine content may decrease the efficacy of levodopa.

Administration Usual dosage: 1 capsule po daily.

Available Drug Forms Generic contents in each capsule: *Vitamins:* E: 30 IU; C: 300 mg; thiamine mononitrate (B_1): 2 mg; riboflavin (B_2): 2 mg; niacinamide (B_3): 30 mg; calcium pantothenate (B_5): 10 mg; pyridoxine (B_6): 5 mg. *Minerals:* iron (fumarate): 30 mg; zinc sulfate: 80 mg.

TRADE NAME Vi-Zac (OTC)

CLASSIFICATION Geriatric multivitamin and mineral preparation

Indications for Use Clients who do not need supplemental amounts of B-complex vitamins and appetite stimulation, and for those clients who cannot tolerate magnesium in zinc supplements.

Administration Usual dosage: 1 capsule po daily or bid.

Available Drug Forms Generic contents in each capsule: *Vitamins:* A: 5000 IU; E: 50 IU; C: 500 mg; *Mineral:* zinc sulfate: 80 mg.

ORAL THERAPEUTIC

Multivitamin Preparations

TRADE NAME Allbee with C (OTC)

CLASSIFICATION Therapeutic oral multivitamin preparation

Indications for Use Vitamin B-complex and C deficiencies: febrile diseases, infections, fractures, surgery, alcoholism, GI disorders, physiologic stress, geriatrics; nutritional supplement for clients on special or restricted diets.

Warnings and Precautions Contains FD&C yellow No. 5 (tartrazine) which may cause allergic reactions (bronchial asthma); not recommended for children under 12 years.

Administration Usual dosage: 1 capsule po daily.

Available Drug Forms Generic contents in each capsule: *Vitamins:* C: 300 mg; thiamine mononitrate (B_1): 15 mg; riboflavin (B_2): 10.2 mg; niacinamide (B_3): 50 mg; calcium pantothenate (B_5): 10 mg; pyridoxine (B_6): 5 mg.

TRADE NAME Allbee-T (OTC)

CLASSIFICATION Therapeutic oral multivitamin preparation

Indications for Use Vitamin deficiency states involving B-complex and C vitamins: severe burns, alcoholism, hyperthyroidism, infections, fractures.

Warnings and Precautions Not recommended for children under 12 years; not intended for the treatment of pernicious anemia.

Drug Interactions Pyridoxine content may decrease the efficacy of levodopa.

Administration Usual dosage: 1 tablet po daily.

Available Drug Forms Generic contents in each tablet: *Vitamins:* C (sodium ascorbate): 500 mg; thiamine mononitrate (B_1): 15.5 mg; riboflavin (B_2): 10 mg; niacinamide (B_3): 100 mg; calcium pantothenate (B_5): 23 mg; pyridoxine (B_6): 8.2 mg; cyanocobalamin (B_{12}): 5 mcg.

TRADE NAME Becotin-T (OTC)

CLASSIFICATION Therapeutic oral multivitamin preparation

Indications for Use Vitamin B-complex and C deficiencies; convalescence from a prolonged disorder or surgery.

Administration Usual dosage: 1 to 2 tablets po daily.

Available Drug Forms Generic contents in each tablet: *Vitamins:* C (sodium ascorbate): 300 mg; thiamine mononitrate (B_1): 15 mg; riboflavin (B_2): 10 mg; niacinamide (B_3): 100 mg; calcium pantothenate (B_5): 20 mg; pyridoxine (B_6): 5 mg; cyanocobalamin (B_{12}): 4 mcg.

TRADE NAME Beminal-500 (OTC)

CLASSIFICATION Therapeutic oral multivitamin preparation

Indications for Use Surgery, infection, chronic illness, debilitating diseases; geriatric clients with physiologic stress; nutritional supplement for clients on restricted diets.

Drug Interactions Pyridoxine content may decrease the efficacy of levodopa.

Administration Usual dosage: 1 tablet po daily.

Available Drug Forms Generic contents in each tablet: *Vitamins:* C (sodium ascorbate): 500 mg; thiamine mononitrate (B_1): 25 mg; riboflavin (B_2): 12.5 mg; niacinamide (B_3): 100 mg; calcium pantothenate (B_5): 20 mg; pyridoxine (B_6): 10 mg; cyanocobalamin (B_{12}): 5 mcg.

Nursing Management Does not contain saccharin or other sweeteners.

TRADE NAME Al-Vite (OTC)

CLASSIFICATION Therapeutic oral multivitamin preparation

See Al-Vite (page 359) for Indications for use, Warnings and precautions, Drug interactions, Administration, and Available drug forms.

TRADE NAME B-C-Bid (RX)

CLASSIFICATION Therapeutic oral multivitamin preparation

See B-C-Bid (page 359) for Indications for use, Administration, Available drug forms, and Nursing management.

TRADE NAME Berocca (RX)

CLASSIFICATION Therapeutic oral multivitamin preparation

See Berocca (page 359) for Indications for use, Warnings and precautions, Administration, and Available drug forms

---

TRADE NAME Cefol (RX)

CLASSIFICATION Therapeutic oral multivitamin preparation

Indications for Use Vitamin B-complex, folic acid, or E deficiencies.

Warnings and Precautions Contains inadequate quantities of folic acid for pregnancy; folic acid content may mask the progressive neurologic damage in clients with pernicious anemia.

Administration Usual dosage: 1 tablet po daily.

Available Drug Forms Generic contents in each tablet: *Vitamins:* E: 30 IU; C (sodium ascorbate): 750 mg; thiamine mononitrate (B_1): 15 mg; riboflavin (B_2): 10 mg; niacinamide (B_3): 100 mg; calcium pantothenate (B_5): 20 mg; pyridoxine (B_6): 5 mg; cyanocobalamin (B_{12}): 6 mcg; folic acid: 500 mcg.

TRADE NAME Mega-B (OTC)

CLASSIFICATION Therapeutic oral multivitamin preparation

See Mega-B (page 359) for Indications for use, Drug interactions, Administration, Warnings and precautions, and Available drug forms.

TRADE NAME Orexin Softab (RX)

CLASSIFICATION Therapeutic oral multivitamin preparation

See Orexin Softab (page 360) for Indications for use, Administration, and Available drug forms.

TRADE NAME Therabid (OTC)

CLASSIFICATION Therapeutic oral multivitamin preparation

Indications for Use Malnutrition, multivitamin deficiency.

Warnings and Precautions Prolonged use may cause vitamin A and D toxicity.

Drug Interactions Pyridoxine content may decrease the efficacy of levodopa.

Administration Usual dosage: 1 to 2 tablets po daily. Dosage should not exceed 4 tablets daily.

Available Drug Forms Generic contents in each tablet: *Vitamins:* A (acetate): 5000 IU; D_2: 200 U; E: 30 IU; C: 500 mg; thiamine mononitrate (B_1): 15 mg; riboflavin (B_2): 10 mg; niacinamide (B_3): 100 mg; calcium pantothenate (B_5): 20 mg; pyridoxine (B_6): 10 mg; cyanocobalamin (B_{12}): 5 mcg.

TRADE NAME Theracebrin (RX)

CLASSIFICATION Therapeutic oral multivitamin preparation

Indications for Use Multivitamin deficiency: GI surgery, severe burns, infections, hepatitis.

Warnings and Precautions Prolonged use may cause vitamin A and D toxicity.

Administration Usual dosage: 1 to 2 Pulvules po daily.

Available Drug Forms Generic contents in each Pulvule: *Vitamins:* A: 25,000 IU; D: 1,500 IU; E: 18.5 IU; C: 150 mg; thiamine mononitrate (B_1): 15 mg; riboflavin (B_2): 10 mg; niacinamide (B_3): 150 mg; *d*-calcium pantothenate (B_5): 20 mg; pyridoxine (B_6): 2.5 mg; cyanocobalamin (B_{12}): 10 mcg.

TRADE NAME Vio-Bec (OTC)

CLASSIFICATION Therapeutic oral multivitamin preparation

Indications for Use Vitamin B-complex and C deficiencies. Stress conditions: alcoholism, chronic illnesses, malnutrition, surgery.

Warnings and Precautions Not intended for the treatment of anemias.

Drug Interactions Pyridoxine content may decrease the efficacy of levodopa.

Administration Usual dosage: 1 capsule po daily.

Available Drug Forms Generic contents in each capsule: *Vitamins:* C: 500 mg; thiamine mononitrate (B_1): 25 mg; riboflavin (B_2): 25 mg; niacinamide (B_3): 100 mg; calcium pantothenate (B_5): 40 mg; pyridoxine (B_6): 25 mg.

Nursing Management Usually well tolerated and does not produce an unpleasant aftertaste.

Multivitamin and Mineral Preparations

TRADE NAME Berocca Plus (RX)

CLASSIFICATION Therapeutic oral multivitamin and mineral preparation

See Berocca Plus (page 360) for Indications for use, Warnings and precautions, Drug interactions, Administration, and Available drug forms.

TRADE NAME Eldercaps (RX)

CLASSIFICATION Therapeutic oral multivitamin and mineral preparation

See Eldercaps (page 360) for Indications for use, Warnings and precautions, Administration, and Available drug forms.

TRADE NAME Enviro-Stress with Zinc and Selenium (OTC)

CLASSIFICATION Therapeutic oral multivitamin and mineral preparation

Indications for Use Nutritional supplement for physiologic stress.

Warnings and Precautions Folic acid content may mask the progressive neurologic damage in clients with pernicious anemia.

Drug Interactions Pyridoxine content may decrease the efficacy of levodopa.

Administration Usual dosage: 1 tablet po daily.

Available Drug Forms Generic contents in each slow release tablet: *Vitamins:* E; 30 IU; C: 600 mg; thiamine (B_1): 50 mg; riboflavin (B_2): 50 mg; niacin (B_3): 100 mg; calcium pantothenate (B_5): 50 mg; pyridoxine (B_6): 50 mg; cyanocobalamin (B_{12}): 25 mcg; folic acid: 400 mcg; *p*-aminobenzoic acid: 5 mg. *Minerals:* magnesium (oxide): 100 mg; zinc (sulfate): 30 mg; selenium: 25 mcg.

Nursing Management Contains no sugar, preservatives, or artificial coloring.

TRADE NAME Hep-Forte (OTC)

CLASSIFICATION Therapeutic oral multivitamin and mineral preparation

Indications for Use Alcoholism, hepatic dysfunction from toxic drugs or poisons, infertility due to hepatic dysfunction (assists in the maintenance and support of normal hepatic function).

Warnings and Precautions Folic acid content may mask the progressive neurologic damage in clients with pernicious anemia.

Administration Usual dosage: 3 to 6 capsules po daily.

Available Drug Forms Generic contents in each capsule: *Vitamins:* A (palmitate): 1200 IU; E: 10 IU; C: 10 mg; thiamine mononitrate (B_1): 1 mg; riboflavin (B_2): 1 mg; niacinamide (B_3): 10 mg; pantothenic acid (B_5): 2 mg; pyridoxine (B_6): 0.5 mg; cyanocobalamin (B_{12}): 1 mcg; folic acid: 0.06 mg; choline bitartrate: 21 mg; inositol: 10 mg; biotin: 3.3 mg. *Mineral:* zinc (sulfate): 2 mg; *Other substances:* desiccated liver: 194.4 mg; liver concentrate: 64.8 mg; liver fraction #2: 64.8 mg; yeast: 64.8 mg; *dl*-methionine: 10 mg.

TRADE NAME Megadose (OTC)

CLASSIFICATION Therapeutic oral multivitamin and mineral preparation

See Megadose (page 361) for Indications for use, Warnings and precautions, Drug interactions, Administration, and Available drug forms.

TRADE NAME Mi-Cebrin T (OTC)

CLASSIFICATION Therapeutic oral multivitamin and mineral preparation

Indications for Use Surgical clients, burns, injuries, febrile diseases, malnutrition.

Warnings and Precautions Prolonged use may cause vitamin A and D toxicity.

Administration Usual dosage: 1 tablet po daily.

Available Drug Forms Generic contents in each coated tablet: *Vitamins:* A: 10,000 IU; D: 400 IU; E: 5.5 IU; C: 150 mg; thiamine mononitrate (B_1): 15 mg; riboflavin (B_2): 10 mg; niacinamide (B_3): 100 mg; calcium pantothenate (B_5): 10 mg; pyridoxine (B_6): 2 mg; cyanocobalamin (B_{12}): 7.5 mcg. *Minerals:* copper (sulfate): 1 mg; iron (sulfate): 15 mg; magnesium (hydroxide): 5 mg; manganese (glycerophosphate): 1 mg; zinc (chloride): 1.5 mg; iodine (potassium iodide): 0.15 mg.

TRADE NAME Mission Presurgical (OTC)

CLASSIFICATION Therapeutic oral multivitamin and mineral preparation

Indications for Use Surgical clients.

Administration Usual dosage: 1 tablet po daily at bedtime.

Available Drug Forms Generic contents in each tablet: *Vitamins:* A: 5000 U.S.P. units; D: 400 U.S.P. units; E: 45 IU; C: 500 mg; thiamine (B_1): 2.5 mg; riboflavin (B_2): 2.6 mg; niacin (B_3): 30 mg; calcium pantothenate (B_5): 16.3 mg; pyridoxine (B_6): 3.6 mg. *Minerals:* iron (gluconate): 27 mg; zinc (sulfate): 22.5 mg.

Nursing Management Should be started at least 1 week prior to surgery and continued through convalescence.

TRADE NAME Os-Cal Forte (OTC)

CLASSIFICATION Therapeutic oral multivitamin and mineral preparation

Indications for Use Conditions in which large quantities of calcium are required; vitamin D_2 content aids in the absorption of calcium.

Administration Usual dosage: 1 tablet po tid.

Available Drug Forms Generic contents in each tablet: *Vitamins:* A (palmitate): 1668 U.S.P. units; D_2: 125 U.S.P. units; E: 0.8 IU; C: 50 mg; thiamine mononitrate (B_1): 1.7 mg; riboflavin (B_2): 1.7 mg; niacinamide (B_3): 15 mg; pyridoxine (B_6): 2 mg; cyanocobalamin (B_{12}): 1.6 mcg; *Minerals:* calcium (oyster shell): 250 mg; copper (sulfate): 0.3 mg; iron (fumarate): 5 mg; magnesium (oxide): 1.6 mg; manganese (sulfate): 0.3 mg; zinc (sulfate): 0.5 mg; iodine (potassium iodide): 0.05 mg.

TRADE NAME Os-Cal Plus (OTC)

CLASSIFICATION Therapeutic oral multivitamin and mineral preparation

Indications for Use Conditions in which large quantities of calcium are required; vitamin D_2 content aids in the absorption of calcium.

Administration Usual dosage: 1 tablet po tid.

Available Drug Forms Generic contents in each tablet: *Vitamins:* A (palmitate): 1666 U.S.P. units; D_2: 125 U.S.P. units; C: 33 mg; thiamine mononitrate (B_1): 0.5 mg; riboflavin (B_2): 0.66 mg; niacinamide (B_3): 3.33 mg; pyridoxine (B_6): 0.5 mg; cyanocobalamin (B_{12}): 0.03 mcg. *Minerals:* calcium (oyster shell): 250 mg; copper (sulfate): 0.036 mg; iron (fumarate): 16.6 mg; manganese (sulfate): 0.75 mg; zinc (sulfate): 0.75 mg; iodine (potassium iodide): 0.036 mg.

TRADE NAME Theragran Hematinic (RX)

CLASSIFICATION Therapeutic oral multivitamin and mineral preparation

Indications for Use Iron deficiency states: anemia, sprue, convalescence, advanced age, menorrhagia, pregnancy

Warnings and Precautions Contains FD&C yellow No. 5 (tartrazine) which may cause an allergic reaction (bronchial asthma). Not intended to treat pernicious anemia and other megaloblastic anemias where vitamin B_{12} is deficient; folic acid content may mask the progressive neurologic damage in clients with pernicious anemia. Not intended to provide adequate quantities of calcium and other substances required during pregnancy and lactation.

Drug Interactions Pyridoxine content may decrease the efficacy of levodopa.

Administration Usual dosage: 1 tablet po tid.

Available Drug Forms Generic contents in each tablet: *Vitamins:* A (acetate): 8333 IU; D: 133 IU; E: 5 IU; C (sodium ascorbate): 100 mg; thiamine mononitrate (B_1): 3.3 mg; riboflavin (B_2): 3.3 mg; niacinamide (B_3): 33.3 mg; calcium pantothenate (B_5): 11.7 mg; pyridoxine (B_6): 3.3 mg; cyanocobalamin (B_{12}): 50 mcg; folic acid: 0.33 mg. *Minerals:* copper (sulfate): 0.67 mg; iron (fumarate): 66.7 mg; magnesium (carbonate): 41.7 mg.

Nursing Management Store at room temperature, away from excessive heat.

TRADE NAME Total Formula (OTC)

CLASSIFICATION Therapeutic oral multivitamin and mineral preparation

Indications for Use Malnutrition, physiologic stress.

Warnings and Precautions Not intended for children 12 years and under. Folic acid content may mask the progressive neurologic damage in clients with pernicious anemia.

Drug Interactions Pyridoxine content may decrease the efficacy of levodopa.

Administration Usual dosage: 1 tablet po daily.

Available Drug Forms Generic contents in each tablet: *Vitamins:* A: 10,000 IU; D_3: 400 IU; E: 30 IU; K: 70 mcg; C: 100 mg; thiamine mononitrate (B_1): 15 mg; riboflavin (B_2): 15 mg; niacinamide (B_3): 40 mg; pantothenic acid (B_5): 25 mg; pyridoxine (B_6): 25 mg; cyanocobalamin (B_{12}): 25 mcg; folic acid: 400 mcg; choline bitartrate: 10 mcg; inositol: 10 mg; biotin: 300 mcg; *p*-aminobenzoic acid: 8 mg; hesperidin complex: 10 mg; citrus bioflavonoids: 10 mg; rutin: 10 mg. *Minerals:* calcium: 100 mg; copper: 2 mg; iron: 20 mg; magnesium: 100 mg; manganese: 6 mg; zinc: 30 mg: iodine: 100 mcg; potassium: 25 mg; phosphorus: 52 mg; chromium: 500 mcg; molybdenum: 100 mcg; selenium: 10 mcg.

TRADE NAME Vicon Forte (RX)

CLASSIFICATION Therapeutic oral multivitamin and mineral preparation

See Vicon Forte (page 362) for Indications for use, Warnings and precautions, Administration, and Available drug forms.

TRADE NAME Vicon-C (OTC)

CLASSIFICATION Therapeutic oral multivitamin and mineral preparation

See Vicon-C (page 361) for Indications for use, Drug interactions, Administration, and Available drug forms.

TRADE NAME Vicon-Plus (OTC)

CLASSIFICATION Therapeutic oral multivitamin and mineral preparation

See Vicon-Plus (page 361) for Indications for use, Drug interactions, Administration, and Available drug forms.

TRADE NAME Vio-Bec Forte (RX)

CLASSIFICATION Therapeutic oral multivitamin and mineral preparation

Indications for Use Improper diet; tissue injury from burns, trauma, and surgery; febrile illnesses, infections, alcoholism; oral and GI disorders.

Warnings and Precautions Not intended for the treatment of pernicious anemia and other megaloblastic anemias where vitamin B_{12} is deficient; folic acid content may mask the progressive neurologic damage.

Drug Interactions Pyridoxine content may decrease the efficacy of levodopa.

Administration Usual dosage: 1 tablet po daily.

Available Drug Forms Generic contents in each film-coated tablet: *Vitamins:* E: 30 IU; C: 500 mg; thiamine mononitrate (B_1): 25 mg; riboflavin (B_2): 25 mg; niacinamide (B_3): 100 mg; calcium pantothenate (B_5): 40 mg; pyridoxine (B_6): 25 mg; cyanocobalamin (B_{12}): 5 mcg; folic acid: 0.5 mg. *Minerals:* copper (sulfate): 3 mg; zinc (sulfate): 25 mg.

TRADE NAME Vicon with Iron (OTC)

CLASSIFICATION Therapeutic oral multivitamin and mineral preparation

See Vicon with Iron (page 362) for Indications for use, Drug interactions, Administration, and Available drug forms.

TRADE NAME Vi-Zac (RX)

CLASSIFICATION Therapeutic oral multivitamin and mineral preparation

See Vi-Zac (page 362) for Indications for Use, Administration, and Available drug forms.

PARENTERAL THERAPEUTIC

Multivitamin Preparations

TRADE NAME Albafort (RX)

CLASSIFICATION Parenteral multivitamin and mineral preparation

Indications for Use Hypochromic and macrocytic anemia, pernicious anemia and sprue, secondary anemia due to blood loss.

Untoward Reactions Transient toxic reactions include nausea, vomiting, hypotension, and pallor.

Administration Adults: 1 to 2 ml IM once or twice weekly; Children: 0.5 to 1 ml IM once or twice weekly.

Available Drug Forms Multidose vials containing 10 ml. Generic contents in 1 ml of liquid: *Vitamins:* thiamine (B_1): 12.5 mg; riboflavin (B_2): 0.5 mg; niacinamide (B_3): 12.5 mg; panthenol (B_5): 1 mg; pyridoxine (B_6): 2 mg; cyanocobalamin (B_{12}): 100 mcg. *Mineral:* iron (gluconate): 50 mg. *Other substances:* 20% liver extract (10mEq of B_{12} per ml).

Nursing Management

1. Do not use if sedimentation or precipitation occurs.
2. Solution does not stain the skin; but the Z-track method is recommended.

TRADE NAME Berocca-C (RX)

CLASSIFICATION Parenteral multivitamin preparation

Indications for Use Surgery, fever, severe burns; disorders that increase metabolism (pregnancy, GI disorders, prolonged wasting disorders, alcoholism).

Warnings and Precautions May cause pain at injection site.

Untoward Reactions Occasional hypersensitivity reaction to thiamine has occurred.

Drug Interactions Pyridoxine content may decrease the efficacy of levodopa.

Administration Usual dosage: 2 to 4 ml added to client's daily IV infusions; Range: 2 to 20 ml daily.

Available Drug Forms Ampules containing 2 ml; multidose vials containing 20 ml. Generic contents in

2 ml of liquid: *Vitamins:* C: 100 mg; thiamine (B_1): 10 mg; riboflavin (B_2): 10 mg; niacinamide (B_3): 80 mg; calcium pantothenate (B_5): 20 mg; pyridoxine (B_6): 20 mg; *d*-biotin: 0.2 mg.

Nursing Management

1. Must be given slowly via IV push or IM.
2. Riboflavin causes darkening of solution but does not affect safety.
3. Check expiration date (stable for 18 months without refrigeration).
4. Should be stored in refrigerator.

TRADE NAME Berocca-C 500 (RX)

CLASSIFICATION Parenteral multivitamin preparation

Indications for Use Severe burns, shock or trauma.

Warnings and Precautions May cause pain at injection site.

Untoward Reactions Occasional hypersensitivity reaction to thiamine has occurred.

Drug Interactions Pyridoxine content may decrease the efficacy of levodopa.

Administration Contents from duplex package (both ampules) added to client's daily IV infusion.

Available Drug Forms Duplex packages containing 1 ampule of Berocca-C (2 ml) and 1 ampule of ascorbic acid 400 mg in 1 ml. Generic contents in each duplex package: *Vitamins:* C: 500 mg; thiamine (B_1): 10 mg; riboflavin (B_2): 10 mg; niacinamide (B_3): 80 mg; calcium pantothenate (B_5): 20 mg; pyridoxine (B_6): 20 mg; *d*-biotin: 0.2 mg.

Nursing Management

1. Riboflavin causes darkening of solution but does not affect safety.
2. Check expiration date (stable for 18 months without refrigeration).
3. Should be stored in refrigerator.

TRADE NAMES MVI; MVI Concentrate (RX)

CLASSIFICATION Parenteral multivitamin preparation

Indications for Use Surgery, severe burns, fractures, and other traumas; severe infectious diseases; comatose states.

Untoward Reactions Occasional hypersensitivity reaction to thiamine has occurred.

Drug Interactions Pyridoxine content may decrease the efficacy of levodopa.

Administration 10 ml of MVI or 5 ml of MVI concentrate are added to at least 500 ml of client's daily IV infusion.

Available Drug Forms Ampules containing 10 ml of solution; ampules containing 5 ml of concentrated solution. Generic contents in 10 ml of liquid: *Vitamins:* A: 10,000 IU; D: 1,000 IU; E: 5 IU; C: 500 mg; thiamine (B_1): 50 mg; riboflavin (B_2): 10 mg; niacinamide (B_3): 100 mg; dexpanthenol (B_5): 25 mg; pyridoxine (B_6): 15 mg.

Nursing Management

1. Do not give via IV push or IM.
2. Should be refrigerated.

TRADE NAME MVI-12 (RX)

CLASSIFICATION Parenteral multivitamin preparation

Indications for Use Surgery, severe burns, fractures, and other traumas; severe infectious diseases; comatose states.

Warnings and Precautions Folic acid content may mask the progressive neurologic damage in clients with pernicious anemia. Not recommended for children under 12 years.

Untoward Reactions Occasional hypersensitivity reaction to thiamine has occurred.

Drug Interactions Pyridoxine content may decrease the efficacy of levodopa.

Administration 10 ml (contents of both ampules) are added to at least 500 ml of client's daily IV infusion.

Available Drug Forms Two ampules each containing 5 ml. Ampule #2 contains biotin, folic acid, and B_{12}. Generic contents in 10 ml of liquid: *Vitamins:* A: 3300 IU; D: 200 IU; E: 10 IU; C: 100 mg; thiamine (B_1): 3 mg; riboflavin (B_2): 3.6 mg; niacinamide (B_3): 40 mg; dexpanthenol (B_5): 15 mg; pyridoxine (B_6): 4 mg; cyanocobalamin (B_{12}): 5 mcg; folic acid: 400 mcg; biotin: 60 mcg.

Nursing Management

1. Do not use if discolored or precipitation occurs.
2. Do not mix with other IV drug solutions; several incompatibilities have been known to occur, including sodium cefazolin (Ancef, Kefzol) and alkaline solutions.
3. Do not give via IV push or IM.
4. Should be refrigerated.

TRADE NAME Neuro B-12 (RX)

CLASSIFICATION Parenteral multivitamin preparation

Indications for Use Vitamin B_{12} deficiency pernicious anemia, beriberi.

Administration 1 ml IM daily, weekly, or monthly, as needed.

Available Drug Forms Multidose vials containing 10 ml. Generic contents in 1 ml of liquid: *Vitamins:* thiamine (B_1): 100 mg; cyanocobalamin (B_{12}): 1000 mcg.

Nursing Management See Vitamin B_{12} for further details.

TRADE NAME Neuro B-12 Forte (RX)

CLASSIFICATION Parenteral multivitamin preparation

Indications for Use Deficiency of vitamins B_1, B_6, or B_{12}; pernicious anemia; beriberi; dietary anorexia.

Drug Interactions Pyridoxine content may decrease the efficacy of levodopa.

Administration 1 ml IM daily, weekly, or monthly, as needed.

Available Drug Forms Multidose vials containing 10 ml. Generic contents in each 1 ml of liquid: *Vitamins:* thiamine (B_1): 100 mg; pyridoxine (B_6): 100 mg; cyanocobalamin (B_{12}): 1000 mcg.

Nursing Management See Vitamin B_{12} for further details.

TRADE NAME Tia-Doce (RX)

CLASSIFICATION Parenteral multivitamin preparation

Indications for Use Deficiency of vitamin B_1, pernicious anemia, beriberi, dietary anorexia.

Administration 0.5 to 1 ml IM daily or as needed. May be added to 500 ml of dextrose solution.

Available Drug Forms 10-ml univials with freeze-dried vitamin B_1 in the lower chamber and vitamin B_{12} in bacteriostatic water in the upper chamber. Generic contents in 1 ml of liquid: *Vitamins:* thiamine (B_1): 100 mg; cyanocobalamin (B_{12}): 1000 mcg.

Nursing Management

1. Place univial on a hard surface. Remove outer cap and press rubber stopper downward firmly. The diluent from the upper chamber will mix with the dry powder.
2. Shake the reconstituted solution gently until dissolved.
3. As with other parenteral solutions, remove desired amount using aseptic technique.

TRADE NAME Vitamin B Complex with B_{12} (RX)

CLASSIFICATION Parenteral multivitamin preparation

Indications for Use Deficiency of B-complex vitamins, anorexia.

Drug Interactions Pyridoxine content may decrease the efficacy of levodopa.

Administration 1 ml IM daily or as needed.

Available Drug Forms Available in tube with 1.25 in. 22-gauge needle. Generic contents in 1 ml of liquid: *Vitamins:* thiamine (B_1): 10 mg; riboflavin (B_2): 5 mg; niacinamide (B_3): 100 mg; *d*-pantothenyl alcohol (B_5): 5 mg; pyridoxine (B_6): 5 mg; cyanocobalamin (B_{12}): 7.5 mcg.

TRADE NAME Vita-Numonyl (RX)

CLASSIFICATION Parenteral multivitamin preparation

Indications for Use Expectorant and antiseptic for the respiratory tract.

Administration Adults: 2 ml IM daily for 5 days; Children: 1 ml IM daily for 5 days.

Available Drug Forms Ampules containing 1 or 2 ml. Generic contents in 1 ml of liquid: *Vitamins:* A (palmitate): 2500 IU; D_2: 250 IU. *Other substances:* eucalyptol: 75 mg; oil of Niaouli: 15 mg; oil of Arachida (CSH): 1 ml.

OTHER NUTRITIONAL SUPPLEMENTS

Multivitamin Preparations

TRADE NAME Alba-Lybe (OTC)

CLASSIFICATION Nutritional supplement

Action Appetite stimulant.

Administration Adults: 1 tbsp po tid; Children: $\frac{1}{2}$ tsp po tid.

Available Drug Forms Generic contents in 5 ml of liquid: *Vitamins:* thiamine (B_1): 5 mg; riboflavin (B_2): 4 mg; niacinamide (B_3): 35 mg; calcium pantothenate (B_5): 7 mg; pyridoxine (B_6): 1 mg; cyanocobalamin (B_{12}): 10 mcg. *Other substances:* lysine: 275 mg; sorbitol q.s.

Nursing Management

1. Has an imitation sherry wine flavor.
2. Can be given to diabetics.

TRADE NAME Becotin (OTC)

CLASSIFICATION Nutritional supplement

Indications for Use Mild B-complex deficiency.

Warnings and Precautions Not intended for the treatment of anemias.

Administration

- *Prophylaxis:* 1 Pulvule po daily;
- *Therapeutic:* 2 to 3 Pulvules po daily.

Available Drug Forms Generic contents in each Pulvule: *Vitamins:* thiamine (B_1): 10 mg; riboflavin (B_2): 10 mg; niacinamide (B_3): 50 mg; pantothenic acid (B_5): 25 mg; pyridoxine (B_6): 4.1 mg; cyanocobalamin (B_{12}): 1 mcg.

TRADE NAME Becotin with Vitamin C (OTC)

CLASSIFICATION Nutritional supplement

Indications for Use Prevention of vitamin B-complex and C deficiencies.

Administration

- *Prophylaxis:* 1 Pulvule po daily;
- *Therapeutic:* 2 to 3 Pulvules po daily.

Available Drug Forms Generic contents in each Pulvule: *Vitamins:* C: 150 mg; thiamine (B_1): 10 mg; riboflavin (B_2): 10 mg; niacinamide (B_3): 50 mg; pantothenic acid (B_5): 25 mg; pyridoxine (B_6): 4.1 mg; cyanocobalamin (B_{12}): 1 mcg.

TRADE NAME Beminal Forte (OTC)

CLASSIFICATION Nutritional supplement

Indications for Use Prevention of vitamin B-complex and C deficiencies.

Administration Usual dosage: 1 capsule po daily.

Available Drug Forms Generic contents in each capsule: *Vitamins:* C: 250 mg; thiamine mononitrate (B_1): 25 mg; riboflavin (B_2): 12.5 mg; niacinamide (B_3): 50 mg; calcium pantothenate (B_5): 10 mg; pyridoxine (B_6): 3 mg; cyanocobalamin (B_{12}): 2.5 mcg.

TRADE NAME Dayalets (OTC)

CLASSIFICATION Nutritional supplement

Indications for Use Dietary supplement for adults and children over 4 years.

Warnings and Precautions Folic acid content may mask the progressive neurologic damage in clients with pernicious anemia.

Administration Usual dosage: 1 tablet po daily.

Available Drug Forms Generic contents in each tablet: *Vitamins:* A: 5000 IU; D: 400 IU; E: 30 IU; C: 60 mg; thiamine (B_1): 1.5 mg; riboflavin (B_2): 1.7 mg; niacinamide (B_3): 20 mg; pyridoxine (B_6): 2 mg; cyanocobalamin (B_{12}): 6 mcg; folic acid: 0.4 mg.

Nursing Management Does not contain sugar; can be given to diabetics.

TRADE NAME Larobec (OTC)

CLASSIFICATION Nutritional supplement

Indications for Use Nutritional supplement for clients receiving levodopa (no pyridoxine).

Warnings and Precautions Not intended for the treatment of pernicious anemia or other primary and secondary anemias; folic acid content may mask the progressive neurologic damage in clients with pernicious anemia.

Administration Usual dosage: 1 tablet po daily.

Available Drug Forms Generic contents in each tablet: *Vitamins:* C: 500 mg; thiamine mononitrate (B_1): 15 mg; riboflavin (B_2): 15 mg; niacinamide (B_3): 100 mg; calcium pantothenate (B_5): 20 mg; cyanocobalamin (B_{12}): 5 mcg; folic acid: 0.5 mg.

Nursing management May be used on clients taking levodopa since tablet does not contain pyridoxine.

TRADE NAME Multicebrin (OTC)

CLASSIFICATION Nutritional supplement

Indications for Use Multiple vitamin deficiencies.

Warnings and Precautions Prolonged use may cause vitamin A and D toxicity.

Administration Usual dosage: 1 tablet po daily.

Available Drug Forms Generic contents in each tablet: *Vitamins:* A: 10,000 IU; D: 400 IU; E: 6.6 IU; C: 75 mg; thiamine (B_1): 3 mg; riboflavin (B_2): 3 mg; niacinamide (B_3): 25 mg; pantothenic acid (B_5): 5 mg; pyridoxine (B_6): 1.2 mg; cyanocobalamin (B_{12}): 3 mcg.

TRADE NAME Surbex (OTC)

CLASSIFICATION Nutritional supplement

Indications for Use Mild vitamin B-complex deficiency.

Administration Usual dosage: 1 tablet po bid.

Available Drug Forms Generic contents in each tablet: *Vitamins:* thiamine mononitrate (B_1): 6 mg; riboflavin (B_2): 6 mg; niacinamide (B_3): 30 mg; calcium pantothenate (B_5): 10 mg; pyridoxine (B_6): 2.5 mg; cyanocobalamin (B_{12}): 5 mcg.

TRADE NAME Surbex C (OTC)

CLASSIFICATION Nutritional supplement

Indications for Use Mild vitamin B-complex and C deficiencies.

Administration Usual dosage: 1 tablet po bid.

Available Drug Forms Generic contents in each tablet: *Vitamins:* C (sodium ascorbate): 250 mg; thiamine mononitrate (B_1): 6 mg; riboflavin (B_2): 6 mg; niacinamide (B_3): 30 mg; calcium pantothenate (B_5): 10 mg; pyridoxine (B_6): 2.5 mg; cyanocobalamin (B_{12}): 5 mcg.

TRADE NAME Thera-Combex H-P (OTC)

CLASSIFICATION Nutritional supplement

Indications for Use Mild vitamin B-complex and C deficiencies in adults and children over 12 years.

Administration Usual dosage: 1 to 2 capsules po daily.

Available Drug Forms Generic contents in each capsule: *Vitamins:* C: 500 mg; thiamine mononitrate (B_1): 25 mg; riboflavin (B_2): 15 mg; niacinamide (B_3): 100 mg; *dl*-panthenol (B_5): 20 mg; pyridoxine (B_6): 10 mg; cyanocobalamin (B_{12}): 5 mcg. *Other substances:* FD&C yellow No. 5.

TRADE NAME Theragran Tablets (OTC)

CLASSIFICATION Nutritional supplement

Administration Usual dosage: 1 tablet po daily.

Indications for Use For adults and children over 12 years.

Available Drug Forms Generic contents in each tablet: *Vitamins:* A: 10,000 IU; D: 400 IU; E: 15 IU; C: 200 mg; thiamine (B_1): 10.3 mg; riboflavin (B_2): 10 mg; niacin (B_3): 100 mg; pantothenic acid (B_5): 18.4 mg; pyridoxine (B_6): 4.1 mg; cyanocobalamin (B_{12}): 5 mcg.

Nursing Management Store at room temperature; avoid excessive heat.

TRADE NAME Theragran Liquid (OTC)

CLASSIFICATION Nutritional supplement

Indications for Use For adults and children over 12 years.

Warnings and Precautions Contains saccharin.

Administration Usual dosage: 1 tsp (5 ml) po daily.

Available Drug Forms Generic contents in 5 ml of liquid: *Vitamins:* A: 10,000 IU; D: 400 IU; C: 200 mg; thiamine (B_1): 10 mg; riboflavin (B_2): 10 mg; niacin (B_3): 100 mg; pantothenic acid (B_5): 21.4 mg; pyridoxine (B_6): 4.1 mg; cyanocobalamin (B_{12}): 5 mcg.

Nursing Management Store at room temperature; avoid excessive heat.

TRADE NAME Vigran (OTC)

CLASSIFICATION Nutritional supplement

Indications for Use For adults and children over 4 years.

Warnings and Precautions Folic acid content may mask the progressive neurologic damage in clients with pernicious anemia.

Administration Usual dosage: 1 tablet po daily.

Available Drug Forms Generic contents in each tablet: *Vitamins:* A: 5000 IU; D: 400 IU; E: 30 IU; C: 60 mg; thiamine (B_1): 1.5 mg; riboflavin (B_2): 1.7 mg; niacin (B_3): 20 mg; pyridoxine (B_6): 2 mg; cyanocobalamin (B_{12}): 6 mcg; folic acid: 0.4 mg.

Nursing Management Store at room temperature; avoid excessive heat.

Multivitamin and Mineral Preparations

TRADE NAME Beminal Stress Plus with Iron (OTC)

CLASSIFICATION Nutritional supplement with minerals

Indications for Use Prevention of anemia, useful for women of childbearing age.

Administration Usual dosage: 1 tablet po daily.

Available Drug Forms Generic contents in each tablet: *Vitamins:* E: 45 IU; C: 700 mg; thiamine (B_1): 25 mg; riboflavin (B_2): 12.5 mg; niacinamide (B_3): 100 mg; calcium pantothenate (B_5): 20 mg; pyridoxine (B_6): 10 mg; cyanocobalamin (B_{12}): 25 mg; folic acid: 400 mcg. *Mineral:* iron (fumarate): 27 mg.

TRADE NAME Beminal Stress Plus with Zinc (OTC)

CLASSIFICATION Nutritional supplement with minerals

Indications for Use Stress related to infections and surgery.

Administration Usual dosage: 1 tablet po daily.

Available Drug Forms Generic contents in each tablet: *Vitamins:* E: 45 IU; C: 700 mg; thiamine (B_1): 25 mg; riboflavin (B_2): 12.5 mg; niacinamide (B_3): 100 mg; calcium pantothenate (B_5): 20 mg; pyridoxine (B_6): 10 mg; cyanocobalamin (B_{12}): 25 mg. *Mineral:* zinc (sulfate): 45 mg.

TRADE NAME Clusivol (OTC)

CLASSIFICATION Nutritional supplement with minerals

Indications for Use Inadequate diet.

Administration Usual dosage: 1 tablet po daily.

Available Drug Forms Generic contents in each tablet: *Vitamins:* A (palmitate): 10,000 U.S.P. units; D_2: 400 U.S.P. units; E: 0.5 IU; C (sodium ascorbate): 150 mg; thiamine mononitrate (B_1): 10 mg; riboflavin (B_2): 5 mg; niacinamide (B_3): 50 mg; *d*-panthenol (B_5): 1 mg; pyridoxine (B_6): 0.5 mg; cyanocobalamin (B_{12}): 2.5 mcg. *Minerals:* calcium (carbonate): 120 mg; iron (fumarate): 15 mg; magnesium (oxide): 3.0 mg; manganese (gluconate): 0.5 mg; zinc (oxide): 0.6 mg.

TRADE NAME Clusivol syrup (OTC)

CLASSIFICATION Nutritional supplement with minerals

Indications for Use Candy-flavored syrup base for children and adults.

Administration Usual dosage: 1 tsp (5 ml) po daily.

Available Drug Forms Generic contents in 5 ml of syrup: *Vitamins:* A (palmitate): 2500 U.S.P. units; D_3: 400 U.S.P. units; C: 15 mg; thiamine (B_1): 1 mg; riboflavin (B_2): 1 mg; niacinamide (B_3): 5 mg; *d*-panthenol (B_5): 3 mg; pyridoxine (B_6): 0.6 mg; cyanocobalamin (B_{12}): 2 mcg. *Minerals:* magnesium (gluconate): 3 mg; manganese (gluconate): 0.5 mg; zinc (lactate): 0.5 mg.

TRADE NAME Compete (OTC)

CLASSIFICATION Nutritional supplement with minerals

Indications for Use Prevention of deficiencies in women of childbearing age.

Warnings and Precautions Folic acid content may mask the progressive neurologic damage in clients with pernicious anemia.

Drug Interactions Pyridoxine content may decrease the efficacy of levodopa.

Administration Usual dosage: 1 tablet po at bedtime.

Available Drug Forms Generic contents in each tablet: *Vitamins:* A: 5000 IU; D: 400 IU; E: 45 IU; C: 90 mg; thiamine (B_1): 2.25 mg; riboflavin (B_2): 2.6 mg; niacinamide (B_3): 30 mg; pyridoxine (B_6): 25 mg; cyanocobalamin (B_{12}): 9 mcg; folic acid: 0.4 mg. *Minerals:* iron (gluconate): 27 mg; zinc sulfate: 22.5 mg.

TRADE NAME Dayalets Plus Iron (OTC)

CLASSIFICATION Nutritional supplement with minerals

Indications for Use For adults and children over 4 years; prevention of deficiencies in women of child-bearing age.

Warnings and Precautions Folic acid content may mask the progressive neurologic damage in clients with pernicious anemia.

Drug Interactions Pyridoxine content may decrease the efficacy of levodopa.

Administration Usual dosage: 1 tablet po daily.

Available Drug Forms Generic contents in each tablet: *Vitamins:* A (acetate and palmitate): 5000 IU; D: 400 IU; E: 30 IU; C: 60 mg; thiamine (B_1): 1.5 mg; riboflavin (B_2): 1.7 mg; niacinamide (B_3): 2.0 mg; pyridoxine (B_6): 2 mg; cyanocobalamin (B_{12}): 6 mcg; folic acid: 0.4 mg. *Mineral:* iron (sulfate): 18 mg.

Nursing Management Does not contain sugar; can be used for diabetics.

TRADE NAME Mi-Cebrin (OTC)

CLASSIFICATION Nutritional supplement with minerals

Indications for Use Multiple vitamin and mineral deficiencies.

Administration Usual dosage: 1 tablet po daily.

Available Drug Forms Generic contents in each tablet: *Vitamins:* A: 10,000 IU; D: 400 IU; E: 5.5 IU; C: 100 mg; thiamine (B_1): 10 mg; riboflavin (B_2): 5 mg; niacinamide (B_3): 30 mg; pantothenic acid (B_5): 10 mg; pyridoxine (B_6): 1.7 mg; cyanocobalamin (B_{12}): 3 mcg. *Minerals:* iron (sulfate): 15 mg; copper (sulfate): 1 mg; magnesium (hydroxide): 5 mg; manganese (glycerophosphate): 1 mg; zinc (chloride): 1.5 mg; iodine (potassium iodide): 0.15 mg.

Nursing Management Does not cause unpleasant aftertaste.

TRADE NAME Myadec (OTC)

CLASSIFICATION Nutritional supplement with minerals

Indications for Use High potency supplement with vitamins and minerals for adults.

Warnings and Precautions Folic acid content may mask the progressive neurologic damage in clients with pernicious anemia.

Administration Usual dosage: 1 tablet po daily.

Available Drug Forms Generic contents in each tablet: *Vitamins:* A (acetate): 10,000 IU; D_2: 400 IU; E: 30 IU; C (sodium ascorbate and ascorbic acid): 250 mg; thiamine mononitrate (B_1): 10 mg; riboflavin (B_2): 10 mg; niacinamide (B_3): 100 mg; calcium pantothenate (B_5): 20 mg; pyridoxine (B_6): 5 mg; cyanocobalamin (B_{12}): 6 mcg; folic acid: 0.4 mg. *Minerals:* copper (sulfate): 2 mg; iron (fumarate): 20 mg; magnesium (oxide): 100 mg; zinc (sulfate): 20 mg; iodine (potassium iodide): 150 mcg; manganese (sulfate): 1.25.

TRADE NAME Optilets-M-500 (OTC)

CLASSIFICATION Nutritional supplement with minerals

Indications for Use High potency supplement with vitamins and minerals for adults.

Administration Usual dosage: 1 tablet po daily.

Available Drug Forms Generic contents in each tablet: *Vitamins:* A (acetate and palmitate): 10,000 IU; D: 400 IU; E: 30 IU; C (sodium ascorbate): 500 mg; thiamine mononitrate (B_1): 15 mg; riboflavin (B_2): 10 mg; niacinamide (B_3): 100 mg; calcium pantothenate (B_5): 20 mg; pyridoxine (B_6): 5 mg; cyanocobalamin (B_{12}): 12 mcg. *Minerals:* copper (sulfate): 2 mg; iron (sulfate): 20 mg; magnesium (oxide): 80 mg; manganese (sulfate): 1 mg; zinc (sulfate): 1.5 mg; iodine (calcium iodate): 0.15 mg.

TRADE NAME Stuart Formula (OTC)

CLASSIFICATION Nutritional supplement with minerals

Indications for Use For adults and children over 4 years.

Warnings and Precautions Folic acid content may mask the progressive neurologic damage in clients with pernicious anemia.

Administration Usual dosage: 1 tablet po daily.

Available Drug Forms Generic contents in each tablet: *Vitamins:* A (palmitate): 5000 IU; D: 400 IU; E: 15 IU; C: 60 mg; thiamine mononitrate (B_1): 1.5 mg; riboflavin (B_2): 1.7 mg; niacinamide (B_3): 20 mg; pyridoxine (B_6): 2 mg; cyanocobalamin (B_{12}): 6 mcg; folic acid: 0.4 mg. *Minerals:* calcium: 160 mg; iron (fumarate): 18 mg; magnesium: 100 mg; phosphorus: 125 mg; iodine: 150 mcg.

TRADE NAME Theragran-M (OTC)

CLASSIFICATION Nutritional supplement with minerals

Indications for Use For adults and children over 12 years.

Administration Usual dosage: 1 tablet po daily.

Available Drug Forms Generic contents in each tablet: *Vitamins:* A: 10,000 IU; D: 400 IU; E: 15 IU; C: 200 mg; thiamine (B_1): 10.3 mg; riboflavin (B_2): 10 mg; niacin (B_3): 100 mg; pantothenic acid: 18.4 mg; pyridoxine (B_6): 4.1 mg; cyanocobalamin (B_{12}): 5 mcg. *Minerals:* copper: 2 mg; iron: 12 mg; magnesium: 65 mg; manganese: 1 mg; zinc: 1.5 mg; iodine: 150 mcg.

TRADE NAME Theragran-Z (OTC)

CLASSIFICATION Nutritional supplement with minerals

Indications for Use For adults and children over 12 years.

Administration Usual dosage: 1 tablet po daily.

Available Drug Forms Generic contents in each tablet: *Vitamins:* A: 10,000 IU; D: 400 IU; E: 15 IU; C: 200 mg; thiamine (B_1): 10.3 mg; riboflavin (B_2): 10 mg; niacin (B_3): 100 mg; pantothenic acid (B_5): 18.4 mg; pyridoxine (B_6): 4.1 mg; cyanocobalamin (B_{12}): 5 mcg. *Minerals:* copper: 2 mg; iron: 12 mg; manganese: 1 mg; zinc: 22.5 mg; iodine: 150 mcg.

TRADE NAME Vigran plus Iron (OTC)

CLASSIFICATION Nutritional supplement with minerals

Indications for Use For adults and children over 4 years.

Warnings and Precautions Folic acid content may mask the progressive neurologic damage in clients with pernicious anemia.

Administration Usual dosage: 1 tablet po daily.

Available Drug Forms Generic contents in each tablet: *Vitamins:* A: 5000 IU; D: 400 IU; E: 30 IU; C: 60 mg; thiamine (B_1): 1.5 mg; riboflavin (B_2): 1.7 mg; niacin (B_3): 20 mg; pyridoxine (B_6): 2 mg; cyanocobalamin (B_{12}): 6 mcg; folic acid: 0.4 mg; *Mineral:* iron: 27 mg.

TRADE NAME Z-Bec (OTC)

CLASSIFICATION Nutritional supplement with minerals

Indications for Use Stress-related situations, including injury or surgery.

Warnings and Precautions Not intended for the treatment of pernicious anemia.

Drug Interactions Pyridoxine content may decrease the efficacy of levodopa.

Administration Usual dosage: 1 tablet po daily.

Available Drug Forms Generic contents in each tablet: *Vitamins:* E: 45 IU; C (sodium ascorbate): 600 mg; thiamine mononitrate (B_1): 15 mg; riboflavin (B_2): 10.2 mg; niacinamide (B_3): 100 mg; calcium pantothenate (B_5): 25 mg; pyridoxine (B_6): 10 mg; cyanocobalamin (B_{12}): 6 mcg. *Mineral:* zinc (sulfate): 22.5 mg.

PART VI

HORMONAL AGENTS

HORMONES ARE CHEMICAL substances that are produced by the various tissues and glands of the body and have specific regulatory effects. The *endocrine glands* are also called *ductless glands* because their secretions (hormones) are released directly into the bloodstream (that is, without passing through ducts).

Individual hormones exert both long- and short-term effects on specific target organs. Most hormones are always present in the blood highly bound to plasma proteins. Once a hormone is freed from its protein-binding site in order to exert a physiologic action, it is inactivated by the liver or kidneys, by intravascular or extracellular enzymes, or by tissues in the target glands.

The onset and duration of action of hormones varies considerably. Most hormones in the unbound, or free state, have half-lives of less than 20 minutes. The thyroid hormones, however, have half-lives of many days and cause long-term physiologic effects.

Hormones are divided into three basic chemical classes: (1) proteins—insulin, growth hormone; (2) amines—thyroxine, epinephrine, norepinephrine; and (3) steroids—cortisol, aldosterone. Although hormones affect virtually every physiologic process, their regulatory effect is especially prominent in the following major areas:

1. Reproduction, growth, and development
2. Digestion and metabolism (energy production)
3. Fluid and electrolyte balance
4. Body defenses (adaptation and immunity)

The *pituitary gland,* often called the *master gland,* is primarily responsible for overall control of the endocrine system. It secretes several important hormones that act directly on the target glands.

Hormone secretion by the endocrine glands is controlled largely by a process called *negative feedback;* that is, hormonal secretions are controlled by inhibitory responses from other glands. For example, when the plasma concentration of a target gland hormone is sufficiently high, the secretory activity of the regulatory endocrine gland (usually the pituitary) is decreased. This, in turn, results in a reduction of the target gland's secretion, which eventually provides a stimulus for the regulatory gland to again increase its hormone secretion. The endocrine system also interacts closely with the nervous system, and each system is capable of affecting the other. The familiar *flight or flight response,* for example, is a result of the very rapid release of epinephrine into the bloodstream when the sympathetic nervous system is stimulated. Other methods of control are exerted by plasma levels of glucose (via insulin), calcium (via parathyroid hormone), or other substances.

Many hormones are now produced synthetically and are widely available for medical use. Exogenous administration of hormones is used therapeutically for (1) replacement therapy when sufficient quantities of a hormone are lacking (for example, insulin for diabetes); and (2) treatment of conditions that respond to concentrations of hormones larger than the normal endogenous secretions (for example, hydrocortisone for rheumatoid arthritis).

Chapter 21

Gonadotropic Agents: Sex Hormones

INTRODUCTION

The male reproductive system consists of a pair of male gonads or testes; excretory ducts, including the epididymis and ductus (vas) deferens; and ejaculatory ducts, including the seminal vesicles (secretory glands), prostate, bulbourethral glands, and the penis. Spermatogenesis, which takes place within the seminiferous tubules of the testes, begins at puberty and continues throughout life. Testosterone, the most significant male sex hormone (androgen), is secreted by the interstitial cells of the testes. This hormone is essential for the development and maintenance of male secondary sex characteristics; that is, the distinguishing features of the male physique and functional reproductive system. Although a very small quantity of testosterone is produced during fetal development and childhood, it is not until puberty that significant amounts of testosterone are secreted. The rate of testosterone secretion, which is sustained at its highest levels during the years before 40, diminishes after 40 until approximately one-fifth of the peak value is reached by old age.

The female reproductive system consists of the uterus, two fallopian tubes, a pair of ovaries (female gonads), and the vagina. Associated structures include the external genitalia and the mammary glands. Oogenesis, after being dormant since the fifth or sixth month of fetal life, proceeds in the ovaries during the reproductive years with the maturation of a primary follicle (which houses the maturing oocyte) into a graafian follicle and an ovum. During the years from puberty to menopause, a graafian follicle ruptures cyclically, extruding an ovum and follicular fluid. Exceptions to this cyclic process, called *ovulation,* are pregnancy and possibly lactation. Beginning a few years prior to puberty and lasting until menopause, the primary ovarian hormone, estrogen (follicular hormone), is produced by the cells of the graafian follicle; the secondary ovarian hormone, progesterone (luteal hormone), is produced following ovulation by the follicular cells of the corpus luteum. Estrogen is essential for the development of female secondary sex characteristics and for the functioning of the reproductive organs. Progesterone is responsible for the implantation and nourishment of the embryo should conception occur. In addition, progesterone suppresses ovulation and menstruation during pregnancy, decreases the irritability of the uterine muscles, and promotes the development of secretory tissue in the breast.

The male and female reproductive systems are regulated by negative feedback by gonadotropic hormones—follicle-stimulating hormone (FSH) and luteinizing hormone (LH), or interstitial cell-stimulating hormone (ICSH)—secreted by the anterior pituitary gland. FSH stimulates follicular growth in the ovaries and spermatogenesis in the testes. LH promotes the formation of the ovarian corpus luteum and stimulates the interstitial cells (Leydig cells) in the testes to produce testosterone.

During pregnancy, the placenta produces several gonadotropic hormones, including chorionic gonadotropin (HCG) and chorionic somatomammotropin (HCS), or placental lactogen (HPL). HCG enhances and prolongs the secretion of the corpus luteum during early pregnancy. HCS causes deposition of protein tissues and produces a diabetogenic glucose-tolerance curve similar to that of growth hormone. In addition, it brings about the same effect that prolactin from the anterior pituitary gland has on the breasts; that is, it stimulates breast development and milk production during pregnancy.

Prostaglandins (PG), which are oxygenated fatty acids, are now classified as hormones. Prostaglandins are produced in most organs of the body, most notably the prostate and the endometrium, and increase selected smooth muscle contractibility and modulate hormonal activity. Their functions and uses continue to be researched as additional effects of these hormones are uncovered.

ANDROGENS

GENERIC NAME Testosterone (RX)

TRADE NAMES Delatestryl, Oreton

CLASSIFICATION Androgen

SOURCE Natural

Action

Androgenic effects Stimulates and maintains the growth and function of the penis, epididymis, seminal vesicles, prostate, Cowper's gland, Littre's glands, and promotes pigmentation of the scrotum. Increases seminal fluid and its fructose, citrate, and acid phosphatase content via action on the seminal vesicles and the prostate. Is essential for seminal fluid and normal numbers of spermatozoa. Excessive amounts cause reversible atrophy of the testes and azoospermia in the normal male because of its inhibitory action on the pituitary. Effects on male secondary sex characteristics include hair development of the head, face, body, and pubis; increased secretion of the sebaceous glands and the apocrine sweat glands of the axillae and genital region; growth of the larynx and deepening of the voice; growth of bones and development of musculature characteristic of the male form, including broad shoulders, long and narrow pelvis, and developed arm and leg muscles; accelerates epiphyseal line closure. In the female, it causes a virilizing effect with the appearance of male sexual characteristics such as hirsutism, deepening of the voice, growth of the clitoris, and forehead baldness.

Anabolic effects Promotes protein synthesis with increased retention of nitrogen, sodium, electrolytes, phosphate, and sulfate. Increased amounts of protein are deposited in the accessory sexual organs, liver, kidneys, and musculature.

Miscellaneous effects Elevates low-density lipoproteins in the plasma. High doses given over a long period of time promote erythropoiesis leading to elevated hemoglobin values and erythrocyte counts. In the sexually mature male, increases erythropoiesis perhaps by stimulating production of renal or extrarenal erythropoietin, thereby accounting for the approximately 20% higher hemoglobin levels in males than in females. Promotes vascularization and darkening of the skin. Antagonizes effects of estrogen excess on female breast and endometrium. High doses usually cause an increase in female libido and euphoria of short duration.

Indications for Use

Virilizing or masculinizing actions Replacement therapy in hypogonadism or castration; management of cryptorchidism (without anatomical obstructions); induction of puberty; maintenance of secondary sex characteristics; male climacteric; oligospermia.

Anabolic protein actions Promotion of the growth of long bones in selected cases of dwarfism; stimulation of erythropoiesis in certain anemic states; management of osteoporosis and osteomalacia in the elderly; after trauma, burns, extensive surgery, debilitating disease, prolonged immobilization.

Antiestrogenic actions Treatment of certain premenopausal mammary carcinomas; hormone-dependent tumors of the prostate gland; palliation of androgen-responsive, inoperable female breast cancer.

Contraindications Carcinoma of the male breast; suspected carcinoma of the prostate; cardiac, hepatic, or renal decompensation; hypercalcemia; prepubertal males; pregnancy; breast-feeding mothers; persons easily stimulated sexually; undiagnosed vaginal bleeding; hypersensitivity to testosterone.

Untoward Reactions

General Edema; retention of sodium, potassium, nitrogen, and phosphorus; creatinuria; steroid fever; skin flushing; diarrhea; occasional nausea and vomiting; GI irritation; acne; priapism; hypercalcemia; increased or decreased libido; cholestatic hepatitis; stomatitis occurring after buccal or sublingual administration.

Males Prostatic enlargement with Leydig cell failure in elderly males. Toxic reactions from over dosage include priapism, excessive masculinization, fluid retention, edema, precordial pain, biliary stasis or hepatic dysfunction, and creatinuria.

Females Hirsutism, deepened voice, masculinization, baldness, clitoral hypertrophy, menstrual irregularities.

Children Premature epiphyseal closure, precocious development of sexual characteristics.

Parameters of Use

Absorption Well absorbed into most tissues and serum. Half-life is about 2 hours.

Crosses the placenta and is found in breast milk.

Metabolism In the liver.

Excretion Primarily by the kidneys with small amounts passing through the enterohepatic route.

Drug Interactions Increases the effects of barbiturates, phenylbutazone, oxyphenbutazone, chlorcyclizine, oral anticoagulants, oral antidiabetic drugs. Concomitant use with adrenal steroids or ACTH may increase testosterone-induced edema.

Laboratory Interactions Causes increased values of bilirubin, bromsulphalein clearance, calcium, cholesterol, acid phosphatase in females, alkaline phosphatase, total protein, serum glutamic-oxaloacetic transaminase, sodium, uptake of triiodothyronine by red blood cells, clotting factors II, V, VII, and X, and 17-ketosteroid excretion. Causes decreased values of corticosteroids, estrogens, thyroid hormones, protein-bound iodine, glucose tolerance, creatinine excretion, response to metyrapone test.

Administration

- *Male eunuchism, climacteric, impotency, cryptorchidism:* 5 to 20 mg by buccal route daily; 10 to 40 mg orally daily.
- *Female postpartum breast engorgement:* 40 mg by buccal route daily; 80 mg orally daily.
- *Female breast cancer:* 100 mg by buccal route daily; 200 mg orally daily.
- *Hypogonadism and oligospermia in males:* 100 to 400 mg IM every 4 to 6 weeks; 2 to 6 pellets may be implanted subc every 3 to 4 months after oral or parenteral dosage has been established.

Available Drug Forms Tablets containing 10 or 25 mg; pellets containing 75 mg. Potency not affected by fading of color. Multidose vials and prefilled syringes containing 200 mg/ml. Should be stored at room temperature; any crystals that form during storage may be dissolved by warming and shaking the vial.

Nursing Management

Planning factors

1. Collect a complete health assessment in order to establish a data base. Particularly, investigate con-

ditions contraindicating use of the drug, use of other medications concurrently, signs or symptoms of adverse effects to the medication, general response to therapy, appetite, and GI response to food ingestion.
2. When used for its anabolic effects, plan a dietary regimen with client and/or responsible family member that is high in protein, calories, vitamins, and minerals. The diet may be better tolerated if offered in frequent small feedings. Evaluate whether GI upset is due to drug therapy. Drug may be given before or with meals to minimize GI distress.

Administration factors

1. Follow usual precautions for IM administration. Observe for local reactions at injection site.
2. With implantation, observe aseptic technique. Observe implantation site for signs of inflammation, infection, sloughing, or signs of hypersensitivity.
3. For subcutaneous implantation, the sites usually selected are the infrascapular area or the posterior axillary line.

Evaluation factors

1. Carefully observe for side effects and progression of disease during the initial 6 to 8 weeks of therapy; discontinue drug if side effects occur.
2. Emotional support is important during therapy, particularly during the trial period of drug use.
3. Dosages of certain medications may need to be adjusted in order to maintain therapeutic levels. Check for synergistic effects of medications used concurrently.
4. Follow diabetics carefully. Insulin or oral hypoglycemic dosage may require adjustment.
5. Diuretics may be used to control edema. Inspect for signs of fluid retention. Weigh client daily and monitor intake-output records.
6. Do periodic tests for serum calcium and cholesterol and liver and cardiac function.
7. Provide fluids to prevent renal calculi and withdraw the drug in patients with high calcium levels.
8. Because increased libido in female patients may be an early sign of serious toxicity, report its manifestation to physician and offer the patient explanations and emotional support.
9. Observe and report onset of deepening of the voice and clitoral enlargement, both of which may be indicative of permanent signs of virilization.
10. Observe for pruritis which may occur before jaundice of the sclera, mucous membranes, and skin.

Client teaching factors

1. Explain possible side effects to patient.
2. Explain that the drug may cause menstrual cycle irregularities in premenopausal women and withdrawal bleeding in postmenopausal women.
3. Reassure female patients that acne and growth of facial hair can be reversed when the drug is discontinued.
4. With use of buccal tablets, teach proper hygienic measures. Instruct patient not to eat, drink, chew, or smoke when the buccal tablet is in place. Caution patient not to swallow the buccal tablet. Instruct proper placement of the medication.

GENERIC NAME Methyltestosterone (RX)

TRADE NAMES Android, Metandren, Neo-Hombreol-M, Oraviron, Oreton Methyl, Synadrotabs, Testred

CLASSIFICATION Synthetic androgen, anabolic

Action Less effective than testosterone esters, but similar to testosterone with a 1:1 androgenic/anabolic activity ratio. When administered to prepubertal males with complete testicular failure, it does not produce full sexual maturation unless preceded by testosterone therapy. Short-acting drug. (See testosterone.)

Indications for Use

Males Impotence resulting from androgen deficiency; male climacteric when symptoms are secondary to androgen deficiency; postpubertal cryptorchidism with evidence of hypogonadism; eunuchoidism, eunuchism.

Females Palliation of androgen-responsive, advancing inoperable cancer in women who are more than 1 year but less than 5 years postmenopausal or who have been proven to have a hormone-dependent tumor; treatment of menopausal symptoms and functional menstrual disorders alone or combined with estrogen; prevention of postpartum breast pain and engorgement in the nonbreast-feeding mother, although there is no conclusive evidence that lactation is prevented or suppressed by this medication.

Contraindications Carcinoma of the male breast; known or suspected carcinoma of the prostate; cardiac, hepatic, or renal decompensation; hypercalcemia; prepubertal males; pregnancy; breast-feeding mothers; patients easily stimulated sexually; history of hypersensitivity to the drug.

Untoward Reactions Hypersensitivity reactions (including rash and dermatitis), anaphylactoid reactions (rare), acne, hypercalcemia, cholestatic jaundice, edema, gynecomastia, oligospermia, decreased ejaculatory volume, priapism, female virilization, hepatocellular neoplasms and peliosis hepatitis (associated with long-term therapy).

Parameters of Use

Absorption From GI tract and oral mucosa.
Metabolism In the liver.
Excretion In the urine.

Drug Interactions Causes an increase in oxyphenbutazone and phenylbutazone plasma levels, sensitivity to oral anticoagulants, and hypoglycemic response to antidiabetic drugs. Barbiturates decrease androgenic effect by increasing rate of hepatic metabolism.

Laboratory Interactions Increases bromsulphalein retention and serum glutamic-oxaloacetic transaminase level; decreases protein-bound iodine; creatinuria is a frequent finding but its significance is not clear.

Administration

- *Male eunuchism, climacteric, impotency, postpubertal cryptorchidism:* 5 to 20 mg by buccal route daily; 10 to 40 mg orally daily.
- *Female breast cancer:* 100 mg by buccal route daily; 200 mg orally daily.
- *Female postpartum breast engorgement:* 40 mg by buccal route daily; 80 mg orally daily for 3 to 5 days.

Available Drug Forms Buccal tablets containing 5 or 10 mg; oral tablets containing 2.5, 10, or 25 mg.

Nursing Management

Planning factors

1. Collect a complete history to rule out contraindications to use of drug.
2. Determine serum calcium and alkaline phosphatase levels before and periodically during therapy.

Administration factors

1. Administer oral doses with food to minimize GI distress.
2. For buccal administration, change location of absorption site with each dose.
3. Advise client that buccal tablets require 30 to 60 minutes to dissolve.

Evaluation factors

1. Monitor carefully those clients who are immobilized, have cardiac, hepatic, or renal disease, or those with breast cancer.
2. Monitor client's weight and check for signs of fluid retention.
3. Discontinue drug if client develops jaundice accompanied by altered liver function tests.

Teaching factors

1. Instruct female clients to report hirsutism or voice change.
2. Instruct male clients to report signs of excess sexual stimulation.
3. Use of any other medication concurrently should be reported.

GENERIC NAME Ethylestrenol (RX)

TRADE NAME Maxibolin

CLASSIFICATION Synthetic androgen, anabolic

See testosterone for Drug interactions and Nursing management.

Action Relatively strong anabolic and weak androgenic activity. Enhances body tissue-building and inhibits tissue-depleting processes. Supports nitrogen, potassium, chloride, and phosphorus conservation. Stimulates bone growth, aids bone matrix reconstitution, and supports calcification of metastatic lesions of breast cancer. (See testosterone for further details.)

Indications for Use Palliatively in female breast cancer; as an adjunct in osteoporosis, selected types of refractory anemias, arthritis, pituitary dwarfism, and marked maturational delay; reverses catabolic effects due to prolonged immobilization and debilitative states.

Contraindications Prostate cancer, benign prostatic hypertrophy with obstruction, male carcinoma of breast, lactation, pregnancy, menstrual disorders, nephrosis, hypercalcemia, infancy, hepatic disorders, renal disorders, hypersensitivity to the drug.

Warnings and Precautions Use with caution in diabetes mellitus; coronary disease; prepubertal males; persons easily stimulated sexually; clients receiving ACTH, anticoagulant, or corticosteroid therapy.

Untoward Reactions

General Gastric irritation, nausea, vomiting, diarrhea, burning of tongue, skin flushing, acne, hypercalcemia, hypersensitivity (rare), anaphylactoid reaction, habituation, excitation, insomnia, increased or decreased libido, leukopenia (rare), hepatocellular carcinoma, sodium and water retention, edema, chills, jaundice.

Males Prepubertal: Growth of facial and body hair, phallic enlargement, premature epiphyseal closure, acne, priapism. Postpubertal: Testicular atrophy, inhibition of testicular function, epididymitis, bladder irritability, impotence, gynecomastia.

Females Signs of virilization, including hirsutism, hoarseness, oily skin, acne, enlarged clitoris, stimulated libido, male-pattern baldness, menstrual irregularities.

Parameters of Use

Absorption From GI tract.

Crosses the placenta and has been found in breast milk.

Metabolism In the liver.

Excretion In the urine.

Administration Adults: 4 to 8 mg po daily (daily dosage not to exceed 0.1 mg/kg body weight); Children: 1 to 3 mg po daily (highly individualized). A single course of therapy should not exceed 6 weeks.

Available Drug Forms Tablets containing 2 mg.

GENERIC NAME Oxymetholone (RX)

TRADE NAMES Androyd, Anadrol

CLASSIFICATION Synthetic androgen, anabolic

See ethylestrenol for Untoward reactions, Parameters of use, and Drug interactions.

Action Actions are similar to those of ethylestrenol with an androgenic/anabolic activity ratio of approximately 1:3. Enhances body tissue-building and inhibits tissue-depleting processes. Supports nitrogen, potassium, chloride, and phosphorus conservation. The production of erythropoietin is intensified in clients with anemias due to bone marrow failure. Erythropoiesis is frequently stimulated in anemias due to deficient red cell production.

Indications for Use Treatment of anemias caused by deficient red cell production: acquired aplastic anemia, congenital aplastic anemia, myelofibrosis, hypoplastic anemias due to administration of myelotoxic drugs; osteoporosis.

Contraindications Carcinoma of prostate or breast in males, pregnancy, infancy, nephrosis or the nephrotic phase of nephritis, hypersensitivity, hepatic dysfunction.

Administration Duration of therapy varies from several weeks to a year. Therapy should be intermittent. Adults: 2 mg po bid or tid (higher doses may be used in clients with bone marrow damage and those on corticosteroid therapy); Children: under 6 years: 1 mg po bid; Ages 6 to 12 years: 2 mg po tid.

Available Drug Forms Tablets containing 2 mg.

Nursing Management Plan a dietary regimen with client that is high in protein, calories, vitamins, and minerals. (See testosterone and ethylestrenol.)

GENERIC NAME Stanozolol (RX)

TRADE NAME Winstrol

CLASSIFICATION Synthetic androgen, anabolic

See testosterone for Parameters of use, Drug interaction, and Nursing management. See testosterone and ethylestrenol for Contraindications and Untoward reactions. See oxymetholone for Administration.

Action Relatively strong anabolic and weak androgenic activity. With sufficient intake of calories and protein, nitrogen balance is improved; it has not been established whether this positive nitrogen balance is of primary benefit in the utilization of protein-building dietary substances. (See testosterone and ethylestrenol.)

Indications of Use With established diagnosis of aplastic (congenital and idiopathic) anemia to enhance increases in hemoglobin levels; female disseminated breast carcinoma; as an adjunct (with probable effectiveness) in senile and postmenopausal osteoporosis and pituitary dwarfism. (See testosterone and ethylestrenol.)

Warnings and Precautions Use with caution in clients with benign prostatic hypertrophy. Athletic ability is not enhanced by this drug. There is the possibility of causing serious disturbances of growth and sexual development if given to young children (The gonadotropic functions of the pituitary are suppressed.)

Available Drug Forms Scored tablets containing 2 mg.

GENERIC NAME Dromostanolone propionate

TRADE NAMES Drolban, Masterone (RX)

CLASSIFICATION Synthetic androgen, antineoplastic

See testosterone for Contraindications, Untoward reactions, Parameters of use, and Drug interactions.

Action Chemically related to testosterone with similar pharmacologic action. It has prominent anabolic effects with low androgenicity. (See testosterone.)

Indications for Use Palliative treatment of androgen-responsive, advanced inoperable metastatic carcinoma of the breast in women who are 1 to 5 years postmenopausal at the time of diagnosis or who have been proven to have hormone-dependent cancer by previous beneficial response to castration.

Administration 100 mg IM three times weekly.

Available Drug Forms Ampules containing 50 mg/ml in sesame oil, with 0.5% phenol as a preservative.

Nursing Management (See testosterone.)

1. At least 2 to 4 months of therapy may be needed to evaluate effectiveness of treatment.
2. Significant advancement of disease during first 6 to 8 weeks of treatment warrants consideration of another form of therapy.
3. Do not refrigerate.

GENERIC NAME Fluoxymesterone (RX)

TRADE NAMES Halotestin, Ora-Testryl, Ultandren

CLASSIFICATION Synthetic androgen

See methyltestosterone for Contraindications, Untoward reactions, Parameters of use, and Drug interactions.

Action Stimulates and maintains secondary sex characteristics associated with the adult male. Androgens influence closure of the epiphyseal lines. Additionally, excretion of nitrogen, sodium, potassium, chloride, phosphorus, and water is reduced. A short-acting drug, but has up to five times the androgenic/anabolic activity of methyltestosterone. (See methyltestosterone.)

Indications for Use

Males Primarily, as replacement therapy in conditions associated with a deficiency or absence of endogenous testicular hormone; following castration; eunuchism and eunuchoidism; climacteric symptoms secondary to androgen deficiency; symptoms of panhypopituitarism related to hypogonadism (appropriate adrenocortical and thyroid hormone replacement therapy are still necessary, and of primary importance); impotence due to androgen deficiency; delayed puberty when it has been established that this is not a family trait.

Females Prevention of postpartum breast pain and engorgement (there is no evidence that lactation is prevented or suppressed by this drug); palliation of androgen-responsive, advanced inoperable breast cancer in women who are more than 1 year, but less than 5 years postmenopausal, and who have been proven to have a hormone-dependent tumor as shown by previous beneficial response to castration. (See methyltestosterone.)

Administration

- *Male hypogonadism, climacteric:* 2 to 10 mg po daily (highly individualized). Dosage later adjusted to individual requirements. Dosage may be divided into 3 or 4 doses.
- *Female breast cancer:* 15 to 30 mg po daily in divided doses for 1 to 3 months.
- *Female postpartum breast engorgement:* 2.5 mg po when active labor begins; then 5 to 10 mg po daily in divided doses for 3 to 4 days.

Available Drug Forms Tablets containing 2, 5, or 10 mg.

Nursing Management Gastric disturbances are more frequent than with other androgens. (See methyltestosterone.)

GENERIC NAME Danazol (RX)

TRADE NAME Danocrine

CLASSIFICATION Synthetic androgen, anterior pituitary suppressant

See testosterone for Contraindications, Parameters of use, and Drug interactions.

Action Derived from ethinyl testosterone, danazol suppresses the pituitary-ovarian axis by inhibiting the output of gonadotropins from the pituitary gland, resulting in anovulation and amenorrhea. Hormonally, it exerts weak androgenic and no estrogenic or progestational activity. Normal and ectopic endometrial tissue becomes inactive and atrophic due to the suppression of ovarian function, resulting in regression of endometriosis and its accompanying pain. Danazol has no effect on large endometriomas or anatomic deformities associated with pain of dysmenorrhea. Vaginal cytology and cervical mucus changes occur due to the suppressive effect on the pituitary-ovarian axis. Suppressive effects are usually reversible, with ovulation and cyclic bleeding returning in 60 to 90 days, when therapy is discontinued.

Indications for Use Palliative treatment of endometriosis amenable to hormonal management for those women for whom other hormonal therapy is intolerable, ineffective, or contraindicated.

Untoward Reactions Nervousness, flushing, sweating, emotional lability, vaginal itching, burning, and bleeding, (hypoestrogenic effects); dizziness, headaches, sleep disorders, appetite changes, fatigue, irritability, chills, tremors, visual disturbances; muscle cramps in back, legs, neck; hematuria (rare); hair loss, decreased libido, elevated blood pressure, pelvic pain, increased possibility of cholestatic jaundice, conjunctival edema. (See testosterone.)

Administration 800 mg po daily in 2 divided doses, for 3 to 9 months.

Available Drug Forms Capsules containing 200 mg.

Nursing Management

1. Therapy should be instituted during menstruation if possible. Otherwise, test for pregnancy before beginning drug.
2. If symptoms recur after termination of therapy, treatment can be reinstated.
3. Danazol-induced amenorrhea is reversible. Ovulation and cyclic bleeding usually return within 60 to 90 days.

ESTROGENS AND PROGESTOGENS

GENERIC NAMES Estrogens; progestogens (RX)

TRADE NAMES See individual drugs following this general information.

Action *Estrogenic agents* influence the normal pattern of ovulation through their effects on the hypothalmus and the subsequent suppression of follicle-stimulating hormone (FSH) and luteinizing hormone (LH). This suppression contributes to the absence of the midcycle surge of estrogen, blocking of ovulation, absence of midcycle peaks of FSH and LH, and the suppression of the expected postovulation increases in serum progesterone and urinary pregnanediol. Ovulation is not suppressed by doses of less than 50 mcg of estrogen.

Progestin affects endometrial structure and secretions, resulting in a pseudodecidual condition of the endometrium as found during pregnancy. The cervical network becomes thick, scanty, cellular, and hostile to the transport of sperm. There is also a decreased ferning of cervical secretions. Furthermore, the capacitation process (the activation of the hydrolytic spermatic enzymes required for sperm to penetrate the cells and investments surrounding the ovum) is inhibited by these changes in the cervical secretions.

The relative estrogenic and progestational activity of the various combination contraceptives is extremely complex. Estrogens affect many organ systems, producing multiple symptoms. The response of these organ systems also varies with respect to the different estrogens and estrogen-progestogen combinations.

Indications for Use See individual drugs.

Contraindications Thromboembolic disorders, pulmonary embolism, cerebral or coronary vascular disease, known or suspected pregnancy, carcinoma of breast or reproductive system, estrogen-dependent neoplasia, abnormal genital bleeding, hepatic tumors, impaired liver function, breast-feeding mothers, essential hypertension.

Warnings and Precautions Risks and benefits must be seriously weighed in the presence of severe vascular or migraine headaches, hypertension with resting diastolic pressure of 110 or greater, termination of pregnancy within past 4 weeks, diabetes or strong family history of diabetes, gall bladder disease, cholecystectomy, previous cholestasis during pregnancy, acute mononucleosis, sickle cell disease, fibrocystic breast disease, elective surgery such as hysterectomy or orthopedic procedures planned for the next month, major injury to lower leg, age over 35 especially if obese, neuro-ocular lesions such as optic neuritis or retinal thrombosis, hypercholesterolemia, cigarette smoking, history of preeclampsia, renal or cardiac diseases, varicosities, a client profile suggestive of anovulation or fertility problems such as failure to establish regular menses, late onset of menses, and very irregular and painful menses.

Untoward Reactions Nausea, weight gain, edema, mild to moderate infrequent headaches, spotting between menstrual periods, changes in menstrual flow, missed menstrual periods, amenorrhea during and after use, chloasma that may be exacerbated by exposure to the sun, vaginal yeast infections, decreased sex drive, mild depression, mood changes, fatigue, hirsutism, dysmenorrhea, allergic rash.

Other effects include the following:

1. Preexisting uterine leiomyomas may increase in size.
2. Disturbances in tryptophan metabolism may result in a pyridoxine deficiency.
3. Serum folate levels may be depressed. Since the pregnant woman is predisposed to the development of folate deficiency, which increases with progressing gestation, it is possible that if a woman becomes pregnant shortly after discontinuing oral contraceptives, she may have a greater chance of developing folate deficiency.
4. Smoking and oral contraceptives have a synergistic effect on the occurrence of circulatory diseases. The risk increases with age, heavy smoking, and duration of contraceptive use.
5. There is no link between oral contraceptive use before pregnancy and congenital malformations. However, contraceptive use during pregnancy may be associated with malformations such as limb reduction, heart defects, and a syndrome of multiple malformations of vertebrae, anus, heart, trachea, esophagus, kidneys, and limbs (acronym: VACTREL).
6. The quantity and quality of breast milk may be decreased.
7. Women with a history of oligomenorrhea or young women with irregular cycles may tend to remain amenorrheic after discontinuing contraceptives. Anovulation may also occur in women without previous irregularities after discontinuation.
8. Studies suggest that women using oral contraceptives for more than 4 years face twice the risk of developing malignant melanoma.

Toxic Effects Serious ill effects have not been reported following ingestion of large doses of oral contraceptives by young children. Overdosage may cause nausea and withdrawal bleeding in women. There may be an allergic reaction to the dye used in some preparations.

Parameters of Use

Absorption Both hormones are freely absorbed from the GI tract. Information concerning half-life is incomplete.

Crosses the placenta and found in breast milk.

Distribution Estroproteins circulate in extracellular fluids.

Excretion Approximately one-fifth of the conjugated products of estriol are excreted in the bile; larger quantities are excreted in the urine; small amounts eliminated in the feces.

Metabolism Estradiol is oxidized to estriol in the liver and also, to a slight extent, elsewhere in the body.

Drug Interactions The following drugs reduce the effectiveness of oral contraceptives: barbiturates, phenylbutazone and other antiinflammatory agents, diphenylhydantoin, primidone, phenytoin sodium, oral antidiabetics, meperidine and some other narcotics, anticoagulants, tranquilizers, rifampin, ampicillin, antihistamines.

Laboratory Interactions Oral contraceptives may cause the following to decrease: serum folate, vitamin B_2, B_6, B_{12}, and C, magnesium, zinc; glucose tolerance; triiodothyronine resin, free thyroxine; antithrombin III, erythrocyte count, hematocrit, prothrombin time; alkaline phosphatase, etiocholanone and urobilinogen excretion, haptoglobin; serum renin, tetrahydrocortisone, estradiol, estriol, FSH, LH, excretion of gonadotropin, 17-hydroxycorticosteriod, 17-ketosteroids, and pregnandiol; alpha-amino nitrogen, calcium, complement-reactive protein, immunoglobulins A, G, and H. Oral contraceptives may cause the following to increase: vitamin A, copper, iron, iron binding capacity, transferrin; FBS and 2-hour postprandial insulin level; cholesterol, lipoproteins, total lipids, triglycerides; butanol extractable iodine, protein-bound iodine, thyroid-bound globulin and triiodothyronine; coagulation factors II, VII, VIII, IX, X, and XII, erythrocyte sedimentation rate, euglobulin lysis, fibrinogen, leukocyte count, partial thromboplastin time, plasma volume, plasmin, plasminogen, platelet count, platelet aggregation, platelet adhesiveness, prothrombin time; alkaline phosphatase, bilirubin, serum glutamic-oxaloacetic transaminase, serum glutamic-pyruvic transaminase, cephalin flocculation, forminoglutamic acid excretion, leucine aminopeptidase, 5-nucleotidase, proporphyrin, bromsulphalein retention; aldosterone, angiotensin, cortisol, growth hormone, testosterone, total estrogens; alpha-I antitrypsin, antinuclear antibody, bilirubin, complement-reactive protein globulins A-1 and A-2, lactate, lupus erythematosus cell preparation, pyruvate, sodium.

Nursing Management

Planning factors

1. The possibility of ovulation and conception should be considered if the oral contraceptive is first initiated at times other than day 5 of the menstrual cycle; an additional contraceptive should be used until after the first 7 consecutive days of taking the oral contraceptive.
2. A woman whose menses begin on the day of, or 1 to 4 days before taking the first tablet, should expect a diminution of flow and fewer menstrual days. The initial cycle may be shortened by 1 to 5 days. Thereafter, cycles should be about 28 days in length.
3. If spotting or breakthrough bleeding occur, the client should be instructed to take her medication as directed. The incidence of spotting or breakthrough bleeding is minimal, most frequently occurring in the first cycle and ceasing within a week. Within 2 or 3 cycles of oral contraceptive use, cycles usually regulate.
4. Taking contraceptives by associating them with some regularly scheduled activity, such as eating and/or going to bed, makes it easier to remember to take them and keep a constant level of medication in the blood.
5. It is recommended that women who discontinue oral contraceptives with the intent of becoming pregnant use an alternative form of contraception for at least 3 months.
6. Because of the relative risk of contraceptive use contributing to thromboembolism, the drug should be discontinued for 4 weeks prior to, and following surgery.

Administration factors Taking tablets after a meal or at bedtime may decrease nausea.

Evaluation factors

1. If dosage schedule is correctly followed, failure of withdrawal bleeding does not mean that the client is pregnant. The possibility of pregnancy should be considered and ruled out before continuing the contraceptive regimen.
2. Withdrawal menses normally occur 2 to 3 days after the last estrogen-progestogen tablet is taken. The schedule for the next cycle should be followed whether or not menses occur as expected, or whether spotting or breakthrough bleeding occur.
3. The first intermenstrual interval after discontinuing the tablets is usually prolonged. Ovulation in such prolonged cycles will occur correspondingly later in the cycle. After the first cycle, however, subsequent posttreatment cycles are usually typical for the client in question.

Client teaching factors

1. If a tablet is missed, it should be taken as soon as possible, and the next tablet at the regular time. An additional method of contraception is recommended for the remainder of the cycle.
2. If 2 consecutive tablets are missed, the dosage should be doubled for the next 2 days. The regular schedule should then be resumed, but an additional method of contraception is recommended for the remainder of the cycle. The possibility of pregnancy increases with each successive day that tablets are omitted.
3. If 3 or more consecutive tablets are missed, an additional method of contraception should be started immediately. The partially used package of tablets should be discarded, and a new package of tablets started on the Sunday after it is realized that 3 or more tablets have been missed (even if bleeding occurs).
4. Tablets should be kept out of the reach of children, who may mistake them for candy. The attractive packaging may tempt curious children.

Estrogens

GENERIC NAME Conjugated estrogens (RX)

TRADE NAME Premarin

CLASSIFICATION Estrogen

SOURCE Natural

Indications for Use Moderate to severe vasomotor symptoms associated with the menopause; atrophic vaginitis; kraurosis vulvae; female castration; primary ovarian failure; female hypogonadism; breast cancer (for palliation only in appropriately selected women and men with metastatic disease); palliative therapy of advanced prostatic carcinoma; postpartum breast engorgement; estrogen deficiency-induced osteoporosis, when used in conjunction with other therapeutic measures such as diet, calcium, and physiotherapy.

Administration

- *Menopause:* 1.25 mg po daily, then 0.625 mg or less for maintenance.
- *Atrophic vaginitis, kraurosis vulvae:* 1.25 to 3.75 mg po daily.
- *Female hypogonadism:* 2.5 to 7.5 mg po daily for 20 days, then none for 10 days. Cycle is repeated if no bleeding occurs.
- *Breast cancer:* 30 mg po daily in divided doses.
- *Prostatic cancer:* 1.25 to 2.5 mg po tid. May be given IM or IV in 5 to 25 mg doses, and/or topically.

Available Drug Forms Tablets containing 0.3, 0.625, 1.25, or 2.5 mg; tubes containing 1.5 oz (0.625 mg/g) vaginal cream; ampules with diluent for reconstitution.

GENERIC NAME Estradiol (RX)

TRADE NAMES Estrace, Progynon

CLASSIFICATION Estrogen

Indications for Use Moderate to severe vasomotor symptoms associated with the menopause, atrophic vaginitis, kraurosis vulvae, female castration, primary ovarian failure, female hypogonadism, palliative therapy of advanced prostatic carcinoma.

Administration 1 to 2 mg po daily, for cyclical short-term use. One 25-mg pellet implanted subc every 3 months. Pellets are usually implanted in the infrascapular region or the posterior axillary line.

Available Drug Forms Tablets containing 1 mg; pellets containing 25 mg.

GENERIC NAMES Estriol; estradiol; estrone (RX)

TRADE NAMES Hormonin No. 1, Hormonin No. 2

CLASSIFICATION Estrogen

Indications for Use Moderate to severe vasomotor symptoms associated with the menopause; female hypogonadism; breast cancer (for palliation only in women who are more than 5 years postmenopausal and have progressive inoperable or radiation-resistant disease); palliative therapy of advanced prostatic carcinoma; postpartum breast engorgement.

Administration

- *Menopause:* 0.02 to 0.05 mg po daily.
- *Female hypogonadism:* 0.05 mg po daily or tid for 2 weeks followed by progesterone on the last half-day of the arbitrary menstrual cycle. After repeating this cycle for 3 to 6 months, therapy is discontinued for 2 months to determine if the client can maintain the menstrual cycle without hormonal therapy. If not, additional cycles of therapy may be prescribed.
- *Breast cancer:* 1 mg po tid.
- *Prostatic cancer:* 0.05 mg po tid or qid.
- *Postpartum breast engorgement:* 0.5 mg po daily for 3 days, then gradual reduction to 0.05 mg bid after 7 days; then discontinued.

Available Drug Forms Tablets containing 0.02, 0.05, or 0.5 mg.

GENERIC NAME Esterified estrogens (RX)

TRADE NAMES Evex, Menest

CLASSIFICATION Estrogen

See conjugated estrogens for Indications for use.

Administration

- *Menopause:* 0.3 to 1.25 mg po daily for 3 weeks; then 1 week off.
- *Female hypogonadism:* 2.5 to 7.5 mg po daily for 21 days, followed by 5 days of progestogen therapy, and then a 7-day rest period. Schedule may be repeated.
- *Atrophic vaginitis, kraurosis vulvae:* 0.3 to 3.75 mg po daily.
- *Breast cancer:* 30 mg po daily for up to 5 months.
- *Prostatic cancer:* 1.25 to 2.5 mg po tid.
- *Postpartum breast engorgement:* 5 mg po daily for 2 to 7 days.

Available Drug Forms Tablets containing 0.3, 0.625, 1.25, or 2.5 mg.

GENERIC NAME Estrone piperazine sulfate (RX)

TRADE NAME Ogen

CLASSIFICATION Estrogen

See estradiol for Indications for use.

Administration

- *Menopause, atrophic vaginitis, kraurosis vulvae:* 0.625 to 5 mg po daily, cyclically.
- *Female hypogonadism, primary ovarian failure:* 1.25 to 7.5 mg po daily, cyclically. For cyclic use, a progestogen is given with the estrogen during the 3rd week of the cycle.

Available Drug Forms Tablets containing 0.625, 1.25, 2.5, or 5 mg.

GENERIC NAME Chlorotrianisene (RX)

TRADE NAME Tace

CLASSIFICATION Estrogen

See esterified estrogens for Indications for use.

Administration

- *Menopause:* 12 to 25 mg po daily, cyclically.
- *Female hypogonadism:* 12 to 25 mg po daily for 21 days, followed by 100 mg progesterone.
- *Prostatic cancer:* 12 to 25 mg po daily.
- *Postpartum breast engorgement:* 12 mg po qid for 7 days; 50 mg po q6h for 6 doses; 72 mg po bid for 2 days.

Available Drug Forms Capsules containing 12 or 25 mg.

GENERIC NAME Diethylstilbestrol (RX)

TRADE NAME DES

CLASSIFICATION Synthetic estrogen

Indications for Use Estrogen deficiency states, female hypogonadism, amenorrhea, female castration, primary ovarian failure, menopausal symptoms, advanced prostatic carcinoma, postpartum breast engorgement.

Administration

- *Estrogen deficiency states:* 0.2 to 0.5 mg po daily, cyclically.
- *Atrophic vaginitis:* Up to 2 mg po daily; vaginal suppositories of 1 mg may be used concomitantly. Vaginal suppositories alone may be used in dosages of 5 to 7 mg weekly.
- *Prostatic cancer:* 1 to 3 mg po daily; may be increased in advanced disease.
- *Postpartum breast engorgement:* 5 mg po daily or tid up to a total of 30 mg.

Available Drug Forms Tablets containing 0.1, 0.25, 0.5, 1, or 5 mg; vaginal suppositories containing 0.1 or 0.5 mg.

GENERIC NAME Polyestradiol phosphate (RX)

TRADE NAME Estradurin

CLASSIFICATION Estrogen

Indications for Use Principally, for palliation of advanced prostatic carcinoma.

Administration Usual dosage: 40 to 80 mg IM every 2 to 4 weeks.

Available Drug Forms Ampules containing 40 mg with a separate ampule of 2 ml sterile diluent. Solution is stable at room temperature for 10 days. Discard solution if cloudiness or precipitate are present.

Progestogens

GENERIC NAMES Norethindrone; norethindrone acetate

TRADE NAMES Norlutin; Norlutate (RX)

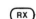

CLASSIFICATION Synthetic progestogen

Indications for Use Secondary amenorrhea, abnormal uterine bleeding due to hormonal imbalance in the absence of organic pathology, endometriosis.

Administration

- *Amenorrhea, abnormal uterine bleeding: Norlutin:* 5 to 20 mg po daily starting on day 5 of the menstrual cycle and ending on the day 25. *Norlutate:* Exactly one-half the dosage of Norlutin.
- *Endometriosis: Norlutin:* 10 mg po daily for 2 weeks; then increments of 5 mg per day every 2 weeks up to 30 mg daily. May be continued for 6 to 9 months, or until annoying breakthrough bleeding demands temporary termination. *Norlutate:* Exactly one-half the dosage of Norlutin.

Available Drug Forms Tablets containing 5 mg.

GENERIC NAME Dydrogesterone (RX)

TRADE NAME Gynorest

CLASSIFICATION Synthetic progestogen

See norethindrone for Indications for use.

Administration

- *Amenorrhea, abnormal uterine bleeding:* 10 to 20 mg po daily in divided doses from day 15 to day 25 of menstrual cycle. Clients should be cycled for 3 to 6 months, and then drug should be discontinued to determine whether a spontaneous menstrual pattern has been established.

Available Drug Forms Tablets containing 5 or 10 mg.

Nursing Management

1. Does not prevent ovulation, so conception can occur during treatment.
2. Does not alter basal body temperature, so basal body temperatures can be taken to determine day of ovulation.
3. Vaginal candidiasis or cystitislike syndrome secondary to drug excess may occur. Instruct client to report to physician for treatment.
4. Any visual changes should be promptly reported; if ophthalmic examination reveals papilledema or retinal lesions, medication will be withdrawn.

GENERIC NAME Medroxyprogesterone acetate

TRADE NAME Provera (RX)

CLASSIFICATION Synthetic progestogen

See norethindrone for Indications for use. See dydrogesterone for Nursing management.

Administration Usual dosage: 5 to 10 mg po daily for 5 to 10 days, beginning on day 16 to day 21 of menstrual cycle. Used following endometrial priming with estrogen.

Available Drug Forms Tablets containing 2.5 or 10 mg.

GENERIC NAME Medroxyprogesterone acetate suspension

TRADE NAME Depo-Provera (RX)

CLASSIFICATION Synthetic progestogen

Indications for Use Endometrial carcinoma. (See norethindrone.)

Depo-Provera was rejected by the FDA for use as a long-acting contraceptive in 1978. The pharmaceutical industry is again campaigning for approval of Depo-Provera as a long-acting contraceptive. It is widely used for this purpose in other countries.

Administration

- *Endometrial carcinoma:* 400 mg to 1g IM weekly. Client may be maintained on as little as 400 mg per month. Used as adjunctive and palliative treatment in advanced, operable cases.

Available Drug Forms Sterile, aqueous suspension containing 100 mg/ml in 5-ml vials or 400 mg/ml in 2.5- or 10-ml vials; disposable syringes containing 400 mg/ml.

Chapter 22

Oral Contraceptives

Loestrin Fe 1.5/30
Norlestrin 1/50-21
Norlestrin 1/50-28
Norlestrin Fe 1/50
Norlestrin 2.5/50-21
Norlestrin Fe 2.5/50
Norinyl 1 + 50-21
Norinyl 1 + 50-28
Norinyl 1 + 80-21
Norinyl 1 + 80-28
Norinyl 2-20
Brevicon 21
Brevicon 28

COMBINATION HORMONAL AND ANTIANXIETY AGENTS

PMB 200
PMB 400
Milprem 200
Milprem 400
Menrium 5-2
Menrium 5-4
Menrium 10-4

HORMONES IN ORAL CONTRACEPTIVES

Although there are numerous estrogen and estrogen-containing preparations, most combined estrogen-progestogen contraceptives are based on two orally active estradiol derivatives: ethinyl estradiol and mestranol. Ethinyl estradiol, a very potent semisynthetic preparation, has a prolonged biologic half-life attributable to the esterified ethinyl group which delays absorption of the hormone. Ethinyl estradiol 50 mg is equal to mestranol 80 mg in suppressing ovulation. However, mestranol has a more potent effect on the endometrium. The incidence of nausea, fluid retention, and headaches is similar for both derivatives. It can be demonstrated that these two estrogens show fewer differences in activity than do the progestogens. Estrogens are not used alone for contraceptive effect because of the tendency for "escape" ovulations to occur after a few courses of treatment, and because of the increased association with undesirable side effects when not combined with progestogens. Estrogen in combination oral contraceptives is used primarily to prevent breakthrough bleeding (intermenstrual bleeding).

Of the two steroid components present in oral contraceptives, the progestogen element is relatively more important for contraception. The natural hormone progesterone has limited appeal as a practical contraceptive because of its very low oral activity. Progestogens (progestational agents with chemically modified molecular structure) have prolonged biologic half-lives and are orally active; as such, they are useful as components of oral contraceptives. Two chemical classes of progestogens are used clinically: (1) progesterone derivatives (17-α - hydroxyprogesterones such as megestrol acetate and medroxyprogesterone acetate); and (2) steroids related to testosterone, including the 19-norsteroids such as norethynodrel, norethindrone, norethisterone, ethynodiol diacetate, dimethisterone, norgestrel, and lynestrenol. Biologically, progestogens can be classified as: (1) true progestogens (progesterone, megestrol acetate, chlormadinone acetate); (2) true progestogens with androgenic effects (medroxyprogesterone acetate, norgestrel); (3) androgens with progestational effects (norethisterone); (4) estrogens with progestational effects (norethynodrel); and (5) steroids of uncertain status (ethynodiol diacetate). The 19-norsteroids are used principally as components of oral contraceptives; progesterone derivatives are more widely used for various gynecological disorders.

SIDE EFFECTS OF ORAL CONTRACEPTIVES

Symptoms of Excess

Estrogen

Symptoms commonly associated with early pregnancy: nausea, vomiting, dizziness, syncope. Symptoms related to reproductive organs: uterine enlargement, fibroid growth, cervical extrophia, clear mucorrhea, vaginal discharge, cystic breast changes, increase in breast size (ductal and fatty tissue). Symptoms related to sodium retention: edema, irritability, cyclic weight changes, bloating, leg cramps, hypertension, visual changes. Symptoms due to vascular alterations: telangiectasia, vascular headache. Miscellaneous symptoms: increased female fat deposition, chloasma, hypermenorrhea, menorrhagia (also related to progesterone deficiency.)

Progesterone

Symptoms similar to those associated with mid to late pregnancy: increased tiredness, decreased libido, depression, increased breast size due to alveolar growth, smooth muscle relaxation accounting for dilated leg veins and decrease in dysmenorrhea. Symptoms related to androgenic and anabolic activity (similar to symptoms seen in Stein-Leventhal syndrome): weight gain associated with increased appetite, hirsutism, acne, oily scalp, rash or pruritus, increased libido, cholestatic jaundice, monilial vaginitis.

Symptoms of Deficiency

Estrogen

Symptoms similar to those associated with menopause: uterine prolapse, small uterus, pelvic relaxations (cystocele, rectocele), vasomotor symptoms, atrophic vaginitis, dyspareunia. Symptoms seen most commonly: breakthrough bleeding and spotting on pill days 1 through 14, decreased menstrual flow, hypomenorrhea.

Progesterone

Symptoms similar to those seen with anovulatory periods and corpus luteum deficiency: heavy menstrual flow and clots, dysmenorrhea, breakthrough bleeding beginning after the 14th pill day, decreased breast size, weight loss.

GENERAL MANAGEMENT PROTOCOL

Assessment and Initiation of Regimen

1. Take a complete medical, family, and sexual history.
   - **(a)** Investigate past and present history for contraindications to oral contraceptive usage and for general health status.
   - **(b)** Investigate for past or present use of any contraceptive methods to establish relevancy of chosen contraceptive method.
   - **(c)** Review sexual history to establish appropriateness of chosen contraceptive method relative to sexual patterns.
2. Check age of client. It is recommended that if client is over 40 years, oral contraceptives should not be used because of possible increased risk of heart attacks.
3. Investigate the following conditions in order to assess the appropriateness and safety related to oral contraceptive use. Use terminology understood by client or clarify language used.
   - **(a)** Family history of breast cancer
   - **(b)** Breast nodules, fibrocystic disease, abnormal mammogram or thermogram, recurrent cystic mastitis
   - **(c)** Diabetes mellitus
   - **(d)** History of high blood pressure, stroke
   - **(e)** History of high blood cholesterol
   - **(f)** Cigarette smoking
   - **(g)** Migraine headaches, recurring headaches
   - **(h)** History of heart or kidney disease, pains in chest (pectoris angina)
   - **(i)** Asthma
   - **(j)** Epilepsy
   - **(k)** History of mental depression
   - **(l)** Fibroid tumors of the uterus
   - **(m)** History of jaundice (yellowing of whites of eyes or skin)
   - **(n)** Gallbladder disease
   - **(o)** Tuberculosis
   - **(p)** Plans for elective surgery (including dental)
   - **(q)** Previous problems with menstrual periods (irregularities)
   - **(r)** Use of any of the following kinds of drugs which might interact with the "pill"; antibiotics, sulfa drugs, drugs for epilepsy or migraine, pain killers, tranquilizers, sedatives or sleeping pills, blood-thinning drugs, vitamins, drugs being used for the treatment of depression, high blood pressure, or high blood sugar (diabetes)
   - **(s)** History of preeclampsia
   - **(t)** Obesity
   - **(u)** History of fetal exposure to diethylstilbestrol
   - **(v)** Varicosities

4. Perform a thorough physical exam prior to initiating the use of oral contraceptives to establish a baseline for evaluation. Include special reference to:
   (a) Blood pressure, vital signs
   (b) Chest and heart sounds
   (c) Breasts
   (d) Abdomen (including liver) for signs or symptoms of pain, tenderness, masses
   (e) Pelvic organs, including a Pap smear
   (f) Weight
   (g) Eyes (particularly for unexplained, gradual, sudden, partial, or complete loss of vision, proptosis or diplopia, papilledema or any evidence of retinal vascular lesions)
   (h) Rule out the possibility of pregnancy
   (i) Hematocrit/hemoglobin
   (j) Urinalysis
   (k) Culture for gonorrhea
   (l) Serologic test for syphilis
5. Teach client how to do self-breast examination, explaining its importance and the need for investigation if a mass is palpated.
6. Discuss other methods of contraception. Review completely the advantages and risks of using oral contraceptives, what oral contraceptives are, how they work, and their approximate cost.
7. Investigate whether client has problems taking pills. (Does she have difficulty swallowing pills? Does she remember to take pills regularly? Is she taking any pills presently? If so, what kind and for what?) Also determine if client can afford the cost of the pills (if oral contraceptives are not provided free of cost).
8. Informed consent. Provide client with literature and review its contents, explaining the effects and side effects of oral contraceptives. The client should know the following:
   (a) Oral contraceptives, *taken as directed*, are about 99% effective in preventing pregnancy. Forgetting to take the "pill" or not taking it as directed increase the chance of pregnancy.
   (b) If the use of oral contraceptives is discontinued with the intent of becoming pregnant, an alternative form of contraception should be utilized for a period of time (at least 3 months recommended by some authorities) before attempting to conceive, because of increased risk of spontaneous abortion (miscarriage) and deformity to the baby.
   (c) There may be an increased risk of ectopic pregnancy after discontinuance of oral contraceptives due to contraception failure.
   (d) Clients with past histories of oligomenorrhea, secondary amenorrhea or young clients who have not established regular ovarian-menstrual cycles have a tendency to remain anovulatory or to become amenorrheic after discontinuing oral contraceptives. (Clients with these problems should be informed of the possible effects and encouraged to use other contraceptive methods.) Clients without previous menstrual irregularities may also experience anovulation, possibly prolonged, after discontinuing oral contraceptives, and should be so informed.
   (e) The use of female sex hormones, both estrogen and progesterone, during early pregnancy may seriously damage the fetus. (If pregnancy is confirmed during the use of oral contraceptives, the client should be informed of the potential risks to the fetus. The advisability of continuing the pregnancy should be discussed in light of these risks.) *Note:* For this reason, the administration of progestogen only or progestogen-estrogen combinations to induce withdrawal bleeding should not be used as a test of pregnancy because of the increased risks of birth defects in offspring.
   (f) Oral contraceptives given in the postpartum period may interfere with lactation by decreasing the amount and quality of breast milk. Also, the hormonal agents in oral contraceptives have been found in mother's milk when oral contraceptives are used. The effects on the breast-feeding baby is unknown. (Recommend that the use of oral contraceptives be deferred until the infant is weaned. Another form of contraception should be utilized during this period if pregnancy is to be avoided.)
   (g) While taking the "pill", exposure to the sun may worsen chloasma.
   (h) There is also an increased risk of the following:
      (i) Recurrence of jaundice in clients with a past history of jaundice during pregnancy.
      (ii) Circulatory system diseases, such as myocardial infarction, pulmonary

embolism, cerebral hemorrhage, subarachnoid hemorrhage, malignant hypertension, cardiomyopathy, mesenteric-artery thrombosis. (This risk increases tenfold in clients using the "pill" for 5 years or more. Clients over 35 years of age and those who smoke face the greatest hazards. Factors predisposing to the development of circulatory diseases, hypertension, high cholesterol levels, diabetes and obesity, play important roles in mortality among oral contraceptive users.)

(iii) Melanoma with exposure to sunlight.

(iv) Benign tumors of the liver, gallbladder disease.

(v) Neuro-ocular lesions, such as optic neuritis or retinal thrombosis.

(vi) An increase in triglycerides and total phospholipids.

(vii) A decrease in glucose tolerance.

(viii) Elevated blood pressure, especially in clients using the "pill" for 5 years or more, those with a history of elevated blood pressure during pregnancy, and those 35 years or more.

(ix) Ectopic pregnancies or oral contraceptive failures.

(x) Cancer in clients with a strong family history of cancer of the breast or of selected reproductive organs.

(i) There are side effects of one kind or another experienced by approximately 40% of "pill" users, some of which are:

(i) *Probably life-threatening:* severe, sharp chest pains or sensation of heaviness in chest; weakness, numbness, or pain in arm(s) or leg(s); coughing up blood; difficulty in breathing; severe headaches or vomiting; disturbances of speech; eye problems, including related symptoms such as blurred vision, flashing lights or blindness; severe leg pains

(ii) *Serious:* gallbladder disease with related symptoms of upper abdominal pain, indigestion, and development of gallstones; liver tumors that can cause jaundice, sudden pain, or shock due to rupture and hemorrhage; undiagnosed vaginal bleeding; breast lumps; unusual swelling

(iii) *Fairly minor:* nausea/vomiting or other stomach or intestinal problems; bleeding (spotting) between menstrual periods; increased vaginal discharge; unusual weight gain or loss; breast tenderness, enlargement or discharge; swollen ankles; mild headaches; decreased menstrual flow; vaginal yeast infections; vaginal itching; depression; mood changes; decreased libido; acne; chloasma; allergic rash

Note: Instruct client to inform physician *immediately* if any of the life-threatening or severe side effects are experienced. Fairly minor side effects should also be reported and attempts made to overcome them, thereby increasing "pill" user effectiveness.

(j) Oral contraceptives must always be taken under the supervision of a clinician or doctor. The importance of regular, periodic return visits (at least once per year) in order to supervise and evaluate the effects of the "pill" on the body and the client's general well-being should be stressed.

(k) Oral contraceptives are of *no* value in the prevention or treatment of venereal disease.

(l) Oral contraceptives may mask the onset of climacteric.

(m) The influence of prolonged oral contraceptive therapy on many body functions has not been established. (These include pituitary, ovarian, adrenal, hepatic, and uterine functions and the immune response.)

(n) The client should be informed that she is free to withdraw from using this or any method of contraception at any time.

9. Investigate client's receptiveness to a second method of contraception, which should be used until the "pill" is protecting her from conception or when there is a break in the "pill" schedule leading to increased risk of pregnancy. If chosen, make sure the client knows how to use the backup method.

10. Explain schedule for taking "pills," including what to do if one, two, or more consecutive tablets are forgotten.

11. Provide opportunities for client to ask questions, clarify what has been said, or to reinforce understanding of facts.

12. New users of oral contraceptives should be started on preparations containing 50 mcg or less of estrogen. Discuss the importance of taking oral contraceptives regularly at the same time each day, explaining why the level of the hormones must be maintained.

Return Visits

1. Early follow-up: approximately 6 to 12 weeks.
   - (a) Check client's health status including:
     - (i) General physical and emotional status with special reference to blood pressure and cardiovascular system.
     - (ii) Determine if client is experiencing signs or symptoms suggestive of warning signals of possible problems, including leg, abdominal, or chest pains; headaches, visual complaints, such as blurred vision; or any other complaints or problems about which the client may volunteer information. Explain that minor side effects tend to disappear after a few cycles of oral contraceptive use. If they persist, instruct client to report them because dose adjustments or a different preparation may be needed to relieve the symptoms.
   - (b) Validate that oral contraceptives are being taken correctly.
   - (c) Rule out the possibility of pregnancy.
   - (d) Review, reinforce, supplement, or clarify information relative to "pill" use, signs or symptoms of side effects, or any concerns expressed by the client that may affect the use of the "pill" or the chosen backup contraceptive method.
   - (e) Unless contraindicated, give client a one-year prescription for oral contraceptives (a 13-month supply is recommended to allow for unavoidable rescheduling of appointments and to ensure continuity of "pill" use). Schedule a visit sooner if indicated by problems with "pill" use, client's need for reassurance or support, or physical side effects influencing the effectiveness of "pill" use.
   - (f) Make appointment for client's next visit; follow with reminder shortly before scheduled date of appointment.
2. Refill visits: at least annually.
   - (a) Physical examination with special reference to weight, blood pressure, breasts, heart and lungs, abdomen, eyes, extremities, and pelvic organs (including Pap smear annually).
   - (b) Laboratory tests, including urinalysis, CBC, Pap smear, hemoglobin/hematocrit, and other tests depending on information obtained through history and or physical examination. (Gonorrhea culture and serologic tests for syphilis are recommended.)
   - (c) Check for signs or symptoms of side effects, general well-being, problems with the "pill" schedule, and onset of problems relating to data from history review. Refer for appropriate diagnostic and therapeutic measures and discontinue oral contraceptives if serious symptoms occur.
   - (d) Review, reinforce, supplement, or clarify information relative to "pill" use, signs or symptoms of side effects, or any concerns expressed by the client that may affect the use of the "pill" or the chosen backup contraceptive method.
   - (e) Rule out the possibility of pregnancy before continuing contraceptive regimen. Consider pregnancy if withdrawal bleeding does not occur (missing two or more periods). Consider the possibility of pregnancy if client has not adhered to the prescriptive schedule.
   - (f) Carefully check for decreased glucose tolerance, particularly in prediabetic and diabetic clients; order glucose-tolerance tests and triclycerides and total phospholipids tests prn.
   - (g) If pathologic reasons for bleeding irregularities are ruled out, the passage of time or a change to another formulation may correct the bleeding problem. A change to an oral contraceptive with a higher estrogen content, while potentially useful in minimizing menstrual irregularities, should be made only when considered necessary since this may increase the risk of thromboembolic disease. Amount, duration of flow, and time of occurrence within the cycle are critical data needed for assessment.
   - (h) Discontinue oral contraceptives at least four weeks before elective surgery or during periods of long immobilization. Oral contraceptive use should not be resumed until at least four weeks after surgery.
   - (i) Because certain endocrine and liver function tests may be affected by the

estrogen in oral contraceptives, it is recommended that any abnormal tests be repeated after the "pill" has been withdrawn for two months.

(j) Instruct client to return before her appointment if two periods are missed, even if the "pill" was taken every day on schedule. A pregnancy test should be taken.

(k) Instruct client to mention that she is using birth control pills if seen by a doctor for other problems. This is particularly important if admitted to the hospital.

(l) Unless contraindicated, give client a one-year prescription for oral contraceptives (a 13-month supply is recommended to allow for unavoidable rescheduling of appointments and to ensure continuity of "pill" use). Schedule a visit sooner if indicated by problems with "pill" use, client's need for reassurance or support, or physical side effects influencing the effectiveness of "pill" use.

(m) Make appointment for client's next visit; follow with reminder shortly before scheduled date of appointment.

(n) Additional noncontraceptive benefits may include:

- (i) Relief of symptoms related to menstrual cycles (minimizes menstrual cramps, decreases the number of days of bleeding and amount of blood loss, produces regular menstrual periods, eliminates the pain of mittelschmerz in most instances)
- (ii) Decreased iron-deficient anemia
- (iii) Diminished premenstrual tension, anxiety, or depression
- (iv) Control of symptoms of estrogen deficiency
- (v) Treatment of medical conditions, such as endometriosis and idiopathic thrombocytopenic purpura
- (vi) Decreased incidence of functional ovarian cysts, fibroadenomas, and fibrocystic breast diseases
- (vii) Improved acne (although certain oral contraceptives may aggravate this condition)
- (viii) Weight gain and/or increase in breast size (which can be beneficial or adverse)
- (ix) Increased enjoyment of sexual intercourse (perhaps related to the fact that fear of pregnancy is diminished)

PROGESTATIONAL AGENTS

GENERIC NAME Progesterone (RX)

TRADE NAME Progestasert

CLASSIFICATION Progestational contraceptive

Action A continuous release of progesterone at an average rate of 65 mg/day into the uterine cavity. The mechanism by which progesterone enhances the contraceptive effectiveness of the T intrauterine device is local, not systemic. The concentrations of luteinizing hormone, estradiol, and progesterone in systemic venous plasma follow regular cyclic patterns indicative of ovulation during use of the Progestasert system. Blood chemistry studies related to liver, kidney, and thyroid function also reveal no changes. During use of the system, the endometrium shows progestational influence. Following removal of the system, the endometrium rapidly returns to its normal cyclic pattern and can support pregnancy. The local mechanism by which continuously released progesterone enhances the contraceptive ability of the T intrauterine device has not been conclusively demonstrated. The hypotheses that have been offered are progesterone-induced inhibition of sperm capacitation or survival and alteration of the uterine milieu so as to prevent nidation.

Indications for Use Prevention of Pregnancy.

Contraindications Pregnancy or suspicion of pregnancy, abnormalities of the uterine cavity, acute pelvic inflammatory disease, history of repeated pelvic inflammatory disease, postpartum endometriosis, infected abortion in past 3 months, uterine or cervical malignancy, unexplained genital bleeding until cancer is ruled out, acute cervicitis.

Warnings and Precautions Women should be reexamined and evaluated within 3 months after insertion of Progestasert system. A routine annual examination with removal of the Progestasert system and appropriate medical and laboratory evaluations should be carried out. If pregnancy occurs with a Progestasert system in situ, it should be removed if the thread is visible, or if removal proves to be (or would be) difficult, interruption of the pregnancy should be considered. If the client chooses to maintain the pregnancy and the system remains in situ, she should be warned of the increased risk of sepsis and be followed with close vigilance. A pregnancy occurring during use of an IUD (intrauterine device) is much more likely to be ectopic; therefore, IUD users who become pregnant should be carefully evaluated.

Untoward Reactions Endometriosis, spontaneous abortion or septic abortion, septicemia, perforation of uterus and cervix, pelvic infection, cystic masses in pelvis, abdominal adhesions, intestinal obstruction, cervical erosion, vaginitis, leukorrhea, cystitis, pregnancy and ectopic pregnancy, uterine embedment, difficult removal, complete or partial expulsion, intermenstrual spotting, prolongation of menstrual flow, anemia, amenorrhea or delayed menses, pain and cramping, backaches, dyspareunia, leg pain or soreness, weight loss or gain, nervousness, bradycardia and syncope secondary to insertion pain. Occasionally, serious pelvic infections may occur with an IUD in situ. If so, the IUD should be removed, appropriate bacteriologic studies done, and antibiotic treatment instituted. Perforation of the uterus may occur. If so, the IUD should be removed. If the IUD is not removed, local inflammatory reaction with abscess formation is possible.

Parameters of Use

Absorption Locally in uterus.
Excretion Locally in uterus.
Metabolism Locally in uterus.

Administration Uterine insertion of the T device that contains progesterone, which is released at about 65 mg/day for 1 year.

Available Drug Forms In cartons containing 6 sterile systems and inserters. The Progestasert Intrauterine Progesterone Contraceptive System is a white, T-shaped unit constructed of ethylene/vinyl acetate copolymer (EVA) containing titanium dioxide. The 36-mm tubular vertical stem of the T unit contains a reservoir of 38 mg progesterone together with barium sulfate for radiopacity; both are dispersed in medical grade silicone oil. The 32-mm horizontal crossarms are solid EVA. Two monofilament nylon indicator/retrieval threads are fastened to the base of the T stem.

Nursing Management

Planning factors

1. Inform client of adverse reactions.
2. Prior to insertion, a pelvic and breast examination, Pap smear, and gonorrhea culture should be done. Sound the uterus prior to insertion and exercise care not to perforate the uterus. Do not use excessive force.
3. Rule out the possibility of pregnancy before inserting IUD. Insert during or shortly following menstrual period. Do not insert postabortally or postpartum until uterine involution is complete.
4. Assess the relevance of this method of contraception for particular clients. Discuss available methods of contraception with client.
5. Allow time for client to ask questions.

Administration factors

1. Inform client that some bleeding or cramps may occur during the first few days after insertion. If these symptoms continue and are severe, they should be reported.
2. Prepare client for insertion:
   a. Warn the client that a moderate degree of pain or nausea may be experienced immediately following insertion of the IUD.
   b. Suggest someone be with them in case of the need for someone to drive them home.

Evaluation factors

1. Inform client of importance of reexamination and evaluation within 3 months after insertion. Also, that the IUD should be replaced annually because the progesterone gradually loses its effectiveness.
2. A second method of birth control should be used for the first 3 months after the IUD is inserted because of the greater possibility of its expulsion during this time.

Client Teaching Factors

1. Teach client how to check for correct placement of IUD.
2. Inform client not to pull on the thread, which would displace the system, and not to remove the IUD by herself.
3. Instruct the client to notify her doctor or clinician immediately anytime fever, pelvic pain or tenderness, severe cramping, or unusual vaginal bleeding occur because these are signs of infections and infections from IUDs, if untreated, can lead to hysterectomy (removal of uterus) or even death.

GENERIC NAME Norethindrone (RX)

TRADE NAMES Nor-Q.D., Micronor

CLASSIFICATION Progestational contraceptive

See page 387 for Indications for use, Contraindications, Warnings and precautions, and Untoward reactions.

Available Drug Forms Tablets containing 0.35 mg

Nursing Management

Planning Factors The administration of medications containing only progestogen to induce withdrawal bleeding should not be used as a test of pregnancy.

Administration factors

1. For maximum contraceptive effectiveness, daily tablets must be taken exactly as directed and at intervals not exceeding 24 hours.
2. Client should take 1 tablet each day without interruption, beginning on the first day of menstruation.
3. The risk of pregnancy is higher than that of combined oral contraceptives and increases with each tablet missed.

Evaluation factors Investigate the cause of breakthrough or irregular bleeding from the vagina. If pathology is excluded, a change to another formulation may solve the problem.

Client teaching factors

1. If 1 tablet is missed it should be taken as soon as remembered. The next tablet should be taken at the regular time, totalling 2 tablets for that day.

2. If 2 tablets are missed on 2 consecutive days, 1 tablet should be taken as soon as remembered, the other missed tablet should be discarded, and the regular tablet for that day taken at the proper time.
3. In addition, another contraceptive method should be used until 14 tablets have been taken or until menses has occurred and pregnancy ruled out.
4. If tablets have been taken as directed and menses does not occur within 60 days from the last period, a method of nonhormonal contraception should be substituted until pregnancy has been ruled out.
5. Micronor users should discontinue taking tablets if 1 tablet is missed and use a nonhormonal contraceptive until menses occurs.

COMBINATION ORAL CONTRACEPTIVES

Trade Name	Composition
Ortho-Novum 1/50-21	Norethindrone 1 mg, mestranol 0.05 mg
Ortho-Novum 1/80-21	Norethindrone 1 mg, mestranol 0.08 mg
Ortho-Novum 1/50-28	Norethindrone 1 mg, mestranol 0.05 mg
Ortho-Novum 1/80-28	Norethindrone 1 mg, mestranol 0.08 mg
Ortho-Novum 2	Norethindrone 2 mg, mestranol 0.10 mg
Ortho-Novum 10	Norethindrone 10 mg, mestranol 0.06 mg
Modicon	Norethindrone 0.5 mg, ethinyl estradiol 0.035 mg
Modicon 28	Norethindrone 0.5 mg, ethinyl estradiol 0.035 mg
Ovral	Norgestrel 0.5 mg, ethinyl estradiol 0.05 mg
Ovral 28	Norgestrel 0.5 mg, ethinyl estradiol 0.05 mg
Lo Ovral	Norgestrel 0.3 mg, ethinyl estradiol 0.03 mg
Lo Ovral 28	Norgestrel 0.3 mg, ethinyl estradiol 0.03 mg
Ovulen	Ethynodiol diacetate 1 mg, mestranol 0.1 mg
Ovulen 21	Ethynodiol diacetate 1 mg, mestranol 0.1 mg

Trade Name	Composition
Ovulen 28	Ethynodiol diacetate 1 mg, mestranol 0.1 mg
Demulen	Ethynodiol diacetate 1 mg, ethinyl estradiol 0.05 mg
Demulen 28	Ethynodiol diacetate 1 mg, ethinyl estradiol 0.05 mg
Enovid 5	Norethynodrel 5 mg, mestranol 0.075 mg
Enovid 10	Norethynodrel 10 mg, mestranol 0.075 mg
Enovid-E	Norethynodrel 2.5 mg, mestranol 10 mg
Ovcon-50	Norethindrone 1 mg, ethinyl estradiol 0.05 mg
Ovcon-35	Norethindrone 0.4 mg, ethinyl estradiol 0.035 mg
Zorane 1/20	Norethindrone 1 mg, ethinyl estradiol 0.02 mg
Zorane 1/50	Norethindrone 1 mg, ethinyl estradiol 0.05 mg
Zorane 1.5/30	Norethindrone 1.5 mg, ethinyl estradiol 0.03 mg
Loestrin 1/20-21	Norethindrone 1 mg, ethinyl estradiol 0.02 mg
Loestrin Fe 1/20	Norethindrone 1 mg, ethinyl estradiol 0.02 mg, ferrous fumarate 75 mg in 7 tablets
Loestrin 1.5/30-21	Norethindrone 1.5 mg, ethinyl estradiol 0.03 mg
Loestrin Fe 1.5/30	Norethindrone 1.5 mg, ethinyl estradiol 0.03 mg, ferrous fumarate 75 mg in 7 tablets
Norlestrin 1/50-21	Norethindrone 1 mg, ethinyl estradiol 0.05 mg
Norlestrin 1/50-28	Norethindrone 1 mg, ethinyl estradiol 0.05 mg
Norlestrin Fe 1/50	Norethindrone 1 mg, ethinyl estradiol 0.05 mg, ferrous fumarate 75 mg in 7 tablets
Norlestrin 2.5/50-21	Norethindrone 2.5 mg, ethinyl estradiol 0.05 mg
Norlestrin Fe 2.5/50	Norethindrone 2.5 mg, ethinyl estradiol 0.05 mg, ferrous fumarate 75 mg in 7 tablets
Norinyl 1 + 50-21	Norethindrone 1 mg, mestranol 0.05 mg

Trade Name	Composition
Norinyl 1 + 50-28	Norethindrone 1 mg, mestranol 0.05 mg
Norinyl 1 + 80-21	Norethindrone 1 mg, mestranol 0.08 mg
Norinyl 1 + 80-28	Norethindrone 1 mg, mestranol 0.08 mg
Norinyl 2-20	Norethindrone 2 mg, mestranol 0.1 mg
Brevicon 21	Norethindrone 0.5 mg, ethinyl estradiol 0.035 mg
Brevicon 28	Norethindrone 0.5 mg, ethinyl estradiol 0.035 mg

Administration Schedules vary according to how a cycle of tablets is packaged. The numbers following the trade name indicate the dosage of progestogen and estrogen per tablet. In addition, the numbers 20, 21, or 28 indicate the number of tablets per package. The packages labeled 28 contain 7 placebo or iron tablets, which are taken in place of the hormone tablets for 7 days during each menstrual cycle.

20-Day schedule Client takes 1 tablet daily for 20 consecutive days, beginning each course on day 5 of the menstrual cycle, or 8 days after taking the last tablet from the previous cycle, whichever occurs first. The first day of menstruation is counted as day 1.

21-Day schedule (method A) *Initial cycle:* Client takes 1 tablet daily starting on the first Sunday after the onset of menstruation. If menses begins on a Sunday, the first tablet is taken that same day. The 21st tablet will then be taken on a Sunday. *Subsequent cycles:* A new 21-day cycle is begun on Sunday, the 8th day after taking the last tablet. All subsequent cycles will also begin on Sunday with 1 tablet taken each day for 3 weeks, followed by a week of no tablets.

21-Day schedule (method B) *Initial cycle:* Client takes 1 tablet daily starting on day 5 of the menstrual cycle, for a total of 21 tablets. *Subsequent cycles:* A new 21-day cycle is begun on the 8th day after taking the last tablet. All subsequent cycles will begin on the same day, with 1 tablet taken each day for 3 weeks, followed by a week of no tablets.

28-Day schedule *Initial cycle:* Client takes 1 tablet daily, starting on the first Sunday after the onset of menstruation. If menses begins on Sunday, the first tablet is taken that same day. The 28th tablet will then be taken on a Saturday. *Subsequent cycles:* A new 28-day cycle begins on the next day (Sunday), with 1 tablet taken each day for 28 days.

Available Drug Forms Dialpak tablet dispensers containing 20, 21, or 28 tablets; Pilpak tablet dispensers containing 20, 21, or 28 tablets; Compack tablet dispensers containing 20, 21, or 28 tablets; Memorette tablet dispensers containing 20, 21, or 28 tablets; packages of 20, 21, and 28 tablets in cartons of 6 packages.

COMBINATION HORMONAL AND ANTIANXIETY AGENTS

Trade Name	Composition
PMB 200	Premarin 0.45 mg, meprobamate 200 mg
PMB 400	Premarin 0.45 mg, meprobamate 400 mg
Milprem 200	Conjugated estrogens 0.45 mg, meprobamate 200 mg
Milprem 400	Conjugated estrogens 0.45 mg, meprobamate 400 mg
Menrium 5-2	Chlordiazepoxide 5 mg, esterified estrogens 0.2 mg
Menrium 5-4	Chlordiazepoxide 5 mg, esterified estrogens 0.4 mg
Menrium 10-4	Chlordiazepoxide 10 mg, esterified estrogens 0.4 mg

Indications for Use Treatment of moderate to severe vasomotor symptoms associated with menopause and accompanied by emotional symptoms, such as anxiety and tension.

Administration The lowest dose possible for controlling symptoms should be used and the medication discontinued as soon as possible. (See Chapter 35 for other information on specific drugs in these combination agents.)

Chapter 23

Antidiabetics and Hyperglycemic Agents

THERE ARE TWO general categories of antidiabetic drugs: insulin and oral hypoglycemics. Insulin is synthesized and secreted by the beta cells of the pancreatic islands of Langerhans. When these cells fail to function or are destroyed, little or no insulin is available for physiologic processes. Insulin regulates the metabolism of carbohydrates, proteins, and fats, and enhances glucose uptake in most cells. When insulin secretion is deficient or ineffective, hyperglycemia or diabetes result due to excess levels of glucose in the blood. The symptoms of diabetes are polyphagia, polyuria, polydipsia, weight loss, and glucosuria.

Diabetes falls into two types of categories: juvenile and maturity-onset diabetes. Juvenile diabetes usually has an abrupt onset and is due to a decrease in the number of beta cells with little or no secretion of insulin. This form of diabetes is treated with insulin injections and a diabetic regime. In maturity-onset or mild diabetes, the beta cells still produce some insulin, and clients with this type of diabetes can usually be maintained on a diabetic diet and/or oral hypoglycemics.

Nursing management of diabetes involves giving emotional support to help the client and family accept the medical diagnosis and educating them about the disease process, urine testing, administering antidiabetics, the signs and symptoms of complications of diabetes, personal hygiene to decrease infection, the diabetic diet, and exercise. The goal of the nurse is to give good health teaching to the client so that he or she will comply with the diabetic regimen and reach the highest possible level of health.

CHARACTERISTICS OF INSULIN

Insulin is a hormone whose use in the treatment of diabetes was discovered in 1922 by Frederick Banting. Although several types of insulin are available, they all have the same basic pharmacologic action. Insulins with different rates of action (rapid acting, intermediate acting, long acting) can be combined to produce the most effective preparation for a particular client. For example, lente insulins can be mixed with each other and regular insulin can be mixed with NPH, globin, and protamine zinc insulin. The dosage of insulin is determined by the individual needs of each client, and is usually administered subcutaneously. Only regular insulin can be given intravenously for very quick action.

Insulin is available in U 40 and U 100 concentrations and insulin syringes (U-40, U-100) come in disposable or reusable glass types. Although the choice of syringe depends on the client's preferences, U-40 insulin must be used with a U-40 syringe and U-100 insulin with a U-100 syringe to obtain the correct amount of medication. In the future, only U-100 insulin will be available and this will help decrease medication errors.

Insulin can be stored in a refrigerator for 36 months or at room temperature for a month. (Insulin given at room temperature decreases lipodystrophy and discomfort.) Regular and globin insulins are clear whereas the other insulins are cloudy. All insulins should be clear from clumps or aggregations after rolling the bottle of insulin between the hands.

Client Education

Once a client is familiar with all the equipment, he or she should be shown how to prepare an insulin syringe. The best approach is to let the client practice drawing up insulin under supervision. One of the main problems involved in withdrawing the insulin is the "dead space" in the syringe hub and shaft of needle. All air bubbles should be expelled from the syringe and when the medicine is withdrawn there should be no "dead space." To mix two insulins in one syringe, the air should be injected into the first bottle (5 U) and the needle withdrawn; the air (15 U) injected into the second bottle and the medication (15 U) withdrawn; then the medication (5 U) taken from the first bottle.

The client should also be taught to rotate injection sites. An easy and effective way to rotate injection sites is to write the dates of the month on a picture of the body that shows the thighs, upper arms, abdomen, and buttocks. (These sites are used because they have increased vascularity.) When injecting the insulin, the following procedure should be followed by the client: (1) wipe the skin with alcohol and allow the site to dry; (2) pinch the skin and fat and insert the needle at a 45-degree angle; (3) inject the insulin and pull the needle out while holding the skin with an alcohol swab.

Diabetic clients should be educated about the signs and symptoms of insulin overdose, hyperinsulinism, or hypoglycemia. Hypoglycemic reactions start with symptoms of fatigue, nervousness, sweating, faintness, and headache. If such symptoms arise, a fast-acting carbohydrate, such as orange juice or candy, should be taken. If the client is unconscious, a hyperglycemic agent will have to be given intravenously. The client also must be able to recognize the signs and symptoms of ketoacidosis or hyperglycemia. This can be caused by physical or psychologic stressors such as infection, surgery, injury, pregnancy, or shock. The early symptoms of diabetic ketoacidosis (DKA) are thirst, anorexia, vomiting, abdominal pain, drowsiness, hot dry flushed appearance, and fruity odor to the breath. If possible, urine should be checked for spillage of sugar when these symptoms occur and regular insulin used according to the amount needed. Insulin is administered subcutaneously if the client is conscious and intravenously if the person is unconscious. Solutions of normal saline are given intravenously to expand plasma volume and establish renal output. Care should be taken to observe the client for insulin shock because he or she can go from ketoacidosis to hyperinsulinism without regaining consciousness.

CHARACTERISTICS OF ORAL HYPOGLYCEMIC AGENTS

Oral antidiabetic agents have been available for public use since 1956 and are used by clients who have some residual pancreatic function in maturity-onset diabetes. There are two types of oral hypoglycemics: sulfonylureas and biquanides. Sulfonylureas stimulate the beta cells in the islands of Langerhans to synthesize and secrete insulin. Biguanides do not act by increasing the release of insulin, but by enhancing glycolysis. These oral preparations are convenient and long acting. Client education should stress that both diet and medication must be followed carefully.

Several other factors must be considered when oral hypoglycemics are used. Namely, since additional amounts of insulin are needed by diabetics in certain situations, such as pregnancy, surgery, or severe stress, clients using oral hypoglycemics should be instructed on parenteral insulin administration and the signs and symptoms of hypoglycemic reactions. In addition, clients should be informed that sulfonylureas can cause alcohol intolerance and are incompatible with barbiturates, sedatives, and hypnotics.

ANTIDIABETICS

Rapid-Acting Insulins

GENERIC NAME Insulin (RX)

TRADE NAMES Regular Iletin, Regular Insulin

CLASSIFICATION Antidiabetic

Source Obtained from beef and/or pork pancreas.

Action This is the shortest acting insulin. It stimulates glycogen synthesis in the liver by promoting the conversion of glucose to glycogen, enhances the cellular utilization of glucose, promotes triglyceride formation, and stimulates protein synthesis by facilitating the transport of amino acids across cell membranes.

Indications for Use Management of juvenile diabetes mellitus and complicated forms of maturity-onset diabetes. May be used to stimulate appetite and weight gain in selected cases of malnutrition. Sometimes used to induce hypoglycemic shock for treatment of psychotic states. The only insulin that can be given IV in ketoacidotic emergencies.

Contraindications Sensitivity to animal protein.

Untoward Reactions Hypoglycemia from overdose (hyperinsulinism): diaphoresis, tremor, weakness, hunger, nausea, palpitations, tachycardia, paresthesias, circumoral pallor, blurred vision, irritability, confusion, convulsions, coma. Allergic reaction: urticaria, anaphylaxis, angioneurotic edema, atrophy at injection site.

Parameters of Use

Absorption Absorbed quickly into plasma from subc injection site. Circulates in extracellular fluid as free hormone. Onset of action is 20 to 30 minutes: administer 15 to 30 minutes before a meal. Duration of action is 5 to 8 hours.

Metabolism Primarily in the liver and kidneys.

Excretion Mainly in the feces, with negligible amounts in urine.

Drug Interactions Insulin effect is intensified with concurrent use of alcohol, anabolic steroids, anticoagulants, guanethidine, MAO inhibitors, propanolol, salicylates, sulfonamides, some antineoplastics, phenylbutazone, and methamphetamine. Insulin effect is antagonized with concurrent use of corticosteroids, diazoxide, epinephrine, estrogens, ethacrynic acid, thyroid preparations, furosemide, glucagon, phenothiazines, thiazides, and phenytoin.

Laboratory Interactions Can cause decreases in serum calcium, cholesterol, phosphate, potassium, and urinary sodium; can cause increases in serum corticosteroids, glucagon, and proteins.

Administration Subcutaneous: Highly individualized. Never use cloudy or discolored solution; regular insulin should be clear. Should be at room temperature; cold insulin can cause local adverse reactions and reduce absorption rate. Can be mixed with NPH, globin, and PZI insulins. Intravenous (ketoacidosis): 50 to 150 U. Add only to glass IV containers, since insulin reacts chemically with plastic.

Available Drug Forms 10-ml vials containing 40 or 100 U/ml of clear solution. Mix by rolling vial in palms of hands. Refrigerate stock supplies. Stable at room temperature for 1 month. Avoid sunlight and temperature extremes.

Nursing Management

Planning factors

1. Warn client that visual disturbances may occur during first few weeks of dosage regulation. Vision is usually stabilized by 6th week.
2. Client should always keep extra insulin and syringes on hand.
3. Administer no more than 30 minutes before a meal so peak action coincides with postprandial elevated glucose.
4. Instruct client to advise health care team of any changes in normal living patterns, any sudden illness, or pregnancy, all of which will alter insulin requirements.
5. Client should always have some type of candy, orange juice, honey, or sugar available in the event of a hypoglycemic reaction. If symptoms do not abate within 30 minutes, physician should be contacted.
6. Client should always wear medical identification bracelet or other ID stating diagnosis, drug used, and physician's name and phone number.

Administration factors

1. Strength of insulin and syringe used must be coordinated.
2. If local allergic reaction occurs at injection site, an antihistamine may be prescribed or the insulin preparation may be changed from pork to beef, or vice versa.
3. In acute hyperglycemia or ketoacidosis, regular insulin only is used until client is stabilized.
4. If alcohol is used to cleanse injection site, wait for site to dry before injecting insulin, since alcohol causes precipitation of the insulin.
5. Aspirate needle before subc injection; inadvertent IV administration can cause acute hypoglycemic response.

Evaluation factors

1. Brittle or labile diabetics should test urine several times a day. The goal is to keep the urine as sugar-free as possible while avoiding hypoglycemia.
2. Because renal thresholds vary greatly, some clients need frequent blood glucose monitoring to determine appropriate insulin dosages. Home measurement of hemoglobin A_1C (a more accurate measure of control than urine testing) is now available for these labile diabetics. These clients should be taught to adjust insulin dosages according to the daily Hgb A_1C results.
3. Accurate record-keeping by the client of food intake, insulin dosages, and urine testing is important in long-term management of diabetes and in delaying or minimizing complications of the disease.
4. The indicators of good diabetic control include: normal serum glucose and lipid levels; weight within normal range; no hypoglycemic reactions; urine negative for glucose, acetone, and protein; normal growth in juvenile diabetics.

Client teaching factors

1. Teach client a systematic approach to rotation of injection sites. There should be a 6 week time interval before a site is reused.
2. Teach client the importance of adherence to diet, urine testing, dosage accuracy, and appropriate personal hygiene to minimize the development of complications.
3. Instruct client to avoid all OTC drugs, since many have high sugar contents, and excessive alcohol intake, which can result in a hypoglycemic reaction.
4. If insulin is temporarily unavailable when the required dose is due, instruct client to increase fluid intake but refrain from eating.

GENERIC NAME Prompt insulin zinc suspension

TRADE NAMES Semilente Iletin, Semilente Insulin

CLASSIFICATION Antidiabetic (RX)

See insulin for Untoward reactions, Parameters of use, Drug interactions, and Nursing management.

Action This is a rapid-acting insulin. (See insulin.)

Indications for Use Management of diabetes mellitus in clients who are allergic to other types of insulin because no modifying protein is added.

Absorption Absorbed quickly into plasma from subc injection site. Onset of action is 30 to 60 minutes; administer 30 minutes before breakfast. Peak action occurs in 5 to 7 hours and duration of action is 14 hours.

Administration Subcutaneous: Highly individualized. Do not give IV. Lente insulins can be mixed together. (See insulin.)

Available Drug Forms 10-ml vials containing 40 or 100 U/ml of suspension. Mix by rolling vial in palms of hands. If precipitate forms, discard vial. (See insulin.)

Intermediate-Acting Insulins

GENERIC NAME Isophane insulin suspension

TRADE NAMES Isophane Insulin, NPH Iletin NPH Insulin

CLASSIFICATION Antidiabetic (RX)

See insulin for Untoward reactions, Parameters of use, and Drug interactions.

Action This is an intermediate-acting insulin. Suspension of modified protamine zinc insulin crystals in a neutral buffer. (See insulin.)

Indications for Use Management of diabetes mellitus.

Absorption Absorbed at a moderate rate into plasma. Onset of action is 60 to 90 minutes: administer 1 hour before breakfast. Peak action occurs in 8 to 12 hours and duration of action is 24 hours.

Administration Subcutaneous: Highly individualized. Do not give IV. Can be mixed with regular insulin, but not with lente insulins. (See insulin.)

Available Drug Forms 10-ml vials containing 40 or 100 U/ml of suspension. (See insulin.)

Nursing Management Instruct client to be alert for hypoglycemic reaction in the afternoon. (See insulin.)

GENERIC NAME Insulin zinc suspension (RX)

TRADE NAMES Lente Iletin, Lente Insulin

CLASSIFICATION Antidiabetic

See insulin for Untoward reactions, Parameters of use, and Drug interactions.

Action This is an intermediate-acting insulin. (See insulin.)

Indications for Use Management of diabetes mellitus in clients allergic to other types of insulin, since it contains no foreign protein.

Absorption Absorbed at a moderate rate into plasma. Onset of action is 60 to 90 minutes; administer 30 to 60 minutes before breakfast. Peak action occurs in 8 to 12 hours and duration of action is 24 hours.

Administration Subcutaneous: Highly individualized. Do not give IV. Lente insulins can be mixed with each other, but not with other modified insulins. (See insulin.)

Available Drug Forms 10-ml vials containing 40 or 100 U/ml of suspension. (See insulin.)

Nursing Management Hypoglycemic symptoms may appear midafternoon or later. (See insulin.)

GENERIC NAME Globin zinc insulin injection

TRADE NAME Globin Zinc Insulin (RX)

CLASSIFICATION Antidiabetic

See insulin for Untoward reactions, Parameters of use, and Drug interactions.

Action This is an intermediate-acting insulin, composed of globin, zinc, and insulin. (See insulin.)

Indications for Use Management of diabetes mellitus in clients who cannot be controlled with other insulins or who are sensitive to protamine.

Absorption Absorbed at a moderate rate into plasma. Onset of action is 2 hours: administer 30 to 60 minutes before breakfast. Peak action occurs in 8 to 16 hours and duration of action is 18 to 24 hours.

Administration Subcutaneous: Highly individualized. Do not give IV or IM. Can be mixed with regular insulin. (See insulin.)

Available Drug Forms 10-ml vials containing 40 or 100 U/ml of clear, yellowish solution. Mix by rolling vial in palms of hands. (See insulin.)

Nursing Management Teach client to be alert for hypoglycemic reaction in the late afternoon. (See insulin.)

Long-Acting Insulins

GENERIC NAME Protamine zinc insulin suspension

TRADE NAMES Protamine, Zinc and Iletin, Protamine, Zinc Insulin, PZI

CLASSIFICATION Antidiabetic

See insulin for Untoward reactions, Parameters of use, and Drug interactions.

Action This is a long-acting insulin composed of protamine, zinc, and insulin. (See insulin.)

Indications for Use Management of diabetes mellitus in clients who cannot be controlled with unmodified insulins.

Absorption Absorbed very slowly from subc injection site into plasma. Onset of action is 4 to 8 hours; administer 30 to 60 minutes before breakfast. Peak action occurs in 14 to 20 hours and duration of action is 24 to 36 hours or more.

Administration Subcutaneous: Highly individualized. Do not give IV. Can be mixed with regular insulin only. (See insulin.)

Available Drug Forms 10-ml vials containing 40 or 100 U/ml of suspension. (See insulin.)

Nursing Management (See insulin.)

1. Teach client to be alert for hypoglycemic reactions in the evening.
2. Regular mealtimes are essential.
3. At beginning of treatment with PZI, full effect may be delayed for 2 to 3 days. During this time, supplemental doses of regular insulin may be required.

GENERIC NAME Extended insulin zinc suspension

TRADE NAMES Ultralente Iletin, Ultralente Insulin

CLASSIFICATION Antidiabetic (RX)

See insulin for Untoward reactions, Parameters of use, and Drug interactions.

Action This is as long-acting insulin. (See insulin.)

Indications for Use Management of diabetes mellitus in clients who are allergic to other types of insulin, since it contains no proteins.

Absorption Absorbed slowly from subc injection site into plasma. Onset of action is 4 to 8 hours; administer 30 to 90 minutes before breakfast. Peak action occurs in 16 to 18 hours and duration of action is 36 hours or more.

Administration Subcutaneous: Highly individualized. Do not give IV. Can be mixed with lente insulins, but not with other modified insulins. (See insulin.)

Available Drug Forms 10-ml vials containing 40 or 100 U/ml of suspension. (See insulin.)

Nursing Management Teach client to be alert for hypoglycemic reactions at night or early morning. (See insulin.)

Oral Hypoglycemic Agents—Sulfonylureas

GENERIC NAMES Tolbutamide; tolbutamide sodium

TRADE NAMES Orinase; Orinase Diagnostic (RX)

CLASSIFICATION Oral hypoglycemic, sulfonylurea

See insulin for Nursing management.

Action Stimulates pancreatic beta cells to synthesize and release insulin. (Effective only if functional beta cells are present in pancreas.)

Indications for Use Maturity-onset diabetes, mild to moderately severe diabetes. Sometimes used with insulin. Also used for diagnosis of islet cell tumor.

Contraindications Labile diabetes; pregnancy; sulfa drug allergy; stress, infection; severe renal, liver, or thyroid deficiency.

Untoward Reactions GI disturbances, dermatologic reactions, photosensitivity reactions, headaches, hypoglycemic symptoms, cholestatic jaundice (rare), blood dyscrasias (rare).

Parameters of Use

Absorption Rapidly absorbed from GI tract; binds to plasma proteins. Onset of action is 30 minutes; administer before breakfast or in divided doses during the day. Peak action occurs in 3 to 5 hours and duration of action is 6 to 12 hours. Half-life is 5 hours.

Metabolism In liver to carboxytolbutamide.

Excretion Primarily by the kidneys within 24 hours.

Drug Interactions The following drugs prolong the effect of oral hypoglycemics: allopurinol, chloramphenicol, oral anticoagulants, MAO inhibitors, oxyphenbutazone, phenylbutazone, phenyramidol, phenytoin, probenicid, salicylates, sulfonamides, alcohol, insulin. The following drugs reduce the effect of oral hypoglycemics: beta-blockers, thiazide diuretics.

Laboratory Interactions Causes reduced radioactive iodine uptake and altered liver function test values.

Administration Oral: Usual dosage: 1000 mg/daily; Maximum dosage: 2000 mg daily. Give with food to minimize GI upset. Intravenous (tolbutamide sodium): 1 g in sterile water over 1 to 3 minutes. IV infusion may produce local irritation or phlebitis.

Available Drug Forms White tablets containing 250 or 500 mg; vials of 1 g with diluent.

Planning factors Instruct client to avoid excessive sunlight until drug effects are determined.

Administration factors

1. Drug should not be taken at bedtime.
2. Drug should always be taken with food to minimize GI upset.

Evaluation factors

1. Teach client that compliance with diabetic diet is imperative for best results.
2. Client's weight should be monitored weekly. Progressive weight gain calls for discontinuance of tolbutamide.
3. Client should be taught to report immediately any signs of liver dysfunction.

GENERIC NAME Chlorpropamide (RX)

TRADE NAME Diabinese

CLASSIFICATION Oral hypoglycemic, sulfonylurea

See tolbutamide for Drug interactions and Nursing management.

Action Longest acting oral hypoglycemic. May potentiate antidiuretic hormone. Is six times more potent than tolbutamide. (See tolbutamide.)

Indications for Use In adults with diabetes mellitus who are stabilized and cannot be controlled by diet alone. Also for polyurea of diabetes insipidus.

Contraindications Pregnancy; Raynaud's disease; juvenile diabetes; renal, liver, or thyroid dysfunction; diarrhea.

Warnings and Precautions Used with caution in elderly clients and those with congestive heart failure.

Untoward Reactions Generally, more toxic than other oral hypoglycemic agents. GI distress, diarrhea, rashes, photosensitivity, cholestatic jaundice (rare), agranulocytosis (rare). (See tolbutamide.)

Parameters of Use

Absorption Rapidly absorbed from GI tract and distributed in extracellular fluid. Onset of action is 1 hour; administer in morning with food. Peak action occurs in 3 to 6 hours and duration of action is up to 72 hours. Half-life is 36 hours. Is bound to plasma proteins and is not metabolically changed to any great extent.

Excretion Slowly by the kidneys in 96 hours.

Administration Oral: Usual dosage: 100 to 500 mg daily; Maximum dosage: 750 mg daily. Give with food to minimize GI upset.

Available Drug Forms Blue tablets containing 100 or 250 mg.

GENERIC NAME Acetohexamide (RX)

TRADE NAME Dymelor

CLASSIFICATION Oral hypoglycemic, sulfonylurea

See tolbutamide for Untoward reactions, Drug interactions, and Nursing management.

Action Longer action than tolbutamide. Has moderate uricosuric effect. (See tolbutamide.)

Indications for Use In stable, mild adult diabetics.

Contraindications Pregnancy, unstable diabetes. (See tolbutamide.)

Parameters of Use

Absorption Rapidly absorbed from GI tract. Onset of action is 30 minutes. Peak action occurs in 3 hours and duration of action is 12 to 14 hours. Half-life is 6 to 8 hours.

Metabolism In liver to hydroxyhexamide.

Excretion By the kidneys within 24 hours (50%) and in the bile (15%).

Administration Oral: Usual dosage: 500 mg daily; Maximum dosage: 1500 mg daily. Give with food to minimize GI upset.

Available Drug Forms White tablets containing 250 mg; yellow tablets containing 500 mg.

GENERIC NAME Tolazamide (RX)

TRADE NAME Tolinase

CLASSIFICATION Oral hypoglycemic, sulfonylurea

See tolbutamide for Contraindications, Untoward reactions, Drug interactions, and Nursing management.

Action Five times more potent than tolbutamide. (See tolbutamide.)

Indications for Use In maturity-onset diabetes of mild to moderate severity. May be effective in clients with intolerance to similar drugs.

Parameters of Use

Absorption Slowly absorbed from the GI tract and bound to plasma protein. Onset of action is 4 to 6 hours. Peak action occurs 4 to 8 hours and duration of action is 10 hours. Half-life is 7 hours.

Metabolism In liver to a number of hypoglycemic substances.

Excretion About 85% of drug in urine.

Administration Oral: 100 to 500 mg daily. Dosage over 500 mg given in divided doses bid.

Available Drug Forms White tablets containing 100, 250, or 500 mg.

Oral Hypoglycemic Agents—Biguanides

GENERIC NAME Phenformin hydrochloride (RX)

TRADE NAMES DBI, Meltrol

CLASSIFICATION Oral hypoglycemic, biguanide

Action Increases glucose utilization by enhancing anaerobic glycolysis. It requires some insulin to be present in body. Has some fibrinolytic activity.

Indications for Use Maturity-onset diabetes; useful in children in conjunction with insulin.

Contraindications Liver and renal impairment, alcoholism, acidosis, pregnancy, surgery, trauma, infection, Raynaud's disease.

Warnings and Precautions Used with caution in elderly clients and those with cardiovascular disease.

Untoward Reactions GI irritation, nausea, vomiting, anorexia, diarrhea, headache, weakness, weight loss, ketonuria.

Parameters of Use

Absorption From the GI tract. Onset of action is 1 to 2 hours. Peak action occurs in 4 to 6 hours and duration of action is 9 to 10 hours.
Metabolism In the liver to glucuronide.
Excretion In urine.

Drug Interactions Client may have increased tendency to hemorrhage if also taking oral anticoagulants. (See tolbutamide.)

Administration Oral: 50 to 150 mg daily in 3 to 5 divided doses; 25 to 50 mg daily as an adjunct to insulin. Should be taken with meals.

Available Drug Forms Tablets containing 25 mg; timed-release capsules containing 50 or 100 mg.

Nursing Management (See tolbutamide.)

1. If client complains of metallic taste or exhibits nausea or vomiting, drug should be withheld and physician notified.
2. Observe elderly clients carefully for signs of hypoglycemia.

HYPERGLYCEMIC AGENTS

GENERIC NAME Glucagon (RX)

CLASSIFICATION Insulin Antagonist, hyperglycemic agent

Action Promotes amino acid uptake by the liver; mobilizes hepatic glycogen producing an increase in blood glucose concentration; increases heart rate and force of contraction.

Indications for Use Treatment of insulin-induced hypoglycemia.

Warnings and Precautions Used with caution in debilitated clients and those with renal or hepatic dysfunction.

Untoward Reactions Nausea, vomiting, hypersensitivity reactions, circulatory collapse.

Parameters of Use

Absorption In 5 to 20 minutes from parenteral administration site. Duration of action is 1 to 2 hours; oral carbohydrates should be given as soon as client awakens.
Metabolism Primarily in liver.

Drug Interactions Potentiates the anticoagulant effects of warfarin and oral anticoagulants. Has additive effects when given in conjunction with other hyperglycemic agents.

Administration Intramuscular, intravenous, subcutaneous: 0.5 to 1.0 mg; may be repeated in 25 to 30 minutes if no response. Do not mix with solutions containing sodium, potassium, or calcium since precipitation will occur. May be mixed in IV dextrose solutions.

Available Drug Forms Vials of powdered drug in 1 or 10 mg, with solution for reconstitution. Must be refrigerated after reconstitution. Will remain stable for 3 months.

Nursing Management

1. Watch for hypersensitivity reaction, since drug is a protein.
2. Teach family members how to give subc or IM in the event of loss of consciousness from hypoglycemic reaction.

GENERIC NAME Diazoxide (RX)

TRADE NAMES Hyperstat I.V., Proglycem

CLASSIFICATION Hyperglycemic agent, antihypertensive

Action Inhibits pancreatic secretion of insulin; increases glycogen synthesis. Causes hyperuricemia, decreased sodium and water excretion, tachycardia. Relaxes vascular smooth muscle, causing decrease in blood pressure.

Indications for Use Management of hyperinsulinism from islet cell hyperplasia or malignancy. Emergency treatment of malignant hypertension crisis.

Contraindications Functional hypoglycemia, hypersensitivity to thiazides or sulfonamides.

Warnings and Precautions Use with caution in diabetes, renal dysfunction, circulatory dysfunction, gout, pregnancy, and in patients taking corticosteroids.

Untoward Reactions Retention of sodium and water, hirsutism, GI upset, tachycardia, hyperuricemia, dermatologic reactions, herpes, headache, weakness. Less common reactions include hypotension, chest pain, congestive heart failure, anxiety, dizziness, insomnia, blood dyscrasias, bleeding tendency, visual disturbances, transient cataracts, nephrotic syndrome, oliguria, hematuria, albuminuria, glycosuria, fever, lymphadenopathy, pancreatitis, paresthesias, and ketoacidosis.

Parameters of Use

Absorption From GI tract in 60 minutes. About 90% bound to plasma proteins. Half-life is 10 to 24 hours in children and 24 to 36 hours in adults.

Crosses placental barrier and appears in breast milk.

Excretion In urine.

Drug Interactions Antihypertensives and diuretics may intensify hypotensive effects of diazoxide. Chlorpromazine and thiazides may intensify hyperglycemic and hyperuricemic effects. Any other protein-bound drug may enhance all the effects of diazoxide.

Laboratory Interactions May cause increased plasma alkaline phosphatase and serum glutamic-oxaloacetic transaminase levels and decreased hemoglobin, hematocrit, and IgB levels. The presence of hypokalemia in the client will enhance the effects of diazoxide.

Administration Oral: 3 to 8 mg/kg/day in divided doses for treatment of hypoglycemia. (Infants: 3 to 15 mg/kg/day in 2 or 3 divided doses.) Intravenous: 300 mg over 30 seconds for treatment of hypertension emergency. Dose may be repeated in 30 minutes if no response.

Available Drug Forms Capsules containing 50 or 100 mg; Suspension containing 50 mg/ml (shake well before use); 300 mg in a 20-ml ampule. Protect from light and extreme temperatures.

Nursing Management Treatment of hypoglycemia.

Planning factors Instruct client to immediately report any visual changes or hirsutism; both are reversible when drug is withdrawn.

Administration factors

1. Clients taking liquid suspension may show higher diazoxide blood levels. This should be considered when changing dosage forms.
2. Urine should be tested daily for glucose and ketones. Changes should be reported immediately in order to prevent hyperglycemia progressing to ketoacidosis.

Evaluation factors

1. Input and output and the development of edema must be monitored carefully, especially in clients with cardiovascular disease.
2. After treatment for overdosage (ketoacidosis), clients must be monitored closely for 1 week, since diazoxide has a long half-life.
3. If the desired response is not evident within 3 weeks, the drug should be discontinued.
4. Vital signs should be checked regularly, although oral administration has minimal effect on blood pressure.

Chapter 24

Pituitary Hormones

CHARACTERISTICS OF PITUITARY HORMONES

ANTERIOR PITUITARY HORMONES

Adrenocorticotrophic hormone injection, repository adrenocorticotrophic hormone injection, adrenocorticotrophic hormone zinc hydroxide suspension

Thyrotropin

Clomiphene citrate

Menotropins

Chorionic gonadotropin

POSTERIOR PITUITARY HORMONES

Vasopressin, vasopressin tannate

Oxytocin, oxytocin citrate

Posterior pituitary hormone

CHARACTERISTICS OF PITUITARY HORMONES

The pituitary gland hormones, which regulate the performance of all other endocrine glands of the body, are subdivided into two major categories: the hormones of the adenohypophysis (anterior pituitary hormones) and the hormones of the neurohypophysis (posterior pituitary hormones).

The anterior pituitary hormones are:

1. Growth hormone (GH), or somatotropin (STH)
2. Prolactin, or luteotropin (LTH)
3. Thyroid-stimulating hormone (TSH)
4. Adrenocorticotrophic hormone (ACTH), or corticotropin
5. Follicle-stimulating hormone (FSH)
6. Luteinizing hormone (LH).

Of these six anterior pituitary hormones, only three are available commercially as purified preparations from animal or human pituitary gland. Thyroid-stimulating hormone and adrenocorticotrophic hormone, which are extracted from animal glands, have a direct effect on their target organs, namely, the thyroid and the adrenal cortex. Since thyroid and adrenocortical steroid hormones are available commercially, the products of the target gland are often used for replacement therapy in simple deficiency states. However, growth hormone deficiencies must be treated with the pituitary hormone itself, which is extracted from human pituitary glands. As this hormone is in short supply, it is available only for well-documented deficiency states. Follicle-stimulating hormone and luteinizing hormone are available commercially and are obtained from the urine of pregnant or postmenopausal females. Luteotropin is not yet available for therapeutic use.

The posterior pituitary hormones are:

1. Antidiuretic hormone (ADH), or vasopressin
2. Oxytocin

Antidiuretic hormone (ADH) has several effects. First, it enhances the renal reabsorption of water and is therefore used in treating primary (neurohypophyseal) diabetes insipidus. Second, it stimulates contraction of gastrointestinal smooth muscle and is therefore used in treating abdominal distention. ADH also has a vasoconstricting effect, especially on gastrointestinal blood vessels. It is being used experimentally for its hemostatic effects in certain types of gastrointestinal bleeding. ADH and its two analogs, desmopressin and lypressin, are available as synthetic drugs.

Oxytocin has a direct effect on the smooth muscle of the uterus, stimulating contractions. It also causes contraction of the mammary ducts, thereby stimulating release of breast milk. It is available as a synthetic drug and is used primarily to stimulate uterine contractions during labor.

In addition Pituitrin, an extract of animal posterior pituitary glands, is available and combines the properties of both ADH and oxytocin.

ANTERIOR PITUITARY HORMONES

GENERIC NAME Adrenocorticotrophic hormone injection; repository adrenocorticotrophic hormone injection; adrenocorticotrophic hormone zinc hydroxide suspension

TRADE NAMES ACTH, Acthar; Cortigel, Cortrophin Gel, Depo-ACTH, H.P. Acthar Gel; Cortrophin Zinc

SOURCE Natural (RX)

CLASSIFICATION Anterior pituitary corticotrophic hormone

Action Stimulates the adrenal cortex to produce and secrete all adrenocortical hormones of a functioning adrenal gland

Indications for Use Diagnostic testing of adrenocortical function; treatment of panhypopituitarism, acute gout, idiopathic hypoglycemia.

Contraindications Sensitivity to porcine proteins; scleroderma, osteoporosis, fungal infections, ocular herpes simplex, peptic ulcer, congestive heart failure, hypertension, recent surgery; not for IV use.

Untoward Reactions Hypersensitivity; prolonged use can produce cataracts and/or glaucoma; sodium and fluid retention, potassium and calcium loss; musculoskeletal weakness, fractures; nausea, vomiting, peptic ulcer, pancreatitis; impaired wound healing; hirsutism, hypopigmentation; hypertension, congestive heart failure; dizziness, shock, increased intracranial pressure, psychotic reactions; menstrual irregularities, suppression of growth.

Parameters of Use

Absorption Concentrates in adrenal cortex, placenta, and kidneys. Binds to plasma proteins. Half-life is less than 20 minutes. (Repository dosage forms are present for 18 to 24 hours.)

Excretion Some in urine.

Drug Interactions Enhanced effect of ACTH in patients with cirrhosis or hypothyroidism. Existing emotional instability may be exacerbated with ACTH. May increase need for hypoglycemic agents in diabetic patients. Patients on ACTH should not be immunized because of lack of antibody response and possible neurologic complications.

Administration ACTH: 20 U subc or IM qid; Repository solutions: 40 to 80 U every 34 to 72 hours; Zinc solution: 10 to 160 U daily or bid; Diagnostic testing: 10 to 25 U in 500 ml of 5% dextrose IV.

Available Drug Forms Gel solution: 5-ml multidose vials containing 40 or 80 U.S.P. units/ml; 1-ml ampules containing 40 or 80 U.S.P. units/ml. Powder: 25 or 40 U.S.P. units/vial; reconstitute at time of use; refrigerate and discard after 24 hours.

Nursing Management

Planning factors

1. Skin testing is recommended before treatment.
2. A low-sodium, high-potassium, high-protein diet counteracts edema.

Administration factors

1. Reduction in dosage must be done gradually over a 5-day period.
2. When used in conjunction with other drugs (except for diagnostic testing), the lowest effective dose should not be exceeded.

Evaluation factors As the drug may mask signs of infection, the patient should be checked frequently.

GENERIC NAME Thyrotropin (RX)

TRADE NAMES Thytropar, TSH

SOURCE Natural

CLASSIFICATION Anterior pituitary thyrotropic hormone

Action Increases iodine uptake by thyroid gland and stimulates the production and secretion of thyroid hormone. May cause hyperplasia of thyroid cells.

Indications for Use Diagnosis of thyroid disease; as an adjunct in treating thyroid carcinoma and metastases; assessment of need for thyroid medication.

Contraindications Hypersensitivity to TSH, coronary thrombosis, untreated Addison's disease. Use with caution in clients with heart disease and hypopituitarism.

Untoward Reactions Menstrual irregularities, nausea, vomiting, headache, fever; hypotension, cardiac irregularities, tachycardia, angina, congestive heart failure; urticaria, anaphylactic syndrome; symptoms of hyperthyroidism (excess doses); thyroid storm and shock (acute excess doses).

Parameters of Use

Absorption Half-life is 35 minutes; longer in hypothyroidism, shorter in hyperthyroidism.

Excretion In urine.

Drug Interactions Levodopa lowers TSH levels.

Administration Diagnostic testing: 10 IU subc or IM daily for 1 to 3 days; Therapy: 10 IUs subc or IM daily for 1 to 8 days.

Available Drug Forms Sterile powder in one vial with a second vial of physiologic saline for diluting. Refrigerate after mixing; may be kept for 2 weeks.

Nursing Management

1. With normal thyroid function, diagnostic levels of TSH (10 IU daily for 1 to 3 days) will cause elevated serum thyroxine levels and increased radioactive iodine (RAI) uptake.
2. In primary hypothyroidism, this dose will cause no change in RAI.
3. In hypothyroidism secondary to hypopituitarism, RAI uptake will increase following this dose.

GENERIC NAME Clomiphene citrate (RX)

TRADE NAME Clomid

CLASSIFICATION Synthetic anterior pituitary gonadotropic hormone

---

Action Not clear, but seems to stimulate release of pituitary gonadotropins (FSH and LH). May also be directly involved in the biosynthesis of ovarian hormones. Requires functioning pituitary gland and ovary for therapeutic effect.

Indications for Use Induction of ovulation in women who do not ovulate regularly and desire pregnancy. Is not effective in panhypopituitarism or ovarian failure.

Contraindications Pregnancy, liver disease, abnormal bleeding, ovarian cyst. Use with caution in clients with enlarged ovaries, pelvic discomfort, or sensitivity to pituitary gonadotropins.

Untoward Reactions Multiple births, congenital anomalies, early abortion, hot flushes, abdominal and pelvic discomfort; visual disturbances; nausea, vomiting, weight gain; urinary frequency, polyuria; dermatologic symptoms; tension headache, depression, insomnia, dizziness, fatigue, alopecia.

Parameters of Use

Absorption From GI tract.
Metabolism In liver; stored in body fat.
Excretion About 50% in feces after 5 days.

Administration 50 mg po daily for 5 days. If ovulation does not occur, then after 30 days, dosage is increased to 100 mg daily for 5 days. Total dosage in a single course of treatment should not exceed 600 mg.

Available Drug Forms Tablets containing 50 mg.

Nursing Management

1. If liver function tests are abnormal, therapy should not be given.
2. Teach client to record basal temperatures for determining day of ovulation.
3. If visual symptoms occur, drug should be discontinued, and ophthalmologic evaluation done.
4. Client usually responds after first course of treatment. If no response occurs after 3 courses, then clomiphene citrate will not be effective.

GENERIC NAME Menotropins (RX)

TRADE NAME Pergonal

CLASSIFICATION Anterior pituitary gonadotropic hormone

Source A purified preparation extracted from urine of postmenopausal women.

Action It has both FSH and LH activity. Promotes growth and maturation of graafian follicles. Does not require pituitary gonadotropin secretion for its effect. Menotropins does not induce ovulation; it is given prior to the sequential administration of HCG, which induces ovulation after follicular maturation has occurred.

Indications for Use Treatment of infertility in women with primary or secondary amenorrhea, irregular menses, anovulatory cycles, and polycystic ovary syndrome.

Contraindications Primary ovarian failure, pregnancy, thyroid or adrenal dysfunction, intracranial lesion, abnormal bleeding of unknown origin, ovarian cysts or enlargement not due to polycystic ovary syndrome, infertility due to factors other than anovulation.

Untoward Reactions Dose-related ovarian enlargement, abdominal pain, ovarian hyperstimulation syndrome (abdominal pain, sudden ovarian enlargement accompanied by ascites and/or pleural effusion); nausea, vomiting, fever, diarrhea, hemoperitoneum, thromboemboli (rare), ovarian cysts, hypovolemia, multiple ovulations.

Parameters of Use

Absorption Unknown.
Excretion About 8% is excreted unchanged in urine. Amount of urinary estrogen excretion is an indicator of follicular enlargement.

Administration Highly individualized. Usual dosage: 75 to 100 IU IM daily for 9 to 12 days, followed by HCG. If ovulation occurs without pregnancy, regimen may be repeated twice. If ovulation does not occur, regimen may be repeated with 150 IU for 3 to 12 days. Do not exceed 150 IU/day.

Available Drug Forms Ampules containing 75 IU of FSH and 75 IU of LH. Dissolve ampule contents in 1 to 2 ml of sterile saline. Unused portions must be discarded.

Nursing Management

Planning factors

1. Treatment should be preceded by a thorough gynecologic and endocrine examination. Pregnancy, primary ovarian failure, and neoplasm must be ruled out.
2. Couple should be instructed to have intercourse daily beginning on day prior to HCG administration, until ovulation is apparent.
3. Client should be aware that statistics indicate a 20% incidence of multiple births, with 5% of total pregnancies resulting in 3 or more fetuses.

Administration factors If total urinary estrogen excretion is more than 100 mcg/24 hours, HCG should not be administered because of the danger of ovarian hyperstimulation.

Evaluation factors

1. Client should be examined for excessive ovarian stimulation at least every other day after administration of HCG. Usually, ovarian hyperstimulation is evident 7 to 10 days after ovulation.
2. Client should record weight daily to detect sudden weight gain. Hyperstimulation occurs over a 3 to 4-day period within 2 weeks following treatment.

Client teaching factors

1. Teach client signs of ovulation: rise in basal body temperature, menstruation following drop in basal temperature, increase in watery vaginal secretions.
2. Instruct client to report immediately any signs of ovarian hyperstimulation. Hospitalization, as well as cessation of intercourse, may be necessary.

GENERIC NAME Chorionic gonadotropin (RX)

TRADE NAMES Antuitrin-S, Follutein, Pregnyl, Riogon

CLASSIFICATION Anterior pituitary gonadotropic hormone

Source A placental hormone purified from the urine of pregnant women.

Action Promotes production of gonadal hormones by stimulating testes to produce androgen and ovaries to produce progesterone. Causes ovulation of follicles stimulated by FSH. Promotes corpus luteum development.

Indications for Use Prepubertal cryptorchidism and male hypogonadism, secondary to pituitary failure. With menotropins, to induce ovulation and pregnancy in infertile women who have secondary anovulation.

Contraindications Hypersensitivity, pituitary enlargement, androgen-dependent neoplasms, precocious puberty. Use with caution in epilepsy, migraine, asthma, and cardiac or renal disease.

Untoward Reactions Irritability, restlessness, fatigue, headache, depression, gynecomastia, edema, ascites, increased steroid excretion in urine, pain at injection site, sexual development in prepubertal clients, ovarian enlargement, rupture of ovarian cysts, arterial thromboembolism.

Parameters of Use

Absorption Concentrates in testes or ovaries. Half-life is 8 to 24 hours.
Excretion In urine over 3 to 4 days.

Administration Highly individualized.

- *Prepubertal cryptorchidism:* 4000 U.S.P. units IM three times weekly; then 5000 U.S.P. units every other day for 4 doses; then 500 to 1000 U.S.P. units for 15 doses over 6 weeks; then 500 U.S.P. units three times weekly for 4 to 6 weeks.
- *Anovulatory women:* 5,000 to 10,000 U.S.P. units IM on day following menotropins.

Available Drug Forms Vial containing 10,000 U.S.P. units of powder and 1 ampule of diluent. When reconstituted, 1 ml equals 1000 U.S.P. units. Refrigerate after mixing; stable up to 3 months.

Nursing Management

1. In prepubescent males, HCG will cause testicular descent if no anatomical barrier is present. In most cases, this response is temporary until puberty.
2. If edema develops as indicated by sudden weight gain, dose should be reduced.
3. If vaginal bleeding develops, drug should be discontinued.

POSTERIOR PITUITARY HORMONES

GENERIC NAMES Vasopressin; vasopressin tannate

TRADE NAMES Pitressin, Lypressin (RX)

CLASSIFICATION Synthetic posterior pituitary antidiuretic hormone

Action Antidiuretic, by increasing reabsorption of water by renal tubules. Causes smooth muscle contraction in GI tract, gall bladder, and urinary tract. Causes contraction of all parts of vascular bed.

Indications for Use Treatment of postoperative abdominal distention and diabetes insipidus. Dispels gas shadows in abdominal x-rays.

Contraindications Anaphylaxis or hypersensitivity to drug, coronary artery disease. Use with caution in epilepsy, migraine, asthma, congestive heart failure, chronic nephritis with nitrogen retention, in the elderly, children, and in pregnancy.

Untoward Reactions Water intoxication, tremor, sweating, vertigo, abdominal cramps, headache, nausea, vomiting, bronchial constriction, pallor, hypertension, arrhythmias, anaphylactic syndrome.

Parameters of Use

Absorption Cumulative for tannate IM preparation. Duration of action is 48 to 96 hours. Duration of action for aqueous preparation is 1 to 8 hours.
Distribution Throughout extracellular fluid. Half-life is 10 to 20 minutes.
Metabolism In liver and the kidneys.
Excretion In the kidneys.

Drug Interactions Ganglionic blocking agents cause increased pressor effects of vasopressin. Lithium, heparin, alcohol, demeclocycline, epinephrine, and cyclophosphamide decrease or block antidiuretic activity of vasopressin. Chlorpropamide, urea, fludrocortisone, and acetaminophen increase antidiuretic response.

Administration Usual dosage: 5 to 10 U subc or IM q3h or q4h. Tannate injection is painful. Give with 1 to 2 glasses of water to reduce GI side effects. Dosages for intranasal spray or drops are highly individualized. Do not give IV.

Available Drug Forms Ampules (aqueous) containing 0.5 (10 U) or 1 ml (20 U); ampules (suspension in oil) containing 1 ml (5 U). Shake before using. Should be warmed to body temperature. If refrigerated, can be used for 2 years.

Nursing Management

1. For relief of abdominal distention, a rectal tube should be inserted after drug is administered.
2. Urinary specific gravity, weight, and blood pressure should be monitored during therapy.
3. Drug can cause myocardial infarction or coronary insufficiency in the elderly. Be alert for signs of water intoxication. If present, discontinue drug and restrict fluids.

GENERIC NAMES Oxytocin; oxytocin citrate (RX)

TRADE NAMES Pitocin, Syntocinon; Pitocin Citrate

CLASSIFICATION Synthetic posterior pituitary hormone

Action Increases permeability of uterine cells to sodium ions, thereby augmenting the number of contracting myofibrils. (Enables uterus to produce the necessary number of contractions.) The uterus is increasingly sensitive to oxytocin as gestation progresses; it reaches maximum sensitivity just before labor begins. Has antidiuretic effect. Promotes letdown reflex in nursing mothers thereby promoting flow of milk.

Indications for Use Induction of labor in selected patients and management of incomplete abortion; control of postpartum bleeding and hemorrhage; relief of pain from breast engorgement; promotion of letdown reflex.

Contraindications Cephalopelvic disproportion, abnormal fetal positions, fetal distress when delivery is not imminent, severe toxemia, hypertonic uterus, any condition where vaginal delivery is contraindicated.

Untoward Reactions Fetal bradycardia, anaphylactic syndrome, postpartum hemorrhage, pelvic hematoma, cardiac arrhythmia, nausea, vomiting, premature ventricular contractions. Uterine hypertonicity, spasms, tetanic contractions, and uterine rupture may occur with excess doses.

Parameters of Use

Absorption Uterine response occurs in: 1 minute (IV); 3 to 7 minutes (IM); 30 minutes (buccal). Duration of action is 30 to 60 minutes. Absorbed into plasma. Half-life is 1 to 3 minutes.

Distribution In mammary gland, kidneys, and liver.

Excretion Some by the kidneys.

Drug Interactions Oxytocin is incompatible with IV fibrinolysin, levarterenol, prochlorperazine, protein hydrolysate, warfarin. Severe hypertension can result with vasopressors.

Administration Determined by uterine response. Intravenous: 1 ml in 1000 ml solution; begin with flow rate of 14 gtt/min. Infusion pump is essential for accurate control. Must be given in secondary IV unit, with unmedicated solution in primary unit. Intramuscular: 1 ml (10 U) after delivery of placenta. Buccal: 1 to 3 tablets every 30 minutes; alternate cheek pouches. Intranasal: single spray 2 to 3 minutes before breast feeding.

Available Drug Forms Ampule containing 0.5 (5 U) or 1 ml (10 U); vials containing 10 ml (10 U/ml); tablets containing 200 U; nasal spray. Refrigerate for long-term storage.

Nursing Management

1. Client on IV oxytocin must be continuously observed; watch especially for water intoxication (convulsions, coma).
2. Fetal heart rate, uterine tone, and duration and frequency of contraction force must be constantly monitored.
3. If caudal or spinal anesthesia is used, watch for hypertensive crisis.
4. If contraction is prolonged, stop infusion, turn patient on side, and administer oxygen if necessary.

GENERIC NAME Posterior pituitary hormone

TRADE NAME Pituitrin (RX)

CLASSIFICATION Complete posterior pituitary hormone

See vasopressin and oxytocin for Action, Contraindications, Untoward reactions, Drug interactions, and Nursing management.

Indications for Use Treatment of diabetes insipidus, stimulation of smooth muscle.

Administration 3 to 10 U subc tid or qid; 5 to 20 mg prn intranasally.

Available Drug Forms Ampules containing 10 or 20 U/ml.

Chapter 25

Adrenocorticosteroids

CHARACTERISTICS OF ADRENOCORTICOSTEROIDS

GLUCOCORTICOIDS AND MINERALOCORTICOIDS

- Hydrocortisone, hydrocortisone acetate, hydrocortisone sodium succinate
- Methylprednisolone, methylprednisolone acetate, methylprednisolone sodium acetate
- Prednisolone, prednisolone acetate, prednisolone sodium succinate, prednisolone sodium phosphate
- Prednisone
- Dexamethasone, dexamethasone acetate, dexamethasone sodium phosphate
- Betamethasone, betamethasone benzoate, betamethasone dipropionate, betamethasone valerate, betamethasone sodium phosphate, betamethasone acetate
- Triamcinolone, triamcinolone acetonide, triamcinolone diacetate, triamcinolone hexacetonide
- Paramethasone acetate
- Flumethasone pivalate
- Desonide
- Fludrocortisone acetate
- Desoxycorticosterone acetate

STEROID HORMONE COMBINATION PREPARATIONS

- Allersone
- Alphosyl-HC
- Anusol-HC
- Barseb HC
- Corticaine
- Cortisporin
- Derma Medicone-HC
- HCV Creme
- Komed HC
- Loroxide-HC
- Mantadil
- Mycolog
- Pramosone
- Proctofoam-HC

Racet
Rectal Medicone-HC
Terra-Cortril
Vanoxide-HC
Vioform-Hydrocortisone
Vytone
Wyanoids HC

CHARACTERISTICS OF ADRENOCORTICOSTEROIDS

The adrenal cortex secretes a number of compounds that can be classified as follows:

1. Glucocorticoids
2. Mineralocorticoids
3. Adrenogenital corticoids (see Chapters 22 and 23)

Glucocorticoids profoundly affect carbohydrate, fat, and protein metabolism. These compounds are best known for their antiinflammatory and antipruritic effects. In addition, they cause vasoconstriction, sodium and water retention, and suppression of the body's immune response. The natural forms, hydrocortisone and cortisone, are used primarily as replacement therapy for deficiency states. The synthetic derivatives generally have a more potent antiinflammatory action and cause less sodium and water retention than the natural products. The available synthetic glucocorticoids include prednisolone, prednisone, methylprednisolone, triamcinolone, paramethasone, flumethasone, dexamethasone, betamethasone, and desonide.

Mineralocorticoids act primarily by increasing sodium and water reabsorption in the distal renal tubules. The natural steroid, aldosterone, is not available for therapeutic use. The synthetic derivatives, desoxycorticosterone and fludrocortisone, are used chiefly in treating salt-losing adrenogenital syndrome and as partial replacement agents in adrenal deficiency states.

Because there is considerable overlap of activity between glucocorticoids and mineralocorticoids, it is prudent to consider nursing management from an overall point of view. The untoward effects in the client receiving high doses or long-term therapy are, in fact, quite similar. Fortunately, the serious adverse effects are usually reversible when the dosage is decreased or the drug is discontinued. The following is a list of adverse effects:

1. Steroids cause gluconeogenesis and conversion of glycogen to glucose, and glycosuria and hyperglycemia can result.
2. Steroids cause increased catabolism, and negative nitrogen balance can result.
3. Steroids cause deposits of fat in the shoulders, face, and abdomen, resulting in "moonface" and obesity.
4. The increased retention of water and sodium and excretion of potassium, calcium, and phosphorus can result in edema, hypokalemia, alkalosis, and hypertension.
5. Suppression of the immune system causes delayed wound healing and increased risk of infection.
6. In children, development of pseudo–brain tumor is possible, causing headache, papilledema, and oculomotor paralysis. Normal bone growth may also be inhibited.

Clients on steroid therapy must be carefully and consistently monitored for adverse effects that necessitate dosage adjustment and should be instructed to follow a low-sodium, high-potassium diet. Arthritic clients must be warned about the dangers of overusing joints that are pain-free because of the underlying arthritic process which can result in permanent joint damage. Rapid weight changes, which indicate edema, must be promptly reported, and blood pressure and serum glucose should be routinely monitored. Any signs of infection or gastric distress merit immediate medical attention, since steroid therapy masks the severity of infections and is known to cause peptic ulcer, pancreatitis, and esophagitis. Finally, under no circumstances should steroid drugs be abruptly withdrawn; gradual dosage reductions will facilitate resumption of normal adrenal gland activity in the client.

GLUCOCORTICOIDS AND MINERALOCORTICOIDS

GENERIC NAMES Hydrocortisone; hydrocortisone acetate; hydrocortisone sodium succinate

TRADE NAMES Alphaderm, Cortef, Cetacourt, Cort-Dome, Cortenema, Cortril, Cotacort, Dermacort, Heb-Cort MC, Hytone, Proctocort, Rectoid, Texacort, Westcort; Cortifoam, Orabase-HCA; A-Hydrocort, Solu-Cortef

CLASSIFICATION Adrenocortical steroid (glucocorticoid)

Action Promotes synthesis of glucose and protein by liver, but inhibits protein synthesis in other organs, resulting in negative nitrogen balance. Causes sodium and fluid retention and increased excretion of potassium, calcium, phosphorus, creatinine, and uric acid. Has a marked antiinflammatory effect. Also suppresses lymphatic activity and the production of antibodies. Increases appetite.

Indications for Use Replacement therapy for adrenocortical insufficiency; collagen diseases, including arthritis, lupus, scleroderma, pemphigus; chronic kidney disease; severe allergic reactions; chronic ulcerative colitis; inflammatory diseases of the eye; shock and central nervous system emergencies; neoplastic diseases, especially of lymphatics.

Contraindications Any suspected infection, peptic ulcer, psychoses, acute glomerulonephritis, ocular herpes simplex, systemic fungal diseases, viral dermatoses, Cushing's syndrome, myasthenia gravis, tuberculosis unless combined with appropriate anti-TB medication in fulminating TB. Use with caution in pregnancy.

Untoward Reactions Short-term treatment or replacement therapy doses seldom cause side effects. Major side effects include "moon face" in which excess fat is deposited on face, neck, shoulders, and abdomen (Cushingoid state); and hirsutism. Adverse effects are: muscle wasting, osteoporosis, pathologic fractures; hyperglycemia, glycosuria; hypertension; edema (sodium retention), potassium and calcium depletion, alkalosis; GI symptoms including peptic ulcer, esophagitis, pancreatitis; thinning of skin and nails, purpura, loss of pigmentation; increased intracranial pressure with papilledema, headache, insomnia, mood changes, exacerbation of existing psychiatric disorders; increased intraocular pressure, glaucoma, cataracts, exophthalmos; obesity, negative nitrogen balance, impaired healing, masked infections; amenorrhea, suppression of growth in children; increased sweating, facial erythema; secondary adrenocortical unresponsiveness in trauma or illness.

Parameters of Use

Absorption From skin, synovial membranes, GI tract, and muscles. Binds to transcortin in the circulation. Half-life is 60 to 90 minutes. Peak action occurs in 2 to 8 hours after oral dose. Crosses placenta and appears in breast milk.

Metabolism In liver.

Excretion In urine as 17-hydroxycorticosteroids and 17-ketogenic steroids, within 12 hours.

Drug Interactions May increase renal excretion of salicylates. Causes increased need for antidiabetic agents in diabetic patients. Has enhanced effect in patients with cirrhosis or hypothyroidism. Causes increased potassium depletion when given with amphotericin B, ethacrynic acid, furosemide, and thiazide diuretics. Can lead to development of resistant bacterial strains when given with antibiotics and tetracyclines. Increased intraocular pressure will exacerbate glaucoma when given with anticholinergics. Decreases effects of anticoagulants. Barbiturates and phenytoin decrease hydrocortisone effect and estrogens increase antiinflammatory effect. Salicylates and indomethacin increase risk of GI ulceration.

Laboratory Interactions Can increase levels of serum amylase, sodium, uric acid, carbon dioxide, cholesterol, triglycerides, and glucose; can decrease levels of serum calcium, potassium, platelets, and erythrocyte sedimentation rate.

Administration Emergency treatment: 0.5 to 2 g IV every 2 to 6 hours. High-dose therapy should not continue beyond 72 hours. Administer dose over 1 to 3 minutes. Usual intravenous dosage: 100 to 500 mg every 1 to 10 hours. Administer over a period of at least 30 seconds. May be infused over a period of 2 to 10 hours. Intramuscular: 50 to 300 mg. Oral: Large initial dose, then 10 to 80 mg divided into 4 daily doses. Intraarticular: 5 to 50 mg. Topical: 0.125 to 1%. Dosage requirements are variable, and depend on disease and individual patient.

Available Drug Forms Topical spray 0.5% solution; ointment, cream, and lotion 0.125, 0.25, 0.5, or 1%; scored tablets containing 5, 10, 20, or 25 mg; retention enema of 60 ml solution containing 100 mg hydrocortisone; rectal suppositories; powder in vials of 100, 250, 500, or 1000 mg with diluent. After mixing, must be stored at room temperature and used within 72 hrs. Use solution only if clear. Store drug in light-resistant containers.

Nursing Management

Planning factors

1. Diet should be high in potassium and low in sodium. Alcohol and caffeine should be avoided.
2. Surgery or other trauma may require an increase in dosage.
3. Immunizations are contraindicated because of lack of antibody response and potential for neurologic complications.

Administration factors

1. When giving IM, inject deep into gluteal region. Subcutaneous administration can cause tissue damage.
2. For topical applications, use care in cleansing site and applying medication, because of poor healing.

Occlusive dressing will increase percutaneous penetration and absorption. Medication should be gently massaged into affected area.
3. Give tablets with meals to minimize GI distress.
4. Blood pressure should be checked twice a day until client is stabilized on maintenance dose.
5. Drug must be withdrawn gradually to prevent adrenal crisis.
6. Mothers on corticosteroids should not breast-feed infants.

Evaluation factors

1. Check client frequently for signs of other illness that may be masked by drug.
2. Client should be weighed daily, since sudden large weight gain indicates edema.
3. Appropriate laboratory values should be checked frequently, as should intraocular pressure.
4. Muscle wasting and weakness indicate negative nitrogen balance.

Client teaching factors

1. Teach appropriate passive and active exercises to prevent further damage to joints (in arthritic diseases) and pathologic fractures.
2. Instruct client to report signs of GI distress and to adhere to scheduled follow-up appointments.
3. Instruct client to carry identification containing appropriate information, such as drug name, dosage, and physician's name.

GENERIC NAMES Methylprednisolone; methylprednisolone acetate; methylprednisolone sodium succinate (RX)

TRADE NAMES Medrol; Depo-Medrol; A-Metha-Pred, Solu-Medrol

CLASSIFICATION Synthetic adrenocortical steroid (glucocorticoid)

See hydrocortisone for Indications for use, Contraindications, Untoward reactions, Parameters of use, and Drug interactions.

Action Antiinflammatory effect more potent than prednisolone. Less likely to cause sodium and water retention than either prednisolone or hydrocortisone. The acetate preparation has more rapid onset of action and longer duration of action than sodium preparation. (See hydrocortisone.)

Absorption Half-life is 3 to 4 hours.

Administration Oral: 2 to 48 mg every day or every other day. Intraarticular: 4 to 80 mg. Intramuscular: 4 to 120 mg daily or weekly; 10 to 40 mg every 6 to 24 hours by deep gluteal injection only. Intralesional: 20 to 60 mg; multiple small injections are preferred to minimize tissue atrophy. Intravenous (IV bolus or continuous drip): 10 to 500 mg. Topical: 0.25 to 1%. Retention enema: 40 mg three to seven times weekly; as an adjunct in the treatment of ulcerative colitis.

Available Drug Forms Powder in vials of 40, 125, 500, or 1000 mg; mix only with diluent provided. Sterile aqueous suspension containing 20, 40, or 80 mg/ml; store at room temperature, protect from light, and use within 48 hours of mixing. Tablets containing 2, 4, 8, 16, 24, or 32 mg; retention enema containing 40 mg; topical use tubes 0.25 or 1%.

Nursing Management Alternate day therapy is often effective in preventing suppression of normal adrenal-pituitary function. Since the maximum activity of the adrenal cortex normally occurs in the early morning hours, the drug should be given before 8 A.M. in order to cause the least suppression of normal adrenal activity. (See hydrocortisone.)

GENERIC NAMES Prednisolone; prednisolone acetate; prednisolone sodium succinate; prednisolone sodium phosphate (RX)

TRADE NAMES Delta-Cortef, Meti-Derm, Sterane; Meticortelone; Meticortelone Soluble; Metreton

CLASSIFICATION Synthetic adrenocortical steroid (glucocorticoid)

See hydrocortisone for Indications for use, Contraindications, Parameters of use, Drug interactions, and Nursing management.

Action Five times more potent than hydrocortisone. (See hydrocortisone for further details.)

Untoward Reactions Same as hydrocortisone, but with a greater tendency to produce gastric, dermatologic, and vasomotor symptoms.

Administration Oral, intramuscular: Initial dosage: 5 to 60 mg daily in divided doses; Maintenance dosage: 5 to 20 mg daily in divided doses. (Alternate day therapy: See methylprednisolone.) Intraarticular, intralesional: 10 to 30 mg. Intravenous: 25 to 50 mg as IV bolus; 100 mg ql2h as continuous drip. Topical: 0.5% tid or qid. Ophthalmic use: 0.5% bid or tid.

Available Drug Forms Tablets containing 5 mg; aerosol 0.5%; cream 0.5%; sterile powder in 50-mg vial; after mixing, refrigerate and use within 24 hours. Aqueous suspension in vial containing 25 mg/ml; do not freeze and shake before use. Ophthalmic solution 0.5%; protect from light and store away from heat.

GENERIC NAME Prednisone (RX)

TRADE NAMES Deltasone, Meticorten, Orasone

CLASSIFICATION Synthetic adrenocortical steroid (glucocorticoid)

See hydrocortisone for Indications for use, Contraindications, Untoward reactions, Parameters of use, Drug interactions, and Nursing management.

Action Five times more potent than hydrocortisone. (See hydrocortisone.)

Administration Adults: Initial dosage: 20 to 60 po qid; maintenance dosage: 5 to 20 mg qid. Children: Initial dosage: 2 mg/kg po qid; Maintenance dosage: 1.5 mg/kg qid. (Alternate day therapy: See methylprednisolone.)

Available Drug forms Tablets containing 1, 2.5, 5, 10, 20, or 50 mg. Store in airtight, light-resistant containers.

GENERIC NAMES Dexamethasone; dexamethasone acetate; dexamethasone sodium phosphate RX

TRADE NAMES Aeroseb-D, Decaderm, Decadron, Deronil, Dexone, Hexadrol; Decadron-LA; Decadron Phosphate

CLASSIFICATION Synthetic adrenocortical steroid (glucocorticoid)

See hydrocortisone for Indications for use, Contraindications, Parameters of use, Drug interactions, and Nursing management.

Action Rarely causes sodium and water retention. (See hydrocortisone.)

Untoward Reactions Intranasal aerosol can cause irritation and dryness, epistaxis, and perforation of nasal septum. (See hydrocortisone.)

Administration Oral: 1.5 to 4.5 mg daily. Intramuscular, intravenous: 0.5 to 9 mg daily, do not give IV with lidocaine. Intraarticular: 4 to 16 mg. Intralesional: 0.8 to 1.6 mg. Ophthalmic or otic use: 1 to 2 gtt tid or qid; do not administer to ear if ear drum is perforated. Intranasal: 2 metered sprays bid or tid; Maximum dosage: 12 sprays daily.

Available Drug Forms Aerosol spray 0.023 mg or 0.084 mg/spray; store away from heat. Gel (topical) 0.1%; elixir containing 0.5 mg/ml; tablets containing 0.5, 0.75, 1.5, or 4 mg. Suspension containing 8 mg/ml; shake before use and protect from heat. Vials and prefilled syringes containing 4 or 24 mg/ml; ophthalmic ointment and solution 0.05 or 0.1%.

GENERIC NAMES Betamethasone; betamethasone benzoate; betamethasone dipropionate; betamethasone valerate; betamethasone sodium phosphate; betamethasone acetate RX

TRADE NAMES Celestone; Benisone, Uticort; Diprosone; Valisone

CLASSIFICATION Synthetic adrenocortical steroid (glucocorticoid)

See hydrocortisone for Contraindications, Untoward reactions, Parameters of use, and Drug interactions.

Action Causes very little sodium and water retention or potassium depletion. (See hydrocortisone.)

Indications for Use Dermatoses, psoriasis. Not used for replacement therapy in adrenal insufficiency. (See hydrocortisone.)

Administration Oral: 0.6 to 7.2 mg daily in divided doses. Intramuscular: 0.5 to 9 mg daily in divided doses; do not inject into deltoid. Intraarticular, intralesional: 1.5 to 6 mg. Topical: 0.01 to 0.2% bid or tid.

Available Drug Forms Cream 0.01, 0.025, 0.05, 0.1, or 0.2%; syrup containing 0.6 mg/5 ml. Tablets containing 0.6 mg; store away from heat and protect from light. Suspension containing 6 mg/ml; shake well before using. Gel, ointment, and lotion 0.025, 0.05, or 0.1%. Aerosol 0.1 or 0.15%; store away from heat.

Nursing Management Do not apply aerosol preparation if area is to be covered by occlusive dressing. Treated areas should not be exposed to sunlight. (See hydrocortisone.)

GENERIC NAMES Triamcinolone; triamcinolone acetonide; triamcinolone diacetate; triamcinolone hexacetonide RX

TRADE NAMES Aristocort, Kenacort; Aristocort Acetonide, Kenalog, Triacet; Aristocort, Kenacort, Tracilon; Aristospan

CLASSIFICATION Synthetic adrenocortical steroid (glucocorticoid)

See hydrocortisone for Indications for use, Contraindications, Parameters of use, Drug interactions, and Nursing management.

Action Causes little sodium and water retention or potassium depletion. Does not increase appetite. Five to ten times more potent than hydrocortisone. (See hydrocortisone.)

Absorption Half-life is 5 hours.

Administration Initial dosage: 4 to 48 mg po daily. (Alternate day therapy: see Methylprednisolone.) Intramuscular: 40 mg once per week deep into gluteal muscle; depot or sustained action. Intraarticular: 5 to 40 mg. Intralesional: Maximum dosage: 12.5 mg/site; may be repeated every 1 to 8 weeks as necessary.

Available Drug Forms Tablets containing 1, 2, 4, 8, or 16 mg. Syrup containing 2 mg/5 ml or 4 mg/5 ml; protect from light. Cream, Lotion, Ointment, and Spray 0.025, 0.1, or 0.5%; store at room temperature, do not freeze. Suspension containing 5, 20, 25, or 40 mg/ml; may be diluted with sterile saline and/or lidocaine 1 to 2%.

GENERIC NAME Paramethasone acetate (RX)

TRADE NAME Haldrone

CLASSIFICATION Synthetic adrenocortical steroid (glucocorticoid)

See hydrocortisone for Indications for use, Contraindications, Untoward reactions, Parameters of use, Drug interactions, and Nursing management.

Action Causes little sodium and water retention or potassium depletion. (See hydrocortisone.)

Administration Initial dosage: 2 to 24 mg po daily. Maintenance dosage: 1 to 8 mg po daily; highly variable.

Available Drug Forms Tablets containing 1 or 2 mg.

GENERIC NAME Flumethasone pivalate (RX)

TRADE NAME Locorten

CLASSIFICATION Synthetic adrenocortical steroid (glucocorticoid)

See hydrocortisone for Contraindications, Untoward reactions, Parameters of use, Drug interactions, and Nursing management.

Action Has a strong local antiinflammatory effect. (See hydrocortisone.)

Indications for Use Various dermatoses, topical use only.

Administration Topical: Apply tid or qid; occlusive dressings may be used.

Available Drug Forms Cream 0.03%.

GENERIC NAME Desonide (RX)

TRADE NAME Tridesilon

CLASSIFICATION Synthetic adrenocortical steroid (glucocorticoid)

See hydrocortisone for Contraindications, Untoward reactions, Parameters of use, Drug interactions, and Nursing management.

Action Has a strong local antiinflammatory effect. (See hydrocortisone.)

Indications for Use Topical use only. (See hydrocortisone.)

Administration Topical: Apply bid or tid; occlusive dressings may be used. Otic use (external auditory canal): 3 to 4 gtt tid or qid; do not administer if tympanic membrane is perforated.

Available Drug Forms Cream 0.05%; ointment 0.05%; solution 0.05%.

GENERIC NAME Fludrocortisone acetate (RX)

TRADE NAME Florinef

CLASSIFICATION Synthetic adrenocortical steroid (glucocorticoid, mineralocorticoid)

See hydrocortisone for Contraindications, Untoward reactions, Parameters of use, Drug interactions, and Nursing management.

Action Causes marked sodium retention and potassium excretion and elevated blood pressure. (See hydrocortisone.)

Indications for Use Partial replacement therapy of adrenocortical insufficiency in Addison's disease, treatment of salt-losing adrenogenital syndrome.

Absorption Half-life is 30 minutes.

Administration Oral: 0.1 to 0.2 mg daily; usually administered in conjunction with hydrocortisone.

Available Drug Forms Tablets containing 0.1 mg. Store at room temperature, avoid excessive heat, and protect from light.

GENERIC NAME Desoxycorticosterone acetate

TRADE NAME Percorten Acetate (RX)

CLASSIFICATION Synthetic adrenocortical steroid (mineralocorticoid)

See hydrocortisone for Drug interactions.

Action Major action is increased sodium and water retention and excretion of potassium. Promotes fat and glucose absorption from GI tract. Has no antiinflammatory effect. (See hydrocortisone.)

Indications for Use Partial replacement therapy of adrenocortical insufficiency in Addison's disease, treatment of salt-losing adrenogenital syndrome.

Contraindications Hypertension, cardiac disease. (See hydrocortisone.)

Untoward Reactions Severe hypoglycemia. (See hydrocortisone.)

Parameters of Use

Absorption Diffuses into tissue fluids; binds to serum proteins.
Metabolism In Liver.
Excretion In urine.

Administration Intramuscular: 1 to 5 mg daily of oil preparation; 25 to 100 mg every 4 weeks of suspension deep into gluteal region. Subcutaneous: 1 pellet for each 0.5 mg of maintenance dose; must be done in Operating Room using strict aseptic technique; duration of action is 8 to 12 months.

Available Drug Forms Vials (oil preparation) containing 5 mg/ml; aqueous suspension containing 25 mg/ml; pellets containing 125 mg. Long-acting repository; only used after client has been regulated on maintenance doses for 2 to 3 months.

Nursing Management (See hydrocortisone.)

1. Any soreness at pellet implantation site should be promptly reported to physician.
2. When administering IM, withdraw with large needle; change to 23-gauge needle for deep gluteal injection.

STEROID HORMONE COMBINATION PREPARATIONS

TRADE NAME Allersone (RX)

CLASSIFICATION Topical steroid antiinflammatory agent

Indications for Use Atopic dermatitis, contact dermatitis, pruritus ani, vulvae, eczema, hemorrhoids.

Contraindications Herpes simplex of the eye, skin tuberculosis.

Untoward Reactions May induce skin irritation.

Administration Apply locally to affected areas bid or tid.

Available Drug Forms Generic contents in ointment: hydrocortisone: 0.5%; diperodon HCL: 0.5%; zinc oxide: 5%.

TRADE NAME Alphosyl-HC (RX)

CLASSIFICATION Topical steroid antiinflammatory agent

Indications for Use Psoriasis.

Warnings and Precautions External use only, avoid contact with the eyes.

Untoward Reactions May induce skin irritation.

Administration Apply locally to affected areas, massaging it into the lesions bid, tid, or qid as needed.

Available Drug Forms Generic contents in lotion or cream: hydrocortisone: 0.5%; coal tar extract: 5%; allantoin: 1.7%.

TRADE NAME Anusol-HC (RX)

CLASSIFICATION Topical steroid antiinflammatory agent

Indications for Use Relief of pain and discomfort associated with hemorrhoids, proctitis, papillitis, cryptitis, and anal fissures, and following anorectal surgery.

Warnings and Precautions Use with extreme caution in the presence of an infection and cautiously in children and infants. Do not use for the eyes.

Untoward Reactions May induce skin irritation.

Administration 1 rectal suppository bid or apply cream locally to affected areas tid or qid for 3 to 6 days, or until inflammation subsides.

Available Drug Forms Suppositories or cream. Generic contents in each suppository: hydrocortisone acetate: 10 mg; bismuth subgallate: 2.25%; bismuth resorcin compound: 1.75%; benzyl benzoate: 1.2%; peruvian balsam: 1.8%; zinc oxide: 11%. Generic contents in each gram of cream: hydrocortisone acetate: 5 mg; bismuth subgallate: 22.5 mg; bismuth resorcin L: 17.5 mg; benzyl benzoate: 12 mg; peruvian balsam: 18 mg; zinc oxide: 110 mg.

TRADE NAME Barseb HC (RX)

CLASSIFICATION Topical steroid antiinflammatory agent

Indications for Use Dermatoses of the scalp.

Warnings and Precautions Use with extreme caution in the presence of an infection. Avoid inhalation, ingestion, or contact with the eyes or nose.

Untoward Reactions May induce burning, itching, dryness, acne form eruptions, hypopigmentation, secondary infection, or skin atrophy.

Administration Part hair, apply sparingly with gentle rubbing daily or bid.

Available Drug Forms Generic contents in scalp lotion: hydrocortisone: 1%; salicylic acid: 0.5%; isopropyl alcohol: 45%.

TRADE NAME Corticaine (RX)

CLASSIFICATION Topical steroid antiinflammatory agent

Indications for Use Relief of the inflammatory manifestations of corticosteroid-responsive dermatosis.

Contraindications Presence of local tuberculosis, fungal and viral infections, pemphigus, and discoid lupus erythematosus.

Warnings and Precautions Use with extreme caution in the presence of an infection. Do not use for the eyes.

Untoward Reactions May induce itching, irritation, dryness, secondary infection, or skin atrophy

Administration Every A.M., at hs, and after each bowel movement for 2 to 6 days. Topical: Apply locally to affected areas bid or qid for 2 weeks.

Available Drug Forms Washable, nongreasy, metholated cream base. Generic contents in cream: hydrocortisone: 0.5%; dibucaine: 0.5%.

Nursing Management

1. Cleanse and dry rectal area thoroughly.
2. Attach plastic applicator to tube, fill with cream, and lubricate applicator with cream.
3. Insert applicator into rectum and squeeze an applicatorful into the rectum.
4. Apply after bowel movement.

TRADE NAME Cortisporin (RX)

CLASSIFICATION Topical antibiotic and antiinflammatory agent

Indications for Use Possibly effective in the treatment of topical bacterial infections in burns, wounds, and skin grafts caused by sensitive organisms.

Contraindications Do not use for the eyes or in the external ear canal if the ear drum is perforated.

Warnings and Precautions Nephrotoxicity and ototoxicity are potential hazards because of the presence of neomycin.

Untoward Reactions May induce striae.

Administration Apply a small quantity to affected areas bid, tid, or qid.

Available Drug Forms Generic contents in each gram of cream: polymyxin B sulfate: 10,000 units; neomycin sulfate: 5 mg; gramicidin; 0.25 mg; hydrocortisone acetate: 5 mg; methylparaben (preservative): 0.25%.

TRADE NAME Derma Medicone-HC (RX)

CLASSIFICATION Topical steroid antiinflammatory agent

Indications for Use Relief of discomfort during the treatment of severely inflammed dermatoses.

Contraindications Do not use for the eyes or if tuberculosis of the skin is present.

Warnings and Precautions Use with extreme caution if an infection is present or if a rash or irritation develop.

Untoward Reactions May induce itching, irritation, dryness, secondary infection, or skin atrophy.

Administration Apply to affected areas bid, tid, or as needed.

Available Drug Forms Generic contents in each gram of ointment: hydrocortisone acetate: 10 mg; benzocaine: 19.8 mg; oxyquinoline sulfate: 10.4 mg; ephedrine HCL: 1.1 mg; menthol: 4.8 mg; ichthammol: 9.9 mg; zinc oxide: 135.8 mg.

TRADE NAME HCV Creme (RX)

CLASSIFICATION Topical antifungal and antiinflammatory agent

Indications for Use Treatment of various inflammatory skin disorders when antifungal action is desired.

Contraindications Do not use for the eyes, viral skin lesions, or if tuberculosis of the skin is present.

Warnings and Precautions Use with extreme caution in the presence of an infection.

Untoward Reactions May induce burning, itching, dryness, secondary infection, skin atrophy, or striae.

Laboratory Interactions The ferric chloride test for PKU can yield a false-positive result if HCV creme is present on the diaper or in the urine. Iodochlorhydroxyquin can be absorbed through the skin and interfere with thyroid function tests.

Administration Apply a thin layer to affected areas tid or qid.

Available Drug Forms Generic contents in each gram of creme: hydrocortisone alcohol: 1%; iodochlorhydroxyquin: 3%.

TRADE NAME Komed HC (RX)

CLASSIFICATION Topical steroid antiinflammatory agent

Indications for Use Acne conditions accompanied by inflammation.

Contraindication Do not use for the eyes.

Warnings and Precautions Use with extreme caution in the presence of an infection. Discontinue use if irritation develops.

Untoward Reactions May induce burning, itching, irritation, dryness, folliculitis, secondary infection, skin atrophy, or striae.

Administration Apply to affected areas bid.

Available Drug Forms Generic contents in lotion: hydrocortisone acetate: 0.5%; sodium thiosulfate: 8%; salicylic acid: 2%; isopropyl alcohol: 25%.

Nursing Management

1. Cleanse and dry affected area thoroughly.
2. Shake lotion well before using.
3. Apply a thin coating to affected areas.

TRADE NAME Loroxide-HC (RX)

CLASSIFICATION Topical steroid antiinflammatory agent

Indications for Use Acne vulgaris, oily skin.

Contraindications Do not use for the eyes, mucous membranes, or viral diseases of the skin.

Warnings and Precautions Discontinue use if itching, redness, or swelling develop. May bleach colored fabrics.

Untoward Reactions May induce irritation and contact dermatitis.

Administration Apply to affected areas daily, bid, or tid.

Available Drug Forms Generic contents in each gram of lotion: hydrocortisone: 0.5%; benzoyl peroxide: 5.5%; chlorhydroxyquinoline: .025%.

Nursing Management

1. Shake lotion well before using.
2. Apply a thin coating to affected areas with gentle massage.

TRADE NAME Mantadil (RX)

CLASSIFICATION Topical steroid antiinflammatory agent

Indications for Use Pruritic skin eruptions, eczema, dermatitis, sunburn, and anogenital pruritus.

Contraindications Do not use for the eyes, viral skin lesions, or if tuberculosis of the skin is present.

Warnings and Precautions Discontinue use if irritation develops. Use with extreme caution in the presence of an infection.

Untoward Reactions May induce allergic contact dermatitis, irritation, acneiform eruptions, secondary infection, or skin atrophy.

Administration Apply locally to affected areas two to five times daily.

Available Drug Forms Generic contents in cream: hydrocortisone acetate: 0.5%; chlorcyclizine HCL: 2%; methylparaben (preservative): 0.25%.

TRADE NAME Mycolog (RX)

CLASSIFICATION Topical antibacterial and antiinflammatory agent

---

Indications for Use Possibly effective in cutaneous candidiasis, superficial bacterial infections, infantile eczema, lichen simplex chronicus, and forms of dermatitis complicated by candidal and/or bacterial infection.

Contraindications Do not use for viral infections, fungal lesions, the eyes, or the external ear canal if the ear drum is perforated.

Warnings and Precautions Prolonged use may cause nephrotoxicity and ototoxicity because of the presence of neomycin.

Untoward Reactions May induce burning, itching, irritation, dryness, secondary infection, or skin atrophy.

Administration Apply a thin layer to affected areas bid or tid.

Available Drug Forms Generic contents in each gram of cream or ointment: nystatin: 100,000 units; neomycin sulfate: 2.5 mg; gramicidin: 0.25 mg; triamcinolone acetonide (0.1%): 1 mg.

TRADE NAME Pramosone (RX)

CLASSIFICATION Topical steroid antiinflammatory agent

Indications for Use Relief of inflammatory manifestations of cortisteroid-responsive dermatoses.

Contraindications Do not use for viral diseases of the skin or if marked impairment of the circulation is present.

Warnings and Precautions Discontinue use if irritation develops. Use with extreme caution in the presence of an infection.

Untoward Reactions May induce burning, itching, acneiform eruptions, secondary infection, skin atrophy, or striae.

Administration Apply to affected areas tid or qid.

Available Drug Forms Generic contents in lotion or cream: hydrocortisone acetate: 0.5, 1, 2.5%; pramoxine HCl: 1%.

TRADE NAME Proctofoam-HC (RX)

CLASSIFICATION Topical steroid antiinflammatory agent

Indications for Use Relief of inflammatory manifestations of cortisteroid-responsive dermatoses of the anogenital area.

Contraindications Do not use for the eyes.

Warnings and Precautions Use with extreme caution in the presence of an infection. Discontinue use if irritation develops.

Untoward Reactions May induce burning, itching, dryness, allergic contact dermatitis, secondary infection, or skin atrophy.

Administration

- *Rectal lesions:* Apply to affected areas with special rectal applicator bid or tid.
- *Perianal lesions:* Apply a small amount to affected areas gently tid or qid.

Available Drug Forms Aerosol container with a special rectal applicator. Generic contents in foam: hydrocortisone acetate: 1%.

TRADE NAME Racet (RX)

CLASSIFICATION Topical steroid antiinflammatory agent

Indications for Use Possibly effective in the treatment of contact and atopic dermatitis, eczema, and various forms of dermatitis.

Contraindications Do not use for the eyes, the external ear canal if the ear drum is perforated, viral skin lesions, or if tuberculosis of the skin is present.

Warnings and Precautions Discontinue use if irritation develops.

Untoward Reactions May induce burning and itching and may stain hair, fabric, or skin.

Laboratory Interactions Do not perform thyroid function tests until 1 month after discontinuing use of this medication as it can interfere with the results. The ferric chloride test for PKU can yield a false-positive result if Racet cream is present on the diaper or in the urine.

Administration Apply a thin layer to affected areas tid or qid.

Available Drug Forms Generic contents in cream: hydrocortisone: 0.5%; iodochlorhydroxyquin: 3%.

TRADE NAME Rectal Medicone-HC (RX)

CLASSIFICATION Topical steroid antiinflammatory agent

Indications for Use Hemorrhoids, acute and chronic proctitis, postoperative edema, cryptitis, pruritus ani.

Contraindications Presence of tuberculosis of the rectum.

Warnings and Precautions Discontinue use if rash or irritation develop. Use with extreme caution in the presence of an infection.

Untoward Reactions May induce burning or itching.

Administration 1 rectal suppository bid for 3 to 6 days.

Available Drug Forms Generic contents in each suppository: hydrocortisone acetate: 10 mg; benzocaine: 130 mg; oxyquinoline sulfate: 15 mg; zinc oxide: 195 mg; menthol: 1 mg; balsam Peru: 65 mg.

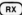

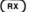

TRADE NAME Terra-Cortril (RX)

CLASSIFICATION Topical antibiotic and antiinflammatory agent

Indications for Use Possibly effective in the treatment of cutaneous infections, atopic and contact dermatitis, and nonspecific pruritus of the anus, vulva, and scrotum.

Contraindications Do not use for the eyes, acute herpes simplex, viral infections, tuberculosis, or fungal disease.

Warnings and Precautions Discontinue use if rash or irritation develop. Use with extreme caution in the presence of an infection.

Untoward Reactions May induce burning, itching, dryness, hypopigmentation, secondary infection, skin atrophy, or striae.

Administration Apply to affected areas bid, tid, or qid.

Available Drug Forms Generic contents in each gram of ointment: oxytetracycline HCl: 30 mg, hydrocortisone: 1%.

Nursing Management

1. Cleanse and dry affected areas thoroughly.
2. Gently apply a thin layer of ointment.

TRADE NAME Vanoxide-HC (RX)

CLASSIFICATION Topical steroid antiinflammatory agent

Indications for Use Acne vulgaris, oily skin.

Contraindications Do not use for the eyes, mucous membranes, or viral diseases of the skin.

Warnings and Precautions Discontinue use if itching, redness, or swelling develop. May bleach colored fabrics.

Untoward Reactions May induce irritation and contact dermatitis.

Administration Apply to affected areas daily, bid or tid.

Available Drug Forms Generic contents of lotion: hydrocortisone: 5 mg; benzoyl peroxide: 55 mg.

Nursing Management

1. Shake lotion well before using.
2. Apply a thin coating to affected areas with gentle massage.

TRADE NAME Vioform-Hydrocortisone (RX)

CLASSIFICATION Topical steroid antiinflammatory agent

Indications for Use Possibly effective in the treatment of contact and atopic dermatitis, eczema, acne urticaria, and bacterial dermatoses.

Contraindications Eye lesions, viral skin lesions, tuberculosis of the skin

Warnings and Precautions Discontinue use if irritation develops. Use with extreme caution in the presence of an infection. May stain hair, fabric, nails, or skin.

Untoward Reactions May induce burning, itching, dryness, allergic contact dermatitis, secondary infection, skin atrophy, or striae.

Laboratory Interactions May interfere with thyroid function tests. The ferric chloride test for PKU can yield a false-positive result if Vioform-Hydrocortisone is present on the diaper or in the urine.

Administration Apply a thin layer to affected areas tid or qid.

Available Drug Forms Generic contents in cream, ointment, or lotion: hydrocortisone: 1%; iodochlorhydroxyquin: 3%.

TRADE NAME Vytone (RX)

CLASSIFICATION Topical steroid antiinflammatory agent

Indications for Use Possibly effective in the treatment of contact and atopic dermatitis, eczema, acne urticaria, and bacterial dermatoses.

Contraindications Do not use for the eyes, viral diseases of the skin, or if marked impairment of the circulation is present.

Warnings and Precautions Discontinue use if irritation develops. May stain skin, hair, nails, or fabric.

Untoward Reactions May induce burning, itching, dryness, allergic contact dermatitis, secondary infection, skin atrophy, or striae.

Laboratory Interactions May interfere with thyroid function tests. The ferric chloride test for PKU can yield a false-positive result if Vytone cream is present on the diaper or in the urine.

Administration Apply to affected areas tid or qid.

Available Drug Forms Generic contents in cream: hydrocortisone: 0.5, 1%; diiodohydroxyquin: 1%.

TRADE NAME Wyanoids HC (RX)

CLASSIFICATION Topical steroid antiinflammatory agent

Indications for Use Possibly effective in the treatment of proctitis secondary to ulcerative colitis.

Contraindications History of glaucoma or organic pyloric stenosis.

Warnings and Precautions Use with caution in clients who have a history of prostatism or urinary retention, elderly clients, and children under 6 years.

Untoward Reactions May induce dry mouth, tachycardia, blurred vision, or dizziness.

Administration 1 rectal suppository bid for 6 days or as required.

Available Drug Forms Generic contents in each suppository: hydrocortisone acetate: 10 mg; belladonna extract: 15 mg; ephedrine sulfate: 3 mg; zinc oxide: 176 mg; boric acid: 543 mg; bismuth oxyiodide: 30 mg; bismuth subcarbonate: 146 mg; peruvian balsam: 30 mg.

Chapter 26

Thyroid Hormones, Antithyroid Agents, and Parathyroid Hormones

CHARACTERISTICS OF THYROID HORMONES

Thyroid preparations, both natural and synthetic, are used for replacement therapy when normal thyroid function is absent or impaired. The natural endogenous hormones, thyroxine (T4) and triiodothyronine (T3), normally affect cellular metabolism in every body system. Plasma levels of thyroid hormones are controlled by TSH (thyroid-stimulating hormone), which is secreted by the pituitary gland, intrinsic thyroid gland mechanisms, and the bioavailability of iodine. When thyroid hormones are released into plasma, they quickly bind to globulin, prealbumin, and albumin. The PBI (protein-bound iodine) test is a measure of the extent of this binding, and will be lower than normal in the presence of drugs (for example, phenytoins, salicylates) that compete for the same protein-binding sites. Conversely, high plasma estrogen levels tend to elevate plasma protein levels, and so the PBI will be increased.

THYROID DISORDERS

Symptoms of Deficiency

Thyroid hormones are essential for controlling the body's overall metabolic rate and normal physical and mental growth. The effects of a decrease or absence of thyroid hormones are therefore profound, particularly in juveniles. Hypothyroidism in adults is known as myxedema, and in infants cretinism.

The initial symptoms of myxedema include intolerance to cold, dry skin, thin dry hair and nails, and fatigue. Progressive hypothyroidism leads to weight gain, peripheral edema, pallor, dyspnea, slow speech, bradycardia, and anginal pain. If the condition is not treated, pericardial effusion, anemia, and organic psychosis may result.

Signs and symptoms of cretinism include thick dry skin, a protruding tongue, and umbilical hernia. Lethargy and apathy are also common symptoms. Mental retardation and dwarfism result if hypothyroidism is untreated.

Symptoms of Excess

Excessive release of thyroid hormones (hyperthyroidism or thyrotoxicosis) is characterized by nervousness, restlessness, tremors, intolerance to heat, diaphoresis, and weight loss even though appetite is increased. Rapid pulse and systolic hypertension are also common symptoms. When toxic goiter is present, exophthalmos and elevated basal metabolic rate (Grave's disease) are additional symptoms.

USE OF ANTITHYROID AGENTS

Hyperthyroidism is treated with antithyroid drugs which interfere with the synthesis of thyroxine and triiodothyronine by the thyroid gland. The effects of antithyroid drugs may not be apparent for several weeks after the initiation of therapy, since the amount of circulating hormone is not affected by these drugs. Similarly, any thyroid hormone administered concurrently will not be affected by antithyroid drugs. For this reason, small amounts of thyroid hormones are sometimes given in conjunction with antithyroid drugs, so that the amount of circulating hormone is sufficient to prevent excessive release of TSH (thyroid-stimulating hormone) from the pituitary adenohypophysis. Excessive TSH will cause a goitrogenic action; that is, an increase in vascularity and size of the thyroid gland.

CHARACTERISTICS OF PARATHYROID HORMONES

Parathyroid hormone (PTH) is one of several substances responsible for the mobilization of calcium into the circulation. When released from the parathyroid glands in response to a reduction in calcium levels, PTH stimulates increased calcium absorption from the gastrointestinal tract and resorption of calcium from the bones. Vitamin D_2 and D_3 have similar effects on calcium metabolism (see Chapter 18). Calcitonin from the thyroid gland, on the other hand, acts to decrease serum calcium by inhibiting bone resorption and by stimulating renal excretion of calcium.

Hypoparathyroidism results in symptoms of hypocalcemia, which include muscle twitching, tetany, and convulsions. Hyperparathyroidism causes symptoms of hypercalcemia, which include vomiting, diarrhea, weakness, calcium deposits in soft tissues, and abnormal cardiac function.

PTH is never used for long-term treatment of hypocalcemia, since the client quickly develops antibodies to the drug. It is used primarily for the treatment of acute hypoparathyroidism/hypocalcemia. Calcitonin is used to treat moderate to severe Paget's disease, because of its inhibition of bone resorption. With long-term use, there may be actual enhancement of bone formation in some clients. Calcium and vitamin D supplements are often prescribed concurrently.

THYROID HORMONES

GENERIC NAME Thyroid hormone (RX)

TRADE NAMES Armour Thyroid, Delcoid, S-P-T, Thyroid, Thyroid Strong

CLASSIFICATION Thyroid hormone

Source Prepared from desiccated animal glands and contains T_4 (levothyroxin) and T_3 (levotriiodothyronine).

Action Increases cellular metabolism in all body systems. Effects include increases in oxygen consumption, respiratory rate, heart rate and cardiac output, circulatory volume, protein, fat, and carbohydrate metabolism, body temperature, enzyme activity, and growth. The exact mechanism of action is unknown. Onset of action is slow, but effects are prolonged.

Indications for Use Replacement therapy in thyroid deficiency states, especially cretinism and myxedema, and simple goiter. As an adjunct to thyroid-inhibiting drugs to decrease release of thyrotropic hormones. Also used to compensate for hypothyroid effects of surgery, radiation, and antithyroid drugs.

Contraindications Uncorrected adrenal insufficiency; acute myocardial infarction without hypothyroidism, thyrotoxicosis, nephrosis, hypogonadism. Use with caution in cardiovascular disease, angina, hypertension, renal insufficiency, pregnancy, and in patients receiving catecholamines. Not used for treatment of obesity, depression, or reproductive disorders.

Untoward Reactions Thyrotoxicosis due to overdosage: tremors, headache, nervousness, insomnia, palpitations, tachycardia, arrhythmias, angina, fever, warm skin, diaphoresis, heat intolerance, weight loss, diarrhea, menstrual irregularities, congestive heart failure, shock. Allergic dermatological reactions are possible, because drug is an animal protein. Chronic overdosage causes emaciation.

Parameters of Use

Absorption Variable rate from GI tract. About 99% binds to plasma proteins. Onset of action is: 3 to 6 hours (T_3); 2 to 3 days (T_4). Half-life is: 12 hours (T_3); 6 to 7 days (T_4). Peak action occurs in: 1 to 2 days (T_3); 9 to 12 days (T_4). Duration of action is: 4 to 6 days (T_3); 3 weeks (T_4). A minimal amount crosses placenta.

Metabolism In liver.

Excretion About 70 to 80% in urine; 20 to 30% in feces.

Drug Interactions Estrogens and cholestyramine decrease thyroid action. Phenytoin and tricyclic antidepressants potentiate effects of thyroid hormone. Thyroid hormone enhances cardiovascular effects of catecholamines. Thyroid hormone potentiates effects of anticoagulants, digitalis, ketamine, and indomethacin.

Laboratory Interactions Causes an increase in serum protein-bound iodine and serum glucose in diabetics. Decreases serum cholesterol.

Administration Dosage is highly individualized. Adults and children over 3 years: Initial dosage: 7.5 to 15 mg po daily for 2 weeks; then 30 mg daily for 2 weeks; then 60 mg daily; Maintenance dosage: 60 to 195 mg daily.

Available Drug Forms Tablets containing 15 to 325 mg; chewable tablets containing 195 mg; sustained-release capsules containing 65, 130, 195, 260, or 325 mg. Store in light-resistant, moisture-proof containers.

Nursing Management

Planning factors Explain that response to thyroid treatment in growing children is dramatic and includes hair loss, initial weight loss followed by rapid growth, and increased assertiveness. As treatment continues, these responses abate.

Administration factors

1. Entire dosage is given all at once; effects are cumulative, so there is no advantage to dividing dosage.
2. Stress that drug must be taken regularly, even though client feels dramatically better. For most clients, replacement therapy is a lifetime requirement.
3. During dosage adjustments, a pulse rate over 100 and/or any changes in heart rhythm should be reported to physician immediately.
4. In clients with hypothyroidism without myxedema, therapy is started with very small doses, since they are very sensitive to thyroid hormone. Pulse rate and rhythm should be closely monitored during dosage adjustments.

Evaluation factors

1. Diabetic clients should test urine regularly, since increased doses of hypoglycemic drugs may be necessary.

2. Initial response to drug in adult hypothyroid clients usually includes diuresis, increased appetite, and increased pulse rate.
3. Growth rate of children must be closely monitored; rapid bone growth can result in premature epiphyseal closure.
4. Clients should have a physical examination monthly during dosage adjustment period.
5. Any signs of aggravated cardiovascular disease, including chest pain, should be reported to physician at once.
6. Clients on concomitant anticoagulant therapy should have prothrombin time monitored more frequently than usual. Anticoagulant dosage may need reduction within 1 to 2 weeks after initiation of thyroid therapy. Teach client signs of excess anticoagulant: ecchymoses, petechiae, purpura, bleeding.

Client teaching factors Clients whose protein-bound iodine is being monitored during dosage adjustments should be taught to avoid any extra iodine intake to ensure accurate assessments. Client should avoid topical iodine applications, any OTC medications containing iodides, dentifrices with iodides, and iodine-rich foods, such as turnips, cabbage, and soybean products.

GENERIC NAME Sodium levothyroxine (RX)

TRADE NAMES Letter, T_4, Synthroid

CLASSIFICATION Synthetic thyroid hormone

See thyroid hormone for Indications for use, Contraindications, Untoward reactions, Parameters of use, Drug interactions, and Nursing management.

Action Administration of T_4 alone is sufficient for complete physiologic thyroid replacement.

Administration Adults: 0.1 to 0.2 mg po daily; 0.2 to 0.5 mg IM or IV daily. Children: 0.3 to 0.4 mg po daily.

Available Drug Forms Scored tablets containing 0.025, 0.05, 0.1, 0.15, 0.2, or 0.3 mg. 10-ml vials containing 0.5 or 10 mg mannitol. Must be reconstituted with 5 ml sodium chloride and shaken thoroughly. Do not use bacteriostatic sodium chloride. Solution must be used immediately and any unused portion discarded.

GENERIC NAME Sodium liothyronine (RX)

TRADE NAMES Cytomel, T_3

CLASSIFICATION Synthetic thyroid hormone

See thyroid hormone for Contraindications, Untoward reactions, Drug interactions, and Nursing management.

Action T_3 is less firmly bound to plasma proteins and therefore more rapidly available to body cells. (See thyroid hormone for further details.)

Indications for Use Can be used for clients allergic to desiccated animal thyroid. (See thyroid hormone.)

Parameters of Use (See thyroid hormone for further details.)

Absorption Onset of action occurs within a few hours. Peak action occurs in 2 to 3 days. Half-life is 2.5 days.

Laboratory Interactions Protein-bound iodine levels will remain below normal throughout drug therapy.

Administration Adults and children over 3 years: Initial dosage: 5 to 25 mcg po daily; Maintenance dosage: 25 to 75 mcg daily.

Available Drug Forms Tablets containing 5, 25, or 50 mcg.

GENERIC NAME Liotrix (RX)

TRADE NAMES Euthroid, Thyrolar

CLASSIFICATION Synthetic thyroid hormone

See thyroid hormone for Indications for use, Contraindications, Untoward reactions, Parameters of use, Drug interactions, and Nursing management.

Action A synthetic combination of T_4 and T_3 in a 4:1 ratio. (See thyroid hormone.)

Laboratory Interactions Thyroid function tests including protein-bound iodine will be normal.

Administration Adults: 15 to 60 mg po daily.

Available Drug Forms Tablets containing 16, 32, 65, 130, 200, or 325 mg.

GENERIC NAME Thyroglobulin (RX)

TRADE NAME Proloid

CLASSIFICATION Thyroid hormone

See thyroid hormone for Action, Indications for use, Contraindications, Untoward reactions, Parameters of use, Drug interactions, and Nursing management.

Source A purified extract of hog thyroid containing T_4 and T_3.

Laboratory Interactions Protein-bound iodine will be normal with appropriate dosage.

Administration Adults: 0.5 to 3 gr (32 to 200 mg) po daily.

Available Drug Forms Tablets containing 16, 32, 65, 100, 130, 200, or 325 mg.

GENERIC NAME Sodium dextrothyroxine (RX)

TRADE NAME Choloxin

CLASSIFICATION Synthetic thyroid hormone

Action Major effect is reduction of serum cholesterol levels in clients with hyperlipidemia. Lipoprotein and triglyceride levels may also be reduced. Drug probably stimulates the liver to increase catabolism and excretion of cholesterol.

Indications for Use As an adjunct to diet for reduction of serum cholesterol in euthyroid clients with no cardiac disease. Treatment of hypothyroidism in clients with cardiac disease who cannot tolerate other thyroid drugs.

Contraindications Euthyroid clients with organic cardiac disease, history of myocardial infarction, arrhythmias or tachycardias, congestive heart failure, hypertension, kidney or liver impairment, pregnancy, lactation, history of iodism.

Untoward Reactions Iodism: rash, pruritus, coryza, conjunctivitis, stomatitis, laryngitis, bronchitis, metallic taste. (See thyroid hormone.)

Parameters of Use (See thyroid hormone.)

Excretion In urine and feces in equal amounts.

Drug Interactions May have additive effects in clients receiving digitalis. Potentiates effects of anticoagulants; dosage may need reduction by as much as 30%. (See thyroid hormone.)

Laboratory Interactions Protein-bound iodine greatly increased. ^{131}I uptake is depressed.

Administration Adults: Initial dosage: 1 to 2 mg po daily; Maintenance dosage: 4 to 8 mg po daily. The maximum dose for clients receiving digitalis is 4 mg/day. Children: 0.1 mg/kg po daily; Maximum dosage: 4 mg/day.

Available Drug Forms Scored tablets containing 1, 2, 4, or 6 mg.

Nursing Management

Planning factors Drug should be discontinued at least 2 weeks before elective surgery.

Administration factors Prescribed dosage and attention to adverse effects is important, since margin of safety is narrow.

Evaluation factors

1. Serum lipid values should be determined at monthly intervals. Client should consume normal diet for several days before testing. Maximum decrease in cholesterol levels occurs 2 to 3 months after initiation of therapy.
2. Symptoms of iodism call for discontinuance of drug.

Client teaching factors

1. Strict birth control measures are advised for women of childbearing age; teratogenic studies are still incomplete.
2. Clients with any cardiovascular disease should immediately report any new or exacerbated signs and symptoms.

ANTITHYROID AGENTS

GENERIC NAME Propylthiouracil (RX)

TRADE NAME PTU

CLASSIFICATION Antithyroid agent

Action Inhibits synthesis of thyroid hormones without inactivating already existing thyroid hormones. May inhibit conversion of T_4 to T_3 (see thyroid hormone). Pituitary TSH release will increase in response to a decrease in circulating thyroid hormone, and thyroid gland will enlarge.

Indications for Use Treatment of mild hyperthyroidism with no significant thyroid enlargement; preoperative preparation for subtotal thyroidectomy to decrease hyperthyroidism; control of toxic goiter.

Contraindications Hypersensitivity; last trimester of pregnancy, lactation; concurrent administration of sulfonamides or coal tar derivatives. Use with caution with any drugs known to cause agranulocytosis.

Untoward Reactions Rash, pruritis, nausea, vomiting, loss of taste. Adverse reactions: paresthesias, dizziness, lethargy, neuritis, edema, lymphadenopathy, skin pigmentation, hair loss. Agranulocytosis, hypoprothrombinemia, other blood dyscrasias, jaundice, and hepatitis rarely occurs.

Parameters of Use

Absorption From GI tract. Onset of action is 30 to 40 minutes. Duration of action is 2 to 4 hours. Half-life is 2 hours.

Excretion In urine; about 35% in 24 hours.

Drug Interactions Potentiates effects of oral anticoagulants by causing hypothrombinemia.

Administration Adults: Initial dosage: 300 to 600 mg po daily in divided doses; Maintenance dosage: 100 to 150 mg po daily. Children: Ages 6 to 10 years: 50 to 150 mg po daily; Over 10 years: 150 to 300 mg po daily.

Available Drug Forms Scored tablets containing 50 mg. Must be stored in light-resistant containers.

Nursing Management

Planning factors

1. When used prior to thyroid surgery, propranolol or iodine is also administered to reduce thyroid size and vascularity.
2. Antithyroid action of drug may be delayed for several weeks until already circulating thyroid hormones are metabolized and excreted.
3. Initial signs of response to drug are weight gain and reduced pulse rate.

Administration factors

1. Give with meals to minimize GI distress.
2. When client begins to respond, a thyroid hormone preparation is often added to suppress TSH production.
3. In pregnancy, thyroid hormone should be given concurrently to prevent cretinism and goiter in the fetus.

Evaluation factors

1. Blood studies should be done every 2 to 3 months, especially prothrombin time.
2. Alert client to report early signs of hypothyroidism (goiter): periorbital edema, intolerance to cold, edema, mental depression.
3. Alert client to report signs of agranulocytosis: sore throat, fever, rash.
4. Alert client to report signs of hypoprothrombinemia: ecchymoses, purpura, petechiae, unusual bleeding.

Client teaching factors

1. In severe thyroid enlargement, response may not be evident for several months. Instruct client that treatment usually takes 1 to 2 years, after which drug is stopped and natural remission may occur.
2. Instruct client not to use any OTC drugs containing iodides. Iodized salt and seafood may also be contraindicated.
3. Client should be taught to check pulse regularly and to record pulse and weight weekly.

GENERIC NAME Methimazole (RX)

TRADE NAME Tapazole

CLASSIFICATION Antithyroid agent

See propylthiouracil for Indications for use, Contraindications, Untoward reactions, Parameters of use, Drug interactions, and Nursing management.

Action Ten times more potent than propylthiouracil. (See propylthiouracil.)

Administration Adults: Initial dosage: 15 to 60 mg po daily; Maintenance dosage: 5 to 15 mg po daily in divided doses. Children: Initial dosage: 0.4 mg/kg po daily; Maintenance dosage: ½ initial dose po daily in divided doses.

Available Drug Forms Scored tablets containing 5 or 10 mg.

GENERIC NAME Sodium iodide ^{131}I, ^{125}I (RX)

TRADE NAMES Iodotope, Oriodide, Radiocaps, Theriodide, Tracervial

CLASSIFICATION Antithyroid agent

Action Inhibits release of thyroid hormones. ^{131}I emits beta-radiation that, in large quantities, destroys thyroid tissue. ^{125}I has low radiation and emits no beta-rays.

Indications for Use Hyperthyroidism (Grave's disease), thyroid carcinoma and metastases, thyroid disorders.

Contraindications Pregnant and nursing mothers; children under 18 years; clients with recent myocardial infarction; acute hyperthyroidism, large nodular goiter, iodine sensitivity. Use with caution in impaired renal or cardiac function.

Untoward Reactions Hypothyroidism, thyroid nodules, thyroiditis (tender, swollen gland with fever, headache, pain), alopecia, cough, nausea, gastritis, angioedema, and bone marrow depression rarely occur.

Parameters of Use

Absorption From GI tract. Concentrates quickly in thyroid gland, salivary glands, and stomach within 3 to 6 minutes. Half-life is: 8 days (^{131}I); 57 to 60 days (^{125}I).

Metabolism ^{131}I disintegrates by emitting beta-particles. Its final product is xenon 131.

Excretion In the kidneys. Small amounts in feces and sweat.

Drug Interactions ^{131}I uptake is impaired by recent iodine intake (any form).

Laboratory Interactions In presence of cirrhosis, and in clients on low-sodium diets, uptake of sodium iodide by thyroid is increased. In clients with congestive heart failure, uptake is decreased.

Administration Dosage measured in millicuries. Dosage highly variable.

- *Diagnosis:* 2 to 10 mCi po or IV.
- *Hyperthyroidism:* 4 to 10 mCi po or IV.
- *Carcinoma:* 50 to 150 mCi po or IV.

Treatment may be repeated every 3 to 4 months.

Available Drug Forms Solution and capsules. Glass storage containers may darken from radiation, but this does not affect strength or safety of drug.

Nursing Management

Planning factors

1. Alert clients to signs of hypothyroidism. Thyroid hormone replacement therapy is indicated in most clients after administration of radioactive iodine.
2. Discontinue any antithyroid drug treatment 4 days prior to administration.
3. Therapeutic response is evident in 3 to 6 weeks.

Administration factors

1. Administer in water; drug is colorless and tasteless. Add more water to glass and administer again to assure total dosage.
2. In women of childbearing age, drug should be administered during menses.
3. For control of hyperthyroidism, several treatments may be necessary over a period of many months.
4. Clients receiving 30 mCi or more should be isolated and radiation levels monitored. Appropriate radiation precautions are instituted according to agency policy.

Evaluation factors Thyroid function tests should be done routinely to detect possible hypothyroidism, which is insidious in onset and can develop over a period of years.

GENERIC NAMES Potassium iodide; potassium iodide solution; strong iodide solution

TRADE NAMES KI-N, Pima; SSKI; Lugol's Solution

CLASSIFICATION Iodine supplement (RX)

Action In enlarged thyroid, the excess iodide temporarily inhibits secretion of thyroid hormone and decreases vascularity of the gland. Also acts directly on bronchial tissue to increase secretion of respiratory fluids, thereby decreasing viscosity.

Indications for Use Short-term treatment of hyperthyroidism; treatment of thyrotoxicosis in conjunction with antithyroid drugs and propanolol; preoperative preparation for subtotal thyroidectomy to decrease vascularity and size of gland.

Contraindications Iodine sensitivity, tuberculosis, hypothyroidism, hyperkalemia, bronchitis. Use with caution in pregnancy.

Untoward Reactions Goiter, hypothyroidism (rare), small bowel lesions, hypersensitivity reactions. Iodism: metallic taste, stomatitis, sneezing, coryza, salivary gland soreness, headache, vomiting, bloody diarrhea.

Parameters of Use

Absorption From GI tract. Onset of action is within 24 hours. Duration of action is 10 to 14 days. Taken up by thyroid and used in hormone synthesis.
Metabolism In liver.
Excretion By the kidneys and in feces.

Drug Interactions Lithium potentiates hypothyroid effects. Estrogens and progestogens may increase protein-bound iodine.

Laboratory Interactions Elevated protein-bound iodine and altered urinary 17-hydroxycorticosteroids.

Administration Solution: 0.3 ml po tid or qid for 2 weeks before thyroidectomy. Strong solution: 0.1 to 0.3 mg po tid for 2 weeks before thyroidectomy.

Available Drug Forms Tablets; enteric-coated tablets containing 300 mg; solution containing 300 mg/0.3 ml; syrup containing 5 gr/tsp. Store in airtight, light-resistant containers. Do not leave uncovered as solution will evaporate. Slight discoloration will not affect strength.

Nursing Management

Planning factors Cannot be preceded or followed by radioactive iodine because thyroid gland will be saturated and cannot take up additional iodine.

Administration factors

1. Administer diluted in juice, milk, or water before meals.
2. When given before thyroidectomy, strict adherence to administration schedule is necessary to minimize possibility of "escape" from drug effects or return of thyrotoxicosis.

Evaluation factors Clients should be assessed frequently for development of goiter. Administration of thyroid hormone or discontinuing the iodide will reverse goiter development.
Client teaching factors Instruct client to avoid OTC drugs containing iodides and foods rich in iodine. Teach signs of iodism.

PARATHYROID HORMONES

GENERIC NAME Calcitonin-salmon (RX)

TRADE NAME Calcimar

CLASSIFICATION Synthetic parathyroid hormone, antihypercalcemic

Action Decreases serum calcium by inhibiting osteoclastic bone resorption and by blocking tubular reabsorption of calcium, sodium, and phosphorus. May initially induce new bone formation by increasing osteoblastic activity and deposition of calcium in bones, but there is no long-term increase in new bone deposition. Short-term administration causes decreased gastric juice volume and acidity and pancreatic trypsin and amylase. About one-half of clients with Paget's disease will develop antibodies to calcitonin with prolonged treatment.

Indications for Use Treatment of Paget's disease and hypercalcemia.

Contraindications Allergy to salmon calcitonin or gelatin; osteoporosis; children.

Untoward Reactions Nausea and/or vomiting; usually disappears with continued administration. Local inflammatory reactions at injection site, skin rash, facial flushing, paresthesias, diuresis, diarrhea. Systemic allergic reaction: anaphylaxis, hypocalcemic tetany.

Parameters of Use

Absorption Into circulation from injection site. Onset of action is 2 hours. Peak action occurs in 4 to 6 hours and duration of action is 12 to 24 hours.

Does not cross placental barrier.

Metabolism In the kidneys to inactive metabolites.

Excretion Small amount in urine.

Drug Interactions Effects potentiated by androgens.

Laboratory Interactions Causes decreased alkaline phosphatase and urinary hydroxyproline.

Administration Expressed in Medical Research Council units. Initial dosage: 100 MRC subc or IM daily; Maintenance dosage: 50 to 100 MRC subc or IM daily.

Available Drug Forms Vial of powder containing 400 MRC with 20 mg hydrolyzed gelatin. Must be reconstituted with 16% gelatin solution packaged with drug. Agitate gently for 2 to 3 minutes. After reconstitution, is stable for 2 weeks under refrigeration.

Nursing Management

Planning factors

1. Skin testing for allergic response should precede first dose.
2. Parenteral calcium should be available in case hypocalcemic tetany develops.

Evaluation factors

1. Serum alkaline phosphatase and 24-hour urine hydroxyproline levels should be checked periodically to assess therapeutic effect.
2. Clients who develop antibodies to drug may exhibit signs and symptoms of hypercalcemia: muscle hypotonicity, renal calculi, bone pain, nausea, vomiting, thirst, polyuria, bradycardia, lethargy, psychosis.
3. Clients who relapse should be tested for antibody titer as follows.
   a. After an overnight fast, serum calcium is measured.
   b. 100 MRC calcitonin is administered IM.
   c. 3-hour and 6-hour blood samples are tested for calcium. A decrease of 0.3 mg/100 ml or less indicates antibody presence.

Client teaching factors

1. Instruct client in handling and storage of drug at home.
2. Teach client importance of continuing drug administration even though symptoms have lessened.
3. Client must be taught sterile technique for self-administration.

GENERIC NAME Parathyroid hormone (RX)

TRADE NAME Parathormone

CLASSIFICATION Parathyroid hormone

Source Prepared from beef glands.

Action Increases renal excretion of phosphorus and stimulates tubular calcium reabsorption and release of calcium and phosphates from bone to serum. Serum calcium levels rise within 4 hours of administration. Increases renal excretion of water, sodium, and bicarbonate. Facilitates renal conversion of vitamin D to its active form thereby enabling increased calcium absorption from GI tract.

Indications for Use Treatment of acute hypoparathyroidism with tetany; oxalic acid and radiophosphorus poisoning. Diagnosis of hypoparathyroidism.

Contraindications Above normal serum calcium levels. Use with caution in clients with renal or cardiac disease. Use in pregnancy is not established.

Untoward Reactions Local reaction at injection site, vasodilation, hypotension, bradycardia, cardiac arrhythmias. Overdosage (symptoms of hypercalcemia): anorexia, vomiting, diarrhea, weakness, lethargy, bone pain, headache, tinnitus, vertigo. Allergic reaction possible in sensitive clients.

Parameters of Use

Absorption Into circulation from injection site. Onset of action is: 15 minutes (IV); 4 hours (subc, IM). Peak action occurs in 12 to 18 hours and duration of action is 20 to 24 hours. Half-life is 20 minutes. Binds to plasma proteins.

Metabolism Probably in the kidneys and liver.

Excretion Only 1% in urine.

Drug Interactions Action is potentiated by thiazides; watch for hypercalcemia. Action is antagonized by dactinomycin, corticosteroids, anticonvulsants, calcitonin, and androgens.

Administration Adults: 20 to 40 U subc, IM, or IV q12h for acute tetany; IV and oral calcium are given concurrently. Infants: 25 to 50 U subc, IM, or IV q12h.

Available Drug Forms 5-ml ampules containing 100 U/ml. Should be stored in refrigerator, but not frozen.

Nursing Management

Planning factors Seizure precautions should be followed until serum calcium returns to normal levels.

Administration factors

1. Preliminary skin test is advised before IV injection. IV administration must be slow.
2. Epinephrine solution should be available in case of sensitivity reaction.
3. Add only to IV dextrose solutions; saline solution will cause precipitation of drug.
4. Administer only for a few days; clients will not respond to it for longer periods.
5. For prolonged treatment of hypoparathyroidism, vitamin D supplements are indicated.

Evaluation factors

1. Frequent serum calcium and phosphorus levels must be done to assess effectiveness of dosage.
2. Intake and output must be monitored. An increased fluid intake may prevent the formation of renal calculi.

PART VII

CENTRAL NERVOUS SYSTEM DEPRESSANTS

THE MAJOR ANATOMICAL components of the central nervous system are the brain, brain stem, and spinal cord. The billions of neurons in the central nervous system act to maintain body functions. They are grouped into functional systems that regulate motor activity, memory, and sensory and autonomic functions. These systems do not function in isolation but interact to elicit a series of responses; therefore, drug effects may not be limited to a particular system.

Central nervous system depressants are used for inducing unconsciousness and for treating a variety of disorders, including pain, insomnia, epilepsy, and muscle spasms. Although each of these agents is intended to act on a specific functional system, generalized central nervous system depression may occur. Drug tolerance and addiction are serious consequences of these agents.

Narcotic analgesics, related to opium, are used to alleviate pain from all sources. Morphine, the most active constituent of opium, is the standard against which all other narcoticanalgesics are compared. Because of their central nervous system depressant action, these agents are also used to induce sedation and to treat cough and diarrhea. Unfortunately, narcotics can cause serious untoward reactions, including respiratory depression and dependency.

Nonnarcotic analgesics can relieve mild to moderate pain, particularly pain associated with the musculoskeletal system, but they are ineffective in alleviating deep visceral or severe pain. These agents have other properties that make them useful in controlling fever and combating inflammation.The major action of barbiturates is central nervous system depression, making them useful for sedation, inducing sleep, relieving anxiety, providing light anesthesia, and controlling convulsions (phenobarbital). As with narcotics, tolerance can develop with continuous use, but unlike narcotics, these agents do not relieve pain. When these drugs are withdrawn after prolonged use, a rebound effect occurs. The liability of excessive central nervous system depression is present, which may result in cardiovascular collapse, respiratory depression, and coma. There are no known antagonists for barbiturates; toxicity must be treated symptomatically.

Anticonvulsants do not induce a generalized central nervous system depression, but increase the brain's seizure threshold and prevent the spread of seizure discharges to other parts of the brain. These agents do not cure epilepsy, but are able to control seizure activity effectively so that the client is able to live normally. Continuous daily use of the drug is required to prevent seizure activity. Unfortunately, chronic toxicity and tolerance to the drug may develop.

Skeletal muscle relaxants decrease muscle spasms, either by depressing the brain's motor areas or by blocking motoneuron impulse transmission. A few of these agents act by blocking impulses at the neuromuscular junction. The central-acting drugs induce untoward reactions similar to other central nervous system depressants. Those relaxants that act peripherally to the brain may also induce respiratory depression by excessive skeletal muscle relaxation.

General anesthetics are used to provide controlled depression of the central nervous system. Most of these agents induce unconsciousness, analgesia, and, when given in large doses, muscle relaxation. They are used to induce unconsciousness so that major and minor surgery can be tolerated in relative safety and comfort. A short-acting barbiturate may be given the evening prior to surgery, and a narcotic may be used an hour before surgery. These central nervous system depressants help to relieve anxiety and reduce the amount of anesthesia required during the operation. Most anesthetic agents are irritating to the respiratory tract and may increase the production of mucus. Anticholinergic agents, such as atropine, are used to control this side effect. As with other central nervous system depressants, respiratory depression and cardiovascular collapse may occur.

Chapter 27

Narcotic Analgesics

Codimal PH	Percocet-5
Colrex Compound	Percodan
Copavln	Pseudo-Hist
Dia-Quel	P-V Tussin
Dimetane Expectorant-DC	Robitussin A-C
Duradyne DHC	Robitussin-DAC
Emprazil-C	Ryna-C
Hycodan	S-T Forte
Innovar	Talwin Compound
Isoclor	Tussanil DH
Norcet	Tussar-2
Novahistine Expectorant	Tussend Expectorant
Nucofed	Tussi-Organidin
Parepectolin	Vicodin
Pediacof	Zactirin Compound

CHARACTERISTICS OF NARCOTIC ANALGESICS

All narcotic analgesics, whether natural or synthetic, are related to opium, which has been used for many centuries. In fact, the term *opiate* or *opioid* is often used as a more accurate and descriptive title for this important group of drugs. Until the early 19th century, opium, which comes from the seeds of the Asian poppy plant, was smoked or ingested in its crude form. Morphine was the first opium alkaloid to be isolated in 1803, and by the latter half of the 19th century, the pure alkaloids of opium were widely used in medical practice. Although over 20 alkaloids have been isolated from crude opium, only a few are used clinically. A number of semi-synthetic opiates, produced by simple modification of the morphine molecule, and true synthetic opiates are also available.

The alkaloids of opium are divided into two chemical categories: phenanthrenes and benzylisoquinolines, which have quite different effects in the body. Papaverine and noscapine belong to the benzylisoquinoline group, but neither of these drugs have addictive properties or significant analgesic potential. Papaverine is used for smooth muscle relaxation and vasodilation and noscapine is used for its antitussive effects; hence, they will not be described in this chapter.

Of the opiate analgesics, morphine is still the standard to which all other opiates are compared. The semisynthetic and synthetic narcotics were developed as part of the search for a potent morphinelike analgesic without the addictive liability and other side effects of the opiates. This search still continues as the most effective analgesics available today all carry the danger of tolerance and addiction when used injudiciously.

Morphine (and related drugs) is effective against all types and sources of pain, including deep visceral pain. Smaller doses are effective for continuous dull pain, whereas larger doses may be needed for relief of intense stabbing pain. Therefore, when pain can be anticipated, as in the postoperative surgical client, it is advisable to administer the prescribed opiate before pain becomes severe.

There is still some difference of opinion as to whether morphine actually alters the *physiologic sensation* of pain or whether it only increases the ability to tolerate painful sensations—that is, raises the pain threshold. Studies seem to indicate that the opiates act selectively on those neurologic centers responsible for the affective reactions associated with the painful stimulus. In other words, if the capability to feel fear, anxiety, terror, suffering, and so on is diminished or eliminated, then the physical pain stimulus can be tolerated. Many clients, in fact, after receiving morphine for pain, report that they continue to perceive the pain but feel much more comfortable.

The major effects of morphine on the central nervous system are related to the drug's depressant effects. In addition to analgesia, other manifestations are drowsiness, mental clouding, and sometimes euphoria (an exaggerated sense of well-being). Although the analgesic effect occurs first, it is often not followed by sleep even though drowsiness, lethargy, and apathy are induced. Morphine also has a pronounced depressant effect on the respiratory center in the medulla, causing a decrease in rate and depth of respirations. In morphine poisoning, death is caused by complete respiratory failure. Other effects on the central nervous system include pupillary constriction, depression of the cough center, and stimulation of the emetic zone in the medulla, which may cause nausea and vomiting.

The effects of morphine on the gastrointestinal tract include increased smooth muscle tone in the sphincters, which causes a delay in stomach emptying, and decreased peristalsis. The defecation reflex is depressed, and constipation may result from continued morphine use. Glandular secretions are also diminished, slowing down the digestive process. Urinary bladder tone is similarly affected, and may cause difficulty in voiding. Urinary output may also be decreased as morphine causes antidiuretic hormone to be released.

In therapeutic doses, morphine has no significant effects on blood pressure or heart rate and rhythm. However, the small blood vessels in the head, neck, and chest may dilate, causing a flushed appearance, diaphoresis, and possibly itching. These manifestations are probably a result of morphine-induced histamine release.

The major clinical use of morphine is for severe pain that is not expected to recur indefinitely. Because of the addictive potential of morphine, it is not prescribed for chronically painful conditions. The exception to this is for the treatment of an incurable terminal illness, where drug dependence is an insignificant consideration, and the client can be kept quite comfortable on continuous doses of morphine. Opiates are often used as preanesthetic medications prior to surgical procedures as they allay anxiety and decrease resistance to the anesthetic. Whole opium preparations (Paregoric) are still used for intractable diarrhea because of their slow absorption.

Addictive Liability

Addiction, or tolerance to opiates, varies with the individual and with the pattern of drug use. The more frequently the drug is used, the more frequently the dose must be increased to produce the desired effects. Tolerance develops to the drug's euphoric, respiratory, analgesic, and sedative effects, but not to the gastrointestinal or pupillary effects; hence, an addict will still exhibit contracted pupils and constipation. When a narcotic analgesic is used continually, tolerance may develop in as little as two weeks. Moreover, if a client is addicted to one opiate, he or she will be just as tolerant to another, so that changing the prescription from one narcotic to another will not delay or prevent addiction.

Symptoms of narcotic withdrawal vary in intensity, depending on the individual, the drug, and the daily dosage. The morphine (or heroin) addict will direct all purposeful activity toward obtaining more drug just before the next scheduled dose is due. The physiologic manifestations of withdrawal begin about eight hours after the last drug dose. These include tearing of the eyes and nose, perspiration, and yawning. Several hours later, the addict may fall into a very restless sleep, from which he or she awakens even more agitated. The symptoms then progress to include dilated pupils, anorexia, irritability, muscle tremors, insomnia, constant yawning, and continued tearing of the eyes and nose with sneezing. Usually, nausea, vomiting, abdominal cramps, and diarrhea also occur. Pulse and blood pressure are elevated, and the client feels alternately cold and flushed, and sweats profusely. Bone and muscle pain accompanied by spasms and kicking are not uncommon, nor are the characteristic waves of gooseflesh seen in untreated withdrawal. All these physical effects contribute to profound weight loss, acid-base imbalance, and dehydration that may lead to vascular collapse. When withdrawal from opiate addiction is medically supervised, appropriate doses of narcotics are given to suppress the most severe withdrawal symptoms.

OTHER OPIATES

Low addiction liability synthetics are generally considered to be nonnarcotic and are not subject to the provisions of the federal Narcotic Law; however, since they are chemically related to the opiates they are included in this chapter.

Narcotic antagonists are chemical derivatives of certain opiates and are used as part of the treatment for narcotic poisoning.

NATURAL OPIUM ALKALOIDS

GENERIC NAME Morphine sulfate, morphine hydrochloride

TRADE NAME MS (Cii)

CLASSIFICATION Narcotic analgesic

Action Depresses cerebral cortex; causes sleep; depresses respiratory center and cough center; causes blood vessel dilatation in face, head, and neck (causes pruritus and sweating); stimulates contraction of ureters, bladder, and other smooth muscles; decreases GI secretions and motility, increases biliary tract pressure; releases ADH and histamine; promotes contraction of bronchial musculature; may cause nausea and vomiting through stimulation of emetic center in medulla.

Indications for Use Relief of severe pain, anxiety; preanesthetic agent; relief of pain and dyspnea in myocardial infarction.

Contraindications Urethral stricture, head injuries, craniotomy, acute alcoholism, bronchial asthma, prostatic hypertrophy, convulsive disorders, undiagnosed abdominal disorders, pancreatitis, ulcerative colitis, hypersensitivity to opiates.

Warnings and Precautions Use with caution in clients with reduced blood volume or those with reduced respiratory reserve; in the presence of hepatic or renal insufficiency; toxic psychosis; arrhythmias; in the elderly or very young children.

Untoward Reactions Slow and shallow respirations, coma, pinpoint pupils, cyanosis, hypothermia, weak pulse, hypotension, nausea, vomiting, dizziness, mental clouding, constipation, cough center depression, urinary retention, dysuria, biliary colic, bradycardia, allergic dermatologic reactions. Coma, severe respiratory depression, pulmonary edema, hypothermia, and cardiac arrest occur with acute intoxication.

Parameters of Use

Absorption From GI tract, nasal mucosa, lungs, and vascular system. Peak action occurs in: 20 minutes (IV), 60 to 90 minutes (subc, IM). Duration of action is 3 to 7 hours.

Crosses placenta and small amounts appear in breast milk.

Distribution Concentrated in the kidneys, lungs, liver, spleen, and skeletal muscles.

Metabolism In the liver.

Excretion Mostly in urine by glomerular filtration. Also in feces via biliary tract (about 7 to 10%).

Drug Interactions Effects are exaggerated and/or prolonged by tricyclic antidepressants, antianxiety agents, phenothiazines, MAO inhibitors, alcohol, general anesthetics, barbiturates, and other sedatives and hypnotics. Morphine can potentiate the effects of other CNS depressants and skeletal muscle relaxants. Narcotic antagonists block the effects of morphine.

Laboratory Interactions Possible false-positive results of serum amylase, lipase, and urine glucose with Benedict's solution. May cause decreased urinary vanilmandelic acid excretion and elevated serum glutamic-oxaloacetic transaminase.

Administration Adults: Oral: 5 to 30 mg every 3 to 4 hours; oral forms are seldom used because GI absorption is not reliable. Intramuscular, subcutaneous: 5 to 15 mg every 3 to 4 hours; 10 mg/70 kg for initial dose. Intravenous: 2.5 to 15 mg in 4 to 5 ml of sterile water. Children: 0.1 to 0.2 mg/kg per dose subc; single dose not to exceed 15 mg.

Available Drug Forms Tablets and capsules containing 10, 15, or 30 mg; oral solution containing 10 mg/5 ml or 20 mg/5 ml; 1-ml ampules containing 2, 8, 10, or 15 mg/ml; 20-mg vials containing 15 mg/ml; prefilled cartridges containing 2, 8, 10, or 15 mg/ml. Store in light-resistant containers.

Nursing Management

Planning factors

1. The most effective analgesia is achieved before client's pain becomes intense. Evaluate client's need for medication carefully and be aware that smaller doses are effective in controlling continuous dull pain.
2. Morphine has a high abuse potential. Clients, except for those who are terminally ill, should be transferred to a less potent analgesic as soon as possible.
3. Oxygen and narcotic antagonists should be readily available.

Administration factors

1. For IV route, administer slowly over a 4-to-5-minute period.
2. Assess pupillary size and vital signs, particularly respirations, before each dose. Withhold medication if respirations are below 12 per minute and notify physician.
3. Do not mix with other medications, since morphine is incompatible with many drugs.

Evaluation factors

1. Elderly clients may become restless because of paradoxical CNS stimulation.
2. Bedrails should be instituted for all clients during first few days of morphine therapy and maintained until effects are ascertained.
3. Intake and output should be monitored and client assessed for urinary retention.
4. Assess client frequently for abdominal distention, decreased peristalsis, and constipation.
5. Clients with acute myocardial infarction may experience temporary hypotension after administration.

Client teaching factors

1. Instruct client not to ambulate without assistance after receiving drug. Postural hypotension, dizziness, and syncope are common side effects.
2. Movement and ambulation often enhance the emetic effect of morphine. Client should be instructed to remain supine following administration until effects are ascertained.

GENERIC NAMES Codeine; codeine phosphate; codeine sulfate (Cii)

CLASSIFICATION Narcotic analgesic and antitussive agent

See morphine for Contraindications, Warnings and precautions, Untoward reactions, and Parameters of use.

Action Similar actions to morphine, but one-tenth the analgesic activity. Less side effects than morphine (gastrointestinal, pupillary, respiratory). Depresses cough center. Addictive, but tolerance develops much more slowly than with morphine. (See morphine.)

Indications for Use Relief of mild to moderate pain; suppression of cough. Used in patients sensitive to morphine.

Drug Interactions Aspirin and codeine have a synergistic effect. (See morphine.)

Administration Adults: 15 to 60 mg po or subc every 3 to 4 hours; Children— 3 mg/kg daily.

Available Drug Forms Tablets containing 15, 30, or 60 mg; vials containing 15, 30, or 60 mg/ml; elixir and syrup for coughs (combination preparation); prefilled cartridges containing 15, 30, or 60 mg/ml.

Nursing Management Large doses may stimulate nerve center causing restlessness. (See morphine for further details.)

WHOLE OPIUM DRUGS

GENERIC NAME Opium tincture (Cv)

TRADE NAME Laudanum

CLASSIFICATION Narcotic (antiperistaltic)

See morphine for Contraindications, Warnings and precautions, Untoward reactions, Parameters of use, and Drug interactions.

Action Similar actions to morphine, but contains only 1% morphine (10 mg/ml). Major effect is gastrointestinal (decreases propulsive peristalsis).

Indications for Use Diarrhea.

Administration 0.3 to 1.5 ml po qid.

Available Drug Forms Liquid alcoholic solution (combination preparation).

Nursing Management (See morphine.)

1. Dilute drug in about 50 ml of water before administering.
2. When diarrhea is controlled, drug should be discontinued, since it has addictive potential.

GENERIC NAME Camphorated opium tincture

TRADE NAME Paregoric (Cv)

CLASSIFICATION Narcotic (antiperistaltic)

See morphine for contraindications, Warnings and precautions, Untoward reactions, Parameters of use, and Drug interactions. See morphine and opium tincture for Nursing management.

Action Opium with camphor, benzoic acid, and anise oil. Similar actions to morphine, but contains 0.25 mg morphine per millileter. Major effect is to decrease peristalsis. (See morphine.)

Indications for Use Diarrhea.

Administration 4 to 8 ml po qid.

Available Drug Forms Liquid in light-resistant bottle containing 0.25 mg/ml.

SEMISYNTHETIC OPIATES

GENERIC NAME Diacetylmorphine (Ci)

TRADE NAME Heroin

CLASSIFICATION Narcotic

Action Similar actions to morphine, but produces greater euphoria. Highly addictive. (See morphine.)

Indications for Use Illegal.

GENERIC NAME Apomorphine hydrochloride

CLASSIFICATION Narcotic (emetic) (Cii)

See morphine for Parameters of use, Drug interactions, and Nursing management.

Action Produced by treating morphine with acids. Has reduced analgesic potency. Stimulates emetic center in medulla causing vomiting.

Indications for Use Oral ingestion of poisons.

Contraindications Corrosive poison ingestion, shock, CNS depression for any reason.

Warnings and Precautions Acts within 10 to 15 minutes. If first dose does not produce emesis, subsequent doses will be ineffective. Do not repeat dosage.

Administration Adults: 5 mg subc; Children: 0.1 mg/kg subc.

Available Drug Forms Powder; hypodermic tablets containing 6 mg. Packaged in airtight, light-resistant containers. Must be dissolved in sterile water and sterilized before use. Once dissolved, solution deteriorates rapidly. Discolored solutions should be discarded.

GENERIC NAME Hydrocodone bitartrate (Cii)

TRADE NAMES Dicodid, Mercodinone (an ingredient of Hycodan)

CLASSIFICATION Narcotic analgesic (antitussive)

See morphine for Warnings and precautions, Untoward reactions, and Parameters of use. See morphine and codeine for Drug interactions.

Action Similar actions to morphine and codeine, but with greater antitussive activity. (See morphine and codeine.)

Indications for Use Primarily for cough.

Contraindications Not to be used in patients with glaucoma. (See morphine.)

Administration Adults: 5 to 15 mg po every 4 hours; always taken after meals. Children: Under 2 years: 1.25 mg po every 4 hours; Ages 2 to 12 years: 2.5 to 5 mg po every 4 hours.

Available Drug Forms Tablets containing 5 mg; syrup containing 5 mg/ml.

Nursing Management (See morphine and codeine.)

1. Addictive liability is greater than for codeine.
2. Warn clients not to operate machinery if drowsiness occurs.

GENERIC NAME Hydromorphone hydrochloride

TRADE NAMES Dilaudid, Hymorphan (Cii)

CLASSIFICATION Narcotic analgesic

See morphine for Contraindications, Warnings and precautions, Untoward reactions, Parameters of use, and Drug interactions.

Action Similar actions to morphine, but five times more effective for pain relief. Less hypnotic effect than morphine. (See morphine)

Indications for Use Relief of moderate to severe pain.

Administration 1 to 4 mg po, IM, subc, or IV every 4 to 6 hours, whenever necessary; Rectal suppository: 3 mg.

Available Drug Forms Tablets containing 1, 2, 3, or 4 mg; ampules containing 1, 2, 3, or 4 mg/ml; vials of 10 or 20 ml containing 2 mg/ml; suppositories containing 3 mg.

Nursing Management (See morphine.)

1. For IV route, administer slowly over a 3- to 5-minute period.
2. Less tendency than morphine to produce nausea, vomiting, and constipation.

GENERIC NAME Methyldihydromorphinone

TRADE NAME Metopon (Cii)

CLASSIFICATION Narcotic analgesic

See morphine for Contraindications, Warnings and precautions, Untoward reactions, Parameters of use, and Drug interactions.

Action Similar actions to morphine, but more potent. Effective with oral administration. Side effects are rare. (See morphine.)

Indications for Use Relief of pain.

Administration 3 mg po every 3 hours, whenever necessary.

Available Drug Forms Tablets containing 3 mg.

Nursing Management Less addictive liability than morphine. (See morphine)

GENERIC NAME Oxycodone hydrochloride (Cii)

TRADE NAME (An ingredient of Percodan)

CLASSIFICATION Narcotic analgesic

See morphine for Warnings and precautions, Untoward reactions, and Parameters of use. See morphine and codeine for Drug interactions. See codeine for Indications for use.

Action Similar actions to morphine and codeine. Effective with oral administration. (See morphine and codeine.)

Contraindications Not to be used in pregnancy or children under 6 years.

Administration Adults: 3 to 20 mg po every 6 hours, whenever necessary. Children: Ages 6 to 12 years: 0.5 mg po every 6 hours, whenever necessary; Over 12 years: 1 mg po every 6 hours, whenever necessary.

Available Drug Forms Tablets (combination preparation).

Nursing Management Addictive liability is greater than for codeine. (See morphine and codeine for further details.)

GENERIC NAME Oxymorphone hydrochloride

TRADE NAME Numorphan (Cii)

CLASSIFICATION Narcotic analgesic

See morphine for Action, Warnings and precautions, Untoward reactions, Parameters of use, and Drug interactions.

Indications for Use Relief of severe pain.

Administration 0.75 to 1.5 mg IM or subc every 4 to 6 hours; Rectal suppository: 2 to 5 mg every 4 to 6 hours.

Available Drug Forms Powder for injection containing 0.5 mg/ml; suppositories containing 2.5 mg. Store in refrigerator

Nursing Management (See morphine.)

1. Less tendency than morphine to produce GI symptoms and respiratory depression.
2. Peak action occurs in 10 to 20 minutes when administered parenterally.

GENERIC NAME Pantopium (Cii)

TRADE NAME Pantopon

CLASSIFICATION Narcotic analgesic

See morphine for Contraindications, Warnings and precautions, Untoward reactions, and Parameters of use. See morphine and codeine for Drug interactions and Nursing management.

Action Similar actions to morphine and codeine. Purified opium alkaloids containing about 50% morphine. (See morphine and codeine)

Indications for Use Relief of pain in patients hypersensitive to morphine.

Administration 5 to 20 mg IM or subc.

Available Drug Forms Ampules containing 20 mg/ml.

SYNTHETIC OPIATES

GENERIC NAMES Meperidine hydrochloride; pethidine hydrochloride

TRADE NAMES Demerol, Dolantin, Dolosal (Cii)

CLASSIFICATION Narcotic analgesic

See morphine for Contraindications, Warnings and precautions, Untoward reactions, and Parameters of use.

Action Similar actions to morphine, but one-tenth the analgesic activity. Less hypnotic, antitussive, and pupillary effects than morphine. Less likely to cause nausea, vomiting, or respiratory depression. (See morphine.)

Indications for Use Relief of moderate or intermittent pain; preanesthetic agent; obstetric analgesic.

Drug Interactions Amphetamines enhance analgesic effect. (See morphine.)

Administration Adults: 50 to 100 mg po or IM every 3 to 4 hours, whenever necessary; Children: 6 mg/kg po or IM daily. Intravenous: 25 mg.

Available Drug Forms Tablets containing 50 or 100 mg; syrup containing 50 mg/5 ml; ampules of 0.5, 1, 1.5, or 2 ml; vials of 30 ml containing 50 mg/ml.

Nursing Management (See morphine.)

Planning factors

1. Constipation and urinary retention are unlikely with Demerol.
2. Addictive liability is less than for morphine.

Administration factors

1. For IV route, administer very slowly over a 3- to 5-minute period.
2. Demerol solution is not compatible with barbiturate solution; do not mix together.

3. Syrup should be diluted in 4 fl oz of water for oral administration.

GENERIC NAME Alphaprodine hydrochloride

TRADE NAME Nisentil (Cii)

CLASSIFICATION Narcotic analgesic

See morphine for contraindications, Warnings and precautions, Untoward reactions, Parameters of use, and Drug interactions.

Action Similar actions to morphine. Analgesic activity is between that of meperidine and morphine, but acts more quickly, and over a shorter duration (2 hours). (See morphine.)

Indications for Use Relief of moderate to severe pain; preanesthetic agent for minor surgery and diagnostic procedures; obstetric analgesic (early labor).

Administration Subcutaneous: 20 to 60 mg every 2 hours; Maximum dosage: 240 mg daily. Intravenous: 20 to 30 mg every 3 to 6 hours.

Available Drug Forms 1-ml ampules containing 40 or 60 mg/ml; 10-ml vials containing 40 or 60 mg/ml.

Nursing Management Less danger of respiratory depression than with morphine. (See morphine.)

GENERIC NAME Anileridine, anileridine phosphate

TRADE NAME Leritine (Cii)

CLASSIFICATION Narcotic analgesic

See morphine for Contraindications, Warnings and precautions, Untoward reactions, Parameters of use, and Nursing management. See morphine and meperidine hydrochloride for Drug interactions. See meperidine hydrochloride for Indications for use.

Action Similar actions to meperidine, but three times the analgesic activity. Unlike meperidine, anileridine seldom causes constipation.

Administration 25 to 50 mg po, IM, or subc every 3 to 4 hours; not to exceed 200 mg daily. Intravenous: 5 to 10 mg every 3 to 4 hours.

Available Drug Forms Ampules and vials containing 25 mg/ml, tablets containing 25 mg.

GENERIC NAME Diphenoxylate hydrochloride with atropine sulfate

TRADE NAMES Colonil, Lomotil (Cii)

CLASSIFICATION Narcotic (antidiarrhetic)

See morphine for Warnings and precautions, Untoward reactions, and Parameters of use. See morphine and meperidine hydrochloride for Drug interactions.

Action Similar actions to meperidine. Strong constipating effect.

Indications for Use Diarrhea.

Contraindications Not to be used for children under 2 years. (See morphine.)

Administration Adults: 20 mg po daily in divided doses; Children: 0.3 to 0.4 mg/kg po daily in divided doses.

Available Drug Forms Tablets and liquid (5 ml) containing 2.5 mg diphenoxylate with 0.025 mg atropine sulfate.

Nursing Management (See morphine.)

1. Exempt from restrictions of federal Narcotic Law.
2. May cause slight sedation with therapeutic doses. In doses over 40 mg/day, client can be expected to exhibit side effects like those of morphine.
3. For children 2 to 12 years, use liquid preparation only.

GENERIC NAME Fentanyl citrate (Cii)

TRADE NAME Sublimaze

CLASSIFICATION Narcotic analgesic

See morphine for Contraindications, Warnings and precautions, Untoward reactions, Parameters of use, Drug Interactions, and Nursing management.

Action Similar actions to morphine. Analgesic activity is equivalent to 10 mg morphine or 75 mg meperidine. Respiratory depression may last longer than analgesic effect.

Indications for Use Primarily as preanesthetic agent or anesthetic supplement.

Administration Intramuscular, intravenous: 0.025 to 0.1 mg.

Available Drug Forms Ampules of 2 or 5 ml containing 0.05 mg/ml.

GENERIC NAME Levorphanol tartrate (Cii)

TRADE NAMES Levo-Dromoran, Methorphinan

CLASSIFICATION Narcotic analgesic

See morphine for Contraindications, Warnings and precautions, Untoward reactions, Parameters of use, Drug interactions, and Nursing management.

Action Similar actions to morphine, but more potent. (See morphine.)

Indications for Use Relief of severe pain; preanesthetic agent.

Administration Oral: 2 to 3 mg every 3 to 4 hours; Subcutaneous: 1 to 3 mg every 3 to 4 hours.

Available Drug Forms Tablets containing 2 mg; 1-ml ampules containing 2 mg/ml; 10-ml vials containing 2 mg/ml.

GENERIC NAME Methadone hydrochloride (Cii)

TRADE NAMES Adanon, Amidone, Dolophine, Methadon, Miadone, Polamidon

CLASSIFICATION Narcotic analgesic

See morphine for Contraindications, Warnings and precautions, Untoward reactions, Parameters of use, and Drug interactions.

Action Similar actions to morphine, but longer duration of action (up to 72 hours). (See morphine.)

Indications for Use Relief of pain; treatment of narcotic withdrawal symptoms, heroin users; antitussive.

Administration

- *Relief of pain:* 2.5 to 10 mg po or IM every 3 to 4 hours.
- *Treatment of narcotic withdrawal symptoms:* 15 to 20 mg po or IM every 3 to 4 hours.
- *Cough:* 1.5 to 2 mg po.

Available Drug Forms Tablets containing 5 or 10 mg; ampules containing 10 mg/ml; vials containing 10 mg/ml; elixir or syrup containing 0.34 to 1 mg/ml.

Nursing Management Withdrawal from methadone addiction is more prolonged than for other opiates, but symptoms are less severe. (See morphine.)

GENERIC NAME Phenazocine (Cii)

TRADE NAMES Prinadol, Xenagol

CLASSIFICATION Narcotic analgesic

See morphine for Contraindications, Warnings and precautions, Untoward reactions, Parameters of use, and Drug interactions.

Action Similar actions to morphine, but causes less sedation. Effective in smaller doses than morphine. (See morphine.)

Indications for Use Relief of severe pain; preanesthetic agent; obstetric analgesic.

Administration Intramuscular: 1 to 3 mg every 4 to 6 hours; Intravenous: 0.5 to 1 mg every 4 to 6 hours.

Available Drug Forms 10-ml vials containing 2 mg/ml; 1-ml vials containing 2 mg/ml.

Nursing Management (See morphine.)

1. Greater danger of respiratory depression than with morphine.
2. Do not mix with other medications, since phenazocine is incompatible with many drugs.

GENERIC NAME Piminodine (Cii)

TRADE NAME Alvodine

CLASSIFICATION Narcotic analgesic

See morphine for Contraindications, Warnings and precautions, Untoward reactions, Parameters of use, and Nursing management. See morphine and meperidine hydrochloride for Drug interactions.

Action Similar actions to meperidine, but with slightly shorter duration of action. Less likely to cause constipation.

Indications for Use Relief of moderate to severe pain.

Administration Oral: 25 to 50 mg every 4 to 6 hours; Intramuscular, subcutaneous: 10 to 20 mg every 4 to 6 hours.

Available Drug Forms Tablets containing 25 mg; vials containing 50 mg/ml. Store in light-resistant containers.

SYNTHETIC OPIATES WITH LOW POTENCY AND LOW ADDICTIVE LIABILITY

GENERIC NAME Propoxyphene hydrochloride

TRADE NAMES Darvon, Dolene, Progesic (Civ)

CLASSIFICATION Analgesic (mild narcotic)

See codeine for Warnings and precautions, Untoward reactions, and Parameters of use.

Action Similar actions to codeine, but only half as potent. With aspirin, is as effective as codeine and aspirin. Has no antitussive effect.

Indications for Use Relief of mild to moderate pain in chronic or recurring diseases.

Contraindications Hypersensitivity; not to be used for children.

Drug Interactions Has synergistic effect with aspirin. Has additive effect with alcohol, tranquilizers, and other CNS depressants.

Administration 65 mg po q4h.

Available Drug Forms Capsules containing 32 or 65 mg.

Nursing Management

1. Exempt from restrictions of federal Narcotic Law.
2. Has very slight addictive liability, but can produce psychic and physical dependence.
3. Client should not drive or operate machinery until effect of drug is evaluated.
4. Drowsiness usually occurs only with very large doses (300 mg or more).
5. Client should not consume alcohol or any other sedatives or hypnotics while taking propoxyphene.

GENERIC NAME Ethoheptazine citrate (C IV)

TRADE NAME Zactane

CLASSIFICATION Analgesic (mild narcotic)

See morphine for Warnings and precautions, Untoward reactions, and Parameters of use. See morphine and meperidine hydrochloride for Drug interactions.

Action Acts on CNS to produce analgesia. Has no antitussive, sedative, or respiratory effects. Structurally related to meperidine.

Indications for Use Relief of mild to moderate musculoskeletal pain. Not effective for headaches.

Contraindications Not used in first trimester of pregnancy. Itching, dizziness, GI distress.

Administration 75 to 150 mg po qid.

Available Drug Forms Tablets containing 75 mg.

Nursing Management (See morphine.)

1. Exempt from restrictions of federal Narcotic Law.
2. Drug is nonaddictive and rarely causes side effects, except with prolonged use.

GENERIC NAME Pentazocine hydrochloride (C IV)

TRADE NAME Talwin

CLASSIFICATION Analgesic (mild narcotic)

See morphine for Warnings and precautions, Untoward reactions, Parameters of use, and Drug interactions.

Action GI and CNS effects similar to morphine and codeine. Is a weak narcotic antagonist and has no antitussive effect. High doses cause elevation in blood pressure and heart rate.

Indications for Use Relief of moderate pain.

Contraindications Not to be used for children under 12 years. Safety in pregnancy has not been established.

Administration Oral: 50 to 100 mg q4h; Intramuscular, subcutaneous, intravenous: 30 to 60 mg q4h. Total dosage should not exceed 600 mg.

Available Drug Forms Tablets containing 50 mg.

Nursing Management (See morphine.)

Planning factors Exempt from restrictions of federal Narcotic law.

Administration factors Do not mix with barbiturates as the drugs are incompatible in solution.

Evaluation factors

1. May cause dependence in clients with a history of drug abuse.
2. Clients should not operate machinery while taking drug.
3. In respiratory depression produced by pentazocine, narcotic antagonists are not effective. Artificial respiration and respiratory stimulants are preferred methods of treatment.

NARCOTIC ANTAGONISTS

GENERIC NAME Nalorphine hydrochloride (RX)

TRADE NAMES Lethidrone, Nalline Hydrochloride

CLASSIFICATION Narcotic antagonist

Action Displaces other narcotics from cellular receptor sites. An effective antagonist against depressant effects of all narcotics. Causes abrupt withdrawal symptoms in narcotic addicts. Is not effective against other CNS depressants, barbiturates, or alcohol. May cause respiratory depression when given alone.

Indications for Use Acute narcotic toxicity with respiratory depression; diagnosing narcotic addiction; prevention of respiratory depression in newborns after narcotic given to mother.

Contraindications CNS depression from sources other than narcotics. Not to be used for the treatment of addiction.

Warnings and Precautions When used on narcotic-free clients, effect is similar to that of a small dose of morphine.

Untoward Reactions Large doses cause drowsiness, sweating, dysphoria, nausea, and vomiting.

Parameters of Use

Absorption From tissues after subc injection.
Metabolism Detoxified in liver.
Excretion In urine.

Drug Interactions Can aggravate the effects of barbiturates and other hypnotics on the respiratory system.

Administration Adults: 2 to 10 mg IM, subc, or IV as needed; Newborns: 0.1 to 0.2 mg IM or IV as needed.

Available Drug Forms Adults: Ampules of 1, 2, or 10 ml containing 5 mg/ml; Children: 1-ml ampules containing 0.2 mg/ml. Store in light-resistant containers.

Nursing Management

Planning factors Exempt from restrictions of federal Narcotic Law.

Administration factors Respiratory rate and volume and blood pressure should increase within 2 minutes after IV administration in clients with severe narcotic depression. Additional doses may be required to prevent recurrence of respiratory depression.

GENERIC NAME Levallorphan tartrate (RX)

TRADE NAME Lorfan

CLASSIFICATION Narcotic antagonist

See nalorphine hydrochloride for Indications for use, Contraindications, Warnings and precautions, Untoward reactions, Parameters of use, Drug interactions, and Nursing management.

Action Similar actions to nalorphine, but ten times more potent. (See nalorphine hydrochloride.)

Administration 0.5 to 1 mg IM, subc, or IV as needed.

Available Drug Forms Adults: 10-ml vials containing 1 mg/ml; 1-ml ampules containing 1 mg/ml. Children: Vials containing 0.05 mg/ml. Store in light resistant containers.

GENERIC NAME Naloxone hydrochloride (RX)

TRADE NAME Narcan

CLASSIFICATION Narcotic antagonist

See nalorphine hydrochloride for Indications for use, Contraindications, Warnings and precautions, Untoward reactions, Parameters of use, Drug interactions, and Nursing management.

Action Similar actions to nalorphine, but 10 to 30 times more potent. When given alone, does not cause morphinelike effects and does not aggravate respiratory depression of barbiturates and hypnotics. (See nalorphine hydrochloride.)

Administration Adults: 0.2 to 1 mg IM, subc, or IV as needed; Children: 0.01 mg/kg IM, subc, or IV as needed.

Available Drug Forms 2-ml ampules containing 0.4 mg/ml; 10-ml vials containing 0.4 mg/ml.

COMBINATION PREPARATIONS

Trade name	Composition
Actifed-C	Codeine 10 mg, tripolidine 2 mg, pseudoephedrine 30 mg, guaifenesin 100 mg
Ambenyl Expectorant	Codeine 10 mg, bromodiphenhydramine 3.75 mg, diphenhydramine 8.75 mg, ammonium chloride 80 mg, potassium guaiacolsulfonate 80 mg
Ascodeen-30	Codeine 30 mg, aspirin 325 mg.
Calcidrine	Codeine 8.4 mg, calcium iodide 152 mg
Codalan	Codeine $\frac{1}{8}$, $\frac{1}{4}$, or $\frac{1}{2}$ gr, acetaminophen $2\frac{1}{2}$ gr, salicylamide $3\frac{1}{2}$, caffeine $\frac{1}{2}$ gr
Codimal PH	Codeine 10 mg, phenylephrine 5 mg, pyrilamine 8.33 mg, Potassium guaiacol sulfonate 83.3 mg
Colrex Compound	Codeine 16 mg, acetaminophen 325 mg, phenylephrine 10 mg, chlorpheniramine 2 mg
Copavin	Codeine 15 mg, papaverine 15 mg
Dia-Quel	Opium tincture 0.03 ml, homatropine 0.15 mg, pectin 24 mg
Dimetane Expectorant-DC	Codeine 10 mg, brompheniramine 2 mg, guaifenesin 100 mg, phenylephrine 5 mg, phenylpropanolamine 5 mg
Duradyne DHC	Hydrocodone 5 mg, aspirin 230 mg, acetaminophen 150 mg, caffeine 30 mg
Emprazil-C	Codeine 15 mg, pseudoephedrine 20 mg, phenacetin 150 mg, aspirin 200 mg, caffeine 30 mg
Hycodan	Hydrocodone 5 mg, homatropine 1.5 mg
Innovar	Fentanyl 0.05 mg, droperidol 2.5 mg
Isoclor	Codeine 10 mg, pseudoephedrine 30 mg, guaifenesin 100 mg
Norcet	Hydrocodone 7.5 mg, acetaminophen 650 mg
Novahistine Expectorant	Codeine 10 mg, phenylpropanolamine 18.75 mg, guaifenesin 100 mg
Nucofed	Codeine 20 mg, pseudoephedrine 60 mg
Parepectolin	Paregoric 3.7 ml, pectin 162 mg, Kaolin 5.5 g
Pediacof	Codeine 5 mg, phenylephrine 2.5 mg, chlorpheniramine 0.75 mg, potassium iodide 75 mg
Percocet-5 Tylox	Acetaminophen 500 mg, Oxycodone 4.88 mg
Percodan	Oxycodone 4.88 mg, aspirin 325 mg

COMBINATION PREPARATIONS

Trade name	Composition
Pseudo-Hist	Hydrocodone 2.5 mg, chlorpheniramine 2 mg, pseudoephedrine 15 mg, glyceryl guaiacolate 100 mg
P-V Tussin	Hydrocodone 2.5 mg, phenylephrine 5 mg, pyrilamine 6 mg, chlorpheniramine 2 mg, phenindamine 5 mg
Robitussin A-C	Codeine 10 mg, guaifenesin 100 mg
Robitussin-DAC	Codeine 10 mg, guaifenesine 100 mg, pseudoephedrine 30 mg
Ryna-C	Codeine 10 mg, pseudoephedrine 30 mg, chlorpheniramine 2 mg
S-T Forte	Hydrocodone 15 mg, phenylephrine 30 mg, phenylpropanolamine 30 mg, pheniramine 80 mg, guaifenesin 480 mg
Talwin Compound	Pentazocine 12.5 mg, aspirin 325 mg
Tussanil DH	Dihydrocodeinone 1.66 mg, phenylephrine 10 mg, phenylpropanolamine 5 mg, pyralimine 3.33 mg, chlorpheniramine 1.66 mg
Tussar-2	Codeine 10 mg, carbetapentane 7.5 mg, Chlorpheniramine 2 mg
Tussend Expectorant	Hydrocodone 5 mg, pseudoephedrine 60 mg, guaifenesin 200 mg
Tussi-Organidin	Codeine 10 mg, glycerol 30 mg, chlorpheniramine 2 mg
Vicodin	Hydrocodone 5 mg, acetaminophen 500 mg
Zactirin Compound	Ethoheptazine citrate, phenacetin, aspirin, caffeine

Chapter 28

Nonnarcotic Analgesics and Antirheumatic Agents

CHARACTERISTICS OF NONNARCOTIC ANALGESICS

SALICYLATES

- Aspirin (acetylsalicylic acid)
- Calcium carbaspirin
- Choline salicylate
- Magnesium salicylate
- Methyl salicylate
- Salicylamide
- Salicylic acid
- Sodium salicylate
- Sodium thiosalicylate

PHENOL DERIVATIVE

- Acetaminophen

PYRAZOLONES

- Phenylbutazone, oxyphenbutazone

ERGOT DERIVATIVES

- Ergotamine tartrate, dihydroergotamine mesylate

ANTIRHEUMATICS

- Indomethacin
- Aurothioglucose
- Fenoprofen
- Ibuprofen
- Meclofenamate
- Naproxen
- Penicillamine
- Piroxicam
- Sulindac
- Tolmetin
- Zomepirac

ANTIGOUT AGENTS

- Allopurinol
- Colchicine
- Probenecid
- Sulfinpyrazone

MISCELLANEOUS ANALGESICS

- Mefenamic acid

COMBINATION ANALGESICS CONTAINING SALICYLATES

- Alka-Seltzer Effervescent
- Anacin
- APC
- Arthritis Pain Formula
- Arthrogesic
- Ascripten
- Bufferin
- Cama Inlay-Tabs

Excedrin
Goodys Headache Powders
Hyalex
Midol
Norgesic
Os-Cal-Gesic
Pabalate
Pabalate-SF
Percodan
Quiet World
Synalgos
Trilisate
Vanquish

TOPICAL SALICYLATE PREPARATIONS

Acnaveen Bar
Acne-Dome
Banalg Liniment
Compound W
Dry and Clear
Duofilm
Exzit
Fostex Medicated Cleansing Bar
Freezone
Ger-O-Foam
Klaron
Komed
Oxipor VHC
P&S Shampoo
Panalgesic
Panscol
Pernox
Pragmatar Ointment
Sebucare
Sebulex Shampoo
Sebutone Shampoo
Stri-Dex
Tinver

COMBINATION ANALGESICS CONTAINING ACETAMINOPHEN

Arthralgen
Bancap
Blanex
Capital
Cetased
Codalan
Darvocet-N
Demerol APAP
Duradyne DHC
Empracet
Esgic
Excedrin
Gaysal-S
Gemnisyn
Maxigesic
Medigesic Plus
Midrin
Migralam
Norcet
Parafon Forte
Percocet-5
Percogesic
Phenaphen with Codeine
Phrenilin
Saroflex
Sedapap-10
Sunril
Supac
Tylenol with Codeine
Tylox
Vanquish
Vicodin
Wygesic

COMBINATION ANALGESICS CONTAINING PHENACETIN

Darvon Compound-65
Fiorinal
Soma Compound

COMBINATION ANALGESICS CONTAINING ERGOT DERIVATIVES

Cafergot
Migral
Wigraine

COMBINATION PREPARATIONS CONTAINING PROBENECID

ColBENEMID, Col-Probenecid, Probenecid with Colchicine
Polycillin-PRB
Principen with Probenecid
Wycillin and Probenecid

CHARACTERISTICS OF NONNARCOTIC ANALGESICS

The nonnarcotic analgesics are among the most widely used drugs in the world today. Many of these agents also possess antipyretic activity and are invaluable for reducing fever in situations where body temperature elevations are likely to cause convulsions—for example, in infants. Those with antiinflammatory activity are important adjuncts in the treatment of rheumatoid arthritis, and still others find their place in controlling gout. The advantage of these drugs in controlling mild to moderate pain lies in the fact that they do not lead to the central nervous system effects common to narcotics; namely, respiratory depression and physical dependence. The nonnarcotic analgesics are most effective in relieving musculoskeletal pain and are of little use in managing deep visceral pain.

Because these drugs are so readily available, and are contained in so many commercial OTC preparations, it is not surprising that accidental ingestion and/or overdose occurs frequently. Aspirin is the leading cause of drug poisoning in children, and long-term use by adults can result in a variety of serious untoward effects. Therefore, long-term use of any of the nonnarcotic analgesics mandates medical supervision with careful monitoring of clinical response, including periodic laboratory tests to detect early signs of significant untoward reactions.

The nursing management of clients in need of analgesia should be directed at helping to relieve pain by other supportive measures, whenever possible. Steps that make the client comfortable—for example, positioning—are often helpful in reducing the frequency at which a prn analgesic must be administered for pain control. On the other hand, personal and cultural factors are closely related to individual pain experiences, and often the client who is most in need of analgesic medication is the least likely to request it. Therefore, the nurse should not administer analgesics haphazardly, but use interviewing and observational skills in carefully assessing the need for, and the effect of, the prescribed medication.

Salicylates Salicylic acid was one of the first chemotherapeutic agents to be isolated from its natural source, which is the bark of the willow tree. Most salicylates are now manufactured synthetically from phenol. All salicylates have antiinflammatory properties; however, the different salicylate salts vary in solubility and extent of local or systemic tissue irritation. The most widely used salicylate is aspirin, which is found in a great number of nonprescription drugs. Aspirin should not, however, be used indiscriminately or for long periods without medical supervision, since adverse effects can be severe and dangerous.

Phenol derivatives The two drugs in this category are acetaminophen and phenacetin. Phenacetin is used only in combination with other drugs, particularly aspirin and caffeine. Because it has been implicated as a cause of blood dyscrasias and renal damage, it is no longer included in most OTC analgesic preparations. Acetaminophen, on the other hand, is a widely used substitute for aspirin and has a lower incidence of toxicity and hypersensitivity reactions. Acetaminophen is almost identical to aspirin in analgesic and antipyretic activity, but does not have any antiinflammatory properties. Other advantages of acetaminophen over aspirin include the following: it does not cause gastrointestinal irritation, does not interfere with platelet production or bleeding time, and does not interact with anticoagulants or most other drugs.

Pyrazolones There are three drugs in this group: phenylbutazone, oxyphenbutazone, which is a metabolite of phenylbutazone, and sulfinpyrazone, which is used as a uricosuric agent in gout therapy. Phenylbutazone and oxyphenbutazone are extremely potent antiinflammatory drugs, but are also very toxic and are used only when other drugs are ineffective.

Ergot derivatives These drugs do not share the analgesic properties of the other drugs discussed in this chapter, but are included because they are used primarily for the relief of headache of vascular origin (migraine). Prolonged use is not recommended because of potential serious untoward reactions.

Antirheumatics The search for antiinflammatory drugs with less potential for causing adverse effects than the salicylates or pyrazolones has led to the development of a number of new drugs. Of these, indomethacin is the prototype and is also the most toxic of the group. In addition to these newer drugs, gold and penicillamine are still used for clients who do not respond to other antirheumatic drug therapy.

Antigout agents The symptoms of acute gout appear when excess uric acid is deposited in the skin, joints, and other tissues. The disorder is treated with antiinflammatory agents and with uricosuric agents, which either interfere with uric acid synthesis in the body or promote urinary excretion of uric acid by blocking its reabsorption in the kidneys. Many of the antiinflammatory agents (salicylates, antirheumatics) used for gout are described early in this chapter; the exception is colchicine whose use is confined to the treatment of gout. The uricosuric agents include probenecid, sulfinpyrazone, and allopurinol.

SALICYLATES

GENERIC NAME Aspirin, Acetylsalicylic acid

TRADE NAMES A.S.A., Aspergum, Decaprin, Ecotrin

CLASSIFICATION Analgesic, antipyretic, antirheumatic

OTC

ACTION The exact mechanism is not known, although the latest clinical evidence suggests that prostaglandin synthesis is blocked, thereby raising the pain threshold. Reabsorption of fluid from swollen tissues and joints is also increased. Furthermore, there may be some interference with the transmission of pain impulses at the thalamic level. Fever is reduced by a reduction in vasoconstrictor impulses from the hypothalamus, thereby promoting vasodilatation and sweating. The antiinflammatory action is a result of decreased capillary permeability and inhibition of the synthesis of prostaglandin E. Other actions include reduction of prothrombin levels, inhibition of platelet aggregation, and mild respiratory stimulation. In low doses, urate excretion is decreased, but in large doses there is an increased excretion of uric acid. It is also hypocholesterolemic and hypoglycemic in large doses.

Indications for Use Mild to moderate musculoskeletal pain, headache, dysmenorrhea, reduction of elevated body temperature. In large doses, for controlling pain from inflammatory conditions, such as rheumatoid arthritis, osteoarthritis, and bursitis. Also used for symptomatic treatment of uncomplicated rheumatic fever. Most recently, salicylates have been used to prevent thromboembolism in high-risk clients; research indicates that benefits are greater for men than for women.

Contraindications Hypersensitivity; any history of GI disorders, such as ulcer, hemorrhage, gastritis, and diverticulosis; vitamin K deficiency; severe anemia; infants under 1 year. Use with caution in diseases of the ear, asthma, nasal polyps, allergies, glucose-6-phosphate dehydrogenase deficiency, Hodgkin's disease, acute carditis, clients undergoing surgery, and in children who are dehydrated from fever.

Untoward Reactions The most common side effects are heartburn, GI distress, and nausea. Hypersensitivity reactions are characterized by vasomotor rhinitis, urticaria, asthma, and nasal polyps. More significant reactions are usually dose related and are classified into mild intoxication, or salicylism, and severe intoxication. Mild intoxication: mental confusion, nausea, vomiting, tinnitus, dizziness, sweating, palpitations, diarrhea, hyperventilation, impaired vision, fever, thirst, drowsiness. Other symptoms may include anorexia, prolonged bleeding time, anemia, decreased protein-bound iodine and prothrombin time, and elevated serum amylase, serum glutamic-oxaloacetic transaminase, serum glutamic-pyruvic transaminase, and carbon dioxide. Severe intoxication: CNS stimulation characterized by delirium and hallucinations, respiratory alkalosis, metabolic acidosis, petechiae, hyponatremia, hypokalemia, renal impairment, pancreatitis , hepatotoxicity, and eventually coma and death.

Parameters of Use

Absorption Rapidly absorbed from stomach and upper GI tract. The rate of absorption depends on the particular preparation, the pH of stomach and bowel, and the stomach emptying time. Detectable in the plasma within 30 minutes after oral administration. Peak action occurs in 1 to 2 hours and duration of action is 4 to 6 hours.

Crosses the placenta and appears in breast milk.

Distribution Widely distributed to most body tissues and crosses the blood-brain barrier.

Metabolism Rapidly hydrolyzed to salicyclic acid primarily in the liver.

Excretion At low doses, 50% is excreted in the urine within 4 hours; at high doses, excretion is much slower. Alkalization of the urine increases the rate of excretion by decreasing reabsorption in the renal tubules. In clients with renal and/or hepatic dysfunction, action is prolonged.

Drug Interactions Action prolonged by urinary acidifiers and P-aminobenzoic acid. By competing for protein-binding sites, large doses of salicylates may enhance the effects of oral anticoagulants, heparin, oral antidiabetics, phenytoin, sulfonamides, penicillin, methotrexate, and indomethacin. Salicylates in small doses inhibit the uricosuric effects of probenecid and sulfinpyrazone. The risk of GI bleeding is increased by concurrent use of alcohol, corticosteroids, indomethacin, and the pyrazolones.

Laboratory Interactions May interfere with urinary 5-hydroxyindoleacetic acid, vanilmandelic acid, ketones, and phenolsulfonphthalein excretion. With large doses, urine glucose determinations by Clinistix and Tes-Tape may give false-negative readings, while Clinitest may give a false-positive reading.

Administration Adults: 325 to 650 mg po or rectally q4h; Children: 65 mg/kg/day po or rectally in divided doses every 6 hours. Antiinflammatory: 2.6 to 7.8 g po or rectally daily.

Available Drug Forms Tablets containing 5 gr (324 mg); timed-release tablets containing 10 gr (650 mg); chewing gum tablets containing $3\frac{1}{2}$ gr (260 mg); suppositories containing 2, 5, or 10 gr. Store in airtight containers.

Nursing Management

Planning factors

1. If tablets are exposed to air, moisture, or heat, they rapidly hydrolyze, and should be discarded if they have a strong acetic odor.
2. All salicylates should be kept out of the reach of children.

Administration factors

1. For clients with a history of allergy, antihistamines and epinephrine should be available.
2. The buffered effervescent peparations are absorbed more rapidly and are less irritating to the GI tract; however, constant use can alkalinize the urine. These preparations are contraindicated in cardiac clients because of their high sodium content.
3. APC tablets (aspirin, phenacetin, caffeine), although popular, should be avoided since the combination is no more effective than aspirin and is responsible for a higher incidence of renal damage.
4. Although the various brands may differ in the binding agents used, they are equally effective in their action.
5. Oral forms should be administered with food, milk, or antacids to reduce GI irritation.
6. For antiinflammatory response, a consistent dosage schedule is important in maintaining therapeutic serum drug levels.
7. Enteric-coated drug forms are indicated for clients who experience GI upset even when taking the drug with food or milk.
8. Tablets may harden with age, and disintegration time will be increased.

Evaluation factors

1. For clients on long-term or high-dose therapy, careful monitoring of prothrombin and hemoglobin is necessary.
2. Hypersensitivity reactions are possible even in clients who have taken salicylates without difficulty in the past.
3. Salicylate intoxication should be treated promptly by the following means: prompt emesis, or gastric lavage; administration of supplementary fluids and electrolytes (IV, if necessary); oxygen administration and artificial respiration, if necessary; and renal dialysis in cases of severe intoxication.

Client teaching factors

1. Instruct clients who are hypersensitive to salicylates to carefully read the labels on all OTC preparations, since many contain salicylates.
2. Caution client that long-term self-medication with salicylates is dangerous and may mask serious underlying diseases.
3. Inform clients taking large doses that urine may be green-brown in color. This is a harmless side effect.

GENERIC NAME Calcium carbaspirin (RX)

TRADE NAME Calurin

CLASSIFICATION Analgesic, antipyretic

See aspirin for Action, Indications for use, Contraindications, Untoward reactions, Parameters of use, and Drug interactions.

Administration Adults: 300 to 600 mg po q4h; children: 150 to 300 mg po q4h.

Available Drug Forms Tablets containing 300 mg.

Nursing Management May be more soluble than aspirin, therefore less irritating to the gastric mucosa. (See aspirin.)

GENERIC NAME Choline salicylate (OTC)

TRADE NAME Arthropan

CLASSIFICATION Analgesic, antipyretic

See aspirin for Action, Indications for use, Contraindications, Untoward reactions, Parameters of use, Drug interactions, and Nursing management.

Administration Adults and children over 12 years: 870 mg po every 3 to 4 hours; Maximum dosage: 5220 mg in 24 hours.

Available Drug Forms Oral liquid (mint-flavored) containing 10 gr/tsp.

GENERIC NAME Magnesium salicylate (RX)

TRADE NAMES Arthrin, Magan, Mobidin, Triact

CLASSIFICATION Analgesic, antipyretic

See aspirin for Action, Indications for use, Contraindications, Untoward reactions, Parameters of use, Drug interactions, and Nursing management.

Administration Adults and children over 12 years: 600 to 650 mg po q4h. For rheumatic fever, as much as 16 tablets (9.6 g) a day may be prescribed to relieve joint pains.

Available Drug Forms Tablets containing 600 or 650 mg.

GENERIC NAME Methyl salicylate (OTC)

TRADE NAME Oil of Wintergreen

CLASSIFICATION Topical analgesic

See aspirin for Contraindications, Untoward reactions, Parameters of use, and Drug interactions.

Action A counterirritant.

Indications for Use Relief of muscular and rheumatic pain.

Administration Apply to affected areas daily or bid.

Available Drug Forms Liniment and ointment 10 to 50%.

Nursing Management (See aspirin.)

Administration factors

1. Should not be used on irritated skin.
2. Systemic absorption occurs if large areas are treated.

Client teaching factors Highly toxic if ingested. Preparations over 10% strength must be stored in child-proof containers.

GENERIC NAME Salicylamide (OTC)

TRADE NAME Salrin, Uromide

CLASSIFICATION Analgesic, antipyretic

See aspirin for Indications for use, Contraindications, Untoward reactions, Parameters of use, and Drug interactions.

Action Similar actions to aspirin, but shorter duration of action and much less toxic.

Administration Adults: 325 to 650 mg po q4h; Children: 65 mg/kg po in a 24-hour period.

Available Drug Forms Tablets containing 325 or 650 mg.

Nursing Management May cause drowsiness, caution client against driving or operating machinery. (See aspirin.)

GENERIC NAME Salicylic acid (OTC)

TRADE NAMES Derma-Soft, Fomac, Keralyt, NP-27, Saligel, Wart-Off

CLASSIFICATION Topical analgesic

See aspirin for Contraindications, Untoward reactions, Parameters of use, Drug interactions.

Action Aids in removing skin scales. Has weak bacteriostatic and fungistatic action.

Indications for Use Psoriasis, acne, and other conditions requiring removal of dead skin.

Administration Apply to affected areas daily or bid.

Available Drug Forms Cream 5 or 10%; ointment 25 or 60%; gel 5 or 6%; soap 3.5%; collodion preparations for corns, warts, and calluses; powder.

Nursing Management (See aspirin.)

Administration factors

1. Before applying, hydrate skin for 5 minutes with wet soaks. This enhances effect of medication.
2. Avoid contact with eyes and mucous membranes, since drug will cause irritation to normal skin surfaces.
3. Systemic absorption occurs if large areas are treated.

Client teaching factors Should not be used for clients with diabetes or peripheral vascular disease.

GENERIC NAME Sodium salicylate (RX)

TRADE NAME Uracel

CLASSIFICATION Analgesic, antipyretic

See aspirin for Action, Indications for use, Contraindications, Untoward reactions, Parameters of use, and Drug interactions.

Administration 325 to 640 mg po or IV q4h.

Available Drug Forms Tablets containing 325 or 650 mg; enteric-coated tablets containing 325 or 650 mg; solution for injection containing 1 or 1.5 mg/10 ml.

Nursing Management (See aspirin.)

1. Liberates free salicylic acid, so is irritating to the gastric mucosa.
2. Not used for clients on low-sodium diets.
3. When given IV, avoid extravasation, since drug can cause tissue necrosis.

GENERIC NAME Sodium thiosalicylate (RX)

TRADE NAMES Asproject, Thiodyne

CLASSIFICATION Analgesic, antipyretic

See aspirin for Action, Indications for use, Contraindications, Untoward reactions, Parameters of use, and Drug interactions.

Administration

- *Rheumatic fever:* 100 to 150 mg IM every 4 to 6 hours for 3 days; then 100 mg bid.
- *Acute gout:* 100 mg IM every 3 to 4 hours for 2 days; then 100 mg daily.

Available Drug Forms Solution for injection containing 50 mg/ml.

Nursing Management Observe injection site for irritation, since tissue necrosis may occur. (See aspirin.)

PHENOL DERIVATIVES

GENERIC NAME Acetaminophen (OTC)

TRADE NAMES Anuphen, APAP, Dapa, Datril, Liquiprin, Phenaphen, Proval, Tempra, Tylenol, Valadol

CLASSIFICATION Analgesic, antipyretic

Action Interferes with the transmission of pain impulses at the thalamic level, raising the pain threshold, and reduces impulses from the hypothalamic temperature-regulating center, as do the salicylates. The major difference between acetaminophen and salicylates is that the former does not inhibit prostaglandin synthesis, and so has no antiinflammatory action.

Indications for Use Mild to moderate pain, reduction of elevated body temperature associated with viral or bacterial infections.

Contraindications Hypersensitivity; glucose-6-phosphate dehydrogenase deficiency; repeated administration to clients with anemia or cardiac, pulmonary, renal, or hepatic disease.

Untoward Reactions None from intermittent low dosages. Prolonged administration can cause methemoglobinemia, which is a serious complication in infants. Hypersensitivity reactions are rare and are usually confined to the skin, but may include angioneurotic edema and fever. Long-term use may cause the following adverse reactions: blood dyscrasias, GI disturbances, psychologic changes, bleeding, renal and hepatic damage, hypoglycemia, cerebral edema, hemolytic anemia, methemoglobinemia. Acute toxicity is characterized by the following: abdominal pain; nausea; vomiting; methemoglobinemia; sulfhemoglobinemia; dizziness; sweating; palpitations; CNS stimulation characterized by excitement, delirium and convulsions and followed by CNS depression characterized by hypothermia, shock, and coma. Hepatic injury may occur if the toxic dose results in a plasma half-life of 4 hours or more, but the extent of hepatic damage may not be apparent for several days. Prompt supportive treatment is essential for acute toxicity to prevent permanent hepatic and renal damage. Treatment is similar to that for salicylism, including gastric lavage and hemodialysis.

Parameters of Use

Absorption Readily absorbed from GI tract. Onset of action occurs within 15 to 30 minutes. Duration of action is 3 to 5 hours. About 25 to 50% bound to plasma proteins. Plasma half-life is 1 to 3 hours.

Distribution Distributed to most body tissues, including cerebrospinal fluid.

Metabolism In the liver.

Excretion Primarily in urine within 24 hours.

Drug Interactions Slightly enhances the effects of oral anticoagulants, but only in large doses. Concurrent administration of phenothiazine and/or other antipyretic drugs may cause severe hypothermia.

Laboratory Interactions May cause false increases in urine 5-hydroxyindoleacetic acid determinations. May produce false-positive results for urine glucose determinations with Benedict's solution or Clinitest.

Administration Adults: 325 to 650 mg po or rectally qid; total dosage not to exceed 2.6 g. Children: Ages 7 to 12 years: 162.5 to 325 mg po or rectally qid; total dosage not to exceed 1.3 g. Ages 3 to 6 years: 120 mg qid; total dosage not to exceed 480 mg.

Available Drug Forms Tablets containing 325 or 500 mg; liquid containing 1 g/30 ml; suspension containing 120 mg/2.5 ml; suppositories containing 120 or 650 mg; drops containing 60 mg/0.6 ml; syrup containing 120 mg/5 ml; chewable tablets containing 80 mg. All preparations should be stored in light-resistant containers.

Nursing Management

Planning factors Only for temporary use; unlike salicylates which are often prescribed for long-term use in rheumatic diseases.

Administration factors

1. If client has ingested a toxic dose, hospitalization is necessary, since hepatic damage may not be evident for 2 to 4 days. Hepatic damage may be prevented by administration of acetylcysteine, which prevents the oxidation of acetaminophen to its toxic metabolites and may combine with the metabolites. This treatment is indicated for clients who have ingested 10 g or more of acetaminophen.
2. Should not be used for children under 6 years without medical supervision.

Evaluation factors Careful observation and evaluation of history by the nurse are important in assessing possible abuse.

Client teaching factors

1. Client should be cautioned not to exceed recommended dosage or duration of administration.

2. Acetaminophen is an ingredient of many OTC preparations, and the danger of indiscriminate use or accidental poisoning is as great as for the salicylates.

PYRAZOLONES

GENERIC NAMES Phenylbutazone; oxyphenbutazone

TRADE NAMES Azolid, Butazolidin, Oxalid, Tandearil

CLASSIFICATION Antiinflammatory (RX)

Action Not determined, but action is similar to that of the salicylates. Inhibits prostaglandin synthesis, leucocyte migration, and lysosomal enzyme activity. Antiinflammatory and antipyretic activity is strong; uricosuric activity is weak. Causes sodium and water retention.

Indications for Use Short-term treatment of pain associated with active rheumatoid arthritis, spondylitis, osteoarthritis, and other acute joint conditions; symptomatic treatment of acute superficial thrombophlebitis. Treatment with these drugs is generally limited to 1 or 2 weeks.

Contraindications Any GI disease, including peptic ulcer; blood dyscrasias; hypertension; renal, hepatic, or cardiac disease; thyroid disease; temporal arteritis; polymyalgia rheumatica; clients with drug allergies and those on anticoagulants or potent chemotherapeutic agents; children under 14 years. Use with caution in clients with glaucoma and those over 40 years.

Untoward Reactions Common reactions are nausea, vomiting, GI distress, rash, diarrhea, vertigo, insomnia, nervousness, blurred vision, sodium and water retention. May also cause GI ulceration with bleeding, abdominal distention, hematemesis, renal dysfunction including stones and obstruction, metabolic acidosis, hyperglycemia, toxic goiter, thyroid hyperplasia, hypertension, pericarditis, myocarditis, cardiac decompensation, and visual and otic pathology. Allergic reactions include petechiae, pruritus, erythema, serum sickness, polyarteritis, arthralgia, fever, anaphylactic shock, and Stevens-Johnson syndrome. Any sign of allergic response calls for immediate discontinuation of drug. CNS symptoms are generally seen only in drug overdoses and include agitation, confusion, lethargy, depression, hallucinations, convulsions, psychosis, and hyperventilation.

Parameters of Use

Absorption Readily and completely absorbed from GI tract. Onset of action is 30 to 60 minutes. Peak action occurs in 2 hours and duration of action is 3 to 5 days. Drugs are highly bound to plasma albumin (90 to 98%). Half-life is 2½ to 4 days.

Crosses placenta and appears in breast milk.

Metabolism In the liver.

Excretion Slowly in urine.

Drug Interactions May potentiate the effects of any other protein-bound drugs, including oral anticoagulants, sulfonamides, phenytoin, oral hypoglycemics, salicylates, and indomethacin. Decreases effect of digitalis by enhancing its metabolism. Tricyclic antidepressants and cholestyramine inhibit the absorption of pyrazolones, thereby decreasing their effects. Androgens may increase the effects of pyrazolones.

Administration 200 to 400 mg po daily in 3 to 4 divided doses; maintenance dosage should not exceed 400 mg/day.

Available Drug Forms Tablets or capsules containing 100 mg.

Nursing Management

Planning factors

1. Complete history and baseline laboratory tests should be done before and during drug therapy.
2. These drugs should never be used as first-line treatment of inflammatory diseases. They are indicated only if salicylates or other antirheumatic agents are ineffective or contraindicated.

Evaluation factors

1. Any significant changes in white blood cell count call for discontinuation of drug.
2. Blood counts should be taken for several weeks after cessation of therapy, since abnormalities may not appear until after treatment has been discontinued.
3. If no clinical response occurs after 1 week, drug should be discontinued. If drug is effective in reducing symptoms, dosage should then be lowered to the minimum effective level.

Client teaching factors

1. Teach client the early signs of blood dyscrasias, such as fever, sore throat, and stomatitis, as well as other adverse reactions, such as edema, tarry stools, and dermatitis. Drug should be discontinued if any of these symptoms appear.
2. Instruct client to maintain prescribed dosage only.
3. Client should restrict sodium intake while on drug therapy. Warn client that compensatory diuresis may occur when drug is discontinued because of sodium retention during drug therapy.

ERGOT DERIVATIVES

GENERIC NAMES Ergotamine tartrate; dihydroergotamine mesylate

TRADE NAMES Ergomar, Ergostat, Gynergen, Medihaler Ergotamine; Circanol, D.H.E. 45

CLASSIFICATION Analgesic (RX)

Action Constricts smooth muscle of the cerebral arteries and depresses central vasomotor centers. The oxytocic effect is evident only with large doses. Continued use leads to damage of vascular endothelium, resulting in thrombosis and gangrene.

Indications for Use Relief of pain from headache of vascular origin. Most effective if used in the early stages of the headache; often used in combination with caffeine.

Contraindications Peripheral vascular diseases, renal or hepatic disease, hypertension, severe pruritus, coronary artery disease, anemia, infection, malnutrition, pregnancy, children. Use with caution in lactation and elderly clients.

Untoward Reactions Numbness and tingling in extremities, muscle weakness, diarrhea, bradycardia. Symptoms of ergotism, which include intermittent claudication, Raynaud's phenomenon, paresthesias, vomiting, diarrhea, and confusion, are less common.

Parameters of Use

Absorption Erratically absorbed from GI tract; therefore, oral doses are often 10 times greater than parenteral doses. Onset of action is 20 to 30 minutes following IM or subc injection. Duration of action may be as long as 24 hours.

Metabolism In the liver.

Excretion Unknown.

Drug Interactions Beta blockers (propanolol and vasopressor drugs potentiate the vasoconstriction.

Administration *Ergotamine:* Sublingual: 2 to 6 mg per attack; Maximum dosage: 10 mg weekly. Intramuscular, subcutaneous: 0.25 to 0.5 mg; may be repeated once. Inhalation: 0.36 mg; repeat every 5 minutes, as needed; Maximum dosage: 6 doses/day. *Dihydroergotamine:* 1 mg q1h IM or IV; total dosage not to exceed 3 mg.

Available Drug Forms *Ergotamine:* tablets containing 0.5, 1, or 2 mg; ampules of 0.5 and 1 ml containing 0.25 and 0.5 mg, respectively; inhaler containing 0.36 mg per inhalation. *Dihydroergotamine:* Ampules of 1 ml containing 1 mg; do not use if discolored.

Nursing Management

Planning factors

1. Drug treatment should be accompanied by other measures, such as rest in a quiet, dark room and avoidance of other stresses.
2. Pregnant women should not take ergot preparations because of oxytocic effects.

Administration factors

1. If an oral dose of more than 8 mg is needed for pain relief, subc injection is advisable.
2. If drug is given early in a migraine attack, sublingual administration is preferred, since it is absorbed more rapidly.
3. IM injection is sometimes used to confirm the diagnosis of vascular headache; client will have pain relief within 15 to 30 minutes.
4. If ergot drugs are administered during the prodromal symptoms of migraine headache, pain relief will be more rapid and more effective.
5. IM administration of ergotamine can cause precordial pain within 5 to 10 minutes; sublingual nitroglycerin is effective in relieving this pain.

Client teaching factors

1. Caution client to avoid long-term use of ergot drugs, since dangerous untoward effects are much more common with prolonged use or excessively high doses.
2. Instruct client to report promptly any of the signs of vascular insufficiency, which call for discontinuation of drug.

ANTIRHEUMATICS

GENERIC NAME Indomethacin (RX)

TRADE NAME Indocin

CLASSIFICATION Antiinflammatory, analgesic

Action Similar to aspirin; probably blocks prostaglandin synthesis. Decreases vascular permeability and movement of leukocytes in injured tissue. Has no uricosuric action.

Indications for Use Palliation in moderate to severe rheumatoid arthritis, ankylosing spondylitis, acute gouty arthritis, and osteoarthritis of hip or shoulder. Only for clients unable to tolerate other drug therapy.

Contraindications Hypersensitivity to aspirin, pregnancy, lactation, children under 14 years, GI diseases, nasal polyps with angioedema. Use with caution in renal or hepatic disease, infections, psychiatric illness, epilepsy, parkinsonism, and elderly clients.

Untoward Reactions Common reactions are headache, dizziness, nausea, dyspepsia, epigastric pain, heartburn, and diarrhea. Other reactions: GI ulceration and perforation, gastroenteritis, rectal bleeding; CNS symptoms, such as confusion, syncope, involuntary movements, peripheral neuropathy, psychic disturbances, depression; blood dyscrasias, hypertension, tachycardia, precordial pain, visual and hearing disturbances, hematuria, vaginal bleeding, hepatitis, edema. Hypersensitivity reactions include dermatologic symptoms, angioedema, hypotension, dyspnea, and asthma syndrome in aspirin-sensitive clients.

Parameters of Use

Absorption Readily absorbed from GI tract. Onset of action is 1 to 2 hours. Peak action occurs in 3 hours and duration of action is 4 to 6 hours. About 90% bound to plasma proteins.

Crosses placenta and appears in breast milk.

Distribution Widely distributed to all body tissues, with lower concentrations in cerebrospinal fluid.

Metabolism In the liver and kidneys.

Excretion In urine, with some in bile and feces.

Drug Interactions Corticosteroids, phenylbutazone, and salicylates increase the risk of GI bleeding. Aspirin in large doses delays absorption of indomethacin. Probenecid increases serum levels of indomethacin, increasing the risk of toxicity. Indomethacin may interfere with the action of furosemide and may impair excretion of lithium, increasing the risk of lithium toxicity. Indomethacin may alter dosage requirements of oral anticoagulants by elevating anticoagulant serum levels and/or causing GI bleeding.

Laboratory Interactions Increases blood urea nitrogen, serum glutamic-oxaloacetic transaminase, serum glutamic-pyruvic transaminase, alkaline phosphatase, cephalin flocculation, thymol turbidity, and serum amylase.

Administration

- *Rheumatoid arthritis:* 25 mg po bid or tid; may be increased by 25 mg at weekly intervals; total dosage not to exceed 200 mg/day.
- *Acute gout:* 50 mg po tid; decrease dose rapidly after pain is tolerable; therapy should not be given for more than 5 days.

Available Drug Forms Capsules containing 25 or 50 mg. Store in airtight, light-resistant containers.

Nursing Management

Planning factors Obtain a history of all drug use; do not administer to clients with aspirin sensitivity.

Administration factors

1. Give with meals or antacid to minimize GI distress.
2. For clients with night pain and morning stiffness, the largest portion of the daily dose should be taken at bedtime. This may also alleviate morning headache, which is the most common CNS side effect.

Evaluation factors

1. Blood counts, renal and hepatic function tests, ophthalmoscopic examinations, and hearing tests should be done at regular intervals.
2. If the symptoms of rheumatoid arthritis do not improve within 3 weeks, drug should be discontinued.
3. Assess client carefully for any signs of infection, which may be masked by drug.

Client teaching factors

1. Instruct client thoroughly in all signs and symptoms of untoward effects, so they can be promptly reported. The serious effects are often dose related, so it is important to establish the lowest possible effective dosage.
2. Advise client to avoid any hazardous activities, since drug may cause dizziness.

GENERIC NAME Aurothioglucose (RX)

TRADE NAMES Gold Thioglucose, Solganal

CLASSIFICATION Antirheumatic

Action Mechanism is unknown. Reduces inflammatory process in early arthritic disease.

Indications for Use Early, active rheumatoid arthritis, nondisseminated lupus erythematosus, pemphigus.

Contraindications Severe diabetes, renal and hepatic disease, hypertension, cardiac disease, systemic lupus erythematosus, blood dyscrasias, eczema, colitis, tuberculosis, recent radiation therapy, pregnancy, elderly clients.

Untoward Reactions Common reactions are dermatitis, erythema, pruritus, stomatitis, metallic taste, flushing, dizziness, and sweating. Less common reactions are pharyngitis, gastritis, colitis, vaginitis, inflammation due to upper respiratory infection, blood dyscrasias, renal dysfunction, hepatitis, peripheral neuritis, and EEG abnormalities. Dermatologic reactions and Stevens-Johnson syndrome are also possible.

Parameters of Use

Absorption Slowly absorbed from injection site. Peak action occurs in 4 to 6 hours. Half-life is 3 to 7 days, so cumulative effects are possible.

Distribution Widely distributed to all body tissues, especially liver, spleen, kidneys, and skin.

Excretion Slowly in urine, with lesser amounts in feces.

Drug Interactions Pyrazolones, antimalarial drugs, and immunosuppressants increase the risk of blood dyscrasias. Corticosteroids reduce effectiveness and increase the potential for toxicity from gold.

Administration Adults: 10 to 25 mg IM weekly for 3 weeks; then 50 mg weekly until the total dosage is 0.8 to 1 g; Maintenance dosage: 25 to 50 mg IM every 3 to 4 weeks. Children: Ages 6 to 12 years: ¼ of adult dosage.

Available Drug Forms Vials of 10 ml containing 50 mg/ml. Shake well to suspend active material. Do not use if darker than a pale yellow. Vial should be warmed to body temperature to facilitate withdrawal of medication.

Nursing Management

Planning factors The antidote for aurothioglucose is dimercaprol, which should be available in the event of overdose.

Administration factors

1. Inject deep into gluteal muscle using an 18-gauge 1½- or 2-inch needle.
2. Urinalysis should be done prior to each dose to detect early signs of nephrotoxicity.
3. Client should be assessed prior to each dose to detect early signs of toxicity.

Evaluation factors

1. Pruritus is an early sign of toxicity. If accompanied by rash, treatment may be discontinued.
2. Skin and mucous membranes may develop a grayish blue pigmentation.
3. Blood counts should be done every 2 weeks; if platelet count is below 100,000/cu ml or leukopenia occurs, drug should be discontinued.
4. Clinical response may not be evident for several months, but once symptoms ameliorate, the improvement may last for a year or longer. Treatment regime may be repeated in a year.

Client teaching factors

1. Instruct client to remain recumbent for 20 minutes after administration because of possible dizziness.
2. Caution client to avoid exposure to sunlight, which exacerbates dermatologic symptoms.
3. Instruct client in scrupulous oral hygiene to relieve painful stomatitis.

GENERIC NAME Fenoprofen (RX)

TRADE NAME Nalfon

CLASSIFICATION Antirheumatic

See indomethacin for Untoward reactions, Parameters of use, and Drug interactions.

Action Antiinflammatory action is similar to that of indomethacin or the salicylates, but is less toxic. Causes less GI distress. (See indomethacin.)

Indications for Use Not used for simple analgesia or antipyresis. Sometimes prescribed for moderate pain from dysmenorrhea, dental surgery, and athletic injury. No advantages over salicylates, except for clients who cannot tolerate continual high doses of salicylates.

Contraindications Should not be used concurrently with salicylates. (See indomethacin.)

Administration 300 to 600 mg po qid.

Available Drug Forms Tablets containing 600 mg; capsules containing 200 or 300 mg.

Nursing Management (See indomethacin.)

1. Administer between meals if no GI distress; otherwise, give with milk or antacids.
2. Drowsiness is common.
3. Periodic hepatic function tests are recommended.

GENERIC NAME Ibuprofen (RX)

TRADE NAME Motrin, Advil, Nuprin

CLASSIFICATION Antirheumatic

See indomethacin for Action, Indications for Use, Contraindications, Untoward reactions, Parameters of use, and Drug interactions.

Administration 200 to 600 mg po qid.

Available Drug Forms Tablets containing 200, 300, 400, or 600 mg.

Nursing Management (See indomethacin.)

1. GI upset is the most common side effect; but drug is usually well tolerated.
2. If blurred vision occurs, drug should be discontinued.
3. 200 mg tablets are now available OTC.

GENERIC NAME Meclofenamate (RX)

TRADE NAME Meclomen

CLASSIFICATION Antirheumatic

See indomethacin for Action, Indications for use, contraindications, Untoward reactions, Parameters of use, and Drug interactions.

Administration 200 to 400 mg po daily in 3 to 4 divided doses.

Available Drug Forms Capsules containing 50 or 100 mg.

Nursing Management (See indomethacin.)

1. Should not be used for initial therapy in rheumatic disorders.
2. Hemoglobin and hematocrit tests should be done periodically.
3. Associated with a high incidence of GI disorders, including severe diarrhea.

GENERIC NAME Naproxen (RX)

TRADE NAME Naprosyn

CLASSIFICATION Antirheumatic

See indomethacin for Indications for use, Contraindications, Untoward reactions, Parameters of use, and Drug Interactions.

Action Naproxen is longer acting because of a prolonged half-life (13 hours).

Administration 250 to 375 mg po bid.

Available Drug Forms Tablets containing 250, 275, or 375 mg.

Nursing Management Maximum clinical response may take up to 1 month after initiation of therapy. (See indomethacin.)

GENERIC NAME Penicillamine (RX)

TRADE NAME Cuprimine

CLASSIFICATION Antirheumatic

Action Mechanism is unknown. Acts as a chelating agent.

Indications for Use Active, severe rheumatoid arthritis that is unresponsive to other therapies; promotion of copper excretion in Wilson's disease; promotion of cystine excretion in cystinuria.

Contraindications Kidney disease; pregnancy; young children; blood dyscrasias; concurrent use with other antiinflammatory, antimalarial, or cytotoxic drugs.

Untoward Reactions Common reactions include indigestion, loss of taste, rash, pruritus, and proteinuria. Other reactions: GI irritation, including activation of peptic ulcer; blood dyscrasias; renal and hepatic dysfunction; tinnitus; optic neuritis; thrombophlebitis; fever; polymyositis; systemic lupuslike syndrome; alveolitis and bronchiolitis; mammary hyperplasia; epidermal necrolysis. Allergic reactions are possible and include arthralgia, dermatologic reactions, lymphadenopathy, synovitis, and thyroiditis.

Parameters of Use

Absorption Readily absorbed from GI tract. Peak action occurs in 1 to 2 hours.
Excretion In urine, within 24 hours.

Administration Initial dosage: 125 to 250 mg po daily for 4 weeks; increase by 125 to 250 mg/day at 4- to 12-week intervals. Maintenance dosage: 500 to 750 mg po daily for 3 to 4 months; Maximum dosage: 1000 to 1500 mg/day.

Available Drug Forms Capsules containing 125 or 250 mg.

Nursing Management

Administration factors

1. Give on an empty stomach only.
2. When client has been in remission for 6 months, dosage may be gradually reduced at 3-month intervals.

Evaluation factors

1. Clinical response is seldom evident until 3 months after initiation of therapy; dosage should not be increased faster than recommended.
2. Blood counts, urinalysis, hemoglobin, and platelet counts should be done every 2 weeks for the first 6 months of treatment. Drug should be discontinued if significant abnormalities occur.
3. Some clients develop increased skin friability at pressure points, and bleeding and skin wrinkling may occur. These effects do not require discontinuation of drug and may disappear when the dosage is reduced.

Client teaching factors Teach client the signs and symptoms of blood dyscrasias and allergic reactions. If promptly treated with dosage reduction and/or antihistamines (for dermatologic symptoms), they will often disappear. If drug-induced fever occurs, drug must be discontinued.

GENERIC NAME Piroxicam (RX)

TRADE NAME Feldene

CLASSIFICATION Antirheumatic

See indomethacin for Indications for use, Contraindications, Untoward reactions, Parameters of use, and Drug interactions.

Action A new drug with a long half-life (50 hours).

Administration 20 mg po daily in 1 or 2 doses.

Available Drug Forms Capsules containing 10 or 20 mg.

Nursing Management (See indomethacin.)

1. GI upset is the most common side effect.
2. Not used for children.
3. Hemoglobin and hematocrit tests should be done periodically.
4. Maximum clinical response may take 8 to 12 weeks after initiation of therapy.

GENERIC NAME Sulindac (RX)

TRADE NAME Clinoril

CLASSIFICATION Antirheumatic

See indomethacin for Indications for use, Contraindications, Untoward reactions, Parameters of use, and Drug interactions.

Administration 150 to 200 mg po bid.

Available Drug Forms Tablets containing 150 or 200 mg.

Nursing Management (See indomethacin.)

1. GI upset is the most common side effect. Drug should be administered with food.
2. Monitor hepatic function tests periodically.

GENERIC NAME Tolmetin (RX)

TRADE NAME Tolectin

CLASSIFICATION Antirheumatic

See indomethacin for Action, Indications for use, Contraindications, Untoward reactions, Parameters of use, and Drug interactions.

Administration Adults: 400 mg po tid; Children: 20 mg/kg daily in 3 to 4 divided doses.

Available Drug Forms Tablets containing 200 mg; capsules containing 400 mg.

Nursing Management (See indomethacin.)

1. Not for children under 2 years.
2. Incidence of GI irritation is less than with salicylates or indomethacin. May be given with food.
3. May cause headache and retention of sodium and water.

GENERIC NAME Zomepirac (RX)

TRADE NAME Zomax

CLASSIFICATION Antirheumatic

See indomethacin for Indications for use, Contraindications, Untoward reactions, Parameters of use, Drug interactions.

Action Prolongs bleeding time. (See indomethacin.)

Administration 50 to 100 mg po every 4 to 6 hours.

Available Drug Forms Tablets containing 100 mg.

Nursing Management (See indomethacin.)

1. Not used for children or for long-term therapy.
2. GI upset is the most common side effect.

ANTIGOUT AGENTS

GENERIC NAME Allopurinol (RX)

TRADE NAME Zyloprim

CLASSIFICATION Antigout agent

Action Inhibits action of xanthine oxidase, an enzyme necessary for uric acid synthesis. Reduces both serum and urinary levels of uric acid. No analgesic, antiinflammatory, or uricosuric actions.

Indications for Use Control of hyperuricemia due to gout or advanced renal failure; recurrent uric acid stone formation; as an adjunct to chemotherapy or radiotherapy for malignancies (to prevent high uric acid plasma levels).

Contraindications Children, lactation, pregnancy. Use with caution in hepatic or renal disease.

Untoward Reactions Hypersensitivity reactions, including fever, nausea, rash, and malaise. Other reactions: severe dermatologic reactions (Stevens-Johnson syndrome), blood dyscrasias, vasculitis, necrotizing angiitis, GI distress (vomiting, diarrhea, abdominal pain), peripheral neuritis, cataract formation, hepatotoxicity, drowsiness, vertigo, precipitation of acute gouty attacks early in therapy.

Parameters of Use

Absorption About 80% absorbed from GI tract. Peak action occurs in 2 to 6 hours. Half-life is 2 to 3 hours.

Distribution Distributed to all body tissues except the brain.

Metabolism Is converted to oxypurinol, which inhibits xanthine oxidase.

Excretion Oxypurinol is excreted slowly in urine (half-life is 18 to 30 hours), so accumulation may occur with prolonged administration.

Drug Interactions May potentiate action of oral anticoagulants, oral hypoglycemics, azathioprine, and mercaptopurine. Thiazide and loop diuretics, salicylates, sulfinpyrazone, probenecid, and xanthines may reduce effects of allopurinol. Allopurinol may increase iron storage in the liver; oral iron supplements should not be administered concurrently. Ampicillin and other penicillins increase the risk of skin rash.

Administration Adults: 200 to 600 mg po daily in 2 divided doses; Maximum dosage: 800 mg/day. Children: Over 6 years: 100 mg po tid; Under 6 years: 50 mg po tid.

Available Drug Forms Tablets containing 100 or 300 mg.

Nursing Management

Planning factors

1. Baseline blood counts and hepatic and renal function tests should be done and repeated periodically during therapy.
2. Acute attacks of gout are likely to occur during the first 6 weeks of treatment; colchicine is often prescribed prophylactically.

Administration factors

1. Give with meals.
2. Transfer from a uricosuric agent to allopurinol should be gradual, with small decreases of the uricosuric drug accompanied by small increases of allopurinol.

Evaluation factors Any decrease in urinary output should be promptly reported, since drug accumulation can occur.

Client teaching factors

1. Inform client to be alert for signs of skin rash, which is an early sign of hypersensitivity and necessitates discontinuation of drug.
2. During the early weeks of treatment, drug may cause drowsiness and vertigo; caution client to avoid hazardous activities.
3. Fluid intake should be at least 2000 ml/day to prevent crystalluria.

GENERIC NAME Colchicine (RX)

CLASSIFICATION Antigout agent

Action Inhibits leukocyte migration and phagocytosis in affected joints. Lactic acid produced by phagocytosis is reduced, thereby decreasing deposition of uric acid.

Indications for Use Relief of pain and inflammation of acute gout; prophylactically for recurrent gout. Experimental uses in leukemia, adenocarcinoma, sarcoid arthritis, mycosis fungoides, and acute calcific tendinitis.

Contraindications Hypersensitivity; severe renal, hepatic, cardiac, or GI disease; subcutaneous or intramuscular use. Use with caution in elderly and debilitated clients and early evidence of renal, hepatic, cardiac, or GI disease.

Untoward Reactions Nausea, vomiting, abdominal pain, and diarrhea are fairly common reactions. Other reactions (at high doses): severe diarrhea, muscle weakness, hematuria, oliguria, vascular damage, alopecia, hepatomegaly. Long-term administration may lead to blood dyscrasias, peripheral neuritis, and aplastic anemia.

Parameters of Use

Absorption Readily absorbed from GI tract. Plasma half-life is 20 minutes.

Distribution Metabolized in the liver. Metabolites and unchanged drug are recycled into the GI tract via biliary and intestinal secretions. Deposited in most body tissues, with higher concentrations in the kidneys, liver, spleen, and intestinal tract. Drug may persist for 9 days in leukocytes after one IV dose.

Excretion Primarily in feces, with small amounts in urine.

Drug Interactions May potentiate effects of CNS depressants and sympathomimetics. Alkalizing agents enhance the effects of colchicine and acidifying agents inhibit the effects. Prolonged administration may reduce GI absorption of vitamin B_{12}.

Laboratory Interactions May interfere with urinary steroid (17-hydroxycorticosteroids) determinations.

Administration

- *Gout:* Oral: 1 to 1.2 mg initially, then 0.5 to 0.6 mg qlh until relief of pain or diarrhea. Acute attacks of gout usually require a total dosage of 4 to 8 mg. Intravenous: 1 to 2 mg initially, then 0.5 mg every 6 hours. Maximum dosage; 4 mg in 24 hours.
- *Prophylaxis:* Usual dosage: 0.5 to 0.6 mg three to four times weekly. Severe cases may require up to 1.8 mg daily.

Available Drug Forms Tablets containing 0.6 mg; ampules containing 1 mg/2 ml.

Nursing Mangement

Planning factors Baseline blood count, hemoglobin, and serum uric acid determinations should be done and repeated periodically during treatment.

Administration factors

1. Give with meals or milk.
2. Drug is most effective if administered in the early stages of a gout attack.
3. May cause local irritation at injection site.
4. Extravasation may cause tissue necrosis. A fresh needle should be used for each injection to avoid contact of skin with solution.
5. Courses of treatment should be at least 3 days apart to prevent cumulative toxicity.
6. Drug should be administered before and after surgical procedures, since an acute attack may be caused by even minor procedures.
7. Colchicine is often prescribed with uricosuric agents in the initial stages of treatment, since the large quantities of uric acid mobilized can precipitate an acute attack.

Evaluation factors

1. Intake and output should be monitored during treatment. High fluid intake is necessary to promote excretion of uric acid and to prevent crystalluria.
2. Clinical response should be evident in 8 to 12 hours; pain and swelling disappear within 24 to 72 hours.

Client teaching factors

1. During acute attack, client should avoid weight-bearing and heat to affected joints.
2. Teach client the signs and symptoms of blood dyscrasias and early toxicity; if symptoms appear, drug should be discontinued until they subside.
3. Treatment for gout should include a purine-restricted diet; high fluid intake; avoidance of beer, ale, and wine; and weight reduction if indicated.

GENERIC NAME Probenecid (RX)

TRADE NAME Benemid

CLASSIFICATION Antigout agent

Action A uricosuric with no analgesic or antiinflammatory actions. Inhibits the renal reabsorption of urates and tubular secretion of weak organic acids, including penicillins and cephalosporins.

Indications for Use Treatment of hyperuricemia associated with gout; as an adjunct to penicillin and cephalosporin therapy, to prolong plasma levels of the drugs.

Contraindications Children under 2 years, blood dyscrasias, uric acid kidney stones, acute gout attack, severe renal impairment. Use with caution in clients with peptic ulcer.

Untoward Reactions Common reactions are GI distress, rash, headache, anorexia. Other reactions: diarrhea, urinary frequency, dizziness, anemia, hepatic necrosis, nephrotic syndrome, exacerbations of acute gout. Hypersensitivity reactions range from dermatologic to anaphylactic shock. Overdosage is characterized by CNS stimulation, convulsions, and respiratory depression.

Parameters of Use

Absorption Readily absorbed from GI tract. Peak action occurs in 2 to 4 hours. About 95% bound to plasma proteins. Half-life is 8 to 10 hours.

Metabolism In the liver.

Excretion Slowly in urine; excretion is increased by alkaline urine.

Drug Interactions Prolongs action of penicillins and cephalosporins by prolonging plasma levels. May enhance action of methotrexate, oral anticoagulants, oral hypoglycemics, indomethacin, sulfinpyrazone, sulfonamides, and thiazide diuretics. Salicylates in small doses, xanthines, and diuretics antagonize uricosuric effects of probenecid.

Laboratory Interactions May decrease urinary 17-ketosteroids; may interfere with hepatic excretion of Bromsulphalein and affect results of urinary phenolsulfonphthalein excretion test. False-positive results of urinary glucose may occur with Benedict's solution or Clinitest.

Administration

- *Gout:* 250 mg po daily for 1 week, then 500 mg bid.
- *Antibiotic therapy:* Adults: 500 mg po qid; Children: 25 mg/kg po to 40 mg/kg/day in 4 divided doses.

Available Drug Forms Tablets containing 0.5 g.

Nursing Management

Administration factors

1. Give with meals or antacid to minimize GI distress.
2. Dosage may be increased every 4 weeks in 500-mg amounts, but should not exceed 2 g/day.

Evaluation factors

1. When client has been free of attacks for 6 months and uric acid levels are stabilized, daily dosage may be decreased by 500 mg every 6 months to lowest effective dosage.
2. Clients with hyperuricemia generally require lifelong probenecid therapy.

Client teaching factors

1. Warn client that acute attacks of gout may increase during the first several months of therapy.
2. Instruct client to follow prescribed dosage regimen carefully; reduction of dosage may precipitate an acute attack of gout.
3. High fluid intake is important to prevent crystalluria.
4. Clients should be cautioned against taking any OTC medications without the advice of physician.
5. Low-purine diet may be recommended. Alcohol should be avoided.

GENERIC NAME Sulfinpyrazone (RX)

TRADE NAME Anturane

CLASSIFICATION Antigout agent

See phenylbutazone for Untoward reactions. See probenecid for Nursing management.

Action A pyrazolone with uricosuric activity. (See phenylbutazone.)

Indications for Use Maintenance therapy in chronic gout.

Contraindications Hypersensitivity to pyrazolones, active peptic ulcer, concurrent administration of salicylates. (See phenylbutazone.)

Parameters of Use

Absorption Readily absorbed from GI tract. Peak action occurs in 1 to 2 hours and duration of action is 4 to 6 hours, although it may persist for 10 hours. About 98% bound to plasma proteins. Half-life is 1 to 9 hours.

Metabolism In the liver.

Excretion In urine.

Drug Interactions May potentiate effects of protein-bound drugs. Salicylates, caffeine, and theophylline may reduce uricosuric effects of sulfinpyrazone. Concurrent administration of colchicine, other pyrazolones, or indomethacin increases the risk of blood dyscrasias. (See phenylbutazone.)

Laboratory Interactions Decreases urinary excretion of aminohippuric acid and phenolsulfonphthalein.

Administration 200 to 400 mg po daily in divided doses intially; then gradually increase to a maximum dosage of 800 mg/day and continue without interruption. Acute attacks are treated with colchicine, phenylbutazone, or indomethacin.

Available Drug Forms Tablets containing 100 or 200 mg.

MISCELLANEOUS ANALGESICS

GENERIC NAME Mefenamic acid (RX)

TRADE NAME Ponstel

CLASSIFICATION Analgesic

Action Not established. Has analgesic, antipyretic, and antiinflammatory actions similar to the salicylates. Indicated only for short-term therapy because of potential for serious toxicity.

Indications For Use Short-term relief of mild to moderate pain (1 week).

Contraindications GI tract ulceration or inflammation, pregnancy, children under 14 years. Use with caution in renal or hepatic disease, blood dyscrasias, asthma, and diabetes.

Untoward Reactions Diarrhea, drowsiness, nervousness. Prolonged use causes hematologic abnormalities, including hemolytic anemia. CNS symptoms include dizziness, visual disturbances, insomnia, confusion, and headache. Can cause renal toxicity, dermatologic reactions, hepatotoxicity, dyspnea, and palpitations.

Parameters of Use

Absorption Absorbed slowly from GI tract. Peak action occurs in 2 to 4 hours and duration of action is up to 6 hours. Bound to plasma proteins.
Metabolism In the liver.
Excretion In urine and feces.

Drug Interactions May enhance effects of oral anticoagulants, salicylates, pyrazolones, corticosteroids, indomethacin, and oral hypoglycemics. May increase insulin requirements in diabetics.

Laboratory Interactions May cause false-positive reactions for urinary bilirubin.

Administration 500 mg po initially, then 250 mg q6h. Therapy should not be given for more than 1 week.

Available Drug Forms Capsules containing 250 mg.

Nursing Management

Administration factors

1. Give with food or milk.
2. Drug should never be used for more than 1 week because of risk of toxicity.

Evaluation factors

1. If diarrhea occurs, drug should be immediately discontinued. Client should not take drug again.
2. Development of rash, petechiae, ecchymoses, dark stools, and hematemesis indicate hypoprothrombinemia; drug should be immediately discontinued.

Client teaching factors May cause drowsiness; caution client to avoid hazardous activities.

COMBINATION ANALGESICS CONTAINING SALICYLATES

TRADE NAME Alka-Seltzer Effervescent (OTC)

CLASSIFICATION Analgesic, antacid

Indications for Use Relief of acid indigestion, sour stomach, or heartburn associated with headache or body aches and pains.

Contraindications Clients on sodium restricted diets or those who have a history of coagulation disorders.

Untoward Reactions Mild salicylism may occur, but is dose related.

Administration 2 tablets in 4 oz water every 4 hours as needed.

Available Drug Forms Generic contents in each tablet: aspirin: 324 mg; sodium bicarbonate (heat treated): 1904 mg; citric acid: 1000 mg. Total sodium content: 551 mg.

Nursing Management

1. Dissolve each tablet in 3 fl oz or more of water.
2. Medicated liquid should be swallowed while effervescents are still present.

TRADE NAME Anacin (OTC)

CLASSIFICATION Analgesic

Indications for Use Relief of pain associated with headache, neuralgia, neuritis, sprains, muscular aches, toothache, menstrual cramps, and minor aches and pains associated with arthritis and rheumatism.

Untoward Reactions Mild salicylism may occur, but is dose related.

Administration 2 tablets or capsules po q4h prn.

Available Drug Forms Generic contents in each tablet or capsule: aspirin: 400 mg; caffeine: 32 mg.

TRADE NAME A.P.C. (OTC)

CLASSIFICATION Analgesic

Indications for Use Relief of headache, minor muscular pains, toothache, and discomfort and fever of colds.

Untoward Reactions Mild salicylism may occur, but is dose related.

Administration 1 to 2 tablets po q4h prn.

Available Drug Forms Generic contents in each tablet: aspirin: 22.6 mg; caffeine: 32 mg.

TRADE NAME Arthritis Pain Formula (OTC)

CLASSIFICATION Analgesic

Indications for Use Relief of minor aches and pains associated with arthritis, rheumatism, and low back pain.

Untoward Reactions Mild salicylism may occur, but is dose related.

Administration 2 tablets po tid or qid.

Available Drug Forms Generic contents in each tablet: microfined aspirin: 487.5 mg; dried aluminum hydroxide gel: 20 mg; magnesium hydroxide: 60 mg.

TRADE NAME Arthrogesic (OTC)

CLASSIFICATION Analgesic

Indications for Use Relief of the signs and symptoms associated with rheumatoid arthritis, osteoarthritis, and other acute joint pains.

Warnings and Precautions Use with caution in clients with chronic renal insufficiency or peptic ulcers and those receiving anticoagulants.

Untoward Reactions May induce salicylism.

Administration 1 to 2 tablets po tid or qid.

Available Drug Forms Generic contents in each tablet: magnesium salicylate: 600 mg; phenyltoloxamine citrate: 30 mg.

TRADE NAME Ascriptin (OTC)

CLASSIFICATION Analgesic

Indications for Use Relief of pain associated with headache, neuralgia, dysmenorrhea, arthritis, and rheumatism. Also used as an inhibitor of platelet aggregation in men who present the risk of recurrent transient ischemic attacks.

Untoward Reactions Mild salicylism may occur, but is dose related.

Administration 2 to 3 tablets po tid or qid.

Available Drug Forms Generic contents in each tablet: aspirin: 325 mg; magnesium hydroxide: 75 mg; dried aluminum hydroxide gel: 75 mg.

TRADE NAME Bufferin (OTC)

CLASSIFICATION Analgesic

Indications for Use Relief of pain associated with simple headache, minor arthritic pain, menstrual cramps, and toothache.

Untoward Reactions Mild salicylism may occur, but is dose related.

Administration 2 tablets po q4h prn.

Available Drug Forms Generic contents in each tablet: aspirin: 324 mg; aluminum glycinate: 48.6 mg; magnesium carbonate: 97.2 mg.

TRADE NAME Cama Inlay-Tabs (OTC)

CLASSIFICATION Analgesic

Indications for Use Relief of pain associated with arthritis and rheumatism.

Untoward Reactions Mild salicylism may occur, but is dose related.

Administration 1 tablet po q4h.

Available Drug Forms Generic contents in each tablet: aspirin: 600 mg; magnesium hydroxide: 150 mg; dried aluminum hydroxide gel: 150 mg.

TRADE NAME Excedrin (OTC)

CLASSIFICATION Analgesic

Indications for Use Relief of pain associated with headache, sinusitis, colds, muscular aches, menstrual discomfort, arthritis, and toothache.

Untoward reactions Mild salicylism may occur, but is dose related.

Administration 2 tablets or capsules po q4h prn.

Available Drug Forms Generic contents in each tablet or capsule: aspirin: 250 mg; acetaminophen: 250 mg; caffeine: 65 mg.

TRADE NAME Goodys Headache Powders (OTC)

CLASSIFICATION Analgesic

Indications for Use Relief of pain associated with simple headache and muscular aches.

Untoward Reactions Mild salicylism may occur, but is dose related.

Administration 1 powder with water every 3 to 4 hours; total dosage not to exceed 4 powders in a 24-hour period.

Available Drug Forms Generic contents in each powder: aspirin: 520 mg; acetaminophen: 260 mg; caffeine: 32.5 mg.

Nursing Management Dissolve powder in 4 fl oz or more of water.

TRADE NAME Hyalex (OTC)

CLASSIFICATION Analgesic

Indications for Use Relief of minor aches and pains associated with arthritis, neuritis, bursitis, and rheumatism, and for nutritional support of affected areas.

Untoward Reactions Mild salicylism may occur, but is dose related.

Administration 1 to 2 tablets po with meals.

Available Drug Forms Generic contents in each tablet: magnesium salicylate: 260 mg; magnesium *p*-aminobenzoate: 162.5 mg; vitamin A (palmitate): 1500 IU; vitamin D: 100 IU; vitamin E: 3 IU; vitamin C: 30 mg; calcium pantothenate (B_5): 5 mg; vitamin B_{12}: 2 mcg; zinc (gluconate): 0.7 mg; magnesium oxide: 5 mg.

TRADE NAME Midol (OTC)

CLASSIFICATION Analgesic

Indications for Use Relief of pain and discomfort associated with menstruation.

Untoward Reactions Mild salicylism may occur, but is dose related.

Administration 2 caplets po q4h prn.

Available Drug Forms Generic contents in each caplet: aspirin: 454 mg; cinnamedrine hydrochloride: 14.9 mg; caffeine: 32.4 mg.

TRADE NAME Norgesic (RX)

CLASSIFICATION Analgesic

Indications for Use Relief of mild to moderate pain associated with acute musculoskeletal disorders.

Contraindications Clients with glaucoma, pyloric or duodenal obstruction, prostatic hypertrophy, or myasthenia gravis.

Warnings and Precautions Use with caution in clients with peptic ulcers or coagulation abnormalities.

Untoward Reactions May induce tachycardia, palpitations, urinary retention, dry mouth, weakness, nausea, vomiting, headache, and drowsiness.

Administration 1 to 2 tablets po tid or qid.

Available Drug Forms Generic contents in each tablet: orphenadrine citrate: 25 mg; aspirin: 385 mg; caffeine: 30 mg.

Nursing Management Warn clients that their mental and/or physical abilities may be impaired.

TRADE NAME Os-Cal-Gesic (OTC)

CLASSIFICATION Analgesic

Indications for Use Relief of symptoms associated with arthritis.

Untoward Reactions Mild salicylism may occur, but is dose related.

Administration 1 to 2 tablets po qid.

Available Drug Forms Generic contents in each tablet: salicylamide: 400 mg; calcium: 100 mg; ergocalciferol (D_2: 50 USP units).

TRADE NAME Pabalate (OTC)

CLASSIFICATION Analgesic

Indications for Use Relief of mild to moderate pain.

Warnings and Precautions Salicylate therapy should be stopped at least 1 week before surgery as it may interfere with blood clotting. Do not use concurrently with sulfonamides as it inhibits their action.

Untoward Reactions May induce GI disturbances. Mild salicylism may occur, but is dose related.

Administration 2 tablets po q4h prn.

Available Drug Forms Generic contents in each enteric-coated tablet: sodium salicylate: 300 mg; sodium aminobenzoate: 300 mg.

Nursing Management Inform clients to avoid taking tablets within an hour of ingesting milk or antacids because of its enteric coating.

TRADE NAME Pabalate-SF (RX)

CLASSIFICATION Analgesic

Indications for Use Relief of mild to moderate pain in those cases where it is desirable to limit the intake of sodium.

Warnings and Precautions Use with extreme caution in clients with chronic renal disease. Do not administer to clients receiving a potassium-sparing diuretic. Discontinue use if symptoms of abdominal pain, distention, nausea, vomiting, or GI bleeding occur as nonspecific small bowel lesions have been known to occur with this medication. Discontinue use at least 1 week prior to surgery as it may interfere with blood clotting. Do not use concurrently with sulfonamides as it inhibits their action.

Untoward Reactions May induce hyperkalemia and/or GI disorders. Mild salicylism may occur, but is dose related.

Administration 2 tablets po q4h prn.

Available Drug Forms Generic contents in each enteric-coated tablet: potassium salicylate: 300 mg; potassium aminobenzoate: 300 mg. Total potassium content: 131.5 mg.

Nursing Management Inform clients to avoid taking tablets within an hour of ingesting milk or antacids because of its enteric coating.

TRADE NAME Percodan (CII)

CLASSIFICATION Analgesic

Indications for Use Relief of moderate to moderately severe pain.

Warnings and Precautions May induce drug dependence of the morphine type. Use with caution in clients with head injuries, increased intracranial pressure, or acute abdominal conditions.

Untoward Reactions May induce dizziness, sedation, nausea, vomiting, and constipation.

Administration 1 tablet po q6h prn.

Available Drug Forms Generic contents in each yellow scored tablet: oxycodone hydrochloride: 4.50 mg; oxycodone terephthalate: 0.38 mg; aspirin: 325 mg.

Nursing Management

1. Warn clients that their mental and/or physical abilities may be impaired.
2. Use cautiously with other CNS depressants because of their additive effect.

TRADE NAME Quiet World (OTC)

CLASSIFICATION Analgesic

Indications for Use Relief of sleeplessness due to pain of headache, sinusitis, muscular aches, and menstrual discomfort.

Untoward Reactions Mild salicylism may occur, but is dose related.

Administration 2 tablets po hs prn.

Available Drug Forms Generic contents in each blue tablet: aspirin: 227 mg; acetaminophen: 162 mg; pyrilamine maleate: 25 mg.

Nursing Management Caution client to avoid operating hazardous equipment.

TRADE NAME Synalgos (RX)

CLASSIFICATION Analgesic

Indications for Use Possibly effective for relief of mild to moderate pain when a sedative effect is desired.

Contraindications Clients with peptic ulcers or coagulation abnormalities.

Warnings and Precautions Use with caution in clients with cardiovascular or hepatic disease.

Untoward Reactions May induce drowsiness, dizziness, sedation, skin reactions, nausea, vomiting, and constipation.

Administration 2 capsules po q4h prn.

Available Drug Forms Generic contents in each maroon and gray capsule: promethazine hydrochloride: 6.25 mg; aspirin: 356.4 mg; caffeine: 30 mg. Synalgos-DC capsules containing 16 mg dihydrocodeine bitartrate are also available.

Nursing Management

1. Warn clients that their mental and/or physical abilities may be impaired.
2. Use cautiously with other CNS depressants because of their additive effect.

TRADE NAME Trilisate (RX)

CLASSIFICATION Analgesic

Indications for Use Relief of signs and symptoms associated with rheumatoid arthritis, osteoarthritis, and other acute joint pains.

Contraindications Not to be given to children under 12 years.

Warnings and Precautions Use with caution in clients with chronic renal insufficiency or peptic ulcers and those receiving anticoagulants.

Untoward Reactions May induce salicylism.

Administration 1500 to 2500 mg po initially in divided doses; then administer according to the client's therapeutic response. The daily dosage must be determined by salicylate blood levels.

Available Drug Forms Generic contents in each pink 500-mg tablet: choline salicylate: 293 mg; magnesium salicylate: 362 mg. Generic contents in each white 750-mg tablet: choline salicylate: 440 mg; magnesium salicylate: 544 mg.

TRADE NAME Vanquish (OTC)

CLASSIFICATION Analgesic

Indications for Use Relief of pain associated with muscular aches, neuralgia, dental procedures, menstrual discomfort, arthritis, rheumatism, and sciatica.

Untoward Reactions Mild salicylism may occur, but is dose related.

Administration 2 caplets po q4h prn.

Available Drug Forms Generic contents in each caplet: aspirin: 227 mg; acetaminophen: 194 mg; caffeine: 33 mg; dried aluminum hydroxide gel: 25 mg; magnesium hydroxide: 50 mg.

TOPICAL SALICYLATE PREPARATIONS

TRADE NAME Acnaveen Bar (OTC)

CLASSIFICATION Antiacne agent

Indications for Use A cleansing bar for acne.

Administration Wash affected areas daily.

Available Drug Forms A sudsing soap-free base containing a mild surfactant. Generic contents in each bar: colloidal oatmeal: 50%; sulfur: 2%; salicylic acid: 2%.

TRADE NAME Acne-Dome (OTC)

CLASSIFICATION Antiacne agent

Indications for Use A skin cleanser used in the treatment of acne.

Untoward Reactions May induce skin irritation or dryness.

Administration Apply to affected areas bid.

Available Drug Forms Supplied in Dispensajar with applicator sponge so fingers never touch the cleanser. Generic contents in lotion: colloidal sulfur, salicylic acid.

Nursing Management

1. Keep away from eyes.
2. Wet skin, apply cleanser to moist sponge, work into a lather, massage for 5 minutes, then rinse.

TRADE NAME Banalg Liniment (OTC)

CLASSIFICATION Analgesic

Indications for Use Relief of minor pain caused by arthritis, sore muscles, and low back pain.

Untoward Reactions May induce skin irritation.

Administration Apply to affected areas several times daily, as needed.

Available Drug Forms Generic contents in lotion: methyl salicylate, menthol, camphor, and eucalyptus oil in a green-colored, nongreasy base.

Nursing Management

1. Avoid contact with the eyes or mucous membranes
2. Apply generously with gentle massage to painful areas.

TRADE NAME Compound W (OTC)

CLASSIFICATION Wart remover

Indications for Use Removal of warts

Contraindications Clients with diabetes or impaired circulatory conditions.

Warnings and Precautions Flammable, do not use near flame or fire.

Administration Apply to affected areas bid for 6 to 7 days.

Available Drug Forms Generic contents in each drop by weight: salicylic acid: 14.2%; glacial acetic acid (in a flexible collodion vehicle): 9%; ether: 57%.

Nursing Management

1. Do not use on the face, mucous membranes, moles, or birthmarks.
2. Soak affected areas in hot water for 5 minutes, dry thoroughly, and apply with the glass rod supplied. Allow to dry, then reapply.

TRADE NAME Dry and Clear (OTC)

CLASSIFICATION Antiacne agent

Indications for Use A skin cleanser used in the treatment of acne; effective in removing oil and dirt from the skin.

Untoward Reactions May induce skin irritation or dryness.

Administration Apply to affected areas daily or bid.

Available Drug Forms Generic contents in lotion: alcohol: 50%; salicylic acid: 0.5%; benzoic acid: 0.5%; benzethonium chloride: 0.1%.

Nursing Management

1. Avoid contact with the eyes, lips, and mouth.
2. Apply with cotton pad after washing face, concentrating on oily areas; do not rinse after application.

TRADE NAME Duofilm (RX)

CLASSIFICATION Wart remover

Indications for Use Removal of warts.

Contraindications Clients with diabetes or impaired circulatory conditions.

Warnings and Precautions Flammable, do not use near flame or fire.

Untoward Reactions May induce skin irritation on tissue surrounding wart.

Administration Apply 3 to 4 drops to affected areas daily until warts are resolved (6 to 12 weeks).

Available Drug Forms A base of flexible collodion. Generic contents in liquid: salicylic acid: 16.7%; lactic acid: 16.7%.

Nursing Management

1. Avoid contact with the eyes or mucous membranes.
2. Do not use on moles or birthmarks.
3. Soak affected areas in hot water for 5 minutes, dry thoroughly, and apply with plastic applicator supplied. Allow each drop to dry thoroughly before applying next one and cover loosely with a Band-Aid.

TRADE NAME Exzit (OTC)

CLASSIFICATION Antiacne agent

Indications for Use A skin cleanser used in the treatment of acne.

Untoward Reactions May induce skin irritation or dryness.

Administration Apply to affected areas bid.

Available Drug Forms Supplied in Dispensajar with applicator sponge so fingers never touch the cleanser. Generic contents in lotion: colloidal sulfur, salicylic acid.

Nursing Management

1. Avoid contact with the eyes.
2. Wet skin, apply cleanser to moist sponge, work into a lather, massage for 5 minutes, then rinse.

TRADE NAME Fostex Medicated Cleansing Bar

CLASSIFICATION Antiacne agent (OTC)

Indications for Use A skin cleanser used in the treatment of acne.

Untoward Reactions May induce skin irritation or dryness.

Administration Wash affected areas bid or tid and rinse well.

Available Drug Forms Generic contents in each bar: salicylic acid: 2%; sulfur: 2%. Also contains a combination of soapless cleansers and wetting agents.

Nursing Management Avoid contact with the eyes.

TRADE NAME Freezone (OTC)

CLASSIFICATION Corn remover

Indications for Use Removal of corns or calluses.

Contraindications Clients with diabetes or impaired circulatory conditions.

Warnings and Precautions Flammable, do not use near flame or fire. Do not use if corn or callus is infected.

Administration Apply, drop by drop, to affected areas bid.

Available Drug Forms Generic contents in liquid by weight: zinc chloride: 2.18%; salicylic acid (in a collodion vehicle): 13.6%; alcohol: 20.5%; ether: 64.8%.

Nursing Management

1. Apply liquid with glass applicator supplied.
2. After 3 to 6 days of drug therapy, soak affected areas in warm water until corn or callus is easily removable.

TRADE NAME Ger-O-Foam (OTC)

CLASSIFICATION Analgesic

Indications for Use Relief of minor pains associated with musculoskeletal conditions, such as rheumatoid arthritis, osteoarthritis, and low back pain.

Untoward Reactions May induce skin irritation.

Administration Apply to affected areas bid or tid.

Available Drug Forms A specially processed oil emulsion base. Generic contents in foam: methyl salicylate: 30%; benzocaine: 3%.

Nursing Management

1. Avoid contact with eyes or mucous membranes.
2. Massage into affected areas.

TRADE NAME Klaron (OTC)

CLASSIFICATION Antiacne agent

Indications for Use A drying lotion used in the treatment of acne.

Untoward Reactions May induce skin irritation or dryness.

Administration Apply a thin layer to affected areas daily or bid.

Available Drug Forms Generic contents in lotion: salicylic acid, colloidal sulfur.

Nursing Management

1. Avoid contact with the eyes.
2. Wash, rinse, and dry affected areas thoroughly before applying lotion.

TRADE NAME Komed (OTC)

CLASSIFICATION Antiacne agent

Indications for Use Treatment of acne associated with oily skin.

Untoward Reactions May induce skin irritation or dryness.

Administration Apply a thin layer to affected areas bid.

Available Drug Forms Generic contents in lotion: sodium thiosulfate: 8%; salicylic acid: 2%; isopropyl alcohol: 25%. Also contains menthol, camphor, colodial alumina, edetate disodium, and purified water.

Nursing Management

1. Do not use on or near the eyes.
2. Wash, rinse, and dry affected areas thoroughly before applying lotion.

TRADE NAME Oxipor VHC (OTC)

CLASSIFICATION Antipsoriasis agent

Indications for Use Relief of symptoms and treatment of psoriasis.

Warnings and Precautions Flammable; do not use near fire or flame.

Administration Apply to affected areas bid.

Available Drug Forms Generic contents in lotion by volume: coal tar solution: 48.5%; salicylic acid: 1%; benzocaine: 2%; alcohol: 81%.

Nursing Management

1. Do not apply to the eyes or mucous membranes.
2. Wash affected areas, then apply lotion with a cotton wad. If the scalp has patches, apply to affected areas with fingertips, then shampoo.
3. Warn clients to avoid unnecessary exposure to sunlight after applying.

TRADE NAME P&S Shampoo (OTC)

CLASSIFICATION Antiseborrheic agent

Indications for Use Helps control the scaling problems of the scalp associated with psoriasis and severe seborrhea.

Untoward Reactions May induce skin irritation.

Administration Shampoo daily, as needed.

Available Drug Forms Generic contents in lotion: salicylic acid: 2%; lactic acid: 0.5%.

Nursing Management

1. Avoid contact with the eyes or mucous membranes.
2. Wet hair, apply shampoo, lather, then rinse; repeat once.

TRADE NAME Panalgesic (OTC)

CLASSIFICATION Analgesic

Indications for Use Relief of arthritic pain and muscle stiffness.

Untoward Reactions May induce skin irritation.

Administration Rub externally to affected areas with gentle massage tid or qid.

Available Drug Forms Generic contents in liquid by weight: methyl salicylate: 50%; aspirin: 8%; menthol and camphor: 4%; emollient oils: 20%; alcohol: 18%.

Nursing Management Avoid contact with the eyes or mucous membranes.

TRADE NAME Panscol (OTC)

CLASSIFICATION Antiseborrheic agent

Indications for Use Relief of symptoms associated with dry, scaly skin.

Untoward Reactions May induce skin irritation.

Administration Apply to affected areas bid.
Available Drug Forms

Available Drug Forms Generic contents in lotion or ointment: salicylic acid: 3%; lactic acid: 2%; phenol: 1%.

Nursing Management

1. Avoid contact with the eyes or mucous membranes.
2. Wash, rinse, and dry affected areas thoroughly before applying ointment or lotion.

TRADE NAME Pernox (OTC)

CLASSIFICATION Antiacne agent

Indications for Use A skin cleanser used in the treatment of acne.

Contraindications Acute inflammation, nodular or cystic acne.

Untoward Reactions May induce skin irritation.

Administration Apply to affected areas bid.

Available Drug Forms Generic contents in lotion; sulfur: 2%; salicylic acid: 1.5%. Also contains a combination of soapless cleansers, wetting agents, and abradant polyethylene granules.

Nursing Management

1. Avoid contact with the eyes or mucous membranes.
2. Wash, rinse and dry affected areas thoroughly before applying lotion.

TRADE NAME Pragmatar Ointment (OTC)

CLASSIFICATION Antiseborrheic agent

Indications for Use Wide range of common skin disorders in adults and children, particularly scalp disorders, chronic dermatitis, and fungus infections, including athlete's foot.

Untoward Reactions May induce skin irritation.

Administration Apply to affected areas daily.

Available Drug Forms An oil-in-water emulsion base. Generic contents in ointment: cetyl alcohol-coal tar distillate: 4%; precipitated sulfur: 3%; salicylic acid: 3%.

Nursing Management

1. Do not use in the eyes, on eyelids, or on blistered areas. Use with caution near the groin or on acutely inflamed areas.
2. Scalp: Apply sparingly to affected areas hs; shampoo out in the morning.
3. Skin: Apply a thin layer to affected areas daily.
4. Discontinue use if skin irritation develops.

TRADE NAME Sebucare (OTC)

CLASSIFICATION Antiseborrheic agent

Indications for Use As an aid in the treatment of dandruff, seborrhea capitis, and other scaling conditions of the scalp.

Warnings and Precautions Flammable; do not use near fire or flame.

Administration Apply daily or bid.

Available Drug Forms Generic contents in lotion: salicylic acid: 1.8%; alcohol: 61%. Also contains water, PPG-40 butyl ether, laureth-4, dihydroabietyl alcohol, and fragrance.

Nursing Management

1. Avoid contact with eyes.
2. Apply directly to scalp and massage with fingertips.

TRADE NAME Sebulex Shampoo (OTC)

CLASSIFICATION Antiseborrheic agent

Indications for Use Treatment of dandruff.

Untoward Reactions May induce skin irritation.

Administration May be used daily.

Available Drug Forms Generic contents in lotion: salicylic acid: 2%; sulfur: 2%. Also contains water, sodium octoxynol-3-sulfonate, sodium lauryl sulfate, lauramide DEA, acetamide MEA, amphoteric-2, hydrolyzed animal protein, magnesium aluminum silicate, propylene glycol, methylcellulose, PEG-14 M, fragrance, disodium EDTA, dioctyl sodium sulfosuccinate, FD&C No. 1 blue, and D&C No. 10 yellow.

Nursing Mangement

1. Avoid contact with the eyes.
2. Massage shampoo into wet scalp, work into a lather, leave for 5 minutes, then rinse; repeat once.
3. Once symptoms are under control, use once or twice weekly.

TRADE NAME Sebutone Shampoo (OTC)

CLASSIFICATION Antiseborrheic agent

Indications for Use Treatment of dandruff and seborrheic dermatitis.

Untoward Reactions May induce skin irritation.

Administration Use two to three times weekly.

Available Drug Forms Generic contents in lotion: sulfur: 2%; salicylic acid: 2%. Also contains coal tar, surface-active cleansers, and wetting agents.

Nursing Management

1. Avoid contact with the eyes.
2. Massage shampoo into wet scalp, work into a lather, leave for 5 minutes, then rinse; repeat once.

TRADE NAME Stri-Dex (OTC)

CLASSIFICATION Antiacne agent

Indications for Use Topical treatment of acne vulgaris.

Untoward Reactions May induce skin irritation.

Administration Apply every morning and night.

Available Drug Forms Generic contents in liquid: salicylic acid: 0.5%; alcohol: 28%. Also contains water, sulfonated alkyl benzenes, citric acid, sodium carbonate, fragrance, and simethicone. Supplied in containers containing 42 or 75 medicated pads.

Nursing Management

1. Avoid contact with the eyes.
2. Wash and dry face; wipe medicated pad over face.

TRADE NAME Tinver (RX)

CLASSIFICATION Antifungal agent

Indications for Use Topical treatment of tinea versicolor infections.

Untoward Reactions May induce skin irritation.

Administration Apply a thin layer to affected areas bid.

Available Drug Forms Generic contents in lotion: sodium thiosulfate: 25%; salicylic acid: 1%; isopropyl alcohol: 10%. Also contains propylene glycol, menthol, edetate disodium, colloidal alumina, and purified water.

Nursing Management

1. Avoid contact with the eyes.
2. Wash, rinse, and dry affected areas thoroughly before applying lotion.

COMBINATION ANALGESICS CONTAINING ACETAMINOPHEN

TRADE NAME Arthralgen (OTC)

CLASSIFICATION Analgesic

Indications for Use Relief of pain associated with arthritis, colds, flu, and myalgia.

Untoward Reactions May induce nausea and other GI disturbances, but rarely. Mild salicylism may occur, but is dose related.

Administration 1 to 2 tablets po qid.

Available Drug Forms Generic contents in each white scored tablet: acetaminophen: 250 mg; salicylamide: 250 mg.

TRADE NAME Bancap (OTC)

CLASSIFICATION Analgesic

Indications for Use Relief of pain associated with arthritis, colds, flu, and myalgia.

Untoward Reactions May induce nausea and other GI disturbances, but rarely. Mild salicylism may occur, but is dose related.

Administration 1 to 2 capsules po qid.

Available Drug Forms Generic contents in each capsule: acetaminophen: 300 mg; salicylamide: 200 mg. Capsules containing 30 mg codeine are also available.

TRADE NAME Blanex (RX)

CLASSIFICATION Analgesic

Indications for Use Relief of pain and stiffness associated with musculoskeletal conditions.

Untoward Reactions Hypersensitivity to the drug may induce drowsiness, dizziness, malaise, or excessive CNS stimulation. Hepatotoxicity may occur.

Administration 2 capsules po qid.

Available Drug Forms Generic contents in each capsule: acetaminophen: 300 mg; chlorzoxazone: 250 mg.

TRADE NAME Capital (C iv)

CLASSIFICATION Analgesic

Indications for Use Relief of mild to moderate pain.

Warnings and Precautions May induce drug dependence of the morphine type. Do not give to clients with head injuries or increased intracranial pressure.

Untoward Reactions May induce lightheadedness, dizziness, sedation, nausea, vomiting, euphoria, dysphoria, constipation, and pruritus.

Drug Interactions Additive effect with CNS depressants.

Administration 1 to 2 tablets every 4 to 6 hours.

Available Drug Forms Generic contents in each pale blue scored tablet: acetaminophen: 325 mg; codeine phosphate: 30 mg.

TRADE NAME Cetased (C iii)

CLASSIFICATION Analgesic

Indications for Use Relief of symptoms associated with muscular contraction or tension headache.

Warnings and Precautions May induce drug dependence. Use with caution in client with peptic ulcers or coagulation abnormalities.

Untoward Reactions May induce drowsiness and dizziness.

Administration 1 to 2 tablets po q4h.

Available Drug Forms Generic contents in each oval-shaped tablet: butalbital: 50 mg; aspirin: 200 mg; acetaminophen: 130 mg; caffeine: 40 mg.

TRADE NAME Codalan (C iii)

CLASSIFICATION Analgesic

Indications for Use Relief of pain.

Warnings and Precautions May be habit forming.

Untoward Reactions May induce sedation, nausea, vomiting, constipation, and dizziness. Mild salicylism may occur, but is dose related.

Administration 1 tablet po every 4 to 6 hours, as needed.

Available Drug Forms Generic contents in each No. 1 orange tablet: codeine phosphate: 7.5 mg; acetaminophen: 160 mg; salicylamide: 225 mg; caffeine: 30 mg. Generic contents in each No. 2 white tablet: codeine phosphate: 15 mg; acetaminophen: 160 mg; salicylamide: 225 mg; caffeine: 30 mg. Generic contents in each No. 3 green tablet: codeine phosphate: 30 mg; acetaminophen: 160 mg: salicylamide: 225 mg; caffeine: 30 mg.

TRADE NAME Darvocet-N (C iv)

CLASSIFICATION Analgesic

Indications for Use Relief of mild to moderate pain.

Contraindications Clients who are suicidal.

Warnings and Precautions May induce drug dependence. Use with caution in clients taking tranquilizers or those who use alcohol in excess. Instruct client not to exceed the recommended prescribed dose and to limit alcohol intake.

Untoward Reactions May induce dizziness, sedation, nausea, and vomiting.

Administration 1 tablet po q4h prn.

Available Drug Forms Generic contents in each dark orange Darvocet-N 50 tablet: propoxyphene napsylate: 50 mg; acetaminophen: 325 mg. Generic contents in each dark orange Darvocet-N 100 tablet: propoxyphene napsylate: 100 mg; acetaminophen: 650 mg.

TRADE NAME Demerol APAP (C iii)

CLASSIFICATION Analgesic

Indications for Use Relief of moderate to severe pain.

Contraindications Clients with head injuries or increased intracranial pressure.

Warnings and Precautions May be habit forming. Use with caution in clients with supraventricular tachycardia or respiratory disorders. Use with extreme caution in clients receiving other CNS depressants.

Untoward Reactions May induce euphoria, weakness, headache, tremor, dizziness, sedation, dry mouth, constipation, flushing of the face, hypotension, respiratory depression, urinary retention, and skin rashes.

Administration 1 to 2 tablets po every 3 to 4 hours, as needed.

Available Drug Forms Generic contents in each tablet: meperidine HCl: 50 mg; acetaminophen: 300 mg.

TRADE NAME Duradyne DHC (C iii)

CLASSIFICATION Analgesic

Indications for Use Relief of mild, moderate, or moderately severe pain.

Contraindications Clients with glaucoma, head injuries, or increased intracranial pressure.

Warnings and Precautions May induce drug dependence. Use with caution in clients receiving other CNS depressants.

Untoward Reactions May induce dizziness, sedation, nausea, and vomiting. Mild salicylism may occur, but is dose related.

Administration 1 to 2 tablets po every 4 to 6 hours, as needed.

Available Drug Forms Generic contents in each green scored tablet: hydrocodone bitartrate: 5 mg; aspirin: 230 mg; acetaminophen: 150 mg; caffeine: 30 mg.

TRADE NAME Empracet (RX)

CLASSIFICATION Analgesic

Indications for Use Relief of mild, moderate, or severe pain.

Contraindications Clients with head injuries or increased intracranial pressure.

Warnings and Precautions May induce drug dependence of the morphine type. Use with caution in clients receiving other CNS depressants.

Untoward Reactions May induce dizziness, sedation, nausea, vomiting, and constipation.

Administration 1 to 2 tablets po q4h prn.

Available Drug Forms Generic contents in each orange No. 3 tablet: codeine phosphate: 30 mg; acetaminophen: 300 mg. Generic contents in each orange No. 4 tablet: codeine phosphate: 60 mg; acetaminophen: 300 mg.

TRADE NAME Esgic (RX)

CLASSIFICATION Analgesic

Indications for Use Relief of symptoms associated with the stress headache syndrome.

Contraindications Do not use during pregnancy as it can damage fetus.

Warnings and Precautions May be habit forming. Hepatotoxicity may occur. Use with caution in clients receiving other CNS depressants. Can decrease the effects of anticoagulants and corticosteroids.

Untoward Reactions May induce drowsiness and dizziness.

Administration 1 to 2 tablets or capsules po q4h prn.

Available Drug Forms Generic contents in each tablet or capsule: butalbital: 50 mg; caffeine: 40 mg; acetaminophen: 325 mg.

TRADE NAME Excedrin (OTC)

CLASSIFICATION Analgesic

See Excedrin (page 467) for further details.

TRADE NAME Gaysal-S (OTC)

CLASSIFICATION Analgesic

Indications for Use Relief of pain associated with rheumatoid arthritis, osteoarthritis, fibrositis, and bursitis.

Untoward Reactions Mild salicylism may occur.

Administration 2 tablets po pc and hs.

Available Drug Forms Generic contents in each tablet: sodium salicylate: 300 mg; acetaminophen: 180 mg; aluminum hydroxide gel: 60 mg.

TRADE NAME Gemnisyn (OTC)

CLASSIFICATION Analgesic

Indications for Use Relief of mild to moderate pain.

Warnings and Precautions Use with caution in clients with peptic ulcers, asthma, hepatic damage, or those receiving anticoagulants.

Untoward Reactions Mild salicylism may occur, but is dose related.

Administration 1 to 2 tablets po every 4 to 6 hours, as needed.

Available Drug Forms Generic contents in each tablet: aspirin: 325 mg; acetaminophen: 325 mg.

TRADE NAME Maxigesic (C iii)

CLASSIFICATION Analgesic

Indications for Use Possibly effective in the relief of moderate to moderately severe pain. Preoperative, postoperative, or obstetric sedation.

Contraindications Clients with head injuries, increased intracranial pressure, or acute abdominal conditions.

Warnings and Precautions May induce drug dependence of the morphine type. Use with caution in clients receiving other CNS depressants.

Untoward Reactions May induce dizziness, nausea, vomiting, sedation, and dry mouth.

Administration 1 to 2 capsules po every 4 to 6 hours, as needed.

Available Drug Forms Generic contents in each gray and white capsule: codeine phosphate: 30 mg; acetaminophen: 325 mg; promethazine HCl: 6.25 mg.

TRADE NAME Medigesic Plus (C iii)

CLASSIFICATION Analgesic

Indications for Use Relief of pain where physician feels mild sedation is also indicated.

Warnings and Precautions May be habit forming.

Untoward Reactions May induce dizziness, nausea, and vomiting.

Administration 1 capsule po q4h prn.

Available Drug Forms Generic contents in each capsule: butalbital: 50 mg; acetaminophen: 325 mg; caffeine: 40 mg.

TRADE NAME Midrin (RX)

CLASSIFICATION Analgesic

Indications for Use Relief of tension or a vascular headache.

Contraindications Clients with glaucoma, hypertension, organic heart disease, hepatic or renal disease, and those receiving MAO inhibitors.

Untoward Reactions May induce transient dizziness and skin rash.

Administration

- *Migraine headache:* 2 capsules po stat, followed by 1 capsule qlh until relieved; Maximum dosage: 5 capsules within 12 hours.
- *Tension headache:* 1 to 2 capsules po q4h prn.

Available Drug Forms Generic contents in each red capsule with pink band: isometheptene mucate: 65 mg; dichloralphenazone: 100 mg; acetaminophen: 325 mg.

TRADE NAME Migralam (RX)

CLASSIFICATION Analgesic

Indications for Use Relief of tension or vascular headache.

Contraindications Clients with glaucoma, hypertension, organic heart disease, hepatic or severe renal disease, and those receiving MAO inhibitors.

Untoward Reactions May induce transient dizziness and skin rash.

Administration

- *Migraine headache:* 2 capsules po stat, followed by 1 capsule po qlh until relieved; Maximum dosage: 5 capsules in 12 hours.
- *Tension headache:* 1 to 2 capsules po q4h prn.

Available Drug Forms Generic contents in each white capsule: isometheptene mucate: 65 mg; caffeine: 100 mg; acetaminophen: 325 mg.

TRADE NAME Norcet (C iii)

CLASSIFICATION Analgesic

Indications for Use Relief of mild to moderate pain.

Warnings and Precautions May be habit forming. Use with caution in clients receiving other CNS depressants.

Untoward Reactions May induce sedation, nausea, vomiting, and constipation.

Administration 1 to 2 tablets po every 4 to 6 hours, as needed.

Available Drug Forms Generic contents in each tablet: acetaminophen: 650 mg; hydrocodone bitartrate: 7.5 mg.

TRADE NAME Parafon Forte (RX)

CLASSIFICATION Analgesic

Indications for Use Relief of pain, stiffness, and limitation of motion associated with most musculoskeletal disorders.

Untoward Reactions May induce malaise or GI disturbances.

Administration 2 tablets po qid.

Available Drug Forms Generic contents in each green tablet: chlorzoxazone: 250 mg; acetaminophen: 300 mg.

TRADE NAME Percocet-5 (C iii)

CLASSIFICATION Analgesic

Indications for Use Relief of moderate to moderately severe pain.

Contraindications Clients with head injuries, increased intracranial pressure, or acute abdominal conditions (since it may obscure the proper diagnosis.)

Warnings and Precautions May induce drug dependence of the morphine type. Use with caution in clients receiving other CNS depressants.

Untoward reactions May induce lightheadedness, sedation, nausea, vomiting, constipation, and skin rash.

Administration 1 tablet po q6h prn.

Available Drug Forms Generic contents in each tablet: oxycodone hydrochloride: 5 mg; acetaminophen: 325 mg.

TRADE NAME Percogesic (OTC)

CLASSIFICATION Analgesic

Indications for Use Relief of mild to moderate pain associated with simple headache, muscle and joint soreness, neuralgia, menstrual cramps, and minor aches of arthritis and rheumatism.

Untoward Reactions May induce drowsiness.

Administration 1 to 2 tablets po q4h prn.

Available Drug Forms Generic contents in each tablet: acetaminophen: 325 mg; phenyltoloxamine citrate: 30 mg. Tablets containing 32.4 mg codeine are also available.

TRADE NAME Phenaphen with Codeine (C iii)

CLASSIFICATION Analgesic

Indications for Use No. 2 and No. 3: Relief of mild to moderate pain; No. 4: Relief of moderate to severe pain.

Contraindications Clients with head injuries, increased intracranial pressure, or acute abdominal conditions.

Warnings and Precautions May induce drug dependence of the morphine type. May impair the mental and/or physical abilities of clients.

Untoward Reactions May induce dizziness, nausea, vomiting, constipation, and pruritus.

Administration No. 2 and No. 3: 1 to 2 capsules po q4h prn; No. 4: 1 capsule po q4h prn.

Available Drug Forms Generic contents in each black-yellow No. 2 capsule: codeine phosphate: 15 mg; acetaminophen: 325 mg. Generic contents in each black-green No. 3 capsule: codeine phosphate: 30 mg; acetaminophen: 325 mg. Generic contents in each green-white No. 4 capsule: codeine phosphate 60 mg; acetaminophen: 325 mg. Phenaphen-650 with Codeine tablets containing 30 mg codeine and 650 mg acetaminophen are also available.

TRADE NAME Phrenilin (RX)

CLASSIFICATION Analgesic

Indications for Use Relief of pain associated with tension headache.

Contraindications Clients with porphyria.

Warnings and Precautions May be habit forming. May impair the mental and/or physical abilities of clients.

Untoward Reactions May induce dizziness, drowsiness, nausea, vomiting, constipation, and skin rash.

Administration 1 to 2 tablets po q4h prn.

Available Drug Forms Generic contents in each pale violet tablet: butalbital: 50 mg; acetaminophen: 325 mg; caffeine: 40 mg.

TRADE NAME Saroflex (RX)

CLASSIFICATION Analgesic

Indications for Use Relief of pain associated with musculoskeletal conditions.

Untoward Reactions May induce malaise or GI disturbances.

Administration 2 capsules po qid.

Available Drug Forms Generic contents in each tan capsule: chlorzoxazone: 250 mg; acetaminophen: 300 mg.

TRADE NAME Sedapap-10 (RX)

CLASSIFICATION Analgesic

Indications for Use Relief of pain associated with tension headache.

Contraindications Clients with hepatic disease.

Warnings and Precautions May be habit forming.

Untoward Reactions May induce drowsiness and/or GI disturbances.

Administration 1 tablet po tid or qid.

Available Drug Forms Generic contents in each tablet: acetaminophen: 648 mg; butalbital: 50 mg.

TRADE NAME Sunril (OTC)

CLASSIFICATION Analgesic

Indications for Use Relief of premenstrual pain, tension, and edema.

Untoward Reactions May induce drowsiness.

Administration 1 capsule po every 3 to 4 hours, as needed.

Available Drug Forms Generic contents in each pink and lavender capsule: acetaminophen: 300 mg; pamabrom: 50 mg; pyrilamine maleate: 25 mg.

TRADE NAME Supac (OTC)

CLASSIFICATION Analgesic

Indications for Use Relief of pain associated with simple head colds, menstruation, headache, tooth extraction, and arthritis.

Untoward Reactions Mild salicylism may occur, but is dose related.

Administration Adults: 1 to 2 tablets po every 4 hours, as needed. Children 7 to 12 years: $\frac{1}{2}$ to 1 tablet po every 4 hours, as needed. Children 3 to 6 years: $\frac{1}{4}$ to $\frac{3}{4}$ tablet po every 4 hours, as needed.

Available Drug Forms Generic contents in each white scored tablet: acetaminophen: 160 mg; aspirin: 230 mg; caffeine: 33 mg; calcium gluconate: 60 mg.

TRADE NAME Tylenol with Codeine #1, #2, #3, #4

CLASSIFICATION Analgesic (C iii)

Indications for Use No. 1, No. 2, and No. 3: Relief of mild to moderate pain; No. 4: Relief of moderate to severe pain.

Contraindications Clients with head injuries, increased intracranial pressure, or acute abdominal conditions.

Warnings and Precautions May be habit forming. Use with caution in clients receiving CNS depressants. May impair the mental and/or physical abilities of clients.

Untoward Reactions May induce sedation, nausea, vomiting, dizziness, and constipation.

Administration No. 1, No. 2, and No. 3: 1 to 2 tablets po q4h prn; No. 4: 1 tablet po q4h prn.

Available Drug Forms Generic contents in each No. 1 tablet: acetaminophen: 300 mg; codeine phosphate: 7.5 mg. Generic contents in each No. 2 tablet: acetaminophen: 300 mg; codeine phosphate: 15 mg. Generic contents in each No. 3 tablet: acetaminophen: 300 mg; codeine phosphate: 30 mg. Generic contents in each No. 4 tablet: acetaminophen: 300 mg; codeine phosphate: 60 mg.

TRADE NAME Tylox (RX)

CLASSIFICATION Analgesic

Indications for Use Relief of moderate to moderately severe pain.

Contraindications Clients with head injuries, increased intracranial pressure, or acute abdominal conditions.

Warnings and Precautions May induce drug dependence of the morphine type. Use with caution in clients receiving other CNS depressants. May impair the mental and/or physical abilities of clients.

Untoward Reactions May induce dizziness, sedation, nausea, vomiting, constipation, and skin rash.

Administration 1 capsule po q6h prn.

Available Drug Forms Generic contents in each capsule: oxycodone hydrochloride: 4.5 mg; oxycodone terephthalate: 0.38 mg; acetaminophen: 500 mg.

TRADE NAME Vanquish (OTC)

CLASSIFICATION Analgesic

See Vanquish (page 469) for further details.

TRADE NAME Vicodin (C iii)

CLASSIFICATION Analgesic

Indications for Use Relief of moderate to moderately severe pain.

Warnings and Precautions May be habit forming. Since it may suppress the cough reflex and depress respiration, it should be used with caution in postoperative clients and clients with respiratory conditions. May impair the mental and/or physical abilities of clients. Use with caution in clients with head injuries, increased intracranial pressure, or acute abdominal conditions.

Untoward Reactions May induce sedation, dizziness, mood changes, constipation, nausea, vomiting, ureteral spasm, and dose-related respiratory depression.

Administration 1 tablet po q6h prn.

Available Drug Forms Generic contents in each tablet: hydrocodone bitartrate: 5 mg; acetaminophen: 500 mg.

TRADE NAME Wygesic (C iv)

CLASSIFICATION Analgesic

Indications for Use Relief of mild to moderate pain.

Contraindications Clients who are suicidal or prone to addiction.

Warnings and Precautions May induce drug dependence. Instruct clients to limit alcohol intake. May impair the mental and/or physical abilities of clients. Use with caution in clients receiving other CNS depressants.

Untoward Reactions May induce dizziness, sedation, nausea, vomiting, constipation, abdominal pain, and skin rash.

Administration 1 tablet po q4h prn.

Available Drug Forms Generic contents in each scored tablet: propoxyphene hydrochloride: 65 mg; acetaminophen: 650 mg.

COMBINATION ANALGESICS CONTAINING PHENACETIN

TRADE NAME Darvon Compound-65 (C iv)

CLASSIFICATION Analgesic

Indications for Use Relief of mild to moderate pain, either alone or accompanied by fever.

Contraindications Clients who are suicidal or prone to addiction.

Warnings and Precautions May be habit forming. Use with caution in clients receiving other CNS depressants. Instruct clients to limit alcohol intake. Use with caution in clients with renal disease, peptic ulcers, or coagulation abnormalities. Phenacetin taken in large doses for a long period of time with other antiinflammatory analgesics is associated with severe renal disease and cancer of the kidney.

Untoward Reactions May induce dizziness, nausea, vomiting, sedation, skin rash, headache, and abdominal pain.

Administration 1 capsule po q4h prn.

Available Drug Forms Generic contents in each capsule: propoxyphene hydrochloride: 65 mg; aspirin: 227 mg; phenacetin: 162 mg; caffeine: 32.4 mg.

TRADE NAME Fiorinal (C ii)

CLASSIFICATION Analgesic

Indications for Use Relief of pain associated with muscular contraction or tension headache.

Warnings and Precautions May be habit forming. Use with caution in clients with peptic ulcers or coagulation abnormalities.

Untoward Reactions May induce drowsiness or GI disturbances. May induce mild salicylism, but is dose related.

Administration 1 to 2 tablets or capsules po q4h prn.

Available Drug Forms Generic contents in each tablet or capsule: butalbital: 50 mg; aspirin: 200 mg; phenacetin: 130 mg; caffeine: 40 mg.

TRADE NAME Soma Compound (RX)

CLASSIFICATION Analgesic

Indications for Use Relief of pain associated with acute musculoskeletal conditions.

Warnings and Precautions Use with caution in clients receiving other CNS depressants. Use with caution for long-term therapy in clients who have anemia or those who have a history of cardiac, pulmonary, hepatic, or renal disease. Phenacetin taken in large doses for a long period of time with other antiinflammatory analgesics is associated with severe renal disease and cancer of the kidney.

Untoward Reactions May induce drowsiness, dizziness, itching, nervousness, and palpitations.

Administration 1 to 2 tablets po every 4 hours, as needed.

Available Drug Forms Generic contents in each orange scored tablet: carisoprodol: 200 mg; phenacetin: 160 mg; caffeine: 32 mg.

COMBINATION ANALGESICS CONTAINING ERGOT DERIVATIVES

TRADE NAME Cafergot (RX)

CLASSIFICATION Analgesic

Indications for Use Relief or prevention of pain associated with vascular or migraine headache.

Contraindications Clients with a history of peripheral vascular disease, coronary heart disease, hypertension, or impaired renal or hepatic function. Do not use during pregnancy.

Warnings and Precautions May induce ergotism.

Untoward Reactions May induce weakness, muscle pain, transient tachycardia or bradycardia, nausea, vomiting, localized edema, and itching.

Administration 2 tablets po at start of attack, then 1 tablet po every 30 minutes, as needed; do not exceed 6 tablets per attack.

Available Drug Forms Generic contents in each pink tablet: ergotamine tartrate: 1 mg; caffeine: 100 mg.

TRADE NAME Migral (RX)

CLASSIFICATION Analgesic

Indications for Use Possibly effective for the treatment of vascular headache.

Contraindications Clients with a history of peripheral vascular disease, coronary heart disease, hypertension, thrombophlebitis, impaired renal or hepatic function, and sepsis. Do not use during pregnancy.

Warnings and Precautions May induce ergotism.

Untoward Reactions May induce nausea, vomiting, diarrhea, polydipsia, and muscle pains and cramps.

Administration 1 tablet po at start of attack, then 1 tablet po every 30 to 60 minutes, as needed; do not exceed 6 tablets per attack or 10 tablets per week.

Available Drug Forms Generic contents in each sugar-coated tablet: ergotamine tartrate: 1 mg; cyclizine hydrochloride: 25 mg; caffeine: 50 mg.

TRADE NAME Wigraine (RX)

CLASSIFICATION Analgesic

Indications for Use Relief of symptoms associated with vascular headache, such as migraine or histamine cephalalgia.

Contraindications Clients who have a history of peripheral vascular disease, coronary heart disease, hypertension, impaired renal or hepatic function, or sepsis. Do not use during pregnancy.

Warnings and Precautions May induce ergotism. Phenacetin taken in large doses for a long time with other antiinflammatory analgesics is associated with severe renal disease and cancer of the kidney.

Administration 1 to 2 tablets po at start of attack, then 1 to 2 tablets po every 15 minutes, as needed; do not exceed 6 tablets per attack or 12 tablets per week.

Available Drug Forms Generic contents in each green tablet: ergotamine tartrate: 1 mg; caffeine: 100 mg; belladonna alkaloids: 0.1 mg; phenacetin: 130 mg.

COMBINATION PREPARATIONS CONTAINING PROBENECID

TRADE NAMES ColBENEMID, Col-Probenecid, Probenecid with Colchicine

CLASSIFICATION Uricosuric (RX)

Indications for Use Treatment of chronic gouty arthritis complicated by frequent, recurrent acute attacks of gout.

Contraindications Clients who have a history of blood dyscrasias or uric acid kidney stones. Do not use during pregnancy.

Warnings and Precautions Use with caution in clients with a history of peptic ulcers.

Untoward Reactions May induce headache, GI disorders, dermatitis, pruritus, sore gums, flushing, dizziness, and anemia. Hematuria, renal colic, costovertebral pain, and the formation of uric acid stones can occur. These disorders can be prevented by encouraging a liberal fluid intake and alkalization of the urine.

Drug Interactions Probenecid increases plasma concentrations of methotrexate; therefore, its dosage should be reduced and serum levels monitored in clients receiving both medications concurrently. Salicylates antagonize the uricosuric action of probenecid.

Administration 1 tablet po daily for 1 week, then 1 tablet po bid.

Available Drug Forms Generic contents in each tablet: probenecid: 500 mg; colchicine: 0.5 mg.

TRADE NAME Polycillin-PRB (RX)

CLASSIFICATION Long-acting penicillin

Indications for Use Uncomplicated infections due to *Neisseria gonorrhoeae.*

Contraindications Hypersensitivity to penicillins; clients with blood dyscrasias or uric acid kidney stones; during an acute attack of gout; severe renal impairment.

Administration 1 bottleful of suspension po (one single dose).

Available Drug Forms Generic contents in each single-dose bottle: ampicillin trihydrate: 3.5 g; probenecid: 1 g.

Nursing Management (See ampicillin in Chapter 60.)

1. Reconstitute drug by adding 20 ml or more of water in 2 portions and shaking well.
2. Use oral suspension within 24 hours.
3. Reculture infected site (male) or endocervical and anal canal (female) in 7 to 14 days.

TRADE NAME Principen with Probenecid (RX)

CLASSIFICATION Long-acting penicillin

Indications for Use Uncomplicated infections due to *Neisseria gonorrhoeae.*

Contraindications Hypersensitivity to penicillins; clients with blood dyscrasias or uric acid kidney stones; during an acute attack of gout; severe renal impairment.

Administration All 9 capsules po (one single dose).

Available Drug Forms Single-dose bottles containing 9 capsules. Generic contents in each capsule: ampicillin trihydrate: 389 mg; probenecid: 111 mg. Generic contents in 9 capsules: ampicillin trihydrate: 3.5 g; probenecid: 1g.

Nursing Management (See ampicillin in Chapter 60.)

1. Reconstitute drug by adding 20 ml or more of water in 2 portions and shaking well.
2. Use oral suspension within 24 hours.

TRADE NAME Wycillin and Probenecid (RX)

CLASSIFICATION Long-acting penicillin

Indications for Use Uncomplicated infections due to *Neisseria gonorrhoeae.*

Contraindications Hypersensitivity to penicillins; clients with blood dyscrasias or uric acid kidney stones; during an acute attack of gout; severe renal impairment.

Administration Inject both syringefuls of penicillin IM and give prolonged probenecid tablets po.

Available Drug Forms Two disposable syringes containing 2 ml of penicillin with 1,200,000 U/ml; 2 tablets of probenecid containing 500 mg each. Generic contents in each container: penicillin G procaine (syringe): 2,400,000 U; probenecid (tablets): 500 mg. Total generic contents: penicillin G procaine: 4,800,000 U; probenecid: 1 g.

Nursing Management (See ampicillin in Chapter 60.)

1. Administer injections deep into upper outer quadrant of the buttocks.
2. Use 2 different injection sites and aspirate for accidental injection into the bloodstream; otherwise the result could be fatal.
3. Give tablets with a full glass of water.
4. Reculture infected site (male) or endocervical and anal canal (female) in 7 to 14 days.

Chapter 29

Barbiturates

CHARACTERISTICS OF BARBITURATES

THE FIRST BARBITURATES to be introduced for medical use in the early part of the 20th century were barbital (Veronal) and phenobarbital (Luminal). Since then, about 2500 barbiturates have been synthesized, of which only a few are in general use.

The major action of barbiturates is central nervous system depression. When used within prescribed dosage ranges, the effects can range from mild sedation to coma, depending on the particular barbiturate used, its duration of action, route of administration, and the client's clinical status. When used in high concentrations, however, barbiturates have a generalized depressant effect on most other body systems. With prompt treatment, these effects are reversible, but the danger of cardiovascular collapse in acute barbiturate intoxication poses a serious threat until the drug is cleared from the body.

When barbiturates are used to induce sleep, several side effects should be anticipated. Initially, the amount of REM sleep is reduced, but this gradually returns to normal within two or three weeks following the initiation of therapy. A rebound effect occurs when the drug is finally withdrawn, which results in markedly increased REM sleep often associated with nightmares, restlessness, and a feeling of fatigue upon awakening.

Barbiturates also have more subtle, long-lasting effects. There is evidence of impairment of fine motor functions and of judgment for as long as 20 hours after ingestion of a sleep-inducing dosage. Many individuals become irritable and/or emotionally labile during this period.

Although all barbiturates have anticonvulsant properties when given in sufficient doses, phenobarbital has a specific effect on the motor cortex when given in small, nonsedative doses. It is most effective for the control of grand mal seizures, either alone, or in combination with other anticonvulsant drugs.

Very-short-acting barbiturates are often used intravenously to induce light anesthesia, for minor surgical procedures, or first-stage anesthesia, which is then followed with an inhalation anesthetic, for more prolonged procedures. Since barbiturates have no analgesic properties, they must be supplemented with other agents for surgical procedures that are lengthy and/or require deep muscle relaxation. Although the dosage required for anesthesia is highly individualized, the anesthetic effect is very rapid (within 30 seconds after slow intravenous administration). Symptoms of respiratory depression are common.

Tolerance

Barbiturates can produce both physical and psychologic dependence and tolerance. Physical tolerance develops for two reasons: (1) the production of enzymes in the liver is increased and results in more rapid metabolism of the drug; and (2) the central nervous system adapts to the drug. As tolerance develops, higher doses are required to maintain effective tissue concentrations of the drug. The tolerance to a lethal dose does not increase proportionately, so that as physical tolerance escalates, the gap between the effective intoxicating dose and the fatal dose is narrowed. Another danger is that barbiturates, alcohol, and many other sedative drugs are cross-tolerant. Therefore, failure to decrease the barbiturate dose when alcohol or another cross-tolerant drug is ingested can have serious consequences. The presence of barbiturates in the body can also alter the intended therapeutic effects of certain other drugs.

Overdosage

Barbiturate overdose produces symptoms that can range from lethargy and slurred speech to cardiovascular collapse, respiratory depression, and coma. Unless the overdosed client is known to the health agency it is often difficult to determine whether the symptoms are caused by barbiturates alone, by other drugs, or by a combination of agents. In any case, there is no known antagonist for barbiturates, so the treatment for overdose is supportive, and depends on the severity of the client's symptoms. Many experts feel that stimulants should *not* be administered to counteract barbiturate intoxication because the central nervous system is then subjected to a double assault, which results in greater instability. The greatest dangers of barbiturate poisoning are circulatory collapse, respiratory insufficiency, and renal failure. Emergency treatment is, therefore, directed at preventing these complications. Intravenous fluids are started in order to maintain cardiovascular function, and plasma expanders and vasopressor drugs are administered, as needed. In the comatose client, an endotracheal tube is inserted and mechanical respiratory assistance is used when necessary.

Gastric lavage may be performed if the drug was ingested recently (within four hours). However, many experts feel that the danger of aspiration in the semicomatose client is too great to warrant gastric lavage. When renal function is still adequate, excretion of the drug can be hastened by alkalizing the urine and by forcing diuresis. When renal function is already impaired, hemodialysis is the most effective method of clearing the drug from the body.

Most clients who overdose on barbiturates do so because they have ingested a single massive dose or because they have taken several cross-tolerant drugs without being aware of the cumulative effects. For treatment purposes, these individuals must be distinguished from those who are chronic, long-term users and are, therefore, physically dependent on high doses of barbiturates. Addicted individuals will experience withdrawal symptoms that can culminate in convulsions and death if the drug is abruptly withdrawn. These individuals should be treated in a safe, medically supervised, drug treatment facility that offers a wide range of supportive services (see Chapter 6).

Despite the potential dangers of barbiturate use, there are a number of legitimate therapeutic indications for these drugs.

ULTRA-SHORT-ACTING BARBITURATES

GENERIC NAME Methohexital sodium (C IV)

TRADE NAME Brevital sodium

CLASSIFICATION Barbiturate anesthetic

Action CNS depressant. Induction dose with 1% solution will provide anesthesia for 5 to 7 minutes.

Indications for Use Induction of anesthesia, anesthetic for short procedures, as a supplement to other anesthetic agents.

Contraindications Known hypersensitivity, severe cardiac disease, hepatic or renal impairment, Addison's disease, myxedema, anemia, asthma, increased intracranial pressure, history of porphyria.

Warnings and Precautions May be habit forming. Use with caution in clients with impaired circulatory, respiratory, endocrine, hepatic, or renal function. Use with caution in pregnancy. Use with extreme caution in status asthmaticus.

Untoward Reactions Circulatory depression, arrhythmias, respiratory depression, bronchospasm, nausea, vomiting, twitching, headache, hiccups, hypotension, rash, sneezing, coughing, hypersensitivity reactions.

Parameters of Use

Absorption Onset of action is 30 to 40 seconds after IV administration.

Crosses placenta.

Distribution Stored in fatty tissues.

Metabolism In the liver.

Excretion By the kidneys.

Drug Interactions An increase in CNS depression occurs with concurrent use of alcohol, other sedatives, narcotics, antihistamines, phenothiazines, disulfiam, MAO inhibitors, procarbazine, and methotrimeprazine. By interfering with absorption and increasing liver enzyme activity barbiturates can decrease the effects of oral anticoagulants, corticosteroids, digitalis glycosides, estrogens, oral contraceptives, griseofulvin, lidocaine, phenytoin, carbamazepine, and methyldopa. Sulfonamides increase the effect of barbiturates by inhibiting protein binding.

Laboratory Interactions May affect Bromsulphalein retention because of accelerated hepatic metabolism and excretion.

Administration 5 to 12 ml (50 to 120 mg) of a 1% solution IV at a rate of 1 ml/5 seconds for induction; then 20 to 40 mg every 4 to 7 minutes for maintenance.

Available Drug Forms Ampules and vials containing 250 or 500 mg of dry powder.

Nursing Management

Planning factors Oxygen and resuscitative equipment should be readily available.

Administration factors

1. Administration must be performed only by qualified anesthetists. Close observation of patient is necessary, since reactions to drug are highly individualistic.
2. Contact with nonvascular tissues can cause necrosis. Intraarterial injection can cause gangrene.
3. Incompatible in solution with lactated Ringer's solution and acid solutions, such as succinylcholine chloride, atropine, and metocurine iodide. Dilute only in sterile water, 5% dextrose, or 0.9% sodium chloride IV solutions.
4. When reconstituted, solution should be clear. If dissolved in sterile water, solution is stable at room temperature for 6 weeks. If dissolved in dextrose or saline, solution is stable at room temperature for 24 hours only.

5. Solution should not contact rubber stoppers or silicone-treated syringes because of incompatibility with silicone.

GENERIC NAME Thiamylal sodium (RX) (C iii)

TRADE NAMES Surital, Thiosceconal

CLASSIFICATION Barbiturate anesthetic

See methohexital sodium for Indications for use, Contraindications, Warnings and precautions, Untoward reactions, Parameters of use, and Drug interactions.

Action CNS depressant.

Administration 3 to 6 ml of a 2.5% solution IV at a rate of 1 ml/5 seconds for induction; then 1 drop/second for maintenance.

Available Drug Forms Ampules and vials containing 1, 5, or 10 g.

Nursing Management Solutions may be stored in refrigerator for 6 days or at room temperature for 24 hours. (See methohexital sodium.)

GENERIC NAME Thiopental sodium (C iii)

TRADE NAMES Intraval, Pentothal

CLASSIFICATION Barbiturate anesthetic

See methohexital sodium for Contraindications, Warnings and precautions, Untoward reactions, Parameters of use, and Drug interactions.

Action CNS depressant.

Indications for Use Control of convulsions following other anesthetics, reducing intracranial pressure during neurosurgical procedures, narcoanalysis and narcosynthesis in psychiatric disorders.

Administration 2 to 3 ml (50 to 75 mg) of a 2.5% solution IV for induction; then use a continuous drip of a 0.2 to 0.4% solution for maintenance or additional IV injections of 25 to 50 mg as necessary.

Available Drug Forms Ampules and vials in a variety of dosages.

Nursing Management (See methohexital sodium.)

1. Reconstituted solutions should be used within 24 hours.
2. After induction of anesthesia, shivering sometimes occurs because of client's increased sensitivity to cold. Client should be warmed with blankets, and room temperature should be maintained at 72 F.

SHORT-ACTING BARBITURATES

GENERIC NAME Pentobarbital sodium (RX)

TRADE NAMES Nebralin, Nembutal, Pental

CLASSIFICATION Barbiturate sedative and hypnotic

See methohexital sodium for Contraindications, Warnings and precautions, Untoward reactions, Parameters of use, and Drug interactions.

Action CNS depressant. Onset of action is 15 to 30 minutes after oral administration. Duration of action is up to 4 hours.

Indications for Use Sedation, hypnosis, preanesthesia, acute convulsive states.

Administration

- *Sedation:* Adults: 30 mg po tid or qid.
- *Hypnosis:* Adults: 100 to 500 mg IV; 150 to 200 mg IM; 120 to 200 mg rectally.

Dosage is individually adjusted according to age, weight, general condition, and purpose of administration.

Available Drug Forms Elixir (5 ml unit dose) in pint and gallon bottles (20 mg/5 ml); capsules containing 30, 50, or 100 mg in bottles and unit-dose packages; tablets containing 100 mg; 2-ml ampules; vials of 20 or 50 ml; suppositories containing 30, 60, 120, or 200 mg.

Nursing Management

Planning factors

1. Client should be warned that mental and/or physical abilities may be impaired for a 24-hour period following dosage.
2. Oxygen and resuscitative equipment should be readily available when drug is administered IV.

Administration factors

1. Parenteral solutions should be clear
2. Extravasation and intraarterial administration must be avoided, since tissue necrosis can result.
3. When administering IM, inject into large muscle mass with no more than 5 ml delivered to a site.

Evaluation factors

1. Since reactions to drug are highly individualistic, clients should be assessed carefully for adverse effects.
2. Vital signs should be monitored every 3 to 5 minutes when drug is administered IV.

3. Some clients, particularly the elderly, may become restless and irritable after administration; appropriate precautions, including bedrails, should be instituted.

Client teaching factors

1. Client should be aware that prolonged use can lead to physical and psychologic dependence.
2. Drug must be stored in a safe place that is not accessible to children.
3. Clients on prolonged therapy must be cautioned against discontinuing the drug abruptly, since withdrawal symptoms can be life threatening.

GENERIC NAME Secobarbital sodium (RX) (C iii)

TRADE NAME Seconal

CLASSIFICATION Barbiturate sedative and hypnotic

See methohexital sodium for Contraindications, Warnings and precautions, Untoward reactions, Parameters of use, and Drug interactions.

Action CNS depressant. Duration of action is up to 4 hours.

Indications for Use Sedation, hypnosis, preanesthesia, acute convulsive states.

Administration

- *Sedation:* Adults: 30 to 50 mg po tid.
- *Hypnosis:* Adults: 100 to 200 mg IV (up to 250 mg); 50 to 150 mg IM; 150 to 250 mg rectally.

Dosages are adjusted for children according to age and body weight.

Available Drug Forms Elixir in 16-oz bottles (22 mg/5 ml); capsules containing 30, 50, or 100 mg in bottles and unit-dose packages; tablets containing 100 mg; 20-ml ampules (50 mg/ml); suppositories containing 30, 60, 120, or 200 mg.

Nursing Management (See pentobarbital sodium.)

1. Ampules and suppositories must be refrigerated.
2. Aqueous solution must be used within 30 minutes after container is opened. Solution is mixed by rotating vial; do not shake. Solution should be clear.

INTERMEDIATE-ACTING BARBITURATES

GENERIC NAME Amobarbital sodium (C iii)

TRADE NAMES Amytal, Tuinal

CLASSIFICATION Barbiturate sedative and hypnotic

See methohexital sodium for Contraindications, Warnings and precautions, Untoward reactions, Parameters of use, and Drug interactions.

Action CNS depressant. Duration of action is up to 8 hours.

Indications for Use Sedation, relief of anxiety, hypnosis, acute convulsive states, narcoanalysis and narcotherapy in psychiatric disorders.

Administration Oral: 30 to 50 mg tid or 65 to 200 mg in one dose; Maximum dosage: 1 g in adults. Intramuscular: 65 to 500 mg (10 to 20% solution); Maximum dosage: 0.5 g in adults. Intravenous: 1 ml/min. of a 10% solution; must not exceed 1 ml/min.

Available Drug Forms Elixir in 16-oz bottles; capsules containing 65 or 200 mg in bottles and unit-dose packages; tablets containing 15, 30, 50, or 100 mg. Ampules containing 125, 250, or 500 mg of dry powder; dissolve in sterile water; may dissolve slowly.

Nursing Management Aqueous solution must be used within 30 minutes after container is opened. Solution is mixed by rotating vial; do not shake. Solution should be clear. (See pentobarbital sodium.)

GENERIC NAME Aprobarbital (C iii)

TRADE NAME Alurate

CLASSIFICATION Barbiturate sedative and hypnotic

See methohexital sodium for Contraindications, Warnings and precautions, Untoward reactions, Parameters of use, and Drug interactions. See pentobarbital sodium for Nursing management.

Action CNS depressant. Duration of action is up to 8 hours.

Indications for Use Sedation, insomnia.

Administration Adults: 5 ml (40 mg) po tid, 5 to 20 ml hs for sedation or insomnia.

Available Drug Forms Elixir in 16-oz and gallon bottles (40 mg/5 ml).

GENERIC NAME Butabarbital sodium (RX) (C iii)

TRADE NAMES Butisol, Butal, Buticaps, Sarisol

CLASSIFICATION Barbiturate sedative and hypnotic

See methohexital sodium for Contraindications, Warnings and precautions, Untoward reactions, Parameters of use, and Drug interactions. See pentobarbital sodium for Nursing management.

Action CNS depressant. Duration of action is 5 to 8 hours.

Indications for Use Sedation, hypnosis.

Administration

- *Sedation:* Adults: 15 to 30 mg po tid or qid; 50 to 100 mg preoperatively.
- *Hypnosis:* Adults: 50 to 100 mg hs.

Available Drug Forms Elixir in pint and gallon bottles (30 mg/5 ml); capsules and tablets containing 15, 30, 50, or 100 mg.

LONG-ACTING BARBITURATES

GENERIC NAME Mephobarbital (C IV)

TRADE NAME Mebaral

CLASSIFICATION Barbiturate sedative

See methohexital sodium for Contraindications, Warnings and precautions, Untoward reactions, Parameters of use, and Drug interactions.

Action Duration of action is 10 hours or more.

Indications for Use Sedation, acute convulsive states (epilepsy).

Administration

- *Sedation:* Adults: 50 mg po tid or qid; Children: 16 to 32 mg po tid or qid.

Available Drug Forms Tablets containing 32, 50, 100, or 200 mg.

Nursing Management (See pentobarbital sodium.)

1. Does not generally cause clouding of mental faculties.
2. Possibility of cumulative drug action increases with the long-acting barbiturates. Client should be instructed to be alert for adverse reactions.
3. Drug should not be withdrawn abruptly, but tapered over a period of 1 to 2 weeks.

GENERIC NAMES Phenobarbital; phenobarbital sodium

TRADE NAMES Eskabarb, Luminal, Solfoton; Sodium Luminal (C IV)

CLASSIFICATION Barbiturate sedative and hypnotic

See methohexital sodium for Contraindications, Warnings and precautions, Untoward reactions, Parameters of use, and Drug interactions.

Action CNS depressant. Onset of action is 10 to 60 minutes and duration of action is 10 to 16 hours. Lowers bilirubin by stimulating production of glucuronyl transferase.

Indications for Use Sedation, hypnosis, acute convulsive states, neonatal hyperbilirubinemia.

Administration

- *Sedation:* Adults: 15 to 120 mg po bid or tid; Children: 15 to 50 mg po
- *Hypnosis:* Adults: 100 to 320 mg po daily; 100 to 300 mg IM or IV daily. Children: 2 to 5 mg/kg IM or IV; 2 to 3 mg/kg rectally bid or tid.

Available Drug Forms Elixir containing 20 mg/5 ml; capsules (prolonged action) containing 65 or 100 mg; tablets containing 8, 16, 32, 65, or 100 mg. Vials containing dry powder must be reconstituted with sterile water. Solution should be clear; stable for 2 days.

Nursing Management (See pentobarbital sodium and mephobarbital.)

Administration factors

1. Drowsiness may occur during early weeks of treatment.
2. Elderly patients may exhibit restlessness or excitability.
3. When administering IV, dose should not exceed 60 mg/min.
4. When administering IM, inject into large muscle mass with no more than 5 ml delivered to a site.

Evaluation factors

1. Long-term treatment may cause blood dyscrasias. Be alert for signs of infection or bleeding.
2. Hepatic function tests and blood counts should be done routinely for clients on prolonged therapy.

BARBITURATE COMBINATION PREPARATIONS

TRADE NAME Antrocol (RX)

CLASSIFICATION Anticholinergic

Indications for Use Peptic ulcer, GI disturbances.

Warnings and Precautions May be habit forming. Do not use in glaucoma. Use with caution in clients who have a history of prostatic hypertrophy.

Untoward Reactions May induce flushing, dry mouth, tachycardia, or urinary retention.

Administration 2 to 8 tablets or capsules po daily.

Available Drug Forms Generic contents in each tablet or capsule: atropine sulfate: 0.195 mg; phenobarbital: 16 mg.

TRADE NAME Arco-Lase Plus (RX)

CLASSIFICATION Anticholinergic

Indications for Use Peptic ulcer, GI disturbances.

Warnings and Precautions May be habit forming. Do not use in clients who have a history of glaucoma or prostatic hypertrophy.

Untoward Reactions May induce dry mouth, tachycardia, or blurred vision.

Administration 1 tablet po pc.

Available Drug Forms Generic contents in each tablet: amylolytic enzyme: 30 mg; proteolytic enzyme: 6 mg; cellulolytic enzyme: 2 mg; lipase: 25 mg; hyoscyamine sulfate: 0.1 mg; atropine sulfate: 0.02 mg; phenobarbital: 7.5 mg.

TRADE NAMES Bellermine-O.D.; Bellergal-S (RX)

CLASSIFICATION Anticholinergic

Indications for Use Management of disorders characterized by nervous tension and exaggerated autonomic response.

Contraindications History of peripheral vascular disease, coronary heart disease, impaired renal or hepatic function, or glaucoma; porphyria; pregnancy and lactation.

Warnings and Precautions May be habit forming.

Untoward Reactions May induce tingling in the extremities, dry mouth, tachycardia, blurred vision, urinary retention, decreased sweating, or flushing.

Drug Interactions Do not give concurrently with dopamine, since hypertension will occur. Additive effects occur if taken with other CNS depressants, alcohol, or sedatives. Phenobarbital content may lower plasma levels of dicumarol. Concomitant administration of tricyclic antidepressants may result in additive anticholinergic effects.

Administration 1 tablet po A.M., 1 tablet po at noon, and 2 tablets po hs.

Available Drug Forms Generic contents in each capsule or tablet: phenobarbital: 40 mg; ergotamine tartrate: 0.6 mg; belladonna alkaloids: 0.2 mg; Bellergal-S also contains FD&C No. 5 yellow.

TRADE NAME Bentyl with Phenobarbital (RX)

CLASSIFICATION Anticholinergic

Indications for Use Possibly effective in the treatment of irritable bowel syndrome and acute enterocolitis.

Contraindications History of obstructive uropathy, paralytic ileus, severe ulcerative colitis, or myasthenia gravis.

Warnings and Precautions May be habit forming. Use with caution in clients who have a history of glaucoma, prostatic hypertrophy, autonomic neuropathy, hyperthyroidism, or cardiac disease.

Untoward Reactions May induce urinary hesitancy, tachycardia, blurred vision, drowsiness, headache, nausea, or urticaria.

Drug Interactions Additive effects occur if taken with other CNS depressants, alcohol, or tranquilizers.

Administration 1 capsule po tid or qid.

Available Drug Forms Generic contents in each capsule: dicyclomine hydrochloride: 10, 20 mg; phenobarbital: 15 mg.

Nursing Management Caution client that heat prostration can occur in warm climates.

TRADE NAME Cantil with Phenobarbital (RX)

CLASSIFICATION Anticholinergic

Indications for Use Peptic ulcer.

Contraindications History of obstructive uropathy, paralytic ileus, severe ulcerative colitis, or myasthenia gravis; lactation.

Warnings and Precautions May be habit forming. Use with caution in clients who have a history of renal or hepatic disease, autonomic neuropathy, mild ulcerative colitis, glaucoma, hyperthyroidism, or cardiac disease.

Untoward Reactions May induce tachycardia, blurred vision, decreased sweating, urinary retention, drowsiness, headache, nausea, or urticaria.

Drug Interactions Additive effects occur if taken with other anticholinergic drugs.

Administration 1 to 2 tablets po qid with meals and hs.

Available Drug Forms Generic contents in each yellow tablet: mepenzolate bromide: 25 mg; phenobarbital: 16 mg. Also contains FD&C No. 5 yellow.

Nursing Management Caution client that heat prostration can occur in warm climates.

TRADE NAME Chardonna-2 (C IV)

CLASSIFICATION Anticholinergic

Indications for Use Possibly effective in the treatment of irritable bowel syndrome.

Contraindications History of glaucoma, prostatic hypertrophy, or porphyria.

Warnings and Precautions May be habit forming. Use with caution in clients who have a history of hepatic or renal disease.

Untoward Reactions May induce tachycardia, dry mouth, blurred vision, vertigo, flushing, drowsiness, headache, nausea, vomiting, or skin eruptions.

Drug Interactions Additive effects occur if taken with other CNS depressants, alcohol, or sedatives.

Administration 1 to 2 tablets po qid, given 30 minutes before meals and hs.

Available Drug Forms Generic contents in each tablet: belladonna extract: 15 mg; phenobarbital: 15 mg.

TRADE NAME Isordil with Phenobarbital (C IV)

CLASSIFICATION Antianginal

Indications for Use Possibly effective in the treatment of angina pectoris.

Warnings and Precautions May be habit forming. Tolerance to this and other nitrates and nitrites may occur.

Untoward Reactions May induce flushing, headache, dizziness, nausea, vomiting, or drug rash.

Drug Interactions Alcohol may enhance the hypotensive effects of this drug. Can act as a physiologic antagonist to norepinephrine, acetylcholine, and histamine.

Administration 1 tablet po qid before meals and hs.

Available Drug Forms Generic contents in each orange scored tablet: isosorbide dinitrate: 10 mg; phenobarbital: 15 mg.

TRADE NAME Phazyme-PB (RX)

CLASSIFICATION Antiflatulent

Indications for Use Relief of gas pain associated with anxiety, as seen in aerophagia, postoperative distention, dyspepsia, and food intolerance.

Warnings and Precautions May be habit forming.

Untoward Reactions May induce drowsiness.

Administration 1 to 2 tablets po qid with meals and hs.

Available Drug Forms Generic contents in each yellow-coated, two-phase tablet: Outer-layer (releases in the stomach): simethicone: 20 mg; phenobarbital: 15 mg. Enteric-coated core (releases in the small intestine): simethicone: 40 mg; protease: 3000 U.S.P. units; lipase: 240 U.S.P. units; amylase: 2000 U.S.P. units.

TRADE NAME Pro-Banthine with Phenobarbital

CLASSIFICATION Anticholinergic (RX)

Indications for Use Possibly effective as adjunctive therapy in the treatment of peptic ulcer and irritable bowel syndrome.

Contraindications History of glaucoma, obstructive uropathy, paralytic ileus, severe ulcerative colitis, or myasthenia gravis.

Warnings and Precautions May be habit forming. Use with caution in clients who have a history of autonomic neuropathy, hepatic, cardiac, or renal disease, hyperthyroidism, or hypertension.

Untoward Reactions May induce tachycardia, dry mouth, blurred vision, drowsiness, headache, urticaria, or GI disturbances.

Drug Interactions Concurrent use of Pro-Banthine with slow-dissolving tablets of digoxin may cause increased serum digoxin levels. Additive effects occur if taken with other anticholinergic drugs or belladonna alkaloids.

Administration 1 tablet po 30 minutes before each meal and 2 tablets po hs.

Available Drug Forms Generic contents in each tablet: propantheline bromide: 15 mg; phenobarbital: 15 mg.

Nursing Management Caution client that heat prostration can occur in warm climates.

TRADE NAME Pyridium Plus (RX)

CLASSIFICATION Antispasmodic

Indications for Use Relief of pain associated with irritation of the lower urinary tract mucosa.

Warnings and Precautions May be habit forming. Do not give to clients who have a history of glaucoma, renal or hepatic insufficiency, or porphyria.

Untoward Reactions May induce methemoglobinemia, hemolytic anemia, and renal and hepatic toxicity; may also induce dry mouth, blurred vision, drowsiness, or GI disturbances.

Administration 1 tablet po pc and hs.

Available Drug Forms Generic contents in each dark maroon tablet: phenazopyridine hydrochloride: 150 mg; hyoscyamine hydrobromide: 0.3 mg; butabarbital: 15 mg.

Nursing Management

1. Inform client that urine will turn a reddish orange.
2. Discontinue use if a yellowish tinge appears in the skin or sclera.

TRADE NAME Valpin 50-PB (RX)

CLASSIFICATION Anticholinergic

Indications for Use Possibly effective as adjunctive therapy in the treatment of peptic ulcer and irritable or neurologic bowel disorders.

Contraindications History of glaucoma, obstructive uropathy, paralytic ileus, severe ulcerative colitis, myasthenia gravis, or porphyria.

Warnings and Precautions May be habit forming. Use with caution in clients who have a history of autonomic neuropathy, hepatic, cardiac, or renal disease, hyperthyroidism, or hypertension.

Untoward Reactions May induce tachycardia, blurred vision, urinary retention, drowsiness, headache, excitement, GI disturbances, or drug rash.

Drug Interactions Phenobarbital may decrease the prothrombin time response to oral anticoagulants. Additive effects occur if taken with other anticholinergic drugs.

Administration 1 tablet po tid.

Available Drug Forms Generic contents in each white scored tablet: anisotropine methylbromide: 50 mg; phenobarbital: 15 mg.

Nursing Management Caution client that heat prostration can occur in warm climates.

TRADE NAME WANS #1, #2 (C iii)

CLASSIFICATION Antiemetic

Indications for Use Relief of nausea and vomiting.

Contraindications Pregnancy and lactation; infants under 6 months; clients with a history of drug dependence or suicidal tendencies; history of porphyria or CNS injury.

Warnings and Precautions May be habit forming. There is some suspicion that central-acting antiemetics in combination with viral illnesses may contribute to the development of Reye's syndrome. Use with caution in clients who have a history of hepatic disease, fever, diabetes, hyperthyroidism, severe anemia, or congestive heart failure.

Untoward Reactions May induce tachycardia, dry mouth, blurred vision, drowsiness, urinary retention, GI disturbances, vertigo, tinnitus, or drug rash.

Drug Interactions Do not give with MAO inhibitors. Additive effects occur if taken with other CNS depressants, alcohol, or tranquilizers.

Administration Adults: No. 1 and No. 2: 1 suppository rectally every 4 to 6 hours, as needed; Maximum dosage: 4 doses. Children: Ages 6 months to 2 years: $\frac{1}{2}$ suppository rectally every 6 to 8 hours, as needed; Ages 2 to 12 years: 1 suppository rectally every 6 to 8 hours, as needed; Maximum dosage: 3 doses.

Available Drug Forms Generic contents in each blue suppository for children: pyrilamine maleate: 25 mg; pentobarbital sodium: 30 mg. Generic contents in each pink No. 1 suppository: pyrilamine maleate: 50 mg; pentobarbital sodium: 50 mg. Generic contents in each yellow No. 2 suppository: pyrilamine maleate: 50 mg; pentobarbital sodium: 100 mg. Also contains FD&C No. 5 yellow.

Chapter 30

Anticonvulsants

SEIZURE DISORDERS ARE characterized by a temporary disturbance in the normal brain waves, which may or may not result in overt-chemical signs. Seizure disorders are a major health problem, since they occur in nearly 1% of the population. Involuntary contractions of muscles, called *convulsions,* are a symptom of seizure disorders. Any sudden or severe alteration (brain injury, infection) in the brain's metabolism may precipitate a convulsion. Common causes of convulsions include temperatures above 105 F, particularly in children (febrile convulsion), hypoxia, intracranial hemorrhage, severe electrolyte disturbances (tetany), infections (meningitis), eclampsia, certain poisons (strychnine, organophosphorus insecticides), and excessive doses of certain drugs (amphetamines, MAO inhibitors, antihistamines). Convulsions are a symptom in several types of *epilepsy,* a seizure disorder that is characterized by brief alterations in consciousness as a result of excessive paroxysmal neuron activity in the brain. Unfortunately, the cause of epilepsy is unknown or idiopathic in most adult epileptics; however, it may be due to minute brain lesions or metabolic disturbances that are inborn or induced by trauma. Brain tumors or defects may precipitate epilepsy in some clients. The clinical signs and symptoms of epilepsy vary according to the location of neuron discharge and how the electrical activity spreads across the brain.

TYPES OF SEIZURE

Historically seizures were classified into three groups: grand mal, petit mal, and psychomotor. Table 30-1 describes the characteristics of these types of seizures. However, seizure disorders are not as distinct as this classification indicates.

Status epilepticus is the term used for grand mal seizures that occur consecutively without a return to consciousness. Clients with this condition require immediate attention to maintain the function of vital organs. Diazepam IV is considered the drug of choice, but IV phenobarbital, phenytoin, or paraldehyde can be used.

Some types of seizure disorders originate in one part of the brain and usually remain localized. These are called *focal seizures* and are characterized by twitching or contractions in specific muscles, which may or may not spread to other muscles. *Jacksonian* seizures are focal seizures characterized by twitching in specific muscle groups, usually in one extremity, and tend to spread over only one side of the body. Occasionally, jacksonian seizures develop into a grand mal seizure involving both sides of the body.

Petit mal seizures are subdivided into *absence* and *complex* petit mal seizures. Absence refers to a very brief (2 to 15 minutes) sensory clouding or loss of consciousness that is accompanied by specific electroencephalogram (EEG) activity and no other clinical symptoms. Complex seizures are accompanied by muscular twitching or other symptoms.

Since paroxysmal disturbances in the temporal lobe of the brain cause the signs and symptoms of psychomotor seizures, the term *temporal lobe seizure* is sometimes used.

Clients manifesting symptoms of more than one seizure disorder are said to have a *mixed seizure disorder.*

The newest international classification of epilepsy groups seizure disorders into broad categories, which are further subdivided according to the area of the brain involved. *Generalized seizures* refer to disorders that affect the brain bilaterally and symmetrically. These seizures are characterized by motor disturbances or changes in consciousness and include grand mal and petit mal seizures. Focal and psychomotor seizures are grouped under *partial seizures,* since they are localized.

ANTICONVULSANT THERAPY

The nature of seizure disorders is complex and as yet there is no specific agent that will cure these disorders. Occasionally, surgical excision of a brain tumor or defect will effect a cure; but more often the seizure must be treated symptomatically. Anticonvulsants can cause central nervous system depression, increase the seizure threshold, and/or prevent the spread of seizure discharges to other parts of the brain.

When a physiologic reason for the convulsion can be identified, the appropriate corrective measures are instituted. For example, tepid baths and aspirin are given to prevent febrile convulsions; appropriate antibiotics are administered for meningitis; antidotes are given for poisoning; and careful administration of IV drugs, such as norepinephrine (levarterenol), will prevent drug-induced convulsions.

TABLE 30-1 Characteristics of Seizures

Type	Loss of Consciousness	Muscular Activity	Other
Grand mal	Unconscious: 2 to 5 minutes	Tonic-clonic contractions	Often preceded by an aura (lights flashing, auditory sounds); collapse to the ground if upright; urinary and fecal incontinence
Petit mal (onset in childhood)	Unconscious: 5 to 30 seconds (may only be 2 to 5 seconds)	Usually absent; may have facial, eye, or general twitching of muscles	Apparent inattentiveness
Psychomotor	Mental clouding or confusion: 1 to 2 minutes	Repetitive, meaningless limb movements; grimacing; bizarre behavior; utterances	Apparent mood alterations followed by forgetfulness

Salts of hydrochloric acid are collectively called *bromides* and they depress the motor cortex and reflexes. These substances are rapidly absorbed and their excretion is relatively prolonged though the kidneys begin to eliminate them immediately. Bromides have been used as anticonvulsants since the middle of the 19th century, but are seldom used today. These substances have been used as sedatives to control grand mal, myoclonic, and poison-induced seizures and for Sydenham's chorea and motion sickness.

Barbiturates, particularly phenobarbital, were found to have anticonvulsant properties and were the drug of choice during the beginning of the 20th century. These agents are effective in controlling grand mal seizures but they cause sedation, and tolerance can develop. The quest for an anticonvulsant that controls seizure activity without causing sedation culminated in the introduction of *phenytoin* in 1938. This hydantoin derivative is the most widely used anticonvulsant. Today, there are numerous nonsedative anticonvulsants available, each of which is used to treat specific seizure disorders (see Table 30-2).

Each type of seizure disorder responds differently to the various classes of anticonvulsants. Barbiturates, analogs of barbiturates, and hydantoin derivatives are effective for grand mal, focal, and other generalized seizure disorders. Valproic acid, succinimides, and oxazolidinedione derivatives are effective for petit mal seizures. Psychomotor seizures can be controlled with hydantoin derivatives, phenobarbital, and primidone. Mixed seizures may require a combination of the appropriate anticonvulsants and may be difficult to treat as many of these drugs interact and alter each other's therapeutic serum drug levels.

CONTROLLING SEIZURE ACTIVITY

Anticonvulsants are administered daily to control the frequency, severity, and duration of seizure activity. The objective is to maintain a serum drug level high enough to prevent seizure activity but low enough to prevent drug toxicity. The range of therapeutic serum drug levels is relatively narrow for some anticonvulsants—for

TABLE 30-2 Drug of Choice for Treating Seizure Disorders

Seizure Disorder	Anticonvulsant Used in Emergencies
Eclampsia	Magnesium Sulfate IV
Status epilepticus	Diazepam IV
Febrile poisoning or drug-induced convulsions	Diazepam or phenobarbital IV
Head injury-induced convulsions	Phenytoin IV

example, phenytoin 10 to 20 mcg/ml. Drug dosage is highly individualized and numerous factors can cause marked fluctuations in serum drug levels. Most anticonvulsants are metabolized in the liver and the rate of metabolism can vary widely from client to client. Furthermore, clients with hepatic impairment or a low metabolic rate may rapidly develop drug toxicity. The potential for drug toxicity can also be increased by agents that displace phenytoin and some other anticonvulsants from their protein-binding sites. In addition, clients with renal impairment may excrete the drug slower than expected. Consequently, treatment is initiated at a low dosage and the client is assessed until a steady-state drug level is achieved. The dosage is then gradually increased over the next few weeks while the client is monitored for seizure control drug toxicity. Occasionally, seizures persist despite high dosages and so a second anticonvulsant is progressively introduced (phenytoin and phenobarbital).

Client compliance in maintaining the dosage schedule is essential because loss of seizure control can occur if serum drug levels drop and abrupt drug withdrawal can precipitate severe seizure activity. As these drugs are often taken for very long periods or as lifelong therapy, clients need to be involved in the development of a drug schedule that he or she can adhere to. Alterations in diet and the use of OTC preparations by the client must also be considered. There is some evidence to indicate that mild dehydration and acidosis decrease grand mal seizure activity. Therefore, the client needs to be cautioned against the excessive ingestion of water. The client should also be warned about factors that may precipitate seizure activity with certain anticonvulsants, including ingestion of alcohol, folic acid supplements, and some OTC drugs. Explanations about these factors may assist in obtaining client compliance.

BIRTH DEFECTS AND OTHER SEVERE UNTOWARD REACTIONS

The long-term use of most anticonvulsants can cause severe, even fatal, untoward reactions. Blood dyscrasias, hepatic impairment, and certain skin reactions have been fatal. Periodic monitoring of laboratory tests and clinical status are essential every 1 to 6 months.

Case-controlled studies have shown a higher than expected incidence of birth defects in infants whose mothers received anticonvulsants, particularly phenytoin and phenobarbital, during pregnancy. Cleft lip or palate, heart malformations, and retardation have been reported. Anticonvulsants cross the placenta and fetal serum drug levels may be the same as the mother's. However, a cause-and-effect relationship has not been proven. Birth defects may be inborn or the result of other factors characteristic of epileptics. The risk of withdrawing anticonvulsant therapy during pregnancy may be fatal as grand mal seizures may cause hypoxia in the fetus. Factual information can be given to the client so that she can participate in the decision whether to continue the anticonvulsant during pregnancy.

Neonatal coagulation defects resembling those of vitamin K deficiency have been reported in newborns of mothers who received certain anticonvulsant drugs during pregnancy. Vitamin K_1 supplements during the last month of pregnancy and the administration of the vitamin to the newborn after delivery is usually effective in correcting these defects.

Although the newer anticonvulsant drugs are effective without producing sedation, central nervous system depression can occur, particularly with large doses. Clients may develop drowsiness, malaise, fatigue, dizziness, slurred speech, ataxia, and respiratory depression. Visual disturbances are known to occur with hydantoin and oxazolidinedione derivatives and the succinimide derivatives can cause behavioral changes ranging from night terrors and mild depression to frank psychosis and suicidal tendencies. Clients receiving anticonvulsants should be warned against engaging in activities that require constant attention, such as driving a car. Resumption of activities, such as the operation of heavy equipment, should be discussed with the physician.

DURATION OF THERAPY

Many clients with seizure disorders must remain on anticonvulsant therapy for the rest of their lives. Clients who are well controlled on anticonvulsants and have been seizure free for one to three years may be gradually tapered off the drug, and remain seizure free. Clients with seizures induced by head trauma may only require two or three years of drug therapy whereas clients who have status epilepticus may require lifelong drug therapy. Some children with petit mal disorders, particularly absence, may become seizure free in adulthood. However, many clients with psychomotor and mixed seizure disorders may require lifelong therapy. The nurse needs to emphasize the client's need for the drug, the importance of regular laboratory and medical checkups, and the necessity for prompt treatment of untoward reactions, so that the client can lead a normal, productive life.

HYDANTOIN DERIVATIVES

GENERIC NAMES Phenytoin; phenytoin sodium

TRADE NAMES Dihycon, Dilantin, Diphentoin, Ekko; Dilantin Sodium

CLASSIFICATION Anticonvulsant (RX)

Action Although chemically related to the barbiturates, phenytoin has little or no sedative effect, but is very effective in controlling grand mal seizures. Phenytoin inhibits the spread of seizure activity in the motor cortex. The exact mechanism of action is unknown, but phenytoin is thought to promote the loss of sodium from neurons and thereby tends to stabilize the threshold against hyperexcitability. The maximal activity of the brain stem centers responsible for the tonic phase of grand mal seizures is reduced. Because phenytoin decreases myocardial contractility and ventricular automaticity it has been used to treat ectopic arrhythmias.

Indications for Use Status epilepticus (often in combination with other anticonvulsants); grand mal seizures (generalized tonic-clonic seizures); psychomotor seizures (temporal lobe); prevention and control of seizures induced by neurosurgery or head trauma. Has been used to treat Reye's syndrome, arrhythmias, and certain types of migraine headache.

Contraindications Hypersensitivity to hydantoin derivatives, sinus bradycardia, S-A block, 2nd and 3rd degree heart block, Adams-Stokes syndrome.

Warnings and Precautions Use with caution in clients with hypotension, severe myocardial insufficiency, acute heart failure, impaired hepatic or renal function, diabetes (since plasma glucose levels may be altered), and the elderly. Not intended for use in seizure due to hyperglycemia or other types of easily identified and corrected seizure activity. Not effective for petit mal (absence) seizures, but has been used in combination with other anticonvulsant drugs. Safe use during pregnancy has not been established; may cause birth defects.

Untoward Reactions Toxicity can occur with IV drug administration or ingestion of an overdose. The most common symptoms include hypotension that progresses to cardiovascular collapse; life-threatening arrhythmias, including ventricular fibrillation and depressed A-V conduction; and CNS depression that may induce ataxia, drowsiness, and nystagmus. Vertigo, circumoral tingling, and nausea have occurred. Death may result from respiratory depression or apnea. Supportive treatment is given since there is no antidote. Dialysis is of some value. Gingival hyperplasia, nausea, and vomiting are common. Gum overgrowth is irreversible and occurs most frequently in children. Although the gum condition may be annoying, the drug is usually continued. Meticulous oral hygiene may prevent further gum overgrowth. Neonatal hemorrhage can be prevented or minimized if the pregnant woman receives prophylactic vitamin K_1 for 1 month prior to and during delivery. The neonate should also receive vitamin K_1 if necessary. Hepatic dysfunction may occur, particularly in the elderly and clients who are critically ill. Toxic hepatitis has been reported. Allergic skin reactions can occur, particularly exfoliative dermatitis. Purpuric or bullous dermatitis, lupus erythematosus, and Stevens-Johnson syndrome have occurred. The drug should be discontinued promptly. Blood dyscrasias, including agranulocytosis, thrombocytopenia, and leukopenia have occurred and usually respond to folic acid supplements. Lymphadenopathy, pseudolymphoma, lymphoma, and Hodgkin's disease have been reported. Osteomalacia has been reported and may be due to phenytoin's interference with vitamin D metabolism. CNS disturbances, including dizziness, insomnia, transient nervousness, twitching, and headache, have occurred. Chorea, dystonia, tremor, and asterixis have been reported, but rarely. Local irritation and pain may occur at injection sites.

Parameters of Use

Absorption Slowly absorbed from GI tract; absorption may vary with the drug dosage, form, and manufacturer. Slow and erratic absorption from IM sites due to drug precipitation; IM injections are avoided. Onset of action is 3 to 5 minutes after IV administration. Peak plasma levels occur in 3 to 12 hours. Therapeutic plasma concentration is 10 to 20 mcg/ml; steady-state therapeutic levels may take 7 to 10 days of therapy. Half-life is 22 hours (ranges from 7 to 42 hours), but varies greatly due to hepatic metabolism. About 70 to 95% bound to plasma proteins, but may be displaced or cause displacement of other drugs from protein-binding sites.

Crosses placenta; risk of birth defects is often outweighed by risk of convulsion. Enters breast milk; lactating mothers should bottle-feed their babies. Crosses blood-brain barrier.

Metabolism By saturable liver enzyme system; hypermetabolizers may have low serum drug levels. Excessive serum drug levels may be induced by hepatic disorders, congenital enzyme deficiencies, or drug interactions.

Excretion Inactive metabolites enter bile, are reabsorbed, and then excreted by the kidneys, primarily by tubular excretion. About 5% excreted as unchanged drug. Severe renal impairment may cause retention of drugs or metabolites.

Drug Interactions There are numerous drug interactions reported for phenytoin, primarily because of the drug's high plasma protein binding and its method of metabolism and excretion. Clients should be monitored carefully for phenytoin toxicity. Drugs that may displace phenytoin from its protein-binding sites include salicylates, sulfonamides, phenothiazines, phenylbutazone, and phenyramidol. Drugs that inhibit the metabolism of phenytoin by the liver include oral anticoagulants, oral contraceptives, aminosalicylic acid, chloramphenicol, disulfiram (antabuse), and isoniazid. Phenytoin decreases the body's supply of folic acid and the two substances are antagonistic. Supplemental use of folic acid may decrease the anticonvulsant action of phenytoin. Phenytoin and other anticonvulsants interact with barbiturates. Concurrent therapy has an additive CNS depressant effect. Barbiturates tend to alter the hepatic metabolism and excretion of phenytoin. Tricyclic antidepressants may induce seizure activity if administered in high dosages. The ingestion of alcohol increases the hepatic metabolism of phenytoin and may induce seizure activity. Phenytoin and lidocaine have additive cardiac depressant effects; however, phenytoin may decrease the action of lidocaine through enzyme induction.

Laboratory Interactions May interfere with metyrapone and dexamethasone tests and cause a decrease in serum levels of protein-bound iodine; the T_3 test remains normal. Serum glucose, alkaline phosphatase, and gamma glutamyl transpeptidase may be elevated.

Administration Highly individualized to provide maximum benefit and maintain therapeutic serum drug levels. Adults: Initial dosage: 100 mg po tid; then increase to 200 mg po tid after 7 to 10 days. Children: Initial dosage: 5 mg/kg/day in 2 or 3 divided doses; then increase as necessary after 7 to 10 days; Usual dosage range: 4 to 8 mg/kg/day; Maximum dosage: 300 mg/day.

- *Status epilepticus:* Adults: 150 to 250 mg slowly via IV bolus initially; then 100 to 150 mg via IV bolus in 30 minutes if necessary; Usual dosage: 15 mg/kg. Children: 250 mg/m^2 of body surface.
- *Prophylaxis during neurosurgery:* 100 to 200 mg IM q4h during surgery and postoperatively.
- *Arrhythmias:* Initial dosage: 125 to 250 mg via IV bolus over 3 to 5 minutes if necessary; Maintenance dosage: 100 mg po bid, tid, or qid.

Available Drug Forms Capsules containing 100 or 300 mg; 300-mg capsules are reserved for noncompliant clients who are willing to take 300 mg daily, but forget to take 100 mg tid. Suspension (Dilantin-125) containing 125 mg/5 ml; pediatric suspension (Dilantin-30) containing 30 mg/5 ml. Chewable tablets (Infatabs) containing 50 mg; yield higher serum drug levels than capsules; switch dosage form with caution. 2-ml ampules of ready-mixed solution containing 50 mg/ml; 2-ml prefilled syringes of ready-mixed solution containing 50 mg/ml; 5-ml ampules of ready-mixed solution containing 50 mg/ml. Capsules containing 100 mg phenytoin and 16 mg phenobarbital; capsules containing 100 mg phenytoin and 32 mg phenobarbital.

Nursing Management

Planning factors

1. Obtain history of seizure disorder. A neurologic flowchart can be helpful. Institute seizure precautions when necessary.
2. Baseline data on vital signs, cardiac status, hepatic (blood urea nitrogen), and renal (creatinine) function should be obtained.
3. Obtain history of cardiac, hepatic, and renal disorders. Notify physician as indicated.
4. When administering IV, have oxygen and vasopressors readily available.
5. Store drug at room temperature away from moisture. Discard all parenteral solutions that are cloudy or have a precipitate. If a faint yellow color occurs, the solution can be used (does not affect potency).

Administration factors

1. Administer oral preparations with 4 fl oz of water or more.
2. Avoid administering oral preparations with other drugs or food. If GI irritation occurs, phenytoin can be given 30 minutes before meals or 60 minutes after meals.
3. Shake suspension vigorously before measuring dosage.
4. When administering IM,
   - **(a)** Inject deep into large muscle mass with good circulation.
   - **(b)** Rotate injection sites.
   - **(c)** Check previous injection sites for irritation.
   - **(d)** Switch to oral drug administration if drug is needed for more than 1 week after neurosurgery; decrease oral dose by 50% for 7 days, since IM drug sites will still be releasing drug. Note: This method of drug administration is no longer recommended.
5. When administering IV,
   - **(a)** Do not dilute in IV solution, such as 5% D/W, as precipitation may occur. A precipitate will form immediately in dextrose solutions. Microcrystallization occurs within 20 to 120 minutes in normal saline solutions.
   - **(b)** Inject IV bolus directly into IV line or use Y port closest to IV site.
   - **(c)** Never mix with other drugs.
   - **(d)** Flush IV line with 1 to 5 ml of normal saline solution.
   - **(e)** Administer at the rate of 25 mg/min. Do not exceed 50 mg/min. when administering IV. A syringe pump is recommended.
   - **(f)** Constantly monitor the client for signs of toxicity when administering drug. EKG monitoring is highly recommended. Discontinue drug if hypotension occurs, PR intervals become prolonged (greater than 0.2), or if QRS complex widens (greater than 0.1).

Evaluation factors

1. Elderly clients and clients with coronary insufficiency (history of angina) are susceptible to rapid toxicity when drug is administered IV.
2. Serum drug levels should be monitored frequently (daily) when drug is administered IV. Periodic (every 2 to 3 days) measurements of drug levels should be taken when drug is first initiated or the dosage form is changed.

3. Maintain a flowchart showing the type, duration, and time (date) of convulsion.
4. Serum drug levels should be obtained every 3 to 6 months for clients on prolonged drug therapy.
5. Assess client for toxicity periodically (daily) when oral and IM preparations are administered. Constant monitoring is required with IV drug administration.
6. Periodic assessment of gums is recommended. Encourage frequent brushing of teeth (after meals), flossing daily, and regular checkups.
7. Serum glucose levels should be obtained daily for diabetic clients when drug is first initiated. Insulin adjustment may be necessary.
8. Complete blood cell counts should be done yearly or twice a year for clients on prolonged drug therapy. Megaloblastic anemia and other blood dyscrasias may occur. Folic acid deficiency may also occur. Folic acid supplements of 0.1 to 0.5 mg/day are usually adequate, but watch the client for loss of seizure control.
9. Duration of therapy is variable. If client is seizure free for 3 to 5 years, the physician may taper the dosage gradually over 3 to 6 months and then discontinue the drug. Abrupt withdrawal of drug may cause seizures.

Client teaching factors

1. The client's need for the drug should be stressed. Emphasize the importance of maintaining dosage schedule to maintain serum drug levels, thereby avoiding loss of seizure control. Warn client to avoid taking drug dosages too close together since toxicity may occur; there is a fine margin between lack of seizure control and drug toxicity.
2. Urge client to eat a well-balanced diet regularly. Some foods rich in folic acid, calcium, and vitamin D should be eaten daily. Consult dietitian and physician, as needed. A vitamin supplement may be indicated.
3. Caution client that adequate hydration is essential, but excessive intake of fluids should be avoided. A state of slight dehydration has been associated with a decrease in the frequency of seizures.
4. Instruct client to avoid activities requiring constant attention (driving a car) until seizure disorder is well controlled (seizure free for 1 year or longer). Some states require epileptics to have a physician's certificate before a driver's license can be issued.
5. Warn client that a harmless pinkish red discoloration of the urine may occur.
6. Caution client to avoid changing dosage form or drug manufacturer, since lack of seizure control or toxicity may occur.
7. Caution client against using OTC drugs and home remedies, since drug interactions may occur. Advise client to seek medical assistance for the treatment of common ailments.
8. Instruct client to avoid ingesting alcohol, as seizures may occur.
9. Instruct family members in the care of a client having a convulsion: Insert a firm but soft object (wallet) between back teeth; do not restrain client but protect client from objects he or she may strike. After seizure, turn head to side, wipe secretions, and keep in a quiet room. Duration and type of seizure should be recorded and the physician notified.
10. Advise client to carry identification indicating seizure disorder and anticonvulsant being used.

GENERIC NAME Ethotoin (RX)

TRADE NAME Peganone

CLASSIFICATION Anticonvulsant

See phenytoin for Warnings and precautions and Drug interactions.

Action Similar to phenytoin, but less effective. The drug is said to be less toxic than phenytoin and lacks its arrhythmic activity. (See phenytoin.)

Indications for Use Grand mal, psychomotor, and jacksonian seizures.

Contraindications Hepatic impairment, hematologic disorders, hypersensitivity to hydantoin derivatives.

Untoward Reactions Lymphadenopathy and systemic lupus erythematosus may occur. Ataxia and gum hypertrophy occur, but rarely.

Parameters of Use

Absorption Half-life is 3 to 9 hours. Therapeutic serum drug levels: 15 to 50 mg/l.
Metabolism In the liver.
Excretion In bile, urine, and some in saliva.

Administration Adults: Initial dosage: 250 mg po qid after meals; then increase slowly every 3 to 7 days until desired effect; Maintenance dosage: 2 to 3 g daily. Children: Initial dosage: 250 mg po bid; then increase, if necessary, to tid or qid; Maintenance dosage: 500 to 1000 mg daily.

Available Drug Forms Scored tablets containing 250 or 500 mg.

Nursing Management GI disturbances are decreased if drug is given after meals. (See phenytoin.)

GENERIC NAME Mephenytoin (RX)

TRADE NAME Mesantoin

CLASSIFICATION Anticonvulsant

See phenytoin for Contraindications and Warnings and precautions.

Action Hydantoin homolog of the barbiturate mephobarbital with characteristics similar to barbiturates and phenytoin.

Indications for Use Refractory seizure disorders only, since drug causes severe untoward reactions: grand mal, focal, jacksonian, psychomotor.

Untoward Reactions May cause severe blood dyscrasias, including neutropenia, leukopenia, and agranulocytosis. May cause severe hypersensitivity reactions, including exfoliative dermatitis.

Parameters of Use

Absorption Onset of action is about 30 minutes and duration of action is 24 to 48 hours. Therapeutic serum drug levels: 5 to 20 mcg/ml.
Metabolism In the liver.
Excretion By the kidneys.

Drug Interactions Additive effects may occur if taken with other CNS depressants or alcohol. (See phenytoin.)

Administration Adults: Initial dosage: 50 to 100 mg po daily; then increase by 50 to 100 mg every 7 to 10 days until desired effect; Maintenance dosage: 200 to 600 mg po daily; Maximum dosage: 200 mg po tid. Children: Initial dosage: 50 to 100 mg po daily; then increase by 50 mg every 7 to 10 days until desired effect; Maintenance dosage: 100 to 400 mg po daily in divided doses.

Available Drug Forms Scored tablets containing 100 mg.

Nursing Management It is recommended that complete blood cell counts (white blood cell and differential) be done initially, then every 2 weeks until desired effect is achieved, then monthly for 1 year. If neutrophils drop below 1600/mm^3, the drug should be discontinued. Notify physician of abnormalities. (See phenytoin.)

BARBITURATES AND DERIVATIVES

GENERIC NAME Phenobarbital (C iv)

TRADE NAMES Eskabarb, Luminal, SK-Phenobarbital

CLASSIFICATION Anticonvulsant

Action CNS depressant that increases the threshold of the motor cortex to stimuli. (See Chapter 29.)

Indications for Use Grand mal and focal seizures; other forms of epilepsy.

Warnings and Precautions Use with caution in the elderly, young children, debilitated clients, diabetics, clients with hyperthyroidism, and clients with multiple allergies.

Untoward Reactions Prolonged use may cause folic acid deficiency and osteomalacia. Abrupt withdrawal may precipitate seizures.

Parameters of Use

Absorption Duration of action is 6 to 10 hours. Half-life is 2 to 5 days. Therapeutic serum drug levels: 10 to 25 mcg/ml; Maximum: 40 mcg/ml; full therapeutic effect occurs in 2 to 3 weeks. About 50% bound to plasma proteins.

Drug Interactions There are numerous drug interactions reported for phenobarbital and other barbiturates, primarily because of the drug's high plasma protein binding and its method of metabolism and excretion. Client should be monitored carefully for drug toxicity. Barbiturates interact with phenytoin and other anticonvulsants. Concurrent therapy has an additive CNS depressant effect. Barbiturates tend to alter the hepatic metabolism and excretion of phenytoin. An increase in CNS depression occurs with concurrent use of alcohol, narcotics, other sedatives, antihistamines, phenothiazines, disulfiram, MAO inhibitors, procarbazine, and methotrimeprazine. Sulfonamides increase the effect of barbiturates by inhibiting protein binding. By interfering with absorption and increasing liver enzyme activity, barbiturates can decrease the effects of oral anticoagulants, corticosteroids, digitalis glycosides,estrogens, oral contraceptives, griseofulvin, lidocaine, carbamazepine, and methyldopa.

Laboratory Interactions May affect bromsulphalein retention because of accelerated hepatic metabolism and excretion.

Administration Adults: 100 to 200 mg po daily administered once hs or given in 2 (q12h) or 3(q8h) divided doses; Children: 4 to 6 mg/kg po daily in 2 divided doses(q12h).

Available Drug Forms Elixir containing 20 mg/5 ml; tablets containing 15, 30, or 120 mg; capsules (prolonged action) containing 65 or 100 mg.

GENERIC NAME Phenobarbital sodium (C iv)

TRADE NAME Luminal Sodium

CLASSIFICATION Anticonvulsant

See phenobarbital for Warnings and precautions, Parameters of use, and Drug interactions.

Indications for Use Status epilepticus; febrile convulsions in children.

Untoward Reactions Symptoms of toxicity include confusion, vomiting, nystagmus, coughing, hiccups, and coma. Extravasation causes pain and necrosis.

Absorption Therapeutic serum drug levels: 10 to 40 mcg/ml.

Administration Adults: 90 to 120 mg IV bolus; then 30 to 60 mg IV every 15 minutes, as needed; Maximum dosage: 500 mg. Children: 5 to 10 mg/kg IV bolus; then repeat every 15 minutes, as needed; Maximum dosage: 20 mg/kg.

Available Drug Forms Injectable solutions containing 30, 50, 65, or 130 mg/ml.

Nursing Management

1. When administering IV bolus, do not exceed 60 mg/min.
2. Several drug incompatibilities can occur; flush IV line with 1 to 3 ml of normal saline before and after drug administration.

GENERIC NAME Amobarbital sodium (Cii)

TRADE NAME Amytal Sodium

CLASSIFICATION Anticonvulsant

See phenobarbital for Drug interaction.

Action Intermediate-acting barbiturate with sedative and hypnotic effects. (See Chapter 29.)

Indications for Use Seizures due to eclampsia, meningitis, tetanus, chorea, procaine reactions, poisoning (strychnine), and picrotoxin; status epilepticus.

Contraindications Porphyria, hypersensitivity to barbiturates, severe respiratory disorder, hepatic impairment.

Warnings and Precautions CNS depression, including apnea, may occur in newborns if the drug was used during labor.

Parameters of Use

Absorption Onset of action is 5 minutes and duration of action is 3 to 6 hours after IV administration.
Metabolism In the liver.
Excretion By the kidneys.

Administration Adults and children over 6 years: 65 to 500 mg slow IV bolus, repeat if necessary; Maximum dosage: 1000 mg. Children under 6 years: 3 to 5 mg/kg slow IV bolus; sometimes given IM.

Available Drug Forms Ampules containing 125, 250, or 500 mg of powder for reconstitution.

Nursing Management

1. Reconstitute powder with sterile water for injection only.
2. Prepare a 10% or more dilute solution:
   (a) 125-mg ampule—add 1.25 ml or more of diluent
   (b) 250-mg ampule—add 2.5 ml or more of diluent
   (c) 500-mg ampule—add 5 ml or more of diluent
3. Rotate ampule to dissolve powder; do not shake.
4. Do not use solution if there is a precipitate.
5. Inject IV bolus slowly; do not exceed 1 ml/min.
6. Monitor blood pressure, pulse, and respiration continuously. Observe for toxicity (apnea, hypotension, sluggish or absent reflexes, coma).
7. Check IV site frequently for irritation; embolism has been reported.
8. Drug deterioration occurs rapidly; discard unused portion.

GENERIC NAME Mephobarbital (Civ)

TRADE NAMES Mebaral, Menta-Bal, Mephoral

CLASSIFICATION Anticonvulsant

See phenobarbital for Nursing management.

Action Mephobarbital is a long-acting barbiturate with anticonvulsant properties similar to phenobarbital. Larger dosages of mephobarbital are required to produce the same effect as phenobarbital. Sedation occurs but the drug is considered a weak hypnotic. Sedative effect is reported to be less than phenobarbital.

Indications for Use Grand mal and petit mal (absence) seizures.

Contraindications Porphyria, hypersensitivity to barbiturates.

Untoward Reactions Prolonged use may cause folic acid deficiency and osteomalacia. Abrupt cessation of drug may precipitate seizures or result in withdrawal symptoms (tremor, insomnia, confusion, weakness).

Parameters of Use

Absorption About 50% absorbed from GI tract. Onset of action is 30 to 60 minutes and duration of action is 10 to 16 hours. Half-life is unknown.
Metabolism About 85% metabolized in the liver to phenobarbital in 24 hours.

Administration Low initial dosage, then increased every 4 to 5 days. Adults: 400 to 600 mg po daily in divided doses; Children: Over 5 years: 32 to 40 mg tid or qid (6 to 12 mg/kg/day); Under 5 years: 16 to 32 mg tid or qid.

Available Drug Forms Tablets containing 32, 50, 100, or 200 mg.

GENERIC NAME Metharbital (Ciii)

TRADE NAME Gemonil

CLASSIFICATION Anticonvulsant

See phenobarbital for Warnings and precautions and Drug interactions.

Action A long-acting barbiturate with anticonvulsant properties that has less toxic and fewer sedative effects than phenobarbital.

Indications for Use Grand mal, petit mal (absence), and mixed seizure disorders.

Contraindications Porphyria, hypersensitivity to barbiturates.

Parameters of Use

Absorption Onset of action is 2 to 4 hours and duration of action is 6 to 12 hours.

Metabolism Demethylated in the liver to barbital.

Excretion In urine.

Administration Adults: Initial dosage: 100 mg po daily, bid, or tid; Maintenance dosage: 300 to 600 mg daily in divided doses; Maximum dosage: 800 mg/day. Children: Initial dosage: 50 mg po daily, bid, or tid; Maintenance dosage: 5 to 15 mg/kg/day in divided doses.

Available Drug Forms Scored tablets containing 100 mg.

Nursing Management Divided doses should be administered around the clock (q8h or q12h). (See phenobarbital.)

ANALOG OF PHENOBARBITAL

GENERIC NAME Primidone (RX)

TRADE NAMES Mysoline, Primidone, Sertan

CLASSIFICATION Anticonvulsant

Action Synthetic analog of phenobarbital whose mechanism of anticonvulsant action is unknown; but primidone is known to increase the seizure threshold and alter the seizure patterns in experimental animals. The drug potentiates the action of phenobarbital and may be used concurrently with other anticonvulsants, particularly for refractory seizure disorders. The sedative effects that occur in almost one-quarter of the clients during the early weeks of drug therapy are attributed to the metabolite phenobarbital. The drug is considered to have a relatively low toxicity.

Indications for Use Grand mal, psychomotor, and focal seizures. May control refractory grand mal seizures. May be used alone or concurrently with other anticonvulsants.

Contraindications Hypersensitivity to phenobarbital, porphyria (group of disorders that alter the metabolism of porphyrin and result in excessive production and urinary excretion of porphyrin).

Warnings and Precautions Abrupt withdrawal may precipitate status epilepticus or other seizure disorders. Safe use during pregnancy has not been established; may cause birth defects. Neonatal hemorrhage due to a coagulation defect resembling vitamin K deficiency has occurred.

Untoward Reactions Ataxia, vertigo, and drowsiness are common during the first few weeks of drug therapy, but tend to subside with continued treatment. If the symptoms persist, dosage reduction is usually effective. GI disturbances, including anorexia, nausea, and vomiting, occur occasionally. Other reactions: fatigue, hyperirritability, emotional disturbances, sexual impotence, diplopia, nystagmus, moribilliform rash. Megaloblastic anemia has occurred, but rarely; the anemia responds to supplements of folic acid without discontinuation of the drug. Neonatal hemorrhage can be prevented or minimized if the pregnant woman receives prophylactic vitamin K_1 for 1 month prior to and during delivery.

Parameters of Use

Absorption About 75% absorbed from GI tract. Peak levels occur in about 4 hours. Therapeutic serum drug levels: 5 to 12 mcg/ml. Half-life varies widely (3 to 24 hours) and largely depends on rate of metabolism. There is little or no binding to plasma proteins.

Crosses placenta and substantial quantities enter breast milk; lactating mothers should bottle-feed their babies.

Metabolism Slowly in the liver to two active metabolites, phenobarbital and phenylethylmalonamide.

Excretion By the kidneys as unchanged drug (about 20%), active metabolites, and inactive metabolites.

Drug Interactions Potentiates the action of phenobarbital. Lower dosages of phenobarbital can be used when drugs are administered concurrently. Phenytoin stimulates the metabolism of primidone to phenobarbital. Toxic effects of phenobarbital may occur. The anticonvulsant effect of primidone may be reduced by folic acid supplements.

Administration Dosage varies according to the individual and severity of seizure disorder. Adults and children over 8 years: Initial dosage: 100 to 125 mg po hs for 3 days; then 100 to 125 mg po bid for 3 days; then 100 to 125 mg po tid for 3 days; Maintenance dosage: 250 mg po tid; Maximum dosage: 2000 mg/day. Children under 8 years: Initial dosage: 50 mg po hs for 3 days; then 50 mg po bid for 3 days; then 100 mg po bid for 3 days; Maintenance dosage: 125 to 250 mg tid; Usual maintenance dosage: 10 to 25 mg/kg/day in divided doses.

Available Drug Forms Scored tablets containing 50 or 250 mg; suspension containing 250 mg/ml.

Nursing Management

Planning factors

1. Obtain history of seizure disorder. A neurologic flowchart can be helpful.
2. Baseline complete blood cell count and SMA-12 should be obtained.

3. Porphyria should be ruled out before instituting drug therapy.
4. When primidone is added to client's anticonvulsant therapy, the dosage of primidone is gradually increased while the dosage of the other anticonvulsant is gradually decreased until the desired balance is achieved.

Administration factors

1. Administer on an empty stomach with 4 fl oz of water or more.
2. GI disturbances may be prevented by administering drug 1 hour after meals.

Evaluation factors

1. Serum drug levels should be monitored frequently when drug is first initiated or the dosage adjusted. Serum phenobarbital levels (therapeutic levels: 15 to 40 mcg/ml) may also be ordered. Steady-state therapeutic drug levels and therapeutic effectiveness usually take several weeks of therapy.
2. Sedative effects may occur during the first 2 weeks or more of therapy. Sedative effects tend to subside as treatment is continued.
3. Anorexia and sedative effects may cause the client to eat inadequately. Encourage client to eat a well-balanced diet and to eat foods rich in folic acid regularly.
4. Maintain a seizure disorder flowchart.
5. Assess client daily for toxicity and other untoward reactions.
6. Complete blood cell counts and SMA-12 should be done periodically (every 3 to 6 months). If anemia occurs, folic acid supplements may be ordered. Observe client for lack of seizure control.
7. Duration of therapy is variable. Dosage may be gradually reduced if the client remains seizure free for 1 to 3 years.
8. Abrupt withdrawal of drug may cause seizures.

Client teaching factors

1. The client's need for the drug should be stressed. Emphasize the importance of adherence to dosage schedule to maintain serum drug levels, thereby avoiding drug toxicity or loss of seizure control.
2. Advise client against abrupt withdrawal of drug.
3. Instruct client to avoid activities requiring constant attention (driving a car) during the first few weeks of drug therapy, since sedative effects occur. Physician should be consulted before resuming these activities.
4. Stress the importance of periodic laboratory and medical checkups to avoid serious untoward reactions.
5. Advise client to carry identification indicating seizure disorder and anticonvulsant being used.

SUCCINIMIDE DERIVATIVES

GENERIC NAME Ethosuximide (RX)

TRADE NAME Zarontin

CLASSIFICATION Anticonvulsant

Action Ethosuximide is considered the most effective succinimide for the control of petit mal (absence) seizures. Although it is less effective than trimethadione, it is often preferred because it causes fewer serious untoward reactions. The exact mechanism of action is unknown but the drug is thought to act by causing depression of the motor cortex and elevation of the CNS threshold to stimuli. The drug decreases the paroxysmal spike and brain wave activity associated with absence seizures. The drug is ineffective against grand mal seizures and may even increase the frequency of such seizures in clients with mixed seizure disorders.

Indications for Use Control of petit mal (absence) epilepsy.

Contraindications Hypersensitivity to succinimides.

Warnings and Precautions Use with caution in clients with hepatic or renal impairment, since ethosuximide is capable of producing morphologic and functional changes in these organs. Lupus erythematosus and fatal blood dyscrasias have been associated with ethosuximide; periodic blood counts are recommended. Safe use in pregnancy and lactation has not been established; birth defects may occur. Impairment of mental and physical abilities required for the performance of potentially hazardous tasks may occur. When used alone, ethosuximide may increase the frequency of grand mal seizures in clients with mixed seizure disorders. Abrupt withdrawal of drug may precipitate absence seizures.

Untoward Reactions GI disturbances are common. Anorexia, vague GI upset, nausea, vomiting, cramps, diarrhea, and epigastric and abdominal pain may occur. Blood dyscrasias, including leukopenia, agranulocytosis, pancytopenia, aplastic anemia, and eosinophilia, may occur, but rarely. CNS disturbances, including ataxia, drowsiness, headache, dizziness, euphoria, hiccups, irritability, lethargy, and fatigue, may occur; these symptoms may be dose related. Psychologic disturbances, including night terrors, inability to concentrate, and aggressiveness, have occurred, particularly in clients with preexisting psychologic abnormalities. Paranoid psychosis, increased libido depression, and suicidal tendencies have been reported, but rarely. Skin reactions, including urticaria, Stevens-Johnson syndrome, systemic lupus erythematosus, and pruritic erythematous rashes, occur, but rarely. Other reactions: myopia, vaginal bleeding, swelling of the tongue, gum hypertrophy, hirsutism. May cause a positive Coombs' test.

Parameters of Use

Absorption Readily absorbed from GI tract. May cause GI disturbances. Therapeutic serum drug levels: 40 to 100 mcg/ml. Steady-state plasma concentration occurs within 1 week. Half-life varies widely (24 to 60 hours). There is little or no binding to plasma proteins.

Crosses placenta and enters breast milk; lactating mothers should bottle-feed their babies. Crosses blood-brain barrier.

Distribution Widely distributed in body tissues.

Metabolism In the liver to inactive metabolites. Rate of metabolism in liver is variable; drug-induced hepatic impairment may occur.

Excretion By the kidneys as unchanged drug (about 10%) and as metabolites. Excretion may be delayed in the elderly and in clients with renal impairment.

Drug Interactions Concurrent ingestion of amphetamines may decrease GI absorption. Drugs that induce or retard liver enzyme systems may alter the metabolism of ethosuximide.

Administration Highly individualized. Do not exceed 1500 mg daily unless close medical supervision is available. Adults and children over 6 years: Initial dosage: 500 mg po daily; then increase by 250 mg daily every 4 to 7 days until desired effect. Children 3 to 6 years: Initial dosage: 250 mg po daily; then increase, if necessary, after 4 to 7 days; Optimal dosage: 20 mg/kg/day. If excessive dosages are required, the drug can be combined with other anticonvulsants.

Available Drug Forms Capsules containing 250 mg; raspberry-flavored syrup containing 250 mg/5 ml.

Nursing Management

Planning factors

1. Obtain history of seizure disorder. A neurologic flowchart can be helpful.
2. Baseline data on hepatic (blood urea nitrogen) and renal (creatinine) function should be obtained.
3. Obtain history of hepatic and renal disorders. Notify physician as indicated.
4. Store drug at room temperature away from moisture.

Administration factors

1. Administer with 4 fl oz of water or more.
2. Shake suspension well before measuring dose.
3. GI disturbances may be prevented by administering drug after breakfast.

Evaluation factors

1. Elderly clients and clients with hepatic or renal impairment are susceptible to rapid toxicity.
2. Serum drug levels should be monitored frequently when drug is first initiated or dosage adjusted.
3. Maintain a seizure disorder flowchart.
4. Assess client daily for toxicity, hypersensitivity, and other untoward reactions.
5. Complete blood cell count, blood urea nitrogen, serum creatinine levels, and urinalysis should be obtained periodically.
6. Duration of therapy is variable. If the client is seizure free for 1 to 3 years, the physician may taper the dosage gradually.
7. Abrupt withdrawal of drug may cause seizures.

Client teaching factors

1. The client's need for the drug should be stressed. Emphasize the importance of adherence to dosage schedule to maintain therapeutic serum drug levels, thereby avoiding loss of seizure control.
2. Advise client against abrupt withdrawal of drug.
3. Instruct client to avoid activities requiring constant attention (driving a car) until seizure disorder is completely controlled (seizure free).
4. Advise client to carry identification indicating seizure disorder and anticonvulsant being used.
5. Teach client and family members untoward reactions and instruct them to report symptoms to health professionals immediately. Stress the importance of regular laboratory and medical checkups.

GENERIC NAME Methsuximide (RX)

TRADE NAME Celontin

CLASSIFICATION Anticonvulsant

See ethosuximide for Action, Contraindications, Warnings and precautions, and Drug interactions.

Indications for Use Refractory petit mal (absence) and psychomotor seizures. May be administered in combination with other anticonvulsants.

Untoward Reactions Nearly one-third of all clients develop untoward reactions, particularly GI disturbances, blood dyscrasias, and CNS disturbances. Behavioral changes may progress to psychosis. (See ethosuximide.)

Parameters of Use

Absorption Peak levels occur in 1 to 3 hours. Therapeutic serum drug levels: 40 to 100 mcg/ml. Half-life is 2 to 4 hours.

Metabolism Rapidly in the liver.

Excretion By the kidneys.

Administration Adults and children: 300 mg po daily the first week; dosage may be increased at weekly intervals by 300 mg; Maximum dosage: 1200 mg daily in divided doses.

Available Drug Forms Capsules containing 150 or 300 mg.

Nursing Management (See ethosuximide.)

1. Complete blood cell count should be done frequently (every 1 to 3 months); hepatic function tests and urinalysis should be done periodically (every 3 to 6 months).
2. Causes harmless pinkish brown color change in urine.
3. Abrupt withdrawal may precipitate seizure activity.

GENERIC NAME Phensuximide (RX)

TRADE NAME Milontin

CLASSIFICATION Anticonvulsant

See ethosuximide for Contraindications, Warnings and precautions, and Drug interactions.

Action Less effective in controlling seizure activity than other succinimide derivatives, but causes fewer severe untoward reactions. (See ethosuximide.)

Indications for Use Petit mal (absence) seizures. May be administered in combination with other anticonvulsants.

Untoward Reactions Frequently causes nausea and other GI disturbances. (See ethosuximide.)

Parameters of Use

Absorption Peak levels occur in 1 to 4 hours. Therapeutic serum drug levels: 40 to 80 mcg/ml. Half-life is about 4 hours.
Metabolism Rapidly metabolized in the liver.
Excretion By the kidneys.

Administration Adults and children: 500 to 1000 mg po bid or tid; Maximum dosage: 3 g/day.

Available Drug Forms Capsules containing 500 mg.

Nursing Management (See ethosuximide.)

1. Complete blood cell count should be done every 3 months and hepatic function tests and urinalysis should be done every 3 to 6 months.
2. Causes harmless pinkish brown color change in urine.
3. Abrupt withdrawal may precipitate seizure activity.

OXAZOLIDINEDIONE DERIVATIVES

GENERIC NAME Paramethadione (RX)

TRADE NAME Paradione

CLASSIFICATION Anticonvulsant

Action Ineffective against grand mal seizures but may be used in conjunction with other anticonvulsants for mixed seizures.

Indications for Use Petit mal (absence) refractory seizure disorders only, since drug causes severe toxic and other untoward reactions.

Warnings and Precautions Use with caution in clients with retinal or optic nerve disorders. Use with caution in clients of childbearing age, since birth defects may occur. An appropriate contraceptive should be used.

Untoward Reactions May cause severe nephrosis and blood dyscrasias, including aplastic anemia and agranulocytosis. Photophobia may occur; clients should be warned to wear screening sunglasses. Hypersensitivity reactions to FD&C No. 5 yellow, including bronchial asthma, may occur with 300-mg capsules.

Parameters of Use

Absorption Therapeutic serum drug levels: 6 to 71 mcg/ml.

Drug Interactions No significant interactions known.

Administration Adults: Initial dosage: 300 mg po tid; then increase by 300 mg every 7 to 10 days until desired effect; Maintenance dosage: 300 to 600 mg po tid or qid. Children: Initial dosage: 300 mg po bid; then increase every 7 to 10 days until desired effect; Maintenance dosage: Infants: 150 mg po bid; Ages 2 to 6 years: 150 mg po tid or qid; Over 6 years: 300 mg po tid.

Available Drug Forms Capsules containing 150 or 300 mg. Bottles of oral solution with a calibrated dropper containing 300 mg/ml (also contains 65% alcohol).

Nursing Management (See phenytoin.)

1. Dilute oral solution in water before giving to children.
2. Administer with at least 4 fl oz of water.
3. Routine complete blood cell count and urinalysis should be done weekly, then monthly for a year, then periodically.

GENERIC NAME Trimethadione (RX)

TRADE NAME Tridione

CLASSIFICATION Anticonvulsant

See paramethadione for Warnings and precautions.

Action Ineffective against grand mal seizures, but may be used in conjunction with other anticonvulsants for mixed seizures.

Indications for Use Petit mal (absence) refractory seizure disorders only, since drug causes severe toxic and other untoward reactions.

Untoward Reactions Exfoliative dermatitis and other severe rashes may occur. (See paramethadione.)

Parameters of Use

Absorption Therapeutic serum drug levels: 20 to 40 mcg/ml.

Administration Adults: Initial dosage: 300 mg po tid; then increase by 300 mg every 7 to 10 days until desired effect; Maintenance dosage: 300 to 600 mg po tid or qid. Children: 20 to 50 mg/kg po daily in divided doses every 6 to 8 hours.

Available Drug Forms Capsules containing 300 mg; chewable tablets containing 150 mg; oral solution containing 40 mg/ml.

Nursing Management (See phenytoin.)

1. Administer with at least 4 fl oz of water.
2. Routine complete blood cell count and urinalysis should be done weekly, then monthly for a year, then periodically.
3. If neutrophil count drops below 2500/mm^3, drug should be discontinued.

BENZODIAZEPINE DERIVATIVES

GENERIC NAME Clonazepam (C iv)

TRADE NAME Clonopin

CLASSIFICATION Anticonvulsant

See phenytoin for Nursing management.

Action CNS depressant that also decreases the frequency, amplitude, duration, and spread of discharge in minor seizures. Suppresses the spike and brain wave discharge in petit mal (absence) seizures.

Indications for Use Lennox-Gastuat syndrome (type of petit mal), akinetic and myoclonic petit mal (absence) seizures that do not respond to succinimides.

Contraindications Hypersensitivity to benzodiazepines, hepatic impairment, acute or narrow-angle glaucoma.

Warnings and Precautions Safe use during pregnancy and lactation has not been established; may cause birth defects. Safe use in children has not been established. Abrupt withdrawal may cause status epilepticus or result in withdrawal symptoms, including convulsions, tremor, abdominal and muscle cramps, vomiting, and sweating. May increase the frequency of tonic-clonic (grand mal) seizure activity in clients with mixed seizure disorder. Use with caution in clients with impaired renal function, the elderly, debilitated clients, and clients with respiratory disorders (since drug causes respiratory depression and excessive salivation).

Untoward Reactions Common reactions include drowsiness (50%), ataxia (30%), and behavioral problems (25%). Respiratory disorders include shortness of breath, rales, and respiratory depression. CNS disturbances include abnormal eye movements, diplopia, slurred speech, aphonia, vertigo, and coma.

Parameters of Use

Absorption Peak levels occur in 1 to 2 hours. Therapeutic serum drug levels: 20 to 50 mcg/ml. Half-life is 18 to 50 hours.

Metabolism Oxidized and reduced to metabolites in the liver.

Excretion In urine.

Administration Adults: Initial dosage: 0.5 mg po tid; then increase by 0.5 mg every 3 days until desired effect; Maximum dosage: 20 mg/day. Infants and children: Initial dosage: 0.01 to 0.03 mg/kg/day bid or tid in divided doses; then increase by 0.25 to 0.5 mg every 3 days until desired effect; Maintenance dosage: 0.1 to 0.2 mg/kg/day.

Available Drug Forms Scored tablets containing 0.5, 1, or 2 mg.

GENERIC NAME Diazepam (C iv)

TRADE NAME Valium

CLASSIFICATION Anticonvulsant

Action CNS depressant with anticonvulsant properties similar to chlordiazepoxide (Librium), but has no peripheral autonomic blocking action and induces fewer extrapyramidal side effects. Large doses may cause ataxia. Has a depressant effect on the cardiovascular system and may cause apnea and/or cardiac arrest, particularly in the elderly and debilitated clients.

Indications for Use Short-term control of status epilepticus, severe recurrent seizures.

Contraindications Hypersensitivity to benzodiazepines, acute narrow-angle glaucoma, untreated open-angle glaucoma.

Warnings and Precautions Tonic status epilepticus has been precipitated in clients treated with diazepam IV for petit mal seizure disorders. Causes local vein irritation and may cause thrombosis.

Parameters of Use

Absorption Has a biphasic half-life: 7 to 10 hours; 2 to 8 days.

Crosses placenta and enters breast milk.

Metabolism In the liver. One active metabolite, oxazepam, is produced. Oxazepam has sedative and muscle relaxant properties.

Excretion By the kidneys.

Drug Interactions There are numerous drug interactions reported for diazepam, primarily because of the drug's method of metabolism and slow excretion. Client should be monitored carefully for drug toxicity. Diazepam increases the effects of phenytoin and other anticonvulsants. Concurrent therapy has an additive CNS depressant effect. An increase in CNS depression occurs with concurrent use of alcohol, narcotics, other sedatives, antihistamines, phenothiazines, MAO inhibitors, and tricyclic antidepressants. Respiratory depression may occur when used concurrently with gallamine triethiodide and other neuromuscular blocking agents.

Administration Adults: 5 to 10 mg slow IV bolus, repeat every 10 to 15 minutes times 2 doses, if necessary; Maximum dosage: 30 mg every 2 to 4 hours. Elderly, debilitated clients with hepatic impairment: 2 to 5 mg slow IV bolus, repeat every 10 to 15 minutes, or twice more, if necessary; Maximum dosage: 15 mg every 2 to 4 hours. Children: 0.1 to 0.3 mg/kg slow IV bolus, repeat every 10 to 15 minutes times 2 doses, if necessary; Maximum dosage: Under 5 years: 5 mg; Over 5 years: 10 mg.

Available Drug Forms Scored tablets containing 2, 5 or 10 mg; 2-ml ampules containing 5 mg/ml; 10-ml multidose vials containing 5 mg/ml.

Nursing Management

Administration factors

1. Use large veins (not hand or wrist veins).
2. Do not mix with other drugs or solutions because of incompatibilities.
3. Flush IV line with normal saline before and after drug administration.
4. Administer slowly; do not exceed 5 mg/min.

Evaluation factors

1. Monitor blood pressure, pulse, and respiration continuously. Observe for toxicity (hypotension, apnea, arrhythmias, coma).
2. Check IV site frequently for phlebitis or thrombosis.
3. Complete blood cell count and SMA-12 should be done periodically.
4. Dialysis is of no value for the treatment of toxicity.

MISCELLANEOUS ANTICONVULSANTS

GENERIC NAME Carbamazepine (RX)

TRADE NAME Tegretol

CLASSIFICATION Anticonvulsant

Action Exact mechanism is unknown but this iminostilbene derivative is thought to have actions similar to phenytoin. It is not considered a drug of choice because of serious untoward reactions.

Indications for Use Psychomotor, grand mal, and mixed seizure disorders; trigeminal neuralgia.

Contraindications History of bone marrow depression, hypersensitivity to carbamazepine or any tricyclic compound, concurrent therapy with MAO inhibitors.

Warnings and Precautions Safe use during pregnancy has not been established.

Untoward Reactions Toxicity, including dizziness, ataxia, drowsiness, stupor, restlessness, agitation, disorientation, tremor, and coma, may occur. Nausea, vomiting, mydriasis, nystagmus, cyanosis, urinary retention, and alterations in blood pressure may occur. Known to cause fatal blood dyscrasias, including aplastic anemia, agranulocytosis, thrombocytopenia, and leukopenia.

Parameters of Use

Absorption Half-life: Initially: 25 to 65 hours, then 12 to 17 hours. Therapeutic serum drug levels: 4 to 12 mcg/ml.

Metabolism In the liver.

Excretion Primarily by the kidneys, some in feces.

Administration Adults and children over 12 years: Initial dosage: 200 mg po bid; then increase by 200 mg daily and give in divided doses q8h; Maximum dosage: Ages 12 to 15 years: 1000 mg/day; Over 15 years: 1200 mg/day; Adults: 1600 mg/day. Children 6 to 12 years: Initial dosage: 100 mg po bid; then increase by 100 mg daily and give in divided doses q8h, then q6h; Maximum dosage: 1000 mg/day.

Available Drug Forms Scored tablets containing 200 mg. Chewable tablets containing 100 mg.

Nursing Management

1. Periodic hepatic function tests are recommended, since hepatic impairment and tumors may occur.
2. Periodic eye examinations are recommended, since changes in the eye have occurred.
3. Complete blood cell count should be obtained every week, then monthly.
4. Drug should be discontinued if any of the following occur: red blood cell count less than 4,000,000/mm^3; hematocrit less than 32%; hemoglobin less than 11 g/dl; platelets less than 100,000/mm^3; reticulocytes less than 20,000/mm^3; serum iron greater than 150 mcg/dl.

GENERIC NAME Magnesium sulfate (RX)

CLASSIFICATION Anticonvulsant

Action Elevated serum magnesium levels cause CNS depression by blocking the release of acetylcholine and may desensitize muscles to neurologic impulses. (See Chapter 19.)

Indications for Use Eclampsia, control of pre-eclampsia, hypomagnesemic seizures.

Contraindications Severe renal failure, congestive heart failure, heart block.

Warnings and Precautions Use with caution just prior to delivery because it will cause CNS depression in the newborn; be prepared to resuscitate the newborn. Complete heart block may occur in digitalized clients.

Parameters of Use

Absorption Onset of action occurs in: minutes (IV); about 1 hour (IM). Duration of action is: 30 to 60 minutes (IV); 3 to 4 hours (IM). Therapeutic serum drug levels: up to 12 mEq/l. Normal serum levels: 1.5 to 3 mEq/l.
Crosses placenta.

Excretion By the kidneys.

Drug Interactions Heart block may occur in clients receiving digitalis glycosides. Profound CNS depression can occur if given concurrently with other anticonvulsants, anesthetics, barbiturates, narcotics, and other CNS depressants. Calcium gluconate can be used to counteract hypermagnesemia (antidote).

Administration Loading dosage: 4 g of 10% solution slow IV bolus or in 100 to 250 ml of 5% D/W; then 4 g IM every 4 to 6 hours, as needed. Renal impairment: 1 to 2 g of 10% solution slow IV bolus or in 50 to 100 ml of 5% D/W; then 1 g every 4 to 6 hours, as needed.

Available Drug Forms 10% solution containing 1 g/10 ml; 50% solution containing 5 g/10 ml.

Nursing Management

Administration factors

1. When administering IV,
   (a) Use 10% solution only.
   (b) May be diluted in 50 to 250 ml of 5% D/W.
   (c) Administer slowly; do not exceed 150 mg/min. (1.5 ml 10% solution). Infusion pump is recommended.
2. When administering IM,
   (a) Use 50% solution only.
   (b) Inject deep into large muscle mass.
   (c) Rotate injection sites.

Evaluation factors

1. Monitor serum magnesium levels frequently and have calcium gluconate available for testing magnesium toxicity.
2. Monitor blood pressure, respiration, and cardiac rhythm continuously; hypotension, heart block, and apnea may occur.
3. Monitor intake and output hourly. Output should be 30 ml/hour or more.
4. Check for toxicity frequently (every 30 to 60 minutes); absence of knee jerk reflex precedes toxicity.

GENERIC NAME Paraldehyde (C IV)

TRADE NAME Paral

CLASSIFICATION Anticonvulsant

Action Relatively nontoxic but potent CNS depressant with sedative and hypnotic properties similar to barbiturates. It has a strong odor and taste.

Indications for Use Status epilepticus, seizures due to drug poisoning, refractory grand mal seizures.

Contraindications Asthma or other pulmonary disorders, severe hepatic impairment.

Untoward Reactions Toxicity may cause pulmonary edema, hypotension, and circulatory and respiratory collapse.

Parameters of Use

Absorption Half-life is 8 hours. Crosses placenta.
Metabolism Primarily in the liver.
Excretion In urine and exhaled air.

Drug Characteristics Deteriorates rapidly to acetic acid; refrigerate in airtight jars. Do not use if solution turns brown.

Administration Adults: 5 to 10 g IM; 200 to 400 mg slow IV in normal saline. Children: 15 mg/kg IM every 4 to 6 hours, as needed; 30 mg/kg as retention enema q1h prn (do not exceed 5 g); continuous drip 5 g/hour or less, as needed.

Available Drug Forms Parenteral solution containing 1 g/ml; oral solution containing 1 g/ml.

Nursing Management

Administration factors

1. Dilute rectal retention enema in 50 to 100 ml of cottonseed or olive oil or with 200 ml of normal saline.
2. When administering IM, inject deep into large muscle mass, since drug can be irritating to tissues and may cause abscesses. Do not deliver more than 5 ml to a site and rotate sites.
3. As drug reacts with plastic, use glass syringes and containers.
4. Add parenteral drug solution to 50 to 250 ml of normal saline (0.9% IV solution) and administer slowly.
5. Keep room well ventilated to remove drug in exhaled air.

Evaluation factors Observe client for toxicity frequently.

GENERIC NAME Phenacemide (RX)

TRADE NAME Phenurone

CLASSIFICATION Anticonvulsant

Action Elevates the seizure threshold and abolishes the tonic phase of maximal electroshock seizures. Particularly effective in controlling focal psychomotor seizures, but the drug is very toxic and causes serious, even fatal, untoward reactions.

Indications for Use Refractory psychomotor seizures; grand mal, petit mal, and mixed seizure disorders.

Warnings and Precautions Safe use during pregnancy has not been established; may cause birth defects.

Untoward Reactions GI disturbances (anorexia, weight loss), nephritis, headache, drowsiness, dizziness, ataxia, insomnia, paresthesia, psychotic behavior, and rashes have been reported. Fatal reactions: hepatitis, aplastic anemia, agranulocytosis, leukopenia.

Parameters of Use

Absorption Well absorbed from GI tract. Duration of action about 5 hours.
Excretion By the kidneys.

Administration Adults: Initial dosage: 500 mg po tid at mealtime; then, if seizures are poorly controlled after 7 days, 500 mg po upon awakening (early A.M.) or at bedtime; dosage range: 2 to 3 g po daily. Children: Ages 5 to 10 years: $\frac{1}{2}$ of adult dosage, same schedule.

Available Drug Forms Grooved tablets containing 500 mg.

Nursing Management Complete blood cell count and hepatic and renal function tests should be done periodically (at least monthly).

GENERIC NAMES Valproic acid; valproate sodium

TRADE NAME Depakene (RX)

CLASSIFICATION Anticonvulsant

Action Precise mechanism of action of this carboxylic acid derivative is unknown, but is thought to increase brain levels of gamma aminobutyric acid.

Indications for Use Simple and complex petit mal seizures, as an adjunct in mixed seizures.

Contraindications Hepatic disease or impairment, hypersensitivity to valproic acid or its sodium salt.

Warnings and Precautions Safe use during pregnancy has not been established; may cause birth defects. Abrupt withdrawal may precipitate status epilepticus in clients being treated for grand mal disorders.

Untoward Reactions Fatal hepatotoxicity has occurred within 6 months of initiating drug therapy and is usually preceded by loss of seizure control, malaise, weakness, lethargy, anorexia, and vomiting. Asymptomatic hyperammonemia may occur. Elevated serum transaminase levels are dose related.

Parameters of Use

Absorption Rapidly absorbed from GI tract. If taken with meals there is a slight delay in rate of absorption, but the total amount is absorbed. Peak levels occur in 1 to 4 hours. Therapeutic serum drug levels: 50 to 100 mcg/ml. Half-life is 8 to 12 hours and pKa is 4.8. About 90% bound to plasma proteins.
Metabolism In the liver; glucuronide conjugate and other metabolites are formed.
Excretion Primarily in urine, some in feces and exhaled air.

Drug Interactions Marked CNS depression can occur when taken with barbiturates and alcohol.

Laboratory Interactions May give false-positive results for urinary ketones.

Administration Adults: Initial dosage: 15 mg/kg/day; then increase 5 to 10 mg at 1-week intervals until desired effect; if total daily dose exceeds 250 mg, give in divided doses; Maximum dosage: 60 mg/kg/day.

Available Drug Forms Capsules containing 250 mg; syrup containing 250 mg/5 ml.

Nursing Management Hepatic function tests should be done frequently (monthly).

Chapter 31

Skeletal Muscle Relaxants

CHARACTERISTICS OF SKELETAL MUSCLE RELAXANTS

There are three basic groups of skeletal muscle relaxants. The central-acting and direct-acting muscle relaxants are described in this chapter, but the neuromuscular blocking agents, which have special characteristics, are described in Chapter 45. All three groups of drugs are used to prevent or relieve muscle spasms associated with muscle trauma or inflammation. Spasticity, characterized by intermittent (clonic) or sustained (tonic) muscular contractions, is associated with several neuromuscular disorders, including cerebral palsy, brain injury or tumors, multiple sclerosis, and spinal cord injuries. The underlying cause of muscle spasms must be determined before an appropriate skeletal muscle relaxant can be selected.

Central-acting skeletal muscle relaxants Although the exact mechanism of action is unknown, this group of muscle relaxants either depresses motor areas of the brain and/or blocks transmission of motoneuron impulses through the polysynaptic reflex arcs in the spinal cord. Diazepam and some of the glycol derivatives are thought to depress brain function, thereby relieving muscle spasms. Diazepam, a well-known central nervous system depressant used for the treatment of psychoneurotic states, can also relieve the anxiety and tension associated with muscle spasms. Unfortunately, the use of agents that depress the central nervous system is limited because of the drowsiness they produce when large dosages are given. However, these agents have been useful for certain clients who need central nervous system depression, such as those with particular spastic disorders, and for inflammation and pain.

Other central-acting agents seem to act more directly on the motoneurons within the spinal cord and decrease muscle spasms without causing undo central nervous system depression. Baclofen and chlorzoxazone appear to exert their action on the brain stem and relieve muscle spasms without interfering with muscle function. These drugs are useful in allaying spasms caused by acute musculoskeletal disorders, such as sprains, bursitis, and myositis. Although pain is not alleviated, muscle spasms that can aggravate the pain are prevented or decreased.

Combination preparations Analgesics are often required to relieve the pain associated with acute musculoskeletal injuries and inflammation. Combination skeletal muscle relaxant and analgesic preparations usually contain mild, but effective, analgesics with antiinflammatory properties, such as aspirin. Occasionally, a central nervous system stimulant is added to counteract the secondary effects of skeletal muscle relaxants on the central nervous system.

Direct-acting skeletal muscle relaxants Unlike the central-acting relaxants, dantrolene acts directly on the skeletal muscle fibers to relieve muscle spasms. It is thought to interfere with the release of calcium ions from the sarcoplasmic reticulum and, in so doing, dissociates the muscular excitation-contraction response; the motoneurons are not affected. When administered parenterally, dantrolene is effectual in the previously fatal anesthetic-induced disorder malignant hyperthermia; there was no efficacious treatment for this disorder before dantrolene was discovered. When administered orally, dantrolene has several untoward reactions, including hepatic and respiratory dysfunction. Photosensitivity reactions have also occurred and clients should be cautioned to avoid exposure to direct sunlight.

Quinine, a common antimalarial agent, has been found useful for nocturnal leg cramps. Although it is not a true direct-acting skeletal muscle relaxant, the drug is thought to primarily increase the refractory period of muscle fibers and to decrease the excitability of motor end plates. Some alteration in the calcium content of muscle fibers may also occur.

NURSING MANAGEMENT

Clients should be observed for excessive central nervous system depression as this sets a primary limitation on the dosage and duration of drug therapy. Prolonged drug use may cause severe untoward reactions, including sensory, cardiovascular, and respiratory disturbances due to secondary effects of the drug. Hepatic or renal dysfunction or blood dyscrasias may also occur as a result of the drug's metabolism, excretion, and distribution.

CENTRAL-ACTING SKELETAL MUSCLE RELAXANTS

Glycol Derivatives

GENERIC NAME Methocarbamol (RX)

TRADE NAMES Delaxin, Metho-500, Robaxin, SK-Methocarbamol

CLASSIFICATION Skeletal muscle relaxant

Action Although methocarbamol has no direct action on skeletal muscles, it causes CNS depression by depressing polysynaptic reflexes in the spinal cord. It also has some antianxiety activity and is effective in relieving muscle spasms caused by injury (sprain, strained ligaments) and inflammation (arthritis, bursitis). Parenteral preparations contain polyethylene glycol as a solvent, which may cause the retention of urea in clients with renal impairment.

Indications for Use As an adjunct in the relief of pain associated with acute musculoskeletal disorders and spasms and pain associated with tetanus.

Contraindications Hypersensitivity to any ingredients; parenteral drug is contraindicated in clients with known or suspected renal pathology.

Warnings and Precautions Safe use in children (under 12 years) and during pregnancy or lactation has not been established. Should not be given concurrently with CNS depressants. Parenteral drug preparations are hypertonic and do not mix with blood; use with caution when administering via IV bolus. Use parenteral drug with caution in epileptic clients and those with a suspected seizure disorder.

Untoward Reactions CNS disturbances: lightheadedness, dizziness, drowsiness, headache, blurred vision. Hypersensitivity reactions: urticaria, pruritus, rash, conjunctivitis, nasal congestion, fever; anaphylaxis, nausea, thrombophlebitis, and pain and sloughing at the injection site may also occur following parenteral administration. Intravenous injections may cause toxic drug reactions, including hypotension, syncope, vertigo, GI discomfort, nausea, and a metallic taste; flushing, nystagmus, diplopia, muscle incoordination, and bradycardia have occurred; convulsions may occur in epileptics. Intravenous injections have the potential of causing hemolysis.

Parameters of Use

Absorption Rapidly absorbed from GI tract. Peak levels occur in about 60 minutes after oral administration. Onset of action is about 10 minutes after IV administration. Duration of action is about 24 hours. May enter breast milk; lactating mothers should bottle-feed their babies.

Metabolism In the liver.
Excretion By the kidneys.

Drug Interactions Alcohol will enhance CNS depression; do not use concurrently. Concomitant use of CNS depressants may increase the sedative effects of methocarbamol; respiratory depression may occur. Inhibits the action of pyridostigmine in clients with myasthenia gravis. Barbiturates may alter the action of central-acting muscle relaxants by enhancing sedative effects and altering their metabolism. MAO inhibitors may potentiate the action of central-acting muscle relaxants by inhibiting their metabolism.

Laboratory Interactions Causes color interference in certain screening tests for 5-hydroxyindoleacetic acid and vanilmandelic acid.

Administration Initial dosage may be given po, IM, or IV. Adults: Oral: Initial dosage: 1.5 to 2 g qid for 2 to 3 days; Maintenance dosage: 1 g qid. Intramuscular: Initial dosage: 1 g q8h prn for 1 or 2 days; Maintenance dosage: 1 g po qid. Intravenous (tetanus): Initial dosage: 1 to 2 g IV bolus and 1 g IV drip q6h prn; then up to 2.4 g daily via nasogastric tube. Children: Intramuscular, Intravenous: 15 mg/kg q6h prn.

Available Drug Forms Scored tablets containing 500 or 750 mg; 10-ml single-dose vials containing 100 mg/ml.

Nursing Management

Planning factors

1. Obtain history of musculoskeletal disorder.
2. Obtain history of any seizure disorders and notify physician.
3. Urinalysis and blood urea nitrogen (BUN) should be done prior to instituting drug; if abnormal notify physician.
4. If administering IM, prepare 5 ml or less in each syringe; 2 syringes are required.
5. If administering IV, start continuous IV in a large vein; avoid small vessels of hand and wrist.
6. Epinephrine, antihistamine, and corticosteroids should be readily available.
7. Clients will require assistance with ambulation when parenteral drug preparations are used.
8. Used only as a supportive therapy in clients with tetanus.

Administration factors

1. Give at mealtime with 4 to 8 fl oz of water to avoid nausea; milk can be used if nausea occurs.
2. May be given around the clock (every 4 to 6 hours) when the client experiences severe pain.
3. When administering IM,
   (a) Inject deep into large muscle mass of the gluteal region; accidental subc injections may cause sloughing.
   (b) Do not deliver more than 5 ml to each gluteal area.
   (c) Inject medication slowly, since pain may occur.
   (d) The Z-track method of administration is recommended.

(e) Rotate injection sites.

4. Do not administer drug IV for more than 3 consecutive days.
5. When administering IV bolus,
   (a) Check patency of IV before administration.
   (b) Inject into Y port of continuous IV administration set.
   (c) Inject slowly; do not exceed 300 mg/min. (3 ml/min.).
   (d) Check blood pressure and pulse before starting and monitor pulse continuously during administration. If pulse becomes weak or bradycardia occurs, stop administering the drug and notify physician.
6. When administering via intermittent IV drip,
   (a) Check patency of IV before administration.
   (b) Add drug to 50 to 250 ml of normal saline or 5% D/W solution.
   (c) Administer slowly; rate of 100 ml/hour.
7. When administering via nasogastric tube,
   (a) Crush tablets well.
   (b) Dilute powder with 100 to 200 ml of water or saline and administer by gravity through the tube.
   (c) Flush medication into stomach with 20 to 30 ml of water or saline.

Evaluation factors

1. Check vital signs before administering drug parenterally. If hypotension, bradycardia, or respiratory depression exist, notify physician.
2. Urinalysis and BUN should be obtained periodically; elevated BUN and acidosis may occur in clients with renal impairment.
3. Observe client for toxicity frequently, particularly when drug is given IV. When administering via IV bolus, monitor client's level of consciousness.
4. Observe IM and IV sites frequently for tissue irritation and notify physician if phlebitis occurs.
5. Observe client for hematuria.

Client teaching factors

1. Emphasize the need for rest and physical therapy.
2. Instruct client to avoid rapid changes in position since orthostatic hypotension may occur, particularly when the drug is administered parenterally.
3. Inform client of CNS depression and explain that sedative effects wane with long-term therapy. Caution client against activities requiring constant attention (driving a car).
4. Warn client against the ingestion of alcohol.
5. Warn client that a harmless brown or greenish black discoloration of the urine may occur.

GENERIC NAME Carisoprodol (RX)

TRADE NAMES Rela, Soma

CLASSIFICATION Skeletal muscle relaxant

Action Although the precise mechanism is unknown, carisoprodol (propanediol dicarbamate) is thought to produce skeletal muscle relaxation by blocking interneuronal activity in the descending reticular formation and the spinal cord. It is thought to alter pain perception without affecting peripheral pain reflexes or the skeletal muscles. The drug has a relatively rapid onset of action and the effects will last up to 6 hours.

Indications for Use Acute musculoskeletal disorders that are painful, stiff, and spastic; effective in relieving the spasticity and rigidity associated with cerebral palsy.

Contraindications Porphyria (disorders of porphyrin metabolism); hypersensitivity to carisoprodol or related compounds (meprobamate, mebritamate, tybamate).

Warning and Precautions Safe use in children (under 12 years) and during pregnancy has not been established. Use with caution in addiction-prone clients, clients with hepatic or renal impairment, and clients receiving concurrent CNS depressants or psychotropic drugs.

Untoward Reactions Drowsiness is the most common untoward reaction. Other CNS disturbances include vertigo, ataxia, tremor, agitation, irritability, headache, depression, syncope, and insomnia. Dosage reduction may be required. Toxicity includes stupor, coma, shock, and respiratory depression, particularly when drug is ingested with alcohol, CNS depressants, or psychotropic drugs; death is rare. Idiosyncratic reactions have occurred within minutes or hours of the 1st dose, but rarely. The symptoms, which include extreme weakness, transient quadriplegia, dizziness, ataxia, temporary loss of vision, diplopia, mydriasis, dysarthria, agitation, euphoria, confusion, and disorientation, usually subside within several hours. Allergic reactions include erythema multiforme and other skin rashes; pruritus and eosinophilia have occurred within the 1st day of drug therapy. Anaphylaxis, asthmatic episodes, fever, weakness, dizziness, angioneurotic edema, smarting eyes, and hypotension have also been reported. Postural hypotension, tachycardia, and facial flushing can occur. GI disturbances, including nausea, vomiting, hiccups, and epigastric distress, are relatively common. No serious blood dyscrasias have been reported. Drug dependency is rare but can occur with long-term therapy. Abrupt withdrawal may cause abdominal cramps, insomnia, chills, headache, and nausea.

Parameters of Use

Absorption Rapidly absorbed from GI tract; may cause GI disturbances. Onset of action is about 30 minutes. Peak action occurs in 1 to 2 hours and duration of action is 4 to 6 hours.

High concentrations are found in breast milk (2 to 4 times plasma levels); lactating mothers must bottle-feed their babies.

Metabolism In the liver.

Excretion Primarily by the kidneys.

Drug Interactions Concomitant ingestion of alcohol or CNS depressants will enhance CNS depression; do not use concurrently. Barbiturates may alter the action of central-acting muscle relaxants by enhancing sedative effects and altering their metabolism.

Administration Adults and children over 12 years: 350 mg po qid.

Available Drug Forms Tablets containing 350 mg.

Nursing Management

Planning factors

1. Porphyria should be ruled out before initiating drug therapy.
2. Obtain history of musculoskeletal disorder.
3. Urinalysis, blood urea nitrogen (BUN), and serum creatinine should be done prior to instituting drug; if abnormal notify physician.
4. Epinephrine and antihistamine should be readily available.
5. Client may require assistance with ambulation, particularly when drug is initiated.

Administration factors Give tablets with meals and at bedtime with milk (4 to 8 fl oz of fluid).

Evaluation factors

1. Assess client frequently (qlh) for untoward reactions during the 1st day of therapy. If idiosyncratic or allergic reactions occur, notify physician and institute supportive treatment as indicated.
2. Check vital signs periodically (daily).
3. Urinalysis, BUN, and serum creatinine should be obtained periodically.
4. Record pain relief.
5. Clients with renal impairment may have elevated serum drug levels.

Client teaching factors

1. Emphasize the need for rest and physical therapy.
2. Instruct client to avoid rapid changes in position since orthostatic hypotension may occur.
3. Warn client about drowsiness and explain that sedative effects wane with long-term therapy. Caution client against activities requiring constant attention (driving a car).
4. Warn client against the ingestion of alcohol.

GENERIC NAME Chlorphenesin carbamate (RX)

TRADE NAME Maolate

CLASSIFICATION Skeletal muscle relaxant

Action This analog of mephenesin also has mild sedative properties. (See methocarbamol.)

Indications for Use Relief of pain associated with muscle strain and spasm.

Untoward Reactions Frequently causes drowsiness and dizziness. May cause paradoxic CNS stimulation manifested by agitation, insomnia, and nervousness. Blood dyscrasias can occur.

Administration 400 to 800 mg po tid over 8 weeks or less.

Available Drug Forms Scored tablets containing 400 mg.

Nursing Management Should be given with meals or milk since it may cause nausea. (See methocarbamol.)

GENERIC NAME Mephenesin (RX)

TRADE NAME Tolserol

CLASSIFICATION Skeletal muscle relaxant

See methocarbamol for Nursing management.

Action Mephenesin has a short duration of action. (See methocarbamol.)

Indications for Use Relief of tremors associated with parkinsonism and alcoholism.

Administration 1 to 3 g po tid or qid; 30 to 150 ml of a solution IV, as needed.

Available Drug Forms Tablets containing 0.25 or 0.5 g; elixir containing 0.1 g/ml.

GENERIC NAME Mephenesin carbamate (RX)

TRADE NAME Tolseram

CLASSIFICATION Skeletal muscle relaxant

See methocarbamol for Nursing management.

Action Although it has the same potency as mephenesin, this carbonate salt has a longer duration of action because it is absorbed and metabolized more slowly.

Indications for Use Relief of pain associated with muscle strain and spasm.

Administration 1 to 3 g po tid or qid.

Available Drug Forms Tablets containing 0.5 g; suspension containing 1 g/5 ml.

GENERIC NAME Meprobamate (RX) (C iv)

TRADE NAMES Equanil, Miltown

CLASSIFICATION Skeletal muscle relaxant

See methocarbamol for Nursing management.

Action Meprobamate (propanediol dicarbamate derivative) relaxes skeletal muscles by CNS depression and spinal interneuron blockade.

Indications for Use Pain, tension, and anxiety associated with musculoskeletal disorders; also used for anxiety, tension, petit mal epilepsy, and alcoholism (antianxiety agent).

Untoward Reactions CNS disturbances, including drowsiness, ataxia, slurred speech, and paradoxic excitation, may occur. May cause hypotension, syncope, arrhythmias, respiratory depression, and blood dyscrasias.

Parameters of Use

Absorption Onset of action is: 60 minutes (po); 10 to 15 minutes (IM). Half-life is 6 to 16 hours.
Crosses placenta and enters breast milk.
Excretion By the kidneys, some in feces.

Administration 400 mg po or IM every 3 to 4 hours prn; Maximum dosage: 2.4 g/day.

GENERIC NAME Metaxalone (RX)

TRADE NAME Skelaxin

CLASSIFICATION Skeletal muscle relaxant

Action The precise mechanism of metaxalone, a structural analog of mephenoxalone, is unknown but is thought to depress CNS. No direct action on skeletal muscles.

Indications for Use Acute muscle spasms associated with sprains, strains, fractures, and dislocations.

Untoward Reactions Nausea, vomiting, GI upset, drowsiness, dizziness, headache. May cause hemolytic anemia or leukopenia.

Laboratory Interactions May cause false-positive results for urinary glucose with Benedict's solution.

Administration Adults and children over 12 years: 800 mg po tid or qid.

Nursing Management Should be given with meals or milk since it may cause nausea. (See methocarbamol.)

GENERIC NAME Oxanamide (RX)

TRADE NAME Quiactin

CLASSIFICATION Skeletal muscle relaxant

See methocarbanol for Nursing management.

Action Inhibits polysynaptic reflexes. Large doses cause a hypnotic effect similar to the barbiturates.

Administration 400 mg po qid.

Available Drug Form Tablets containing 400 mg.

GENERIC NAME Phenyramidol (RX)

TRADE NAME Analexin

CLASSIFICATION Skeletal muscle relaxant

See methocarbanol for Nursing management.

Action Also has analgesic properties.

Indications for Use Relief of pain associated with muscle strain and spasms.

Administration 200 to 400 mg po q4h.

Available Drug Forms Tablets containing 200 mg.

GENERIC NAME Styramate (RX)

TRADE NAME Sinaxar

CLASSIFICATION Skeletal muscle relaxant

See methocarbamol for Nursing management.

Action Styramate, which is structurally similar to mephenesin carbamate, also has a mild sedative effect. It has a longer duration of action than mephenesin.

Administration 200 to 400 mg po qid.

Available Drug Forms Tablets containing 200 mg.

Other Central-Acting Agents

GENERIC NAME Cyclobenzaprine hydrochloride

TRADE NAME Flexeril (RX)

CLASSIFICATION Skeletal muscle relaxant

Action Cyclobenzaprine is a synthetic tricyclic amine salt structurally related to tricyclic antidepressants. It relieves skeletal muscle spasms of local origin without interfering with muscle function. Although the drug is ineffective in allaying muscle spasms due to CNS disease, it does reduce tonic somatic motor activity that affects the gamma and alpha motor systems. Cyclobenzaprine acts primarily within the brain stem and may have some action on spinal cord neurons. It has a sedative effect, a potent anticholinergic effect, and may cause tachycardia. The drug reduces local pain and tenderness and increases the range of motion.

Indications for Use Muscle spasms associated with acute, painful musculoskeletal disorders of short duration; concomitant use of MAO inhibitors or within 14 days of their cessation; acute myocardial infarction; arrhythmias; heart block or conduction disturbances; congestive heart failure; hyperthyroidism.

Warnings and Precautions Safe use in children (under 15 years) and during pregnancy has not been established. Use for more than 2 to 3 weeks is not recommended. Use with caution in clients known to be hypersensitive to tricyclic antidepressants (amitriptyline, imipramine); clients with urinary retention, angle closure glaucoma, or increased intraocular pressure (due to anticholinergic properties); clients with hepatic impairment (as dose-related hepatocyte vacuolation with lipidosis has occurred in animal trials); in the elderly; debilitated clients; and clients with cardiovascular disorders.

Untoward Reactions Drowsiness (40%), dry mouth (28%), and dizziness (11%) are common. Tachycardia, weakness, fatigue, paresthesia, blurred vision, an unpleasant taste, and GI disturbances (nausea, dyspepsia) have occurred relatively frequently. Allergic reactions, including skin rashes, urticaria, and edema of the face and tongue have occurred, but rarely. Untoward reactions to tricyclic depressants: hypotension, arrhythmias, heart block, stroke, seizures, extrapyramidal symptoms, disturbances of accommodation, paralytic ileus, photosensitivity, bone marrow depression, hepatitis, testicular swelling, breast enlargement, altered libido, altered serum glucose level, urinary frequency, mydriasis, alopecia. Abrupt cessation of these drugs, after long-term therapy, may cause withdrawal symptoms, including nausea, headache, and malaise. Rare reactions: sweating, myalgia, dyspnea, abdominal pain, constipation, coated tongue, tremors, dysarthria, euphoria, nervousness, disorientation, confusion, headache, urinary retention, ataxia, depression, hallucinations.

Parameters of Use

Absorption Well absorbed from GI tract. Absorption is not affected by aspirin and other analgesics. Plasma levels vary widely. Half-life is 1 to 3 days. Highly bound to serum proteins; drug interactions may occur.

May enter breast milk; lactating mothers should bottle-feed their babies.

Metabolism In the liver.

Excretion Primarily by the kidneys.

Drug Interactions Antagonistic effect with reserpine. Potentiates norepinephrine; do not administer concurrently. As with tricyclic antidepressants, cyclobenzaprine may interact with MAO inhibitors and result in high fever, severe convulsions, and death; do not administer within 14 days of each other. Concomitant ingestion of alcohol, barbiturates, and CNS depressants may enhance CNS depression; do not use concurrently. Due to its own anticholinergic effect, anticholinergic drugs should be administered with caution. May block the antihypertensive action of guanethidine and related compounds.

Administration Usual dosage: 10 mg po tid; Range: 20 to 40 mg daily in divided doses; Maximum dosage: 60 mg/day.

Available Drug Forms Film-coated tablets containing 10 mg; unit-dose packages.

Nursing Management

Planning factors

1. Obtain history of musculoskeletal disorder.
2. Hepatic function tests should be done prior to instituting drug therapy.
3. Obtain history of cardiovascular disorders and urinary retention.
4. Record intake and output.
5. Check vital signs.
6. Drug therapy should not be used for longer than 2 to 3 weeks.
7. Monitor blood pressure of hypersensitive clients receiving reserpine.

Administration factors Give with 4 to 8 fl oz of water.

Evaluation factors

1. Check vital signs periodically (once per shift). If tachycardia, arrhythmias, or hypotension occur, notify physician before administering next dose.
2. Record pain relief.
3. Record intake and output.
4. If constipation occurs, a stool softener may be ordered.

Client teaching factors

1. Emphasize the need for rest and physical therapy.
2. Caution client against activities requiring constant attention (driving a car).
3. Warn client against the ingestion of alcohol.
4. Inform client that chewing sugarless gum may assist in relieving a dry mouth; but that excessive use may cause gastric discomfort.
5. Warn client against abrupt drug withdrawal.

GENERIC NAME Baclofen (RX)

TRADE NAME Lioresal

CLASSIFICATION Skeletal muscle relaxant

Action Similar to cyclobenzaprine.

Indications for Use Spasticity associated with multiple sclerosis and spinal cord injuries.

Warnings and Precautions Use with caution in clients with renal impairment, stroke, and epilepsy.

Untoward Reactions Nausea, drowsiness, dizziness, weakness. May cause hyperglycemia, hypotension, urinary frequency, excessive sweating, and allergic rashes.

Parameters of Use

Absorption Well absorbed from GI tract. Plasma levels vary widely.
Metabolism In the liver.
Excretion Primarily by the kidneys.

Laboratory Interactions May elevate alkaline phosphatase and serum glutamic-oxaloacetic transaminase.

Administration Initial dosage; 5 mg po tid for 3 days; then increase by 5 mg every 3 days, as needed; Maximum dosage: 80 mg/day.

Available Drug Forms Tablets containing 10 mg; unit-dose packages.

Nursing Management (See cyclobenzaprine hydrochloride.)

1. Give with meals or milk to avoid nausea.
2. Abrupt withdrawal may precipitate spasticity and induce hallucinations.
3. Do not induce vomiting for overdose; use supportive measures.
4. Seizure activity may increase in epileptics.

GENERIC NAME Chlorzoxazone (RX)

TRADE NAME Paraflex

CLASSIFICATION Skeletal muscle relaxant

Action Although the exact mechanism is unknown, chlorzoxazone inhibits multisynaptic reflex arcs in the spinal cord and subcortical areas of the brain. It increases mobility and decreases spasms and pain. Often administered with the analgesic acetaminophen.

Indications for Use Acute, painful musculokeletal disorders.

Warnings and Precautions Safe use during pregnancy has not been established. Use with caution in clients with a history of drug allergies and clients with hepatic impairment.

Untoward Reactions Relatively low toxicity, but may cause drowsiness, dizziness, lightheadedness, and GI disturbances (nausea, vomiting, anorexia, GI bleeding). Hepatic dysfunction has been reported, but rarely. Hypersensitivity reactions, including skin rashes, petechiae, ecchymoses, and angioneurotic edema, have occurred, but rarely.

Parameters of Use

Absorption Peak levels occur in 3 to 4 hours.
Metabolism Rapidly metabolized in the liver.
Excretion Rapidly in urine as unchanged drug (1%) and metabolites.

Available Drug Forms Tablets containing 250 mg.

Nursing Management (See cyclobenzaprine hydrochloride.)

1. Give with meals or milk to avoid nausea.
2. Warn client about harmless orange-red color change in urine.
3. Record pain relief and drowsiness.
4. Hepatic function tests should be obtained periodically.

GENERIC NAME Diazepam (C IV)

TRADE NAME Valium

CLASSIFICATION Skeletal muscle relaxant

Action CNS depressant that is thought to relieve skeletal muscle spasms through a sedative effect. It has no peripheral blocking action. Large doses may cause ataxia.

Indications for Use Reflex spasm due to local injury or inflammation, spasticity associated with back strain, cerebral palsy paraplegia.

Contraindications Hypersensitivity to benzodiazepines, acute narrow-angle glaucoma, untreated open-angle glaucoma.

Untoward Reactions Has a cardiovascular depressant effect and may cause apnea and/or cardiac arrest, particularly in elderly or debilitated clients. Causes local vein irritation and may cause thrombosis.

Parameters of Use

Absorption Has a biphasic half-life: 7 to 10 hours; 2 to 8 days.
Crosses placenta and enters breast milk.
Metabolism In liver. One active metabolite, oxazepam, is produced. Oxazepam has sedative and muscle relaxant properties.
Excretion By the kidneys.

Drug Interactions There are numerous drug interactions reported for diazepam, primarily because of the drug's method of metabolism and slow excretion. Client should be monitored carefully for drug toxicity. Diazepam increases the effects of phenytoin and other anticonvulsants. Concurrent therapy has an additive CNS depressant effect. An increase in CNS depression occurs with concurrent use of alcohol, narcotics, other sedatives, antihistamines, phenothiazines, MAO inhibitors, and tricyclic antidepressants. Respiratory depression may occur when used concurrently with gallamine triethiodide and other neuromuscular blocking agents.

Administration Adults: Initial dosage (severe spasms): 5 to 10 mg IM or IV; then 5 to 10 mg IM or IV every 3 to 4 hours, as needed. Usual dosage (mild to moderate spasms): 2 to 10 mg po tid or qid. Children: 1 to 2.5 mg po tid or qid.

Available Drug Forms Tablets containing 2, 5, or 10 mg; 2-ml ampules containing 5 mg/ml; 10-ml multidose vials containing 5 mg/ml.

Nursing Management (See cyclobenzaprine hydrochloride.)

1. Inject deep into large muscle mass and rotate injection sites.
2. Flush IV line tubing with normal saline before and after IV bolus. Administer at the rate of 5 mg/min. or slower.

GENERIC NAME Orphenadrine citrate (RX)

TRADE NAMES Banfles, Myophen, Myotrol, Norflex

CLASSIFICATION Skeletal muscle relaxant

See cyclobenzaprine hydrochloride for Nursing management.

Action Although the exact mechanism is unknown, orphenadrine, which is structurally related to the antihistamine diphenhydramine, reduces spasms in skeletal muscles. The drug is thought to inhibit motor areas of the brain. It has weak antihistamine action but relatively strong anticholinergic effect. The drug has a low incidence of untoward reactions.

Indications for Use As an adjunct in the treatment of acute, painful musculoskeletal disorders; rigidity of Parkinson's disease.

Contraindications Glaucoma, pyloric or duodenal obstruction, prostatic hypertrophy, myasthenia gravis.

Warnings and Precautions Safe use during pregnancy has not been established.

Untoward Reactions Dry mouth, tachycardia, arrhythmias, urinary retention, and increased intraocular pressure may occur.

Drug Interactions Additive effect occurs when given concurrently with propoxyphene. Dosage reduction of one or both drugs is usually required.

Administration 100 mg po bid; 60 mg IM or IV every 12 hours.

Available Drug Forms Tablets containing 100 mg; 2-ml ampules containing 30 mg/ml; multidose vials containing 30 mg/ml.

COMBINATION PREPARATIONS

TRADE NAMES Flexaphen, Lobac, Mus-Lax, Parafon Forte, Saroflex, Spasgesic (RX)

CLASSIFICATION Skeletal muscle relaxant with analgesic

Indications for Use Possibly effective in the symptomatic relief of pain, stiffness, and limitation of motion associated with musculoskeletal disorders.

Administration Adults: 2 capsules po qid.

Available Drug Forms Generic contents: capsules containing acetaminophen: 300 mg; chlorzoxazone: 250 mg.

TRADE NAME Robaxisal (RX)

CLASSIFICATION Skeletal muscle relaxant with analgesic

Indications for Use Acute, painful musculoskeletal disorders.

Warnings and Precautions Avoid giving more than 2 tablets at a time to clients who do not tolerate salicylates.

Administration Adults and children over 12 years: 2 tablets po qid; 3 tablets po qid for 1 to 3 days only for severe pain.

Available Drug Forms Generic contents in each laminated tablet: methocarbamol: 400 mg; aspirin: 325 mg.

TRADE NAMES Carisoprodol Compound, Soma Compound (RX)

CLASSIFICATION Skeletal muscle relaxant with analgesic

Indications for Use Relief of discomfort associated with acute, painful musculoskeletal disorders.

Warnings and Precautions Use in children under 5 years is not recommended. Phenacetin analgesic preparations may cause severe renal disease if taken for prolonged periods of time in high dosages.

Administration Adults: 1 to 2 tablets po qid.

Available Drug Forms Generic contents in each orange scored tablet: carisoprodol: 200 mg; phenacetin: 160 mg; caffeine: 32 mg.

TRADE NAME Soma Compound with Codeine

CLASSIFICATION Skeletal muscle relaxant with analgesic and narcotic (C iii)

Indications for Use Relief of discomfort associated with acute, painful musculoskeletal disorders.

Warnings and Precautions May be habit forming. Use in children under 5 years is not recommended. Phenacetin analgesic preparations may cause renal disease if taken for prolonged periods of time in high dosages.

Administration Adults: 1 to 2 tablets po qid.

Available Drug Forms Generic contents in each white tablet: carisoprodol: 200 mg; phenacetin: 160 mg; caffeine: 32 mg; codeine phosphate: 16 mg.

DIRECT-ACTING SKELETAL MUSCLE RELAXANTS

GENERIC NAME Dantrolene sodium (oral) (RX)

TRADE NAME Dantrium

CLASSIFICATION Skeletal muscle relaxant

Action Dantrolene, a hydrated sodium salt derivative of hydantoin, acts directly on skeletal muscles to produce relaxation. Although the precise mechanism is unknown, the drug is thought to interfere with the release of calcium ions from sarcoplasmic reticulum, thereby uncoupling the excitation-contraction process. Unlike other classes of skeletal muscle relaxants, dantrolene does not affect motoneurons or myoneural junctions. However, it does have an indirect effect on the CNS. Large doses may cause drowsiness, dizziness, and generalized weakness. The drug has a pronounced impact on the liver and fatal hepatotoxicity has occurred, particularly with long-term therapy. Dantrolene should not be given for longer than 45 days unless there is a noticeable improvement in the client's spasticity.

Indications for Use Spasticity resulting from upper motoneuron disorders, such as spinal cord injuries, stroke, cerebral palsy, and multiple sclerosis.

Contraindications Active hepatic disease or disorder, including hepatitis and cirrhosis; disorders that use spasticity to maintain muscle function and an upright position; lactation.

Warnings and Precautions Safe use in children (under 5 years) and during pregnancy has not been established. Not effective in relieving muscle spasms associated with rheumatic disorders. Subclinical hepatic impairment should be determined before initiating drug; if abnormalities exist, the drug should either be used with extreme caution or not at all. Risk versus benefit considerations should be weighed before instituting long-term therapy, particularly in children. Use with caution in females and clients over 35 years, since the incidence of hepatotoxicity is greater in these individuals. Use with caution in clients with impaired pulmonary function (chronic obstructive pulmonary disease) or cardiac function (myocardial infarction) and in clients with a history of previous hepatic disorders or dysfunction.

Untoward Reactions Common reactions: drowsiness, dizziness, weakness, malaise, fatigue, diarrhea. These symptoms can often be avoided by initiating therapy with a low dose and then gradually increasing the dosage. Hepatic dysfunctions (hepatotoxicity), including acute hepatitis, hepatocellular injury, and jaundice, have occurred, particularly in females and clients over 35 years who have taken the drug for longer than 3 to 12 months. Photosensitivity may occur, particularly with long-term therapy. GI disturbances, including anorexia, difficulty in swallowing, GI irritation, abdominal cramps, GI bleeding, and constipation, have occurred. CNS disturbances include headache, lightheadedness, visual disturbances, diplopia, altered sensation of taste, insomnia, speech disturbances, and seizures. Mental depression, confusion, and nervousness have also been reported. Hypersensitivity reactions include pleural effusions, pericarditis, eczematoid dermatitis, urticaria, and pruritus. Genitourinary disturbances include crystalluria, hematuria, urinary frequency, dysuria, urinary retention, incontinence, nocturia, and difficult erection. Other reactions: abnormal hair growth, acnelike rash, myalgia, backache, excessive tearing, a suffocating feeling.

Parameters of Use

Absorption Slowly and incompletely absorbed from GI tract. Serum drug levels depend on the amount of drug absorbed. Duration and intensity of action are related to serum drug levels. Half-life is 8.7 hours after 100 mg po.

Metabolism Probably in the liver microsomal enzyme system; other drugs that affect this system may increase dantrolene metabolism.

Excretion Primarily by the kidneys as unchanged drug and metabolites.

Drug Interactions Increased incidence of hepatotoxicity in female clients receiving estrogen therapy concurrently. Excessive CNS depression may occur if CNS depressants or alcohol or taken concomitantly.

Administration Lowest possible dose is used; optimal effect without untoward reactions is desired. Adults: Initial dosage: 25 mg po daily; then increase frequency of administration bid, tid, or qid every 7 days; then increase by 25 mg every 7 days until desired effect; Maintenance dosage: 400 mg po qid, a dose higher than 400 mg daily is rarely required. Children: Initial dosage: 0.5 mg/kg po daily; then increase frequency of administration bid, tid, or qid every 7 days; then increase by 0.5 mg/kg every 7 days until desired effect; Maximum dosage: 400 mg/day.

Available Drug Forms Capsules containing 25, 50, or 100 mg.

Nursing Management

Planning factors

1. Obtain baseline data on spastic disorder, client's self-care abilities and limitations, and spastic characteristics that annoy client.
2. Obtain baseline hepatic function tests, including serum glutamic-oxaloacetic transaminase, serum glutamic-pyruvic transaminase, alkaline phosphate, and total bilirubin. If any abnormalities exist, notify physician.
3. Determine intake and output.
4. Obtain history of hepatic, renal, pulmonary, and cardiac disorders.

Administration factors

1. Give at mealtime to prevent GI distress. Milk can be used if nausea occurs. The drug should be discontinued if severe diarrhea persists.
2. Avoid administering with other drugs, particularly drugs that affect the CNS.
3. Capsules may be opened and dissolved in 1 to 2 fl oz of acidic fluid (orange juice) for clients who have difficulty in swallowing capsules.

Evaluation factors

1. Maintain a flowchart showing client's abilities and limitations. Assess client and update chart weekly. Notify physician when there is a lack of response.
2. Optimal effect results in reduction of pain and/or disabling spasticity, increase in self-care, and elimination of annoying manifestations.
3. Hepatic function tests should be done periodically (weekly, then biweekly, then monthly). If any abnormalities occur, notify physician.

Client teaching factors

1. Caution client against activities requiring constant attention (driving a car).
2. Warn client against the ingestion of alcohol and CNS depressants.
3. Inform client that capsules can be taken at mealtime or with milk to avoid GI disturbances.
4. Instruct client to wear sunglasses and to use sunscreening agents in order to avoid photosensitivity reactions.
5. Instruct client to notify health professionals immediately of any untoward reactions that occur, particularly jaundice, diarrhea, fever, and/or a rash.

GENERIC NAME Dantrolene sodium (parenteral)

TRADE NAME Dantrium IV (RX)

CLASSIFICATION Skeletal muscle relaxant

Action Dantrolene injection is a sterile lyophilized formulation of dantrolene sodium, pH 9.5. It has the same actions as dantrolene (oral), but the injection also contains mannitol as a vehicle and sodium hydroxide to adjust the pH. Dantrolene is thought to relax skeletal muscles by interfering with the release of calcium ions from the sarcoplasmic reticulum. Anesthetic-induced malignant hyperthermia syndrome is a rare genetic disorder of muscle tissue that is characterized by a sudden rise in myoplasmic calcium. The elevation in muscle calcium accentuates catabolic processes and results in a crisis manifested by fever, tachycardia, tachyphonia, hypercarbia, metabolic acidosis, cyanosis, increased utilization of anesthesia, and skeletal muscle rigidity. This disorder frequently results in death (about 70%). Although the immediate use of dantrolene IV increases the chance of survival, prompt attention to increased oxygen needs, management of fever, metabolic acidosis, and fluid and electrolyte balance are essential.

Indications for Use Malignant hyperthermia crisis.

Contraindications None.

Warnings and Precautions Safe use during pregnancy has not been established. The anesthetic agent (triggering agent) must be discontinued immediately and supportive measures instituted.

Untoward Reactions Extravasation of drug may cause severe tissue irritation and sloughing. Only hypersensitive skin reactions have occurred with short-term therapy. [See dantrolene sodium (oral).]

Parameters of Use See dantrolene sodium (oral) for further details.

Administration Total dosage required depends on severity of disorder, amount of triggering agent used, and the time lapse between onset of symptoms and drug administration. Initially, 1 mg/kg via continuous rapid IV bolus; then repeat as necessary; Maximum dosage: 10 mg/kg. If symptoms reappear, the regime may be repeated.

Available Drug Forms Vials for reconstitution containing 20 mg dantrolene and 3000 mg mannitol.

Nursing Management

Planning factors

1. Drug should be readily available in all locations where anesthetic agents are administered, including operating rooms, clinics, doctors' offices, and dentists' offices.
2. Sterile water without a bacteriostatic agent should be kept with the drug.
3. Protect vials from direct sunlight.

Administration factors

1. The triggering agent (anesthetic) should be discontinued.
2. Reconstitute drug with 60 ml of sterile water (without preservatives) and shake vial until solution becomes clear.
2. Check patency of IV site. Avoid administering into small blood vessels and questionable IV sites.
3. Administer continuously until symptoms subside. An anesthetist will usually administer the drug; a syringe pump can be used.
4. Prepare the next vial of drug as the first dose is being administered, thus preventing lapses in drug administration.

Evaluation factors

1. Monitor vital signs continuously during crisis, then every 10 to 15 minutes. Cardiac monitoring is recommended.
2. Record intake and output hourly.
3. A respirator may be required to maintain ventilation.
4. Frequent monitoring (hourly) of arterial gases is required until all danger has passed.
5. Notify physician immediately if the client's condition begins to deteriorate.

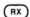

GENERIC NAME Quinine sulfate (RX)

TRADE NAMES Quinamm, Quinite, Quinium Sulfate

CLASSIFICATION Skeletal muscle relaxant

Action Quinine, a cinchona alkaloid, is a well-known antimalarial agent that may have a relaxant effect on skeletal muscles. It is thought to act directly on muscles by three mechanisms: (1) increases refractory period of muscle fibers; (2) decreases excitability of motor end plates; and (3) alters the distribution of calcium ions within muscle fibers. Because of its oxytocic properties, quinine has been used by laymen to induce abortion for years, but toxic or even fatal doses are required for complete abortion. Although the exact mechanism of antimalarial activity is unknown, the drug is thought to inhibit protein synthesis and depress enzyme systems in asexual erythrocytic parasites. It does not affect the exoerythrocytic form. Quinine also has antipyretic and analgesic properties.

Indications for Use Prevention and treatment of nocturnal leg muscle cramps. Malaria due to *Plasmodium falciparum* (chloroquine-resistant malaria).

Contraindications Hypersensitivity to quinine derivatives, pregnancy, glucose-6-phosphate dehydrogenase deficiency, tinnitus, optic neuritis, history of blackwater fever.

Warnings and Precautions Repeated use or excessive doses may cause cinchonism. Hemolysis may occur in clients with a glucose-6-phosphate dehydrogenase deficiency. Known to be a mutagen and potential carcinogenic agent. Use with caution in digitalized clients. Can cause congenital malformations, including deafness (auditory nerve hypoplasia), limb abnormalities, visceral defects, and blindness, particularly when toxic doses are ingested.

Untoward Reactions Cinchonism (hypersensitivity to cinchona alkaloids) is characterized by flushing, tinnitus, slight deafness, and vertigo. Pruritus, fever, GI distress, dyspnea, and visual impairment may also occur. Amblyopia may follow the administration of large doses; tinnitus may occur when serum drug levels exceed 10 mcg/ml. Blood dyscrasias, including hemolysis, thrombocytopenia, agranulocytosis, hypoprothrombinemia, and hemoglobinuria, which progresses to blackwater fever (fever, enlarged spleen and liver, epigastric pain, vomiting, jaundice, sudden shock) may occur. Visual disturbances, including photophobia, diplopia, decreasing visual fields, and disturbed color vision, may also occur. Angina may develop, particularly in clients with impairment of the cardiovascular system. CNS disturbances: deafness, vertigo, headache, nausea, vomiting, apprehension, confusion, syncope; convulsions have also occurred with excessive dosages. Allergic skin reactions, particularly urticaria, and papular or scarlatinal rashes, are common. Sweating and edema of the face may occur. Acute asthmatic episodes may be precipitated, but rarely. Angioneurotic edema has also been reported.

Parameters of Use

Absorption Readily absorbed from small intestine; irritating to GI tract. Completely absorbed, even when diarrhea is present. Peak action occurs in 1 to 3 hours. Average plasma drug levels: 7 mcg/ml (with 1 g po daily). Half-life is 4 to 5 hours. About 70% bound to plasma proteins.

Crosses placenta and enters breast milk; Lactating mothers should bottle-feed their babies.

Metabolism Primarily in the liver; primary metabolites are hydroxy derivatives; may depress enzyme system that synthesizes factors dependent on vitamin K.

Excretion Primarily by the kidneys as unchanged drug (5%) and metabolites; some in feces, bile, gastric juices, and saliva. Excretion is twice as rapid in acidic urine; tubular reabsorption occurs in alkaline urine.

Drug Interactions The simultaneous administration of aluminum-containing antacids may delay or decrease absorption of quinine. The effects of neuromuscular blocking agents, particularly pancuronium, succinylcholine, and tubocurarine, may be potentiated by quinine and result in respiratory depression. Urinary alkalizing agents, such as acetazolamide and sodium bicarbonate, may elevate quinine blood levels and result in toxicity. Urinary acidifiers promote the excretion of quinine and may be useful when treating quinine toxicity. Quinine may enhance the action of oral anticoagulants; but it may also chemically interact with heparin, thereby decreasing its anticoagulation capabilities.

Laboratory Interactions Quinine may alter the determination of urinary catecholamines and elevate the levels of 17-hydroxycorticosteroids when measured by the Timmerman method.

Administration Leg cramps: 260 mg po at bedtime; if ineffective, 260 mg po following evening meal and again at bedtime. Malaria: Adults, 260 mg po q h for 10 consecutive days. As much as 680 mg po 8 h may be required. Children: up to 15 mg/Kg/day in divided doses of q 8 h for 10 consecutive days. May be given concurrently with pyrimethamine or sulfadiazine or tetracycline during the first 3 to 5 days of drug therapy.

Available Drug Forms Tablets containing 260 mg.

Nursing Management

Planning factors

1. Complete blood cell count (CBC), prothrombin time (PT), and visual and hearing tests should be done prior to instituting drug.
2. Check for potential drug interactions.
3. Obtain history of the onset, duration, and severity of leg cramps.
4. Daily doses should be scheduled in the evening.
5. Obtain complete history of drug hypersensitivity.

Administration factors

1. May be given 1 hour after meals and with a snack at bedtime if GI disturbances occur.
2. Administer with a full glass of water.

Evaluation factors

1. When drug is first administered, check client frequently for hypersensitivity reactions. As little as 300 mg may cause tinnitus in hypersensitive clients.
2. Obtain CBC and PT periodically.
3. Check color of urine.
4. Assess the severity and duration of leg cramps. Once leg cramps no longer occur, the drug may be withheld for 1 to 2 days to determine drug's effectiveness.

Client teaching factors

1. Instruct client to report any untoward reactions, such as darkening of urine, tinnitus, and visual disturbances, immediately.
2. Instruct client to store drug away from light or excessive heat.

Chapter 32

General Anesthetics

BEFORE THE INTRODUCTION of anesthetic agents, surgery was a horrible ordeal performed hastily, often within minutes, on conscious clients. The anesthetic properties of nitrous oxide and ether had been accurately described in the 18th century, but it was not until nearly a century later that these properties were successfully demonstrated and the agents were accepted for use in surgery.

General anesthesia is a controlled depression of the central nervous system that renders the client unconscious with a loss of sensation throughout the body. The precise mechanism by which general anesthetics act is unknown, but it is thought that they inhibit the transmission of impulses from the peripheral nervous system to the brain by (1) blocking nerve synapses; (2) mechanically obstructing nerve conduction; and (3) inhibiting nerve cell membrane permeability. There is considerable experimental evidence to indicate that general anesthetics act primarily in the ascending reticular activating system to produce *narcosis,* a general term indicating progressive depression of the central nervous system that eventually leads to unconsciousness.

STAGES OF GENERAL ANESTHESIA

The progressive depression of the central nervous system was first described for the general anesthetic ether and the criteria used to determine the depth of ether anesthesia constitute the general guidelines used today (see Table 32-1).

The client is intubated after muscular and gag reflexes are depressed in stage I. Because stage II can have severe adverse effects on the client, anesthetics, such as thiopental sodium, are often administered intravenously to promote rapid induction of the initial stages of anesthesia. Most operations are performed during plane 2 or 3 of the surgical anesthesia stage (stage III). As some anesthetics do not provide adequate muscle relaxation for abdominal surgery, skeletal muscle relaxants, such as tubocurarine, are often used in addition to the anesthetic. When surgery is completed, the client is brought back up through the various stages of anesthesia, including stage II.

TYPES OF GENERAL ANESTHETIC AGENTS

General anesthetics can be divided into two groups: inhaled anesthetics and intravenous anesthetics. The inhalants can be further divided into gases and volatile liquids. The volatile liquids (chloroform, ether, fluroxene, methoxyflurane, trichloroethylene, vinyl ether) are vaporized and the client breathes a mixture of vapor and oxygen or other gases. When the vaporized gases (cyclopropane, ethylene, halothane, nitrous oxide) are administered, the client's oxygen intake may be altered. Hypoxia is a potential complication, particularly with nitrous oxide.

The absorption, distribution, and elimination of gases and the vapor of volatile liquids are similar. The drug is inhaled with inspired air into the alveoli and diffuses across the membrane into the blood. As long as the partial pressure of the anesthetic agent is greater than that in the tissues, a gradient is formed and the anesthetic enters the tissues until equilibrium occurs. Highly vascular tissues (liver, heart, brain) absorb the anesthetic agent faster than poorly vascularized tissue (fat). Although a few gases are metabolized to some degree (halothane is partially metabolized in the liver), most inhaled anesthetics are eliminated in expired air. Once the anesthetic agent is discontinued, the pressure gradients are reversed and the gas is expired. In general, the longer the gas is administered, the greater is the quantity of anesthetic stored in fatty tissue. Because of its lack of vascularity, fatty tissue liberates the gas slowly and therefore elimination of the gas is prolonged. Encouraging the client to cough and deep breathe postoperatively will assist in the elimination of the anesthetic. Since induction of anesthesia is relatively slow with ether, halothane, methoxyflurane, and trichloroethylene, the recovery from anesthesia is also prolonged.

Other drugs that cause central nervous system depression are synergistic with anesthetic agents. The barbiturates not only induce central nervous system depression, but the ultra-short-acting barbiturates, such as thiopental sodium, are also able to induce anesthesia. These compounds as well as other solutions, such as ketamine and droperidol/fentanyl, are adminis-

TABLE 32-1 Stages of Anesthesia

Stage	Characteristics	Remarks
I: Analgesia	Onset of drug administration until loss of consciousness. No response to painful stimuli. Depression of muscular and gag reflexes.	Endotracheal intubation
II: Delirium or excitement	Loss of consciousness. Depression of cortex but lower brain still functioning and causes involuntary activity, including laughing and restlessness. Increase in skeletal muscle tone. Overactive reflexes resulting in excessive salivation and respiratory secretions, coughing, and vomiting. Dilated pupils. Irregular breathing. Increase in blood pressure and heart rate.	Undesirable stage, ideally this stage is made as short as possible. Ultra-short-acting barbiturates IV cause client to pass through this stage quickly so that symptoms are essentially absent.
III: Surgical anesthesia	Spontaneous respirations (loss of irregular respirations) until cessation of respiratory activity (apnea).	
Plane 1	Regular respirations. Normal pupil size. Some muscular relaxation and facilitating eye movements occur. Inhibition of eyelid reflex.	
Plane 2	Deep, regular but slow respirations. Loss of eyelid and conjunctival reflexes. Fixed eyeballs. Skeletal muscle relaxation.	Desired plane for most operations.
Plane 3	Abdominal breathing due to diminished intercostal muscle action. Dilating pupils.	Lowest desired level for major surgery. Some manual ventilation desirable.
Plane 4	Complete intercostal muscle paralysis. Completely dilated and fixed pupils (do not respond to light).	Mechanical ventilation essential.
Stage IV: Medullary or respiratory paralysis	Complete cessation of respiratory activity (apnea). Severe hypotension that eventually leads to complete cardiovascular collapse.	Undesirable stage, death will ensue.

tered intravenously and induce anesthesia rapidly. Since their duration of action is short, these agents are frequently used to induce anesthesia for minor operations and diagnostic procedures. As these agents also promote the rapid induction of stage II, they are often used to induce anesthesia and a gaseous agent is used to maintain surgical anesthesia.

OTHER SUPPORTIVE DRUGS REQUIRED DURING GENERAL ANESTHESIA

Although all general anesthetic agents induce narcosis, some do not eliminate pain (analgesia), provide adequate skeletal muscle relaxation for abdominal surgery, or control untoward reactions. Halothane and thiopental sodium produce little or no anesthesia. Unfortunately, the client usually regains consciousness before an anesthetic can be safely administered. The nurse must use appropriate measures until the narcotic or analgesic can be safely administered.

During surgery, skeletal muscle relaxants are often required. Ether and methoxyflurane are exceptionally effective in relaxing skeletal muscles, but halothane, nitrous oxide, and thiopental sodium have inadequate muscle relaxation properties; droperidol/fentanyl causes muscular rigidity. Cholinergic neuromuscular blockers, such as gallamine, pancuronium, succinylcholine, and tubocurarine, are often required. These drugs may cause residual muscular weakness and pain during the immediate postoperative period.

Anticholinergic agents, such as atropine and scopolamine, are used preoperatively to diminish respiratory secretions and to block cardiac vagal reflexes stimulated by many of the anesthetics. Thiopental sodium may induce bronchospasms and laryngospasms if these anesthetic-induced effects are not blocked by other agents.

Fear of surgery and severe anxiety can adversely effect the central nervous system and the autonomic nervous system; cardiac arrest has occurred, particularly in children, at the onset of anesthesia. Some anxiety is natural and can be controlled by the administration of a barbiturate or hypnotic the night before. The preoperatively administered narcotic plays a dual role: it allays anxiety and decreases the quantity of anesthetic required to induce narcosis.

NURSING MANAGEMENT

There are a number of essential guidelines to follow in the preoperative care of a client.

1. Describe the anesthetic process and preoperative and postoperative procedures. Answer all questions. Teach coughing and deep breathing.
2. If the client expresses undue fear about surgery, notify physician. Allow the client to talk about his or her concerns. The operation may require postponement or a local anesthetic when possible.
3. Administer the hypnotic at the client's usual bedtime or 10 P.M., whichever comes first.
4. Administer the preoperative medication (usually a narcotic and anticholinergic agent) at the prescribed time, usually 45 to 60 minutes prior to surgery.
5. If surgery is delayed, notify operating room personnel of the time at which the preoperative medication was administered.

Postoperatively, the following guidelines should be observed.

1. Know what drugs were administered during the operation; these are recorded on the operating room sheet.
2. Expect pain with nonanalgesic anesthetics.
3. Expect muscular weakness when skeletal muscle relaxants have been used. Be sure the client's call bell is in his or her hand and that he or she can use it.
4. When the client is moved from stretcher to bed, expect blood pressure to be lower than normal due to the movement. Watch client for depressed respiration for 10 to 15 minutes, then repeat blood pressure measurement. Blood pressure should now be stabilized.
5. Start supplemental oxygen immediately upon return from operating room. Depressed respirations with resultant hypoxia frequently occur.
6. Encourage the client to cough and deep breathe frequently (every 15 minutes).
7. Assess the client's return to consciousness; ask client to tell you his or her name and where they are.
8. Inform client that surgery is over.
9. Administer analgesic as soon as it can be done safely, when nonanalgesic anesthetics have been used. Watch for respiratory depression and hypotension.
10. If an arrhythmia is indicated in the pulse rate and pressure, attach the client to cardiac monitoring equipment and treat accordingly.
11. If excitement occurs (return through stage II), notify surgeon or anesthetist and stay with the client.

INHALED ANESTHETICS

GENERIC NAME Chloroform (RX)

TRADE NAME Chloroform (RX)

CLASSIFICATION Inhaled general anesthetic

See chapter introduction for Nursing management.

Action Chloroform is a volatile liquid that is five times as potent as ether, has a narrow range of safety, and does not irritate the respiratory mucosa. The primary effects of chloroform on the body are:

1. Eliminates pain
2. Relaxes skeletal muscles
3. Progressively depresses respirations
4. Causes hypotension and bradycardia

Indications for Use Has been used for obstetrics and short procedures, but is rarely used today.

Untoward Reactions

Primary postoperative effects Rapid recovery with few ill effects. Toxic to liver and kidneys.

Parameters of Use

Induction Onset of action is 2 to 5 minutes. Induction is rapid.

GENERIC NAME Cyclopropane (RX)

TRADE NAMES Cyclopropane, Trimethylene

CLASSIFICATION Inhaled general anesthetic

See chapter introduction for Nursing management.

Action Cyclopropane is a volatile gas that has a wide margin of safety and does not irritate the respiratory mucosa. The primary effects of cyclopropane on the body are:

1. Eliminates pain
2. Relaxes skeletal muscles
3. Causes respiratory depression at high concentrations
4. Causes little change in blood pressure or heart rate
5. Sensitizes myocardium to catecholamines and causes arrhythmias

Indications for Use Has been used for major and minor operations, but is seldom used today.

Untoward Reactions

Primary postoperative effects Rapid recovery with few or no ill effects.

Parameters of Use

Induction Onset of action is 2 to 3 minutes. Induction is rapid.

Excretion Rapidly eliminated by lungs; allows use of high oxygen concentrations. Some excreted by the kidneys.

GENERIC NAME Ether (RX)

TRADE NAMES Diethyl Ether, Ethyl Ether

CLASSIFICATION Inhaled general anesthetic

See chapter introduction for Nursing management.

Action Ether is a volatile liquid with an unpleasant odor. It has a wide range of safety and does not sensitize the myocardium to catecholamines. Ether is sometimes used after anesthesia has been induced by a shorter-acting anesthetic. When in contact with air, ether will degrade products such as plastics. The primary effects of ether on the body are:

1. Eliminates pain
2. Relaxes skeletal muscles excellently
3. Initially increases, then depresses respiration
4. Causes hypotension and bradycardia during surgical anesthesia

Indications for Use Major operations, obstetric procedures.

Untoward Reactions

Primary postoperative effects Slow recovery with nausea and vomiting. Toxic to liver and kidneys.

Parameters of Use

Induction Onset of action is 10 to 20 minutes. Induction is slow.
Excretion By the lungs and kidneys.

GENERIC NAME Ethylene (RX)

TRADE NAME Ethene

CLASSIFICATION Inhaled general anesthetic

See chapter introduction for Nursing management.

Action Ethylene is a gas with an unpleasant sweet odor and requires the use of a premedication for most operations. It does not sensitize the myocardium to catecholamines or irritate the respiratory mucosa. A mixture of nitrous oxide and ethylene is highly explosive. The primary effects of ethylene on the body are:

1. Relaxes skeletal muscles
2. Causes little or no respiratory and vasomotor depression
3. May produce hypoxia during induction
4. Initially raises blood pressure and then it returns to normal during surgical anesthesia

Indications for Use Short operations, but rarely used due to explosive properties.

Untoward Reactions

Primary postoperative effects Rapid recovery with few or no ill effects. Little or no liver and kidney toxicity.

Parameters of Use

Induction Induction is rapid; after 6 to 8 inhalations. Surgical anesthesia occurs in 2 to 5 minutes.

GENERIC NAME Fluroxene (RX)

TRADE NAME Fluoromar

CLASSIFICATION Inhaled general anesthetic

See chapter introduction for Nursing management.

Action Fluroxene, a volatile liquid, is a fluorine-containing ether that is less flammable than other ethers. It does not sensitize the myocardium to catecholamines. The primary effects of fluroxene on the body are:

1. Produces excellent analgesia
2. Relaxes skeletal muscles
3. Causes little change in blood pressure, pulse, or respirations

Indications for Use Minor operations, induction agent for other anesthetics.

Untoward Reactions

Primary postoperative effects Rapid recovery with nausea and vomiting. Relatively nontoxic to liver and kidneys.

Parameters of Use

Induction Onset of action is about 2 to 3 minutes.

GENERIC NAME Halothane (RX)

TRADE NAME Fluothane

CLASSIFICATION Inhaled general anesthetic

See chapter introduction for Nursing management.

Action Halothane is a gas containing fluorine that is four times as potent as ether. Anesthesia induced by halothane is similar to that induced by chloroform but with considerably less toxicity. It does not irritate the respiratory mucosa and the use of preanesthetic agents reduces induction delirium. Hypoxia is avoided during induction. This agent is often used with nitrous oxide and muscle relaxants. The primary effects of halothane on the body are:

1. Produces poor analgesia
2. Causes some skeletal muscle relaxation
3. Depresses respirations, which progressively deteriorate
4. Causes hypotension and bradycardia
5. Sensitizes myocardium to catecholamines

Indications for Use Major and minor operations.

Warnings and Precautions Use with caution in obstetric procedures as uterine contractions are decreased.

Untoward Reactions

Primary postoperative effects Slow recovery, which is faster than ether, that may be accompanied by respiratory depression. May cause hepatotoxicity.

Parameters of Use

Induction Surgical anesthesia occurs in 2 to 10 minutes.
Metabolism Major products of metabolism are chlorine and bromine, which are excreted by the lungs and kidneys.

GENERIC NAME Methoxyflurane (RX)

TRADE NAME Penthrane

CLASSIFICATION Inhaled general anesthetic

See chapter introduction for Nursing management.

Action Nonflammable anesthetic gas that is very potent and causes anesthesia similar to halothane. However, unlike halothane, methoxyflurane causes some irritation to the respiratory mucosa. The primary effects of methoxyflurane on the body are:

1. Eliminates pain
2. Relaxes skeletal muscles excellently
3. Progressively depresses respirations
4. Causes some hypotension and bradycardia during surgical anesthesia
5. Produces some myocardial sensitization to catecholamines

Indications for Use Obstetric procedures.

Untoward Reactions

Primary postoperative effects Prolonged recovery with analgesia persisting after consciousness regained. Toxic to kidneys.

Parameters of Use

Induction Induction is slow.
Excretion Primarily by the kidneys.

GENERIC NAME Nitrous oxide (RX)

TRADE NAME Nitrogen Monoxide

CLASSIFICATION Inhaled general anesthetic

See chapter introduction for Nursing management.

Action Nitrous oxide is a gas with relatively low potency; but concentrations above 70% may cause hypoxia. Preanesthetic agents are required and skeletal muscle relaxants must be used for abdominal and other surgical procedures. The primary effects of nitrous oxide on the body are:

1. Eliminates pain
2. Produces little skeletal muscle relaxation
3. Causes little or no change in blood pressure, pulse, or respiration
4. May cause hypoxia that can be profound in large doses or with prolonged use

Indications for Use Minor operations; adjunct in major operations, but not recommended for prolonged anesthesia.

Untoward Reactions

Primary postoperative effects Moderately rapid recovery with few ill effects. Hypoxia may occur if oxygen therapy is not given. Prolonged use may cause nausea and vomiting. Return to consciousness may be delayed. Low toxicity.

Parameters of Use

Induction Onset of action is 1 to 2 minutes. Induction is rapid.
Excretion By the lungs.

GENERIC NAME Trichloroethylene (RX)

TRADE NAMES Chlorylen, Trilene

CLASSIFICATION Inhaled general anesthetic

See chapter introduction for Nursing management.

Action Trichloroethylene is a volatile liquid with an odor similar to that of chloroform. It is frequently used because it is nonflammable and nonexplosive. The primary effects of trichloroethylene on the body are:

1. Produces rapid, shallow respirations
2. Sensitizes myocardium to catecholamines
3. Causes arrhythmias, bradycardia, and A-V conduction disturbances

Indications for Use Major and minor operations, obstetric procedures, trigeminal neuralagia.

Untoward Reactions

Primary postoperative effects Slow recovery; toxic to liver.

Parameters of Use

Induction Induction is slow.

GENERIC NAME Vinyl ether (RX)

TRADE NAMES Divinyl Oxide, Vinethene

CLASSIFICATION Inhaled general anesthetic

See chapter introduction for Nursing management.

Action Vinyl ether is a volatile liquid. It is an explosive anesthetic similar to ether, but with a less objectionable odor, and irritates the respiratory mucosa. The primary effects of vinyl ether on the body are:

1. Eliminates pain
2. Relaxes skeletal muscles
3. Initially increases, then depresses respirations
4. Causes hypotension and bradycardia during surgical anesthesia

Indications for Use Minor operations and other short procedures.

Untoward Reactions

Primary postoperative effects Rapid recovery; extensive hepatotoxicity with prolonged use; can cause kidney toxicity.

Parameters of Use

Induction Onset of action is about 30 seconds. Induction is rapid.

INTRAVENOUS ANESTHETICS

GENERIC NAME Droperidol (RX)

TRADE NAME Inapsine

CLASSIFICATION Intravenous anesthetic

Action Droperidol produces marked tranquilization and sedation and has an antiemetic effect. It potentiates CNS depressants and causes a mild alpha-adrenergic blockade, but does not eliminate pain. The primary effects of droperidol on the body are:

1. Causes an indifference to surroundings
2. May decrease pulmonary arterial pressure
3. Causes peripheral vascular dilation and hypotension
4. Desensitizes myocardium to catecholamines (prevents arrhythmias)
5. Decreases incidence of nausea and vomiting

Indications for Use Premedication, short diagnostic or surgical procedures, as an adjunct to general anesthesia.

Warnings and Precautions Safe use in children (under 2 years) and during pregnancy has not been established.

Untoward Reactions

Primary postoperative effects Residual effects may persist for 12 hours. Hypotension, chills (shivering), and hallucinations may occur.

Parameters of Use

Absorption Onset of action is 3 to 10 minutes. Peak action occurs in 30 minutes and duration of action is 2 to 4 hours.

Metabolism In the liver.

Excretion In urine.

Administration Highly individualized.

- *Premedication:* Adults: 2.5 to 10 mg IM 30 to 60 minutes preoperatively; Children, elderly and debilitated clients: About $\frac{1}{2}$ of adult dosage.
- *Adjunct:* Adults: Initial dosage: 0.1 mg/lb IV; Maintenance dosage: 1.25 to 2.5 mg IV bolus; Children, elderly and debilitated clients: About $\frac{1}{2}$ of adult dosage.

Available Drug Forms Ampules of 2 or 5 ml containing 2.5 mg/ml; 10-ml multidose vials containing 2.5 mg/ml.

Nursing Management (See page 526.)

1. IV solutions and other measures to combat hypotension should be readily available.
2. Usually administered with a narcotic analgesic.

GENERIC NAME Fentanyl citrate (RX)

TRADE NAME Sublimaze

CLASSIFICATION Intravenous anesthetic

Action Narcotic analgesic (100 mcg equals about 10 mg morphine or 75 mg meperidine). Large doses may cause apnea. The drug is used with oxygen and skeletal muscle relaxants.

Indications for Use Premedication, induction of anesthesia, as an adjunct to other anesthetic agents, anesthesia for high-risk clients (open heart surgery).

Warnings and Precautions Safe use in children (under 2 years) and during pregnancy has not been established. Effects may be potentiated by MAO inhibitors. May decrease pulmonary artery pressure.

Untoward Reactions May cause nausea, vomiting, muscular rigidity, bradycardia, euphoria, miosis, bronchoconstriction, or hypotension.

Primary postoperative effects Residual effects may persist for 4 hours. Respiratory depression persists after analgesic effect disappears. Reduced dosages of analgesics are used.

Parameters of Use

Absorption Onset of action is: immediate (IV); 7 to 8 minutes (IM). Duration of action is: 30 to 60 minutes (IV); 1 to 2 hours (IM).

Metabolism In the liver.

Excretion By the kidneys.

Administration Highly individualized.

- *Premedication:* 50 to 100 mcg IM 30 to 60 minutes preoperatively.
- *Adjunct:* 2 to 20 mcg/kg IM or IV.
- *Anesthesia:* 50 to 100 mcg/kg IM or IV.

Available Drug Forms Ampules of 2, 5, 10, or 20 ml containing 50 mcg/ml.

Nursing Management (See page 526.)

1. Narcotic antagonist and mechanical ventilation equipment should be readily available in the event of apnea.
2. Protect from light and store at room temperature.

GENERIC NAME Droperidol/fentanyl (Cii)

TRADE NAME Innovar

CLASSIFICATION Intravenous anesthetic

See droperidol and fentanyl citrate for Action, Warnings and precautions, Untoward reactions, and Parameters of use. See page 526 and droperidol and fentanyl for Nursing management.

Indications for Use Premedication, surgical and diagnostic procedures of short duration, as an adjunct to anesthesia, anesthesia.

Administration Highly individualized.

- *Premedication:* Adults: 0.5 to 2 ml IM 45 to 60 minutes preoperatively; Children, elderly and debilitated clients: About $\frac{1}{2}$ of adult dosage.
- *Adjunct:* Adults: 1 ml/20 to 25 lb slow IV bolus or IV drip; Children, elderly and debilitated clients: About $\frac{1}{2}$ of adult dosage.

Available Drug Forms Ampules of 2 or 5 ml. Generic contents: droperidol: 2.5 mg; fentanyl: 50 mcg.

GENERIC NAME Ketamine hydrochloride (RX)

TRADE NAMES Ketaject, Ketalar

CLASSIFICATION Intravenous anesthetic

See chapter introduction for Nursing management.

Action Ketamine is a dissociative anesthetic; that is, it selectively interrupts association pathways in the brain before inducing somesthetic sensory blockade. Since the anesthesia does not affect pharyngeal-laryngeal reflexes or skeletal muscle reflexes, it cannot be used for bronchoscopy or other respiratory tract procedures. The drug has a wide margin of safety and low toxicity. It is usually given with atropine and skeletal muscle relaxants. The primary effects of ketamine hydrochloride on the body are:

1. Eliminates pain
2. Depresses respirations
3. Elevates blood pressure (above 20 to 25%) and increases pulse rate
4. Produces involuntary tonic-clonic movements
5. Elevates cerebrospinal fluid pressure

Indications for Use Sole anesthetic for diagnostic procedures and burn dressings; as an adjunct to other anesthetics; as a supplement to low potency anesthetics, such as nitrous oxide; often used in children as the sole anesthetic.

Contraindications Clients in whom elevated blood pressure would constitute a serious hazard, including clients with hypertension and congestive heart failure.

Warnings and Precautions Safe use in pregnancy has not been established. Use with caution in clients with elevated cerebrospinal fluid pressure.

Untoward Reactions

Primary postoperative effects Confused state may last up to 24 hours. Dreamlike state, hallucinations, and emergence can be minimized if client has reduced verbal and tactile stimulation.

Parameters of Use

Absorption Onset of action is: 30 seconds (IV); 5 to 10 minutes (IM). Duration of action is: 5 to 10 minutes (IV); 12 to 25 minutes (IM). Peak serum levels: 0.75 mcg/ml.

Crosses placenta.

Metabolism In the liver.

Excretion In urine, some in feces.

Administration Highly individualized. Initial dosage: Intramuscular: 6.5 to 13 mg/kg; Intravenous: 1 to 4.5 mg/kg infused over 60 seconds or more. Maintenance dosage: $\frac{1}{2}$ full calculated dosage.

Available Drug Forms Tablets containing 10, 25, or 50 mg; 10-ml vials containing 10 or 20 mg/ml; suspension containing 50 mg/5ml.

GENERIC NAME Methohexital sodium (C iv)

TRADE NAME Brevital Sodium

CLASSIFICATION Intravenous anesthetic

Action Nonsulfur-containing, ultra-short-acting barbiturate (see Chapter 29). The primary effects of methohexital sodium on the body are:

1. Depresses respirations and may cause bronchospasms
2. Produces muscular twitching
3. Causes hypotension and tachycardia
4. Causes excessive salivation, nausea, and vomiting
5. Causes pain at injection site

Indications for Use Induction of anesthesia for short procedures, as an adjunct for other general anesthetics, induction of hypnotic states.

Warnings and Precautions Safe use during pregnancy has not been established. Use with caution in the elderly; debilitated clients; and clients with impaired respiratory, circulatory, renal, hepatic, or endocrine function. Use with extreme caution in clients with status asthmaticus. Extravasation may cause pain, ulceration, and necrosis.

Untoward Reactions

Primary postoperative effects Rapid recovery with nausea and vomiting. Emergence delirium may occur.

Parameters of Use

Absorption Onset of action is immediate and duration of action is 5 to 7 minutes after IV bolus.

Administration Highly individualized. IV bolus: Initial dosage: 50 to 120 mg of a 1% solution; then 20 to 40 mg of a 1% solution every 4 to 7 minutes. Continuous IV drip: 0.2% solution administered at 60 gtt/min.

Available Drug Forms 50-ml vials containing 500 mg; 50-ml vials containing 2500 mg; vials containing 500 mg of dry powder; IV bottles (500 ml) containing 5000 mg of dry powder.

Nursing Management (See page 526.)

1. 0.2% solution (not sterile water) prepared by adding 500 mg of drug to 250 ml of 5% D/W or normal saline.
2. Reconstituted solutions are stable for 24 hours; do not use if cloudy or if precipitate is present.

GENERIC NAME Thiamylal sodium (C iii)

TRADE NAME Surital

CLASSIFICATION Intravenous anesthetic

Action Ultra-short-acting barbiturate (see Chapter 29). The primary effects of thiamylal sodium on the body are:

1. Depresses respirations and may cause bronchospasms
2. Produces muscular twitching

3. Causes hypotension and tachycardia
4. Causes excessive salivation, nausea, and vomiting
5. Causes pain at injection site.

Indications for Use Induction of anesthesia, as an adjunct for other general anesthetics, induction of hypnotic states.

Warnings and Precautions Safe use during pregnancy has not been established. Use with caution in the elderly and clients with impaired respiratory, circulatory, renal, hepatic, or endocrine function. Use with extreme caution in clients with status asthmaticus. Extravasation may cause pain, ulceration, and necrosis.

Parameters of Use

Absorption Onset of action is immediate. Duration of action is 5 to 7 minutes. Recovery occurs within 20 to 30 minutes.

Administration Highly individualized. IV bolus: Initial dosage: 3 to 6 ml of a 2.5% solution at a rate of 1 ml/second; then 0.5 to 1 ml, as needed; Continuous IV drip: 0.3% solution; Maximum dosage: 40 ml of a 2.5% solution.

Available Drug Forms: Vials containing 1, 5, or 10 g for dilution with normal saline or 5% D/W.

Nursing Management (See page 526.)

1. May be used with muscle relaxants.
2. Discard solution if it becomes cloudy or a precipitate is present.

GENERIC NAME Thiopental sodium (C iii)

TRADE NAME Pentothal

CLASSIFICATION Intravenous anesthetic

See chapter introduction for Nursing management.

Action Thiopental sodium, a sulfur analog of sodium pentobarbital, is an ultra-short-acting CNS depressant that induces hypnosis and anesthesia but not analgesia. The primary effects of thiopental on the body are:

1. Does not eliminate pain; there is pain at injection site
2. Causes shivering
3. Depresses respirations and apnea follows each injection
4. Causes hypotension and bradycardia

Indications for Use Sole anesthetic for brief procedures, induction of anesthesia for major surgery, as an adjunct to other anesthetics, induction of hypnotic states, control of convulsions during surgery and postoperatively

Contraindications Status asthmaticus, porphyria.

Warnings and Precautions Use with extreme caution in clients with cardiovascular disorders, hypotension, shock, Addison's disease, hepatic or renal impairment, myxedema, elevated blood urea nitrogen, severe anemia, asthma, or myasthenia gravis. Extravasation may cause tissue necrosis.

Untoward Reactions

Primary postoperative effects Rapid recovery after small dose with somnolence, retrograde amnesia, and shivering.

Parameters of Use

Absorption Onset of action is about 60 seconds. Half-life is 3 to 8 hours. About 80% bound to plasma proteins.

Crosses placenta and enters breast milk. Crosses blood-brain barrier.

Storage Stored in fatty tissues in concentrations 6 to 12 times greater than in plasma; released slowly to cause prolonged anesthesia.

Metabolism In the liver; some in the kidneys and brain.

Excretion In urine.

Administration Highly individualized.

- *Induction:* 210 to 280 mg IV bolus.
- *Anesthesia:* 50 to 75 mg IV bolus infused over 1 minute; may be repeated if necessary.
- *Convulsions:* 75 to 125 mg IV bolus.

Available Drug Forms Vials containing 1, 2, 5, or 10 g.

PART VIII

PSYCHOTROPIC AGENTS

PSYCHOPHARMACOLOGY HAS BEEN revolutionized over the past three decades. Severe mental illness, which formerly doomed people to institutionalized lives, can now be successfully treated with medication and psychotherapy while the client remains in the community.

The role of mental health nurses has also changed dramatically. Today, mental health nurses work increasingly with clients who use outpatient services provided by local community mental health centers. The nurses at these centers are professionally accountable for the administration of psychotropic agents to nearly all the clients who use these services.

Although nurses have welcomed these new opportunities to provide community-based services, added responsibilities have developed as a result of this development. Nurses who administer medications in hospital settings feel secure in the knowledge that skilled nurses, physicians, and allied health personnel are instantly available when patients suddenly develop allergic responses to powerful drugs. However, nurses in community settings, even more than their hospital-based colleagues, must be able to anticipate these emergencies and be able to take quick action. Consequently, extensive knowledge of psychotropic agents, which is constantly updated, is a necessity.

Psychotropic agents have been prescribed so frequently in recent years that great controversy has been aroused. These drugs, in fact, account for more than half of all prescriptions written. Today, these agents are not only used to treat people suffering from hallucinations or delusions, but also to help people adjust to a change in health status or body image following medical or surgical therapy. Women coping with abusive husbands, demanding children, or a restrictive life-style imposed by their culture are more often treated with a quick prescription rather than a leisurely counseling session.[1]

Controversy has also developed concerning the extensive use of psychotropic agents in prisons, nursing homes, and other institutions that serve people who are not mentally ill. Bereaved persons are often given psychotropic agents to help them cope with their normal experience of grief and young children identified as hyperactive are given drugs to help them perform better in school. In addition, the problems of addiction, illicit street use, and suicide attempts that are associated with these drugs are so vast that they cannot be ignored.[2]

Nurses need to play an active role to reverse this alarming trend of inappropriate medication; that is, medication used for social control. Although nurses have always accepted their professional obligation to question an order that gives a medication via the wrong route or involves administering a toxic dose, they now need to accept the responsibility of questioning an order that prescribes a powerful psychotropic agent for a social problem, such as grief, divorce, or unemployment.

Nurses must also query the long-term use of these agents. If an antianxiety agent is prescribed for an individual in an alcohol abuse treatment program, for how long should that drug be taken? A week? A month? Forever? Nurses need to work in partnership with allied health professionals to minimize both the number of prescriptions and the length of time compliance is expected.

[1]Stephenson, P. S., and Walker, G. A. 1980. Psychotropic drugs and women. *Bioethics Quarterly* 2:20.

[2]Martin, E. W. 1978. *Hazards of medication*. Philadelphia: J. B. Lippincott, pp. 10–11, 308–310.

Chapter 33

Antipsychotic Agents

CHARACTERISTICS OF ANTIPSYCHOTIC AGENTS

The five major types of antipsychotic agents are (1) phenothiazines; (2) butyrophenones; (3) thioxanthenes; (4) dihydroindolones; and (5) dibenzoxazepines. Formerly called major tranquilizers, antipsychotic agents are also known as neuroleptics and ataractics.

Antipsychotic agents are also sometimes termed chemical restraints, as they have made such physical restraints as straitjackets and hydrotherapy obsolete. The resulting dramatic reduction in the incidence and duration of violent behavior among the mentally ill receiving these drugs provided the impetus to care for people in the least restrictive environment possible.

Antipsychotic agents effectively decrease the occurrence of hallucinations, delusions, and the accompanying hostility. Clients who take these medications consistently as treatment for psychosis are more amenable to participating in other treatment modalities, such as group therapy.

Properties of Phenothiazines

Chlorpromazine The usefulness of chlorpromazine in treating mental illness was discovered at the time when antihistamine research was in progress, and it has been widely accepted as an effective antipsychotic agent since 1951. A number of derivatives that provide the same therapeutic effects as chlorpromazine while minimizing the toxic side effects have also been developed. The phenothiazines act as sedative antipsychotic agents by depressing the subcortical centers of the brain, which are believed to be the seat of the emotions. Although vital centers of the brain are not depressed, the calmness produced is often sufficient to improve sleep problems. The exact mechanism of action is unknown, but the drugs apparently work by blocking dopamine receptors. Some experts believe that the turnover rate of dopamine in the basal ganglia is increased.

FUTURE DIRECTIONS AND ONGOING RESEARCH

The following drugs have been identified by Patricia Duggan Irons[1] as long-acting antipsychotic agents and are currently under investigation. The federal Food and Drug Administration has not yet approved these drugs for use in the United States:

1. Fluspirilene (Imap)
2. Penfluridol (Semap)
3. Pimozide (Orap)

PHENOTHIAZINES

GENERIC NAME Chlorpromazine hydrochloride

TRADE NAMES Chlor-PZ, Promachel, Promapar, Sonazine, Thorazine

CLASSIFICATION Antipsychotic (RX)

Action Antipsychotic, antiemetic, hypothermic, sedative, antidopaminergic, and anticholinergic actions. Inhibits release of ACTH, growth hormone, and prolactin-inhibiting factor. Not effective in depression or retarded withdrawal states.

Indications for Use Psychoses, hiccups, acromegaly, as an antiemetic. Also, during surgery, labor, and delivery, to enhance action of narcotics and hypnotics. In combination with analgesics for severe cancer pain.

Contraindications Pregnancy, coma, glaucoma, prostatic hypertrophy, cardiovascular disease, convulsive disorders, infants under 6 months.

Warnings and Precautions Use with caution in women of childbearing age, elderly clients, and children (since they are more susceptible to acute dystonia than adults). Clients with cirrhosis are more susceptible to sedative effects. Clients with the following conditions should be evaluated frequently: renal, hepatic, cardiovascular, or respiratory disease, blood dyscrasias, cardiovascular accidents, hypoparathyroidism.

Untoward Reactions Drowsiness is common; tolerance usually develops in 1 to 2 weeks. Hypotension, evidenced by dizziness and weakness on standing, is common. Extrapyramidal symptoms: uncoordinated spasmodic movements, involuntary motor restlessness, parkinsonism. Tardive dyskinesia, which is characterized by hyperkinetic activity in the oral region and for which there is no effective treatment, may appear after long-term use, but has also been reported after low doses given for short periods. Autonomic nervous system effects: dry mouth,

[1] Duggan Irons, P. 1978. *Psychotropic drugs and nursing intervention.* New York: McGraw Hill, p. 14.

blurred vision, constipation, urinary disturbances, weight gain, delayed ovulation, amenorrhea, abnormal lactation, increased libido in women, decreased libido in men. Dermatologic effects: skin rash, skin discoloration on exposure to sunlight, phototoxicity (painful sunburn after brief exposure to sun). Visual changes: corneal and lens opacities. Toxic effects: obstructive jaundice, agranulocytosis, hepatitis, leukopenia.

Parameters of Use

Absorption Readily absorbed from parenteral sites; erratic absorption following oral administration. Peak action occurs in 1 to 3 hours and duration of action is 3 to 6 hours. Half-life is about 6 hours.

Crosses placenta and blood-brain barrier.

Distribution Distributed to all body tissues with some distribution to brain. Concentrated in lungs and keratin structures.

Metabolism In the liver.

Excretion In urine and feces.

Drug Interactions Potentiates hypotensive effects of methyldopa, reserpine, and beta blockers; potentiates the anticholinergic effects of tricyclic antidepressants and antiparkinsonian drugs. Enhances respiratory depression produced by meperidine. Blocks the hypotensive effects of guanethidine. Lithium, trihexyphenidyl, and antacids decrease plasma levels of chlorpromazine. Alcohol and sedatives potentiate sedative effects of chlorpromazine.

Laboratory Interactions False-positive results may occur for urobilinogen, urine bilirubin, and pregnancy tests. May also affect results for urine catecholamines, ketones, and radioactive iodine uptake tests.

Administration Adults: 30 mg to 1 g po, IM, or IV daily in divided doses; Rectal suppository: 100 mg every 6 to 8 hours. Children: 2 mg/kg po daily in divided doses.

Available Drug Forms Tablets containing 10, 25, 50, 100, or 200 mg; sustained-release capsules containing 30, 75, 150, or 200 mg; ampules of 1 or 2 ml containing 25 mg/ml; 10-ml vials containing 25 mg/ml; syrup containing 10 mg/5 ml; suppositories containing 25 or 100 mg.

Nursing Management

Planning factors

1. Drug should be discontinued at least 48 hours prior to surgery.
2. Protect elderly clients with bedrails; these clients are more prone to develop hypotension.
3. Institute measures to prevent hyperthermia or hypothermia.

Administration factors

1. Protect skin, eyes, and clothing from contact with drug.
2. When administering IM, drug should be slowly and deeply injected. The pain from injection can be alleviated by massaging the injection site.
3. Do not mix with other drugs.

Evaluation factors

1. Because orthostatic hypotension is common, the client's blood pressure should be monitored daily. Observe for dizziness and weakness.
2. In severe cases of hypotension, put client in Trendelenburg's position and request administration of plasma expanders.
3. Monitor intake and output; check frequency of bowel movements.
4. Report any visual changes and schedule regular eye examinations.
5. Report sore throat or elevated temperature.
6. Observe client for jaundice.
7. If client develops extrapyramidal symptoms, reduce sensory stimuli.

Client teaching factors

1. Caution client against activities requiring mental alertness and muscular coordination.
2. Advise client to avoid alcohol, sedatives, and hypnotics.
3. Advise client to change position gradually and to dangle legs for 1 minute before getting out of bed.
4. Because of photosensitivity, client should be instructed to protect him- or herself from exposure to sun.
5. Encourage high fluid intake and frequent rinsing of mouth.
6. Advise client not to discontinue drug without medical supervision.

GENERIC NAME Acetophenazine maleate (RX)

TRADE NAME Tindal

CLASSIFICATION Antipsychotic

See Chlorpromazine for Contraindications, Warnings and precautions, Parameters of use, Drug interactions, and Nursing management.

Action Acetophenazine has a stronger sedative effect than chlorpromazine. (See chlorpromazine.)

Indications for Use Management of psychoses in the elderly, such as organic brain syndrome. Large dosages are needed to treat other psychoses.

Untoward Reactions Produces fewer extrapyramidal symptoms than chlorpromazine. (See chlorpromazine.)

Administration Adults: 40 to 80 mg po daily; Children: 0.8 to 1.6 mg/kg po daily in 3 divided doses.

Available Drug Forms Tablets containing 20 mg.

GENERIC NAME Butaperazine maleate (RX)

TRADE NAME Repoise

CLASSIFICATION Antipsychotic

See chlorpromazine for Contraindications, Warnings and precautions, Parameters of use, Drug interactions, and Nursing management.

Action Similar to chlorpromazine. (See chlorpromazine.)

Indications for Use Treatment of paranoia and chronic brain syndrome.

Untoward Reactions Extrapyramidal symptoms occur frequently.

Administration Adults: 15 to 30 mg po daily in divided doses; can be increased to a maximum dosage of 100 mg/day. Geriatrics: $\frac{1}{4}$ to $\frac{1}{2}$ of adult dosage.

Available Drug Forms Tablets containing 5, 10, or 25 mg.

GENERIC NAME Carphenazine maleate (RX)

TRADE NAME Proketazine

CLASSIFICATION Antipsychotic

See chlorpromazine for Indications for use, Contraindications, Warnings and precautions, Untoward reactions, Parameters of use, and Drug interactions.

Action Similar to other phenothiazines in the piperazine group. (See chlorpromazine.)

Administration Adults: 75 to 150 mg po daily in divided doses; can be increased every 1 to 2 weeks by 25 to 50 mg; Maximum dosage: 400 mg/day. Geriatrics: $\frac{1}{2}$ of adult dosage.

Available Drug Forms Tablets containing 12.5, 25, or 50 mg; concentrate containing 50 mg/ml.

Nursing Management Full therapeutic effect may not be apparent for several months. (See chlorpromazine.)

GENERIC NAME Fluphenazine enanthate, fluphenazine decanoate

TRADE NAME Prolixin (RX)

CLASSIFICATION Antipsychotic

See chlorpromazine for Contraindications, Warnings and precautions, Parameters of use, and Drug interactions.

Action Similar to chlorpromazine. (See chlorpromazine.)

Indications for Use Treatment of outpatients whose compliance with a medication regimen is doubtful.

Untoward Reactions This drug is very potent and has a high incidence of extrapyramidal symptoms. (See chlorpromazine.)

Administration Adults: 2.5 to 10 mg po daily in divided doses; under close hospital supervision, clients can receive up to 20 mg daily; 25 mg IM every 1 to 3 weeks. Children: 0.25 to 3 mg po daily in divided doses.

Available Drug Forms Vials of 10 ml containing 2.5 mg/ml; protect from light; if solution is darker than light amber, do not use. Tablets containing 1, 2.5, 5, or 10 mg; protect from light. Elixir containing 0.5 mg/ml; avoid freezing.

Nursing Management (See chlorpromazine.)

1. Antiparkinsonian drugs may be needed to prevent extrapyramidal symptoms.
2. Geriatric clients are at a greater risk of developing extrapyramidal symptoms, especially women who have been medicated with phenothiazines for a long time.

GENERIC NAME Mesoridazine besylate (RX)

TRADE NAME Serentil

CLASSIFICATION Antipsychotic

See chlorpromazine for Indications for use, Contraindications, Warnings and precautions, Untoward reactions, Parameters of use, Drug interactions, and Nursing management.

Action Similar to chlorpromazine. Not effective in treatment of delirium tremens. (See chlorpromazine.)

Administration Adults: 100 to 400 mg po daily in divided doses; 25 to 200 mg IM daily in divided doses. Geriatrics: $\frac{1}{4}$ or $\frac{1}{2}$ of adult dosage.

Available Drug Forms Tablets containing 10, 25, 50, or 100 mg; 10-ml vials containing 25 mg/ml.

GENERIC NAME Perphenazine (RX)

TRADE NAME Trilafon

CLASSIFICATION Antipsychotic, antiemetic

See chlorpromazine for Indications for use, Contraindications, Warnings and precautions, Untoward reactions, Parameters of use, and Drug interactions.

Action Similar to chlorpromazine, but six times more potent. (See chlorpromazine.)

Administration Adults: 16 to 64 mg po or IM daily in divided doses.

Available Drug Forms Tablets containing 2, 4, or 8 mg; syrup containing 2 mg/5 ml; concentrate containing 16 mg/ml (diluted in 60 ml of fluid).

Nursing Management (See chlorpromazine.)

1. May be used IV during surgery for hiccups or vomiting. Should not be given IV as an antipsychotic.
2. Dilute concentrate with water, milk, or orange juice. Do not mix with tea, coffee, cola, apple, or grape juice.

GENERIC NAME Piperacetazine (RX)

TRADE NAME Quide

CLASSIFICATION Antipsychotic

See chlorpromazine for Contraindications, Warnings and precautions, Parameters of use, Drug interactions, and Nursing management.

Action Similar to chlorpromazine. (See chlorpromazine.)

Indications for Use Schizophrenia characterized by agitation; most effective in treating acute rather than chronic schizophrenia.

Untoward Reactions Piperacetazine causes a higher incidence of extrapyramidal symptoms than most phenothiazines. (See chlorpromazine.)

Administration Adults: 20 to 40 mg po daily in divided doses; can be increased to 160 mg daily in divided doses. Geriatrics: $\frac{1}{4}$ to $\frac{1}{2}$ of adult dosage.

Available Drug Forms Tablets containing 10 or 25 mg.

GENERIC NAME Prochlorperazine maleate (RX)

TRADE NAMES Combid, Compazine

CLASSIFICATION Antipsychotic, antiemetic

See chlorpromazine for Indications for use, Contraindications, Warnings and precautions, Parameters of use, Drug interactions, and Nursing management.

Action Prochlorperazine has greater antiemetic activity than most phenothiazines. It is also effective as an antipsychotic agent. (See chlorpromazine.)

Untoward Reactions The risk of developing extrapyramidal symptoms is greater for prochlorperazine than for other phenothiazines. (See chlorpromazine.)

Administration

- *Antipsychotic:* Adults: 5 to 10 mg po or IM bid, tid, or qid; the dosage can be gradually increased to 75 to 150 mg daily in divided doses. Rectal suppository: 25 mg bid. Children: Ages 2 years and older: 0.4 mg/kg daily in divided doses.
- *Antiemetic:* Adults: Preoperative: 5 to 10 mg IM 1 to 2 hours before surgery; 5 to 10 mg IV 30 minutes before anesthesia. Postoperative: 5 to 10 mg IM.

Available Drug Forms Tablets containing 5, 10, or 25 mg; sustained-release capsules containing 10, 15, 30, or 75 mg; 10-ml vials containing 5 mg/ml; 2-ml ampules containing 5mg/ml; suppositories containing 2.5, 5, or 25 mg; syrup containing 5 mg/5 ml; concentrate containing 10 mg/ml.

GENERIC NAME Trifluoperazine hydrochloride

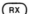

TRADE NAME Stelazine (RX)

CLASSIFICATION Antipsychotic

See chlorpromazine for Contraindications, Warnings and precautions, Parameters of use, and Drug interactions.

Action Trifluoperazine is fast acting and 10 times more potent than chlorpromazine. (See chlorpromazine.)

Indications for Use Treatment of psychoses where the client demonstrates withdrawal and apathy.

Untoward Reactions Extrapyramidal symptoms occur frequently. (See chlorpromazine.)

Administration Adults: Oral: 2 to 5 mg bid or tid initially; then increase to 15 to 20 mg daily in 2 to 3 divided doses. Intramuscular: 1 to 2 mg every 4 to 6 hours; can be increased to 6 to 10 mg daily. Children: Ages 6 to 12 years: 1 to 2 mg po daily; Maximum dosage: 15 mg/day.

Available Drug Forms Tablets containing 1, 2, 5, or 10 mg; 10-ml vials containing 2 mg/ml; concentrate containing 10 mg/ml (dilute in 60 ml of fluid).

Nursing Management The maximum therapeutic effect is reached in 3 weeks and is more prolonged than with chlorpromazine. (See chlorpromazine.)

GENERIC NAME Triflupromazine hydrochloride

TRADE NAME Vesprin (RX)

CLASSIFICATION Antipsychotic

See chlorpromazine for Indications for use, Contraindications, Warnings and precautions, Parameters of use, Drug interactions, and Nursing management.

Action Similar to chlorpromazine; fast acting. (See chlorpromazine.)

Untoward Reactions Extrapyramidal symptoms are the most serious. (See chlorpromazine.)

Administration Adults: Determined individually; up to 150 mg daily. Children: Ages 6 to 12 years: 2 mg/kg po, or 0.25 mg/kg IM daily. Maximum dosage: 150 mg/day po, or 10 mg/day IM.

Available Drug Forms Tablets containing 10, 25, or 50 mg; 10-ml vials containing 10 or 20 mg/ml; suspension containing 50 mg/5 ml.

GENERIC NAME Thiopropazate hydrochloride

TRADE NAME Dartal (RX)

CLASSIFICATION Antipsychotic

See chlorpromazine for Contraindications, Warnings and precautions, Untoward reactions, Parameters of use, Drug interactions, and Nursing management.

Action Similar to chlorpromazine. (See chlorpromazine.)

Indications for Use Psychoses marked by hostility and aggression.

Administration Adults: 10 mg po tid; Maximum dosage: 100 mg/day.

Available Drug Forms Tablets containing 5 or 10 mg.

GENERIC NAME Thioridazine hydrochloride

TRADE NAME Mellaril (RX)

CLASSIFICATION Antipsychotic

See chlorpromazine for Indications for use, Contraindications, Warnings and precautions, Parameters of use, Drug interactions, and Nursing management.

Action Thioridazine is one of the less potent tranquilizers. It has very little antiemetic activity and does not affect the temperature-regulating mechanism. It is considered to be a useful antipsychotic drug and a good basic tranquilizer. (See chlorpromazine.)

Untoward Reactions Produces fewer extrapyramidal symptoms than chlorpromazine. Large dosages have reportedly produced pigmentary retinopathy. Sudden death has been reported following long-term use. (See chlorpromazine.)

Administration Adults: 20 to 800 mg po daily; Children: Over 2 years: 1 mg/kg po daily in 3 to 4 divided doses.

Available Drug Forms Tablets containing 10, 25, 50, 100, 150, or 200 mg; concentrate containing 30 mg/ml.

BUTYROPHENONES

GENERIC NAME Haloperidol (RX)

TRADE NAME Haldol

CLASSIFICATION Antipsychotic, antiemetic

See chlorpromazine for Warnings and precautions and Drug interactions.

Action Similar to phenothiazines. (See chlorpromazine.)

Indications for Use Control of hyperactivity that occurs in the manic phase of manic-depressive illness; acute psychiatric problems.

Contraindications Parkinsonism. (See chlorpromazine.)

Untoward Reactions Generally similar to phenothiazines, but there is a high incidence of extrapyramidal symptoms and less sedation, hypotension, hypothermia, and photosensitivity. Severe depression leading to suicidal tendencies may develop. (See chlorpromazine.)

Parameters of Use (See chlorpromazine.)

Absorption Peak action occurs in 30 to 45 minutes.
Excretion Slowly in urine.

Administration Adults: 2 to 8 mg po or IM daily; can be gradually increased 0.5 to 1 mg every 3 days; Maximum dosage: 15 mg/day.

Available Drug Forms Tablets containing 0.5, 1, or 2 mg; concentrate containing 2 mg/ml; ampules containing 5 mg/ml.

Nursing Management There is a narrow margin between therapeutic and toxic dosages. (See chlorpromazine.)

THIOXANTHENES

GENERIC NAME Chlorprothixene (RX)

TRADE NAME Taractan

CLASSIFICATION Antipsychotic, antiemetic

See chlorpromazine for Contraindications, Warnings and precautions, Drug interactions, and Nursing management.

Action Similar to phenothiazines, but a more powerful inhibitor of motor coordination and produces fewer antihistaminic effects. (See chlorpromazine.)

Indications for Use Schizophrenia, acute depression, neurosis, withdrawal from alcohol, agitation.

Untoward Reactions Drowsiness, orthostatic hypotension, and dry mouth occur frequently. Extrapyramidal symptoms, agranulocytosis, and cholestatic hepatitis are less likely to occur. (See chlorpromazine.)

Parameters of Use (See chlorpromazine.)

Absorption Peak action occurs in 30 minutes.

Administration Adults: 30 to 200 mg po or IM daily in divided doses; Children: 30 to 100 mg po daily.

Available Drug Forms Tablets containing 10, 25, 50, or 100 mg; vials containing 12.5 mg/ml.

GENERIC NAME Thiothixene (RX)

TRADE NAME Navane

CLASSIFICATION Antipsychotic

See chlorpromazine for Contraindications, Warnings and precautions, Parameters of use, and Drug interactions.

Action Similar to phenothiazines, but a more powerful inhibitor of motor coordination and produces fewer antihistaminic effects. (See chlorpromazine.)

Indications for Use Acute and chronic schizophrenia.

Untoward Reactions Insomnia and extrapyramidal symptoms occur frequently. (See chlorpromazine.)

Administration Adults: 6 to 15 mg po or IM daily in divided doses; can be gradually increased to a maximum oral dosage of 60 mg/day or a maximum intramuscular dosage of 30 mg/day.

Available Drug Forms Capsules containing 1, 2, 5, or 10 mg; concentrate containing 5 mg/ml; vials containing 2 mg/ml.

Nursing Management There is a very narrow margin between therapeutic and toxic dosages. (See chlorpromazine.)

DIHYDROINDOLONES

GENERIC NAME Molindone (RX)

TRADE NAMES Lidone, Moban

CLASSIFICATION Antipsychotic

See chlorpromazine for Contraindications and Nursing management.

Action Similar to phenothiazines. (See chlorpromazine.)

Indications for Use Acute schizophrenia.

Warnings and Precautions Clients have experienced profound CNS depression while taking other drugs. (See chlorpromazine.)

Untoward Reactions Excessive weight gain is less of a problem. (See chlorpromazine.)

Administration

- *Mild schizophrenia:* Adults: 5 to 15 mg po daily in divided doses.
- *Moderate schizophrenia:* Adults: 10 to 25 mg po daily in divided doses.
- *Severe schizophrenia:* Adults: Up to 225 mg po daily in divided doses.

Available Drug Forms Tablets and capsules containing 5, 10, or 25 mg.

DIBENZOXAZEPINES

GENERIC NAME Loxapine (RX)

TRADE NAMES Daxolin, Loxitane

CLASSIFICATION Antipsychotic

See chlorpromazine for Contraindications, Warnings and precautions, Parameters of use, Drug interactions, and Nursing management.

Action Newly available tricyclic drug with actions similar to phenothiazines. (See chlorpromazine.)

Indications for Use Schizophrenia.

Untoward Reactions Similar to phenothiazines, but less likely to produce the serious side effects, such as extrapyramidal symptoms. (See chlorpromazine.)

Administration Adults: 60 to 100 mg po daily in divided doses; can be gradually increased to a maximum dosage of 250 mg/day.

Available Drug Forms Capsules containing 5, 10, 25, or 50 mg; concentrate containing 25 mg/ml.

Chapter 34

Antidepressant Agents

TRICYCLIC ANTIDEPRESSANTS

- Amitriptyline hydrochloride
- Desipramine hydrochloride
- Doxepin hydrochloride
- Imipramine hydrochloride
- Nortriptyline
- Protriptyline hydrochloride

MONAMINE OXIDASE INHIBITORS

- Isocarboxazid
- Phenelzine sulfate
- Tranylcypromine sulfate

OTHER ANTIDEPRESSANTS

- Lithium carbonate

THE FOUR MAJOR types of antidepressant agents are (1) tricyclic antidepressants; (2) monoamine oxidase (MAO) inhibitors; (3) psychomotor stimulants; and (4) lithium carbonate. This chapter discusses all of the above categories except psychomotor stimulants, which are discussed in Chapter 36.

Antidepressant agents are used to treat clients with endogenous depression, clients in the depressive phase of manic-depressive illness, and less often for clients with neurotic depression.

TRICYCLIC ANTIDEPRESSANTS

GENERIC NAME Amitriptyline hydrochloride

TRADE NAMES Amitid, Amitril, Elavil, Endep, SK-Amitriptyline

CLASSIFICATION Tricyclic antidepressant (RX)

Action

Amitriptyline is closely related to the phenothiazines and produces an antidepressant effect without the side effects of MAO inhibitors. Although the exact mechanism of action is unknown, amitriptyline is believed to interfere with the reuptake of brain amines by nerves; this action is similar to that of atropine and the antihistamines. In addition, it depresses the effects of epinephrine and serotonin; it is a mild CNS depressant. Amitriptyline is an effective mood elevator and promotes mental acuity and an increased level of physical activity. Its sedative effects help counteract insomnia.

Indications for Use

Treatment of depressive disorders and anxiety neuroses.

Contraindications

Acute phase of myocardial infarction, severe renal or hepatic deficiency, concomitant use of MAO inhibitors, glaucoma.

Untoward Reactions

Dry mouth, constipation, orthostatic hypotension; allergic reactions; CNS symptoms (extrapyramidal signs, anxiety, agitation, disorientation, hallucinations, ataxia, tremors, seizures); cardiovascular symptoms (arrhythmias, congestive heart failure, stroke); GI symptoms (gastric upset); endocrine and hematologic changes; altered blood sugar, blood dyscrasias, altered hepatic function.

Parameters of Use

Absorption Readily absorbed from GI tract. Peak action occurs in 3 to 4 hours. Half-life is 2 days. About 95% bound to plasma proteins.

Distribution Widely distributed in body tissues.

Metabolism In the liver.

Excretion In urine.

Drug Interactions

Enhances the effects of other CNS depressants, catecholamines, adrenergics, anticholinergics, thyroid hormones, disulfiram, anticoagulants, vasodilators, and central-acting skeletal muscle relaxants. Antagonizes the effects of antihypertensives, anticonvulsants, phenylbutazone, and cholinergics. Tricyclic effects are potentiated by phenothiazines, methylphenidate, amphetamines, furazolidone, acetazolamide, MAO inhibitors, and urinary alkalizers. Tricyclic effects are inhibited by urinary acidifiers and barbiturates.

Administration

Adults: 75 mg po or IM daily, usually in divided doses; can be increased gradually to a maximum dosage of 150 mg/day. Geriatrics and teenagers: 10 mg po tid and 20 mg hs.

Available Drug Forms

Tablets containing 10, 25, or 50 mg; vials containing 10 mg/ml.

Nursing Management

(See chlorpromazine in Chapter 33.)

Planning factors

1. Drug should be discontinued at least 48 hours prior to surgery.
2. Baseline vital signs, particularly blood pressure, should be determined prior to institution of therapy.

Administration factors

1. Entire daily dose may be prescribed at bedtime, since drug is long acting and has sedative effects.
2. Monitor blood pressure frequently during initial phase of therapy.

Evaluation factors

1. Assess suicide risk carefully, since all depressed clients are potentially suicidal.
2. Observe for slowing of normal elimination processes, since urinary retention and constipation are common side effects.

Client teaching factors

1. Inform client that the full therapeutic effect may occur 1 to 3 weeks after initiation of therapy.
2. Instruct client that drug must be taken as prescribed, not merely when needed for depression.
3. Instruct client to be alert for development of orthostatic hypotension; the elderly are particularly susceptible.
4. Caution clients to avoid prolonged exposure to sunlight.
5. Warn client not to drive or use heavy machinery while taking drug, since drowsiness is a frequent side effect.
6. Instruct client that alcohol will potentiate the drug's depressant effects, possibly producing extreme drowsiness and ataxia.
7. Advise client to ingest sufficient fluids, rinse the mouth frequently, and chew gum to relieve the unpleasantness of dry mouth.

GENERIC NAME Desipramine hydrochloride

TRADE NAMES Norpramin, Pertofrane (RX)

CLASSIFICATION Tricyclic antidepressant

See amitriptyline hydrochloride for Indications for use, Contraindications, Parameters of use, Drug interactions, and Nursing management.

Action It has been theorized that desipramine is the active metabolite of imipramine and so is at least as therapeutic as imipramine. Desipramine may no longer be as effective after a few weeks, which is the amount of time needed for behavioral changes when other tricyclic antidepressants are administered. (See amitriptyline hydrochloride.)

Untoward Reactions May cause hyperthermia or a bad taste in the mouth. (See amitriptyline hydrochloride.)

Administration Adults: 25 to 50 mg po daily in divided doses; then increase gradually to a maximum dosage of 200 mg/day until desired effect; Maintenance dosage: 50 to 100 mg po daily.

Available Drug Forms Tablets containing 25, 50, 75, 100, or 150 mg; capsules containing 25 or 50 mg.

GENERIC NAME Doxepin hydrochloride (RX)

TRADE NAMES Adapin, Sinequan

CLASSIFICATION Tricyclic antidepressant

See amitriptyline hydrochloride for Contraindications, Untoward reactions, Parameters of use, Drug interactions, and Nursing management.

Action Similar to amitriptyline. (See amitriptyline hydrochloride.)

Indications for Use Treatment of depression in psychoneurotic patients.

Administration Adults: 75 mg po daily in divided doses; Maximum dosage: 150 to 300 mg/day.

Available Drug Forms Capsules containing 10, 25, or 50 mg.

GENERIC NAME Imipramine hydrochloride (RX)

TRADE NAME Tofranil

CLASSIFICATION Tricyclic antidepressant

See amitriptyline hydrochloride for Indications for use, Contraindications, Untoward reactions, Parameters of use, and Drug interactions.

Action Similar to amitriptyline. (See amitriptyline hydrochloride.)

Administration Adults: Outpatients: 75 mg po or IM daily in divided doses. Hospitalized clients: 100 to 150 mg po or IM daily; can be gradually increased to a maximum dosage of 300 mg/day in divided doses until desired effect; Maintenance dosage: 50 to 150 po or IM daily. Geriatrics and teenagers: Initially, 30–40 mg daily, not to exceed 100 mg daily.

Available Drug Forms Tablets containing 10, 25, or 50 mg; vials containing 12.5 mg/ml.

Nursing Management (See amitriptyline hydrochloride.)

1. A change in behavior may be observed as early as 3 days after onset of therapy.
2. Full therapeutic effect may not be apparent for 1 or 2 weeks.

GENERIC NAME Nortriptyline (RX)

TRADE NAME Aventyl

CLASSIFICATION Tricyclic antidepressant

See amitriptyline hydrochloride for Indications for use, Contraindications, Untoward reactions, Parameters of use, and Drug interactions.

Action Similar to amitriptyline. (See amitriptyline hydrochloride.)

Administration Adults: Initial dosage: 20 to 40 mg po daily in divided doses for the 1st week; Maintenance dosage: 30 to 75 mg po daily; Maximum dosage: 100 mg/day. Geriatrics: 30 to 50 mg po daily.

Available Drug Forms Capsules containing 10 or 25 mg; concentrate containing 10 mg/5 ml.

Nursing Management (See amitriptyline hydrochloride.)

GENERIC NAME Protriptyline hydrochloride

TRADE NAME Vivactil (RX)

CLASSIFICATION Tricyclic antidepressant

See amitriptyline hydrochloride for Indications for use, Contraindications, Parameters of use, Drug interactions, and Nursing management.

Action Similar to amitriptyline. (See amitriptyline hydrochloride.)

Untoward Reactions Causes more cardiovascular side effects than other tricyclic antidepressants, but produces less sedation. (See amitriptyline hydrochloride.)

Administration Adults: Initial dosage: 30 to 60 mg po daily in divided doses; Maintenance dosage: 15 to 40 mg po daily.

Available Drug Forms Tablets containing 5 or 10 mg.

MONOAMINE OXIDASE INHIBITORS

GENERIC NAME Isocarboxazid (RX)

TRADE NAME Marplan

CLASSIFICATION Antidepressant (MAO inhibitor)

Action MAO inhibitors interfere with the enzyme, monoamine oxidase, which metabolizes norepinephrine. The direct clinical result is a buildup of norepinephrine in the tissues, with all the attendant complications. These drugs affect blood pressure and hepatic function.

Indications for Use Endogenous depression, manic-depressive psychosis, severe reactive depression. Usually only administered after a trial with tricyclic antidepressants has proven ineffective.

Contraindications Children under 16 years, congestive heart failure, hepatic dysfunction, pheochromocytoma, hyperthyroidism, cardiovascular disease, the elderly, debilitated clients.

Untoward Reactions Orthostatic hypotension, dizziness, insomnia, GI upsets, headache, arrhythmias, tremors, hypomania, euphoria, confusion, memory loss, ataxia, hallucinations, convulsions, dry mouth, blurred vision, dysuria, impotence, palpitations, edema, weight gain, blood dyscrasias, jaundice, photosensitivity reactions, sodium retention, hypoglycemia, glaucoma, anorexia.

Parameters of Use

Absorption Readily absorbed from GI tract.
Metabolism Rapidly metabolized in the liver.
Excretion In urine.

Drug Interactions Potentiates the effects of sympathomimetics, anticholinergics, antihistamines, antiparkinsonian drugs, and antihypertensives. Increases the toxic effects of barbiturates, phenothiazines, and CNS depressants. Increases the hypoglycemic effects of hypoglycemic drugs and the muscle-relaxing effect of succinylcholine. Interferes with the effect of antiepileptics. Foods containing tyramine (cheese, sour cream, yogurt, beer, wine, yeast, herring, chicken livers, aged meats, tenderizers, licorice, caffeine, chocolate) increase the risk of hypertensive crisis. Reserpine or guanethidine administered IV or IM can cause severe hypertension.

Administration Adults: 30 mg po daily in a single dose or in divided doses; Maintenance dosage: 10 to 20 mg po daily.

Available Drug Forms Tablets containing 10 mg.

Nursing Management

Planning factors

1. Drug should be discontinued at least 3 weeks prior to surgery.
2. Baseline blood and hepatic function tests and blood pressure determinations should be done prior to institution of therapy.

Administration factors

1. Give with meals to reduce GI distress.
2. Observe client carefully for toxic reactions, which can occur within hours of the first few doses.
3. Blood pressure should be monitored between doses during initial phase of therapy.

Evaluation factors

1. Observe client for color blindness, which indicates eye damage.
2. Assess lethality of client's suicidal statements, since client's mood improves with continued therapy.
3. Since drug is long acting and may have a cumulative effect, behavioral changes may not be apparent for 1 to 4 weeks.

Client teaching factors

1. Instruct client to take no other drugs, including OTC preparations, concurrently and for 3 weeks following cessation of therapy.
2. Instruct client to avoid tyramine-rich foods.
3. Advise client to change positions slowly to avoid postural hypotension.
4. Instruct client to report promptly any symptoms suggestive of hypertensive crisis (headache, palpitations).
5. Client should report any rapid or unusual weight gain or other unusual symptoms.

GENERIC NAME Phenelzine sulfate (RX)

TRADE NAME Nardil

CLASSIFICATION Antidepressant (MAO inhibitor)

See isocarboxazid for Indications for use, Contraindications, Parameters of use, and Drug interactions.

Action Similar to isocarboxazid. (See isocarboxazid.)

Untoward Reactions Similar to isocarboxazid, but less likely to precipitate a hypertensive crisis. (See isocarboxazid.)

Administration Adults: Initial dosage: 45 mg po daily in divided doses; then gradually increase to a maximum dosage of 75 mg/day, if necessary, until desired effect; Maintenance dosage: 15 mg po every other day.

Available Drug Forms Tablets containing 15 mg.

Nursing Management Therapeutic effect can occur after 1 to 2 weeks. (See isocarboxazid for further details.)

GENERIC NAME Tranylcypromine sulfate (RX)

TRADE NAME Parnate

CLASSIFICATION Antidepressant (MAO inhibitor)

See isocarboxazid for Contraindications, Parameters of use, Drug interactions, and Nursing management.

Action Similar to isocarboxazid, but stimulant effect is stronger. (See isocarboxazid.)

Indications for Use Intractable depression. Should only be administered when other safer medications have been tried.

Untoward Reactions As the peak effect of this drug occurs much sooner than that produced by the other MAO inhibitors, there is a greater chance of precipitating a hypertensive crisis.

Administration Adults: Initial dosage: 20 mg po daily in divided doses for 2 to 3 weeks; then gradually increase to a maximum dosage of 30 mg/day until desired effect; Maintenance dosage: 10 to 20 mg po daily.

Available Drug Forms Tablets containing 10 mg.

OTHER ANTIDEPRESSANTS

GENERIC NAME Lithium carbonate (RX)

TRADE NAMES Eskalith, Lithane, Lithonate, Lithotabs

CLASSIFICATION Antidepressant

Action Precise mechanism is unknown, but seems to act similarly to the sodium ion and enhances the excretion of sodium and potassium. Decreases circulating thyroid hormones, may block renal response to ADH, decreases glucose tolerance, and increases circulating growth hormone levels.

Indications for Use Some controversy abounds concerning the value of lithium in treating manic-depressive illness. It has been found to be extremely effective in controlling acute manic and hypomanic behaviors, such as hyperactivity, poor judgment, flight of ideas, and aggressiveness. May be used in conjunction with phenothiazines.

Contraindications Cardiovascular or renal impairment, dehydration, clients taking diuretics, clients with sodium depletion, pregnancy, lactation, schizophrenia, organic brain disease. Safe use in children (under 12 years) has not been established.

Untoward Reactions Dry mouth, metallic taste, thyroid enlargement, glycosuria, hyperglycemia, weight gain, edema. Lithium poisoning: nausea, diarrhea, diabeteslike symptoms, tremors. More serious symptoms include blurred vision and slurred speech. Dermatologic manifestations may also occur. In acute toxicity, convulsions, shock, coma, and death can occur. (See amitriptyline hydrochloride.)

Parameters of Use

Absorption Rapidly absorbed from GI tract. Peak action occurs in 2 to 4 hours. Half-life is 24 hours.

Crosses the blood-brain barrier slowly. Crosses placenta and appears in breast milk.

Distribution Widely distributed in body water with high concentrations in the kidneys and saliva. Some drug is concentrated in bone, muscles, and liver.

Excretion About 75% in urine within 24 hours; alkalization of the urine enhances excretion.

Drug Interactions Acetazolamide, aminophylline, sodium bicarbonate, and sodium chloride enhance the renal excretion of lithium, thereby decreasing its effect. Phenothiazines may enhance hyperglycemic effects. Iodine-containing agents and tricyclic antidepressants may enhance hypothyroid effects. Thiazide diuretics, haloperidol, and methyldopa may increase lithium toxicity. Lithium may decrease the effects of amphetamines.

Administration Adults: 300 to 600 mg po tid until desired effect; Maintenance dosage: 300 mg po tid.

Available Drug Forms Tablets and capsules containing 300 mg.

Nursing Management

Planning factors Since there is no antidote available for lithium poisoning, every effort must be made to prevent it.

Administration factors

1. Careful monitoring is required because there is a narrow margin between therapeutic and toxic dosages. Blood lithium levels should be determined

before each morning dose during the initial treatment period and then weekly; therapeutic serum drug levels: 0.6 to 1.5 mEq/l.
2. Give with meals to minimize GI upset.

Evaluation factors

1. Therapeutic response is usually evident within 10 days. If no response occurs within 2 weeks, drug should be discontinued.
2. Client should be weighed daily. Report evidence of fluid retention.
3. Assess client regularly for symptoms of hypothyroidism and/or thyroid enlargement.
4. Lithium intoxication begins to develop when serum levels reach 1.5 mEq/l; if such levels occur, therapy should be discontinued for 1 day and then resumed at a lower dosage.

Client teaching factors

1. Emphasize the importance of performing serum lithium determinations as scheduled (monthly).
2. Stress the need to maintain adequate sodium and fluid intake and to avoid the use of diuretics.
3. Advise client not to drive or operate machinery, since drowsiness is common.

Chapter 35

Antianxiety Agents

BENZODIAZEPINES

- Diazepam
- Chlordiazepoxide
- Clorazepate dipotassium
- Oxazepam

PROPANEDIOLS

- Meprobamate

THE FOUR MAJOR types of antianxiety agents are (1) benzodiazepines; (2) propanediols; (3) diphenylmethanes; and (4) sedatives and hypnotics. Benzodiazepines and propanediols are discussed in this chapter; diphenylmethanes and sedatives and hypnotics are discussed in Part VIII. Formerly called minor tranquilizers, antianxiety agents effectively reduce mild to moderate anxiety and the accompanying neurotic symptoms without interfering with the individual's ability to function at an adequate level.

Antianxiety agents have been especially useful in treating people with psychosomatic problems, neuroses, or withdrawal from alcohol intoxication. The use of these drugs is said to enhance the individual's ability to participate effectively in psychotherapy.

BENZODIAZEPINES

GENERIC NAME Diazepam (RX)

TRADE NAME Valium

CLASSIFICATION Antianxiety agent

Action Unlike the barbiturates used as antianxiety agents, diazepam produces only minor circulatory and respiratory depression, while preserving mental acuity even when administered in large dosages. Most of the brain is not depressed, but electrical impulses in the limbic system are inhibited. Diazepam is an effective skeletal muscle relaxant and a powerful anticonvulsant, but its mode of action is not clearly understood. Benzodiazepines depress the polysynaptic reflexes of the spinal cord, which reduces skeletal muscle tension, thereby inhibiting those afferent proprioceptive impulses that might aggravate existing anxiety. Benzodiazepines also inhibit stimulation of the amygdala and the hippocampus structures of the brain, which influence behavior. These drugs therefore have a mild sedative effect but do not alter the level of consciousness or the ability to perform psychomotor tasks.

Indications for Use Anxiety states of organic or functional origin, such as anxiety due to angina pectoris, asthma, premenstrual tension, or menopause; insomnia; preoperative sedation; relaxation of tension due to arthritis and low back pain; status epilepticus; withdrawal from alcohol intoxication.

Contraindications Severe psychoses, glaucoma, shock, children under 6 months.

Untoward Reactions Drowsiness, lethargy, ataxia, confusion, headache, syncope, vertigo, depression, stupor, excitement, dry mouth, constipation, urinary retention, blurred vision, hypotension, weight gain, cardiovascular collapse, blood dyscrasias, hypersensitivity reactions, endocrine abnormalities.

Parameters of Use

Absorption Readily absorbed from GI tract or the bloodstream. Onset of action is: 30 to 60 minutes (po); 15 to 30 minutes (IM). Peak blood levels occur in 2 hours. Half-life is 20 to 50 hours.

Crosses placenta and appears in breast milk.

Metabolism Metabolized in the liver slowly; can still be found in the blood 7 days after discontinuation of therapy.

Excretion In urine, with a small amount in feces.

Drug Interactions Enhances the depressant effects of alcohol, barbiturates, antihistamines, phenothiazines, and narcotics. Potentiates the effects of phenytoin and skeletal muscle relaxants. Antagonizes the effects of levodopa. Smoking may inhibit the effects of benzodiazepines.

Administration Adults: 4 to 40 mg po, IM, or IV daily in divided doses; Elderly patients require a lower dosage; Children: Over 6 months: 1 to 2.5 mg po tid.

Available Drug Forms Tablets containing 2, 5, or 10 mg; vials of 2 to 10 ml containing 5 mg/ml.

Nursing Management

Planning factors Since the effect of diazepam is accumulative, therapeutic results may not be apparent for 5 to 10 days after initiation of therapy.

Administration factors

1. Since diazepam is long acting, 1 dose per day is usually sufficient. The dose should be given at bedtime to promote sleep and relieve anxiety throughout the following day.
2. IM injection must be deep into gluteal muscle.
3. Do not mix drug with other solutions. Do not add to IV fluids.
4. IV injection should not exceed 5 mg/min. Give into a large vein and avoid extravasation.

Evaluation factors

1. Observe client for excessive drowsiness or ataxia. Provide bedrails and assistance with ambulation.
2. Observe client for signs of developing physiologic or psychologic dependence. As dosage and duration of therapy increase, the risk of dependence increases.
3. Observe geriatric clients carefully, since they are more likely to develop side effects.
4. Periodic blood and hepatic function tests should be done during long-term therapy.

Client teaching factors

1. Instruct client not to take alcohol or any other CNS depressant.

2. Instruct client not to drive or operate dangerous machinery.
3. Instruct client to change position slowly to prevent postural hypotension.
4. Instruct client not to discontinue drug without medical supervision.

GENERIC NAME Chlordiazepoxide; chlordiazepoxide hydrochloride

TRADE NAMES Libritabs; Librium (RX)

CLASSIFICATION Antianxiety agent

See diazepam for Contraindications, Parameters of use, Drug interactions, and Nursing management.

Action (See diazepam.)

Indications for Use Management of delirium tremens; treatment of anxiety associated with psychosomatic conditions.

Warnings and Precautions Use with caution in addiction-prone clients.

Untoward Reactions Drowsiness and ataxia are common. Agranulocytosis and jaundice occur, but rarely. (See diazepam.)

Administration Adults: 15 to 40 mg po, IM, or IV daily in divided doses; can be gradually increased to a maximum dosage of 300 mg/day. Geriatrics: 10 to 20 mg po, IM, or IV daily. Children: Over 6 years: 0.5 mg/kg po, IM, or IV daily.

Available Drug Forms Tablets and capsules containing 5, 10, or 25 mg; ampules containing 100 mg of dry powder.

GENERIC NAME Clorazepate dipotassium (RX)

TRADE NAME Tranxene

CLASSIFICATION Antianxiety agent

See diazepam for Action, Indications for use, Contraindications, Untoward reactions, Parameters of use, Drug interactions, and Nursing management.

Administration Adults: 15 to 60 mg po daily in divided doses; Geriatrics: 7.5 to 15 mg po daily; Children: Over 6 years: 7.5 to 60 mg po daily in divided doses.

Available Drug Forms Capsules containing 3.75, 7.5, or 15 mg.

GENERIC NAME Oxazepam (RX)

TRADE NAME Serax

CLASSIFICATION Antianxiety agent

See diazepam for Action, Indications for use, Contraindications, Untoward reactions, Parameters of use, and Drug interactions.

Administration Adults: 30 to 120 mg po daily in divided doses.

Available Drug Forms Tablets containing 15 mg; capsules containing 10, 15, or 30 mg.

Nursing Management Monitor elderly clients carefully for the development of hypotension. (See diazepam.)

PROPANEDIOLS

GENERIC NAME Meprobamate (RX)

TRADE NAMES Equanil, Miltown

CLASSIFICATION Antianxiety agent

See diazepam for Contraindications, Parameters of use, and Drug interactions.

Action Similar to diazepam in that it reduces anxiety. Meprobamate is a skeletal muscle relaxant and an anticonvulsant. Its action is believed to be similar to phenobarbital.

Indications for Use Insomnia, simple nervous tension, petit mal epilepsy.

Untoward Reactions Drowsiness and skin rash occur frequently. (See diazepam.)

Administration Adults: 400 mg po or IM daily in divided doses. Children: Over 6 years: 100 to 200 mg po or IM daily in divided doses; Maximum dosage: 2.4 g/day.

Available Drug Forms Tablets and capsules containing 200 or 400 mg; oral suspension containing 40 mg/ml; vials containing 80 mg/5 ml.

Nursing Management (See diazepam.)

1. Skin rash responds to antihistamines.
2. Drug dependence may develop.

PART IX

CENTRAL NERVOUS SYSTEM STIMULANTS

DRUGS THAT STIMULATE the central nervous system are classified into three groups according to their primary site of action: the cerebral cortex, the medulla, or the spinal cord. Central nervous system stimulants are sometimes referred to as analeptics because they give the appearance of restoring the client's vigor and health. However, since restoration of health can be dramatic when certain central nervous system stimulants are used to treat drug-induced respiratory depression, the term *analeptic* is often reserved for respiratory stimulants. In general, the more stimulating the drug, the more profound the depression that follows as the effects of the drug subside.

Cerebral stimulants affect the cerebral cortex and have extensive therapeutic use today. This group of drugs can be subdivided into (1) central sympathomimetics, such as amphetamines; (2) xanthines, such as caffeine; (3) psychomotor stimulants, such as methylphenidate (Ritalin); (4) tricyclic antidepressants; (5) monoamine oxidase (MAO) inhibitors; and (6) the hallucinogens. Although they have no therapeutic value, the hallucinogens are included in Chapter 36 since a basic understanding of their action and effects are essential for effective medical and nursing management of drug-induced toxicity and untoward reactions.

Unlike the other central nervous system stimulants, tricyclic antidepressants and MAO inhibitors induce a less intense, but more prolonged, stimulation and can therefore be used in relative safety therapeutically for several weeks or even months. However, as the main purpose of these antidepressants is in psychotherapeutics, they are described in Part VIII.

Medullary stimulants exert their action on the brain stem, including the respiratory and vasomotor centers. Few of these drugs are utilized today because they have a narrow margin of safety—there is a fine line between stimulation and convulsion. Furthermore, most of the *respiratory stimulants* have been replaced by respirators; however, those that are still used to treat respiratory depression induced by sedatives, hypnotics, and general anesthetics are described in Chapter 37.

Spinal cord stimulants, such as strychnine, act primarily on the spinal cord. Strychnine, which has been used for centuries as a rat poison, gained popularity as an ingredient in bitter tonics and as a cardiac and respiratory stimulant during the 18th century. Unlike most central nervous system stimulants, strychnine induces excitation by blocking inhibitory influences, thus allowing stimuli from the senses to proceed unchecked. Toxic doses cause rigidity in the neck and facial muscles, excessive reflex response, and eventually a symmetrical thrust of the extensors and opisthotonic convulsions. (It should be remembered that any sensory input, including noise, light, and touch, can induce convulsions.) Unfortunately, strychnine is well absorbed from the gastrointestinal tract and is very slowly excreted from the body. Treatment of strychnine poisoning is therefore directed at preventing convulsions by administering central nervous system depressants, such as short-acting barbiturates, and reducing sensory input. (Neurotoxins produced by *Clostridium tetani* induce convulsions similar to strychnine and are treated in an analogous manner.)

Although most central nervous system stimulants will affect the cerebral cortex, medullary centers, and spinal cord, they tend to affect one of these three structures more markedly than the others. For example, small doses (150 mg) of the cerebral stimulant caffeine cause mild excitation of the cortex; but doses of 500 mg or more stimulate the medullary centers and act as a respiratory stimulant. Toxic doses of any central nervous system stimulant have the potential of causing severe untoward reactions, including convulsions.

Some central nervous system stimulants affect both the respiratory and vasomotor centers of the medulla. The vasomotor center assists in the maintenance of vasoconstriction and stimulation of this center will cause a pressor effect. These stimulants are used with caution in clients with hypertension and marked arteriosclerotic diseases. Some drugs may stimulate the vomiting center and induce vomiting without nausea.

Amphetamines and other central nervous system depressants act mainly on the appetite control center located in the cerebrum. These agents can cause anorexia and may be used for the short-term treatment of exogenous obesity. Unfortunately, tolerance to anorexiants develops within a few weeks and the drug must be discontinued.

Any drug that crosses the blood-brain barrier can potentially bring about either depression or stimulation of the CNS. A large number of sympathomimetics cause CNS stimulation even when given in therapeutic doses, whereas many other drugs, including antimuscarinic agents, local anesthetics, and salicylate analgesics, may act as a stimulant in toxic doses.

Chapter 36

Cerebral Stimulants

TYPES OF CEREBRAL STIMULANTS

AMPHETAMINES

- Amphetamine sulfate
- Amphetamine phosphate
- Dextroamphetamine phosphate
- Dextroamphetamine sulfate
- Benzphetamine hydrochloride
- Levamfetamine succinate
- Methamphetamine hydrochloride

COMBINATION AMPHETAMINE PREPARATIONS

- Biphetamine
- Obetrol

XANTHINES

- Caffeine, citrated caffeine, caffeine and sodium benzoate

SYMPATHOMIMETICS

- Chlorphentermine hydrochloride
- Clotermine hydrochloride
- Deanol acetamidobenzoate
- Diethylpropion hydrochloride
- Fenfluramine hydrochloride
- Mazindol
- Methylphenidate hydrochloride
- Pemoline
- Phendimetrazine tartrate
- Phenmetrazine hydrochloride
- Phentermine hydrochloride

COMBINATION PREPARATIONS

- Efed II

CEREBRAL STIMULANTS WITH LITTLE OR NO KNOWN THERAPEUTIC VALUE

- Bufotenine
- Cocaine
- Cocaine hydrochloride
- Dimethyltryptamine
- Lysergic acid diethylamide
- Mescaline
- Psilocybin

DRUGS THAT STIMULATE the cerebral cortex are called *central* or *cerebral stimulants,* and include amphetamines, xanthines, and some sympathomimetics. All of these drugs cross the blood-brain barrier, which is a prerequiste for any central nervous system stimulant. Cocaine and the hallucinogens are also classified as cerebral stimulants although they have little or no therapeutic value. This class of drugs relieves feelings of fatigue, elevates the mood, suppresses the appetite, and increases alertness.

TYPES OF CEREBRAL STIMULANTS

Amphetamines, which are sympathomimetic amines, are potent cerebral stimulants. The dextro isomers of amphetamine are more potent than the levo isomers. Although chemically similar to ephedrine, tolerance to amphetamines can develop within a few weeks; whereas tolerance to ephedrine preparations can take months. The abuse of amphetamines as "pep pills" has led to the substitution of ephedrine containing preparations for the long-term treatment of obesity. Agents that induce anorexia or suppress the appetite are termed *anorexigenic.*

Amphetamines are useful for the control of *narcolepsy,* a central nervous system disorder manifested by periodic episodes of drowsiness and sleep. It has been found that low dosages of amphetamines are effective in controlling narcolepsy for months or even years without the development of tolerance. Certain *minimal brain dysfunctions* also respond to amphetamines. Although amphetamines are central nervous system stimulants, their use in some young children can produce a paradoxic calming effect, presumably by drug-induced stimulation of underdeveloped centers in the central nervous system. Tolerance to this clinical effect can result in the lack of normal growth, and the child must be assessed periodically. Methylphenidate, which is chemically similar to amphetamines, is effective in the treatment of minimal brain dysfunctions and narcolepsy and produces fewer untoward reactions on growth and the cardiovascular system. This drug is usually the one of choice for small children.

Although xanthines induce central nervous system stimulation, most of these drugs are used more often for their diuretic effect (see Chapter 53). Caffeine is the most commonly used xanthine in OTC preparations as a stimulant. It should be remembered that doses greater than 150 to 200 mg cause nervousness and tremors in most clients. When administered intravenously, as caffeine and sodium benzoate, caffeine is an effective respiratory stimulant and is used to treat barbiturate- and narcotic-induced central nervous system depression.

Some *sympathomimetics* cross the blood-brain barrier and are effective in treating narcolepsy, minimal brain dysfunctions, and as a short-term adjunct for obesity. These agents produce untoward reactions characteristic of other sympathomimetics.

The *hallucinogens* and other central nervous system stimulants have little or no known therapeutic value. Unfortunately, these drugs can be obtained illegally and many clients require treatment because of toxic or other untoward reactions.

AMPHETAMINES

GENERIC NAME Amphetamine sulfate (Cii)

TRADE NAME Benzedrine

CLASSIFICATION Cerebral stimulant

Action Amphetamine is a synthetic sympathomimetic amine (noncatecholamine) similar to ephedrine that has a marked stimulatory effect on the CNS and has alpha- and beta-adrenergic activity. Although the exact mechanism of CNS stimulation is unknown, amphetamine is thought to stimulate alpha receptors in the CNS and to induce the release of norepinephrine and dopamine in the cerebral cortex and the reticular activating system. The drug-induced CNS stimulation results in wakefulness, diminished feelings of fatigue, mood elevation, self-confidence, and an enhanced ability to concentrate. Although work output may increase, the number of work errors seldom decreases. Amphetamine depresses the sense of smell and taste and is an effective appetite suppressant (central anorectic agent), but has limited therapeutic value because drug tolerance develops after a few weeks and the drug must be discontinued. As a result of mild stimulation of the medullary respiratory center, the rate and depth of respirations are increased. Amphetamine may also reverse barbiturate-induced depression of the reticular activating system (arousal sleep system). Peripheral effects include elevation of blood pressure, mild relaxation of bronchial, gastrointestinal and urinary smooth muscles, constriction of the urinary bladder sphincter, mydriasis without cyclopegia, and contraction of the spleen. The plasma concentration of free fatty acids is increased, but there is little or no change in glucose metabolism.

Indications for Use Narcolepsy, hyperkinesis, minimal brain dysfunctions, as a short-term adjunct in exogenous obesity. Has been used to treat nocturnal enuresis and as an adjunct in the treatment of apathy, certain fatigue states, and psychomotor dysfunctions.

Contraindications Advanced arteriosclerosis, moderate or severe hypertension, hyperthyroidism, angina pectoris, symptomatic cardiovascular disorders, glaucoma, hypersensitivity to sympathomimetic amines, history of drug abuse, severe agitated state, concurrently or within 14 days of therapy with MAO inhibitors.

Warnings and Precautions Long-term effects in children have not been established; not recommended for children under 3 years. May inhibit physical growth in children. May exacerbate behavioral disturbances in psychotic children. Amphetamines are not appropriate for all children with minimal brain dysfunctions; careful assessment and evaluation are required. Tolerance, extreme psychologic dependence, and severe social disability have occurred; the lowest feasible dose should be prescribed or dispensed. Safe use during pregnancy has not been established. Insulin requirements in diabetic clients may be altered by drug therapy.

Untoward Reactions Common reactions include tachycardia, palpitations, insomnia, talkativeness, and restlessness. Fatigue and mental depression may occur when drug is discontinued. CNS disturbances include dizziness, euphoria, dysphoria, tremor, and irritability. Psychotic episodes may occur, but rarely at recommended doses. Psychotic disturbances may occur with prolonged doses higher than those recommended. Confusion, schizophreniclike psychosis, combative behavior, delirium, paranoid delusions, vivid hallucinations, and panic states have been reported. Dermatitis and marked weight loss are associated with chronic intoxication. Fatalities from toxicity are a result of convulsions and coma due to cerebral hemorrhages. Cardiovascular disturbances include pallor or flushing, hypertension or hypotension, chills, arrhythmias, dry mouth, and metallic taste. Other reactions include impotence, excessive sweating, and alterations in libido. Hypersensitivity reactions, including urticaria, have been reported.

Parameters of Use

Absorption Rapidly absorbed. Onset of appetite suppression is 30 to 60 minutes. Duration of action varies between 4 and 24 hours.

Distribution Widely distributed. High concentrations are found in the brain and cerebrospinal fluid. Crosses blood-brain barrier.

Metabolism Some in the liver.

Excretion Primarily by the kidneys. Urinary acidifiers increase drug excretion; but urinary alkalizers promote reabsorption of drug.

Drug Interactions Hypertensive crisis may occur if amphetamines are administered concurrently or within 14 days of therapy with MAO inhibitors. Urinary alkalizers, including sodium bicarbonate and acetazolamide, will increase the renal reabsorption of amphetamines. Urinary acidifiers, including ascorbic acid and ammonium chloride, will promote excretion of amphetamines; ammonium chloride is often used to promote drug excretion during toxicity. Amphetamines will decrease the antihypertensive effects of guanethidine. Phenothiazines, reserpine, and haloperidol will decrease the effects of amphetamines. Caffeine and sympathomimetic amines may potentiate the CNS and/or peripheral effects of amphetamines.

Administration

- *Narcolepsy:* Adults: 5 to 60 mg po daily in divided doses; Children: over 12 years: 10 mg po daily in divided doses; Ages 6 to 12 years: 5 mg po daily in divided doses.
- *Brain disorders:* Children: Over 5 years: 5 mg po daily; Ages 3 to 5 years: 2.5 mg po daily; dosage may be increased weekly until desired effect.
- *Obesity:* Adults and children over 12 years: 5 mg po tid 30 to 60 minutes before meals.

Available Drug Forms Tablets containing 5 or 10 mg; sustained-release capsules containing 15 mg.

Nursing Management

Planning factors

1. Obtain history of neurologic, cardiovascular, and renal disorders.
2. When administered as an appetite suppressant, obtain history of obesity.
3. Obtain baseline vital signs. Notify physician if blood pressure is elevated.
4. Determine what OTC and prescription drugs the client has been taking. Notify physician of potential drug interactions and if client has a history of drug addiction or abuse.
5. Protect drug from light.
6. Many individuals with narcolepsy will maintain clinical effectiveness from small doses (5 to 10 mg) for years; but tolerance to anorectic effect often develops within 3 to 6 weeks.

Administration factors

1. Give tablets with a full glass of water.
2. Sustained-release capsules should be given in early A.M.
3. Schedule amphetamine administration in early A.M. (narcolepsy or minimal brain dysfunction) or before meals (appetite suppression). Last dose of day should be given in late afternoon to avoid insomnia.

Evaluation factors

1. Evaluate effectiveness of drug for narcolepsy. A flowchart indicating the client's patterns of sleep, feelings of tiredness, and wakefulness are helpful.
2. Evaluate effectiveness of drug as appetite suppressant. A flowchart showing caloric intake, activity level, and daily weight is helpful.
3. Obtain vital signs periodically, particularly when drug is first initiated or dosage adjusted. If hypertension or arrhythmias occur, notify physician.

4. If euphoria occurs, notify physician, since the potential for abuse is great.
5. Abrupt withdrawal of drug after prolonged use may result in severe psychotic disturbances. Clients must be weaned off drug.
6. Monitor physical growth of children during therapy.

Client teaching factors

1. Emphasize the importance of schedule for drug administration to elicit best response without untoward reactions.
2. Warn client to notify physician if drug tolerance occurs.
3. Caution client against driving a car or engaging in hazardous activity.
4. Emphasize the need for regular medical evaluation of drug's effectiveness. Encourage client to maintain appointments.
5. Instruct client to obtain medical advice before taking OTC preparations.
6. Instruct client to avoid caffeine drinks, since potentiation of drug action may occur.
7. Warn client against drinking large quantities of cranberry juice, since drug excretion will be hampered.

GENERIC NAME Amphetamine phosphate (Cii)

CLASSIFICATION Cerebral stimulant

See amphetamine sulfate for Contraindications, Warnings and precautions, Untoward reactions, Parameters of use, Drug interactions, and Nursing management.

Action The phosphate salt of amphetamine is more soluble than the sulfate salt and can therefore be given parenterally. It can also be given orally in the same dosages as the sulfate salt. (See ampetamine sulfate.)

Indications for Use Narcolepsy, hyperkinesis, minimal brain dysfunctions, as a short-term adjunct in exogenous obesity.

Administration 10 to 15 mg po or IM, as needed.

Available Drug Forms Vials of dry powder for reconstitution.

GENERIC NAME Dextroamphetamine phosphate

CLASSIFICATION Cerebral stimulant (Cii)

See amphetamine sulfate for Contraindications, Warnings and precautions, Untoward reactions, Parameters of use, Drug interactions, and Nursing management.

Action Dextro isomer of amphetamine with greater stimulatory effect than amphetamine sulphate. (See amphetamine sulfate.)

Indications for Use Narcolepsy, hyperkinesis, minimal brain dysfunctions, as a short-term adjunct in exogenous obesity.

Administration 5 mg po every 4 to 6 hours, as needed.

Available Drug Forms Tablets containing 5 mg.

GENERIC NAME Dextroamphetamine sulfate

TRADE NAME Dexedrine (OTC) (RX)

CLASSIFICATION Cerebral stimulant

See amphetamine sulfate for Contraindications, Warnings and precautions, Untoward reactions, Parameters of use, Drug interactions, and Nursing management.

Action Dextro isomer of amphetamine with greater stimulatory effect than amphetamine sulfate. (See amphetamine sulfate.)

Indications for Use Narcolepsy, hyperkinesis, minimal brain dysfunctions, as a short-term adjunct in exogenous obesity.

Administration 2.5 mg po tid.

Available Drug Forms Tablets containing 5 mg; sustained-release tablets containing 5, 10, or 15 mg; elixir containing 5 mg/ml with 10% alcohol.

GENERIC NAME Benzphetamine hydrochloride

TRADE NAME Didrex (Ciii)

CLASSIFICATION Cerebral stimulant

See amphetamine sulfate for Contraindications, Warnings and precautions, Untoward reactions, Parameters of use, Drug interactions, and Nursing management.

Action Less potent than amphetamine sulfate. (See amphetamine sulfate.)

Indications for Use As a short-term adjunct in exogenous obesity.

Administration 25 to 50 mg po daily, bid, or tid.

Available Drug Forms Tablets containing 25 or 50 mg.

GENERIC NAME Levamfetamine succinate (Cii)

TRADE NAME Cydril

CLASSIFICATION Cerebral stimulant

See amphetamine sulfate for Contraindications, Warnings and precautions, Untoward reactions, Parameters of use, Drug interactions, and Nursing management.

Action Levo isomer of amphetamine. Levamfetamine induces less CNS stimulation than the dextroamphetamines, but has a more potent vasopressor effect. It may delay the emptying of the stomach. (See amphetamine sulfate.)

Indications for Use As a short-term adjunct in exogenous obesity.

Administration 7 mg po tid.

Available Drug Forms Tablets containing 7 mg.

GENERIC NAME Methamphetamine hydrochloride

TRADE NAMES Desoxyn, Drinalfa, Methedrine, Obedrin

CLASSIFICATION Cerebral stimulant (RX)

See amphetamine sulfate for Contraindications, Warnings and precautions, Untoward reactions, Parameters of use, Drug interactions, and Nursing management.

Action Methamphetamine is an analog of amphetamine with slightly greater stimulatory effect, but fewer cardiovascular effects. (See amphetamine sulfate.)

Indications for Use Narcolepsy, hyperkinesis, minimal brain dysfunctions, as a short-term adjunct in exogenous obesity.

Administration 2.5 to 5 mg po daily, bid, or tid.

Available Drug Forms Tablets containing 2.5 or 5 mg; sustained-release tablets containing 5, 10, or 15 mg; elixir containing 1 mg/ml.

COMBINATION AMPHETAMINE PREPARATIONS

TRADE NAME Biphetamine (RX)

CLASSIFICATION Cerebral stimulant

See amphetamine sulfate for Contraindications, Warnings and precautions, Untoward reactions, Parameters of use, Drug interactions, and Nursing management.

Action Resin complexes of amphetamine and dextroamphetamine. (See amphetamine sulfate.)

Indications for Use Narcolepsy, minimal brain dysfunctions, as a short-term adjunct in exogenous obesity.

Administration 1 capsule po daily in early A.M.

Available Drug Forms Capsules containing 7.5, 12.5, or 20 mg. Generic contents in each 7.5-mg capsule: dextroamphetamine: 3.75 mg; amphetamine: 3.75 mg. Generic contents in each 12.5-mg capsule: dextroamphetamine: 6.25 mg; amphetamine: 6.25 mg. Generic contents in each 20-mg capsule: dextroamphetamine: 10 mg; amphetamine: 10 mg.

TRADE NAME Obetrol (CII)

CLASSIFICATION Cerebral stimulant

See amphetamine sulfate for Contraindications, Warnings and precautions, Untoward reactions, Parameters of use, Drug interactions, and Nursing management.

Action Combination of neutral salts of amphetamine and dextroamphetamine. (See amphetamine sulfate.)

Indications for Use Narcolepsy, hyperkinesis, minimal brain dysfunctions, as a short-term adjunct in exogenous obesity.

Administration

- *Narcolepsy:* 5 to 60 mg po daily in divided doses.
- *Hyperkinesis:* Children: Ages 3 to 5 years: 2.5 mg po daily; Ages 6 years and older: 5 mg po daily or bid.
- *Obesity:* Adults: 5 to 30 mg po daily in divided doses.

Available Drug Forms Tablets containing 10 or 20 mg. Generic contents in each 10-mg tablet: dextroamphetamine saccharate: 2.5 mg; amphetamine aspartate: 2.5 mg; dextroamphetamine sulfate: 2.5 mg; amphetamine sulfate: 2.5 mg. Generic contents in each 20-mg tablet: dextroamphetamine saccharate: 5 mg; amphetamine aspartate: 5 mg; dextroamphetamine sulfate: 5 mg; amphetamine sulfate: 5 mg.

XANTHINES

GENERIC NAMES Caffeine; citrated caffeine; caffeine sodium benzoate

CLASSIFICATION Cerebral stimulant (OTC) (RX)

Source Caffeine is found in coffee, tea, cocoa, and the kola nut, which is used in soft drinks. The content of caffeine in some dietary substances is: brewed coffee: 100 to 150 mg/cup; instant coffee: 60 to 150 mg/cup; tea: 40 to 100 mg/cup; cola drinks: 17 to 55 mg/80 ml.

Action Caffeine has a poor solubility in water; caffeine sodium benzoate has increased solubility. Caffeine is the most potent xanthine CNS and respiratory stimulant. Like other xanthines, caffeine produces diuresis, dilation of the coronary arteries, and stimulation of the myocardium, but to a lesser extent than theophylline or theobromide. Stimulation of skeletal and smooth muscles also occurs. Caffeine crosses the blood-brain barrier and stimulates the cerebral cortex and medullary respiratory, vasomotor, and vagal centers. Mental alertness and attention span increase while fatigue and drowsiness decrease. The rate and depth of respirations are increased. Vascular resistance decreases peripherally but increases in the cerebral vasculature. Cardiac output and metabolic rate increase. In excessive doses, caffeine will cause arrhythmias, irritability, and possibly convulsions resulting from stimulation of the spinal cord. Even small doses of caffeine stimulate the secretion of gastric juices and may produce epigastric discomfort or aggravate a peptic ulcer. The drug is often included in analgesic preparations to counteract analgesic-induced depression of the cerebral cortex.

Indications for Use Mild to moderate respiratory depression induced by CNS depressants, such as barbiturates and narcotics; as an adjunct in restoring mental alertness and combating lethargy; headache caused by vascular congestion or spinal puncture. Has been used as a mild diuretic.

Contraindications Hypersensitivity to caffeine or caffeine-containing substances, gastric or duodenal ulcer, acute myocardial infarction.

Warnings and Precautions Tolerance to the diuretic and vasodilator effects of caffeine will develop with prolonged use, but cerebral stimulation will still occur. Cross-tolerance between the xanthines may occur. Psychologic dependence may occur with prolonged use. Ineffective for alcohol-induced and other types of severe respiratory depression.

Untoward Reactions Tachycardia, diuresis, and insomnia are common. Acute toxicity causes insomnia, restlessness, excitability, delirium, sensory disturbances (ringing in ears, flashes of light), fine muscular tremors, twitching, tachycardia, arrhythmias, and diuresis; convulsions may follow. Death is unlikely but may be caused by respiratory failure. Short-acting barbiturates are effective in treating toxicity. Gastric irritation is common after oral administration. May aggravate existing gastritis or peptic ulcer. Abrupt withdrawal after chronic ingestion of large doses may cause irritability, nervousness, and headache.

Parameters of Use

Absorption Rapidly absorbed from GI tract and parenteral sites. About 15% bound to proteins.

Crosses placenta and enters breast milk; caffeine should be avoided by pregnant and lactating women. Crosses blood-brain barrier.

Metabolism Unknown but probably oxidized and demethylated.

Excretion In urine; 10% excreted as unchanged drug.

Drug Interactions Not significant.

Administration Adults: Oral: 60 to 200 mg, as needed; Intramuscular, intravenous: 500 mg, as needed; Intravenous: 250 to 100 mg q4h, as needed; Maximum dosage: 1 g.

Available Drug Forms *Caffeine:* Bitter powder. *Citrated caffeine* (caffeine and citric acid): Tablets containing 60 mg. *Caffeine and sodium benzoate:* Ampules containing NoDoz, Stimm 250, and Vivarin. Ingredient in several analgesics, including APC, Buff-A Comp, Cafamine, Cafergot, Rogesic, Soma Compound, and Vanquish.

Nursing Management

Planning factors

1. Determine what medication or chemical substance caused the respiratory depression. If alcohol was ingested, notify physician before administering drug.
2. Gastric lavage is performed simultaneously, when indicated.
3. Obtain baseline vital signs.
4. Obtain history of cardiovascular disorders. Drug is usually avoided if acute myocardial infarction is suspected.
5. Indwelling urinary catheter insertion may be necessary.
6. Start an IV drip.
7. Equipment for mechanical ventilation should be readily available.
8. Cardiac monitoring is recommended.

Administration factors

1. Medication may be injected deep into large muscle mass. Rotate sites when multiple injections are required.
2. May be given via IV bolus over 1 to 5 minutes. Do not mix with other medications.
3. Check expiration date of caffeine and sodium benzoate before administering.

Evaluation factors

1. Assess neurologic signs and ventilation frequently (every 5 to 15 minutes). Remember that caffeine decreases the client's response to superficial pain.
2. Monitor vital signs frequently. If hypotension or hypertension occur, notify physician immediately.
3. If arrhythmias develop, notify physician and treat accordingly.
4. Monitor intake and output.

Client teaching factors

1. Clients should be warned that excessive intake of caffeine can cause gastric irritation and cardiovascular dysfunction.
2. Reassure clients that irritability, nervousness, and headache are common after abrupt withdrawal, but that these symptoms disappear within a few days.

SYMPATHOMIMETICS

GENERIC NAME Chlorphentermine hydrochloride

TRADE NAMES Chlorophen, Pre-Sate (C iii)

CLASSIFICATION CNS stimulant

Action Appetite suppressant similar to amphetamine; but significantly less stimulation of CNS occurs. (See amphetamine sulfate.)

Indications for Use As a short-term adjunct in exogenous obesity.

Contraindications Glaucoma, clients on MAO inhibitors, severe cardiovascular disorders.

Warnings and Precautions Tolerance to anorectic effect may develop within 4 to 8 weeks. Use with caution in clients with hypertension. Not recommended for children under 12 years. Safe use during pregnancy and lactation has not been established.

Untoward Reactions Insomnia, tachycardia, palpitations, and a slight increase in blood pressure are common. GI disturbances include nausea, an unpleasant taste, and either diarrhea or constipation. CNS disturbances include dizziness, nervousness, headache, and paradoxic sedation.

Administration 65 mg po daily before breakfast.

Available Drug Forms Sustained-release capsules containing 65 mg.

Nursing Management (See amphetamine sulfate.) Monitor blood pressure and pulse periodically.

GENERIC NAME Clotermine hydrochloride (C iii)

TRADE NAME Voranil

CLASSIFICATION CNS stimulant

Action A sympathomimetic amine similar to amphetamine. It suppresses the appetite by inducing CNS stimulation and elevates blood pressure. (See amphetamine sulfate.)

Indications for Use As a short-term adjunct in exogenous obesity.

Contraindications Hyperthyroidism, hypersensitivity to sympathomimetic amines, glaucoma, severe hypertension, concurrent use of MAO inhibitors.

Warnings and Precautions Tolerance to anorectic effect may develop within a few weeks. Use with caution in diabetic clients since insulin requirements may change. Safe use during pregnancy and lactation has not been established.

Untoward Reactions Insomnia, tachycardia, palpitations, restlessness, and a slight elevation in blood pressure are common. Hepatitis may develop if the drug is taken for longer than 8 weeks. Hypersensitivity reactions to FD & C No. 5 yellow have occurred. (See amphetamine sulfate.)

Administration Adults: 50 mg po daily in midmorning.

Available Drug Forms Tablets containing 50 mg.

Nursing Management Monitoring blood pressure and pulse periodically. (See amphetamine sulfate.)

GENERIC NAME Deanol acetamidobenzoate (RX)

TRADE NAMES Deaner, Deaner-250

CLASSIFICATION CNS stimulant

Action Psychomotor stimulant which is a nonquaternized precursor to choline. It is thought to cross the blood-brain barrier and serve as the choline precursor of acetylcholine in the brain. It has a low toxicity and induces mild untoward reactions. Unlike amphetamines, this drug does not suppress the appetite or induce nervousness.

Indications for Use Minimal brain dysfunctions, dyskinesia. Has been used for mild depressive states.

Contraindications Grand mal epilepsy.

Warnings and Precautions Use with caution in clients with hypertension or diabetes mellitus.

Untoward Reactions Headache, constipation, muscular tightness, twitching, and insomnia are relatively common. Dyspnea, irritability, rashes, and postural hypotension have been reported. Most untoward reactions disappear after several weeks of therapy.

Administration Children: Over 6 years: initial dosage: 500 mg po daily after breakfast; then 250 to 500 mg po daily. Depression: 25 to 150 mg po daily.

Available Drug Forms Tablets containing 50 or 250 mg.

Nursing Management Beneficial response will not occur until after several weeks of therapy. (See amphetamine sulfate.)

GENERIC NAME Diethylpropion hydrochloride

TRADE NAMES Diethylpropion-TR, Tenuate, Tenuate Dospan, Tepanil, Tepanil Ten-Tab

CLASSIFICATION CNS stimulant (C iv)

See amphetamine sulfate for Nursing management.

Action A sympathomimetic amine similar to amphetamine, but less effective as an anorexiant. It causes CNS stimulation and elevates blood pressure.

Indications for Use As a short-term adjunct in exogenous obesity.

Contraindications Advanced arteriosclerosis, hypersensitivity to sympathomimetic amines, agitated states, history of drug abuse, within 14 days of therapy with MAO inhibitors, epilepsy.

Warning and Precautions Tolerance to anorectic effect may develop after 4 to 8 weeks. Use with caution in diabetic clients since insulin requirements may change.

Untoward Reactions Tachycardia, palpitations, elevation in blood pressure, and nervousness are common. CNS disturbances include dizziness, headache, and precipitation of a preexisting psychosis. Menstrual irregularities may occur. Bone marrow depression has been reported with prolonged use.

Administration Adults: 25 mg po tid 60 minutes before meals; 75 mg sustained-release tablet po daily in midmorning.

Available Drug Forms Tablets containing 25 mg; sustained-release tablets and capsules containing 75 mg.

GENERIC NAME Fenfluramine hydrochloride

TRADE NAME Pondimin (C iv)

CLASSIFICATION CNS stimulant

Action A sympathomimetic amine that differs from amphetamine in that more CNS depression than stimulation occurs.

Indications for Use As a short-term adjunct in exogenous obesity.

Contraindications Glaucoma, severe cardiovascular disorders, history of drug abuse or alcoholism, hypersensitivity to sympathomimetic amines, mental depression, concurrent use of MAO inhibitors.

Warnings and Precautions Tolerance to anorectic effect may develop within a few weeks. Use with caution in clients with hypertension or diabetes mellitus.

Untoward Reactions Insomnia, palpitations, and alterations in blood pressure are common. GI disturbances include dry mouth, nausea, vomiting, diarrhea, and constipation. Genitourinary disturbances, including dysuria, urinary frequency, and impotence, may occur. Urticaria, sweating, fever, and eye irritation have been reported.

Administration Initial dosage: 20 mg po tid before meals; Maximum dosage: 40 mg.

Available Drug Forms Tablets containing 20 mg.

Nursing Management Monitor vital signs and blood sugar periodically. (See amphetamine sulfate.)

GENERIC NAME Mazindol

TRADE NAMES Mazanor, Sanorex (C iv)

CLASSIFICATION CNS stimulant

See amphetamine sulfate for Nursing management.

Action An isoindole anorexiant with action similar to amphetamine. Stimulates the CNS, particularly the limbic system.

Indications for Use As a short-term adjunct in exogenous obesity.

Contraindications Glaucoma, hypersensitivity to mazindol, agitated states, history of drug abuse, within 14 days of therapy with MAO inhibitors.

Warnings and Precautions Tolerance to anorectic effect may develop within a few weeks. Not recommended for children under 12 years. Safe use during pregnancy and lactation has not been established.

Untoward Reactions Nervousness, dry mouth, tachycardia, constipation, and insomnia are common. GI disturbances may occur. Overstimulation or drowsiness may occur. Corneal opacities have occurred with prolonged use in dogs.

Administration 1 mg po tid 60 minutes before meals or 2 mg po daily 60 minutes before lunch.

Available Drug Forms Tablets containing 1 or 2 mg.

GENERIC NAME Methylphenidate hydrochloride

TRADE NAMES Methidate, Ritalin (C iv)

CLASSIFICATION CNS stimulant

See amphetamine sulfate for Nursing management.

Action Piperidine derivative with actions similar to amphetamine. Stimulates the cerebral cortex and exerts mild stimulation of respirations.

Indications for Use Narcolepsy, attention deficit disorder, minimal brain dysfunctions, mild depression, withdrawn senile behavior.

Contraindications Glaucoma, marked anxiety or tension, agitation, within 14 days of therapy with MAO inhibitors, hypersensitivity to piperidine derivatives.

Warnings and Precautions Not effective for children with primary psychosis or secondary environmental behavioral disturbances. Not recommended for children under 6 years. Suppression of growth may occur but no cause and effect relationship has been found. Safe use during pregnancy and lactation has not been established.

Untoward Reactions Insomnia, nervousness, tachycardia, palpitations, alterations in blood pressure, and transient headaches are common. GI disturbances, including dry mouth, nausea, anorexia, and weight loss, can occur. Exfoliative dermatitis, urticaria, and other rashes have occurred. Dyskinesia and blurred vision have been reported. Toxicity may cause convulsions.

Administration Highly individualized. Adults (narcolepsy, depression): 10 mg po bid or tid 30 minutes before meals; Dosage range: 5 to 50 mg daily. Children: Ages 6 years and older: Initial dosage: 5 to 10 mg po daily before breakfast or lunch; then increase weekly, as needed; maximum dosage: 60 mg/day.

Available Drug Forms Tablets containing 5, 10, or 20 mg.

GENERIC NAME Pemoline (C iv)

TRADE NAME Cylert

CLASSIFICATION CNS stimulant

Action Pemoline is an oxazolidinone compound that stimulates the CNS and has minimal sympathomimetic effects. Mechanism of action is unknown, but it is thought to stimulate dopaminergic neurons in the brain.

Indications for Use Minimal brain dysfunctions, attention deficit disorder, hyperkinetic syndrome.

Contraindications History of drug abuse, children under the age of 6.

Warnings and Precautions Use with caution in clients with impaired renal or hepatic function. Safe use during pregancy and lactation has not been established.

Untoward Reactions May exaggerate a preexisting psychotic disturbance. Anorexia, transient weight loss, and insomnia may occur in the first few weeks of therapy. Nausea, stomach pain, irritability, dizziness, headache, depression, and hallucinations have been reported. Elevations in serum glutamic-oxaloacetic transaminase, serum glutamic-pyruvic transaminase, and lactate dehydrogenase have occurred after several months of therapy. Jaundice has also been reported. Dyskinetic movements have been reported and may be due to the drug. Toxicity causes agitation, restlessness, hallucinations, dyskinetic movements, and tachycardia.

Parameters of Use

Absorption Half-life: is 12 hours. Steady-state levels reached in 2 to 3 days.

Excretion By the kidneys as unchanged drug (43%) and metabolites.

Administration Children: Ages 6 years and over: Initial dosage: 37.5 mg po daily; then increase by 18.75 mg weekly; Dosage range: 56.25 to 75 mg; Maximum dosage: 112.5 mg/day.

Available Drug Forms Tablets containing 18.75, 37.5, or 75 mg; chewable tablets containing 37.5 mg.

Nursing Management (See amphetamine sulfate.)

1. Growth should be monitored during therapy.
2. Monitor hepatic function tests periodically.
3. Beneficial effects may not occur for 3 to 4 weeks.

GENERIC NAME Phendimetrazine tartrate (C iv)

TRADE NAMES Bacarate, Bontril PDM, Melfiat, Plegine, Prelu-2, SPRX-105, Trimstat, Trimtabs, Wehless-35

CLASSIFICATION CNS stimulant

See amphetamine sulfate for Nursing management. See phenmetrazine hydrochloride for Contraindications, Warnings and precautions, and Untoward reactions.

Action Phendimetrazine tartrate is an analog of phenmetrazine. (See phenmetrazine hydrochloride.)

Indications for Use As a short-term adjunct in exogenous obesity.

Parameters of Use

Absorption Peak blood levels occur in about 1 hour for the regular tablet and the duration of action is 4 hours. Duration of action is about 12 hours for sustained-release capsules.

Administration Adults: 35 mg po bid or tid 60 minutes before meals; 105 mg sustained-release capsule po daily in midmorning.

Available Drug Forms Tablets containing 35 mg; sustained-release capsules containing 105 mg.

GENERIC NAME Phenmetrazine hydrochloride

TRADE NAME Preludin (RX)

CLASSIFICATION CNS stimulant

See amphetamine sulfate for Drug interactions.

Action Phenmetrazine is a sympathomimetic amine that belongs to the oxazine group of compounds. This drug has anorectic effects, similar to amphetamine. It stimulates the CNS and elevates blood pressure.

Indications for Use As a short-term adjunct in exogenous obesity.

Contraindications Advanced arteriosclerosis, severe cardiovascular disorders, hypertension, hyperthroidism, hypersensitivity to sympathomimetic amines, glaucoma, agitated states, history of drug abuse, within 14 days of therapy with MAO inhibitors.

Warnings and Precautions Tolerance to anorectic effect may develop after a few weeks. Safe use during pregnancy and lactation has not been established.

Untoward Reactions Insomnia, tachycardia, and elevation in blood pressure are common. CNS disturbances include overstimulation, restlessness, dizziness, euphoria, dysphoria, tremors, and headache; psychosis rarely occurs. GI disturbances include dry mouth, unpleasant taste, diarrhea, and constipation. Urticaria has been reported. Impotence and alterations in libido may occur.

Administration Adults and children over 12 years: 25 mg po bid or tid 60 minutes before meals; 50 to 75 mg sustained-release tablets po daily.

Available Drug Forms Tablets containing 25 mg; sustained-release tablets containing 50 or 75 mg.

Nursing Management Monitor vital signs periodically. (See amphetamine sulfate.)

GENERIC NAME Phentermine hydrochloride

TRADE NAMES Adipex-P, Anoxine, Fastin, Ionamine, Parmine, T-Diet, Teramine, Wilpo

CLASSIFICATION CNS stimulant (C iv)

Action Similar to amphetamine.

Indications for Use As a short-term adjunct in exogenous obesity.

Contraindications Hypertension, angina or severe cardiovascular disorders, glaucoma.

Warnings and Precautions Tolerance to anorectic effect may develop. Use with caution in clients with a history of drug addiction or hyperexcitability.

Untoward Reactions Tachycardia, palpitations, nervousness, and insomnia are common. Fatigue may develop as the effects of the drug subside. Dry mouth, nausea, and constipation may occur. Hypertension and dizziness have been reported. Impotence may occur.

Drug Interactions Urinary acidifiers enhance excretion of the drug. Urinary alkalizers enhance reabsorption and may result in prolonged drug effects. (See amphetamine sulfate.)

Administration 8 mg po tid 30 to 60 minutes before meals; 30 or 37.5 mg of sustained-release form 15 to 30 minutes before breakfast.

Available Drug Forms Tablets containing 8 mg; sustained-release capsules containing 30 mg; sustained-release tablets containing 37.5 mg (free base bound to an ion exchange resin for delayed release).

Nursing Management Monitor vital signs periodically. (See amphetamine sulfate.)

COMBINATION PREPARATIONS

TRADE NAME Efed II (OTC)

CLASSIFICATION CNS stimulant

See ephedrine sulfate and phenylpropanolamine hydrochloride in Chapter 39 and caffeine for Contraindications, Untoward reactions, and Nursing management.

Action Produces CNS stimulation, bronchial dilation, and decongestion.

Indications for Use Relieves fatigue, drowsiness, and stiffness; used to increase mental alertness. Has been used for bronchial asthma.

Warnings and Precautions Use with caution in elderly clients with prostatic hypertrophy, since urinary retention may occur, and clients with hypertension, cardiac disease, hyperthyroidism, or diabetes. Not recommended for children.

Untoward Reactions May interfere with sleep if taken within 4 hours of bedtime.

Administration Adults: 1 capsule po q4h; Maximum dosage: 4 capsules daily.

Available Drug Forms Generic contents in each capsule: ephedrine sulfate: 25 mg; phenylpropanolamine hydrochloride: 50 mg; caffeine: 125 mg.

Nursing Management Reduce dosage if nervousness, restlessness, or insomnia occur.

CEREBRAL STIMULANTS WITH LITTLE OR NO KNOWN THERAPEUTIC VALUE

GENERIC NAME Bufotenine (Ci)

CLASSIFICATION Cerebral stimulant

Source Occurs naturally in the skin secretions of toads and in the seeds of *Piptadenia peregrina.*

Action Bufotenine is an indole derivative of serotonin and has been used as a snuff by some South American Indians. It induces vivid hallucinations.

GENERIC NAME Cocaine (Cii)

TRADE NAME Cocaine Topical Solution

CLASSIFICATION Cerebral stimulant

Source Alkaloid obtained from the leaves of *Erythroxylon cocoa* or synthetically produced from ergonine.

Action Exists as levorotatory colorless crystals or a white crystalline powder, hence the street name "snow." Cocaine is an effective topical anesthetic with a duration of action of 60 minutes. It has limited use as an anesthetic for nasal, oral, and ophthalmic examinations or procedures. Little or no absorption occurs through the skin, but it is well absorbed through mucous membranes. Addicts sniff cocaine or inject it intravenously for its systemic effects, which include euphoria, feelings of physical superiority, and self-confidence. Paranoid delusions and hallucinations also occur.

Warnings and Precautions High abuse potential.

Available Drug Forms Topical solution 1%.

GENERIC NAME Cocaine hydrochloride (Cii)

TRADE NAME Cocaine Hydrochloride Topical Solution

CLASSIFICATION Cerebral stimulant

Source Salt of cocaine that is more soluble in water than plain alcohol.

Action Unstable at elevated temperatures; loses potency when sterilized by autoclaving. Bacteriologic filtration is used to remove pathogens. It has limited use as an anesthetic for nasal, oral, and ophthalmic examinations or procedures.

Warnings and Precautions High abuse potential.

Available Drug Forms Topical solutions 2 to 10%.

GENERIC NAME Dimethyltryptamine (~~US~~)

TRADE NAMES DET, DMT

CLASSIFICATION Cerebral stimulant

Action Induces vivid hallucinations for approximately 1 hour.

Untoward Reactions Alterations in blood pressure, pulse, and respirations.

GENERIC NAME Lysergic acid diethylamide (~~US~~)

TRADE NAME LSD

CLASSIFICATION Cerebral stimulant

Action Potent hallucinogenic compound. Contains indole ethylamine and phenylethylamine. Has been taken orally as: a solution containing 100 to 400 mcg; a sugar cube in 100 to 400 mcg; with lactose in capsules or tablets; or in a solution dropped on a sugar cube.

Untoward Reactions Initial reactions (within 30 to 40 minutes): anxiety, sweating, clouding of consciousness; then, psychomimetic effects with disturbances of perception, vivid hallucinations, and euphoria, which last about 8 hours. May induce prolonged psychotic disturbances with flashes of light. Acute episodes can be terminated by phenothiazine tranquilizers.

GENERIC NAME Mescaline (~~US~~)

TRADE NAMES DOM, Peace, Peyote, Serenity, STP, Tranquility

CLASSIFICATION Cerebral stimulant

Source Occurs naturally in the flowering heads (mescal buttons) of the Mexican cactus *Lophophora williamsii.*

Action Mescaline is an amine that is chemically related to lysergic acid diethylamide. It has been used in religious ceremonies by certain Mexican Indian tribes and

Indians in the Southwestern states. Synthetic preparations are considerably more potent than natural ones (peyote).

GENERIC NAME Psilocybin

CLASSIFICATION Cerebral stimulant

Source Active hallucinogenic principle found in certain Mexican mushrooms of the Psilocybe group.

Action Similar to mescaline and lysergic acid diethylamide. It has been used in religious ceremonies by Mexican Indians. Peak effects occur in 2 minutes, but they are of short duration.

Chapter 37

Respiratory Stimulants

RESPIRATORY STIMULANTS

- Pentylenetetrazol
- Aromatic ammonia spirit
- Alpha lobeline
- Bemegride
- Camphor spirit
- Caffeine
- Doxapram hydrochloride
- Ethamivan
- Nikethamide
- Pentylenetetrazol
- Picrotoxin

ANALEPTIC PREPARATIONS CONTAINING PENTYLENETETRAZOL

- Cenalene
- Cerebro-Nicin
- Eldertonic
- Geracin
- Geravite
- Menic
- Meni-D
- Nico-Metrazol
- Nico-Vert
- Nicozol
- Ru-Vert
- Senilezol
- T-Circ
- Verstat
- Vita-Metrazol

AGENTS THAT STIMULATE the respiratory center in the medulla are called *respiratory stimulants*. Like cerebral stimulants, these drugs must cross the blood-brain barrier to exert their action. As most respiratory stimulants must be given in large dosages, the client can be in danger of developing convulsions or hypertension.

Respiratory stimulants are primarily used to treat drug-induced respiratory depression until the client can be intubated with an endotracheal tube and attached to a respirator. As hypoxia and hypercapnia are usually the major causes of death in drug-induced respiratory depression, a respirator, rather than drugs, is used until the depressant's effects subside. Other uses of respiratory stimulants include reversing or terminating the effects of certain anesthetic agents, treating certain types of drug poisoning, and as analeptics in low dosages. Pentylenetetrazol has been found to be particularly useful in enhancing the mental and physical activity of elderly clients.

RESPIRATORY STIMULANTS

GENERIC NAME Pentylenetetrazol (RX)

TRADE NAMES Metrazol, Nelex-100, Nioric, Petrazole

CLASSIFICATION CNS stimulant

Source Pentylenetetrazol is synthesized from cyclohexanone and hydrazoic acid.

Action Pentylenetetrazol is a CNS stimulant that acts at the medullary and cerebral levels; it also affects the spinal cord in large doses. It was originally used parenterally as an antidote for barbiturates and other CNS depressants and to induce convulsive therapy. Although effective, it is less potent than picrotoxin. Because pentylenetetrazol has a narrow margin of safety, the drug is only used orally to enhance the mental and physical activity of elderly clients who are in a state of confusion and have memory defects. Its parenteral use has been replaced by respirators (for drug-induced respiratory depression) and electroshock therapy (for inducing convulsions). Although the precise mechanism of action is unknown, pentylenetetrazol is thought to induce CNS stimulation by decreasing the neuronal recovery time. The myocardium is not directly affected by vagal stimulation. Hypotension may occur as a result of bradycardia, conduction disturbances, and splanchnic vasodilation.

Indications for Use Analeptic agent in elderly clients to enhance their mental and physical activity. Has been used to treat drug-induced respiratory depression.

Contraindications Acute seizure disorders, low convulsive threshold, focal brain lesions.

Warnings and Precautions Use with caution in clients with severe cardiac disease, hypotension, or severe hepatic impairment. Safe use in children and during pregnancy and lactation has not been established.

Untoward Reactions Insomnia and headache are relatively common. GI disturbances, including anorexia, nausea, and vomiting, may occur after oral administration. Bradycardia, conduction disturbances, and splanchnic vasodilation may occur and result in hypotension, particularly when large doses are administered. Overdosage may cause twitching, fasciculations, tremors, agitation, hyperreflexia, confusion, hallucinations, and vomiting. Toxicity results in spontaneous clonic convulsions that may last for several minutes; marked CNS depression and coma may follow. Deaths have been reported from 10 g of drug. Death results from medullary depression, hypoxia, and respiratory paralysis.

Parameters of Use

Absorption Rapidly absorbed from all sites.
Metabolism Primarily in the liver.
Excretion About 75% by the kidneys as inactive metabolites.

Drug Interactions May interact with antihypertensive agents causing severe untoward reactions in elderly clients; concurrent use is not recommended.

Laboratory Interactions May produce a false-positive result for the HCG pregnancy test.

Administration

- *Analeptic agent:* 100 to 200 mg po tid.
- *Drug-induced respiratory depression:* Initial dosage: 100 to 500 mg IV bolus and repeat, if necessary, until corneal and swallowing reflexes return; then 100 to 200 mg IM, as needed.

Available Drug Forms Tablets containing 100 mg. Wine-flavored elixir containing 100 mg/5 ml; also contains 15% alcohol. Ampules containing 100 mg/ml.

Nursing Management

Planning factors

1. Obtain history of cardiovascular, hepatic, GI, and neurologic disorders.
2. Obtain a history of OTC and prescription drugs ingested.
3. When an overdose is suspected, a mechanical respirator should be readily available.

Administration factors

1. When administered orally, give between meals; if local GI disturbances occur, give 1 hour after meals.

2. Parenteral administration should be performed by a physician or specially trained professional.

Evaluation factors

1. Observe client for toxicity periodically when drug is administered orally; monitor vital signs periodically (daily).
2. When used parenterally,
   (a) Client should be continually assessed for return of reflex activity and excessive CNS stimulation; consciousness usually returns soon after reflex activity.
   (b) Monitor vital signs frequently.
   (c) Monitor intake and output.
   (d) Cardiac monitoring is recommended.

GENERIC NAME Aromatic ammonia spirit (OTC)

TRADE NAME Spirit of Ammonia

CLASSIFICATION Respiratory stimulant

Action Respiratory and cerebral stimulant. Stimulates the respiratory and vasomotor centers of the medulla by irritation of sensory (trigeminal) nerve endings in the mucous membranes of the nose and throat.

Indications for Use Fainting.

Untoward Reactions Excessive inhalation may cause irritation of lung tissue and may result in pulmonary edema.

Administration Inhale vapor of broken ampule prn.

Available Drug Forms Cloth-covered ampules containing 70% alcohol, essential oils, and ammonia.

Nursing Management

1. Break ampule in gauze or tissue.
2. Pass a drug-coated tissue under the nose once or twice.
3. Client should remain in recumbent or sitting position until fully alert (5 to 30 minutes).

GENERIC NAME Alpha lobeline (OTC) (RX)

TRADE NAMES Lobeline Hydrochloride (Injection), Lobeline Sulfate (Oral)

CLASSIFICATION Respiratory stimulant

Action Respiratory stimulant that induces physiologic effects similar to nicotine

Indications for Use As an aid to stop smoking. Has been used to treat acute respiratory depression.

Administration Intramuscular subcutaneous: 10 to 20 mg prn; Intravenous (bolus): 3 to 6 mg prn.

Available Drug Forms Vials containing 3 or 10 mg/ml. An ingredient of several antismoking aids.

GENERIC NAME Bemegride (RX)

TRADE NAME Megimide

CLASSIFICATION Respiratory stimulant

See pentylenetetrazol for Contraindications, Warnings and precautions, Untoward reactions, Parameters of use, Drug interactions, and Nursing management.

Action Glutarimide derivative that is similar to pentylenetetrazol in barbiturate antagonist stimulating effects. Bemegride is no longer an official drug in the United States because it has no advantages over pentylenetetrazol. (See pentylenetetrazol.)

Indications for Use Termination of barbiturate-induced anesthesia. Has been used to treat glutethimide poisoning.

Administration 50 mg IV every 5 minutes until reversal occurs.

Available Drug Forms Vials containing 5 mg/ml.

GENERIC NAME Camphor spirit (OTC)

CLASSIFICATION Respiratory stimulant

Action Respiratory irritant that has been used as a stimulant. It is no longer available as an official drug in the United States as it has no pharmacologic effect on the medullary centers.

Indications for Use Previously used as a respiratory stimulant.

Available Drug Forms Cloth-covered ampules containing 10% in alcohol.

GENERIC NAME Caffeine (OTC)

CLASSIFICATION Respiratory stimulant

(See caffeine, page 559.)

GENERIC NAME Doxapram hydrochloride (RX)

TRADE NAME Dopram

CLASSIFICATION Respiratory stimulant

Action Short-acting CNS stimulant that affects all levels of the cerebrospinal axis, but with greater effects on the medulla. Doxapram has a relatively wide margin of safety. It increases respiratory ratio and volume, elevates blood pressure, and increases pulse rate. Respiratory and oral secretions may also be increased.

Indications for Use Postanesthesia respiratory depression, reversal of drug-induced respiratory depression, acute hypercapnia associated with chronic obstructive pulmonary disease.

Contradications Epilepsy, seizure disorders; head trauma; severe cardiovascular disorders, hypertension, cerebrovascular accidents, heart failure; respiratory failure due to flail chest, pulmonary embolism, pneumothorax, neuromuscular disorders, or bronchial asthma.

Warnings and Precautions Use with caution in clients with a history of bronchial asthma, arrhythmias, or pheochromocytoma and those with tachycardia, cerebral edema, or elevated cerebrospinal fluid pressure. Safe use in children and during pregnancy has not been established.

Untoward Reactions Respiratory disturbances, including dyspnea, sneezing, coughing, bronchospasm, and reflex hypoventilation, may occur. Cardiovascular disturbances include dizziness, headache, disorientation, paresthesia, sweating, dilated pupils, flushing, and a positive bilateral Babinski reflex. Convulsions may occur with excessive doses or prolonged use. GI disturbances, including nausea, diarrhea, and vomiting, may occur. Genitourinary disturbances, including urinary retention or incontinence, may occur.

Parameters of Use

Absorption Onset of action is in seconds. Peak action occurs in 1 to 2 minutes and duration of action is about 10 minutes.

Metabolism Rapidly metabolized by the body.

Drug Interactions Cardiovascular effects may be potentiated by MAO inhibitors.

Administration 0.5 to 1.0 mg/kg IV bolus; may be administered IM and repeated as needed or given by continuous IV drip at a rate of 2 to 3 mg/min.; Maximum dosage: 2 mg/kg/day.

Available Drug Forms Vials containing 20 mg/ml.

Nursing Management

1. Establish an airway before administering drug.
2. Evaluate arterial blood gases and vital signs before initiating therapy.
3. IV bolus should be given at a rate of 5 mg/min. or less.
4. Constant assessment is essential.
5. Cardiac monitoring is recommended.

GENERIC NAME Ethamivan (RX)

TRADE NAME Emivan

CLASSIFICATION Respiratory stimulant

Action Ethamivan, a derivative of vanillic acid, induces central and respiratory stimulation. Continuous IV drip increases the rate and depth of respirations.

Indications for Use As an adjunct in the treatment of respiratory depression.

Contraindications Epilepsy, seizure disorders; head trauma; severe cardiovascular disorders, hypertension, cerebrovascular accidents, heart failure; respiratory failure due to flail chest, pulmonary embolism, pneumothorax, neuromuscular disorders, or bronchial asthma.

Warnings and Precautions High doses may cause convulsions.

Untoward Reactions Respiratory disturbances, including dyspnea, coughing, bronchospasm, and reflex hypoventilation may occur. Cardiovascular disturbances include dizziness and disorientation. Convulsions may occur with excessive doses or prolonged use.

Administration Initial dosage: 0.5 to 5.0 mg/kg via slow IV bolus; then continuous IV drip according to client's response.

Available Drug Forms Vials containing 50 mg/ml.

Nursing Management

1. Adjust continuous IV rate according to client's respiratory rate and monitor constantly.
2. IV pump is recommended.
3. Assess client for muscular twitching and hyperreflexia frequently; if observed, change to KVO and notify physician.

GENERIC NAME Nikethamide (RX)

TRADE NAMES Coramine, Nikorin

CLASSIFICATION Respiratory stimulant

See doxapram hydrochloride for Contraindications and Warnings and precautions.

Action Nikethamide, a pyridine derivative, is a respiratory stimulant that acts by reflex stimulation of chemoreceptors (carotid body) and has a weak central effect similar to amphetamines. Large doses stimulate the respiratory center in the medulla. This drug is more effective in clients with drug-induced respiratory depression; it has little effect on the normal respiratory center.

Indications for Use Barbiturate-induced respiratory depression, acute alcoholism, electroshock therapy, carbon monoxide poisoning, as an adjunct in the treatment of neonatal asphyxia. Has been used as an adjunct in cardiac arrest associated with respiratory arrest.

Untoward Reactions Common reactions include burning and itching in nasopharyngeal area. Overdosage may cause coughing, sneezing, hyperpnea, and muscle tremors; blood pressure and pulse rate may be increased. Toxicity may develop and result in muscular twitching, which progresses to convulsions, nausea, and vomiting.

Administration Adults: Initial dosage: 125 to 250 mg IV bolus; then repeat as needed; Maximum dosage: 1000 mg; Maintenance dosage: 75 to 125 mg po every 4 to 6 hours, as needed. Neonates: 375 mg IV into umbilical vein, as needed.

Available Drug Forms Solution 25% (25 mg/ml); ampules containing 25 mg/ml.

Nursing Management

1. Mechanical ventilation should be instituted as soon as possible.
2. IV bolus may be diluted with an equal amount of sterile distilled water.

GENERIC NAME Pentylenetetrazol (RX)

TRADE NAME Metrazol Tablets, Metrazol Liquidum

CLASSIFICATION CNS stimulant, analeptic agent

Action This drug's precise mechanism of action is unknown, but it is thought to act directly on the neurons to decrease neuronal recovery time. The mental and physical activity of elderly clients is enhanced. It was once used intravenously, in large doses, to induce convulsions in clients with psychiatric disorders. Although it has no direct effects on the myocardium, the drug's central-vagal stimulation may induce bradycardia. Hypotension may result from splanchnic vasodilation and cardiac rhythm disturbances.

Indications for Use As an adjunct in the treatment of elderly clients with mental confusion, apathy, and memory defects.

Contraindications Epilepsy or seizure disorders, bradycardia.

Warnings and Precautions Safe use in children, during pregnancy, or during lactation has not been established. Use with caution in clients with cardiovascular disorders.

Untoward Reactions Cardiovascular disturbances include bradycardia and other cardiac arrhythmias. Hypotension has been reported. Gastrointestinal disturbances include anorexia, nausea, and vomiting. Neurologic disturbances include insomnia and headache. Large doses may induce confusion, agitation, and paranoia in susceptible clients. Toxicity may result in convulsions followed by profound depression. Death may result from respiratory paralysis.

Parameters of Use

Absorption Readily absorbed from the gastrointestinal tract.

Metabolism Primarily by the liver.

Excretion 75% via the kidneys as inactive metabolites.

Drug interactions May interact with antihypertensive agents. Use caution when drugs are used concurrently.

Administration 100 to 200 mg po tid.

Available Drug Forms Tablets containing 100 mg. Wine-flavored elixir containing 100 mg/5 ml and 15% alcohol.

Nursing Management

1. Store drug at temperatures between 59°–86°F.
2. Ingestion of 10 g or more has resulted in death.
3. Taking drug after meals will prevent gastric irritation.

GENERIC NAME Picrotoxin (RX)

TRADE NAME Cocculin

CLASSIFICATION Respiratory stimulant

Source Active principle obtained from seeds of *Anamirta cocculus*.

Action Potent respiratory and central stimulant formerly used to treat barbiturate poisoning. Large doses are required for clients in coma. As picrotoxin-induced muscular twitching is often delayed, convulsions may occur. This drug is seldom used today.

Indications for Use Coma due to barbiturate poisoning. Smaller doses are used to treat overdoses of hypnotics, such as paraldehyde.

Administration 1 to 2 mg/min. IV until corneal and swallowing reflexes return.

Available Drug Forms Vials containing 3 mg/ml.

ANALEPTIC PREPARATIONS CONTAINING PENTYLENETETRAZOL

TRADE NAME Cenalene (RX)

CLASSIFICATION Analeptic

See individual generic contents for Warnings and precautions and Untoward reactions.

Action Vitamins are in nontherapeutic quantities, but may assist in preventing deficiencies.

Indications for Use Treatment of elderly clients with mental confusion, apathy, and memory defects.

Administration Initial dosage: 10 ml or 2 tablets po tid for 1 month; then 5 ml or 1 tablet tid.

Available Drug Forms Generic contents in 5 ml of elixir or each coated tablet: pentylenetetrazol: 100 mg; thiamine (B_1): 1.67 mg; niacinamide (B_3): 7.5 mg; cyanocobalamin (B_{12}): 2.5 mcg; alcohol: 15%.

TRADE NAME Cerebro-Nicin (RX)

CLASSIFICATION Analeptic

Action Cerebral and medullary stimulant (pentylenetetrazol) and vasodilator (nicotinic acid). Affects respiratory, vasomotor, and vagal centers.

Indications for Use Analeptic agent for elderly clients.

Contraindications Epilepsy.

Untoward Reactions May cause flushing and tingling sensations (nicotinic acid). GI disturbances, including nausea occur, but rarely.

Administration 1 capsule po tid.

Available Drug Forms Generic contents in each capsule: pentylenetetrazol: 100 mg; vitamin C: 100 mg; thiamine HCl (B_1): 25 mg; riboflavin (B_2): 2 mg; nicotinic acid (B_3): 100 mg; niacinamide (B_3): 5 mg; pyridoxine (B_6): 3 mg; 1-glutamic acid: 50 mg.

TRADE NAME Eldertonic (RX)

CLASSIFICATION Analeptic

See pentylenetetrazol for Contraindications.

Action Mild cerebral stimulant. Vitamins are in nontherapeutic quantities, but may assist in preventing deficiencies.

Indications for Use Treatment of elderly clients with mental confusion, apathy, or memory defects.

Warnings and Precautions Use with caution in clients with bradycardia or hypertension.

Administration 30 ml po tid.

Available Drug Forms Elixir with a sherry wine base. Generic contents in 30 ml of elixir: pentylenetetrazol: 20 mg; thiamine HCl (B_1): 2 mg; riboflavin (B_2): 2 mg; niacinamide (B_3): 10 mg; dexpanthenol (B_5): 5 mg; pyridoxine HCl (B_6): 0.5 mg; cobalamin concentrate (B_{12}): 2 mg; alcohol: 13.5%.

TRADE NAME Geracin (RX)

CLASSIFICATION Analeptic

Action Mild respiratory and cerebral stimulant. Niacin causes transient peripheral vasodilation.

Indications for Use Treatment of elderly clients with mental confusion, apathy, or memory defects; senility.

Contraindications Epilepsy, focal brain lesions, recent cerebral hemorrhage.

Warnings and Precautions Use with caution in clients with severe hepatic impairment, peptic ulcer, or hypotension.

Untoward Reactions May cause transient flushing. Pruritus may occur and the drug should be discontinued. GI disturbances, including nausea, may occur.

Drug Interactions May potentiate hypotensive agents and phenothiazines.

Administration 1 to 2 tablets po bid.

Available Drug Forms Generic contents in each coated tablet: pentylenetetrazol: 50 mg; vitamin C: 30 mg; niacin (B_3): 50 mg.

TRADE NAME Geravite (RX)

CLASSIFICATION Analeptic

See pentylenetetrazol for Contraindications.

Action Respiratory and cerebral stimulant. Lysine is an essential amino acid with glycogenic properties. It assists in the absorption of calcium from the GI tract. Vitamins are in nontherapeutic quantities, but may assist in preventing deficiencies.

Indications for Use Treatment of elderly clients with mental confusion, apathy, and memory defects; analeptic agent for elderly clients.

Warnings and Precautions Use with caution in clients with bradycardia or hypertension.

Administration 15 ml po tid.

Available Drug Forms Generic contents in 15 ml of elixir: pentylenetetrazol: 100 mg; lysine: 150 mg; thiamine HCl (B_1): 1 mg; riboflavin (B_2): 1.2 mg; niacinamide (B_3): 10 mg; cyanocobalamin (B_{12}): 10 mcg; alcohol: 5%.

TRADE NAME Menic (RX)

CLASSIFICATION Analeptic

See Geracin for Contraindications, Warnings and precautions, and Untoward reactions.

Action Respiratory and cerebral stimulant. Nicotinic acid causes transient peripheral vasodilation. Similar to Geracin, but contains twice the amount of pentyleneterazol.

Indications for Use Treatment of elderly clients with mental confusion and memory defects; analeptic and vasodilating agent for elderly clients; senility.

Administration 1 to 2 tablets po tid after meals.

Available Drug Forms Generic contents in each tablet: pentylenetetrazol: 100 mg; nicotinic acid (B_3): 50 mg.

TRADE NAME Meni-D (RX)

CLASSIFICATION Analeptic

See Geracin for Contraindications, Warnings and precautions, and Untoward reactions.

Action Respiratory and cerebral stimulant similar to Geracin. Dimenhydrinate (Dramamine) is an antihistamine that is useful in treating labyrinthitis due to poor circulation.

Indications for Use Treatment of elderly clients with mental confusion, memory defects, and dizziness; analeptic and vasodilating agent for elderly clients; senility.

Administration 1 to 2 capsules po tid after meals.

Available Drug Forms Generic contents in each capsule: pentylenetetrazol: 50 mg; niacin (B_3): 50 mg; dimenhydrinate: 50 mg.

Nursing Management Caution client against driving a car or engaging in hazardous activities, since drowsiness may occur.

TRADE NAME Nico-Metrazol (RX)

CLASSIFICATION Analeptic

See Geracin for Contraindications, Warnings and precautions, and Untoward reactions.

Action CNS stimulant that affects all levels of the cerebrospinal axis. Enhances mental and physical activity in elderly clients. Similar to Geracin, but contains twice the amount of pentylenetetrazol.

Indications for Use Treatment of elderly clients with mental confusion and memory defects; analeptic and vasodilating agent for elderly clients; senility.

Administration 5 to 10 ml or 1 to 2 tablets po tid.

Available Drug Forms Generic contents in 5 ml of elixir or each tablet: pentylenetetrazol: 100 mg; niacin (B_3) 50 mg. Wine-flavored elixir also contains 15% alcohol.

TRADE NAME Nico-Vert (RX)

CLASSIFICATION Analeptic

Action Precise mechanism of action of dimenhydrinate in unknown, but it depresses excessive stimulation of the labyrinth. Nico-Vert also contains a CNS stimulant (pentylenetetrazol) and a peripheral vasodilator (niacin).

Indications for Use Symptomatic treatment of peripheral vestibular disorders (vertigo) associated with Meniere's disease, labyrinthitis, and fenestration procedures; treatment of vertigo associated with senility.

Contraindications Hypersensitivity to any ingredient, acute hypotension, active hemorrhaging.

Warnings and Precautions Use with caution in clients with severe hepatic impairment, epilepsy, focal brain lesions, and those with a history of peptic ulcer or severe diabetes. Safe use during pregnancy has not been established. May mask antibiotic-induced ototoxicity until irreversible damage occurs.

Untoward Reactions Drowsiness is common when therapy is first initiated, but tolerance develops with continued use. Abnormal glucose-tolerance test may occur.

Administration 1 to 2 capsule po qid; Maximum dosage: 8 capsules daily.

Available Drug Forms Generic contents in each capsule: pentylenetetrazol: 25 mg; niacin (B_3): 50 mg; dimenhydrinate: 25 mg.

Nursing Management Caution client against driving a car or engaging in hazardous activities.

TRADE NAME Nicozol (RX)

CLASSIFICATION Analeptic

See Geracin for Contraindications, Warnings and precautions, and Untoward reactions.

Action Respiratory and cerebral stimulant similar to Geracin, but contains twice the amount of pentylenetetrazol.

Indications for Use Treatment of elderly clients with mental confusion and memory defects; analeptic and vasodilating agent for elderly clients; senility.

Administration 2.5 to 5 ml or 1 to 2 capsules po tid.

Available Drug Forms Generic contents in 2.5 ml of elixir or each capsule: pentylenetetrazol: 100 mg; niacin (B_3): 50 mg. Elixir also contains 5% alcohol.

TRADE NAME Ru-Vert (RX)

CLASSIFICATION Analeptic

Action Respiratory and cerebral stimulant. Peripheral vasodilating (nicotinic acid) and antihistaminic (pheniramine acetate) properties are particularly useful in elderly clients with poor peripheral circulation.

Indications for Use Symptomatic treatment of acute or chronic vertigo.

Contraindications Hypersensitivity to any ingredient, hypotension.

Warnings and Precautions Use with caution in clients with epilepsy, focal brain lesions, or severe cardiac disease. Safe use during pregnancy and lactation has not been established. Not recommended for children under 12 years.

Untoward Reactions Acute overdose may cause overstimulation of the CNS and excessive vasodilation. Symptoms include nausea, vomiting, agitation, tremors, hyperreflexia, sweating, confusion, hallucinations, headache, and tachycardia. Convulsions and death can occur from 10 mg of pentylenetetrazol.

Administration 1 to 2 tablets po tid with meals or a light snack.

Available Drug Forms Generic contents in each capsule: pentylenetetrazol: 25 mg; pheniramine maleate: 12.5 mg; nicotinic acid (B_3): 50 mg.

TRADE NAME Senilezol (RX)

CLASSIFICATION Analeptic

See Geracin for Contraindications, Warnings and precautions, and Untoward reactions.

Action Enhances mental and physical activity in elderly clients. Similar to Geracin, but contains twice the amount of pentylenetetrazol.

Indications for Use Analeptic and vasodilating agent for elderly clients, senility.

Administration 1 to 2 capsules po tid.

Available Drug Forms Generic contents in each capsule: pentylenetetrazol; 100 mg; niacin (B_3): 50 mg. Store at room temperature.

TRADE NAME T-Circ (RX)

CLASSIFICATION Analeptic

See Nico-Vert for Contraindications, Warnings and precautions, Untoward reactions, and Nursing management.

Action Similar to Nico-Vert, but contains twice the amount of pentylenetetrazol.

Indications for Use Treatment and prevention of nausea, vomiting, vertigo, and motion sickness.

Administration 1 to 2 capsules po qid; Maximum dosage: 8 capsules daily.

Available Drug Forms Generic contents in each capsule: pentylenetetrazol; 50 mg; niacin (B_3): 50 mg; dimenhydrinate: 25 mg. Store at room temperature.

TRADE NAME Verstat (RX)

CLASSIFICATION Analeptic

See Ru-Vert for Contraindications, Warnings and precautions, and Untoward reactions.

Action Similar to Ru-Vert, but may cause fewer GI disturbances.

Indications for Use Symptomatic treatment of acute or chronic vertigo.

Administration 1 to 2 capsules po tid.

Available Drug Forms Generic contents in each capsule: pentylenetetrazol: 25 mg; pheniramine maleate: 12.5 mg; nicotinic acid (B_3): 50 mg.

TRADE NAME Vita-Metrazol (RX)

CLASSIFICATION Analeptic

See pentylenetetrazol for Contraindications.

Action Respiratory and cerebral stimulant. Enhances mental and physical activity of elderly clients. Vitamins are in nontherapeutic quantities, but may assist in preventing deficiencies.

Indications for Use Analeptic agent for elderly clients.

Warnings and Precautions Use with caution in clients with bradycardia or hypertension.

Administration 5 to 10 ml po tid.

Available Drug Forms Generic contents in 5 ml of elixir: pentylenetetrazol: 100 mg; thiamine HCl (B_1): 1 mg; riboflavin (phosphate sodium) (B_2): 1.4 mg; niacinamide (B_3): 10 mg; pyridoxine HCl (B_6): 1 mg; alcohol: 15%. Store at room temperature.

PART X

ADRENERGIC AND CHOLINERGIC AGENTS

MESSAGES ARE TRANSMITTED to body tissues by nerve fibers. Chemical substances, called neurotransmitters, provide the link from the nerve cell across a space, called a synapse, to the tissue. Nerve fibers that release the neurotransmitter acetylcholine are called *cholinergic* neurons, and the *adrenergic* neurons release norepinephrine.

The adrenergic system transmitter, epinephrine, is made by the body and stored in tiny vesicles in the nerve fiber. Impulses in the nerve fiber stimulate the release of epinephrine; the neurotransmitter crosses the synapse, stimulates the adrenergic receptor site in the tissue (smooth or cardiac muscle or gland), and a response occurs. The adrenergic receptor sites are termed alpha, $beta_1$, and $beta_2$, depending on the tissue innervated. Stimulation of alpha receptor sites induces vasoconstriction, dilation of the pupils, and relaxation of gastrointestinal and other smooth muscles.

$Beta_1$ receptor sites are located in the heart. Stimulation of these sites increases the rate and force of contraction and also causes an increase in free fatty acids. Stimulation of $beta_2$ receptor sites induces relaxation of smooth muscle in the gastrointestinal tract, bronchial tree (bronchodilation), and uterus. Blood vessels in the skeletal muscles also relax, producing vasodilation.

The cholinergic system transmitter, acetylcholine, is released from certain nerve fibers and interacts at muscarinic or nicotinic receptor sites to elicit a response. Once released, acetylcholine is rapidly inactivated by the enzyme acetylcholinesterase.

Stimulation of the cholinergic receptor sites produces essentially the opposite effect as adrenergic stimulation. Cholinergic stimulation induces dilation of peripheral blood vessels, bronchoconstriction, and stimulation of smooth muscle in the gastrointestinal and genitourinary tracts, but relaxation of their respective sphincters. Several exocrine glands, including the salivary, lacrimal, gastric, bronchial, and sweat glands, are stimulated to secrete their fluids. The pupil of the eye is stimulated to constrict and there is a decrease in cardiac rate and contractility.

Unlike the adrenergic system, cholinergic nerve fibers are found in skeletal muscles. Nicotinic receptor sites are located not only in autonomic ganglia but also at the neuromuscular junction. Contractility of skeletal muscles is stimulated by acetylcholine. Therefore, drugs that stimulate cholinergic nicotinic nerve fibers are effective in treating certain neuromuscular disorders, such as myasthenia gravis.

All the drugs in this section are concerned with stimulation of either the adrenergic or cholinergic system. The catecholamines, such as epinephrine, are potent stimulators of the adrenergic system and are used to treat shock, asthma, bronchospasm, allergic reactions, bradycardia, and even cardiac arrest. Adrenergic agents, which lack the catechol nucleus, are presented in the chapter titled Noncatecholamine Adrenergic Agents. Being less potent, many of these drugs are used as local decongestants of the nasal cavity or to treat eye irritations. A relatively new drug called ritodrine, a beta-adrenergic stimulant, is used to prevent premature labor. For convenience to the reader, noncatecholamine drugs commonly used to treat shock are presented in the chapter titled Antishock Agents. These drugs are separated into the alpha-adrenergic vasopressors and beta-adrenergic cardiac stimulants.

The cholinergic agents are useful for treating a variety of human ailments, including certain neuromuscular disorders, urinary retention, paralytic ileus, and to reverse the effects of surgically or drug-induced muscular paralysis.

Chapter 38

Catecholamines

BASED ON THEIR chemical structures, the sympathomimetic agents epinephrine, norepinephrine, dopamine, and isoproterenol are classified as catecholamines. Collectively, these substances are the most potent stimulators of adrenergic neurons known to man. Catecholamines have two basic effects on muscular tissue: they either cause contraction of tissue that is normally in a state of relaxation (alpha response) or relaxation of tissue that is normally in a state of semicontraction (beta response). Although there are some exceptions to this generalization, stimulation of alpha receptors causes contraction of (1) the blood vessels (vasoconstriction of veins and cutaneous, renal, and abdominal visceral arteries and arterioles); (2) the iris (pupil dilation); (3) the pregnant uterus; (4) the ureter and vas deferens; (5) the pyloric, rectal, and other sphincters of the GI tract; (6) the errector muscles (pilomotor response); and (7) the splenic capsule. Stimulation of beta receptors causes relaxation of (1) bronchial and intestinal smooth muscle; (2) the ciliary muscles; (3) the blood vessels (vasodilation of vessels in skeletal muscle and brain); and (4) the uterus. A marked exception is the increase in contractility of the myocardium in response to $beta_1$ stimulation. Catecholamines also elevate blood glucose (both alpha and beta response) and increase free fatty acids (beta response). The differences between the catecholamines, and therefore their clinical usefulness, vary according to which receptor sites are stimulated and the intensity of that stimulation.

CATECHOLAMINES

GENERIC NAME Dopamine hydrochloride (RX)

TRADE NAME Intropin

CLASSIFICATION Catecholamine

Action Dopamine is the naturally occurring immediate precursor of norepinephrine, and acts on alpha- and beta-adrenergic receptors. It increases the rate and force of cardiac output. Peripheral resistance remains unchanged when recommended doses are not exceeded. Systolic and pulse pressures increase, but there is little or no increase in diastolic pressure. The drug also acts on dopamine receptor sites in renal and mesenteric vascular beds. Renal and mesenteric blood vessels are dilated, thereby increasing glomerular filtration, sodium excretion, and urinary output.

Indications for Use Hypotension associated with myocardial infarction, congestive heart failure, renal failure, and endotoxic septicemia. It is also used to increase cardiac output and to improve perfusion of vital organs.

Contraindications Tachycardia, ventricular fibrillation, pheochromocytoma, pregnancy (unless benefits outweigh risks).

Parameters of Use

Absorption Onset of action is within 5 minutes and duration of action is less than 10 minutes.

Distribution Widely distributed in body tissues. Does not cross blood-brain barrier.

Metabolism Inactivated by monoamine oxidase in the liver, kidneys, and plasma.

Excretion Primarily as metabolites in urine.

Drug characteristics Sensitive to light, alkaline solutions, iron salts, and oxidizing agents. Do not add to an alkaline IV solution. Protect from light. Discard if solution becomes discolored.

Drug Interactions If MAO inhibitors have been taken within the last 2 weeks, dopamine must be started at minute doses, since there will be a heightened, prolonged response to dopamine; hypertensive crisis may occur. General anesthetics, including cyclopropane and halogenated hydrocarbons, potentiate the effects of dopamine on the myocardium and increase the risk of cardiac arrhythmias, elevated blood pressure, and other untoward reactions. Diuretics potentiate the effects of dopamine on the renal vascular bed. The analgesic effects of morphine are antagonized by dopamine. Propranolol antagonizes the myocardial effects of dopamine.

Warnings and Precautions Use with caution in children and clients with occlusive vascular diseases, hypothermic injuries, hypothermia, and embolism, since the drug may decrease the blood supply to extremities and result in color and temperature changes; necrosis may ultimately occur.

Untoward Reactions Ectopic beats, tachycardia, angina, headache, dyspnea, and peripheral vasoconstriction occur frequently. GI disturbances, including nausea and vomiting, may occur. Aberrant conduction, widened QRS complex, bradycardia, azotemia, elevated blood pressure, and piloerection may occur, but rarely. Prolonged use may cause a decrease in plasma volume. Extravasation may cause local ischemia and necrosis.

Administration Initial dosage: 2 to 5 mcg/kg/min. by continuous IV infusion; then increase by 5 to 10 mcg/kg/min.; Maintenance dosage: 20 to 50 mcg/kg/min.

Available Drug Forms Ampules of 5 ml containing 40 mg/ml. Store in airtight, light-resistant containers; sensitive to light, alkaline solutions, iron salts, and oxidizing agents.

Nursing Management

Planning factors

1. If signs and symptoms of hypovolemia (central venous pressure below 10 cm H_2O) are present, notify physician; this condition should be corrected before administering drug.
2. Use large vein to avoid extravasation. Avoid a cutdown if possible.
3. Continuous cardiac monitoring is highly recommended.
4. Discard drug if solution is discolored.
5. Phentolamine should be readily available; it may be needed to treat elevated blood pressure or extravasation.

Administration factors

1. Dilute drug in 250 to 500 ml of IV solution; do not add to alkaline IV solutions.
2. Start with a slow IV rate, then increase flow rate in small increments until desired systolic pressure is obtained (usually 90 to 110 mm Hg).
3. Adjust flow rate according to blood pressure response; maintain systolic pressure between 90 to 110 mm Hg.
4. If severe tachycardia, arrhythmias (premature ventricular contractions), or a marked decrease in pulse pressure occur, reduce flow rate or temporarily discontinue therapy and notify physician.
5. If hypotension persists or if urinary output remains low, notify physician: the client may be hypovolemic. Phentolamine should be readily available; it may be needed to treat elevated blood pressure or extravasation.
6. If excessive blood pressure elevation occurs, discontinue drug and monitor blood pressure for 10 minutes. If unresponsive, phentolamine may be given.
7. Mixed solutions remain stable about 24 hours. Time and date bottle when prepared.
8. Keep IV bottle away from direct sunlight.

Evaluation factors

1. The following should be monitored: vital signs (every 15 to 30 minutes); peripheral pulses (q1h); adequacy of nail bed filling (q1h); urinary output (q1h), when possible; central venous pressure (q1h), if available.
2. If there is a marked narrowing of pulse pressure, decrease infusion rate and check for other signs of vasoconstriction.
3. If toxic or untoward reactions occur, reduce flow rate or temporarily discontinue therapy, as needed.
4. Check for peripheral ischemia (weak or absent peripheral pulses, color and temperature changes in extremities); if symptoms occur, notify physician.
5. Check IV site for extravasation frequently (q1h).
6. Other vasopressors (norepinephrine) may be required if a dopamine drip is ineffective in maintaining blood pressure.

GENERIC NAMES Epinephrine hydrochloride; epinephrine in oil

TRADE NAMES Adrenalin, Suprarenalin, Suprarenin; Adrenalin in Oil, Asmolin, Sus-Phrine

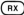

CLASSIFICATION Catecholamine (RX)

Source Naturally occurring catecholamine obtained from the adrenal medulla of animals or prepared synthetically.

Action Epinephrine stimulates the alpha- and beta-adrenergic receptors. It is not only the first hormone isolated by man, but it is also the most potent stimulator known to man. Alpha-adrenergic stimulation causes vasoconstriction of arterioles in most vascular beds, particularly the vessels of the skin, mucosa, and kidneys, thereby increasing blood pressure. When epinephrine stimulates beta-adrenergic receptors it inhibits constriction (causing dilation) of the brain and skeletal muscle blood vessels and stimulates the cardiac pacemaker and cardiac conduction tissue, thereby increasing the heart rate, contractility conduction velocity, and automaticity. Metabolism is also affected. In addition, epinephrine increases glycogenolysis in the liver and muscles; inhibits the release of insulin; raises the concentration of free fatty acids in the blood; and induces the liver to release potassium, which is taken up by muscles causing transient hyperkalemia followed by hypokalemia. There is little excitation of the CNS per se, but apprehension, headache, and tremors may occur. Other actions of epinephrine include inhibition of uterine tone and contractions and lowering of intraocular pressure (probably by reducing the production of aqueous humor and increasing outflow). Little or no mydriasis occurs in normal eyes; however, it does occur in clients with certain pathologies, such as acute pancreatitis, diabetic coma, and hyperthyroidism.

Epinephrine is a potent cardiac stimulant and bronchial dilator, and is therefore useful for restoring cardiac rhythm during cardiac arrest and relieving bronchospasm and anaphylaxis. Cardiac output is increased as a result of a shorter and more powerful cardiac systole. Although epinephrine does not stimulate respirations, it can relax bronchial muscle, thereby increasing vital capacity. Even when inhaled, epinephrine will relieve bronchial congestion, dilate the bronchi, and constrict the pulmonary vessels; thus increasing tidal volume and decreasing alveolar carbon dioxide levels.

Indications for Use Bronchospasm rash (as occurs in bronchial asthma), bronchitis, and hypersensitivities to drugs and other allergens; allergic reactions, such as angioneurotic edema and urticaria; cardiac arrest; syncope due to complete heart block or carotid sinus hypersensitivity. Also used to prolong the action of spinal and intraspinal anesthetics. It is used locally for minor surgery, open-angle glaucoma, and as a decongestant.

Contraindications Shock due to congestive heart failure, hemorrhage, trauma, or cardiogenic shock;

cerebral arteriosclerosis, organic brain syndrome; tachyarrhythmias, severe coronary insufficiency, cardiac hypertrophy; labor (delays second stage); infiltration of poorly vascularized tissues (toes, fingers, nose), since sloughing may occur; narrow-angle glaucoma; children under 6 years.

Warnings and Precautions Use with caution in pregnancy; in clients with diabetes, hyperthyroidism, hypertension, psychoneurosis, angina, chronic obstructive pulmonary disease, or tuberculosis; those receiving general anesthesia with cyclopropane or halogenated hydrocarbons; and elderly and debilitated clients. Use with extreme caution in clients who are hypersensitive to catecholamines.

Untoward Reactions Secondary effects, including anxiety, headache, fear, tremors, weakness, dizziness, palpitations, pallor, and urinary retention, are common. Toxic effects include a sharp rise in blood pressure, which may cause cerebral hemorrhage (pressor effect can be counteracted with nitrates or rapid-acting alpha-adrenergic blockers), severe throbbing headache, and ventricular arrhythmias. Arrhythmias, including tachycardia that may progress to ventricular fibrillation, may occur. Alteration of perception and thought processes can occur and may progress to frank psychosis. Tissue necrosis at the injection site, due to vasoconstriction, can occur.

Parameters of Use

Absorption Onset of action is: 1 to 5 minutes (IM); 3 to 5 minutes (subc); 60 seconds or less (inhalation). Some of the inhaled drug enters the bloodstream and causes a systemic effect. Duration of action is 20 minutes (IM); 20 to 30 minutes (subc, aqueous); 8 to 10 hours (subc, suspension).

Crosses placenta and enters breast milk. Does not cross blood-brain barrier.

Metabolism Primarily in the liver by catechol-O-methyl transferase (COMT) and monoamine oxidase (MAO); if one enzyme is unavailable, then the other enzyme will metabolize epinephrine.

Excretion In urine as unchanged drug (small amounts) and metabolites.

Drug characteristics Changes color (pink to brown) and loses its potency when exposed to air and light due to oxidation; protect containers from sunlight.

Drug Interactions Epinephrine is destroyed by oxidizing agents and alkaline solutions (halogens, nitrates, chromates, sodium bicarbonate); should not be given IV or intracardiac just prior to or immediately following these substances unless the IV line has been flushed with normal saline. Epinephrine is ineffective in treating the toxic effects of adrenergic blocking agents and phenothiazines as severe hypotension may result. Epinephrine may be lethal when it is used to treat clients who have received large doses of sympathomimetic amines. Tricyclic antidepressants potentiate the effects of epinephrine on the cardiovascular system and increase the risk of severe alterations in blood pressure, arrhythmias, convulsions, and other untoward reactions. General anesthetics, such as cyclopropane and halothane, and digitalis preparations potentiate the effects of epinephrine on the myocardium and increase the risk of ventricular tachycardia and fibrillation. Some antihistamines potentiate the effects of epinephrine by inhibiting tissue storage, thereby increasing the amount of epinephrine available at receptor sites. Propranolol potentiates the pressor effects of epinephrine and may cause a severe reflex bradycardia and A-V block. Drugs that inhibit COMT or MAO will potentiate the effects of epinephrine. Cocaine may potentiate the effects of epinephrine.

Concurrent administration with thyroid preparations may precipitate an acute episode of coronary insufficiency. Oral hypoglycemic agents are antagonized by epinephrine; blood sugars should be taken frequently and appropriate precautionary measures taken. Insulin requirements are increased during therapy with epinephrine; there is some indication that insulin antagonizes the cardiac effects of epinephrine. Nitrates and nitrites can be used as an antidote for epinephrine toxicity; rapid-acting nitrites have been effective in counteracting epinephrine's pressor effects.

Phentolamine inhibits the myocardium's sensitivity to epinephrine and may be effective in preventing epinephrine-induced ventricular arrhythmias in anesthetized clients. Alcohol may decrease the client's response to epinephrine by increasing the rate of excretion.

Laboratory Interactions Epinephrine elevates the serum levels of glucose, cholesterol, lactate, and urate; it may cause a false increase in bilirubin. Lactic acidosis may occur in epinephrine toxicity.

Administration Adults: 1:1000 solution for injection: Intramuscular, subcutaneous: 0.1 to 0.5 mg (0.1 to 0.5 ml); Maximum dosage: 1 mg/4 hours. Intravenous (bolus): 0.1 to 0.25 mg (0.1 to 0.25 ml); dilute to 10 ml with normal saline and give slowly (over 5 minutes). Intracardiac: 0.1 to 0.5 mg (0.1 to 0.5 ml); Maximum dosage: 1 mg; can be used in resuscitation. Intraspinal: 0.2 to 0.4 mg (0.2 to 0.4 ml). Local infiltration: 1 to 2 ml 1:10,000 to 1:20,000 solution, as needed. Children: Over 6 years: 1:1000 solution for injection: Subcutaneous: 0.01 mg/kg (0.1 ml/kg); Maximum dosage: 0.5 mg/4 hours. Ophthalmic use: Instill 1 to 5 drops 0.1 to 2% solution into conjunctival sac; do not drop directly into eye. Inhalation: 1:100 (1%) solution by aerosol or nebulizer. Nasal: 1:1000 solution (drops, spray).

Available Drug Forms *Aqueous solutions:* 1-ml ampules containing 1 mg/ml (1:1000 solution); 1-ml disposable syringes containing 1 mg/ml (1:1000 solution) (for IM or subc use only); 10-ml disposable syringes containing 0.1 mg/ml (1:10,000 solution) (available with a $1\frac{1}{2}$-in. (IV) or $3\frac{1}{2}$-in. (intracardiac) needle; 30-ml multidose sterile vials containing 1 mg/ml (1:100 solution); 10-ml multidose sterile vials containing 0.1 mg/ml (1:10,000 solution. *Suspensions* (epinephrine in peanut or sesame oil): 1-ml ampules containing 2 mg/ml (1:500 suspension); 1-ml ampules containing 2.5 mg/ml (1:400 suspension); 1-ml ampules containing 5 mg/ml (1:200 suspension). *Other solutions:* Inhalants, eye drops, nose drops: Available in various strengths and quantities; do not give parenterally.

Nursing Management

Planning factors

1. Promptness is essential when administering drug during emergency situations. Know where drug

and intracardiac needle are located and the strengths available.
2. Store in closed containers away from light.
3. Check drug supply monthly; replace all expired drug packages.
4. Discard drug if solution is discolored or if a precipitate has formed.
5. Rapid-acting nitrates and propranolol should be readily available for treating toxic pressor effects and arrhythmias, respectively.
6. When possible, obtain baseline pulse, respiration, and blood pressure.
7. Date multidose vials when opened and discard after time period indicated by the manufacturers.

Administration factors

1. Triple check drug form and concentration, since fatalities can occur with improper dosage and route of administration.
2. When administering suspensions,
   (a) Give IM or subc only; do not give IV or intracardiac.
   (b) Rotate suspension well, but gently.
   (c) Inject deep into subcutaneous or muscle tissue.
   (d) Initial drug absorption can be enhanced by rubbing the injection site gently for 1 minute.
   (e) If multiple injections are required, rotate injection sites to prevent tissue necrosis from drug's pressor effect.
3. When administering aqueous solution parenterally,
   (a) Inspect for color change; discard if it has turned pink or brown.
   (b) Inject deep into well-vascularized tissue.
   (c) Rotate injection sites. Check injection site for signs of necrosis (such as blanching of skin or cool to touch).
4. Since the dosage is potent, give a small initial dose and increase dose according to client's response.
5. If administered intracardiac, obtain a blood return before injecting and resume external cardiac massage immediately in order to circulate the drug.
6. IV administration is seldom used because extensive local vasoconstriction may occur.
7. Do not mix drug with alkaline solutions. Flush IV line with normal saline before and after drug administration.

Evaluation factors

1. Monitor pulse and blood pressure frequently (every 1 to 3 minutes) until blood pressure stabilizes.
2. Notify physician immediately if hypertension or arrhythmias develop. Rapid-acting nitrates may be required to treat toxicity.
3. Acidosis may develop; be prepared to administer sodium bicarbonate IV, as needed.

GENERIC NAME Isoproterenol hydrochloride

TRADE NAMES Isoproterenol Injection, Isuprel Glossets, Isuprel Hydrochloride (RX)

CLASSIFICATION Catecholamine

Action Isoproterenol, a synthetic catecholamine related to epinephrine, is a potent beta-adrenergic agent; it has little or no effect on alpha receptors. The primary actions are on the heart ($beta_1$) and the bronchial smooth muscle ($beta_2$). Stimulation of $beta_1$-receptor sites accelerates the heart rate, increases conduction velocity and contractility, relaxes intestinal smooth muscle, and raises the levels of free fatty acids in the blood. $Beta_2$ stimulation produces a marked relaxation of bronchial smooth muscle, some vasodilation, and secretion of renin. Renin causes the reabsorption of sodium by the kidneys and tends to elevate blood pressure. While the increase in cardiac output elevates systolic pressure, peripheral vasodilation lowers diastolic pressure, so that the mean pressure remains the same or drops slightly when small doses are administered; but large doses can cause a marked decrease in mean pressure.

Indications for Use As an adjunct in the treatment of shock (hypoperfusion syndrome), cardiac arrest, carotid sinus hypersensitivity, Adams-Stokes disease, heart block and ventricular arrhythmias (which are eliminated by restoring normal conduction pathways), bronchospasm during anesthesia, reversible bronchospasm.

Contraindications Tachycardia caused by digitalis toxicity, preexisting arrhythmias associated with tachycardia, recent myocardial infarction.

Warnings and Precautions Use with caution in pregnancy, elderly and debilitated clients, and in clients with coronary insufficiency, diabetes, hyperthyroidism, or hypersensitivity to sympathomimetic amines. Not recommended for children under 6 years.

Untoward Reactions Tachycardia, palpitations, nervousness, mild tremors, and sweating and flushing of the face are secondary effects of isoproterenol. Drug-induced tachycardia of 130 beats/min. May induce ventricular arrhythmias. Clients with organic disease of the A-V node may develop Adams-Stokes seizures. Nausea, vomiting, and hyperglycemia may occur.

Parameters of Use

Absorption Sublingual and oral absorption are unreliable.

Distribution Widely distributed in tissues; tissue uptake limits drug action.

Metabolism Conjugated in liver, kidneys, and other tissues. Children usually metabolize the drug faster than adults.

Excretion By the kidneys as unchanged drug and metabolites within 24 to 48 hours.

Drug characteristics Gradually darkens on exposure to heat and light. Do not use drug solution that has become discolored.

Drug Interactions Propranolol and other beta blockers antagonize the effects of isoproterenol. Excessive cardiac stimulation will occur if given concurrently with epinephrine.

Administration

- *Shock:* 0.5 to 5 mcg/min. by continuous IV drip.
- *Heart block:* Adults: 0.02 to 0.06 mg IV bolus; then

0.01 to 0.02 mg IV bolus, as needed, or 5 mcg/min. by continuous IV drip. Children: 0.01 to 0.03 mg IV bolus, as needed, or 2.5 mcg/min. by continuous IV drip.

- *Reversible bronchospasm:* Adults: 10 to 20 mg sublingual every 6 to 8 hours, as needed; Children: 5 to 10 mg sublingual every 6 to 8 hours, as needed.
- *Adams-Stokes disease and A-V block:* 30 to 180 mg sustained-release tablet po daily.

Available Drug Forms Sublingual tablets containing 10 to 15 mg; sustained-release tablets containing 30 mg; ampules containing 0.2 mg/ml (1:5000 solution); vials containing 0.2 mg/ml (1:5000 solution). Inhalants, in a variety of strengths, are also available.

Nursing Management

Planning factors

1. Obtain history of cardiovascular and respiratory disorders.
2. Hypovolemia and acid-base imbalances should be corrected before initiating therapy.
3. Continuous cardiac monitoring is highly recommended.
4. Drug may be alternated with epinephrine; but do not administer concurrently.
5. An infusion pump should be available for continuous IV drip.
6. IV drip may be used until a transvenous pacemaker can be inserted; tachycardia and ventricular arrhythmias may occur when catheter touches ventricular myocardium.
7. Electroshock is the preferred method of treating marked ventricular tachycardia associated with heart block.
8. Equipment for administering oxygen mixtures and ventilatory assistance should be readily available, especially for clients with status asthmaticus and abnormal gas tensions.
9. A demand pacemaker is the preferred method of treating Adams-Stokes disease.
10. Discard drug if solution is discolored or a precipitate has formed.

Administration factors

1. Oral inhalation is the preferred method of treating bronchospasm, since sublingual tablets are absorbed erratically.
2. Give oral tablets with a full glass of water. May be taken 30 minutes after breakfast if GI disturbances occur.
3. Sublingual tablet should be held under the tongue until completely dissolved. Instruct client to avoid swallowing tablet or saliva. Mouth should be rinsed with plain water after drug therapy to avoid tooth decay.
4. Initial drug therapy may be given IM or subc in nonemergency situations; usual dosage is 0.2 mg. Inject deep into well-vascularized tissue.
5. When administering via IV bolus,
   (a) Dilute dosage with at least 10 ml of sodium chloride or 5% D/W to make a 1:50,000 solution.
   (b) Give IV bolus over 1 to 15 minutes depending on dosage and client's sensitivity to drug (as shown by pulse rate).
6. When administering via continuous IV drip,
   (a) Dilute 2.0 mg (20 ml of a 1:5000 solution) with 500 ml of 5% D/W to yield 8 mcg/ml (1:500,000 solution).
   (b) An infusion pump is highly recommended, but a microdrip administration set can be used.
   (c) Start IV drip at 2.5 mcg/min. (children) to 5 mcg/min. (adults).

Dose		Rate of Administration	
(mcg/min.)	(ml/min.)	(15 gtt/ml)	(60 gtt/ml)
2.5	0.31	4.7	18.75
5.0	0.625	9.4	37.5
10.0	1.25	18.75	75.0
15.0	1.87	28.0	112.5
20.0	2.5	37.5	150.0

   (d) Adjust rate of IV drip according to response of blood pressure and pulse.

Evaluation factors

1. Constant monitoring (pulse, blood pressure, EKG, central venous pressure, urinary output) is essential when drug is administered IV.
2. Measure central venous pressure and intake and output hourly. Notify physician if output falls below 30 ml/hour or if fluid retention occurs.
3. Maintain pulse rate between 80 to 100 beats/min.
4. Reduce IV rate if pulse rate exceeds 110 beats/min.
5. If anginal or precordial pain occurs, turn IV rate to KVO and notify physician immediately.

Client teaching factors

1. Instruct client to protect tablets from heat and light. Keep stock supply in dark area.
2. Instruct client to carry a small quantity (2 or 3) of sublingual tablets at all times in a small dark medication container.
3. Instruct client to avoid swallowing sublingual tablets or saliva until the tablet has dissolved completely.
4. Instruct clients and their families to seek medical assistance immediately if bronchospasm persists or if fainting occurs.
5. Inform client about common secondary side effects.

GENERIC NAME Norepinephrine (RX)

TRADE NAME Levophed

CLASSIFICATION Catecholamine

Action Norepinephrine, formerly called levarterenol bitartrate, is the catecholamine transmitter naturally found at most postganglionic sympathetic nerve synapses. The drug acts on (a) alpha-adrenergic receptors causing peripheral vasoconstriction, which reduces blood flow to skeletal muscles, brain, kidneys, liver, and spleen; and (2) beta-adrenergic receptors (weak effect) causing inotropic stimulation of the heart and dilation of the coronary arteries. Norepinephrine increases systolic, diastolic, and usually pulse pressure. Cardiac output may remain the same or increase slightly. A compensatory vagal reflex overcomes accelerating action of norepinephrine on the heart; since the heart rate is slowed, stroke volume will increase. The rate of glomerular filtration is maintained unless there is a marked decrease in renal artery flow. Large doses may cause hyperglycemia by stimulating glycogenolysis and inhibiting the release of insulin. Contraction of the pregnant uterus may also occur.

Indications for Use Acute hypotension associated with sympathectomy, spinal anesthesia, pheochromocytomectomy, myocardial infarction, drug reactions, septicemia, and cardiac arrest.

Contraindications Mesenteric or peripheral vascular thrombosis, since the drug will increase ischemia and thereby extend the infarction; profound hypoxia or hypercarbia, since the drug may induce life-threatening arrhythmias; Pregnancy, unless the risks outweigh the benefits.

Warnings and Precautions Severe ischemia and ultimately necrosis may occur in clients with occlusive vascular diseases. Use with caution in the elderly and clients with preexisting hypertension, hyperthyroidism, or severe cardiac disease.

Untoward Reactions Toxic effects include excessive elevation of blood pressure, headache (which may be severe), bradycardia, decreased cardiac output, chest and pharyngeal pain, diabetes, and convulsions. Cerebral hemorrhage may occur, particularly in elderly clients. Photophobia and blurred vision have been reported. Extravasation causes local ischemia and necrosis. Secondary effects include a moderate decrease in urinary output, headache, dizziness, arrhythmias, reflex bradycardia, nodal rhythms, ectopic beats, restlessness, anxiety, tremors, insomnia, and weakness. Life-threatening arrhythmias, including heart block, ventricular tachycardia and fibrillation may occur, particularly in the elderly and clients with preexisting cardiac disease. Ischemia (pallor, cold to touch) and ultimately necrosis of the extremities have occurred, particularly in the legs. Prolonged use may cause a decrease in plasma volume, oliguria, edema, and necrosis of the kidneys, liver, and intestines.

Parameters of Use

Absorption Onset of action is within 30 seconds and duration of action is less than 3 minutes.

Crosses placental barrier.

Distribution Tends to localize at sympathetic nerve endings.

Metabolism Primarily in the liver and kidneys by catechol-O-methyl transferase; some is metabolized by monoamine oxidase in the liver, kidneys, and plasma.

Excretion By the kidneys as unchanged drug (10 to 15%) and metabolites.

Drug characteristics Store in airtight, light-resistant containers as the drug slowly darkens and loses its potency when exposed to air or light, as a result of oxidation.

Drug Interactions Tricyclic antidepressants potentiate the effects of norepinephrine on the cardiovascular system and increase the risk of severe elevations of blood pressure, arrhythmias, convulsions, and other serious untoward reactions. General anesthetics, particularly cyclopropane and halothane, potentiate the effects of norepinephrine on the myocardium and increase the risk of ventricular tachycardia and fibrillation. Some antihistamines weakly potentiate the effects of norepinephrine by inhibiting tissue storage, thereby increasing the amount of norepinephrine available at receptor sites. The effects of norepinephrine may be intensified and prolonged if administered within 2 weeks of therapy with MAO inhibitors; hypertensive crisis may result. Thyroid agents may increase the risk of acute coronary insufficiency. Alcohol ingestion may inhibit the client's response to norepinephrine by increasing the rate of excretion. Thiazide diuretics antagonize the pressor effects of norepinephrine.

Administration Highly individualized according to client's response. Initial dosage: 3 to 12 mcg/min. IV infusion; Maintenance dosage: 2 to 4 mcg/min.

Available Drug Forms Ampules of 4 ml containing 1 mg/ml.

Nursing Management

Planning factors

1. If signs and symptoms of hypovolemia (central venous pressure below 10 cm H_2O) are present, notify physician; this condition should be corrected before administering drug.
2. Use large vein to avoid extravasation. Do not use cut-downs (tie-in technique) unless absolutely necessary, since cut-downs have a tendency to produce venous stasis.
3. Continuous cardiac monitoring is highly recommended.
4. Discard drug if solution is discolored or if a precipitate has formed.
5. Phentolamine (Regitine) and drugs for treating life-threatening arrhythmias should be readily available.
6. Pressor effects can be controlled by decreasing the rate of administration.

Administration factors

1. Dilute drug in 500 to 1000 ml of 5% D/W or 5% D/S; do not use normal saline. (Dextrose inhibits oxidation and loss of potency.)
2. An infusion pump is highly recommended, but a carefully observed microdrip IV administration set can be used.
3. Infusion rate is determined by blood pressure response. Start with a low infusion rate and increase cautiously at 2-minute intervals, while monitoring blood pressure and pulse, until desired systolic pressure is obtained (usually 80 to 100 mm Hg). Blood pressure is generally maintained at 40 mm Hg below client's normal pressure.

4. When therapy is to be discontinued, reduce flow rate slowly, and check blood pressure every 2 to 5 minutes. If hypotension reoccurs, maintain systolic pressure above 80 mm Hg and notify physician.

Evaluation factors

1. The following should be monitored: blood pressure (every 2 to 5 minutes initially, then every 5 minutes); pulse and respiration (every 2 to 5 minutes initially, then every 15 minutes); peripheral pulses, particularly in the legs (q1h); adequacy of nail bed filling, particularly in the toes (q1h); urinary output (q1h), when possible; central venous pressure (q1h), if available.
2. Check for profound peripheral ischemia, particularly in the legs (peripheral pulse, color, temperature).
3. If toxic effects, life-threatening arrhythmias, chest pain, convulsions, or other untoward reactions occur, reduce flow rate and notify physician immediately.
4. If hypotension persists, notify physician; the client may be hypovolemic or may require a more potent solution.
5. Check IV site for extravasation frequently (q1h). Watch for blanching along course of vein and the formation of a hard swelling at IV site. If it occurs, change IV site and notify physician immediately. Extravasation is treated by infiltration, as soon as possible, with 5 to 10 mg of diluted phentolamine; 5 to 10 ml of sterile saline can be used for dilution.

Chapter 39

Noncatecholamine Adrenergic Agents

MANY ADRENERGIC AGENTS lack the catechol nucleus found in catecholamines. The noncatecholamines are less potent adrenergic neuron stimulants than the catecholamines, but a similar response is induced. The primary action of the noncatecholamines is to induce the release of catecholamines (epinephrine and norepinephrine) that are naturally stored in the body. Adrenergic receptor sites are stimulated over a longer period of time by the noncatecholamines than by the catecholamines, but once the body's stores of catecholamines are depleted, the adrenergic stimulation decreases markedly.

The agents in this chapter induce stimulation of either alpha, $beta_1$, or $beta_2$ adrenergic receptor sites. Ephedrine stimulates both alpha- and beta-adrenergic receptor sites and is therefore useful as a long-acting bronchodilator ($beta_2$ and alpha responses), and as a nasal decongestant (alpha response) But since $beta_1$ receptor sites are also stimulated, tachycardia and cardiac arrhythmias may be induced.

Several of the drugs in this chapter stimulate alpha receptor sites and are either administered orally (pseudoephedrine) or locally (propylhexedrine) for their decongestant effect. Due to their vasoconstricting ability, some of these agents, such as naphazoline, are useful for treating both nasal congestion and eye irritations. Great caution must be used to ensure that the stronger nasal solution (0.1%) is never used on the delicate eye tissues (0.012%, 0.015%, or 0.02% solutions only), since eye damage could result.

There is a relatively selective beta-adrenergic agent called ritodrine that induces relaxation of the uterus, a $beta_2$ response. It is useful for preventing premature labor. Unfortunately, beta receptor sites in the heart ($beta_1$ response) are also stimulated. Tachycardia, cardiac arrhythmias, and pulmonary edema are serious untoward reactions to ritodrine therapy.

It should be remembered that the agents presented in this chapter may induce unwanted secondary responses because they stimulate both alpha- and beta-adrenergic responses. Even locally applied drugs may be absorbed through mucous membranes and cause a systemic reaction. Hypertension, tachycardia, cardiac arrhythmias, urinary retention, and gastrointestinal disturbances are common systemic reactions.

EPHEDRINE AND RELATED SUBSTANCES

GENERIC NAMES Ephedrine sulfate; ephedrine hydrochloride

RX

TRADE NAMES Ectasule Minus III, Ephedsol, Slo-Fedrin

CLASSIFICATION Adrenergic agent (indirect)

Source An alkaloid obtained from the stems of Ephedra; but is now commercially prepared by synthetic methods. The L-isomer of ephedrine is usually used therapeutically.

Action Ephedrine causes stimulation of alpha- and beta-adrenergic receptors directly and indirectly. It is believed to act indirectly by stimulating the release of body stores of norepinephrine, which is the adrenergic neurotransmitter that primarily affects alpha-receptor sites; thus its action results in peripheral vasoconstriction and an elevation of blood pressure. Stimulation of $beta_2$-receptor sites causes bronchodilation, the primary clinical application for this drug. The physiologic effects of ephedrine are similar to epinephrine, but it has a slower onset of action and its duration of action is seven times longer than that of epinephrine. The degree of bronchodilation is less than that produced by epinephrine, but because ephedrine can be taken orally and it has a relatively long duration of action, the drug is more effective in preventing bronchoconstriction rather than treating acute episodes. Ephedrine can be used as a respiratory decongestant because it reduces engorgement and edema, which facilitates ventilation and drainage. The drug also produces mydriasis, stimulates the CNS similar to amphetamines, and potentiates the action of acetylcholine. This latter effect may increase skeletal muscle tone in myasthenia gravis. Unlike epinephrine, ephedrine has little or no effect on serum glucose levels and reduces rather than stimulates uterine contractions. It acts directly on smooth muscle to cause relaxation, thus prolonging the stomach emptying time and decreasing mobility. Ephedrine sulfate is the most commonly used salt. Ephedrine hydrochloride is sometimes used in combination with theophylline and other drugs, but is more irritating than the sulfate salt.

Indications for Use Prevention of bronchoconstriction in clients with asthma and other chronic lung diseases; treatment of hypotension, particularly hypotensive states associated with spinal anesthesia; nasal decongestant; as an adjunct in narcotic and barbiturate poisoning (improves ventilation); as an adjunct in the treatment of myasthenia gravis. It is also used in Adams-Stokes disease to increase the ventricular rate.

Contraindications Hypersensitivity to ephedrine, narrow-angle glaucoma, severe coronary artery disease, arrhythmias, porphyria, psychosis, marked neurosis, concurrent therapy with MAO inhibitors.

Warnings and Precautions Use with caution in the elderly and clients with cardiovascular disorders, hypertension, hyperthyroidism, prostatic hypertrophy, and those receiving general anesthesia with cyclopropane or halogenated hydrocarbons. Safe use during pregnancy has not been established.

Untoward Reactions Cardiovascular disturbances, including hypertension, tachycardia, arrhythmias, and precordial pain, may occur, particularly in the elderly and clients with a preexisting cardiovascular disorder. CNS disturbances, including insomnia, nervousness, anxiety, and tremulousness, are common; dizziness, headache, and confusion may also occur. Urinary retention may occur, particularly in elderly males with prostatic hypertrophy; difficult or painful urination may also occur. GI disturbances include nausea, vomiting, anorexia, and excessive thirst. Other reactions include sweating and dry throat. Local application to mucous membranes may cause stinging and excessive dryness.

Parameters of Use

Absorption Well absorbed from GI tract; may cause GI irritation. Peak bronchodilation occurs in about 1 hour and duration of effect is 3 to 4 hours.

Distribution Widely distributed in body tissues. Crosses blood-brain barrier and may induce CNS stimulation.

Excretion Primarily by the kidneys as unchanged drug (10 to 70%).

Drug Interactions Hypertensive crisis may develop if given concurrently with MAO inhibitors or tricyclic antidepressants. The latter drugs increase the quantity of stored norepinephrine, which is released by ephedrine and other indirect adrenergic agents. Methyldopa and reserpine may inhibit the vasopressor and other effects of ephedrine. Arrhythmias may develop if ephedrine is given concomitantly with digitalis, halothane, and many general anesthetics. Excessive CNS stimulation may result if ephedrine is administered concurrently with aminophylline and other drugs that induce CNS stimulation. Phenobarbital and other barbiturates are sometimes given to counteract CNS stimulation by ephedrine. Ephedrine antagonizes the effects of guanethidine and other agents that suppress the alpha- and beta-adrenergic responses, and vice versa.

Administration

- *Hypotension and Adams-Stokes disease:* Adults: Intramuscular, subcutaneous: 25 to 50 mg q6h, as needed; Intravenous: 10 to 25 mg every 4 to 6 hours, as needed; Maximum dosage: 150 mg/day. Children: Subcutaneous, intravenous: 3 mg/kg q4h or q6h in divided doses, as needed; Maximum dosage: 3 mg/kg/day.
- *Bronchoconstriction and congestion:* Adults: 12.5 to 50 mg po bid, tid, or qid; Maximum dosage: 400 mg/day. Children: 2 to 3 mg/kg po every 4 to 6 hours in divided doses; Maximum dosage: 3 mg/kg/day.

Available Drug Forms Tablets containing 25 mg; capsules containing 25 or 50 mg; oral syrup containing 16 mg/4 ml; ampules of sterile solution containing 50 mg/ml; nose drop solution 1 or 3% in sodium chloride and jelly; eye drop solution 3 or 5%.

Nursing Management

Planning factors

1. Obtain baseline pulse, blood pressure, and respirations.
2. Volume deficit should be corrected before administering for vasopressor effect.
3. Cardiac monitoring is essential for clients with arrhythmias.
4. Store drug in airtight containers at room temperature, away from heat.

Administration factors

1. When administered orally, give with a full glass of water.
2. When administering IM or subc,
   (a) Inject deep into well-vascularized tissue.
   (b) Rotate injection sites.
3. When administering IV bolus,
   (a) Inject slowly.
   (b) Observe for hypersensitivity (tachycardia, arrhythmias, excessive vasopressor effect); if symptoms occur, discontinue drug and notify physician.

Evaluation factors

1. Hypoxia, acidosis, and elevated arterial carbon dioxide levels may reduce drug's effectiveness and increase untoward reactions. These disorders should be continually assessed and corrected promptly. If symptoms occur, notify physician.
2. Monitor blood pressure, pulse, and respirations frequently (every 5 to 15 minutes) when drug is administered parenterally.
3. Monitor intake and output. Notify physician if oliguria or urinary retention occur.
4. Drug's effectiveness may decrease after 2 to 3 weeks of continuous use; the dosage may be increased or the drug discontinued for 3 to 4 days, and then reintroduced.

Client teaching factors

1. Warn client about drug-induced CNS stimulation and to avoid taking drug near bedtime.
2. Instruct client to report palpitations, angina, and urinary retention promptly.
3. Caution client against taking OTC drugs containing ephedrine or CNS stimulants. Instruct client to consult physician, as needed.

GENERIC NAME Hydroxyamphetamine hydrobromide

TRADE NAME Paredrine (RX)

CLASSIFICATION Adrenergic agent (indirect)

Action Hydroxyamphetamine causes dilation of the pupil, probably by stimulation of the dilator muscles of the iris, and may increase intraocular pressure. It is similar to ephedrine in that it will cause nasal decongestion, but is a weak bronchodilator and appetite suppressant. Hydroxyamphetamine can cause a marked elevation of blood pressure if accidentally ingested.

Indications for Use When pupil dilation is required, such as during eye examinations.

Contraindications Narrow-angle glaucoma.

Untoward Reactions Photophobia, blurred vision.

Parameters of Use

Absorption Onset of action is about 30 minutes and duration of action is several hours. Some systemic absorption can occur through the nasal mucosa.

Administration Instill 1 to 2 drops in conjunctival sac, as necessary.

Available Drug Forms Solution 1% in distilled water with 2% boric acid.

Nursing Management

1. Notify physician if eye irritation occurs.
2. Store drug in dark area away from light.
3. Caution client against operating hazardous equipment while vision is blurred.
4. Warn client against entering bright sunlight without sunglasses.

GENERIC NAME Phenylpropanolamine hydrochloride

TRADE NAMES Amfed, Propadrine (OTC) (RX)

CLASSIFICATION Adrenergic agent (indirect)

See ephedrine sulfate for Contraindications, Warnings and precautions, Untoward reactions, and Drug interactions.

Action Phenylpropanolamine is a sympathomimetic amine similar to ephedrine, but with greater vasoconstrictor ability, less CNS stimulation, and fewer toxic effects. It is effective when administered orally. Marked vasoconstriction occurs when the drug is administered parenterally.

Indications for Use Nasal congestion. Has been used parenterally to prevent or treat mild shock during spinal anesthesia.

Parameters of Use

Absorption Onset of action is about 30 minutes and peak action occurs in about 2 to 3 hours.

Administration

- *Nasal congestion:* Adults: 25 to 50 mg po q4h, as needed; Children: Ages 6 to 12 years: 12.5 to 25 mg po q4h, as needed; Ages 2 to 5 years: 6.25 to 12.5 mg po q4h, as needed.
- *Shock during spinal anesthesia:* Adults: 37.5 to 75 mg IM, as needed.

Available Drug Forms Tablets containing 25, 50, or 70 mg; ampules containing 75 mg/ml. It is used as a decongestant in several preparations, including Bayer Children's Cold Tablets and Cough Syrup, Brocon C. R., Congespirin, Contrex, Coricidin, Coryban-D, CoTylenol, Daycare, Decon-Aid, Dimetane Expectorant, Dimetapp, Entex, Formula 44D, Hycomine, Novahistine, Ornade, Poly-Histine, Respinol LA, Robitussin-CF, Ru-Tuss, Sine-Aid, Sinubid, Triaminic, and Tuss-Ornade. Phenylpropanolamine is also used as a common ingredient in OTC appetite suppressants, including Anorexin, Appedrine, Cenadex, Dexatrim, Prolamine, and Slender-X.

Nursing Management (See ephedrine sulfate.)

1. When administering IM,
   (a) Fluid balance and acidosis should be corrected before administering drug.
   (b) Inject deep into well-vascularized muscle mass (deltoid).
   (c) Monitor vital signs frequently, since the drug's action may be unpredictable.
   (d) Monitor client closely; nausea and vomiting may occur and ventricular arrhythmias may be induced.
2. When administering orally as a decongestant:
   (a) Give with a full glass of water.
   (b) Observe for hypersensitivity (tachycardia, arrhythmias, excessive vasopressor effect); if symptoms occur, discontinue drug and notify physician.
   (c) Hypoxia and acidosis may increase untoward reactions.
   (d) Notify physician if oliguria or urinary retention occur.
   (e) Drug's effectiveness may decrease with continuous use.
   (f) Warn client about the possibility of drug-induced CNS stimulation and to avoid taking drug near bedtime.
   (g) Warn elderly clients and parents of young children to avoid excessive use of drug. Only 4 doses should be taken in 24 hours.

GENERIC NAME Pseudoephedrine hydrochloride

TRADE NAMES Afrinol, Cenafed, Novafed, Sudabid, Sudafed, Sudafed SA, Suphedrine (OTC)

CLASSIFICATION Adrenergic agent (indirect)

See ephedrine sulfate for Untoward reactions, and Drug interactions.

Action Pseudoephedrine is an indirect sympathomimetic amine similar to ephedrine, but causes less systemic pressor action and milder untoward reactions. It produces a selective pressor effect on blood vessels of the upper respiratory tract, thus reducing tissue inflammation in the upper respiratory tract, including the eustachian tube. Pseudoephedrine causes some peripheral vasodilation.

Indications for Use Nasal congestion associated with the common cold, sinusitis, and allergic rhinitis; decongestion of the eustachian tube in children with middle ear inflammations.

Contraindications Hypersensitivity to ephedrine or pseudoephedrine.

Warnings and Precautions Use with caution in pregnancy and lactation and in clients with hypertension, cardiac disease, diabetes, urinary retention, glaucoma, and hyperthyroidism.

Parameters of Use

Absorption Onset of action is 15 to 30 minutes and peak action occurs in about 2 hours. Half-life is about 5 hours.

Crosses placenta and enters breast milk.

Administration Adults and children over 12 years: 60 mg po every 4 to 6 hours; Children: Ages 6 to 12 years: 30 mg po q4-6h; 60 to 120 mg sustained-release preparations po q12h; Ages 2 to 5 years: 15 mg po every 4 to 6 hours; Maximum dosage: 4 doses daily.

Available Drug Forms Tablets containing 60 or 120 mg; syrup containing 30 mg/5 ml; sustained-release preparations, which are not recommended for children under 12 years.

Nursing Management (See ephedrine sulfate.)

1. Instruct client not to take drug within 2 hours of bedtime, since insomnia may occur.
2. Dosage should be reduced if nervousness, restlessness, dizziness, or nausea occur.

OTHER ADRENERGIC AGENTS

GENERIC NAME Naphazoline hydrochloride

TRADE NAMES Clear Eyes, Naphcon, Privine, Vasoclear, Vasocon

CLASSIFICATION Adrenergic agent (OTC) (RX)

Action Naphazoline, an imidazoline derivative, is a potent vasoconstrictor that is similar to ephedrine in action. It is used as a local decongestant for the nasal mucosa and the eye.

Indications for Use Nasal congestion; ophthalmic congestion due to irritation.

Contraindications Glaucoma.

Warnings and Precautions Safe use during pregnancy has not been established. Use with caution in clients with diabetes, hyperthyroidism, severe arteriosclerosis, or cardiac disease.

Untoward Reactions Transient stinging and irritation are common. Excessive use may cause rebound congestion. (See ephedrine sulfate.)

Drug Interactions Hypertension may occur in clients taking MAO inhibitors concurrently. (See ephedrine sulphate.)

Administration

- *Nasal congestion:* Adults: 2 drops 0.1% solution every 3 to 4 hours, as needed; Children: Ages 6 to 12 years: 1 to 2 drops 0.05% solution every 3 to 6 hours, as needed.
- *Ophthalmic congestion:* Adults: Instill 1 to 2 drops every 3 to 4 hours in lower conjunctival sac, as needed.

Available Drug Forms Nasal spray; nasal drops 0.1% (adult) or 0.05% (pediatric) solution; sterile ophthalmic solution 0.012, 0.015, or 0.02%.

Nursing Management

1. Double check that the right preparation is being used on the right mucous membrane, since the accidental administration of the nasal preparation to the eye can cause serious damage to the eye's delicate membrane.
2. The dosage of nasal solution is instilled in each nostril.
3. Inform client to seek medical advice if irritation does not subside within 5 days.
4. Instruct client not to use preparation for more than 5 days. If congestion persists, physician should be notified.

5. Observe client for vasoconstriction and other systemic effects, since systemic absorption may occur.
6. Instruct client in proper application.
7. Inform client to avoid excessive use and to notify physician if nasal congestion persists.

GENERIC NAME Oxymetazoline hydrochloride

TRADE NAMES Afrin, Nafrine (OTC)

CLASSIFICATION Adrenergic agent

Action Oxymetazoline, an imidazoline derivative, is a long-acting vasoconstrictor and is a decongestant when applied to the nasal mucosa.

Indications for Use Nasal congestion.

Warnings and Precautions Use with caution in clients with hyperthyroidism, hypertension, diabetes, or severe cardiac disease. Safe use during pregnancy has not been established.

Untoward Reactions Headache, palpitations, dizziness, or drowsiness may occur if systemic absorption occurs. Excessive use may cause rebound congestion.

Administration Adults and children over 6 years: 2 to 4 drops 0.5% solution bid; Children: Ages 2 to 6 years: 2 to 3 drops of 0.025% solution bid.

Available Drug Forms Nasal spray; nasal drops 0.05% (adult) or 0.025% (pediatric) solution.

Nursing Management (See naphazoline hydrochloride.) Instruct client not to use preparation for more than 3 to 5 days. If congestion persists, physician should be notified.

GENERIC NAME Propylhexedrine (OTC)

TRADE NAME Benzedrex

CLASSIFICATION Adrenergic agent

Action Propylhexedrine is a volatile sympathomimetic amine that produces vasoconstriction and a decongestant effect when inhaled into the nasal cavities. It induces little or no CNS stimulation, but it will cause a dose-related mild stimulation of the heart.

Indications for Use Nasal congestion associated with the common cold, sinusitis, and allergic rhinitis.

Administration 1 to 2 inhalations q4h, as needed.

Available Drug Forms Nasal inhaler.

Nursing Management (See naphazoline hydrochloride.)

1. Instruct client to clear nasal passages before using inhaler.
2. Warn client that excessive use may cause rebound congestion.

GENERIC NAME Tetrahydrozoline hydrochloride

TRADE NAMES Tyzine, Visine (OTC)

CLASSIFICATION Adrenergic agent

Action Tetrahydrozoline, an imidazol derivative, is closely related to naphazoline in action. It produces vasoconstriction and a decongestant effect when applied locally.

Indications for Use Nasal congestion; ocular redness associated with eye irritation and allergic disorders.

Contraindications Glaucoma.

Warnings and Precautions Not recommended for children under 2 years.

Untoward Reactions May cause transient burning or stinging. Excessive use may cause rebound congestion.

Administration

- *Nasal congestion:* Adults and children over 6 years: 2 to 4 drops of 0.1% solution every 4 to 6 hours, as needed; children: Ages 2 to 6 years: 2 to 3 drops of 0.05% solution every 4 to 6 hours, as needed.
- *Eye irritation:* Adults and children over 2 years: Instill 1 to 2 drops bid or tid in lower conjunctival sac, as needed.

Available Drug Forms Nasal spray; nasal solution 0.1% (adult) or 0.05% (pediatric); sterile ophthalmic solution 0.05%.

Nursing Management (See hydroxyamphetamine for further details about eye instillation; see naphazoline hydrochloride for further details about nasal instillation.)

1. Double check that the right preparation is being used on the right mucous membrane, since the accidental administration of the nasal preparation to the eye can cause serious damage to the eye's delicate membrane.
2. The dosage of nasal solution is instilled in each nostril.
3. Inform client to seek medical advice if irritation persists.

GENERIC NAME Xylometazoline hydrochloride

TRADE NAMES Otrivin, Sine-Off Nasal Spray

CLASSIFICATION Adrenergic agent (OTC)

Action Xylometazoline, an imidazoline derivative, produces vasoconstriction and a decongestant effect when applied locally to the nasal mucosa. It has a relatively long duration of action when compared to other nasal decongestants; however, systemic absorption usually occurs.

Indications for Use Nasal congestion.

Contraindications Narrow-angle glaucoma.

Warnings and Precautions Use with caution in clients with diabetes, hyperthyroidism, severe arteriosclerosis, or cardiac disease. Safe use during pregnancy has not been established.

Untoward Reactions May cause transient stinging or burning. Excessive use may cause rebound congestion or ulceration of the nasal mucosa.

Administration Adults and children over 12 years: 2 to 3 drops of 0.1% solution every 6 to 8 hours, as needed; Children: Under 12 years: 2 to 3 drops 0.05% solution every 8 to 10 hours, as needed.

Available Drug Forms Nasal spray; nasal drops 0.1% (adult) or 0.05% (pediatric) solution.

Nursing Management The dosage of nasal solution is instilled in each nostril. (See naphazoline hydrochloride.)

BETA-ADRENERGIC AGENTS

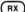

GENERIC NAME Ritodrine hydrochloride (RX)

TRADE NAME Yutopar

CLASSIFICATION Beta-adrenergic agent

Action Inhibits uterine contractions by stimulating beta-adrenergic receptor sites in the uterus. By decreasing the intensity and frequency of uterine contractions, gestation is prolonged in most pregnant mothers. The incidence of neonatal mortality and respiratory distress syndrome is decreased as gestation is lengthened. Prevention of premature labor is more effective when the mother has little or no cervical dilation. The heart rate is increased and the pulse pressure is widened.

Transient elevation of blood sugar and insulin may occur, but levels usually return to normal within 48 to 72 hours after initiating drug therapy. The serum potassium level decreases and there may be an increase in free fatty acids and cyclic AMP.

Indications for Use Pre-term labor in mothers of 20 weeks gestation or longer.

Contraindications Less than 20 weeks of pregnancy when continuation of pregnancy is hazardous to mother or fetus, due to eclampsia, fetal death, chorioamnionitis, or antepartal hemorrhage. Preexisting disorders of the mother that can be seriously affected by the drug including hypovolemia, tachyarrhythmias, uncontrolled hypertension, and pheochromocytoma.

Warnings and Precautions Safe use has not been established when the mother has cervical dilation of 4 cm or more.

Untoward Reactions Circulatory overload and pulmonary edema may occur in the mother after delivery. Deaths have been reported.

Dose-related increases in maternal and fetal heart rates occur frequently. A persistent tachycardia may indicate the onset of pulmonary edema.

Dose-related widening of maternal blood pressure occurs frequently. The systolic pressure increases an average of 12 mm Hg and the diastolic pressure decreases an average of 23 mm Hg.

Palpitations, tremors, nausea, vomiting, headache, and erythema have frequently been reported.

Malaise, nervousness, restlessness, anxiety, or other forms of emotional instability have been reported occasionally.

Cardiac arrhythmias and chest pains have been reported, but rarely.

Parameters of Use

Absorption Only about 30% of drug is available after oral administration.

Crosses the placenta.

Onset of action is about 30 minutes after oral administration; peak action occurs in about 60 minutes. Half-life after oral administration is 1.3 hours and 12 hours. Half-life after IV administration is 6 to 9 minutes; 1.7 to 2.6 hours; 10 hours.

Excretion 90% is excreted within 24 hours. Can be dialyzed.

Drug Interactions Beta-adrenergic blockers antagonize the effects of ritodrine. When corticosteroids are administered concurrently, the mother may develop pulmonary edema after delivery. Additive effect occurs when administered concurrently with other sympathomimetic amines. The potential for hypotension may be increased when anesthetic agents are given.

Administration Dosage is highly individualized according to uterine response and untoward reactions.

Initially, to stop a threatened abortion, dilute 150 mg in 500 ml IV solution (0.3 mg/ml). Give 0.1 mg/min (20 micro gtt/min or 20 ml/hr). Increase drip rate by 0.5 mg/min (10 micro gtt/min or 10 ml/hr) every 10 to 15 minutes until desired response occurs. Usual effective dose: 0.15 to 0.35 mg/min (30 to 70 micro gtt/min or 30 to 70 ml/hr). Uterine contractions usually cease within 12 hours.

When uterine contractions have stopped, give first 10 mg po within 30 minutes of IV drug termination, then 10 mg po every 2 hours for 24 hours. Maintenance dose: 10

to 20 mg every 4 to 6 hours depending on uterine activity and untoward reactions. Maximum daily dose: 120 mg.

Available Drug Forms

5 ml ampules containing 50 mg/ml; tablets containing 10 mg.

Nursing Management

Planning factors

1. Obtain baseline data on rate of uterine contraction and maternal heart rate, blood pressure, and respiratory status.
2. Determine baseline fetal heart rate.
3. When available, a fetal monitor is highly recommended.
4. Baseline data about maternal blood sugar, electrolytes, and hematocrit should be obtained.
5. Volume deficit should be corrected before initiating drug therapy.
6. An IV pump is highly recommended to ensure consistent administration of the drug but a closely monitored microdrip IV administration set can be used.
7. Drug can be diluted in several IV solutions, including sodium chloride, 5% D/W, and Ringer's solution.
8. Store ampules and tablets in a cool area (below 86°F). Protect drug from excessive heat.
9. Freshly prepared IV solutions must be used since drug solution is stable for only 48 hours. Label all IV solutions with date and time.
10. Discard all drug solutions that are discolored or contain a precipitate.

Administration factors

1. Maintain client in a left lateral side-lying position to minimize hypotension when drug is administered IV.
2. Give all other IV medication via a second IV site or piggyback into the primary IV line.
3. Oral medication can be given 1 hour after meals to minimize gastrointestinal disturbances.

Evaluation factors

1. When administering drug IV:
   (a) Monitor maternal blood pressure, pulse rate, and frequency of uterine contractions every 10 to 15 minutes. If excessive tachycardia or hypotension occur, decrease rate of drug administration and notify physician.
   (b) Assess mother's lung status at least hourly. If rales develop, decrease rate of drug administration and notify physician.
   (c) Continue to assess mother's lung status for at least 24 hours after drug is discontinued, since pulmonary edema may occur.
   (d) Assess fetal heart rate every 10 to 15 minutes while drug is being administered. If excessive tachycardia occurs, notify physician immediately.
   (e) Monitor intake and output. Notify physician if oliguria or urinary retention occur.
   (f) Monitor blood sugar, serum potassium, and other electrolytes frequently (every 6 hours).
2. When initially administering drug orally:
   (a) Monitor maternal blood pressure, pulse rate, and uterine contractions.
   (b) Assess mother's lung status frequently. If excessive tachycardia occurs, notify physician.
   (c) Monitor fetal heart rate frequently. If excessive tachycardia occurs, notify physician.
   (d) Monitor blood sugar, serum potassium, and other electrolytes frequently (daily). Once stabilized, these laboratory tests can be done weekly.
   (e) Monitor intake and output.

Client teaching factors

1. Caution client against lifting any objects heavier than 5 to 10 lb.
2. Instruct client to get plenty of rest and to eat a well-balanced diet.
3. Depending on serum potassium levels, encourage client to eat at least 2 servings of potassium-rich foods daily. Provide examples.
4. Caution client that drug must be taken continuously around the clock to prevent premature labor. Help mother plan appropriate times for drug administration.
5. Instruct client to notify physician immediately if uterine contractions resume or if palpitations, tachycardia, difficulty breathing, or urinary retention occur.
6. Caution client to avoid taking OTC drugs unless physician is consulted first. Many OTC drugs contain adrenergic stimulants that may intensify untoward reactions to ritodrine.
7. Instruct client to store drug in a cool place (below 86°F) and to protect drug from excessive heat.

Chapter 40

Antishock Agents

CHARACTERISTICS OF SHOCK

Physiologic shock and its treatment varies according to the causes. Shock is a clinical syndrome manifested by inadequate peripheral blood flow of oxygenated blood to meet tissue demands. Initially, the body compensates by increasing the heart rate to maintain adequate cardiac output and by decreasing urinary output. Also, respiratory rate and depth increase in an attempt to combat metabolic acidosis. As the body endeavors to conserve oxygenated blood for the vital organs, peripheral vasoconstriction occurs and the skin becomes cool to touch. But, as these compensatory mechanisms fail, systolic blood pressure drops below 90 mm Hg (or about 50 mm Hg below normal systolic pressure) and brain cells receive inadequate oxygenation. Finally, agitation and/or semiconsciousness, which eventually lead to a total lapse in consciousness, develop.

Metabolic Acidosis

As a result of the lack of oxygen to skeletal muscles and other tissues, cellular anaerobic metabolism occurs and lactic acid accumulates. This acidic buildup in the body depresses myocardial contractility and the body's peripheral response to further adrenergic stimulation. Death will eventually ensue if the acidosis and shock are untreated. Sodium bicarbonate IV is the drug of choice in most cases.

Causative Factors

Shock may be due to fluid loss (hemorrhage, surgery, trauma, burns), pump failure (myocardial infarction, complete heart block), mechanical obstruction of circulation (pulmonary embolism, dissecting aortic aneurysm), excessive pooling of blood in the peripheral vasculature (infection, toxins, anaphylaxis), or hypoglycemia (metabolic acidosis due to insulin shock).

Treatment of shock is based on identification of the cause. Testing to determine the cause includes arterial blood gases, complete blood cell count, EKG, central venous pressure, vital signs, cardiac monitoring, serum glucose and electrolyte levels, determination of urinary output, and other appropriate tests correlated with the clinical picture. Immediate supportive measures include elevation of the legs and feet above the head, institution of an intravenous infusion so that IV medications can be given for their immediate effects and administration of supplemental oxygen via a mask or other means. Continuous assessment and supportive care are essential.

TREATMENT

Fluid Loss

The loss of red blood cells and other blood elements is treated with whole blood, packed cells, or synthetic blood, as indicated. Albumin may be used to replace protein, and normal saline, Ringer's lactate, or high molecular IV solutions, such as dextran, may be used to replace fluid volume deficits. When indicated, fluid deficits and electrolyte imbalances should be corrected prior to or concurrently with the administration of a vasopressor agent.

Adrenergic Agents

The catecholamine epinephrine is the drug of choice in anaphylactic shock and may be the only adrenergic agent required. Being an indirect stimulator of endogenous catecholamines, ephedrine is seldom used in anaphylaxis because it has a slow onset of action. Alpha-adrenergic vasopressors are useful for the treatment of peripheral pooling of blood; unfortunately, most of these agents may decrease arrhythmias and urinary output. (See Table 40-1). Norepinephrine is generally considered the drug of choice in profound shock. Metaraminol can be used, but tends to produce arrhythmias.

The clinical use of methoxamine and mephentermine is usually restricted to preventing or treating drug-induced peripheral vasodilation. Although effective in counteracting the peripheral vascular effects of spinal anesthesia, these two drugs tend to be weak alpha-adrenergic agents and their effects are sometimes unpredictable.

Dopamine is frequently used for moderate shock due to pump failure as it increases peripheral resistance, renal perfusion (in low dosages), and increases cardiac contractility. However, the newer drug dobutamine is now prescribed by some physicians because of its selective action on the myocardium; it is particularly effective in increasing cardiac output. Some controversy exists regarding the use of dobutamine or any other drug that increases cardiac contractility in clients with recent myocardial infarctions. Some experts believe that the use of these agents may cause extension of the infarcted area while counteracting the cardiogenic shock.

Intracardiac epinephrine is effective in treating cardiac arrest, but isoproterenol is often used to increase the heart rate, and therefore the cardiac output, in clients with heart block. Being a potent beta-adrenergic agent, isoproterenol is also useful in treating bronchospasm, particularly when inhaled. Ephedrine can be used to prevent or treat mild bronchospasm (see Chapter 54).

ALPHA-ADRENERGIC VASOPRESSORS

GENERIC NAME Mephentermine sulfate (RX)

TRADE NAME Wyamine

CLASSIFICATION Adrenergic vasopressor

Action Synthetic noncatecholamine similar to ephedrine in action. Causes beta- and some alpha-adrenergic activity by direct stimulation. Indirectly induces the release of tissue stores of norepinephrine. Elevates blood pressure by increasing cardiac output. Increases blood flow through cerebral and coronary arteries. Depresses A-V conduction time, prolongs arterial refractory time, and slows ventricular conduction; thus preventing arrhythmias.

Indications for Use Hypotension, shock, hyptension caused by ganglionic blockade or spinal anesthesia.

Contraindications Known or suspected hemorrhage; hypotension due to hemorrhage (except in emergency situations); within 2 weeks of therapy with MAO inhibitors; concurrent therapy with phenothiazines.

Warnings and Precautions Use with caution in elderly and disturbed clients and in clients with arteriosclerosis, hyperthyroidism, hypotension, or cardiovascular disorders.

Untoward Reactions Large dosages may cause bradycardia, arrhythmias, and a marked elevation in blood pressure. CNS disturbances, including euphoria, anxiety, nervousness, incoherence, tremors, and convulsions, may occur.

Parameters of Use

Absorption Onset of action is: 5 to 15 minutes (IM); within 1 to 2 minutes (IV). Duration of action is: 30 to 60 minutes (IM); 15 to 30 minutes (IV).

Metabolism Metabolized rapidly.

Excretion By the kidneys; alkaline urine may slow rate of excretion.

Drug Interactions Arrhythmias and other untoward reactions may occur if given concurrently with cyclopropane or halothane. Vasopressor activity may be potentiated in clients receiving MAO inhibitors.

Administration

- *Prevention of hypotension:* Adults: 30 mg IM 10 to 20 minutes prior to spinal anesthesia.
- *Treatment of hypotension:* Adults: 30 to 45 mg IV bolus; then 30 mg IV bolus, as needed. Children: 0.4 mg/kg IV. Can be given by continuous IV drip (0.1% solution).

Available Drug Forms Vials or prefilled syringes containing 30 mg/ml.

Nursing Management (See phenylephrine hydrochloride.)

1. Hypovolemia, hypoxia, and acidosis should be corrected before instituting therapy.
2. Do not mix with other drugs.
3. When administering via continuous IV drip,
   (a) Add to 5% D/W.
   (b) Monitor blood pressure continuously and adjust IV rate accordingly.
4. Monitor blood pressure and pulse frequently. Cardiac monitoring and frequent central venous pressure readings are recommended. Drug effects may last as long as 4 hours in some clients.
5. When administering IM, inject deep into large muscle.

GENERIC NAME Metaraminol bitartrate (RX)

TRADE NAME Aramine

CLASSIFICATION Adrenergic vasopressor

Action Potent synthetic noncatecholamine without CNS stimulation. Less potent than norepinephrine, but longer acting. Direct stimulation of alpha-adrenergic receptor sites results in vasoconstriction. There is some stimulation of beta-receptor sites. Indirectly causes the release of norepinephrine from storage sites. May increase pulmonary and decrease renal blood flow.

Indications for Use Prevention of hypotension associated with spinal anesthesia; treatment of hypotension associated with septicemia, surgery, and other forms of shock.

TABLE 40-1 Comparison of Vasopressor Agents

Generic Name	Trade Name	Action on: Alpha	Beta$_1$ (cardiac)	Beta$_2$
Dobutamine	Dobutrex	Weak	Strong	Some
Dopamine*	Intropin	Strong	Strong	Some
Ephedrine†	Ephedrine	Strong	Moderately strong	Strong
Epinephrine‡	Adrenalin	Strong	Strong	Some
Isoproterenol‡	Isuprel	None	Strong	Strong
Mephentermine	Wyamine	Weak	Moderately strong	Weak
Metaraminol	Aramine	Strong	Some	None
Methoxamine	Vasoxyl	Moderately strong	None	None
Norepinephrine*	Levophed	Strong	Strong	None
Phenylephrine	Neo-Synephrine	Strong	Some	Some

*See Chapter 38.
†See Chapters 39 and 54.
‡See Chapters 38 and 54.

Contraindications Pulmonary edema; peripheral or mesenteric thrombosis; uncorrected acidosis, hypoxia, or hypercarbia.

Warnings and Precautions Use with caution in digitalized clients and clients with hyperthyroidism, hypertension, diabetes, cirrhosis, hepatic disorders, or a history of malaria. Safe use during pregnancy has not been established.

Untoward Reactions Toxicity may induce a sustained elevation of blood pressure. Severe headache, convulsions, arrhythmias, cardiac arrest, dyspnea, and acute pulmonary edema have also occurred. Metabolic acidosis may occur, particularly in clients with hypovolemia. Nausea, vomiting, restlessness, flushing, sweating, hyperglycemia, and decreased urinary output may occur. Arrhythmias, including tachycardia, bradycardia, ectopic beats, and A-V dissociation, have been reported. Extravasation may cause tissue necrosis.

Parameters of Use

Absorption Onset of action is: about 10 minutes (IM); 1 to 2 minutes (IV). Duration of action is: about 90 minutes (IM); about 20 to 30 minutes (IV).

Drug Interactions Hypertensive crisis may occur if given within 2 weeks of therapy with MAO inhibitors. Arrhythmias may occur if used concurrently with cyclopropane or halothane.

TABLE 40-1 *Continued*

	Effect on						
Cerebral Cortex (stimulation)	Systolic Pressure	Diastolic Pressure	Cardiac Output	Heart Rate	Arrhythmogenic	Respiration	Remarks
No	Secondary increase	Secondary increase	Increased	Some increase	Yes	Unchanged	Increases cardiac contractility
Yes	Increased	Little or no increase	Increased	Increased	Yes	Unchanged	Increases cardiac contractility
Yes	Increased	Slightly increased	Increased	Increased	Yes	Slightly increases	May induce atrial fibrillation; bronchodilator
Yes (tremors)	Marked increase	Decreased	Increased	Increased	Yes	Unchanged	May induce ventricular fibrillation; bronchodilator
Yes (tremors)	Increased	Decreased	Increased	Increased	Yes	Littor or no rate change	May induce tachycardia; potent bronchodilator
Little or none	Increased	Increased	Unchanged	Unchanged	No	Little or no rate change	May induce bradycardia
None	Increased	Increased	Unchanged	Reflex	Yes	Some bronchoconstriction	May induce sinus or ventricular arrhythmias
Little or none	Increased	Increased	Unchanged or decreased	Reflex bradycardia	No	Unchanged	
Yes	Increased	Increased	Increased	Decreased (occasional increase)	Yes	Unchanged	Increases cardiac contractility; may induce ventricular fibrillation
Slight	Increased	Increased	Increased	Decreased	No	Reflex depression	

Administration

- *Prevention of hypotension:* Adults: 2 to 10 mg IM, as needed; 0.5 to 5 mg slow IV bolus, as needed. Children: 0.1 mg/kg IM, as needed; 0.01 mg slow IV bolus, as needed.

- *Treatment of hypotension:* Adults: 50 to 100 mg/500 ml of 5% D/W continuous IV drip; Children: 20 mg/500 ml of 5% D/W continuous IV drip.

Available Drug Forms Multidose vials of 10 ml containing 10 mg/ml; prefilled syringes containing 10 mg/ml for rapid preparation of continuous IV drip solutions.

Nursing Management (See phenylephrine hydrochloride.)

1. Hypovolemia, hypoxia, and acidosis should be corrected before instituting therapy.
2. When administering IM, inject deep into large muscle mass. Rotate injection sites.
3. When administering via continuous IV drip,
   (a) Add drug to 5% D/W or normal saline IV solution.
   (b) Do not mix with other drugs, including sodium bicarbonate and multivitamins, since a precipitate will form.
   (c) Use large blood vessels only. Check IV site regularly.

(d) Adjust IV rate every 5 minutes until blood pressure is stable, then every 15 minutes.
4. Cardiac monitoring and central venous pressure readings should be obtained periodically.
5. Monitor intake and output hourly.

GENERIC NAME Methoxamine hydrochloride

TRADE NAME Vasoxyl (RX)

CLASSIFICATION Adrenergic vasopressor

Action Sympathomimetic amine that stimulates alpha-adrenergic receptor sites directly. Causes no beta or CNS stimulation. Cardiac rate decreases as blood pressure increases. Prolongs refractory period of blood flow through renal arteries. Coronary artery blood flow and cardiac output are essentially unchanged.

Indications for Use Prevention of hypotension associated with spinal anesthesia; treatment of hypotension associated with anesthesia; paroxysmal supraventricular tachycardia (atrial and nodal).

Contraindications Severe myocardial disease, congestive heart failure.

Warnings and Precautions Peripheral ischemia and ultimately necrosis may occur in clients with occlusive vascular diseases. Use with caution in the elderly and in clients with a history of hypertension, hyperthyroidism, bradycardia, or partial heart block.

Untoward Reactions Toxic effects include excessive elevation of blood pressure, severe headache, projectile vomiting, and bradycardia (which is reversed by atropine). Paresthesia, a feeling of coldness, metabolic acidosis, a desire to void, and oliguria, which may result in anuria, may occur. Gooseflesh due to a pilomotor response is relatively common. Angina or congestive heart failure may be precipitated.

Parameters of Use

Absorption Onset of action is: 15 minutes (IM); about 1 minute (IV). Duration of action is: 90 minutes (IM); 60 minutes (IV).

Drug Interactions Severe elevation of blood pressure may occur with ergot alkaloids and oxytocic agents. Halothane may cause arrhythmias. MAO inhibitors given within the last 2 weeks may intensify and prolong the effects of methoxamine, resulting in hypertensive crisis.

Administration

- *Prevention of hypotension:* 10 to 15 mg IM about 15 to 20 minutes before spinal anesthesia.
- *Paroxysmal supraventricular tachycardia:* Adults: 15 to 20 mg IM; 5 to 15 mg slow IV bolus.
- *Treatment of hypotension:* Adults: Initial dosage: 3 to 5 mg slow IV bolus; then 10 to 15 mg IM to prolong drug effects. Children: 80 mcg/kg slow IV bolus.

Available Drug Forms Ampules containing 20 mg/ml; 10-ml multidose vials containing 10 mg/ml.

Nursing Management (See phenylephrine hydrochloride.)

1. Hypovolemia, hypoxia, and acidosis should be corrected before instituting therapy.
2. When administering IM, inject deep into large muscle mass. Rotate injection sites.
3. Administer IV bolus over 5 minutes or more while observing client's response.
4. Continuous cardiac monitoring is required in clients with paroxysmal supraventricular tachycardia.
5. Monitor intake and output.

GENERIC NAME Phenylephrine hydrochloride

TRADE NAMES Isophrin, Neo-Synephrine (RX)

CLASSIFICATION Adrenergic vasopressor

Action Phenylephrine, a sympathomimetic amine, is chemically similar to epinephrine, but is less effective in maintaining blood pressure. The drug acts primarily on alpha-adrenergic receptors and causes extensive vasoconstriction in most vascular beds, including the cutaneous, renal, and pulmonary vessels. In addition, it may constrict the cerebral, splanchnic, and peripheral blood vessels of the extremities. Beta-adrenergic receptors are also stimulated, but to a lesser degree. Beta stimulation results in dilation of the coronary arteries; there is little or no inotropic stimulation of the heart. Stimulation of the CNS is minimal. Phenylephrine increases systolic, diastolic, and pulmonary pressures and there is a slight increase in venous pressure. Also, the circulatory time is prolonged. Reflex stimulation of the vagus nerve occurs in response to increased blood pressure, thereby causing the heart rate to decrease (reflex bradycardia). Consequently, cardiac output will decrease.

Indications for Use Prevention or treatment of hypotensive states associated with surgical procedures using spinal or general anesthesia; acute vascular hypotension; toxicity or hypersensitivity to drugs (ganglionic blocking agents, phenothiazines); paroxysmal supraventricular tachycardia (artrial and nodal).

Contraindications Hypertension; ventricular tachycardia; narrow-angle glaucoma; severe coronary artery disease, including myocardial infarction.

Warnings and Precautions Peripheral ischemia and ultimately necrosis may occur in clients with occlusive vascular diseases. Use with caution in the elderly and in clients with preexisting hypertension, hyperthyroidism, bradycardia, partial heart block, myocardial disease, diabetes, or severe arteriosclerosis, particularly cerebral arteriosclerosis.

Untoward Reactions Relatively nontoxic drug, but may cause excessive elevation of blood pressure and headache. Cardiac rhythm disturbances, including tachycardia, extrasystoles, and short bursts of ventricular tachycardia, may occur. Cardiovascular disturbances, including pallor, sweating, paresthesia of extremities, dizziness, angina, lightheadedness, trembling, and weakness, may occur. Blurred vision has been reported. Prolonged use may cause a lack of response (tachyphylaxis). Bradycardia, which can be abolished with atropine, has been reported.

Parameters of Use

Absorption Onset of action is: about 20 minutes (IM, subc); within 5 minutes (IV). Duration of action is: 1 to 2 hours (IM, subc); about 20 minutes (IV).

Distribution Widely distributed in body tissues.

Metabolism In the liver by monoamine oxidase.

Excretion By the kidneys.

Drug Characteristics Slowly darkens and loses its potency when exposed to air or light. Do not use if discolored or if a precipitate forms.

Drug Interactions If MAO inhibitors have been given within the last few weeks, the effects of phenylephrine may be intensified and prolonged and result in hypertensive crisis. Oxytocic agents, tricyclic antidepressants, and guanethidine may potentiate the pressor effects of phenylephrine, and may cause arrhythmias. Concurrent use with halothane or epinephrine can result in arrhythmias or hypertensive crisis.

Administration

- *Prevention of hypotension:* Adults: 2 to 5 mg IM or subc; Dosage range: 1 to 10 mg. Children: 0.1 mg/kg IM or subc. Do not give more than 5 mg initially. Dosage depends on degree of pressor effect desired.

- *Paroxysmal supraventricular tachycardia:* 0.2 mg rapid IV bolus (over 20 to 30 seconds); Dosage range: 0.1 to 0.5 mg; do not exceed 0.5 mg initially. If arrhythmias are unresponsive, dosage may be increased in increments of 0.1 to 0.2 mg; do not give more than 1 mg at any one time and do not repeat more than every 10 to 15 minutes.

- *Treatment of hypotension:* 0.2 mg slow IV bolus; Dosage range: 0.1 to 0.5 mg. Continuous IV drip: Add 1 ampule to 500 ml of IV fluid; Initial flow rate: 100 to 180 gtt/min.; Maintenance flow rate: 40 to 60 gtt/min.; actual dosage depends on client's response.

Available Drug Forms Ampules of 1 ml containing 10 mg/ml. Store in airtight, light-resistant containers.

Nursing Management

Planning factors

1. If signs and symptoms of hypovolemia (central venous pressure below 10 cm H_2O) are present, notify physician; this condition should be corrected prior to or concurrently with phenylephrine.
2. Continuous cardiac monitoring is recommended.
3. Discard drug if solution is discolored or if a precipitate has formed.
4. Atropine should be readily available to treat excessive bradycardia reactions.

Administration factors

1. Give IV bolus over 1 minute for arrhythmias. A disposable insulin or TB syringe can be used to ensure an accurate dosage.
2. Give IV bolus over 1 to 5 minutes for pressor effect.
3. A convenient solution of 1 mg/ml (for IV bolus) can be prepared by adding 9 ml of sterile water to 1 ampule (10 mg).
4. Prepare continuous IV drip by adding 10 to 20 mg to 5% D/W. An IV pump is highly recommended, but a microdrip IV administration set can be used.
5. Adjust flow rate according to blood pressure response; maintain systolic blood pressure between 90 to 110 mm Hg.
6. Monitor blood pressure and pulse frequently (every 2 to 5 minutes if given IV or every 5 to 15 minutes if given IM or subc).

Evaluation factors

1. The following should be monitored: blood pressure (every 15 to 30 minutes); pulse and respiration (every 15 to 30 minutes); urinary output (q1h), when possible.
2. If toxic effects, such as excessive bradycardia or elevation of blood pressure, occur, reduce flow rate and notify physician.
3. If hypotension persists, notify physician; the client may be hypovolemic or require a more potent solution or vasopressor.

BETA-ADRENERGIC CARDIAC STIMULANTS

GENERIC NAME Dobutamine hydrochloride

TRADE NAME Dobutrex (RX)

CLASSIFICATION Adrenergic cardiac stimulant

Action Dobutamine, a synthetic catecholamine, directly stimulates beta-adrenergic receptors of the heart with little or no stimulation of other adrenergic receptor sites. It increases cardiac output by enhancing contractility (inotropic effect) and therefore the stroke volume. Unlike isoproterenol, dobutamine does not induce marked tachycardia with a resulting decrease in stroke volume. The heart rate usually increases 5 to 15 beats/min. and the systolic pressure usually increases 10 to 20 mm Hg above pretreatment pressure at therapeutic drug levels. Dobutamine enhances atrioventricular conduction and may induce ventricular tachycardia in clients with arterial fibrillation. In addition, the drug decreases peripheral vascular resistance, but to a lesser degree than isoproterenol.

Indications for Use Short-term treatment of adults with cardiac decompensation due to reduced contractility associated with organic heart disease or heart surgery.

Contraindications Idiopathic hypertrophic subaortic stenosis.

Warnings and Precautions Use with caution in clients with preexisting hypertension or premature ventricular contractions. No improvement in cardiac output has been observed in clients with marked mechanical obstruction, such as aortic stenosis. Safe use following acute myocardial infarction has not been established; an increase in heart rate and conduction may cause extension of the infarcted area. Safe use in children and during pregnancy has not been established.

Untoward Reactions Toxic effects include an increase in pulse and systolic pressure in excess of 30 beats/min. or 50 mm Hg above pretreatment levels; slowing the IV rate will result in an immediate reversal of symptoms. An increase in the number of premature ventricular beats per minute may occur and is dose related. Nausea, headache, angina, chest pains, and shortness of breath have been reported.

Parameters of Use

Absorption Onset of action is 1 to 2 minutes and peak action occurs in 10 minutes. Plasma half-life is 2 minutes.

Metabolism Methylation of the catechol and conjugation.

Excretion By the kidneys as active and inactive metabolites.

Drug characteristics Reconstituted solutions are oxidized and will produce a color change. If stored at room temperature, use within 6 hours. Refrigerated solutions may be stored for 48 hours.

Drug Interactions Dobutamine may be ineffective if used concurrently with beta-adrenergic blockers; an increase in peripheral vascular resistance has been observed in animal studies. Concomitant use with sodium nitroprusside may result in a higher cardiac output and a lower wedge pressure than when either drug is used alone.

Administration Highly individualized. Adults: 2.5 to 10 mcg/kg/min. via continuous IV infusion. Up to 40 mcg/kg/min. have been used. Has been safely used for as long as 72 hours.

Available Drug Forms Vials containing 250 mcg of dry powder for reconstitution.

Nursing Management

Planning factors

1. Obtain the following baseline data: EKG; blood pressure and pulse; central venous pressure (CVP), if available; pulmonary wedge pressure and cardiac output, if possible.
2. Obtain an infusion pump if at all possible.
3. Notify physician if the client has hypertension, premature ventricular contractions, tachycardia, or a low CVP.
4. Hypovolemia should be corrected before instituting therapy.
5. Start a primary IV line so that the medication can be given via a secondary line.
6. Continuous cardiac monitoring is highly recommended.

Administration factors

1. Determine client's body weight and calculate the approximate starting dosage (mcg/kg).
2. Add 10 ml of sterile water for injection of 5% D/W for reconstitution; 20 ml of diluent can be used if dry powder remains undissolved.
3. Reconstituted solution may be added to 5% D/W, normal saline, or sodium lactated Ringer's solution.
4. Label solution with date and concentration.

Quantity of Diluent (ml)	Concentration of Solution (mcg/ml)
250	1000
500	500
1000	250

5. Check patency of IV before initiating therapy. Add medicated solution as a piggyback to primary IV line.
6. Start with a low IV rate (0.25 to 0.5 mcg/kg/min.) and adjust rate according to blood pressure response every 10 minutes.

Evaluation factors

1. Continuous monitoring of blood pressure, pulse, cardiac monitoring, CVP, pulmonary wedge pressure, and cardiac output is recommended.
2. IV drip rate is maintained when desired response occurs.
3. If the increase in pulse rate exceeds 30 beats/min., frequent PVCs occur, or if the increase in systolic pressure exceeds 50 mm Hg, decrease IV rate until client's response stabilizes at a lower level.
4. Physician should be informed of client's response.

Chapter 41

Cholinergic Agents

THE NEUROTRANSMITTER AT cholinergic neurons is acetylcholine and drugs that either mimic or enhance the effects of acetylcholine are called *cholinergic agents.* Since neurotransmission at both pre- and postparasympathetic synapses is mediated by acetylcholine, the cholinergic agents are also termed *parasympathomimetic agents.* However, this term is imprecise because acetylcholine is also the transmitter at skeletal muscle neuromuscular synapses and some postganglionic sympathetic fibers, sweat glands, and certain peripheral blood vessels. In order to understand how these agents activate cholinergic neurons, it is necessary to know how acetylcholine functions.

ACETYLCHOLINE

Acetylcholine is stored in tiny vesicles at cholinergic nerve endings. Once released from these nerve endings, acetylcholine crosses the synapse and excites its receptor sites. The enzyme acetylcholinesterase inactivates acetylcholine by hydrolyzing it to choline and acetic acid. To resynthesize acetylcholine, the enzyme choline acetyltransferase mediates the transfer of an acetyl group from acetylcoenzyme A to choline. Additional body supplies of choline are obtained from protein foods, such as egg yolks, nuts, cereals, and legumes.

Certain evidence indicates that body stores of acetylcholine decrease during the aging process and that the loss of short-term memory in the elderly may be related to a lack of acetylcholine. Elderly clients who have been given concentrated lecithin, a dietary substance high in acetylcholine precursors, may have some improvement in short-term memory.

Cholinergic receptors are divided into two groups depending on whether they are stimulated by nicotine or muscarine. Nicotinic receptors located at autonomic ganglia are blocked by hexamethonium and those at neuromuscular junctions by curare drugs. The stimulation of muscarinic receptors at postganglionic parasympathetic synapses is blocked by atropine. Both nicotinic and muscarinic receptors are found in the central nervous system.

A wide variety of effects result from cholinergic stimulation by acetylcholine (see Table 41-1); however, acetylcholine is seldom used clinically because it affects all cholinergic neurons and is inactivated by serum and tissue acetylcholinesterase within minutes. Most cholinergic agents have a longer duration of action and are more selective in their action than acetylcholine. These substances are used to treat glaucoma, urinary retention, paralytic ileus induced by drugs or surgery, and myasthenia gravis. Cholinergic agents are usually classified as either direct-acting agents or cholinesterase inhibitors.

PROPERTIES OF DIRECT-ACTING CHOLINERGIC AGENTS

Drugs that mimic the effects of acetylcholine are termed *direct-acting cholinergic agents.* Most of these drugs are chemically similar to acetylcholine and induce stimulation of muscarinic receptors; they also have a longer duration of action because they resist hydrolysis by acetylcholinesterase. Examples of direct-acting cholinergic agents are bethanechol, which selectively affects gastrointestinal and genitourinary smooth muscle, and is used to treat urinary retention and postoperative distention; carbachol, which induces miosis when administered topically to the eye; and methacholine, which selectively affects the cardiovascular system and has been used to treat atrial tachycardia and peripheral vascular disease (PVD). (However, as a result of the advent of more effective therapy for tachycardia and PVD, metacholine is rarely used today.) Pilocarpine and its derivatives, which have a chemical structure similar to muscarine, not acetylcholine, are particularly effective for inducing miosis. Pilocarpine is thought to act directly on the eye's cholinergic receptors rather than disturbing the acetylcholine-cholinesterase relationship. (Pilocarpine and other cholinergic ophthalmic agents are described in Chapter 79).

PROPERTIES OF CHOLINESTERASE INHIBITORS

Drugs that promote cholinergic stimulation by endogenous acetylcholine by inhibiting the breakdown of the transmitter are called *cholinesterase inhibitors* or *anticholinesterase agents.* Since endogenous acetylcholine is not hydrolyzed, both nicotinic and muscarinic receptors are affected

TABLE 41-1 The Effects of Cholinergic Stimulation

Action	Usual Signs and Symptoms	Untoward Reactions
Peripheral vasodilation	Flushing of face; rise in skin temperature; transient fall in blood pressure	Hypotension
Increased secretions from exocrine glands	Increase in bronchial (transient cough) and gastric secretions; lacrimation (tearing); salivation; sweating	Coughing, rales; epigastric distress, nausea, vomiting; drooling; diaphoresis
Bronchoconstriction	Increased respiratory rate	Dyspnea, rhonchi, wheezing, bronchospasm
Decreased heart rate and contractility	Decreased pulse rate	Bradycardia, heart failure
Miosis	Constricted pupils; decrease in elevated intraocular pressure	None known
Stimulation of gastrointestinal and genitourinary smooth muscle (tone and motility) and relaxation of sphincters	Increased peristalsis, defecation, and urination	Abdominal cramps, incontinence of feces and urine
Improved contractility of striated muscle	Increased muscle tone in myasthenia gravis	Cholinergic crisis: muscular twitching, tightness, fasciculations, dysphagia, respiratory insufficiency

by these agents. Cholinesterase inhibitors are effective in treating myasthenia gravis and may be used for glaucoma (if their action is limited by topical administration).

The drug-induced inhibition of cholinesterase may be reversed within hours (*reversible agents*) or may last for days or even weeks (*irreversible agents*). Physostigmines, neostigmines, and other reversible cholinesterase inhibitors exert their action by binding to cholinesterase and blocking the enzyme from acetylcholine receptor sites. As these agents are gradually broken down by cholinesterase, the enzyme begins to hydrolyze acetylcholine again.

Irreversible cholinesterase inhibitors are organophosphates, which are used today as pesticides, and include "nerve gas", or "nerve poison", which was used during World War II. These agents are considered irreversible because they are not broken down by cholinesterase. Their effects are only canceled when enough enzyme has been newly synthesized by the body; thus their duration of action is several days. Organophosphates are absorbed through the skin and mucous membranes and must be handled with extreme caution. The skin must be thoroughly cleansed if it comes into contact with even a drop of the chemical.

Organophosphates have limited therapeutic use, but when applied locally to the eye, they are effective antiglaucoma agents. Unlike other agents used for glaucoma, these substances do not have to be instilled frequently and so are particularly effective for clients who have severe glaucoma and those who are unable (or forget) to instill their "several-times-a-day" antiglaucoma agents.

ORGANOPHOSPHATE POISONING

Organophosphate poisoning can occur from the careless use of these toxic and potentially lethal insecticides. Inhalation of organophosphate vapours or contact with the skin or mucous membranes can cause severe untoward reactions. Hypotension, bradycardia, and cardiac or respiratory arrest will occur as a result of the excessive accumulation of acetylcholine. The antimuscarinic agent atropine is administered intravenously to counteract the effects of poisoning and the cholinesterase reactivator pralidoxime is administered to reverse the organophosphate-cholinesterase bond, thus releasing cholinesterase for inactivation of acetylcholine. Unfortunately, the antidote pralidoxime is unable to cross the blood-brain barrier and so its action is restricted to peripheral organophosphate-cholinesterase bonds. Consequently, both atropine and pralidoxime should be given as soon as possible after poisoning has occurred.

Supportive respiratory therapy is vital to the survival of the poisoned client. Maintaining an airway, mechanical removal of bronchial secretions, and sustaining ventilation via a respirator may be required. Seizure precautions should be instituted and, if convulsions occur, anticonvulsants administered with caution, since the action of barbiturates is potentiated by anticholinesterase agents.

MYASTHENIA GRAVIS

Myasthenia gravis is a chronic progressive disease manifested by skeletal muscle weakness without muscular atrophy; the muscle weakness is due to a lack of acetylcholine at cholinergic neuromuscular synapses (nicotinic receptors). Although the etiology is unknown, the disease may be due to a cellular type of autoimmunity involving immunoglobulin G (IgG) and the thymus gland.

Reversible cholinesterase inhibitors are the primary drugs employed for the treatment of myasthenia gravis. The short-acting drug edrophonium (Tensilon) is used to diagnose the disorder and the hand-grip test is used to determine the absence or presence of the disease. Neostigmine, physostigmine, and related drugs, which are longer acting, are given therapeutically (orally).

Periodically, exacerbations of the disease may occur, which necessitate an increase in the daily drug dosage possibly administered parenterally. Fatigue, upper respiratory infections, and other physical stressors may precipitate an exacerbation. During an exacerbation, it may be difficult to differentiate between a myasthenic crisis and an overdose of a cholinergic agent (cholinergic crisis) (see Table 41-2).

Adrenocorticosteroids may be helpful in myasthenia gravis; but when infection occurs, several antibiotics, including streptomycin, gentamicin, kanamycin, neomycin, and polymyxin, must be avoided since muscular weakness may occur. Narcotics, sedatives, and hypnotics should be used sparingly because respiratory depression and other toxic effects may occur.

DIRECT-ACTING CHOLINERGIC AGENTS

GENERIC NAME Acetylcholine chloride (RX)

TRADE NAME Miochol

CLASSIFICATION Direct-acting cholinergic agent

Action Acetylcholine chloride is a quaternary ammonium compound that stimulates cholinergic receptors in the eye and has a short duration of action. It induces rapid and complete miosis and stimulates local vasodilation; miosis is maintained for up to 60 minutes. The drug is rapidly hydrolyzed to choline and acetic acid.

Indications for Use Applied topically to skin for dermatosis and varicose ulcers. Ophthalmic solution is used as an adjunct in eye surgery, including cataract, keratoplasty, and iridectomy.

Administration Used to irrigate affected tissues or applied as a moist dressing, as indicated by physician. Ophthalmic solution is instilled by physician.

Available Drug Forms Vials containing 20, 50, or 200 mg.

Nursing Management See Chapter 41 introduction.

GENERIC NAME Bethanechol chloride (RX)

TRADE NAMES Duvoid, Myotonachol, Urecholine, Vesicholine

CLASSIFICATION Direct-acting cholinergic agent

Action Bethanechol is an ester of a hygroscopic choline-like compound. It stimulates the parasympathetic nervous system, thus inducing urinary bladder tone and promoting micturition. The drug also stimulates gastric motility and increases gastric tone. Unlike acetylcholine, bethanechol is not destroyed by cholinesterase. It has strong muscarinic but weak nicotinic action.

Indications for Use Acute postoperative or postpartum urinary retention (nonobstructive); neurogenic bladder atony with retention

TABLE 41-2 Characteristics of Myasthenic and Cholinergic Crises

Crisis	Cause	Signs and Symptoms	Response to Tensilon Test	Treatment
Myasthenic	Exacerbation of disease	Muscular weakness; dysphagia; respiratory weakness (which may progress to paralysis)	No change or slight increase in muscular strength; fasciculations usually absent; little or no tearing, sweating, nausea, and diarrhea	Increase dosage of cholinergic agent
Cholinergic	Overdose of cholinergic agent	Generalized weakness; muscular tightness and fasciculations; dysphagia; respiratory weakness due to CNS drug effect	Decreased muscular strength; fasciculations; severe tearing, sweating, nausea, vomiting, and diarrhea	Atropine sulfate (antimuscarinic agent)

Contraindications Hyperthyroidism, pregnancy, peptic ulcer, bronchial asthma, bradycardia, hypotension, coronary artery disease, epilepsy, Parkinsonism, mechanical obstruction of genitourinary or GI tract, muscular rupture of genitourinary or GI tract (recent bladder surgery, bowel resection, acute inflammatory lesions, peritonitis).

Warnings and Precautions Never administer IM or IV since a violent cholinergic reaction may occur (hypotension, shock, cardiac arrest).

Untoward Reactions Toxic reactions include bradycardia, hypotension, bronchoconstriction, and bloody diarrhea. Urinary frequency may occur. GI disturbances include abdominal cramps, diarrhea, nausea, vomiting, and excessive salivation. Flushing, excessive sweating, miosis, and tearing may occur.

Parameters of Use

Absorption Onset of action is: 30 minutes (po); 15 minutes (subc). Peak action occurs in 30 minutes (subc). Duration of action is: about 1 hour (po); about 2 hours (subc).

Administration Highly individualized. Adults: Oral: 10 to 50 mg tid or qid. Subcutaneous: 5 mg repeated at 15- to 30-minute intervals, up to 4 doses; minimum effective dosage may be given 3 or 4 times daily, as needed; Test subc dose: 2.5 mg.

Available Drug Forms Tablets containing 5, 10, or 50 mg; vials containing 5 mg/ml

Nursing Management

1. When administering subc, inject deep into subcutaneous tissue only.
2. Give tablets on an empty stomach with water.
3. Assess vital signs frequently.
4. Atropine (0.6 mg) should be available in a syringe for immediate use when parenteral injection is given.

GENERIC NAME Carbachol (RX)

TRADE NAME Doryl

CLASSIFICATION Direct-acting cholinergic agent

Action Carbachol (choline chloride carbonate) is a hygroscopic substance similar to acetylcholine, but is more stable to hydrolysis and therefore has a prolonged drug effect. It has greater nicotinic than muscarinic activity. Tends to be toxic when injected or absorbed systemically.

Indications for Use Refractory glaucoma.

Administration 1 to 2 drops 0.75 to 3% solution bid or tid instilled in lower conjunctival sac.

Available Drug Forms Sterile ophthalmic solution.

Nursing Management See Chapter 41 introduction.

GENERIC NAME Methacholine bromide (RX)

TRADE NAME Mecholyl Bromide

CLASSIFICATION Direct-acting cholinergic agent

Action Similar to the chloride salt but less hygroscopic. (See methacholine chloride.)

Indications for Use Raynaud's disease, scleroderma, chronic ulcers.

Administration 200 mg po bid or tid.

GENERIC NAME Methacholine chloride (RX)

TRADE NAME Mecholyl Chloride

CLASSIFICATION Direct-acting cholinergic agent

Action Unlike acetycholine, the methyl derivative is relatively stable in the body and induces a sustained stimulation of the parasympathetic nervous system with little or no nicotinic effect. It depresses atrial conduction and induces vasodilation and gastric peristalsis. Toxicity and untoward reactions are dose related; however, this drug is seldom used today.

Indications for Use Raynaud's disease, scleroderma, chronic ulcers. Has been used for paroxysmal atrial tachycardia (less effective than quinidine).

Administration Initial dosage: 10 mg subc; then 25 mg may be given 10 to 30 minutes later; Dosage range: 10 to 40 mg.

ANTICHOLINESTERASE (REVERSIBLE) AGENTS

GENERIC NAMES Neostigmine bromide; neostigmine methylsulfate (RX)

TRADE NAMES Prostigmin Bromide; Prostigmin Methylsulfate

CLASSIFICATION Cholinergic agent (anticholinesterase)

Action Neostigmine is a synthetic quaternary ammonium compound similar to physostigmine. It enhances the effects of acetylcholine at cholinergic synapses by inhibiting the hydrolysis of acetylcholine by the enzyme cholinesterase. Neostigmine exerts its action by competing for enzyme binding sites for acetylcholine and by other means. Neostigmine intensifies and prolongs the effects of endogenous acetylcholine and direct-acting cholinergic agents. This action results in an increase in intestinal muscle tone, miosis, bronchoconstriction, bradycardia, and stimulation of salivary, gastric, lacrimal, and sweat glands. The increase in skeletal muscle tone and contractility may be due to a direct action on muscle fibers and acetylcholine.

Indications for Use Prevention and treatment of abdominal and urinary retention in the absence of mechanical obstruction; diagnosis and treatment of myasthenia gravis; postoperative reversal of nondepolarizing neuromuscular blocking agents (tubocurarine, metocurine, gallamine, pancuronium); postoperative paralytic ileus in the absence of mechanical obstruction; functional amenorrhea.

Contraindications Hypersensitivity to neostigmine or bromides, mechanical obstruction of GI or genitourinary tract, peritonitis, severe bradycardia.

Warnings and Precautions Use with caution in clients with bronchial asthma, bradycardia, recent coronary occlusion, vagotonia, hyperthyroidism, arrhythmias, or peptic ulcer. Differential diagnosis between myasthenic crisis and cholinergic crisis is important since the treatment is different. Anticholinesterase agents may cause uterine irritability and premature labor in pregnant women. Safe use in children and during lactation has not been established.

Untoward Reactions Toxic reactions (cholinergic crises) are dose related and are due to overstimulation of cholinergic neurons. In addition to muscarinic and nicotinic effects, CNS stimulation occurs and results in restlessness, agitation, anxiety, and confusion. GI disturbances, including nausea, vomiting, diarrhea, fecal incontinence, abdominal cramps, and excessive salivation, are common. Cardiovascular disturbances, including hypotension, bradycardia, and reflex tachycardia, may occur. Bronchoconstriction, excessive bronchial secretions, dyspnea, and a productive cough may occur. Bronchospasm and respiratory depression may develop, particularly when large doses are administered. Miosis with a resulting blurring of vision may occur. Tearing may also occur, particularly with large dosages. Skeletal muscle cramps, fasciculations, and tremors have been reported, particularly with large dosages. Muscular weakness may follow as the drug's effects wane. Rashes due to bromide ingestion may occur.

Parameters of Use

Absorption Erratic absorption from GI tract. Bromide salt (oral) absorbed better than methylsulfate salt (parenteral). Onset of action is: about 2 hours (po); 10 to 30 minutes (parenteral). Duration of action is: about 4 hours (po); about 3 hours (parenteral).

Distribution Widely distributed in body tissues. Large dosages may cross blood-brain barrier.

Metabolism In the liver by microsomal enzymes.

Excretion By the kidneys.

Drug Interactions Neostigmine potentiates the action of direct-acting cholinergic agents; concurrent use is not recommended. Parenteral neostigmine antagonizes the neuromuscular effects of depolarizing blocking agents (such as tubocurarine and pancuronium).

Aminoglycoside antibiotics and antiarrhythmic agents (such as quinidine and procainamide) antagonize the action of neostigmine or neuromuscular synapses.

Atropine is an effective antidote for neostigmine's muscarinic effects.

Administration Highly individualized.

- *Abdominal distention:* 0.5 to 1 mg IM or subc every 4 to 6 hours, as needed. Clients with paralytic ileus may be given smaller dosages initially. The smallest dosage needed to provide relief should be given.

- *Myasthenia gravis:* Adults: 15 to 30 mg po tid; 0.5 mg IM or IV every 1 to 3 hours, as needed. Parenteral dosages are usually reserved for severe cases. Children: 7.5 to 15 mg po tid or qid.

Available Drug Forms Tablets containing 15 mg; multidose vials containing 1 mg/ml (1:1000 solution) or 0.5 mg/ml (1:2000 solution); ampules containing 0.5 mg/ml (1:2000 solution) or 0.25 mg/ml (1:4000 solution).

Nursing Management

Planning factors

1. Assess the status of the cardiovascular, intestinal, genitourinary, and respiratory systems.
2. Obtain history of disorders that may be associated with contraindications.
3. Obtain baseline vital signs.
4. Assess baseline neuromuscular function of clients with myasthenia gravis.
5. Atropine (0.5 to 2 mg slow IV bolus) should be available in a syringe for immediate use.

Administration factors

1. Give tablets on an empty stomach with water
2. When administering IM or subc, inject deep into tissue. Rotate injection sites.
3. Administer IV slowly; usually given by a physician or anesthetist.

Evaluation factors

1. Obtain vital signs frequently when drug is first initiated or dosage adjusted.
2. Assess muscular strength of myasthenic clients periodically. If weakness occurs within 60 to 90 minutes after drug administration, notify physician immediately; cholinergic crisis may be occurring.
3. Assess abdominal distention and bowel sounds frequently, when indicated.
4. Monitor intake and output, when indicated.
5. Assess respiratory status periodically. If depression occurs, notify physician immediately.

Client teaching factors

1. Inform myasthenic client and family of drug's action and untoward reactions.
2. Instruct myasthenic client's family to notify physician if lack of drug effect or overstimulation of cholinergic neurons occurs.
3. Instruct myasthenic client to carry an identification card indicating the disease and the drugs being used.
4. Emphasize the need for continued drug use and periodic reevaluation of myasthenia gravis.

GENERIC NAME Ambenonium chloride (RX)

TRADE NAME Mytelase

CLASSIFICATION Cholinergic agent (anticholinesterase)

Indications for Use Myasthenia gravis; often used for clients who are hypersensitive to neostigmine or pyridostigmine.

Contraindications Hypersensitivity to anticholinesterase agents; mechanical obstruction of the gastrointestinal or genitourinary systems.

Untoward Reactions Induces relatively few untoward reactions. GI disturbances, including nausea, vomiting, diarrhea, and cramps, are common. Bronchoconstriction, miosis, bradycardia, hypotension, urinary incontinence, and skeletal muscle cramps may occur.

Parameters of Use

Absorption Relatively long duration of action.

Administration Highly individualized. Initial dosage: 5 mg po every 3 to 4 hours; then increase by 5 mg every other day until desired effect; Maintenance dosage: 5 to 50 mg every 3 to 4 hours.

Available Drug Forms Capsules containing 5 mg.

Nursing Management (See neostigmine bromide for further details.)

1. Monitor vital signs frequently when drug is first initiated or dosage adjusted.
2. Atropine sulfate should be available for immediate use (IV or subc).
3. Toxicity may occur with daily dosages over 200 mg.

GENERIC NAME Edrophonium chloride (RX)

TRADE NAME Tensilon

CLASSIFICATION Cholinergic agent (anticholinesterase)

Action Edrophonium is a synthetic compound chemically related to neostigmine methylsulfate. The primary action of edrophonium is inhibition or inactivation of cholinesterase at cholinergic synapses. It displaces curariform drugs from neuromuscular receptor sites, thus permitting normal transmission of impulses. Because of its short duration of action, edrophonium is seldom used for treating myasthenia gravis, but has replaced neostigmine in differentiating between cholinergic and myasthenic crises.

Indications for Use Respiratory depression caused by curare toxicity; antidote for curare poisoning; reversal of the effects of neuromuscular blocking agents (curare, tubocurarine, gallamine); diagnostic test for myasthenia gravis.

Contraindications Hypersensitivity to anticholinesterase agents, mechanical obstruction of GI or genitourinary tract.

Warnings and Precautions Use with caution in clients with bronchial asthma or arrhythmias; cardiac and respiratory arrest may occur due to vagotonic effect of drug. Safe use during pregnancy and lactation has not been established.

Untoward Reactions A transitory anticholinesterase insensitivity may occur; drug should be withheld or reduced until drug sensitivity returns. Cholinergic crisis (toxicity) is initially manifested by muscular weakness, dysphagia, fasciculations, bronchoconstriction, excessive salivary and bronchial secretions, bradycardia, a decrease in cardiac output (which progresses to respiratory paralysis), profound hypoxia, marked hypotension, ventricular arrhythmias, and convulsions. (See neostigmine bromide.)

Parameters of Use

Absorption Onset of action is 30 to 60 seconds and duration of action is 10 minutes.

Drug Interactions Not only is edrophonium ineffective in reversing the effects of depolarizing neuromuscular blocking agents, such as succinylcholine and decamethonium, but it may even prolong their effects. (See neostigmine bromide.)

Administration

- *Diagnostic test for myasthenia gravis:* Adults: 10 mg IM or 2 mg (0.2 ml) IV injected over 15 to 30 seconds; if no reaction occurs, remaining 8 mg (0.8 ml) is injected. Test can be repeated in 30 minutes. If muscarinic effects (fasciculations, muscular weakness) occur; test is discontinued and atropine 0.4 to 0.5 mg is administered IV. IM route is used if no veins are accessible. Children: Over 34 kg: Initial dosage: 2 mg IV; then 1 mg IV after 45 seconds every 30 to 45 seconds until response occurs; Maximum test dosage: 10 mg IV; or 5 mg can be given IM when no veins are accessible. Under 34 kg: Initial dosage: 1 mg IV; then 0.1 mg IV after 45 seconds every 30 to 45 seconds until response occurs; Maximum test dosage: 5 mg IV; or 2 mg can be given IM when no veins are accessible.

- *Periodic evaluation of myasthenia gravis:* 1 to 2 mg IV bolus 1 hour after usual oral dosage.

- *Myasthenic crisis:* Initial dosage: 1 mg IV bolus; then 1 mg IV after 60 seconds.

- *Curare antagonism:* 10 mg IV given over 30 to 45 seconds; dosage may be repeated as necessary; Maximum dosage: 40 mg.

Available Drug Forms Ampules of 1 ml containing 10 mg/ml; 10-ml multidose vials containing 10 mg/ml.

Nursing Management

Planning factors

1. Obtain baseline data on muscular strength and respiratory status.
2. Atropine (1 mg) should be available in a syringe for immediate use.
3. Equipment for manual ventilation and suctioning should be available for immediate use.
4. Respiratory exchange should be adequate before instituting Tensilon test. Suction as needed. Tracheostomy may be required.

Administration factors

1. Medication is administered IV by a physician or a specially trained health professional.
2. When administering IM, inject deep into large muscle mass.
3. Be prepared to manually suction excessive bronchial secretions and to provide manual ventilation.
4. Monitor client constantly for improvement of muscular weakness.

Evaluation factors

1. Transient improvement of muscular weakness indicates myasthenic crisis; but accentuation of muscular weakness, fasciculations, and bradycardia indicate cholinergic crisis.
2. Suction excess oral and bronchial secretions, as needed. Assess respiratory status frequently.
3. Assess cardiovascular status frequently. Notify physician if bradycardia or hypotension occur. An automatic blood pressure cuff and cardiac monitoring equipment are recommended so that the nurse is free to maintain adequate ventilation.
4. Measure intake and output, as needed (if hypotension occurs).

GENERIC NAME Physostigmine salicylate (RX)

TRADE NAME Antilirium

CLASSIFICATION Cholinergic agent (anticholinesterase)

Source Potent alkaloid obtained from *Physostigma venenosum.*

Action Cholinesterase-inhibiting properties vary with pH: greatest effect below pH of 7.5 (acidic); neutral effect at pH of 8.5 or higher (alkaline). Stimulates intestinal musculature and induces miosis. Only cholinergic that crosses blood-brain barrier and induces a central effect. Effective in reversing life-threatening toxic effects such as tachycardia, arrhythmias, delirium, and coma.

Indications for Use Anticholinergic toxicity or poisoning; tricyclic antidepressant or belladonna (atropine, scopolamine) toxicity.

Contraindications Hypersensitivity to anticholinesterase agents; mechanical obstruction of the gastrointestinal or genitourinary systems.

Warnings and Precautions Use with caution in clients with cardiovascular disorders, epilepsy, peptic ulcer, bronchial asthma, gangrene, or diabetes.

Untoward Reactions CNS disturbances include restlessness, excitability, sweating, ataxia, miosis, nausea, vomiting, diarrhea, excessive salivation, bronchospasm, and dyspnea.

Parameters of Use

Absorption Onset of action is 3 to 8 minutes and duration of action is 30 to 60 minutes.

Administration Test dosage: 2 mg IM; Toxicity: 0.5 to 4.0 mg IM or slow IV bolus; may be repeated q2h, as necessary.

Available Drug Forms 2 ml ampules containing 1 mg/ml.

Nursing Management (See edrophonium.)

1. Atropine (0.5 mg) should be available for immediate use (IV or subc). Equipment for mechanical support of breathing should be readily available.
2. Use clear solution only; red solutions indicate oxidation and are less potent.
3. Administer IV bolus slowly at a rate of 1 mg/min. or less. A syringe pump is recommended.
4. Drug should be administered in the presence of physician.
5. Maintain side rails.
6. Position client for maximum ventilation.

GENERIC NAME Pyridostigmine bromide (RX)

TRADE NAMES Mestinon, Regonal

CLASSIFICATION Cholinergic agent (anticholinesterase)

Action Pyridostigmine is a synthetic analog of neostigmine that is only 20% as effective and has a longer duration of action. The drug may inactivate pseudocholinesterase and facilitates the transmission of impulses across the myoneural junction.

Indications for Use Myasthenic crisis; myasthenia gravis when oral therapy is undesirable (surgery, labor, postpartum); reversal agent for nondepolarizing muscle relaxants (curariform drugs, gallamine).

Contraindications Hypersensitivity to anticholinesterase agents; mechanical obstruction of the gastrointestinal or genitourinary systems.

Warnings and Precautions Use with extreme caution in clients with arrhythmias or bronchial asthma.

Untoward Reactions Induces fewer untoward reactions than neostigmine (bradycardia, salivation, GI secretions).

Parameters of Use

Absorption Timed-release tablets provide 60 mg immediately; duration of action is about $2\frac{1}{2}$ times that of regular 60-mg tablets.

Administration Highly individualized. Oral: Usual dosage: 60 to 120 mg 3 to 6 times a day. 180 mg timed-release tablet daily or bid at least 6 hours apart; Dosage range: 1 to 3 tablets daily or bid. Severe cases may require up to 1500 mg given in divided doses. It is essential that dosage be administered at the same time each day. Intravenous: Adults: 10 to 30 mg, as needed (q2h in myasthenia gravis).

Available Drug Forms Raspberry-flavored syrup containing 60 mg/5 ml and 5% alcohol; tablets containing 60 mg; timed-release tablets containing 180 mg; ampules containing 5 mg.

Nursing Management

1. Atropine (0.5 mg) should be available for immediate use (IV or subc).
2. When treating curare toxicity, atropine (via slow IV bolus) is given prior to the administration of pyridostigmine.
3. Monitor vital signs frequently. Measures to prevent respiratory impairment may be required.
4. Syrup is often used for children and severely affected adults with bulbar involvement.

IRREVERSIBLE CHOLINESTERASE INHIBITORS

GENERIC NAME Echothiophate iodide (RX)

TRADE NAME Phospholine Iodide

CLASSIFICATION Irreversible cholinesterase inhibitor

Action Long-acting organophosphate compound that is stable in peanut oil, but decomposes rapidly in water. (See Chapter 79.)

Indications for Use Glaucoma.

Warnings and Precautions Handle with great care as drug can be absorbed through skin.

GENERIC NAME Isoflurophate (RX)

TRADE NAMES DFP, Floropryl

CLASSIFICATION Irreversible cholinesterase inhibitor

Action Long-acting quaternary salt that is poorly absorbed, but effective when applied topically. (See Chapter 79.)

Indications for Use Glaucoma.

Warnings and Precautions Handle with great care as drug can be absorbed through skin.

GENERIC NAMES Hexaethyltetraphosphate; tetraethylpyrophosphate; parathion; octamethylpyrophosphoramide (RX)

TRADE NAMES HETP; TEPP; Alkron, Niran, Thiophos; OMPA, Pestox III, Sehradan

CLASSIFICATION Irreversible cholinesterase inhibitor

Action Group of phosphate esters (organophosphorus compounds) that irreversibly inhibit cholinesterase. They are highly toxic and can be absorbed by inhalation, through the skin, or by ingestion.

Indications for Use Pesticides. Some have been used as "nerve gases" during warfare.

Warnings and Precautions Individuals who work with these compounds should be warned against direct contact with the chemicals or their vapors.

CHOLINESTERASE REACTIVATORS

GENERIC NAME Pralidoxime chloride (RX)

TRADE NAME Protopam

CLASSIFICATION Cholinesterase reactivator

Action Pralidoxime, a quaternary ammonium compound, reactivates cholinesterase that has been inactivated by the process of phosphorylation due to organophosphates; thus excessive quantities of acetylcholine at neuromuscular junctions can be destroyed by cholinesterase. The drug will also detoxify certain organophosphates by a direct chemical reaction. Since little or no drug crosses the blood-brain barrier, pralidoxime's action is limited to peripheral cholinergic sites and should be used during the early stages of organophosphate toxicity. Depression of the respiratory center must be treated with atropine sulfate. Pralidoxime antagonizes the effects of carbamate anticholinesterases (neostigmine, pyridostigmine, ambenonium); but it is less effective than atropine. Pralidoxime is effective treatment for poisoning with the following: azodrin, diazinon, DOVP with chlordane disulfoton, EPN, isoflurophate, malathion, fenthion, methyl demeton, methyl parathion, mevinphos, parathion, parathion with mevinphos, phosphamidon, sarin, TEPP.

Indications for Use Antidote in the treatment of poisoning due to organophosphate pesticides, drugs, and chemicals with anticholinesterase activity. Also used as an antidote to treat cholinergic crisis (anticholinesterase drug toxicity).

Contraindications Poisoning due to phosphorus, inorganic phosphates, or organophosphates with no anticholinesterase activity, including the insecticide sevin.

Warnings and Precautions Use with caution in clients with renal disorders, since excessive serum drug levels may occur. Use with extreme caution in clients with myasthenia gravis, since myasthenic crisis may be precipitated.

Untoward Reactions Tachycardia, laryngospasm, and muscular rigidity will occur if pralidoxime is administered too rapidly IV. Excitation and manic behavior immediately following recovery of consciousness are common. Hyperventilation, muscular weakness, headache, dizziness, nausea, and tachycardia are relatively common; these effects may be associated with concurrent use of atropine. Visual disturbances, including diplopia, blurred vision, and impaired accommodation, may occur.

Parameters of Use

Absorption Peak serum levels occur 2 to 3 hours after oral administration. Half-life is about 2 hours. Not bound to plasma proteins.

Distribution Widely distributed in extracellular fluid. Little or no drug crosses the blood-brain barrier.

Metabolism Some in the liver.

Excretion Rapidly excreted by the kidneys as unchanged drug and metabolites.

Drug Interactions Pralidoxime potentiates sevin toxicity. Although the following drugs have no direct drug interaction with pralidoxime, they should be avoided in clients with organophosphate poisoning: morphine, theophylline, aminophylline, succinylcholine, reserpine, phenothiazines. The effects of barbiturates are potentiated by anticholinesterases and should be used with extreme caution for the treatment of convulsions.

Administration

- *Organophosphate poisoning:* Adults: Initial dosage: 1 to 2 g in 100 ml of saline IV over 15 to 30 minutes. If pulmonary edema is present, give as diluted IV bolus over 5 minutes or more; then repeat in 1 hour if muscle weakness persists. IM or subc injections can be given if IV is not feasible. When poison is ingested, continued drug therapy may be required every 3 to 8 hours. In mild cases of poisoning (in the absence of GI disturbances) give 1 to 3 g q5h. Children: Initial dosage: 20 to 40 mg/kg via IV infusion.

- *Cholinergic crisis:* Initial dosage: 1 to 2 g IV; then 250 mg every 5 minutes, as needed.

Available Drug Forms Emergency kit containing a 20-ml vial with 1 g of sterile drug powder for reconstitution, a 20-ml ampule of sterile water for injections, a 20-ml disposable syringe with needle, and an alcohol swab. Single-dose vials containing 1 g of powder; tablets containing 500 mg.

Nursing Management

Planning factors

1. Maintain airway and ventilation.
2. Determine amount of chemical or drug ingested, inhaled, or injected, when possible.
3. Determine what drugs the client has ingested in the last 24 hours, when possible.
4. Pralidoxime should be given within a few hours of poisoning.
5. Obtain baseline vital signs. Cardiac monitoring is required in severe cases.
6. Determine intake and output. Insertion of an indwelling catheter may be required.
7. If poison was absorbed through skin, remove clothing (while wearing gloves) and wash affected skin with a large amount of sodium bicarbonate solution.
8. Atropine therapy should be initiated at the same time as pralidoxime therapy. In the absence of cyanosis, administer 2 to 4 mg IV bolus concurrently via a different IV site or just prior to hanging pralidoxime infusion. If cyanosis is present, give atropine IM while instituting measures to improve ventilation. Repeat atropine injection every 5 to 10 minutes until signs of atropine toxicity occur. Smaller dosages of atropine are usually given periodically for 48 hours.

Administration factors

1. Reconstitute dry powder with 20 ml of sterile water for injection.
2. When administering via IV infusion,
   (a) Add reconstituted solution to 100 ml of normal saline.
   (b) Check patency of IV before administering drug.
   (c) Infuse directly into vein over 30 minutes.
   (d) An IV pump is recommended.
   (e) Do not add other medications to IV solution.
3. When administering IV bolus,
   (a) Give directly into vein or in Y port nearest IV site.
   (b) Do not mix with other medications.
   (c) Administer slowly over 5 minutes or more.
   (d) A syringe pump is recommended.
4. Drug should be administered by a physician or a specially trained health professional.

Evaluation factors

1. Assess respiratory status frequently and institute appropriate measures, as needed. Maintain an airway and manual ventilation until client is capable of sustaining adequate ventilation.
2. Monitor intake and output.
3. Obtain vital signs periodically.
4. If convulsions occur, a 2.5% solution of thiopental may be administered with caution. Institute seizure precautions.
5. Notify physician immediately if respiratory depression, hyperventilation, bradycardia, tachycardia, arrhythmias, alterations in consciousness, oliguria, or hypotension occur.
6. When poison is ingested, clients should be kept under close observation for 2 to 3 days, since poison may continue to be absorbed from large intestine. All clients should remain under observation for at least 24 hours.

PART XI

ADRENERGIC AND CHOLINERGIC BLOCKERS

When symptoms occur that would benefit by decreasing adrenergic or cholinergic activity, drugs that inhibit their respective section of the nervous system are used. Inhibition of one system allows the action of the other system to predominate.

The adrenergic system uses endogenous norepinephrine to stimulate its receptor sites, resulting in excitation that mimics sympathetic nervous stimulation. Drugs that inhibit the action of norepinephrine, other catecholamines, or sympathomimetic agents are termed adrenergic blockers, adrenergic blocking agents, or sympatholytic or sympathoplegic agents. Since the advent of drugs that selectively inhibit alpha- or beta-adrenergic receptor sites, the terms alpha blockers and beta blockers have become popular. Another group of drugs, termed adrenergic neuron blockers, actually depletes or prevents the release of endogenous catecholamines; or, they might act by resembling the adrenergic neurotransmitters, and thereby occupying the receptor sites and inducing weak adrenergic stimulation.

Adrenergic blockers are divided into the alpha blockers and the beta blockers. The alpha blockers are used to treat post-partum bleeding, migraine and vascular headaches, senility, and a number of other human ailments. The beta blockers are used for a variety of disorders, including hypertension, angina pectoris, supraventricular tachycardia, and migraine headaches, since these drugs decrease heart rate, cardiac output, and cardiac conduction velocity. They also reduce blood pressure by inducing relaxation of smooth muscle. The adrenergic neuron blockers are primarily used to treat hypertension, since vasodilation is induced. More details on these drugs can be found in Chapters 47, 48, and 50.

Drugs that antagonize or inhibit the effects of the cholinergic neurotransmitter acetylcholine are called cholinergic blockers, anticholinergic agents, or parasympathetic agents. Drugs that inhibit the effects of acetylcholine receptor sites located at parasympathetic postganglionic synapses are antimuscarinic agents. But since nicotinic receptor sites are located at both parasympathetic and sympathetic ganglia, drugs that block these receptors are often called *ganglionic blocking agents*.

Acetylcholine is the neurotransmitter of the voluntary nervous system as well; drugs that inhibit acetylcholine can block transmission of nerve impulses to the skeletal muscles. Therefore, the neuromuscular blocking agents are included in this section. These drugs may act either by competing with acetylcholine for receptor sites (competitive blockers), or by depolarizing the motor and plate of the skeletal muscle (depolarizing blocking agents).

Inhibition of cholinergic stimulation in the brain allows endogenous dopamine to have a greater influence; consequently the anticholinergic agents that cross the blood-brain barrier and induce an anticholinergic effect in the brain have been grouped together in the chapter titled Antiparkinsonian Agents.

Chapter 42

Alpha- and Beta-Adrenergic Blockers

ADRENERGIC BLOCKERS INHIBIT the effects of endogenous norepinephrine, epinephrine, and sympathomimetic drugs at adrenergic receptor sites, which are located at postganglionic sympathetic synapses, and are classified as alpha or beta blockers according to the type of receptor they affect (see Table 42-1). Adrenergic receptor sites are divided into alpha and beta receptors by virtue of the substance that stimulates them. Alpha receptors are very sensitive to the catecholamine epinephrine and least sensitive to isoproterenol (a synthetic catecholamine). Beta receptors are very sensitive to epinephrine. Norepinephrine stimulates both alpha and beta receptors, but not as effectively as epinephrine. The primary effects of activation of alpha receptors are vasoconstriction of peripheral blood vessels, myocardial ectopic excitation, and contraction of the uterus, particularly the gravida uterus. Beta receptors are subdivided into two types according to the body tissue(s) affected. $Beta_1$ activation primarily affects the myocardium, causing an increase in heart rate, contractility, and conduction velocity through the atria and ventricles. The major effects of $beta_2$ activation are vasodilation of peripheral blood vessels, relaxation of bronchial and gastrointestinal smooth muscle, and inhibition of uterine contractions.

TYPES OF ALPHA-ADRENERGIC BLOCKING AGENTS

Although the oxytocic action of Ergot alkaloids has been known since the 16th century, the alpha-adrenergic blocking ability of some of these agents was not identified until the turn of the 20th century. The use of ergot alkaloids varies according to their major effects. For example, ergonovine is primarily used as an oxytocic to control postpartum bleeding, whereas ergotamine is used for its alpha blockade action on cranial vascular smooth muscles—vasoconstriction of previously dilated cranial blood vessels assists in aborting migraine and cluster headaches (histamine cephalalgia). Some ergot alkaloids also antagonize the secretion of serotonin, a central neurohumoral agent that is thought to decrease the pain threshold; thus antagonism of serotonin increases the pain threshold. Unfortunately, ergot alkaloids can cause severe toxic reactions (ergotism), which are characterized by excessive peripheral vasoconstriction, gastrointestinal disturbances, and arrhythmias. The relatively new product ergoloid mesylates is a potent adrenergic blocking agent that causes vasodilation (not vasoconstriction), central sedation, and slowing of the heart rate. Unlike other ergot alkaloids, this product was marketed for the treatment of senility.

Imidazoline derivatives, such as phentolamine and tolazoline, are also effective alpha-adrenergic blockers. Phentolamine, which is a potent blocker of epinephrine, is useful in treating pheochromocytoma-induced hypertension. Pheochromocytoma is a tumor of the adrenal gland that produces excessive quantities of catecholamines (epinephrine and norepinephrine). Although the tumor is usually benign, periods of hypertensive crisis occur. The vasodilator effect of phentolamine is also effective in treating extravasation (IV infiltration) of norepinephrine; but the affected site must be injected with phentolamine as soon as possible, in order to prevent tissue necrosis. Tolazoline blocks both circulating epinephrine and the function of sympathetic nerves. As it causes a type of histamine reaction, it has been found useful for treating vasospastic peripheral vascular disorders.

Other alpha-adrenergic blockers include phenoxybenzamine and azapetine, both of which are used to treat vasospastic peripheral vascular disorders. Phenoxybenzamine is said to cause a "chemical sympathectomy," but it may also cause postural hypotension, tachycardia, and miosis.

TYPES OF BETA-ADRENERGIC BLOCKING AGENTS

Propranolol was the first drug to be introduced that selectively blocks beta-adrenergic receptors. This drug is useful in several cardiovascular disturbances, but it also causes some severe untoward reactions.

Recently, compounds have been found that are selective $beta_1$-adrenergic blockers; that is, they lower blood pressure and decrease heart rate and conduction velocity while causing relatively few effects on bronchial and gastrointestinal smooth muscle. Thus, $beta_1$ blockers are considered relatively safe to use in clients susceptible to bronchospasm. However, it should be remembered that the $beta_1$ blockers are less selective when large dosages are used and bronchospasm may occur. One beta-adrenergic blocker, called timolol maleate, is effective in treating glaucoma, since the drug reduces intraocular pressure when administered topically. See Chapter 79 for further details.

ALPHA-ADRENERGIC BLOCKERS

Ergot Alkaloids and Related Substances

GENERIC NAME Ergotamine tartrate (RX)

TRADE NAMES Ergomar, Ergostat, Gynergen

CLASSIFICATION Alpha-adrenergic blocker

Action Although ergotamine was originally used as an oxytocic agent, it fell into disuse when ergonovine, another ergot alkaloid, was found to be just as effective but less toxic. It is now used for its alpha-adrenergic blockade effect on cranial and peripheral vascular smooth muscle. Ergonovine causes vasoconstriction of previously dilated cerebral blood vessels and antagonizes the effects of serotonin. Unlike many other headache remedies, ergonovine does not cause oxytocic effects. The drug is often combined with caffeine to provide increased relief of migrainetype headaches.

Indications for Use Relief of pain associated with migraine, cluster headache (histamine cephalalgia), and other vascular headaches.

Contraindications Peripheral vascular disease, coronary artery disease, hypertension, impaired hepatic or renal function, sepsis, pregnancy, hypersensitivity to ergot alkaloids.

Warnings and Precautions Use with caution in children, the elderly, and in clients who have been dieting extensively.

Untoward Reactions Acute ergotism can occur, but rarely. The symptoms include vomiting, diarrhea, and thirst. Paresthesia, confusion, and a lowered skin temperature may progress to gangrene of the fingers, toes, ears, and nose. A rapid or weak pulse and convulsions may occur. Chronic ergotism may occur, particularly with prolonged therapy at large doses. The symptoms include intermittent claudication, cold and cyanotic extremities, muscular pains and numbness (Raynaud's phenomenon). Pulses may be absent in the extremities, and precordial pain and arrhythmias may occur. Secondary effects include nausea, vomiting, diarrhea, weakness, muscular pains, numbness or tingling of the digits, and chest pain. Edema and rashes have occurred, but rarely.

Parameters of Use

Absorption Poor and erratic absorption from GI tract Sublingual preparations are absorbed the best. Oral dosage must be 10 times that of parenteral injection to produce the same effect. Duration of action is about 24 hours.

Metabolism In the liver.

Drug Interactions Propranolol and other beta-adrenergic blockers may increase the frequency and severity of migraine headaches; do not use concurrently. Sympathomimetics may cause hypertension; do not use concomitantly.

Administration Drug's effectiveness is greater and the dosage required is less when drug is used at the first sign of a migraine headache. Sublingual: 2 mg every 30 minutes times 3 doses; Maximum dosage: 6 mg day; total weekly dosage should not exceed 10 mg. Oral: 10 mg tid. Intramuscular, subcutaneous: 250 to 500 mcg q1h prn.

Available Drug Forms Sublingual tablets containing 1 or 2 mg; tablets and chewable tablets containing 10 mg; ampules containing 500 mcg/ml.

Nursing Management

Planning factors

1. Drug should be given immediately after symptoms begin.
2. One tablet (sublingual) should be kept at the bedside and the client should be informed to notify health professionals as soon as this tablet is used.
3. Obtain history of the migraine's characteristics, including any prodromal symptoms that occur.
4. Baseline vital signs and blood pressure should be obtained.
5. History of vascular disorders and examination of vascular system should be done before initiating therapy.

Administration factors

1. Sublingual tablets should be held under the tongue until completely dissolved. Warn client to avoid swallowing tablet.
2. Oral tablets should be given on an empty stomach with a full glass of water.
3. Rotate parenteral injection sites.
4. Room should be kept quiet and dark during and immediately following therapy.

Evaluation factors

1. Determine the frequency of drug therapy and the dosage required. Some types of migraine headache do not respond to ergotamine.
2. Obtain and record blood pressure and pulse periodically.
3. Check and record peripheral pulses. If any are absent, notify physician.

Client teaching factors

1. Instruct the client who has frequent migraine headaches to carry the drug at all times and to use it at the first sign of headache.

TABLE 42-1 Summary of Alpha- and Beta-Adrenergic Blockers

Adrenergic receptor	Blocker	Primary Effects	Indications for Use	Primary Untoward Reactions
Alpha	Ergotamine tartrate	Vasoconstriction of previously dilated cerebral blood vessels, antagonizes serotonin	Migraine and vascular headaches	Chronic ergotism; secondary effects include gastrointestinal disturbances and effects of peripheral vascular vasoconstriction
	Dihydroergotamine mesylate	Vasoconstriction of previously dilated cerebral blood vessels; depresses central vasomotor centers; antagonizes serotonin	Migraine and vascular headaches	Chronic ergotism; secondary effects are rare
	Ergoloid mesylates	Vasodilation; central sedation; central inhibition of pressor reflexes	Idiopathic decline in mental capacity	Transient secondary effects; sublingual irritation
	Methysergide maleate	Antagonizes serotonin (weak adrenergic blocker)	Migraine and vascular headaches	Fibrotic changes, cardiovascular disturbances
	Phentolamine hydrochloride Phentolamine mesylate	Potent blocker of epinephrine; vasodilation; increases gastric secretions	pheochromocytoma-induced hypertension; extravasation by norepinephrine	Hypotension, gastrointestinal disturbances (peptic ulcer)
	Tolazoline hydrochloride	Vasodilation; increases heart rate; increases gastric secretions	Vasospastic peripheral vascular disorders	Arrhythmias, gastrointestinal disturbances
	Phenoxybenzamine hydrochloride	Vasodilation; lowers blood pressure	Pheochromocytoma-induced hypertension; vasospastic peripheral vascular disorders	Secondary effects, particularly postural hypotension, tachycardia, nasal congestion, and miosis
	Azapetine phosphate	Vasodilation	Vasospastic peripheral vascular disorders; hypertension	Few and mild
$Beta_1$ and $beta_2$	Propranolol hydrochloride	Decreases heart rate, output, and conduction velocity; prevents relaxation of bronchial and gastrointestinal smooth muscle	Hypertension; angina pectoris; supraventricular tachycardia; migraine headache	Bradycardia, hypotension, congestive heart failure, bronchospasm, gastrointestinal disturbances

TABLE 42-1 *Continued*

Adrenergic receptor	Blocker	Primary Effects	Indications for Use	Primary Untoward Reactions
	Nadolol	Decreases heart rate, output, and conduction velocity; prevents relaxation of bronchial and gastrointestinal smooth muscle	Hypertension	Milder than propanolol
$Beta_1$ (primarily)	Atenolol	Decreases heart rate, output, and conduction velocity; lowers blood pressure	Hypertension	Bradycardia, postural hypotension, tiredness, cold extremities
	Metoprolol tartrate	Decreases heart rate, output, and conduction velocity; lowers blood pressure	Hypertension	Central nervous system disturbances, bradycardia, diarrhea, shortness of breath, peripheral vascular insufficiency

2. Advise client to remain still and quiet for at least 1 hour after the disappearance of the headache.
3. Warn client against excessive use of drug. Client should notify physician before exceeding maximum daily and weekly drug dosages.

GENERIC NAME Dihydroergotamine mesylate

TRADE NAME D.H.E. 45 (RX)

CLASSIFICATION Alpha-adrenergic blocker

Action Dehydroergotamine, a hydrogenated ergot alkaloid derivative, is very similar to ergotamine, but possesses a greater alpha-adrenergic blocking ability and lacks oxytocic action. The drug has a direct vasoconstrictor effect on smooth muscle of peripheral and cranial blood vessels. It also produces depression of central vasomotor centers and antagonizes serotonin. Dihydroergotamine has the advantage of being as effective, if not more effective, than ergotamine in the treatment of migraine headaches and has milder untoward reactions. It causes somewhat less vasoconstriction and fewer GI disturbances than ergotamine.

Indications for Use Prevention and aborting vascular headaches (migraine, histamine cephalalgia).

Contraindications Peripheral vascular diseases, coronary heart disease, hypertension, impaired hepatic or renal function, sepsis, pregnancy, hypersensitivity to ergot alkaloids.

Warnings and Precautions Use with caution in children and the elderly.

Untoward Reactions Secondary effects occur, but rarely. Nausea, vomiting, numbness or tingling of fingers and toes, muscular pains, weakness, precordial pain, and transient tachycardia or bradycardia have been reported. Localized edema and itching around injection sites have been reported. (See ergonovine tartrate.)

Parameters of Use

Absorption Well absorbed from parenteral sites; poorly absorbed from GI tract. Onset of action is 15 to 30 minutes and duration of action is 3 to 4 hours.

Metabolism In the liver.

Drug Interactions Propranolol and other beta-adrenergic blockers may increase the frequency and severity of migraine headaches; do not use concurrently. Sympathomimetics may cause hypertension; do not use concomitantly.

Administration Highly individualized, the lowest effective dose for aborting headache can be determined after 3 to 4 courses of drug therapy. Intramuscular:

1 mg every hour times 3 doses; Maximum dosage: 3 mg/day. Intravenous: 1 mg; repeat in 1 hour, if necessary; Maximum dosage: 2 mg/day. Total weekly dosage should not exceed 6 mg.

Available Drug Forms Ampules of 1 ml containing 1 mg/ml.

Nursing Management (See ergotamine tartrate.)

1. Discard drug if solution is discolored.
2. Store ampules in dark area away from light.
3. IV administration provides faster relief.
4. Exceeding maximum dosages may cause ergotism.

GENERIC NAME Ergoloid mesylates (RX)

TRADE NAMES Circanol, Hydergine

CLASSIFICATION Alpha-adrenergic blocker

Action Ergoloid mesylates contains equal portions of the hydrogenated ergot alkaloids dihydroergocornine, dihydroergocristine, and dihydroergocryptine as the mesylates. These compounds do not cause vasoconstriction like other ergot alkaloids, but vasodilation. They are relatively strong adrenergic blockers and they cause a central sedative effect that results in a slowing of the heart rate. Although the drug was originally used for its vasodilating effects, the drug is marketed as an agent to relieve the symptoms of idiopathic decline in mental capacity (senility). The mechanism by which mental functions are improved is unknown, but it may be related to the drug's ability to increase cerebral blood flow; however, there is no conclusive evidence that the drug affects cerebral arteriosclerosis or cerebrovascular insufficiency. The efficiency of the drug was evaluated by a special rating scale developed by Sandoz called the "Sandoz Clinical Assessment Geriatric" (SCAG). Features that showed significant improvement after 12 weeks of therapy included mental alertness, confusion, recent memory, orientation, emotional lability, self-care, depression, anxiety/fear, cooperation, sociability, appetite, dizziness, fatigue, and bothersomeness. Studies on the drug's long-term effects have not been completed.

Indications for Use Idiopathic decline in mental capacity (cognitive and interpersonal skills, mood, self-care, lack of motivation) associated with senility, primary progressive dementia, Alzheimer's dementia, and multi-infarct dementia.

Contraindications Acute or chronic psychosis (regardless of etiology); mental disorders secondary to systemic primary neurologic disorders; primary disturbances of mood; hypersensitivity to drug.

Untoward Reactions The only secondary effects reported to date include transient nausea, gastric disturbances, and sublingual irritation.

Parameters of Use

Absorption Rapidly but incompletely absorbed from GI tract. Oral tablets result in slightly higher plasma levels than sublingual tablets. Peak plasma levels occur in 1 hour. Duration of action is less than 24 hours.

Metabolism Rapidly in the liver. Nearly 50% of absorbed drug is metabolized in the first pass through the liver.

Drug Interactions No known significant interactions.

Administration 1 mg po or sublingual tid between meals.

Available Drug Forms Oral tablets containing 1 mg; sublingual tablets containing 0.5 or 1 mg; dropper bottles of oral liquid containing 1 mg/ml.

Nursing Management (See ergonovine tartrate.)

1. Careful diagnostic and assessment procedures should be completed to determine the etiology of the disease before prescribing or initiating drug therapy. The SCAG is recommended; but other forms can be used.
2. Oral tablets should be given on an empty stomach with a full glass of water.
3. When sublingual tablet is used, mouth should be rinsed with plain water after the tablet is completely dissolved.
4. Liquid oral preparations may be easier to administer to uncooperative clients.
5. Milk or an antacid may relieve drug-induced nausea or gastric distress.
6. Assess the client's symptoms frequently (weekly).
7. Symptoms are alleviated gradually over 3 to 4 weeks.

GENERIC NAME Methysergide maleate (RX)

TRADE NAME Sansert

CLASSIFICATION Serotonin antagonist, alpha-adrenergic blocker

---

Action Methysergide is a synthetic ergot derivative chemically related to methylergonovine. The primary action of methysergide is antagonism of serotonin, a central neurohumoral agent that is thought to lower the pain threshold. Although the drug is a relatively weak alpha-adrenergic agent, it is effective in preventing migraine headaches. It is ineffective in aborting migraine headaches, but the intensity and frequency of vascular headaches is reduced. Unfortunately, the long-term use of methysergide causes severe untoward reactions, including fibrotic changes in retroperitoneal, pleuropulmonary, cardiac, and other tissues. Methysergide has a slight oxytocic effect.

Indications for Use Prevention of vascular headaches (migraine); as an adjunct in treating (reducing the intensity of) vascular headaches.

Contraindications Pregnancy, children, peripheral vascular disease, severe arteriosclerosis, severe hypertension, coronary artery disease, valvular heart disease, phlebitis or cellulitis of the lower extremities, pulmonary disease, collagen diseases, fibrotic processes, impaired hepatic or renal function, severe infections (sepsis), debilitated clients.

Warnings and Precautions Abrupt withdrawal of drug may cause rebounding headaches. Safe use in children has not been established.

Untoward Reactions Fibrotic changes may occur if the drug is administered for longer than 6 months at any one time (see table). Retroperitoneal and pleuropulmonary fibrosis have been reported. Fibrotic thickening of cardiac valves may also occur. Fibrotic changes usually disappear upon withdrawal of the drug. Symptoms include numb, painful, and cold hands and feet, leg cramps upon walking, chest, pelvic, or flank pain, and shortness of breath. The drug should be withdrawn for 3 to 4 weeks every 6 months.

Area of Fibrosis	Signs and Symptoms
Retroperitoneal connective tissue, usually around pelvic brim (elevated sedimentation rate and blood urea nitrogen)	Backache, general malaise, fatigue, weight loss, low-grade fever, urinary obstruction, vascular insufficiency of lower limbs (pain, edema)
Pleuropulmonary tissue (noted on chest x-ray)	Dyspnea, tightness or pain in the chest, pleural friction rub, pleural effusion
Aorta, aortic and mitral valve	Dyspnea, heart murmurs
Fibrotic plaques causing Peyronie's disease	Distortion or deflection of penis, particularly upon erection

GI symptoms, including nausea, vomiting, diarrhea, epigastric distress, and abdominal pain, have occurred, particularly during the first few weeks of therapy; the symptoms subside gradually. CNS disturbances have been reported, but they may be associated with the vascular headache rather than drug therapy. The symptoms include insomnia, drowsiness, euphoria, dizziness, ataxia, lightheadedness, hyperesthesia, and hallucinations. Weight gain is relatively common. Blood dyscrasias, including neutropenia and eosinophilia, have occurred. Rare reactions include facial flushing, telangiectasia, dermatitis, excessive hair loss, peripheral edema, brawny edema, weakness, arthralgia, and myalgia.

Parameters of Use

Absorption Seems to be well absorbed, may cause GI disturbances if taken on an empty stomach.

Distribution Widely distributed in body tissues.

Metabolism In the liver. Rate of metabolism unknown.

Excretion Probably by the kidneys.

Drug Interactions May antagonize the analgesic action of narcotics.

Administration 4 to 8 mg po daily in divided doses.

Available Drug Forms Tablets containing 2 mg.

Nursing Management

Planning factors

1. Obtain history of frequency, duration, and characteristics of headaches.
2. History of vascular disorders and examination of vascular system should be done before initiating therapy. Record pulse pressures in legs.
3. Baseline vital signs and blood pressure should be obtained.
4. EKG, blood urea nitrogen (BUN), and serum creatinine should be done before instituting therapy.
5. Schedule drugs with meals or with a snack (milk and crackers).
6. Client should be kept under close medical supervision as long as the drug is being used.
7. Recommended maximum duration of therapy is 6 months. Drug can be reinstituted after 3 to 4 weeks of withdrawal.

Administration factors

1. Give with a full glass of water.
2. Administer with meals to prevent GI disturbances.
3. Dosage should be tapered off over 2 to 3 weeks before discontinuing drug.

Evaluation factors

1. Maintain a flowchart on the frequency, duration, and intensity of headaches. If the symptoms are not reduced within 3 to 4 weeks, the drug should be discontinued.
2. Check pulses in legs frequently. If pulse pressure decreases or if dependent edema occurs, notify physician.
3. Heart and lung sounds should be ausculated periodically. If murmurs or extra sounds occur, notify physician.
4. EKG, BUN, complete blood cell count, and serum creatinine should be done periodically (monthly).

Client teaching factors

1. Instruct client in the maintenance of a headache flowchart.
2. Instruct client to notify medical personnel if pain, shortness of breath, leg cramps, leg edema, or cold extremities occur.
3. Advise client that medical supervision during drug therapy is essential.
4. Advise client to take medication with meals or snacks.
5. Inform client that drug therapy should be interrupted every 6 months for 3 to 4 weeks.
6. Warn client against abrupt withdrawal of medication.
7. Caution client against excessive caloric intake.

Imidazolines

GENERIC NAMES Phentolamine hydrochloride; phentolamine mesylate

TRADE NAMES Regitine Hydrochloride; Regitine Mesylate

CLASSIFICATION Alpha-adrenergic blocker (RX)

Action Phentolamine is a relatively potent competitive blocker of alpha-adrenergic receptors and circulating epinephrine. The drug is useful for blocking the effects of injected epinephrine and in the control of pheochromocytoma-induced hypertension, since vasodilation occurs. It also has a direct effect on the heart and may increase cardiac output. Unfortunately, phentolamine causes a type of histamine reaction that results in increased gastric secretions and dilation of peripheral blood vessels. The annoying secondary effects on the GI tract (nausea, vomiting, diarrhea) are caused by drug-induced stimulation of parasympathetic nerves. As the stability and solubility of phentolamine mesylate is greater than phentolamine hydrochloride, the mesylate salt is used for injection.

Indications for Use Diagnosis of pheochromocytoma; prevention and control of pheochromocytoma-induced hypertensive episodes until surgical removal of tumor; prevention and treatment of necrosis and sloughing caused by extravasation of potent vasoconstrictors, particularly norepinephrine.

Contraindications Myocardial infarction, coronary artery disease (coronary insufficiency, angina pectoris), hypersensitivity to phentolamine.

Warnings and Precautions Use with caution in clients with known or suspected peptic ulcer. Save use during pregnancy and lactation has not been established.

Untoward Reactions Acute and prolonged hypotension may occur, particularly in the elderly or other susceptible clients. Arrhythmias, including tachycardia, may occur, particularly after parenteral administration. Secondary effects include postural hypotension, flushing, dizziness, nausea, vomiting, nasal stuffiness, weakness, and diarrhea. Exacerbation of a preexisting peptic ulcer may occur.

Parameters of Use

Absorption Onset of action is: about 30 to 60 minutes (po); 10 to 20 minutes (IM), 2 minutes (IV). Duration of action is: about 4 to 6 hours (po); 30 to 45 minutes (IM); 15 to 30 minutes (IV).

Metabolism Unknown.

Excretion About 10% as unchanged drug in urine.

Drug Interactions Epinephrine is ineffective in counteracting the effects of phentolamine overdosage and may even cause a paradoxic drop in blood pressure. Norepinephrine is an effective antidote in phentolamine-induced shock.

Administration

- *Pheochromocytoma diagnostic test:* Adults: 5 mg IM or IV bolus; Children: 3 mg IM or 1 mg IV bolus.
- *Controlling pheochromocytoma-induced hypertension:* Adults: 50 mg po 4 to 6 times daily; Children: 25 mg po 4 to 6 times daily.
- *Surgical removal of pheochromocytoma:* Adults: 5 mg IV 1 to 2 hours preoperatively; repeat as necessary; 5 mg IV prn during surgery. Children: 1 mg IM or IV 1 to 2 hours preoperatively; repeat as necessary; 1 mg IV prn during surgery.
- *Extravasation due to drug-induced vasoconstriction:* Infiltrate area with 5 to 10 mg mixed with 10 ml of normal saline q12h, as needed.

Available Drug Forms Tablets containing 50 mg; ampules containing 5 mg of dry powder for reconstitution with 1 ml of sterile water.

Nursing Management

Planning factors

1. Store ampules and tablets in a dry dark area.
2. Withhold all medications (including antihypertensive agents, digitalis, and insulin) for 24 to 72 hours before diagnostic test for pheochromocytoma. Client must be in a hypertensive state before test is done. Do not perform test on a normotensive client.
3. Norepinephrine should be readily available in the event of an excessive fall in blood pressure. If hypotension occurs, keep client recumbent and elevate legs. IV fluids and other supportive measures are used until blood pressure returns to a normal level.
4. Baseline vital signs and blood pressure should be obtained before instituting therapy.
5. If arrhythmias occur, digitalis glycosides should not be used until cardiac rhythm returns to normal.

Administration factors

1. Place client in supine position before administering drug parenterally. Client can resume activity after blood pressure restabilizes
2. When diagnostic test is given,
   - **(a)** Place client in supine position in a quiet darkened room.
   - **(b)** Take blood pressure every 10 minutes until it stabilizes at a resting level.
   - **(c)** Dissolve drug in 1 ml of sterile water.
   - **(d)** Physician injects needle of drug-filled syringe into vein; once pressor response to venipuncture has subsided, medication is injected rapidly.
   - **(e)** Record blood pressure immediately after IV injection; then every 30 seconds for 3 minutes; then every minute for the next 7 minutes.
   - **(f)** If medication is injected IM, record blood pressure every 5 minutes for 30 to 45 minutes.

(g) Positive test results for pheochromocytoma include:
 (i) Drop in systolic pressure of 35 mm Hg or more.
 (ii) Drop in diastolic pressure of 25 mm Hg or more.
 (iii) Blood pressure returns to pretest level in 15 to 30 minutes after IV bolus.
 (iv) Maximum drop in blood pressure occurs in about 20 minutes and returns to normal 30 to 45 minutes after IM injection.
(h) False-positive results can occur, particularly in clients with paroxysmal hypertension.

3. Treatment of extravasation:
 (a) Infiltration must be done within 12 hours or less. The sooner phentolamine infiltration is started, the less necrosis occurs.
 (b) Infiltrate area with 5 to 10 mg mixed with 10 ml of normal saline q12h, as needed.
 (c) Infiltrate drug with a 25- to 27-gauge needle into superficial tissues of involved area initially, then with a 21- to 23-gauge needle into deeper tissues. (Usually done by physician).
 (d) Sometimes 1 ampule of reconstituted phentolamine is added directly to the IV bottle containing norepinephrine.
4. Always use freshly prepared solution for parenteral administration. Discard unused portion, since aqueous solution is unstable.

Evaluation factors

1. Check blood pressure every 2 to 5 minutes after parenteral administration.
2. Check blood pressure frequently (q2h) after oral administration.
3. Check infiltrated site for signs of necrosis frequently. If site becomes cold to touch, notify physician.

Client teaching factors

1. Warn client to notify physician immediately if dizziness, chest pain, angina, tachycardia, or stomach pain occurs.
2. Advise client to take tablets after meals or with a snack to decrease gastric irritation.

GENERIC NAME Tolazoline hydrochloride (RX)

TRADE NAMES Priscoline, Toloxan, Tolzol

CLASSIFICATION Alpha-adrenergic blocker

Action Tolazoline is chemically related to phentolamine, but has a greater vasodilating effect due to its direct histaminelike activity, which causes relaxation of vascular smooth muscle. Tolazoline is a weak alpha-adrenergic blocker and also causes cardiac stimulation (tachycardia). Its secondary effects on the GI tract (nausea, vomiting, diarrhea) are due to parasympathetic stimulation. Gastric secretions are increased because of the drug's histaminic activity.

Indications for Use Possibly effective for vasospastic peripheral vascular disorders associated with acrocyanosis, acroparesthesia, arteriosclerosis obliterans, Buerger's disease, causalgia, diabetic arteriosclerosis, gangrene, endarteritis, sequelae to frostbite, thrombophlebitis, Raynaud's disease, and scleroderma.

Contraindications Following cerebrovascular accident, known or suspected coronary artery disease, hypersensitivity to tolazoline.

Warnings and Precautions Use with caution in clients with known or suspected peptic ulcer and those with mitral stenosis (since tolazoline may alter pulmonary artery pressure). Safe use during pregnancy and lactation has not been established.

Untoward Reactions Arrhythmias, anginal pain, and marked changes in blood pressure are relatively common in the elderly and clients with coronary artery disease. GI disturbances include nausea, vomiting, diarrhea, and epigastric distress. Exacerbation of peptic ulcer disease has occurred. Other effects include alterations in blood pressure, tachycardia, flushing, edema, increased pilomotor activity, tingling or chilliness, and rash. Blood dyscrasias, including thrombocytopenia and leukopenia, have been reported, particularly after long-term therapy. Confusion, hallucinations, hepatitis, oliguria, and hematuria have been reported, but rarely. Intraarterial administration may cause a burning sensation in the injected extremity, transient weakness, vertigo, apprehension, palpitations, and formication. A paradoxic decrease in blood supply may precipitate gangrene, but rarely.

Parameters of Use

Absorption Well absorbed. Onset of action is 30 to 60 minutes (IM, subc). Duration of action is: 4 to 6 hours (IM, subc); about 4 hours (IV).

Excretion Primarily by the kidneys as unchanged drug.

Drug Interactions Tolazoline inhibits the metabolism of acetaldehyde, a metabolite of alcohol, and produces a serious untoward reaction.

Administration Highly individualized. Dosage depends on blood pressure response. Therapy is started with low dosages and then increased gradually every few days until desired effect. Oral: 50 mg qid; Dosage range: 25 to 75 mg qid; 80 mg long-acting preparation bid. Intramuscular, subcutaneous: 10 to 40 mg qid. Intraarterial: Test dosage: 25 mg administered slowly; then 25 to 75 mg (depending on response) daily or bid.

Available Drug Forms Tablets containing 25 or 50 mg; long-acting tablets containing 80 mg; multidose vials containing 25 mg/ml.

Nursing Management

Planning factors

1. Baseline vital signs and blood pressure should be monitored for several days before initiating therapy.
2. Obtain a complete history, including GI disturbances, cardiac disorders, and vascular disorders.

3. A baseline complete blood cell count should be obtained.
4. Secondary effects tend to decrease with long-term therapy.

Administration factors

1. Tablets should be taken on an empty stomach with a full glass of water. Can be taken with milk if GI irritation occurs.
2. Intraarterial injections should be done by a physician or specially trained professional. This route should be avoided, if possible, because of the risks involved.
   (a) Place pressure on site for 10 to 15 minutes after injection.
   (b) Observe site q1h for 3 to 4 hours for bleeding.

Evaluation factors

1. Monitor vital signs and blood pressure frequently (q4h and prn) when therapy is first initiated or dosage adjusted.
2. Observe affected limbs for impaired circulation (skin temperature, color).
3. An early sign of toxicity is generalized warmth, piloerection, and a "creeping" or "chilling" sensation of the skin. If symptoms occur, notify physician.

Client teaching factors

1. Caution client against the ingestion of alcohol and explain why.
2. Instruct client in ways of conserving body heat (house temperature, clothing), since drug is more effective when body is kept warm.
3. Instruct client to notify health professionals if epigastric distress, palpitations, postural dizziness, edema, or excessive piloerection occur. (Milk or an antacid are usually effective for epigastric distress.)
4. Instruct client to change position slowly to avoid postural hypotension.

Other Alpha Blockers

GENERIC NAME Phenoxybenzamine hydrochloride

TRADE NAME Dibenzyline (RX)

CLASSIFICATION Alpha-adrenergic blocker

Action Phenoxybenzamine, a beta haloalkylamine, causes a relatively complete noncompetitive blockade of alpha-adrenergic receptors. Although the drug's onset of action is slow, its duration of action is prolonged and not even massive doses of epinephrine will reverse the blockade. Phenoxybenzamine is also effective against other sympathomimetic amines. The drug causes a significant increase in peripheral blood flow and lowers blood pressure. Unlike some other alpha blockers, phenoxybenzamine has no effect on parasympathetic nerves or the GI tract. Beta-adrenergic receptors remain unopposed. Unfortunately, excessive postural hypotension makes the drug undesirable for the treatment of hypertension.

Indications for Use Effective in controlling hypertensive episodes and sweating caused by pheochromocytoma (beta blockers may be required concurrently to control tachycardia); possibly effective against vasospastic peripheral vascular disorders, particularly Raynaud's syndrome, acrocyanosis, causalgia, and sequelae to frostbite.

Contraindications Any disorder in which a fall in blood pressure is undesirable, including cerebral insufficiency and a history of postural hypotension.

Warnings and Precautions Use with caution in the elderly and in clients with cerebral or coronary arteriosclerosis or renal impairment. Adrenergic blockers may aggravate the symptoms of respiratory infections. Direct-acting vasodilators are preferred in diseases involving the larger blood vessels.

Untoward Reactions Secondary effects are common and the severity of symptoms depends on the quantity of drug used to cause adrenergic blockade. Nasal congestion, miosis, postural hypotension, tachycardia, and inhibition of ejaculation may occur; these symptoms tend to decrease as therapy is continued. GI irritation has been reported. Exacerbation of a preexisting peptic ulcer may occur. Toxicity may occur. The symptoms include postural hypotension, dizziness, fainting, tachycardia, vomiting, lethargy, and shock.

Parameters of Use

Absorption Poorly absorbed from GI tract; about one-third enters the bloodstream. Onset of action is about 24 hours. Half-life is about 24 hours.

Excretion In feces; absorbed drug is excreted by the kidneys; some reenters the intestines via bile.

Drug Interactions Epinephrine is ineffective in counteracting the effects of phenoxybenzamine overdosage and induces a further drop in blood pressure. Propranolol and other beta-adrenergic blockers may be useful in controlling tachycardia and other untoward reactions of phenoxybenzamine.

Administration Highly individualized. Initial dosage: 10 mg po daily for 4 days; then increase by 10 mg every 4 days until desired effect; Dosage range: 20 to 60 mg daily.

Available Drug Forms Capsules containing 10 mg.

Nursing Management

Planning Factors

1. Baseline vital signs and blood pressure should be monitored for several days before initiating therapy.
2. Obtain a complete history, including postural

hypotension and other symptoms of cerebral insufficiency, cardiac disorders, and renal impairment. If oliguria or other abnormalities exist, notify physician.
3. Creatinine clearance is recommended.
4. Complete noncompetitive blockade takes about 2 weeks of therapy. No known drug will reverse the blockade.
5. Optimum response is achieved when there is symptomatic relief of impaired circulation with no serious secondary effects.

Administration factors Capsules should be taken on an empty stomach with a full glass of water. Can be taken with milk if GI irritation occurs.

Evaluation factors

1. Monitor vital signs and blood pressure frequently (each shift and prn) when dosage is adjusted; then daily as necessary.
2. Observe affected limbs for impaired circulation (skin temperature, color).
3. Observe for postural hypotension and tachycardia. If symptoms occur notify physician. Beta blockers may be helpful in controlling tachycardia.

Client teaching factors

1. Instruct client in ways of conserving body heat (house temperature, clothing), since drug is more effective when body is kept warm.
2. Instruct client to notify health professionals if epigastric distress, palpitations, or postural dizziness occur. (Milk or an antacid are usually effective for epigastric distress.)
3. Instruct client to change position slowly to avoid postural hypotension.

GENERIC NAME Azapetine phosphate (RX)

TRADE NAME Ilidar

CLASSIFICATION Alpha-adrenergic blocker

See phenoxybenzamine hydrochloride for Warnings and precautions, Untoward reactions, Parameters of use, and Drug interactions.

Action Azapetine is a dibenzazepine derivative and is similar to the beta-haloalkylamine compounds. This drug differs from phenoxybenzamine in that the alpha-adrenergic blockade is reversible when sufficient quantities of epinephrine or other sympathomimetic amines are administered. Azapetine causes direct vasodilation and blocks the vasoconstrictor effects of circulating epinephrine. Few parasympathetic effects have been reported.

Indications for Use Treatment of vasospastic peripheral vascular disorders, including Raynaud's syndrome, acrocyanosis, causalgia, and sequelae to frostbite. May be useful in Buerger's disease and acute arterial occlusion. May prove to be useful in the treatment of moderate to severe hypertension.

Contraindications None known.

Administration Highly individualized. Initial dosage: 25 mg po tid for 7 days; then increase slowly by 25 mg until desired effect; Dosage range: 50 to 70 mg tid.

Available Drug Forms Tablets containing 25 mg.

Nursing Management

Planning factors

1. Baseline vital signs and blood pressure should be monitored for several days before initiating therapy.
2. Obtain a complete history, including postural hypotension and other symptoms of cerebral insufficiency, cardiac disorders, and renal impairment. If oliguria or other abnormalities exist, notify physician.

Administration factors Tablets should be taken on an empty stomach with a full glass of water. Can be taken with milk if GI irritation occurs.

Evaluation factors

1. Monitor vital signs and blood pressure frequently (each shift and prn) when dosage is adjusted; then daily.
2. Observe affected limbs for impaired circulation (skin temperature, color).
3. Observe for postural hypotension and tachycardia. If symptoms occur, notify physician. Beta blockers may be helpful in controlling tachycardia.

Client teaching factors

1. Instruct client in ways of conserving body heat (house temperature, clothing), since drug is more effective when body is kept warm.
2. Instruct client to notify health professionals if epigastric distress, palpitations, or postural dizziness occur. (Milk or an antacid are usually effective for epigastric distress.)
3. Instruct client to change position slowly to avoid postural hypotension.

BETA-ADRENERGIC BLOCKERS

GENERIC NAME Propranolol hydrochloride (RX)

TRADE NAME Inderal

CLASSIFICATION Beta-adrenergic blocker

Action Propranolol is a nonselective beta-adrenergic blocker that has no other autonomic nervous system activity. The drug competes with the body's catecholamines (epinephrine and norepinephrine) for beta-adrenergic sites, thus blocking the stimulation of beta receptors. Propranolol affects the heart (beta$_1$ receptors) by decreasing rate, output, and conduction function. Beta$_2$ blockade prevents relaxation of bronchial, GI, and uterine smooth muscle. Blood pressure is decreased, but the mechanism of action is unknown. Drug-induced factors that affect blood pressure include decreased cardiac output, inhibition of renin secretion (decreases the reabsorption of sodium by the kidneys), and depression of sympathetic innervation from the brain's vasomotor center. Its antimigraine effect may be the result of drug-induced inhibition of spasms in the brain's arterioles.

Indications for Use Hypertension (usually given with a thiazide diuretic); prevention of angina pectoris due to coronary disease; supraventricular tachycardia, including paroxysmal atrial tachycardia induced by catecholamines or digitalis and Wolff-Parkinson-White syndrome; persistent sinus tachycardia and premature atrial contractions; tachycardia and arrhythmias caused by thyrotoxicosis; atrial flutter and fibrillation; persistent tachyarrhythmias due to excessive catecholamine action during anesthesia; prevention of common migraine headaches; management of hypertrophic subaortic stenosis; as an adjunct in the treatment of pheochromocytoma-induced beta stimulation.

Contraindications Bronchial asthma, allergic rhinitis, sinus bradycardia, heart block greater than first degree, cardiogenic shock, right ventricular failure due to pulmonary hypertension, acute congestive heart failure, clients taking adrenergic-augmenting psychotropic agents (such as MAO inhibitors).

Warnings and Precautions Use with caution in the elderly; in clients with a history of cardiac failure, since the drug has the potential of depressing myocardial contractility and thereby precipitating cardiac failure; in clients with hyperthyroidism, since the signs and symptoms of thyrotoxicosis may be masked; in clients susceptible to bronchospasm (chronic bronchitis, emphysema); in clients with impaired hepatic or renal function; in diabetic clients, since the signs and symptoms of hypoglycemia may be masked; and when treating arrhythmias in anesthetized clients. Abrupt withdrawal of drug may precipitate angina pectoris, myocardial infarction, thyroid storm, and other disorders. Clients with Wolff-Parkinson-White syndrome may develop severe bradycardia when drug is first initiated; the insertion of a demand pacemaker may be required. Safe use during pregnancy and lactation has not been established.

Untoward Reactions Bradycardia, congestive heart failure, and excessive hypotension have occurred and may be life threatening. Arterial insufficiency with paresthesias of the hands may occur. Bronchospasm can occur in susceptible clients and may be life threatening. GI disturbances, including nausea, vomiting, epigastric distress, abdominal cramps, diarrhea, and constipation, may occur. Mesenteric arterial thrombosis and ischemic colitis have been reported. Hypoglycemia without tachycardia and hypotension may occur in diabetic clients. Thyrotoxicosis without tachycardia may occur in clients with hyperthyroidism; thyroid function tests are unaffected. Blood dyscrasias, including agranulocytosis, nonthrombocytic purpura, and thrombocytopenic purpura, have been reported. CNS reactions, including lightheadedness, depression, insomnia, weakness, visual disturbances, hallucinations, disorientation, and short-term memory loss, have occurred. Allergic reactions include pharyngitis, agranulocytosis, rashes, fever, sore throat, and laryngospasm. Rare reactions include reversible alopecia and dryness of skin, mucous membranes, and conjunctiva.

Laboratory Interactions Elevated blood urea nitrogen levels have been reported in clients with severe cardiac disease. Elevated serum transaminases, including lactate dehydrogenase and alkaline phosphatase, have occurred.

Parameters of Use

Absorption Well absorbed from GI tract. Onset of action is: about 30 minutes (po); about 2 minutes (IV). Peak plasma levels occur in: 60 to 90 minutes (po); 15 minutes (IV). Duration of action is: about 6 hours (po); 3 to 6 hours (IV).

Plasma half-life Varies from 3.4 to 6 hours; some clients metabolize the drug faster than others. About 90% bound to plasma proteins.

Crosses placenta and enters breast milk; lactating mothers should bottle-feed their babies. Crosses blood-brain barrier and may cause CNS disturbances.

Distribution Widely distributed in body tissues.

Metabolism In the liver.

Excretion By the kidneys as unchanged drug and metabolites. Less than 5% excreted in feces.

Drug Interactions Propranolol does not abolish the inotropic action of digitalis and its glycosides; however, because propranolol has a negative inotropic effect, it will negate some of the inotropic effects of digitalis. Propranolol will further depress AV conduction in digitalized clients, thus enhancing bradycardia; use with great caution concurrently. Propranol antagonizes the action of aminophylline; concurrent drug therapy should be avoided. Propranolol may alter the insulin requirements of clients previously stabilized on oral hypoglycemic agents; watch clients for hypoglycemia. Isoproterenol and norepinephrine antagonize the effects of propranolol and can be used as antidotes. The action of neuromuscular blocking agents, such as tubocurarine, may be prolonged; watch client for respiratory depression. The cardiac depressant action of phenytoin and quinidine may be enhanced. Drugs that deplete catecholamines, such as the antihypertensive agent reserpine, may have an additive effect when given concurrently with beta blockers; observe client closely for hypotension and marked bradycardia, since vertigo, syncope, or postural hypotension may occur. When clonidine is given concurrently with beta blockers, the latter should be discontinued several days before the gradual withdrawal of clonidine. Anesthetic agents that depress the myocardium (ether, cyclopropane, trichloroethylene) may cause severe hypotension, bradycardia, and cardiovascular collapse; discontinue beta blocker 48 hours prior to surgery.

Administration Highly individualized.

- *Hypertension:* Initial dosage: 40 mg po bid; then increase every few days until desired effect; Dosage range: 160 to 480 mg daily in divided doses. Full antihypertensive effect may take several weeks.

- *Angina pectoris:* Initial dosage: 10 to 20 mg po tid or qid before meals and at bedtime; then gradually increase every 3 to 7 days until desired effect; Dosage range: 160 to 320 mg daily.
- *Arrhythmias:* 1 to 3 mg IV bolus for life-threatening arrhythmias at a rate not exceeding 1 mg/min.; a second dose of 1 to 3 mg may be given after 2 to 5 minutes; do not repeat for 4 hours. Transfer to oral therapy as soon as possible: 10 to 80 mg tid or qid before meals and at bedtime.
- *Migraine headaches:* Initial dosage: 80 mg po daily in divided doses; Dosage range: 160 to 240 mg daily in divided doses. Adequate response may take 4 to 6 weeks.
- *Preoperative management of pheochromocytoma:* 60 mg po daily in divided doses for 3 days.
- *Management of inoperable tumor:* 30 mg po daily in divided doses.

Available Drug Forms Tablets containing 10, 20, 40, or 80 mg; 1-ml ampules containing 1 mg/ml.

Nursing Management

Planning factors

1. Baseline data appropriate to the purpose of administration should be obtained.
2. Cardiovascular and respiratory status should be assessed for possible contraindications. Baseline vital signs should be recorded.
3. Hepatic and renal function should be assessed. If blood urea nitrogen (BUN) or serum creatinine are elevated, notify physician. If oliguria exists, notify physician.
4. Drug should be kept on units (emergency room, intensive care unit, coronary care unit, extended coronary care unit) where there are clients who may need it for life-threatening arrhythmias.
5. Store drug in dark area (closet).
6. Appropriate drugs should be readily available for use in the event of toxicity.
7. Drug should be withdrawn temporarily 48 hours prior to surgery that requires general anesthetic agents, with the exception of clients with pheochromocytoma.

Administration factors

1. Check blood pressure and pulse before therapy is first initiated or dosage adjusted. If severe bradycardia or hypotension exist, notify physician before administering drug.
2. Give drug before meals and at bedtime on an empty stomach. Follow with a full glass of water.
3. When administering IV,
   - **(a)** IV bolus given over 1 to 3 minutes is often used to treat life-threatening arrhythmias; diluted IV drug solution q4h (50 or 100 ml) is then used to maintain serum levels.
   - **(b)** Desired dose can be diluted in 50 to 100 ml of normal saline or 5% D/W.
   - **(c)** Do not administer at a rate faster than 1 mg/min.
   - **(d)** Continuous cardiac monitoring is essential.
   - **(e)** Monitor blood pressure and pulse continuously.
   - **(f)** Central venous pressure readings are recommended.
   - **(g)** A second dose may be required.

Evaluation factors

1. When IV therapy is used, monitor blood pressure and pulse every 2 minutes until stable. Cardiac monitoring is essential to determine type of arrhythmia. If no response occurs after 2 doses, another antiarrhythmic agent or cardioversion may be required.
2. Blood pressure and pulse should be taken before each dosage initially; then periodically.
3. Complete blood cell count, BUN, and serum creatinine levels should be obtained periodically.
4. Record intake and output.
5. Dosage must be reduced gradually before discontinuing drug.

Client teaching factors

1. Inform client of potential untoward reactions and to notify physician immediately if any occur, particularly low pulse rate (below 60 beats/min.), shortness of breath, and hypoglycemia.
2. Advise client (particularly if normotensive) to change position slowly to avoid lightheadedness.
3. Advise client to avoid excessive use of CNS depressants and stimulants (alcohol or caffeinated drinks such as coffee, soda, or tea), since untoward reactions may occur.
4. Inform client that adaptation to stressful situation will be altered and to avoid stress if possible.
5. Advise client that untoward reactions may occur if the drug is discontinued abruptly.

GENERIC NAME Nadolol (RX)

TRADE NAME Corgard

CLASSIFICATION Beta-adrenergic blocker

See propranolol hydrochloride for Warnings and precautions and Drug interactions.

Action Nadolol is similar to propranolol, another nonselective beta-adrenergic blocker. Both drugs reduce heart rate, cardiac output, systolic and diastolic blood pressure, and reflex orthostatic tachycardia, and inhibit isoproterenol-induced tachycardia. Whereas the duration of action for propranolol is only 6 hours, that for nadolol is 24 hours. Client compliance with drug therapy is theoretically better with nadolol because it only needs to be given once a day, instead of 4 times a day with propranolol. Toxic and other untoward reactions seem to be milder than with propranolol.

Indications for Use Prevention of hypertension (usually given with a thiazide diuretic). Although not approved as yet, the drug is theoretically useful for other disorders, including the prevention of angina and the treatment of tachyarrhythmias.

Contraindications Bronchial asthma, sinus bradycardia greater than first-degree heart block, cardiogenic shock, acute cardiac failure.

Untoward Reactions Although the reported incidence of untoward reactions to nadolol is less than to propranolol, the same type of reactions occur. (See propranolol hydrochloride.)

Parameters of Use

Absorption Fairly well absorbed from GI tract; food may increase absorption. Onset of action is about 30 to 60 minutes and duration of action is 24 hours.

Crosses placenta and enters breast milk; lactating mothers should bottle-feed their babies.

Distribution Widely; little in cerebrospinal fluid.

Metabolism Probably in the liver. Drug can be removed from circulation by hemodialysis.

Excretion By the kidneys.

Drug Interactions May alter requirements for hypoglycemic agents. Concurrent use with digitalis may cause excessive bradycardia.

Administration Highly individualized.

- *Angina pectoris:* Initial dosage: 40 mg po daily; then increase by 40 to 80 mg every 3 to 7 days until desired effect; Dosage range: 80 to 240 mg daily.
- *Hypertension:* Initial dosage: 40 mg po daily; then increase by 40 to 80 mg over several days or weeks; Dosage range: 80 to 320 mg daily. Lower dosages are required for clients with impaired renal function; dosage is usually administered every other day.

Available Drug Forms Tablets containing 40, 80, 120, or 160 mg.

Nursing Management

Planning factors

1. Baseline data appropriate to the purpose of administration should be obtained.
2. Cardiovascular and respiratory status should be assessed for possible contraindications. Baseline vital signs should be recorded.
3. Hepatic and renal function should be assessed. If blood urea nitrogen (BUN) or serum creatinine are elevated, notify physician. If oliguria exists, notify physician.
4. Appropriate drugs should be readily available for use in the event of toxicity.

Administration factors

1. Check blood pressure and pulse before therapy is first initiated or dosage adjusted. If severe bradycardia or hypotension exist, notify physician before administering drug.
2. Give drug with meals (breakfast).

Evaluation factors

1. Blood pressure and pulse should be taken before each dosage initially; then periodically.

RECOMMENDED TREATMENT FOR TOXICITY

Symptom	Treatment
Bradycardia	Atropine 0.25 to 1.0 mg IV bolus; if no response, give isoproterenol slowly via IV drip
Cardiac failure	Digitalization and diuresis
Hypotension	Epinephrine may be the drug of choice; norepinephrine may be used to maintain blood pressure
Bronchospasm	Administer a $beta_2$-stimulating agent and/or a theophylline derivative

2. Complete blood cell count, BUN, and serum creatinine levels should be obtained periodically.
3. Record intake and output.
4. Dosage must be reduced gradually before discontinuing drug.

Client teaching factors

1. Inform client of potential untoward reactions and to notify physician immediately if any occur, particularly low pulse rate (below 60 beats/min.).
2. Advise client (particularly if normotensive) to change position slowly to avoid lightheadedness.
3. Advise client to avoid excessive use of CNS depressants and stimulants (alcohol or caffeinated drinks such as coffee, soda, or tea), since untoward reactions may occur.
4. Inform client that adaptation to stessful situations will be altered and to avoid stress if possible.
5. Advise client that untoward reactions may occur if the drug is discontinued abruptly.

GENERIC NAME Atenolol (RX)

TRADE NAME Tenormin

CLASSIFICATION Beta-adrenergic blocker

Action Atenolol is a beta-adrenergic blocker that is specific to $beta_1$-receptor sites in the heart when usual dosages are used. However, large dosages inhibit $beta_2$-receptor sites, particularly in the bronchial and vascular musculature. Unlike most beta blockers, atenolol can be cautiously tried in clients with bronchospastic disorders. The drug reduces heart rate, cardiac output, systolic and diastolic blood pressure, and reflex orthostatic tachycardia, and inhibits isoproterenol-induced tachycardia. Atenolol causes a beta blockade of the SA node and prolongs AV conduction. Since atenolol does not affect membrane stabilizing activity, myocardial contractility will not be depressed beyond the effects produced by beta blockade.

Indications for Use Treatment of hypertension either alone or in conjunction with thiazide diuretics.

Contraindications Sinus headache, second- or third-degree heart block (may be used in first-degree heart block, namely when there is a prolonged P-R interval), cardiogenic shock, acute heart failure.

Warnings and Precautions Use with caution in clients known to have a history of congestive heart failure; in clients with asthma or other disorders that cause bronchospasm; in clients with diabetes, since beta-adrenergic blockers may mask the symptoms of hypoglycemia; in clients with hyperthyroidism, since beta-adrenergic blockers may mask the symptoms of hyperthyroidism and precipitate a thyroid storm upon abrupt withdrawal; and in clients with impaired renal function. Abrupt withdrawal of beta-adrenergic blockers in clients with coronary artery disease may precipitate angina pectoris or possibly myocardial infarction. Safe use in children and during pregnancy has not been established.

Untoward Reactions Bradycardia, postural hypotension, dizziness, tiredness, fatigue, cold extremities, and leg pains have been reported and are secondary effects of the drug. GI irritation, including nausea and diarrhea, have been reported. Dyspnea has been reported, but rarely. Although skin rashes and dry eyes have been reported after the use of other beta blockers, none have been reported to date from atenolol; if symptoms occur, drug should be discontinued. Potential toxic reactions include severe bradycardia, second- or third-degree heart block, congestive heart failure, hypotension, bronchospasm, and hypoglycemia; however, none have been reported to date. Other potential untoward reactions include agranulocytosis, purpura, hypersensitivity, fever, generalized aching, sore throat, laryngospasm, respiratory distress, mental depression, visual disturbances, disorientation, short-term memory loss, mesenteric thrombosis, ischemic colitis, alopecia, Raynaud's disease, and oculomucocutaneous syndrome. Although none have been reported from atenolol, these reactions have occurred during therapy with other beta blockers.

Parameters of Use

Absorption Rapid but incomplete; about 50% absorbed. Peak plasma levels occur in 2 to 4 hours. Duration of action is 24 hours. About 6 to 16% bound to plasma proteins. Half-life is 6 to 7 hours; activity persists for at least 24 hours with doses of 50 or 100 mg.

Metabolism Little or none in the liver. Relatively consistent blood levels are maintained.

Excretion Primarily by the kidneys. Excretion not affected until creatinine clearance falls below 35 ml/min./1.73 m^2.

Drug Interactions Drugs that deplete catecholamines, such as the antihypertensive agent reserpine, may have an additive effect when given concurrently with beta blockers; observe client closely for hypotension and marked bradycardia, since vertigo, syncope, or postural hypotension may occur. When clonidine is given concurrently with beta blockers, the latter should be discontinued several days before the gradual withdrawal of clonidine. Anaesthetic agents that depress the myocardium (ether, cyclopropane, trichloroethylene) may cause severe hypotension, bradycardia, and cardiovascular collapse; discontinue beta blocker 48 hours prior to surgery.

Administration Initial dosage: 50 mg po daily; can be increased to 100 mg po daily after 1 to 2 weeks, when necessary. Little or no benefit is achieved with dosages over 100 mg daily.

- *Dosage in clients with renal failure:* Creatinine clearance 15 to 35 ml/min.: 50 mg po daily; Creatinine clearance below 15 ml/min.: 50 mg po every other day. Drug should be administered following hemodialysis.
- *Dosage in clients with asthma:* 25 to 50 mg po bid.

Available Drug Forms Tablets containing 50 or 100 mg.

Nursing Management

Planning factors

1. Cardiovascular and respiratory status should be assessed for possible contraindications. Baseline vital signs should be recorded.
2. Hepatic and renal function should be assessed. If blood urea nitrogen (BUN) or serum creatinine are elevated, notify physician.
3. Appropriate drugs should be readily available for use in the event of toxicity. Toxic effects can be reversed by dobutamine, isoproterenol, and atropine.
4. Drug should be withdrawn temporarily 48 hours prior to surgery that requires general anesthetic agents.

Administration factors

1. Check apical-radial pulse before administering. If bradycardia exists, notify physician before administering drug.
2. Give drug before meals and at bedtime on an empty stomach. Follow with a full glass of water.
3. May be given concurrently with thiazide diuretics or antihypertensive agents.

Evaluation factors

1. Blood pressure and pulse should be taken before each dosage initially; then periodically.
2. Complete blood cell count, BUN, and serum creatinine levels should be obtained periodically.
3. Record intake and output.
4. Dosage must be reduced gradually before discontinuing drug.

Client teaching factors

1. Inform client of potential untoward reactions and to notify physician immediately if any occur, particularly low pulse rate (below 60 beats/min.).

2. Advise client to change position slowly to avoid lightheadedness.
3. Advise client that untoward reactions may occur if the drug is discontinued abruptly.

GENERIC NAME Metoprolol tartrate (RX)

TRADE NAMES Betaloc, Lopressor

CLASSIFICATION Beta-adrenergic blocker

Action Metoprolol is a beta-adrenergic blocker that is specific to $beta_1$-receptor sites in the heart when usual dosages are used. Like atenolol, large dosages will inhibit $beta_2$-receptor sites, particularly in the bronchial and vascular musculature. Low dosages can be used in clients with bronchial disorders. Also like atenolol, metoprolol reduces heart rate, cardiac output, blood pressure, and reflex orthostatic tachycardia, and inhibits isoproterenol-induced tachycardia. Unlike atenolol, metoprolol is rapidly metabolized in the liver and has a highly variable plasma drug level. Metoprolol crosses the blood-brain barrier and high concentrations are found in cerebrospinal fluid. Its antihypertensive effect may be due to (1) the decreased cardiac output from competitive antagonism of catecholamines, (2) a central effect that leads to a reduction in sympathetic transmission to peripheral nerve endings; or (3) suppression of renin activity, which causes a loss of sodium from the body.

Indications for Use Treatment of hypertension either alone or in conjunction with other antihypertensive agents, particularly thiazide diuretics.

Contraindications Sinus headache, second- or third-degree heart block (may be used in first-degree heart block, namely when there is a prolonged P-R interval), cardiogenic shock, acute heart failure.

Warnings and Precautions Long-term animal studies have indicated the possibility of the development of small benign adenomas in the lungs of mice, the formation of localized accumulations of foamy macrophages in the alveoli of rats, and some biliary hyperplasia in rats. (See atenolol.)

Untoward Reactions CNS disturbances, including tiredness, dizziness, and depression, are relatively common, but are usually mild. Headaches, nightmares, and insomnia have been reported. Secondary effects, including bradycardia and shortness of breath, have occurred relatively frequently. Peripheral arterial insufficiency, cold extremities, palpitations, and congestive heart failure have been infrequently reported. Bronchospasm with wheezing and pruritus have been reported in less than 1 client per 100. Diarrhea is relatively common; but nausea, gastric pain, constipation, flatulence, and other GI disturbances have been reported less often. Peyronie's disease has been reported, but rarely. Although none have been reported with metoprolol, the following untoward reactions have been reported with other beta-adrenergic blockers: visual disturbances, hallucinations, disorientation, memory loss, emotional lability, blood dyscrasias, rash, fever, sore throat, respiratory distress, reversible alopecia, and elevation of blood urea nitrogen and serum transaminases. Toxicity has been reported in a 19-year-old who ingested 200 50-mg tablets. Upon hospital admission, he was conscious and had peripheral cyanosis, weak heart sounds, and unmeasurable blood pressure. Femoral pulse was palpable. EKG showed a sinus rhythm of 60 to 70 beats/min. with normal AV conduction, S-T segments, and T waves. Complete recovery occurred within 12 hours after administering Ringer's lactate, metaraminol (vasopressor), glucagon (hyperglycemic agent), and sodium bicarbonate.

Parameters of use

Absorption Rapid and complete. Duration of effect on heart rate is dose related and is: 3.3 hours (20 mg); 5 hours (50 mg); 6.4 hours (100 mg). This data assumes normal liver function, and the relationship is linear. Duration of effect on blood pressure is not dose related; repeated oral doses of 100 mg reduce blood pressure for about 12 hours. Half-life is 3 to 4 hours. About 12% bound to albumin.

Metabolism About 5% serum drug level is metabolized in the liver during the first pass. Variable rates in liver metabolism cause highly variable serum drug levels from client to client.

Drug Interactions Drugs that deplete catecholamines, such as the antihypertensive agent reserpine, may have an additive effect when given concurrently with beta blockers; observe client closely for hypotension and marked bradycardia, since vertigo, syncope, or postural hypotension may occur. When clonidine is given concurrently with beta blockers, the latter should be discontinued several days before the gradual withdrawal of clonidine. Anesthetic agents that depress the myocardium (ether, cyclopropane, trichloroethylene) may cause severe hypotension, bradycardia, and cardiovascular collapse; discontinue beta blocker 48 hours prior to surgery. Excessive bradycardia may occur when metoprolol is given to digitalized clients; extreme caution is warranted when drugs are administered concurrently.

Administration Highly individualized. Initial dosage: 50 mg po bid; can be increased after 1 to 2 weeks until desired blood pressure response; Dosage range: 100 to 450 mg daily in divided doses. If blood pressure tends to be elevated (rises 9 to 12 hours after drug administration), the dosage can be increased or the drug may be administered q8h.

Available Drug Forms Film-coated tablets containing 50 or 100 mg.

Nursing Management

Planning factors

1. Baseline blood pressure and pulse should be obtained before initiating therapy.
2. Cardiovascular and respiratory status should be assessed for possible contraindications. Baseline vital signs should be recorded.
3. Hepatic and renal function should be assessed. If blood urea nitrogen (BUN) or serum creatinine are elevated, notify physician.

4. No reduction in dosage is required when drug is administered concurrently with diuretics.
5. Drug should be withdrawn temporarily 48 hours prior to surgery that requires general anesthetic agents.

Administration factors

1. Check blood pressure and pulse before therapy is first initiated or dosage adjusted. If severe bradycardia or hypotension occur, notify physician before administering drug.
2. Give drug before breakfast and at bedtime on an empty stomach. Follow with a full glass of water.

Evaluation factors

1. A vital sign flowchart should be maintained when therapy is first initiated or dosage adjusted. Check and record blood pressure and pulse q4h. While client is awake, record blood pressure when drug is given and 2 hours before and after a scheduled dose. If blood pressure tends to return to untreated hypertensive state, notify physician, since a dosage adjustment is required.
2. Complete blood cell count, BUN, and serum creatinine should be obtained periodically.
3. Record intake and output.
4. Dosage must be reduced gradually before discontinuing drug.

Client teaching factors

1. Inform client of potential untoward reactions and to notify physician immediately if any occur, particularly low pulse rate (below 60 beats/min.), diarrhea, dizziness, or depression.
2. Advise client to change position slowly to avoid lightheadedness.
3. Advise client to avoid excessive use of CNS depressants and stimulants (alcohol or caffeinated drinks such as coffee, soda, or tea), since untoward reactions may occur.
4. Inform client that adaptation to stressful situations will be altered and to avoid stress if possible.
5. Advise client that untoward reactions may occur if the drug is discontinued abruptly.
6. Instruct client to store medication in tightly covered containers away from moisture (not in bathroom or kitchen).

Chapter 43

Antimuscarinic and Ganglionic Blocking Agents

DRUGS THAT ANTAGONIZE or block the effects of acetylcholine at receptor sites are often called *cholinergic blocking agents, anticholinergic agents*, or *parasympatholytic agents*. There are two types of cholinergic receptor sites: (1) those stimulated by muscarine, called *muscarinic receptor sites;* and (2) those stimulated by nicotine, called *nicotinic receptor sites*. Muscarinic receptor sites are located at parasympathetic postganglionic synapses and are antagonized by atropine and other *antimuscarinic agents*. Nicotinic receptor sites are located at parasympathetic and sympathetic ganglia; since the effects of acetylcholine are antagonized at both the parasympathetic and sympathetic branches of the autonomic nervous system by hexamethonium and related drugs, these drugs are simply termed *ganglionic blocking agents*. The terms anticholinergic agent and antimuscarinic agent are used interchangeably, but the preferred term for an antinicotinic agent is ganglionic blocking agent.

PROPERTIES OF ANTIMUSCARINIC AGENTS

Atropine is a potent antimuscarinic agent that competitively blocks the action of acetylcholine at postganglionic parasympathetic synapses. As atropine, scopolamine, and other related substances are alkaloids found naturally in *Atropa belladonna*, this group of drugs in sometimes referred to as the belladonna alkaloids. Several synthetic antimuscarinic drugs are also available.

Primary Actions

Atropine and related drugs all affect gastrointestinal and urinary tract smooth muscle, ciliary and other muscles of the eye, the cardiovascular, and central nervous systems, and the exocrine glands, but their degree of action varies.

The effect of these drugs on the smooth muscle of the gastrointestinal tract is an antispasmodic one, and they inhibit gastric secretions. Consequently, antimuscarinic agents are frequently used to treat peptic ulcer, diarrhea, and other spastic gastrointestinal disturbances. Unfortunately, the secretions from salivary and sweat glands are also inhibited and this results in an unpleasant dry mouth and an intolerance to heat. The inability to lose body heat through sweating can cause pronounced hyperthermia under toxic conditions. Urinary retention can also occur, particularly in elderly males, because the bladder's smooth muscle is relaxed and the bladder sphincter is constricted. Although bronchial smooth muscle is affected, bronchodilation is minimal when compared to the adrenergic agent isoproterenol.

These agents also produce mydriasis (dilation of pupils) and cycloplegia (paralysis of the ciliary muscles of accommodation) and these effects are desirable for certain diagnostic eye examinations and for treating inflammatory disorders of the iris and other eye structures. Unfortunately, the effects of topically applied atropine on the eye may last as long as 7 to 12 days and cause photophobia and blurred vision. Newer synthetic agents, such as tropicamide, have a short duration of action, only 15-20 minutes. Caution should be used when administering atropine drugs to elderly clients since undiagnosed narrow-angle glaucoma may be precipitated.

Atropine is effective in blocking the cholinergic vagal inhibition of the heart, thus causing an increase in heart rate; but causes little or no effect on blood pressure. Central nervous system disturbances, particularly euphoria, restlessness, and delirium, may occur in the elderly or when excessive dosages are taken. Scopolamine may cause minor stimulation of the central nervous system, but when hypnotic doses are administered, it will induce amnesia, drowsiness, and dreamless sleep.

Therapeutic Uses

In addition to their antispasmodic and ophthalmic effects, antimuscarinic agents are also useful for preparing clients preoperatively, inhibiting parkinsonism or drug-induced tremors and rigidity, preventing motion sickness, and relieving rhinitis. Since these drugs inhibit salivary, gastric, bronchial, pancreatic, and lacrimal secretions, clients are often injected with a narcotic 30 to 60 minutes preoperatively to "dry up" secretions and to counteract the untoward effects of inhaled anesthetic agents. (See Chapters 42, 55, and 79 for details concerning the therapeutic effects of the anticholinergic agents in these disorders.)

Untoward Reactions

Atropine and other antimuscarinic agents produce a number of diverse effects on the body that are responsible for their therapeutic and untoward effects. The untoward effects are a result of undesirable secondary effects. Although inhibition of exocrine secretions is desirable in rhinitis and in preoperative clients, dryness of the mouth is an annoying secondary effect when the drugs are administered for parkinsonism.

The following is a list of common untoward reactions that are related to the secondary effects of the drugs' actions.

- Gastrointestinal disturbances: dry mouth, constipation
- Genitourinary disturbances: urinary retention, impotence
- Eye disturbances: blurred vision, photophobia
- Cardiovascular disturbances: tachycardia, flushing of head and neck, arrhythmias
- Skin disturbances: absence of sweating (heat intolerance), dry hot skin

PROPERTIES OF GANGLIONIC BLOCKING AGENTS

Ganglionic blocking agents antagonize the effects of acetylcholine at ganglionic synapses by (1) inhibiting the synthesis and storage of acetylcholine (hemicholinium); (2) inhibiting the release of acetylcholines (certain anesthetics); (3) competitively blocking nicotinic receptor sites (trimethaphan); or (4) antagonizing ganglionic neurotransmission by a combination of these mechanisms.

Primary Actions and Uses

Blockade of sympathetic pathways causes a decrease in vascular tone which results in a drop in blood pressure. Normotensive clients will experience a minimal drop in blood pressure, but a marked drop will occur in hypertensive clients. As peripheral blood vessels dilate and pool blood, there is a decrease in the venous return to the heart (decreased preload) and cardiac output is decreased. In addition, as the blood vessels dilate, the blood flow increases to certain body regions, particularly the skin. Ganglionic blocking agents are therefore potent antihypertensives and some agents, for example tetraethylammonium, are effective in treating peripheral vascular diseases, such as Buerger's disease.

Limited Therapeutic Usefulness

Although ganglionic blocking agents are of use in treating hypertension and peripheral vascular disorders, their usefulness is limited by (1) the development of orthostatic hypotension in some clients; (2) undesired parasympathetic effects (constipation, urinary retention, decreased salivary, gastric, and pancreatic secretions, inhibition of sweating, mydriasis); (3) the development of drug tolerance; and (4) incomplete or erratic absorption from the gastrointestinal tract. Unfortunately, many of these drugs must be administered parenterally and are limited to the treatment of hypertensive crisis. Antihypertensive agents that are effective orally are now available; therefore the use of parenterally administered ganglionic blocking agents is now limited to the short-term control of hypertensive crisis and to the production of controlled hypotension during certain surgical procedures.

ANTIMUSCARINIC AGENTS

GENERIC NAME Atropine sulfate (RX)

TRADE NAME Atropine

CLASSIFICATION Antimuscarinic agent

Source Poisonous alkaloid obtained from botanical sources such as *Atropa belladonna*.

Action Atropine competitively blocks the action of acetylcholine at muscarinic receptor sites located at postganglionic parasympathetic neurons. It has an antispasmodic effect on the smooth muscles of the GI tract and reduces the frequency and strength of contractions.

The smooth muscle of the bladder is also relaxed, but the bladder sphincter is contracted; this effect can cause urinary retention, particularly in older men. Secretions from exocrine glands—salivary, gastric, sweat, lacrimal, pancreatic, and bronchial—are decreased; this action is of therapeutic value in preoperative clients and clients with peptic ulcer (inhibits gastric secretions), but produces undesirable effects, such as dryness of the mouth (therapeutic doses) and extreme hyperthermia (toxic doses), when the drug is used to treat other conditions. Atropine is useful in certain eye disorders, since it causes mydriasis (dilation of the pupils) and cycloplegia (paralysis of the ciliary muscles of accommodation). Although small dosages of atropine will result in a slight decrease in heart rate, large dosages block inhibitory vagal impulses to the heart and result in an increase in A-V conduction (shortened P-R intervals) and heart rate. In therapeutic dosages, atropine has little or no effect on blood pressure, but may cause flushing of the head and neck due to vasodilation. Some dilation of the bronchial tree also occurs, but this effect is minimal. The CNS is stimulated but behavioral changes—euphoria, restlessness, and delirium—do not occur unless toxic dosages are taken.

Indications for Use Antidote for anticholinesterase insecticide poisoning (organophosphate compounds); preoperative preparation of clients (decreases secretions and blocks vagal cardiac reflex); bradycardia; as an adjunct in the treatment of peptic ulcers, irritable bowel syndrome, neurogenic bowel disturbances, and other spastic GI disorders; eye examination; acute inflammation of the iris.

Contraindications Narrow-angle glaucoma, urinary retention of prostatic hypertrophy, obstruction of the GI or genitourinary tract, paralytic ileus, toxic megacolon, myasthenia gravis.

Warnings and Precautions Use with caution in pregnancy, in clients with hyperthyroidism, coronary artery disease, arrhythmias, congestive heart failure, hypertension, ulcerative colitis, hiatal hernia associated with reflux esophagitis, or hepatic or renal disorders and in debilitated clients with chronic obstructive pulmonary disease, since mucous plugs may occur. Use with extreme caution in clients with acute hemorrhage, since reflex tachycardia may be suppressed and result in shock. May precipitate latent glaucoma or urinary retention in clients over 40 years. Children under 6 years may have an exaggerated response to the drug's action. Heat exhaustion or stroke may be precipitated ın humid environments, since the ability to lose body heat by perspiration is reduced.

Untoward Reactions Common secondary effects include dry mouth, blurred vision, photophobia, and tachycardia; flushing of the head and neck may also occur. Anhydrosis, the absence of sweating, may produce intolerance to heat and may seriously impair body temperature regulation, particularly when high dosages are used. Constipation is a common secondary reaction, particularly in elderly and debilitated clients over 40 years. Impotence has been reported in young males. CNS disturbances, including dizziness, restlessness, tremors, and fatigue, may occur. Allergic skin reactions include various rashes that may progress to exfoliative dermatitis. Toxicity is manifested by tachycardia, arrhythmias, dry and hot skin, impairment of speech and swallowing, headache, restlessness, marked blurring of vision, and difficult micturition. Toxicity may progress to scarlet flushing of skin, weak thready pulse, extreme dilation of pupils, hallucinations, atonia, delirium, and coma.

Parameters of Use

Absorption Rapidly absorbed from GI tract and parenteral sites. Little systemic absorption occurs through skin or mucus membranes of adults, but may occur in children. Crosses placenta and is found in breast milk.

Distribution Rapidly disappears from blood into tissues.

Metabolism Hydrolyzed by enzymes in the liver and other tissues.

Excretion Primarily by the kidneys as unchanged drug and metabolites. Small quantities found in body secretions.

Drug Interactions Atropine antagonizes the action of anticholinesterases and is therefore useful as an antidote. Atropine antagonizes the respiratory depression induced by morphine, but may intensify morphine-induced nausea and vomiting. Atropine delays gastric emptying and may delay or even reduce the amount of orally administered drugs absorbed. Some drugs, such as levodopa, are inactivated in the acidic environment of the stomach, and may produce an inadequate therapeutic response. Drugs that may have some anticholinergic activity, such as tricyclic antidepressants, meperidine, certain antihistamines, and phenothiazines, may have additive or potentiating effects when given concurrently. Meperidine and atropine are frequently given together preoperatively and may cause marked flushing and dryness of the mouth. Respiratory depression may also occur. MAO inhibitors may potentiate the effects of atropine; administer antimuscarinic agents with extreme caution to clients who have received MAO inhibitors within the last 2 weeks. Aluminum-containing antacids inhibit the GI absorption of atropine and homatropine; do not administer simultaneously. Physostigmine salicylate is an effective antidote for atropine toxicity.

Administration

- *Antidote for anticholinesterase:* 2 mg or IV; repeat qlh until symptoms disappear; as much as 6 mg may be required in severe cases.
- *Preoperative preparation:* Adults: 0.4 to 0.6 mg IM 45 to 60 minutes before anesthesia; Children: 0.1 mg/kg IM 45 to 60 minutes before anesthesia; maximum dosage: 0.4 mg.
- *Bradycardia:* Adults: 0.5 to 1.0 mg IV bolus; repeat every 5 minutes, as necessary; Maximum dosage 2 mg; doses less than 0.5 mg may induce bradycardia. Children: 0.01 mg/kg; repeat every 4 to 6 hours, as needed; Maximum dosage 0.4 mg.
- *Adjunct in GI disorders:* Adults: 0.4 to 0.6 mg po every 4 to 6 hours. Children: 3 to 10 kg: 0.1 to 0.15 mg po

every 4 to 6 hours; 11 to 29 kg: 0.12 to 0.3 mg po every 4 to 6 hours; 30 to 40 kg: 0.4 to 0.6 mg every 4 to 6 hours.

Available Drug Forms Vials of 1 ml containing 0.4, 1.0, or 1.2 mg/ml; Prefilled syringes containing 0.5 mg/5 ml or 1 mg/10 ml. Oral tablets; Ophthalmic solution.

Nursing Management

Planning factors

1. Have client void before administering drug.
2. Obtain baseline blood pressure and vital signs.
3. An eye examination for glaucoma should be done before initiating therapy.
4. Obtain history of GI and genitourinary disturbances.
5. Cardiac monitoring is highly recommended when atropine is used for bradycardia.

Administration factors

1. When administering drug orally,
   - (a) Do not administer simultaneously with antacids.
   - (b) Give with a full glass of water.
   - (c) Oral preparation should be given 1 hour after meals, but can be given 30 minutes before meals.
2. Double check dosage when preparing drug for parenteral use. Several dosages are available and a small accidental overdose may result in toxicity.
3. When administering drug parenterally,
   - (a) Most preoperative medications, such as meperidine, can be mixed in the same syringe, but be careful to avoid contamination of a multidose vial.
   - (b) Administer parenteral medication deep into tissues.
   - (c) Inject IV bolus within 1 minute. Bradycardia may occur initially, but usually disappears within 1 to 2 minutes.
   - (d) Bedrest and side rails are recommended when large dosages are used.

Evaluation factors

1. Monitor vital signs frequently (every 1 to 2 hours) when large dosages are used.
2. Continuous cardiac monitoring is necessary when large dosages are used. Notify physician if premature ventricular contractions or excessive tachycardia occur.
3. Measure input and output. If urinary hesitancy occurs, notify physician.
4. Observe children under 6 years, the elderly, and debilitated clients frequently for toxicity. Notify physician if tachycardia, arrhythmias, restlessness, or marked dilation of pupils occur.
5. Eye examinations for glaucoma should be done periodically (monthly)

Client teaching factors

1. Warn client against rapid changes in position for the first 1 to 2 hours following drug administration, since orthostatic hypotension may occur, particularly in the elderly.
2. Instruct client to void before taking drug.
3. Instruct client to inform health professionals immediately if difficulty in voiding or marked blurring of vision occur.
4. Warn client about dryness of mouth. Cold drinks, ice chips, and sugarless gum may help.
5. When appropriate, instruct client to drink at least 2000 ml of fluid daily to avoid constipation.
6. Warn client to avoid excessive exposure to heat, since heat exhaustion may occur.
7. Instruct client to wear sunglasses in bright sunlight.

GENERIC NAME Atropine methyl nitrate (RX)

TRADE NAME Festalan

CLASSIFICATION Antimuscarinic agent

See atropine sulfate for Contraindications, Warnings and precautions, Untoward reactions, Parameters of use, Drug interactions, and Nursing management.

Action Reduces GI muscle tone and spasms. (See atropine sulfate.)

Indications for Use Spastic and hypermobility of GI tract, irritable colon syndrome.

Administration 1 to 2 tablets with meals.

Available Drug Forms Festalan also contains lipase 6000 units, amylase 30,000 units, protease 20,000 units, hemicellulase 50 mg, and bile concentrate 25 mg.

GENERIC NAME Atropine oxide hydrochloride

TRADE NAME X-Tro Genatropin (RX)

CLASSIFICATION Antimuscarinic agent

See atropine sulfate for Contraindications, Warnings and precautions, Untoward reactions, Parameters of use, Drug interactions, and Nursing management.

Action Slow release of atropine for prolonged action. (See atropine sulfate.)

Indications for Use As an adjunct in the treatment of a peptic ulcer, neurogenic bowel disturbances, and other functional GI disturbances.

Administration 0.5 to 1.0 mg po tid or qid.

Available Drug Forms Capsules with or without phenobarbital.

GENERIC NAME Atropine tannate (RX)

TRADE NAME Atratan

CLASSIFICATION Antimuscarinic agent

See atropine sulfate for Contraindications, Warnings and precautions, Untoward reactions, Parameters of use, Drug interactions, and Nursing management.

Action Long-acting salt of atropine that relieves smooth muscle spasms and pain. (See atropine sulfate.)

Indications for Use Ureteral colic, following cystoscopy, renal colic.

Administration 1 to 2 mg po q4h, as needed.

GENERIC NAME Glycopyrrolate (RX)

TRADE NAME Robinul

CLASSIFICATION Antimuscarinic agent

See atropine sulfate for Contraindications, Warnings and precautions, Untoward reactions, Parameters of use, and Drug interactions.

Action Similar to atropine but completely ionized at physiologic pH values and has fewer untoward reactions. (See atropine sulfate.)

Indications for Use Preoperative preparation, as an adjunct in the treatment of peptic ulcer, reversal of neuromuscular blockade.

Administration

- *Preoperative preparation:* Adults and children over 2 years: 0.002 mg/lb IM 30 to 60 minutes before anesthesia; Children: Under 2 years: Up to 0.004 mg/lb may be required.
- *Adjunct in peptic ulcer:* 0.1 to 0.2 mg IM or IV q4h; up to 4 doses daily.
- *Reversal:* 0.2 mg IV for each 1.0 mg neostigmine or 5.0 mg pyridostigmine; may be mixed in same syringe.

Available Drug Forms Tablets containing 1 or 2 mg; vials containing 0.2 mg/ml.

Nursing Management (See atropine sulfate.)

1. Unstable in solutions with a pH of 6 or greater.
2. May be mixed with 5% D/W, 5% D/S, meperidine, morphine, Innovar, or hydroxyzine.
3. Store at room temperature (59 to 86° F).
4. Check injectable solutions for particulate matter and discoloration before administration.
5. Not recommended for continuous use in children.

GENERIC NAME Homatropine methylbromide

TRADE NAMES Homolone, Mesopin, Novatrin, Novatropine

CLASSIFICATION Antimuscarinic agent (RX)

See atropine sullfate for Contraindications, Warnings and Precautions, Untoward reactions, Parameters of use, Drug interactions, and Nursing management.

Source Synthetic quaternary ammonium derivative of belladonna alkaloids.

Action Less CNS stimulation than atropine. Reduces GI muscle spasms and secretions. May cause drowsiness and blurred vision. (See atropine sulfate for further details.)

Indications for Use As an adjunct in the treatment of peptic ulcer.

Administration 1 tablet 30 minutes before meals and at bedtime.

Available Drug Forms Tablets containing 5 or 10 mg.

GENERIC NAME Hyoscyamine (RX)

CLASSIFICATION Antimuscarinic agent

See atropine sulfate for Contraindications, Warnings and precautions, Untoward reactions, Parameters of use, Drug interactions, and Nursing management.

Action Relieves smooth muscle spasms and pain. Toxicity may occur with as little as 0.6 mg. (See atropine sulfate.)

Indications for Use Hypermotility of lower urinary tract.

Administration 0.15 to 0.3 mg po tid or qid.

Available Drug Forms Tablets containing 0.15 mg.

GENERIC NAME Hyoscyamine hydrobromide

CLASSIFICATION Antimuscarinic agent (RX)

See atropine sulfate for Contraindications, Warnings and precautions, Untoward reactions, Parameters of use, Drug interactions, and Nursing management.

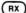

Action Similar to hyoscyamine sulfate, but is not deliquescent. Similar action as atropine, but less CNS stimulation occurs. (See atropine sulfate.)

Indications for Use Urinary antispasmodic (most frequent use), as an adjunct in the treatment of peptic ulcer, spastic GI disorders, diverticulitis, irritable bowel syndrome, neurologic bowel disturbances, infant colic, biliary and renal colic, antidote for anticholinesterase compounds.

Administration 0.25 to 3.0 mg po or IM q4h, as needed.

Available Drug Forms Contained in preparations such as Butabell HMB, Pyridium Plus, and Urogesic.

GENERIC NAME Hyoscyamine sulfate (RX)

TRADE NAMES Cystopaz-M, Levsin, Levsinex

CLASSIFICATION Antimuscarinic agent

See atropine sulfate for Contraindications, Warnings and precautions, Untoward reactions, Drug interactions, and Nursing management.

Action Relieves smooth muscle spasms and pain. Similar to atropine sulfate, but has the disadvantage of rapid deterioration when exposed to moist air (deliquescence). Must be stored away from light and moisture. (See atropine sulfate.)

Indications for Use As an adjunct in the treatment of peptic ulcer, spastic GI disorders, diverticulitis, irritable bowel disturbances, infant colic, biliary and renal colic, antidote for anticholinesterase compounds.

Parameters of Use

Absorption Completely absorbed from GI tract and other sites of administration. Half-life is $3\frac{1}{2}$ hours.

Traces found in breast milk.

Excretion In urine as unchanged drug within 12 hours.

Administration Adults: Oral: 1 to 2 tablets or 5 to 10 ml tid or qid; 1 sustained-release capsule every 8 to 12 hours. Intramuscular, subcutaneous, intravenous: 0.25 to 0.5 mg as needed; up to 4 doses daily. Children: Oral (elixir); 10 lb: 0.5 to 0.75 ml; 20 lb: 1.25 to 2 ml; 30 lb: 2.5 ml; 50 lb: 3.75 to 5 ml; dosage may be repeated q4h, as needed; up to 4 doses daily. Infants: Oral (drops): 5 lb: 3 gtt; 7.5 lb: 4 gtt; 10 lb: 5 gtt; 15 lb: 6 gtt; 20 lb: 7 gtt; dosage may be repeated q4h, as needed. Ages 1 to 10 years: $\frac{1}{2}$ to 1 ml q4h, as needed.

Available Drug Forms Tablets containing 0.125 mg; elixir containing 0.125 mg/5 ml; infant drops containing 0.125 mg/ml; sustained-release capsules (Cystospaz-M, Levsinex) containing 0.375 mg; ampules containing 0.5 mg/ml. Tablets, elixir, drops, and sustained-release capsules containing phenobarbital are also available. Generic contents in each tablet, 5 ml of elixir, and 1 ml of drops: hyoscyamine: 0.125 mg; phenobarbital: 15 mg. Generic contents in each sustained-release capsule: hyoscyamine: 0.375 mg; phenobarbital: 45 mg.

GENERIC NAME Scopolamine hydrobromide

TRADE NAME Hyoscine Hydrobromide (RX)

CLASSIFICATION Antimuscarinic agent

See atropine sulfate for Contraindications, Warnings and precautions, Untoward reactions, Parameters of use, and Drug interactions.

Action Most stable salt of scopolamine. Similar peripheral action as atropine, but different CNS effects. Large dosages will cause dreamless sleep for about 8 hours and client does not remember events that take place. Because it induces "twilight sleep", or temporary amnesia, when given with morphine, the combination has been used in obstetrics during labor.

Indications for Use Postencephalitic parkinsonism, smooth muscle spasms, preoperative preparation, sedation, hypnosis.

Administration 0.3 to 0.6 mg po or parenteral q4h, as needed; may be given tid or qid.

Available Drug Form Ampules containing 0.4 mg/ml.

Nursing Management The client may be disoriented until sedation occurs. (See atropine sulfate.)

GANGLIONIC BLOCKING AGENTS

GENERIC NAME Hexamethonium bromide, hexamethonium chloride (RX)

CLASSIFICATION Ganglionic blocking agent, antihypertensive agent

---

Action Induces competitive blockade by occupying receptor sites in the ganglia. Potent antihypertensive agent that causes a marked and prolonged drop in blood pressure.

Indications for Use Severe malignant hypertension.

Contraindications Severe cardiac disease, recent myocardial infarction, chronic pyelonephritis, uremia, severe renal insufficiency.

Warnings and Precautions Use with caution in clients with prostatic hypertrophy, glaucoma, pyloric stenosis, or renal, coronary, or cerebrovascular insufficiency. Fever, excessive environmental temperatures, and stress may increase the antihypertensive effect. Abrupt withdrawal may cause rebound hypertension.

Untoward Reactions Orthostatic hypotension, nausea, vomiting, constipation, dry mouth, paresthesia, blurred vision, fatigue, and tremors are common. Choreiform movements and weakness may lead to convulsions when high dosages are used. Headaches, sedation, dizziness, and psychotic disturbances may occur.

Parameters of Use

Absorption Incomplete and erratic absorption from GI tract. Crosses blood-brain barrier.

Drug interactions Antihypertensive effect may be potentiated by alcohol, antihypertensive agents, sympathomimetics, and thiazide diuretics.

Administration Adults: 50 to 100 mg parenterally q6h, as needed; 125 to 250 mg po qid; Maximum dosage: 3000 mg/day.

Available Drug Forms Tablets containing 250 mg; vials containing 30 mg/ml.

Nursing Management

1. Give tablets with meals.
2. Sodium-restricted diets are not necessary.
3. Constipation can usually be relieved with diet changes, Milk of Magnesia, and increased fluid intake. Instruct client to notify physician before using an OTC laxative.
4. Instruct client to avoid excessive heat (showers) and to notify physician if fever occurs.
5. Warn client about orthostatic hypotension.

GENERIC NAME Mecamylamine hydrochloride

TRADE NAME Iversine (RX)

CLASSIFICATION Ganglionic blocking agent, antihypertensive agent

---

See hexamethonium for Contraindications, Warnings and precautions, Untoward reactions, Drug interactions, and Nursing management.

Action Induces competitive and noncompetitive blockade of acetylcholine receptors. Potent antihypertensive agent similar to hexamethonium, but has a longer duration of action and development of tolerance takes longer. Fewer severe side effects than other ganglionic blockers. (See Chapter 50.)

Indications for Use Moderate to severe essential hypertension, uncomplicated malignant hypertension.

Parameters of Use

Absorption Well absorbed from GI tract.

Administration Adults: Initial dosage 2.5 mg po bid; then increase by 2.5 mg every 2 days until desired effect; Average daily dosage: 7.5 mg tid.

Available Drug Forms Tablets containing 2.5 or 10 mg.

GENERIC NAME Pentolinium tartrate (RX)

TRADE NAME Ansilysen

CLASSIFICATION Ganglionic blocking agent, antihypertensive agent

---

See hexamethonium for Contraindications, Warning and precautions, Drug interactions, and Nursing management.

Action Potent antihypertensive agent with relatively long duration of action. Optimal effect is measured by the maximum reduction in blood pressure without causing postural hypotension. (See Chapter 50.)

Indications for Use Moderate to severe hypertension.

Untoward Reactions Painful irritation at injection site (See hexamethonium.)

Parameters of Use

Absorption Moderately well absorbed from GI tract.

Administration Adults: Initial dosage: 20 mg po q8h; then increase every 2 to 5 days until desired effect; can be administered IM or subc, but not IV.

Available Drug Forms Tablets containing 20, 100, or 200 mg; vials containing 10 mg/ml.

GENERIC NAME Tetraethylammonium chloride

TRADE NAME Etamon (RX)

CLASSIFICATION Ganglionic blocking agent

See hexamethonium for Contraindications, Untoward reactions, Drug interactions, and Nursing management.

Action Blocks sympathetic vasospasm and results in an increased blood supply to affected tissues and a decrease in blood pressure. Neostigmine is an effective antidote.

Inidications for Use Peripheral vascular diseases (Buerger's disease), diagnosis of pheochromocytoma.

Warnings and Precautions Use with caution in the elderly, since hypotension may occur. (See hexamethonium.)

Parameters of Use

Absorption Short duration of action. Ineffective when administered orally.

Administration Highly individualized. Do not exceed 7 mg/kg; administered IM or IV.

Available Drug Forms Vials containing 100 mg/ml.

GENERIC NAME Trimethaphan camsylate (RX)

TRADE NAME Arfonad

CLASSIFICATION Ganglionic blocking agent, antihypertensive agent

---

Action Induces competitive blockade and stabilizes postsynaptic membrane against acetylcholine. Induces vasodilation. (See Chapter 50.)

Indications for Use Hypertensive crisis, controlled hypertension during surgery occur associated with excessive bleeding (neurosurgical procedures).

Contraindications Pregnancy, hypovolemia, shock, asphyxia, anemia, respiratory insufficiency.

Warnings and Precautions Use with caution in clients with a history of allergic disorders. Use with extreme caution in children, the elderly, debilitated clients, in clients with arteriosclerosis, cardiac, hepatic, or renal disease, Addison's disease or diabetes, and those receiving adrenocorticosteroids.

Untoward Reactions Tachycardia and severe orthostatic hypotension are common. Extreme weakness and respiratory depression may occur. Respiratory arrests have been reported. Urinary retention may occur

Parameters of Use

Absorption Ultra-short duration of action (about 10 minutes). Ineffective when administered orally.

Administration Adults: Initial dosage : 1 to 2 mg/min. via continuous IV drip; then adjust to desired blood pressure response; Dosage range: 0.2 to 6 mg/min.

Available Drug Forms Vials containing 50 mg/ml.

Nursing Management

1. Must be diluted. Add 500 mg (10 ml) to 100 ml or more of 5% D/W. Must be freshly prepared.
2. Position client to avoid cerebral anoxia.
3. Administer oxygen therapy.
4. Constant assessment is essential. Adjust IV rate according to blood pressure response.
5. Use an IV pump.
6. Do not use IV line to administer other drugs.
7. Administered only by specially trained health professionals, usually physicians.

GENERIC NAME Trimethidinium methosulfate

TRADE NAME Ostensin (RX)

CLASSIFICATION Ganglionic blocking agent, antihypertensive agent

---

See hexamethonium for Nursing management.

Action Noncompetitive ganglionic blocker. (See Chapter 50.)

Indications for Use Moderate to severe hypertension.

Contraindications Pyloric stenosis, peptic ulcer, severe cerebral arteriosclerosis.

Warnings and Precautions Use with caution in the elderly and in clients with renal disorders.

Untoward Reactions May cause mydriasis, which can be counteracted with pilocarpine.

Administration Adults: Initial dosage: 20 mg po bid; then increase by 20 mg every 3 days until desired effect; Average daily dosage: 40 to 300 mg in divided doses.

Available Drug Forms Tablets containing 20 mg or 40 mg.

Chapter 44

Neuromuscular Blocking Agents

THE NEUROMUSCULAR BLOCKING agents of the voluntary nervous system are actually cholinergic blocking agents. These drugs block the transmission of nerve impulses to the skeletal muscles and are therefore employed as skeletal muscle relaxants. Neuromuscular blocking agents are usually divided into two groups according to their method of action: the *competitive blockers* and the *depolarizing blocking agents.* A knowledge of motoneuron transmission is helpful in understanding how these agents exert their action.

NEUROMUSCULAR INNERVATION

Motor nerves exit the anterior horn of the spinal cord and terminate in skeletal muscle fibers. When the motor nerve is stimulated, acetylcholine is released from tiny vesicles at the neuromuscular junction and crosses the synapse to stimulate nicotinic receptor sites in the motor end plate. Stimulation of these receptors produces changes in the muscle's membrane that result in depolarization and contraction of the muscle. Acetylcholine is rapidly destroyed (hydrolyzed) by the enzyme acetylcholinesterase.

PROPERTIES OF COMPETITIVE BLOCKERS

The drugs in this group compete with acetylcholine for receptor sites and thereby block depolarization of the skeletal muscles. Curare derivatives, such as tubocurarine, are the primary drugs in this group. (A *curariform* action refers to the ability of curare to block skeletal muscle action.) These drugs are frequently used to produce adequate skeletal muscle relaxation or paralysis during general anesthesia for major operations. Since the intercostal muscles, which assist in respiration, may also be paralyzed, apnea may occur and manual or mechanical ventilation must be instituted immediately to prevent hypoxia. Paralysis of intercostal muscles can be advantageous when caring for clients on a respirator, since the machine will be able to adequately ventilate the client under controlled conditions without the client "forcing" against the machine and causing it to cycle prematurely. Unfortunately, these drugs may cause excessive salivary and respiratory secretions; consequently, clients receiving these drugs must be suctioned frequently to prevent hypoxia.

PROPERTIES OF DEPOLARIZING BLOCKING AGENTS

Succinylcholine and other drugs in this group depolarize the motor end plate membrane of skeletal muscles, thus preventing the spread of a depolarizing wave that causes muscle contraction. As long as the drug remains at the end plate, flaccid paralysis occurs. These drugs have a short duration of action because they are rapidly dissipated by the enzyme pseudocholinesterase. The action of succinylcholine is usually prolonged by anticholinesterase agents, such as physostigmine, neostigmine, and edrophonuim; whereas these agents antagonize the action of curare. There is no known antidote for the depolarizing agents. Since hypoxia and apnea can occur, it is essential that measures for ventilating the client manually or mechanically are available.

Repeated use of depolarizing agents will eventually result in *tachyphylaxis,* desensitization of muscle endplates. Consequently, these drugs can only be used for relatively short periods of time.

They have been found to be useful for orthopedic manipulations, diagnostic procedures, such as bronchoscopy, and other short operations.

COMPETITIVE BLOCKERS

GENERIC NAME Tubocurarine chloride (RX)

TRADE NAMES Tubarine, D-Tubocurarine

CLASSIFICATION Neuromuscular blocking agent

Source Alkaloid of curare obtained from the plant *Chondodendron tomentosum.*

Action Tubocurarine produces relaxation of skeletal muscles by competing with the neuromuscular transmitter acetylcholine at cholinergic receptor sites. The drug is frequently used as an adjunct to general anesthesia in surgical procedures to produce adequate relaxation of abdominal and other muscles without using large quantities of anesthetics. Since low dosages of tubocurarine decrease muscle spasticity and produce muscle relaxation, it has been used during convulsive therapy to reduce the incidence of dislocations and bone fractures arising from drug or electrically induced convulsions. In larger dosages, tubocurarine causes respiratory paralysis, an effect that is useful in preventing intubated clients on a respirator from breathing on their own and interfering with the function of the machine. When very small dosages of tubocurarine are administered to clients with myasthenia gravis, their symptoms are markedly exaggerated; therefore the drug is useful in diagnosing this disease when testing with neostigmine or edrophonium is inconclusive.

Although it has a short duration of action, tubocurarine is a potent drug with a very narrow margin of safety and should be used only by specially trained professionals, such as anesthesiologists. The drug stimulates the release of histamine and can cause bronchospasm. It also has ganglionic blocking properties that can result in hypotension. The drug has no effect on consciousness or pain threshold, but when pain does occur, the drug-induced muscle paralysis prevents the client from stating that pain is present.

Indications for Use As an adjunct to anesthesia during surgical procedures and orthopedic manipulations to induce skeletal muscle relaxation; facilitation of endotracheal intubation and mechanical ventilation; prevention of dislocations and bone fractures during electroshock or drug-induced therapy; diagnostic testing for myasthenia gravis.

Contraindications Hypersensitivity to curare derivatives; clients in whom the release of histamine is a definite hazard, such as asthmatics.

Warnings and Precautions Use with caution in the elderly, debilitated clients, and clients with dehydration, electrolyte disturbances, porphyria, or thyroid, renal, hepatic, pulmonary, or neuromuscular disorders. Use with extreme caution in clients with myasthenia gravis. Safe use during pregnancy has not been established; large dosages during cesarean section may cause respiratory depression in the infant. There is no antidote when large dosages are used.

Untoward Reactions Respiratory depression that progresses to apnea and eventually hypoxia may occur, particularly with rapid IV administration or large dosages. Hypotension that may progress to circulatory collapse can occur, particularly in the elderly and clients with preexisting cardiovascular disorders or renal impairment. Bronchospasm may occur, particularly in clients with a history of respiratory-type allergies. Excessive bronchial secretions may also occur. Prolonged or profound muscular relaxation, including residual muscular weakness and flaccidity, may occur.

Parameters of Use

Absorption Slow and irregular following IM administration. Onset of action is: variable (IM); in seconds (IV). Peak action occurs in 2 to 3 minutes following IV administration. Duration of actions is: variable but greater than 25 to 90 minutes (IM); 25 to 90 minutes (IV). Some bound to serum proteins.

Crosses placenta and probably enters breast milk.

Metabolism Some in the liver.

Excretion Rapidly excreted by the kidneys. Primarily as unchanged drug; some found in bile.

Drug Interactions Quinidine prolongs neuromuscular blockage and when clients receive quinidine postoperatively, recurarization may occur and lead to respiratory paralysis; concurrent use is not recommended. The intensity of blockade and duration of action are increased by inhaled anesthetics (halothane, ether, methoxyflurane, enflurane). Aminoglycoside antibiotics (gentamicin, kanamycin, neomycin, streptomycin) potentiate neuromuscular blockade and may lead to respiratory depression; use these antibiotics cautiously postoperatively. Thiazide diuretics, furosemide, ethacrynic acid, narcotic analgesics, and propranolol may potentiate neuromuscular blockade; use these drugs cautiously postoperatively. Depolarizing muscle relaxants, such as succinylcholine, are sometimes used for endotracheal intubation; delay the use of tubocurarine until the effects of succinylcholine disappear. Injections of edrophonium or neostigmine may be used to antagonize the relaxant action of tubocurarine on skeletal muscles.

Administration Highly individualized.

- *Adjunct to anesthesia:* Dosage varies according to anesthetic agent used. Adults: Initial dosage: 40 to 60 units (2 to 3 ml) IV at time of incision or bone manipulation; then 20 to 30 units (1 to 1.5 ml) IV after 3 to 5 minutes, as needed; then 20 units (1 ml) IV prn. Children: 1 unit/kg ($\frac{1}{2}$ unit/lb), as needed; should be on mechanical ventilation
- *Facilitation of mechanical ventilation:* Initial dosage: 10 units (0.50 ml) IV; then adjust dosage to desired response and administer as needed.
- *Convulsive therapy:* Up to $\frac{1}{2}$ unit/lb IV over 60 to 90 minutes; 20 units of calculated dosage are usually withheld initially.
- *Diagnostic test for myasthenia gravis:* $\frac{1}{15}$ to $\frac{1}{5}$ of adult dosage; this is about 5 to 15 units (0.25 to 0.75 ml) for a 150-lb person.

Available Drug Forms Multidose vials containing 20 units/ml (3 mg/ml); 1 mg equals 7 units and 0.05 ml contains 1 unit.

Nursing Management

Planning factors

1. Equipment for endotracheal suctioning and manual or mechanical ventilation should be readily available.
2. IV fluids, vasopressors, and edrophonium or neostigmine should be readily available.
3. Obtain history of thyroid, renal, hepatic, and cardiovascular disorders. If abnormalities exist, notify physician.
4. Baseline serum electrolytes and urinalysis should be obtained; record intake and output.
5. Discard drug if solution is discolored.

Administration factors

1. Drug should be given only by specially trained personnel.
2. Administer slowly at a rate of 20 to 40 units/min. ($\frac{1}{2}$ ml/min.) or less.
3. Discontinue administration if untoward reactions occur.

Evaluation factors

1. Maintain an airway. Be prepared to institute emergency measures for apnea, excessive respiratory secretions, and other untoward reactions.
2. Monitor intake and output.
3. Monitor serum electrolytes.
4. Warning signs and symptoms of respiratory paralysis include inability to move facial muscles (eyelids, smile, difficulty swallowing); then inability of client to squeeze your hand.
5. Monitor vital signs continuously during administration; then every 5 to 15 minutes until muscle action returns; then periodically. Cardiac monitoring is recommended.
6. Residual muscular weakness may last 24 hours or longer. Assist client with turning and ambulation.

GENERIC NAME Gallamine triethiodide (RX)

TRADE NAME Flaxedil

CLASSIFICATION Neuromuscular blocking agent

See tubocurarine hydrochloride for Warnings and precautions, Untoward reactions, Drug interactions, and Nursing management.

Action Synthetic competitive neuromuscular blocking agent about 20% as potent as tubocurarine. It does not cause ganglionic blockade or histamine release.

Indications for Use As an adjunct to anesthesia to induce relaxation; drug or electrically induced convulsive therapy; facilitation of mechanical ventilation.

Contraindications Hypersensitivity to drug or iodides.

Warnings and Precautions Use with caution in clients with thyroid dysfunction or preexisting pulmonary, hepatic, or renal impairment. Decreases vagal stimulation and may result in tachycardia almost immediately after drug administration. Clients with electrolyte imbalance, dehydration, and hypoalbuminemia may be overly sensitive to the drug's action.

Parameters of Use

Absorption Onset of action is about 3 minutes. Peak action occurs in about 3 minutes and duration of action is 15 to 20 minutes. Some bound to serum albumin.

Excretion Primarily by the kidneys as unchanged drug.

Administration Adults and children: Initial dosage: 1 mg/kg IV; then 0.5 to 1.0 mg/kg IV every 30 to 50 minutes, as needed; Maximum dosage: 100 mg. Neonates: Initial dosage: 0.25 to 0.75 mg/kg IV; then 0.01 to 0.05 mg/kg IV every 30 to 50 minutes.

Available Drug Forms Multidose vials containing 20 or 100 mg/ml.

Nursing Management (See tubocurarine chloride.)

1. Protect drug from light and excessive heat. Store at room temperature.
2. Do not mix with other drugs; flush IV line with normal saline before and after drug administration.
3. Monitor vital signs continuously during administration; then every 15 minutes. Cardiac monitoring is recommended.

GENERIC NAME Metocurine iodide (RX)

TRADE NAME Metubine

CLASSIFICATION Neuromuscular blocking agent

See tubocurarine hydrochloride for Warnings and precautions and Untoward reactions.

Action This methyl analog of tubocurarine is a competitive neuromuscular blocking agent and is three times as potent as tubocurarine. The drug reaches myoneural junctions faster and causes less histamine release than tubocurarine. Repeated doses may have a cumulative effect. Skeletal muscle relaxation may be altered by dehydration, body temperature changes, hypocalcemia, excessive magnesium levels, or acid-base imbalances.

Indications for Use As an adjunct to anesthesia to induce skeletal muscle relaxation; drug or electrically induced convulsive therapy; facilitation of endotracheal intubation.

Contraindications Hypersensitivity to curare derivatives or iodides.

Untoward Reactions Histamine release may cause erythema, edema, flushing, tachycardia, hypotension, bronchospasm, and circulatory collapse.

Parameters of Use

Absorption Onset of action is 1 to 4 minutes. Peak action occurs in $1\frac{1}{2}$ to 10 minutes (maximum twitch inhibition). Duration of peak action is 35 to 60 minutes. Half-life is about 36 hours. About 35% bound to beta- and gamma-globulin.

Crosses placenta rapidly.

Excretion Primarily by the kidneys as unchanged drug (50%); some in bile.

Drug Interactions Certain general anesthetics, aminoglycoside antibiotics, polymyxin B, colistin, clindamycin, tetracyclines, quinidine, and narcotic analgesics may potentiate the neuromuscular blocking action of metocurine.

Administration

- *Surgical procedures;* Initial dosage: 0.2 to 0.4 mg/kg continuous IV bolus over 30 to 60 seconds at onset of intubation (effect lasts about 60 minutes); then 0.5 to 1.0 mg as needed.
- *Convulsive therapy:* 1.75 to 5.5 mg continuous IV bolus over 30 to 60 seconds until head drop response occurs; Average dosage: 2 to 3 mg.

Available Drug Forms Multidose vials containing 2 mg/ml.

Nursing Management Unstable in alkaline solutions; do not mix with other drugs; flush IV line with normal saline before and after drug administration. (See tubocurarine chloride.)

GENERIC NAME Pancuronium bromide (RX)

TRADE NAME Pavulon

CLASSIFICATION Neuromuscular blocking agent

Action Synthetic competitive neuromuscular blocking agent that is five times as potent as tubocurarine. Its onset and duration of action are dose related. Pancuronium causes little or no histamine release or ganglionic blockade (thus little or no bronchospasm or hypotension). It has little effect on the circulatory system. Drug action is altered by dehydration, electrolyte imbalances, acid-base imbalances, renal impairment, and other neuromuscular blocking agents.

Indications for Use As an adjunct to anesthesia to induce skeletal muscle relaxation; facilitation of endotracheal intubation and mechanical ventilation.

Contraindications Hypersensitivity to drug or bromides.

Warnings and Precautions Use with caution in clients with preexisting pulmonary, hepatic, or renal impairment. Safe use during pregnancy has not been established. (See tubocurarine chloride.)

Untoward Reactions Tachycardia (common), excessive salivation, residual muscular weakness, prolonged or profound skeletal muscle relaxation, apnea, and a burning sensation at the IV site may occur.

Parameters of Use

Absorption Onset of action is about 45 seconds. Peak action occurs in about $4\frac{1}{2}$ minutes and duration of action is about 60 minutes.

Excretion Primarily by the kidneys as unchanged drug.

Drug Interactions Drug action is antagonized by acetylcholine, anticholinesterases, and potassium ions. Drug action is potentiated by inhaled anesthetics, quinine, quinidine, magnesium salts, hypokalemia, some carcinomas, aminoglycoside antibiotics, polymyxin B, clindamycin, lithium, and narcotic analgesics.

Administration Highly individualized. Adults: Initial dosage: 0.04 to 0.1 mg/kg IV bolus, then 0.01 mg/kg IV bolus as needed (q1h during anesthesia or every 1 to 2 hours to facilitate clients on respirators). Children: Initial dosage: 0.04 to 0.1 mg/kg IV bolus; then $\frac{1}{5}$ of initial dosage IV bolus, as needed (every 30 to 60 minutes). A test dose of 0.02 mg/kg is recommended for neonates, since they are very sensitive to the drug.

Available Drug Forms Multidose vials of 10 ml containing 1 mg/ml; single-dose ampules of 2 or 5 ml containing 2 mg/ml.

Nursing Management (See tubocurarine chloride.)

1. Do not mix with other drugs; flush IV line with normal saline before and after drug administration.
2. Store in refrigerator; do not store in plastic syringes.

DEPOLARIZING BLOCKING AGENTS

GENERIC NAME Succinylcholine chloride (RX)

TRADE NAMES Anectine, Choline Chloride Succinate, Quelicin

CLASSIFICATION Neuromuscular blocking agent

Action Succinylcholine, a synthetic compound that chemically resembles acetylcholine, depolarizes the end plate membrane of skeletal muscles and makes the end plate insensitive to acetylcholine, thus inducing skeletal muscle paralysis. It competes with acetylcholine for cholinergic receptor sites. Initially, stimulation of the end plate results in muscular twitching, or fasciculations; but this effect is quickly followed by flaccid paralysis of skeletal muscles, which will last as long as adequate quantities of the drug remain at receptor sites. Succinylcholine is considered an ultra-short neuromuscular blocking agent because it is rapidly dissipated by the enzyme pseudocholinesterase. Anticholinesterases, such as physostigmine, neostigmine, and edrophonium, usually prolong the action of succinylcholine, whereas they antagonize tubocurarine. Repeated use of depolarizing agents eventually causes tachyphylaxis, desensitization of the endplates. The secondary effects of succinylcholine include a slight, transient increase in intraocular pressure due to the brief contraction of intraocular muscles during the initial fasciculation phase. The drug should not be used for the surgical repair of acute eye injuries and should be used cautiously in clients with glaucoma. Although the drug has no direct effect on the myocardium, the vagus nerve is stimulated and may result in bradycardia, hypotension, and arrhythmias, particularly during endotracheal intubation of children. Eventually, a reflex tachycardia may occur due to an asphyxial pressor response and mild stimulation of sympathetic ganglia.

Indications for Use When skeletal muscle relaxation is required for short periods of time, such as orthopedic manipulations and endotracheal intubation; as an adjunct to anesthesia to induce skeletal muscle relaxation; to reduce the intensity of skeletal muscle contractions caused by drug or electrically induced convulsions.

Contraindications Hypersensitivity to drug, marked lack of plasma pseudocholinesterase, marked hypovolemia.

Warnings and Precautions Use with caution in clients with severe hepatic disease, cirrhosis, severe anemia, malnutrition, severe dehydration, abnormal body temperature, exposure to insecticides, or receiving antimalarial agents, since depression of serum pseudocholinesterase levels occur; in clients with hyperkalemia, paraplegia, spinal cord injuries, or degenerative neuromuscular disorders, since severe hyperkalemia may occur; in clients with glaucoma and during ocular surgery; and in clients with fractures, since the fasciculation phase may cause further damage. Safe use during pregnancy has not been established. Prolonged use of the drug is not recommended.

Untoward Reactions Prolonged respiratory depression may progress to apnea. Hypoxia may occur if the client is not adequately ventilated. (If caused by nondepolarizing metabolites, neostigmine may be helpful). Postoperative muscular pain is common, particularly after repeated doses. Bradycardia with resulting hypotension and arrythmias may occur, particularly in children. This reaction is enhanced with cyclopropane and halothane and may be followed by tachycardia and hypertension. An increase in intraocular pressure may occur. Hyperkalemia may occur in susceptible clients. Rare reactions include excessive salivation, myoglobinemia, and allergic reactions.

Parameters of Use

Absorption Onset of muscular relaxation (low dosages) is within 1 minute, persists for 2 minutes, and returns to normal in 8 to 10 minutes; initially acts on selective muscle groups of face, then limbs, and finally respiratory muscles. Onset of paralysis (larger dosages) is 2 to 3 minutes.

Does not cross placenta.

Metabolism Rapidly hydrolyzed by pseudocholinesterases to succinylmonocholine and then more slowly to the inactive metabolites succinic acid and choline. Succinylmonocholine causes mild nondepolarizing muscle relaxation.

Excretion By the kidneys as unchanged drug (10%) and metabolites.

Drug Interactions Several antibiotics, including aminoglycosides, polymyxin B, and colistin, potentiate neuromuscular blockade. Drugs that inhibit plasma pseudocholinesterase and thus potentiate depolarizing neuromuscular blockade include antimalarial agents, MAO inhibitors, echothiophate, neostigmine, and edrophonium. Lidocaine increases blockade by displacing succinylcholine from plasma protein binding sites. Digitalis glycosides and quinidine may induce arrhythmias.

Administration Highly individualized.

- *Short surgical procedures:* 40 mg IV bolus; repeat as needed; Dosage range: 20 to 80 mg. A test dose of 10 mg may be used to detect hypersensitivity to drug.
- *Long surgical procedures:* Adults: Intial dosage: 40 mg IV bolus or 0.5 to 10 mg/min., continuous IV infusion until desired effect; then 2.5 mg/min. via continuous IV drip; Average initial dosage: 4.3 mg/min. Children: 1.0 to 2.0 mg/kg IM or IV: Maximum dosage: 150 mg.

Available Drug Forms Single-dose vials containing 20 mg/ml; 10 ml multidose vials containing 20 mg/ml; dry powder (FLO-PACK) for preparing continuous IV drip containing 500 or 1000 mg.

Nursing Management

Planning factors

1. Obtain history concerning factors that decrease plasma pseudocholinesterase.
2. Serum pseudocholinesterase activity should be determined before administering drug. Serum electrolytes should also be obtained.
3. Equipment for maintaining respirations manually or mechanically should be readily available for immediate use.
4. Check expiration date before using drug.
5. A test dose may be given to determine client's response to drug.

Administration Factors

1. Drug should be given only by specially trained personnel.
2. Manufactured prepared solutions are usually used for IM injections, initial administration of drug IV, and short procedures.
3. Use freshly reconstituted solution only, since aqueous solutions lose potency rapidly, particularly when exposed to light.
4. Reconstitute dry powder with water or IV solution and add to 500 or 1000 ml of 5% D/W, normal saline, or lactated Ringer's for continuous drip.
5. Date and time continuous drip.
6. Do not mix IV solution with alkaline drugs as precipitation will occur.
7. An infusion pump should be used for continuous drip.
8. IM injections are usually administered deep into deltoid muscle.
9. Maintain patent airway at all times. Suctioning is usually required.

Evaluation factors

1. Untoward reactions are usually related to the drug's primary action.

2. Apnea may occur during initial peak drug action (within 1 to 2 minutes); breathing usually returns after 15 seconds to 3 minutes.
3. Several factors may contribute to prolonged apnea.
4. Monitor vital signs continuously during drug administration.
5. Residual muscular pain or weakness may occur. When narcotics are administered, observe client for depressed respirations. If symptoms occur, notify physician. Certain antibiotics can also cause depressed respirations.

GENERIC NAME Decamethonium bromide (RX)

TRADE NAME Syncurine

CLASSIFICATION Neuromuscular blocking agent

See succinylcholine chloride for Drug interactions.

Action Action is similar to succinylcholine, but less predictable. (See succinylcholine chloride.)

Indications for Use As an adjunct to anesthesia to induce skeletal muscle relaxation, particularly procedures lasting less than 20 minutes; facilitation of endotrachial intubation; to reduce contractions and complications caused by drug or electrically induced convulsions.

Contraindications Hypersensitivity to bromides, impaired renal function, hypovolemia.

Warnings and Precautions Use with caution in the elderly, debilitated clients, in clients requiring lithotomy or Trendelenburg's position, and in clients with hepatic, renal, or pulmonary impairment or electrolyte imbalances (Na, K, Ca). (See succinylcholine chloride.)

Parameters of Use

Absorption Onset of muscular relaxation is about 4 to 8 minutes. Duration of action is about 20 minutes.

Excretion Primarily by the kidneys as unchanged drug.

Administration Adults: Initial dosage: 0.5 to 3.0 mg slow IV bolus; then 0.5 to 1.0 mg slow IV bolus every 10 to 30 minutes, as needed. Children: Initial dosage: 0.05 to 0.08 mg/kg slow IV bolus; then 0.02 to 0.03 mg/kg every 10 to 30 minutes, as needed.

Available Drug Forms Vials containing 1 mg/ml; dry powder for reconstitution.

Nursing Management (See succinylcholine chloride.)

1. Repeated doses are not recommended since prolonged apnea or reduced muscular relaxation may result.

2. May cause muscular stiffness and pain postprocedure.

GENERIC NAME Hexafluorenium bromide (RX)

TRADE NAME Mylaxen

CLASSIFICATION Neuromuscular blocking agent

See succinylcholine chloride for Warnings and precautions, Parameters of use, Drug interactions, and Nursing management.

Actions Selective inhibitor of plasma cholinesterase with mild competitive neuromuscular blocking action. Prolongs the effect of succinylcholine and decreases fasciculations that occur with this drug. (See succinylcholine chloride.)

Indications for Use To prolong the duration of succinylcholine action. (See succinylcholine chloride.)

Contraindications Hyersensitivity to bromides, clients with bronchial asthma, elderly or debilitated client.

Untoward Reactions May prolong neuromuscular blockade unduly. May cause bronchospasm. (See succinylcholine chloride.)

Administration Initial dosage: 0.4 mg/kg IV followed by succinylcholine 0.2 mg/kg; may be repeated every 20 to 30 minutes; Maximum dosage: 36 mg.

Available Drug Forms Multidose ampules and vials containing 20 mg/ml.

Chapter 45

Antiparkinsonian Agents

PARKINSONISM IS A syndrome that affects more than a million individuals in the United States. It is considered the single most common neurogenic disease that is nonvascular in nature. Parkinsonism may result from (1) poisoning with carbon monoxide, magnesium, or other toxic substances; (2) as a sequela to enchephalitis caused by certain viruses; (3) arteriosclerosis involving the basal ganglia; or (4) the cause may be unknown (idiopathic parkinsonism). Since the advent of tranquilizers for the treatment of mental disorders, drug-induced extrapyramidal symptoms similar to parkinsonism have become a major concern. The long-term use of trifluoperazine, phenothiazines, reserpine, and other drugs will induce symptoms similar to parkinsonism, particularly when high dosages are used.

MANIFESTATIONS OF PARKINSONISM

Parkinsonism is characterized by muscular rigidity, tremors, which are often seen as "pill-rolling" between the fingers and thumb, and impairment of involuntary movements, which is called *dyskinesia*. Early symptoms include stiffness, hesitation before changing position, and impaired handwriting. Although intelligence is not affected and purposeful motions are initially unimpaired, automatic movements become progressively worse. The client develops a lack of facial expression, blepharospasm, periods of involuntary deviation and fixation of the eyeball (oculogyric crisis), speech disturbances, drooling, difficulty in swallowing, and disturbances in the neurons of the brain's basal ganglia.

Imbalance Between Dopamine and Cholinergic Neuron Stimulation

In the corpus striatal region of the basal ganglia, dopamine released from nigrostriatal neurons inhibits cholinergic neuron excitation. Thus stimulation of certain dopamine receptors prevents excessive cholinergic stimulation in the basal ganglia. Idiopathic and encephalitic parkinsonism are associated with degeneration of nigrostriatal neurons, and this results in a lack of dopamine and its inhibitory effects on cholinergic neurons. It is the uninhibited excitation of cholinergic neurons in the basal ganglia that leads to parkinsonism symptoms. Although the nigrostriatal neurons remain intact in drug-induced parkinsonism, reserpine and other central nervous system depressants are thought to decrease the quantity of dopamine present in the striatum. Phenothiazines and other tranquilizers actually block stimulation of dopamine receptor sites by dopamine. Both drug-induced actions result in extrapyramidal symptoms similar to parkinsonism.

TYPES OF ANTIPARKINSONIAN AGENTS

Drugs that decrease the cholinergic activity in the basal ganglia or restore the inhibitory effects of dopamine receptor stimulation are effective in controlling the symptoms of parkinsonism. Until the late 1960s, only drugs with anticholinergic activity were available; as the client's symptoms progressed, the characteristic tremors could only be controlled by brain surgery. Levodopa, the precursor of dopamine, was released for use in 1970. Both levodopa and anticholinergic drugs are used today.

Anticholinergic agents, such as trihexyphenidyl, are effective in controlling the rigidity and tremors of parkinsonism. Drugs that block the brain's muscarinic receptor sites are particularly effective; unfortunately, these atropinelike drugs cause numerous untoward reactions, including dry mouth, constipation, blurred vision, and urinary retention. When necessary, the long-acting drug benztropine can be injected and is used for clients who are unable to take oral medication. The newer synthetic anticholinergic agents are effective in controlling akinesia, as well as rigidity and tremors.

Antihistamines, such as diphenhydramine, and the *phenothiazine derivative* ethopropazine have anticholinergic properties and are therefore useful in controlling symptoms of parkinsonism. The effectiveness of antihistamines and ethopropazine seems to be related to their anticholinergic properties. These drugs tend to cause drowsiness and other central nervous system disturbances.

Levodopa increases the amount of dopamine in the basal ganglia. Dopamine is unable to cross the blood-brain barrier, but levodopa can and is converted to dopamine by the nigrostriatal nerve endings. Although parkinsonism symptoms do not improve immediately, continued use of the drug will first result in improvement of akinesia and then rigidity and tremors. Levodopa is like insulin to diabetes; it does not cure the disease, it only replaces a necessary body substance. If the drug is not taken regularly, symptoms will reappear. Due to the high incidence of untoward reactions, levodopa treatment is initiated at relatively low dosages and the dosage is then gradually increased every 5 to 7 days until the maximum benefit is obtained with the minimum of untoward reactions, particularly nausea and orthostatic hypotension. As the effectiveness of levodopa varies from individual to individual, dosages are highly individualized.

Carbidopa prevents the degradation of levodopa by body tissues so that larger quantities of intact levodopa molecules are available to cross the blood-brain barrier. Carbidopa exerts its action by inhibiting the enzyme dopa decarboxylase, which catalyzes the conversion of levodopa to dopamine. Since carbidopa is unable to cross the blood-brain barrier, its action is limited to tissues outside the brain. When carbidopa is administered concurrently with levodopa, lower dosages of levodopa are required to sustain therapeutic drug levels in the blood and therefore the brain. Other inhibitors of dopa decarboxylase are being investigated.

Amantadine is actually an antiviral agent, but has been found to be effective in treating parkinsonism. Although the exact mechanism of action is unknown, amantadine is thought to stimulate the release of dopamine from nigrostriatal neurons, thus causing increased dopamine levels in the basal ganglia. Unlike levodopa, amantadine is effective therapeutically within 2 to 4 weeks and causes few untoward reactions.

Bromocriptine was introduced as an inhibitor of prolactin secretion from the anterior pituitary gland. The drug has been found to be a potent stimulator of dopamine receptor sites in the corpus striatum and is therefore useful in the treatment of parkinsonism. Unfortunately, the drug is less effective than levodopa and can induce marked behavioral changes. However, combined therapy with levodopa permits smaller dosages of each drug to be used in order to control the symptoms of parkinsonism.

ANTICHOLINERGIC AGENTS

GENERIC NAME Trihexyphenidyl hydrochloride

TRADE NAMES Artane, Hexyphen, Pipanol, Tremin, Trihexidyl

CLASSIFICATION Anticholinergic agent (RX)

Action Trihexyphenidyl, a synthetic tertiary amine, causes relaxation of smooth musculature through a direct action on the muscle tissue and indirectly by inhibiting the parasympathetic nervous system. Its antispasmodic activity is about one-half as effective as atropine; but trihexyphenidyl causes milder secondary effects, such as mydriasis, drying of secretions, and cardioacceleration. The drug is particularly effective in reducing the rigidity associated with all forms of parkinsonism and is effective in treating extrapyramidal disorders caused by CNS drugs, such as dibenoxazepines, phenothiazines, thioxanthenes, and butyrophenones. It is said to partially relieve some of the depression associated with parkinsonism.

Indications for Use Drug-induced extrapyramidal disorders, as an adjunct in the treatment of postencephalitic, arteriosclerotic, and idiopathic parkinsonism.

Contraindications Although it is not contraindicated in hypertensive clients, these clients should be assessed frequently for untoward reactions.

Warnings and Precautions Use with caution in clients with glaucoma, obstructive disorders of the GI tract, and elderly clients with prostatic hypertrophy. Elderly clients (over 60 years) and clients with arteriosclerosis or a history of drug hypersensitivity may be hypersensitive to the drug's action and may require reduced dosages during long-term therapy. Incipient glaucoma may be precipitated.

Untoward Reactions Mild secondary reactions such as dry mouth, blurred vision, dizziness, nausea, and nervousness, are experienced by 30 to 50% of clients. These symptoms tend to disappear during long-term therapy. Untoward reactions characteristic of atropine, including suppurative parotitis, skin rashes, colon dilation, paralytic ileus, delusions, and hallucinations, rarely occur. Dilation of the pupil and increased intraocular tension may progress to angle-closure glaucoma during long-term therapy. GI disturbances, including nausea, vomiting, and constipation, may occur. Urinary hesitancy and retention may occur, particularly in elderly males. Drowsiness, tachycardia, weakness, and headaches may occur. Elderly clients and clients with arteriosclerosis or a history of drug hypersensitivity may develop CNS disturbances, including confusion, amnesia, agitation, paranoid behavior, nausea, and vomiting.

Parameters of Use

Absorption Rapidly absorbed from GI tract; may be irritating to GI tract. Onset of action is about 1 hour. Peak action occurs in 2 to 3 hours and duration of action is 6 to 12 hours.

Metabolism Unknown.

Excretion By the kidneys.

Drug Interactions Concurrent therapy with antihistamines has additive anticholinergic effects and may cause excessive dryness of the mouth, loss of teeth, and suppurative parotitis. Concomitant-therapy with amantadine may cause CNS disturbances, such as confusion, agitation, delusions, and hallucinations. The dosage of trihexyphenidyl should be reduced before instituting amantadine therapy.

Administration Highly individualized. Reduced dosages are required in clients over 60 years.

- *Drug-induced extrapyramidal disorders:* If the dosage of the causative agent is reduced, less trihexyphenidyl is required to eliminate the extrapyramidal symptoms. Initial dosage: 1 mg po daily after a meal; 1 mg po bid after meals; then 1 mg po tid after meals; then increase by 1 to 2 mg po daily; Dosage range: 5 to 15 mg daily. Dosage may be reduced when the symptoms are controlled for several days.
- *Idiopathic and postencephalitic parkinsonism:* Initial dosage: 1 mg po daily after meals; then increase by 2 mg daily every 3 to 5 days; give in 2 to 3 divided doses after meals; Dosage range for idiopathic: 6 to 10 mg daily; Dosage range for postencephalitic: 12 to 15 mg daily. Clients receiving other antiparkinsonian agents, particularly levodopa, may only require 3 to 6 mg daily.

Available Drug Forms Scored tablets containing 2 or 5 mg; elixir containing 2 mg/5 ml; sustained-release capsules containing 5 mg (used after desired dosage has been established).

Nursing Management

Planning factors

1. Assess the amount of muscular rigidity, drooling, and other symptoms before instituting therapy.
2. Gonioscopic evaluation and intraocular pressure should be determined before initiating therapy.
3. Obtain history of drug hypersensitivities and the presence of urinary disturbances, particularly in elderly males.
4. Client may require cool drinks, ice chips, or sugarless gum to control dry mouth.
5. Optimal therapeutic effects may not be apparent for several days.

Administration factors

1. Give after meals with a full glass of water.
2. Provide client with a full pitcher of ice water or other measures to control dry mouth.
3. Drug can be given 3 minutes before meals; but may cause nausea.

Evaluation factors

1. Assess the type and severity of symptoms daily when drug is first instituted or dosage adjusted.
2. Assess the presence of CNS disturbances in elderly clients daily when drug is first instituted or dosage adjusted.
3. Record intake and output. Notify physician if urinary retention occurs.
4. Intraocular pressure should be determined periodically (every 3 to 6 months).
5. Tolerance to the drug may develop with long-term therapy. Assess the symptoms of parkinsonism monthly. A flowchart is helpful.

Client teaching factors

1. Caution client against driving or engaging in other activities that require constant attention until dosage adjustment is complete.
2. Caution client against the use of candy for dry mouth, unless the client can maintain dental hygiene.
3. Advise client to void before taking drug.
4. Instruct client on long-term therapy to report the return of symptoms (muscular rigidity) to health professionals.

GENERIC NAME Benztropine mesylate (RX)

TRADE NAME Cogentin

CLASSIFICATION Anticholinergic agent

See trihexyphenidyl hydrochloride for Warnings and precautions, Untoward reactions, and Drug interactions.

Action Benztropine exhibits anticholinergic and antihistaminic effects. This drug has the advantage of being injectable and can therefore be used in emergency situations for dystonia. (See trihexyphenidyl hydrochloride.)

Indications for Use Parkinsonism, drug-induced extrapyramidal disorders, acute dystonia (except tardive dyskinesia).

Contraindications Children under 3 years, angle-closure glaucoma. May aggravate tardive dyskinesia and may cause paralytic ileus.

Parameters of Use

Absorption Onset of action is: about 1 hour (po); within minutes (IM, IV). Duration of action is about 8 to 12 hours.

Administration

- *Parkinsonism:* Initial dosage: 0.5 to 1 mg po at bedtime; then increase gradually; Usual dosage: 1 to 2 mg daily.
- *Drug-induced extrapyramidal disorders:* 1 to 2 mg IM; then 1 to 2 mg po bid to prevent reoccurrence.
- *Acute dystonia:* 1 to 2 mg IM or IV; then 1 to 2 mg po bid; may be gradually increased by 0.5 mg/day; Maximum dosage: 6 mg/day.

Available Drug Forms Tablets containing 0.5, 1, or 2 mg; 2-ml ampules containing 2 mg/ml.

Nursing Management Protect ampules from light. (See trihexyphenidyl hydrochloride.)

GENERIC NAME Biperiden hydrochloride (RX)

TRADE NAME Akineton Hydrochloride

CLASSIFICATION Anticholinergic agent

See trihexyphenidyl hydrochloride for Parameters of use, Drug interactions, and Nursing management.

Action More effective than atropine in reducing akinesia, rigidity, and tremors. Weak action on intestinal mucosa and blood vessels and little mydriatic activity. Particularly effective in treating drug-induced akathisia, akinesia, dyskinetic tremors, rigidity, oculogyric crisis, and profuse sweating caused by reserpine and phenothiazines. May not be effective for arteriosclerotic parkinsonism.

Indications for Use Drug-induced extrapyramidal disorders, parkinsonism, spastic disorders (multiple sclerosis, cerebral palsy, spinal cord injuries).

Contraindications Hypersensitivity to biperiden preparations.

Warnings and Precautions Safe use in children and during pregnancy and lactation has not been established.

Untoward Reactions Dry mouth and blurred vision are common. GI disturbances may occur, particularly when given on an empty stomach. Hypotension and dizziness may occur.

Absorption Nearly 90% of drug is thought to be absorbed from GI tract.

Administration 2 mg po tid or qid after meals or with food.

Available Drug Forms Scored tablets containing 2 mg.

GENERIC NAME Biperiden lactate (RX)

TRADE NAME Akineton Lactate

CLASSIFICATION Anticholinergic agent

See trihexyphenidyl hydrochloride for Contraindications, Parameters of use, and Drug interactions. See biperiden hydrochloride for Action.

Indications for Use Acute episodes of drug-induced extrapyramidal disorders.

Warnings and Precautions Use with caution in clients with arrhythmias or prostatic hypertrophy.

Untoward Reactions Transient hypotension, confusion, euphoria, and disturbances of coordination may occur.

Administration 5 mg slow IV bolus; may be repeated in 24 hours or 2 mg IM or IV may be repeated every 30 minutes until resolution of symptoms; Maximum dosage: 8 mg/day.

Available Drug Forms Ampules of 1 ml containing 5 mg/ml.

Nursing Management (See trihexyphenidyl hydrochloride.)

1. Do not use if solution is discolored or if a precipitate has formed.
2. Monitor vital signs frequently, particularly in elderly and debilitated clients.
3. Have client void before administering drug, when possible.

GENERIC NAME Chlorphenoxamine hydrochloride

TRADE NAME Phenoxene (RX)

CLASSIFICATION Anticholinergic agent

See trihexyphenidyl hydrochloride for Contraindications, Drug interactions, and Nursing management.

Action Mild anticholinergic activity. Particularly effective in controlling rigidity. Tremors may be augmented.

Indications for Use All forms of parkinsonism.

Warnings and Precautions Use with caution in clients with narrow-angle glaucoma, arrhythmias, or prostatic hypertrophy.

Untoward Reactions Blurred vision, constipation, dry mouth, nausea, and vomiting. May cause drowsiness, particularly in the elderly.

Parameters of Use Similar to trihexyphenidyl, but longer duration. (See trihexyphenidyl hydrochloride.)

Administration 50 to 100 mg po tid or qid after meals.

GENERIC NAME Cycrimine hydrochloride (RX)

TRADE NAME Pagitane Hydrochloride

CLASSIFICATION Anticholinergic agent

See trihexyphenidyl hydrochloride for Parameters of use and Nursing management.

Action Less than half as potent as atropine in reducing neuromuscular symptoms and is slightly more toxic. May not be well tolerated or effective in arteriosclerotic parkinsonism or the elderly. Ineffective for drug-induced extrapyramidal disorders.

Indications for Use Parkinsonism.

Warnings and Precautions Safe use during pregnancy has not been established. Use with caution in the elderly and clients with glaucoma, tachycardia, or urinary retention.

Untoward Reactions Blurred vision, GI disturbances, and dry mouth are common. CNS disturbances may occur.

Administration

- *Postencephalitic parkinsonism:* 5 mg po tid; then increase slowly.
- *Idiopathic and arteriosclerotic parkinsonism:* 1.25 mg po tid; then increase slowly; Maximum dosage: 20 mg/day.

Available Drug Forms Sugar-coated tablets containing 0.25 or 2.5 mg.

GENERIC NAME Procyclidine hydrochloride (RX)

TRADE NAME Kemadrin

CLASSIFICATION Anticholinergic agent

See trihexyphenidyl hydrochloride for Parameters of use, Drug interactions, and Nursing management.

Action Relieves spasticity of voluntary muscles. Particularly effective in reducing rigidity, but may not reduce tremors.

Indications for Use Parkinsonism, drug-induced extrapyramidal disorders, sialorrhea.

Contraindications Angle-closure glaucoma.

Warnings and Precautions Use with caution in clients with mental disorders, since psychotic reactions may be precipitated. Use with caution in the elderly, and in clients with tachycardia, prostatic hypertrophy, or hypotension.

Safe use in children and during pregnancy or lactation has not been established.

Untoward Reactions Low toxicity, but secondary reactions frequently occur with high dosages. Dry mouth, mydriasis, blurred vision, and nausea are common. Suppurative parotitis may occur. Constipation, epigastric distress, and vomiting are relatively common. Allergic skin rashes have occurred. Weakness, confusion, disorientation, agitation, and hallucinations have occurred.

Parameters of Use

Absorption Onset of action is about 30 minutes and duration of action is about 4 hours.

Administration

- *Parkinsonism:* Initial dosage: 2 to 2.5 mg po tid after meals; then increase slowly; usual dosage: 15 to 30 mg daily.
- *Extrapyramidal disorders:* Initial dosage: 2 to 2.5 mg po tid after meals; then increase by 2 to 2.5 mg daily until desired effect; Usual dosage: 10 to 20 mg daily.

Available Drug Forms Scored tablets containing 2 or 5 mg.

ANTIHISTAMINES

GENERIC NAME Diphenhydramine hydrochloride

TRADE NAME Benadryl, Phenamine (RX)

CLASSIFICATION Antiparkinsonian agent

Action Has significant anticholinergic activity. (See Chapter 83.)

Indications for Use Parkinsonism in the elderly who are unable to tolerate other antiparkinsonian agents. Mild parkinsonism in all age groups except newborns. Sometimes used in conjunction with anticholinergic agents for parkinsonism.

Contraindications Neonates, premature infants, breast-feeding mothers, clients with acute bronchial and other lower respiratory tract disorders, clients taking MAO inhibitors.

Warnings and Precautions Use with caution in young children and clients with hyperthyroidism, hypertension, or a history of bronchial asthma. Use with extreme caution in clients with narrow-angle glaucoma, peptic ulcer, pyloric obstruction, or urinary retention. Safe use during pregnancy has not been established.

Untoward Reactions Photosensitivity, diplopia, nausea, dry mouth, constipation, dysuria, and nasal stuffiness are relatively common. Tends to cause drowsiness, particularly in the elderly.

Parameters of Use

Absorption Readily absorbed from GI tract. Peak action occurs in about 60 minutes. Duration of action is 4 to 6 hours. Crosses blood-brain barrier.

Metabolism Mainly by liver; some by other tissues, including the kidneys and lungs.

Excretion In urine, primarily as metabolites.

Drug Interactions Anticholinergic agents and MAO inhibitors may prolong and intensify the anticholinergic effects of antihistamines. Excessive sedation and other CNS disturbances may occur when alcohol, barbiturates, and CNS depressants are used concomitantly.

Administration Adults: 25 to 50 mg po tid or qid; Children under 12 years: 5 mg/kg po daily in 4 divided doses.

Available Drug Forms Capsules containing 25 or 50 mg; Elixir containing 12.5 mg/ml and 14% alcohol; Multidose vials containing 10 mg/ml.

Nursing Management Warn client against concurrent ingestion of alcohol. (See trihexyphenidyl hydrochloride.)

GENERIC NAME Orphenadrine hydrochloride

TRADE NAME Disipal (RX)

CLASSIFICATION Antiparkinsonian agent

See trihexyphenidyl hydrochloride for Nursing management. See diphenhydramine hydrochloride for Indications for use, Contraindications, Warnings and precautions, and Drug interactions.

Action Low antihistaminic, but high anticholinergic action.

Untoward Reactions Dry mouth, constipation, arrhythmias, urinary hesitancy, and paralytic ileus may occur. May cause some drowsiness, but this soon disappears with continued therapy.

Administration 50 mg po qid or 100 mg po bid.

Available Drug Forms Tablets containing 50 mg.

Nursing Management (See trihexyphenidyl hydrochloride.)

PHENOTHIAZINE DERIVATIVES

GENERIC NAME Ethopropazine hydrochloride

TRADE NAME Parsidol (RX)

CLASSIFICATION Antiparkinsonian agent

See trihexyphenidyl hydrochloride for Nursing management.

Action Although the exact mechanism of action is unknown, ethopropazine is effective in controlling the neuromuscular symptoms of all forms of parkinsonism and extrapyramidal disorders induced by reserpine and phenothiazines. The drug exerts a significant anticholinergic and antihistaminic effect. Unlike many of the drugs used in the treatment of parkinsonism, ethopropazine is effective in controlling tremors in most clients. It is also effective in relieving rigidity, spasms, sialorrhea, oculogyric crises, and festination associated with parkinsonism. Unlike phenothiazines, ethopropazine does not potentiate CNS depressants or have an antiemetic effect.

Indications for Use All forms of parkinsonism, drug-induced extrapyramidal disorders (reserpine, phenothiazines).

Contraindications Glaucoma, prostatic hypertrophy.

Warnings and Precautions Use with caution in clients with a history of hypersensitivity to anticholinergic agents. May precipitate toxic psychosis in clients with mental disorders. Safe use during pregnancy and lactation has not been established.

Untoward Reactions Common secondary reactions include drowsiness, inability to think, lassitude, forgetfulness, and confusion. Anticholinergic secondary reactions include dry mouth, nausea, vomiting, blurred vision, diplopia, constipation, and urinary retention. These symptoms tend to disappear with dosage reduction. Mild, transient hypotension may occur when large dosages are administered. Other effects include epigastric distress, muscle cramps, paresthesia, sensation of heavy limbs, and skin rashes. Phenothiazine-related secondary reactions include seizures, slowing of EEG, tachycardia, agranulocytosis, pancytopenia, purpura, jaundice, hallucinations, and pigmentation of the cornea, lens, retina, or skin.

Drug Interactions Unlike other phenothiazines, ethopropazine does not potentiate CNS depressants. Atropine has an additive effect with ethopropazine in the control of oculogyric crises. May mask phenothiazine-induced extrapyramidal disorders, which may become permanent with prolonged phenothiazine therapy.

Administration Highly individualized. Initial dosage: 50 mg po daily or bid; may be gradually increased to 100 to 400 mg po daily in divided doses. Postencephalitic parkinsonism may require as much as 500 to 600 mg daily.

Available Drug Forms Tablets containing 10 or 50 mg.

ANTIPARKINSONIAN AGENTS

GENERIC NAME Levodopa (RX)

TRADE NAMES Dopar, L-Dopa, Larodopa

CLASSIFICATION Antiparkinsonian agent

Action Levodopa is a synthetic levorotatory isomer of dihydroxyphenylalanine (dopa). The symptoms of Parkinson's disease are related to depletion of striatal dopamine in the CNS. Dopamine cannot be given to overcome the deficit since it is unable to cross the blood-brain barrier. However, the precursor of dopamine levodopa is able to penetrate the blood-brain barrier. Levodopa is thought to be converted to dopamine in the basal ganglia, thus relieving the symptoms of parkinsonism by restoring dopamine levels in extrapyramidal centers. Cardiac stimulation may occur due to action on beta-adrenergic receptors and the drug may alter glucose metabolism.

Indications for Use Idiopathic Parkinson's disease (paralysis agitans), postencephalitic parkinsonism associated with carbon monoxide and magnesium poisoning, parkinsonism associated with cerebral arteriosclerosis.

Contraindications Hypersensitivity to levodopa, narrow-angle glaucoma, within 2 weeks of therapy with MAO inhibitors. Levodopa may activate malignant melanoma and should therefore not be used in clients with suspicious or undiagnosed skin lesions.

Warnings and Precautions Use with caution in clients with severe cardiovascular or pulmonary disease, bronchial asthma, wide-angle glaucoma, renal, hepatic, or endocrine disorders, and those receiving antihypertensive drugs. Use with extreme caution in clients with arrhythmias or a history of myocardial infarction. GI hemorrhage may occur in clients with a history of peptic ulcer disease. Psychotic and depressed clients may develop severe depression or suicidal tendencies. Safe use in children under 12 years and during pregnancy has not been established; animal studies indicate abnormal fetal growth and viability.

Untoward Reactions Adventitious movements, such as choreiform and/or dystonia, are common. Involuntary grimacing or head movements, ataxia, tremors, muscular twitching, and body jerks may occur. Bradykinetic episodes in which the adventitious movements are sometimes present and sometimes absent may occur. Other CNS disturbances include loss of memory, delirium, hallucinations, anxiety, nervousness, insomnia, nightmares, fatigue, and euphoria. Cardiac irregularities (arrhythmias) and orthostatic hypotension are relatively common. Changes in mental status are relatively common and include depression, paranoid reactions, and psychotic disturbances. Urinary retention, incontinence, priapism, and excessive or inappropriate sexual behavior may occur. GI disturbances, including nausea, vomiting, and anorexia, are relatively common. Dry mouth, abdominal discomfort, and dysphagia may also occur. Bitter taste, burning sensation of the tongue, diarrhea, and constipation have been reported. Visual disturbances, including blepharospasm, blurring, diplopia, dilated pupils, oculogyric crisis, and activation of latent Horner's syndrome, have occurred. A harmless dark discoloration of urine and sweat may occur. Hepatotoxicity may occur. Leukopenia has occurred and a reduction in hemoglobin and hematocrit has been reported.

Laboratory Interactions Blood urea nitrogen, serum glutamic-oxaloacetic transaminase, serum glutamic-pyruvic transaminase, lactate dehydrogenase, bilirubin, alkaline phosphatase, uric acid, and protein-bound iodine may be elevated. A positive Coombs' test result may occur.

Parameters of Use

Absorption Rapidly and completely absorbed from GI tract; may cause GI disturbances. Peak plasma levels occur in 1 to 3 hours. Therapeutic response lasts about 5 hours.

Metabolism Some converted to dopamine in GI tract and liver; may cause tachycardia and other systemic dopamine effects. Crosses blood-brain barrier; amount entering is variable; then converted to dopa decarboxylase.

Excretion Primarily by the kidneys as metabolites dopamine and homovanillic acid; some excreted in feces.

Drug Interactions Pyridoxine (vitamin B_6) in dosages of 10 to 25 mg will reduce the therapeutic effects of levodopa rapidly. Drugs that decrease the therapeutic effectiveness of levodopa include anticholinergic agents, tricyclic antidepressants, phenothiazines, phenytoin, papaverine, and reserpine. Concomitant administration of antacids or propranolol may increase the therapeutic effects of levodopa. Concurrent therapy with MAO inhibitors is contraindicated within 14 days of levodopa therapy; hypertension may occur. Levodopa may alter the effects of antihypertensive agents and postural hypotension can occur.

Drug Administration Highly individualized; the goal is to induce maximum improvement with the minimum of untoward reactions. Six months of therapy may be required for maximum therapeutic response. Initial dosage: 500 to 1000 mg po daily in 2 or 3 divided doses with food; then increase by 500 to 750 mg daily every 3 to 7 days as tolerated; Maximum dosage: 8 g daily.

Available Drug Forms Scored tablets containing 250, 500, or 1000 mg; capsules containing 250, 500, or 1000 mg.

Nursing Management

Planning factors

1. Obtain history of GI, genitourinary, hepatic, ophthalmic, endocrine, and cardiovascular disorders.
2. Diabetics should be well controlled before instituting drug.
3. Intraocular pressure should be determined before initiating drug. If elevated, notify physician.
4. Determine the potential for drug interactions (include multivitamin preparations).
5. Record symptoms of parkinsonism and their severity.

Administration factors

1. If client is unable to swallow the tablet or capsule, it can be crushed and taken with apple sauce or other food.
2. Give drug with meals.

Evaluation factors

1. Symptoms of parkinsonism should improve in 2 to 4 weeks, but may take up to 6 months. A flow-

chart showing the client's symptoms will demonstrate progress. Assess symptoms weekly.

2. Record all untoward reactions. A flowchart can be helpful. Assess the client every day initially, then weekly.
3. Monitor vital signs periodically (q8h) during dosage adjustments.
4. Muscular twitching and blepharospasm are early warnings of drug toxicity. If symptoms occur, notify physician.
5. Monitor the occurrence of depression. Suicide precautions may be required. Notify physician, as indicated.
6. Clients with glaucoma should have their intraocular pressure checked periodically.
7. Check serum glucose of diabetic clients frequently during dosage adjustments. Urinary testing for sugar content may be unreliable.
8. Dosage should be reduced if drug-induced involuntary muscle movements occur. More than 75% of clients may develop involuntary movements after 1 to 2 years of drug therapy.
9. Clients receiving antihypertensive drugs may require dosage adjustments. Monitor blood pressure and notify physician, as indicated.
10. If surgery is required during levodopa therapy, the drug should be stopped and reinstituted as soon as possible. Lower dosages may be required if client has been off drug for more than a few days.
11. Periodic evaluations of hepatic, renal, hematopoietic, and cardiovascular function are recommended. Complete blood cell count, blood urea nitrogen, and other hepatic function tests should be taken every 1 to 6 months. If hepatotoxicity occurs, the drug should be discontinued.

Client teaching factors

1. Warn client to change position slowly to avoid orthostatic hypotension.
2. Instruct client and family members to administer drug regularly with meals, as prescribed.
3. Warn client that interruptions in drug therapy can cause untoward reactions.
4. Instruct client to consult physician before taking OTC drugs, since many contain drugs that interact with levodopa.
5. Instruct client to consult physician before taking a multivitamin preparation.
6. Inform client that physiotherapy and physical activity will assist in increasing abilities; but warn client to resume activities slowly.
7. Stress the importance of periodic laboratory and medical checkups.

GENERIC NAME Levodopa/carbidopa (RX)

TRADE NAME Sinemet

CLASSIFICATION Antiparkinsonian agent

See Levodopa for Indications for use, Contraindications, and Nursing management.

Action Large dosages of levodopa are required to produce adequate drug levels in the CNS because large quantities are metabolized in the GI tract and liver. Carbidopa is a dicarboxylase inhibitor that is unable to cross the blood-brain barrier. When given in combination, carbidopa inhibits the metabolism of levodopa; thus leaving more intact levodopa available to cross the blood-brain barrier. Carbidopa increases the plasma half-life of both levodopa and homovanillic acid. Consequently, about 75% less levodopa is required to produce a therapeutic effect and fewer untoward reactions (GI disturbances, arrhythmias) occur. An added benefit of the combination drug is that pyridoxine intake does not alter the therapeutic effect of levodopa significantly. Pyridoxine increases the rate of decarboxylation and since carbidopa inhibits this process, pyridoxine supplements do not increase the metabolism of levodopa. Although the combination drug decreases the incidence of GI disturbances and dopamine-related reactions, it does not decrease CNS disturbances. More rapid titration of the drug is also possible.

Warnings and Precautions Levodopa must be discontinued at least 8 hours before instituting the combination drug. (See levodopa.)

Untoward Reactions Choreiform, dystonia, and other involuntary movements are common. Changes in mental status, including depression and psychosis, can occur. Convulsions have been reported, but rarely. Some nausea may occur. (See levodopa.)

Drug Interactions Fewer drug interactions occur with the combination drug than with levodopa. Papaverine, diazepam, clonidine, and phenothiazines may antagonize the therapeutic effects of levodopa. (See levodopa.)

Administration Highly individualized. Initial dosage: 1 to 2 25/250-mg tablets with meals; Maintenance dosage: 3 to 6 25/250-mg tablets daily in divided doses with meals; Maximum dosage: 8 tablets of 25/250 or 25/100 mg daily. If greater quantities of levodopa are needed, plain levodopa is added to the regime. Maximum dosage of carbidopa: 200 mg daily.

Available Drug Forms 10/100 tablets containing 10 mg carbidopa and 100 mg levodopa; 25/100 tablets containing 25 mg carbidopa and 100 mg levodopa; 25/250 tablets containing 25 mg carbidopa and 250 mg levodopa.

GENERIC NAME Amantadine hydrochloride (RX)

TRADE NAME Symmetrel

CLASSIFICATION Antiparkinsonian and antiviral agent

Action Although amantadine was originally released as an antiviral agent, the drug was found to have an antiparkinsonian effect. The exact mechanism of action is unknown, but amantadine is thought to stimulate the release of dopamine from nigrostriatal neurons, since animal studies have demonstrated increased dopamine levels in the brain. Although the drug is less effective than levodopa and lacks anticholinergic activity, amantadine causes relatively fewer serious untoward reactions and therapeutic results occur relatively quickly, usually within 2 to 4 weeks. Amantadine is effective against influenza A virus. The drug apparently prevents the release of infectious viral nucleic acid into the host cell. The drug does not seem to interfere with the vaccine against influenza A virus and can therefore be used prophylactically in conjunction with the vaccine for high-risk clients exposed to the viral infection until adequate antibody formation has occurred.

Indications for Use Idiopathic Parkinson's disease (paralysis agitans), postencephalitic parkinsonism, drug-induced extrapyramidal reactions, parkinsonism associated with head injuries and cerebral arteriosclerosis. Respiratory infections caused by influenza A viral infections in susceptible clients, such as the elderly and debilitated clients.

Contraindications Hypersensitivity to amantadine.

Warnings and Precautions Use with caution in epileptics and clients with seizure disorders, since seizure activity may increase; in clients with a history of congestive heart failure or peripheral edema, since congestive heart failure may be precipitated; in clients with hepatic disorders or with a history of eczematoid rashes. If used concurrently with anticholinergic drugs, the dosage of the latter drug should be reduced if untoward reactions characteristic of atropine occur. Use with caution during pregnancy; embryotoxic and teratogenic effects have occurred in animal studies. Safe use in infants under 1 year has not been established.

Untoward Reactions CNS disturbances include depression, psychosis, hallucinations, confusion, anxiety, irritability, ataxia, dizziness, insomnia, headache, slurred speech, and visual disturbances. Cardiovascular disturbances include the development of peripheral edema, which may progress to congestive heart failure. Orthostatic hypotension occurs relatively frequently, as does urinary retention. GI disturbances include anorexia, nausea, vomiting, constipation, and dry mouth. Livedo reticularis frequently occurs, but eczematoid dermatitis is rare. Rare reactions include convulsions, leukopenia, neutropenia, and oculogyric reactions.

Parameters of Use

Absorption Fairly well absorbed from GI tract. Peak serum levels occur in 4 hours. Mean half-life is about 15 hours. Onset of therapeutic effect occurs in about 48 hours.

Crosses placenta and enters breast milk; lactating mothers should bottle-feed their babies.

Metabolism None.

Excretion By the kidneys as unchanged drug at the rate of 5 mg/hour.

Drug Interactions No significant interactions known. No known antidote.

Administration Highly individualized; drug's effectiveness may subside after a few months necessitating an increase in dosage.

- *Parkinsonism:* Only drug used: 100 mg po bid; Maximum dosage: 400 mg daily in divided doses. Multiple drug therapy: 100 mg po daily for 1 week; then 100 mg po bid, as needed. Lower dosages may be required for debilitated clients.
- *Drug-induced extrapyramidal reactions:* 100 mg po bid; 300 mg daily may be required by some clients.
- *Prevention and treatment of influenza A virus infections:* Adults: 200 mg po daily or 100 mg po bid. Continuous drug therapy for 10 days after exposure to virus is required. When administered concurrently with vaccine it is given for 2 to 3 weeks. Children: Ages 1 to 9 years: 4.4 to 8.8 mg/Kg/day; Ages 9 to 12 years: 100 mg po bid; Maximum dosage: 150 mg/day.

Available Drug Forms Capsules containing 100 mg; syrup containing 50 mg/5 ml.

Nursing Management (See levodopa.)

1. Warn elderly and debilitated clients to change position slowly to avoid orthostatic hypotension.
2. Administer drug early in the day to avoid insomnia.
3. Give with a full glass of water.
4. Warn client about CNS disturbances and to avoid situations that require constant attention until CNS disturbances subside. If CNS disturbances persist with a one-a-day dosage schedule, a split dosage schedule may eliminate them.
5. Instruct client to inform physician of untoward reactions and worsening of parkinsonism (usually around 2 to 6 months after beginning drug).
6. Warn client against abrupt withdrawal of drug, as this may precipitate a parkinsonian crisis (rapid and marked deterioration).
7. Optimal therapeutic effect may not be apparent for 2 weeks.

GENERIC NAME Bromocriptine mesylate (RX)

TRADE NAME Parlodel

CLASSIFICATION Antiparkinsonian and hyperprolactinemia agent

Action Bromocriptine, an ergot derivative, is a potent stimulant of dopamine receptor sites, including those in the corpus striatal region of the brain and in the tubero-infundibular process. Stimulation of the latter receptor sites inhibits the secretion of prolactin from the anterior pituitary gland, so the drug has been found effective in the short-term treatment of amenorrhea, galactorrhea, and infertility associated with hyperprolactinemia. The stimulation of dopamine receptor sites in the corpus striatal region causes an inhibitory response on cholinergic neurons in the area and is therefore effective in minimizing the symptoms of parkinsonism. Although the drug-induced untoward reactions tend to be mild and transient, there is a significantly higher incidence of untoward reactions during long-term therapy of parkinsonism than with levodopa/carbidopa drug therapy.

Indications for Use Short-term treatment of hyperprolactinemia that results in amenorrhea, galactorrhea, and female infertility; prevention of lactation after an abortion, stillbirth, or childbirth when lactation is undesired or contraindicated; Idiopathic or postencephalitic parkinsonism, particularly in clients who experience end-of-dose-failure or on-off phenomenon with levodopa therapy.

Contraindications Hypersensitivity to ergot alkaloids.

Warnings and Precautions The presence of a pituitary tumor (Forbes-Albright syndrome) should be ruled out before instituting drug therapy. Although plasma prolactin levels are decreased by the drug, accepted therapies for destruction of the pituitary tumor must be instituted. Discontinue drug immediately if pregnancy occurs. Client should be assessed frequently for tiny prolactin-secreting adenomas that are not detectable by standard diagnostic measures; but which may grow and cause compression of the optic nerve during pregnancy. Vital signs must be stabilized after abortion or childbirth before the drug can be instituted, since hypotension may occur. Use with caution in clients receiving drugs that lower blood pressure and those with arrhythmias or a history of myocardial infarction. Safe use in children under 15 years and clients with hepatic or renal disorders has not been established. Safe use of drug beyond 2 years for parkinsonism has not been established. Contraceptive measures, other than oral contraceptives, should be used during drug therapy.

Untoward Reactions The incidence of untoward reactions varies according to the purpose of drug administration. Nausea and other GI disturbances occur more frequently in clients being treated for amenorrhea, galactorrhea, and female infertility. Hypotension, headache, and dizziness are common in clients receiving the drug for prevention of lactation. CNS disturbances are more common in parkinsonian clients.

Hypotension is a secondary reaction to the drug and may be symptomatic in some clients. Faintness, dizziness, fatigue, lightheadedness, vertigo, and syncope are common within the first few days of therapy; but the symptoms subside when the dosage is reduced. GI disturbances, including nausea, vomiting, abdominal cramps, diarrhea, and constipation, are common. CNS disturbances, including headache, hallucinations, and confusion, are common. Drowsiness, weakness, insomnia, depression, nervousness, lethargy, nightmares, and paresthesia have been reported. Abnormal involuntary movements and "on-off" phenomenon have emerged in clients being tapered off levodopa/carbidopa. Other reactions, including nasal stuffiness (common), urinary frequency, incontinence or retention, skin rashes, seizures, and ergotism, have occurred, but rarely.

Laboratory Reactions Alterations include transient elevations in blood urea nitrogen, serum glutamic-oxaloacetic transaminase, serum glutamic-pyruvic transaminase, creatine phosphokinase, alkaline phosphatase, and uric acid.

Parameters of Use

Absorption Less than one-third of the oral dose is absorbed from the GI tract; GI disturbances are common. Some bound to serum albumin, but not significantly in vivo. Almost 96% bound to serum albumin in vitro.

Metabolism Completely metabolized in the liver and other tissues.

Excretion Primarily in bile and ultimately excreted in feces. Only 2 to 5.5% in urine. Completely excreted after 5 days.

Drug Interactions Symptomatic hypotension may occur if administered concurrently with antihypertensive agents. Pregnancy may occur if client relies on oral contraceptives.

Administration

- *Ammenorrhea, galactorrhea, infertility:* Initial dosage: 2.5 mg po daily with meals; dosage may be increased within 1 week; then 2.5 mg po bid or tid with meals for 14 days to 6 months. Do not exceed 6 months of therapy.
- *Prevention of lactation:* 2.5 mg po bid with meals for 14 to 21 days.
- *Parkinsonism:* Initial dosage: 1.75 mg po bid with meals; then increase by 2.5 mg every 14 to 28 days until desired effect.

Available Drug Forms Tablets containing 2.5 mg.

Nursing Management

Planning factors

1. Obtain history of symptoms for which the drug is to be administered.
2. Baseline hepatic function tests (blood urea nitrogen, transaminases) should be obtained.
3. Pregnancy test should be performed, when applicable.
4. Obtain baseline blood pressure.

Administration factors

1. Give drug with meals or a snack.
2. Tablet can be crushed and mixed with apple sauce for clients who have difficulty in swallowing.

Evaluation factors

1. Obtain blood pressure before administering dose when drug is first initiated or dosage adjusted.
2. In amenorrhea, menses may resume within 6 to 8 weeks of therapy.
3. In galactorrhea, breast secretions and inflammation are usually reduced by 75% after 8 to 12 weeks of therapy.
4. A pregnancy test is recommended every 4 weeks when drug is administered for hyperprolactinemia.
5. Pregnancy test should be done if menses do not commence within 3 days of expected date.
6. Assess improvement of parkinsonism weekly or biweekly. A flowchart may be helpful.
7. When long-term therapy is required, hepatic, hematopoietic, cardiovascular, and renal function tests should be done periodically.

Client teaching factors

1. Warn client that lightheadedness and fainting may occur when drug is started and when dosage is

increased. Client should change position slowly and report symptoms immediately.
2. Instruct client to take medication with meals to avoid nausea.
3. When appropriate, caution female clients to use contraceptive measures other than oral contraceptives to avoid pregnancy.
4. Caution client against driving a car or engaging in activities that require constant attention until hypotension is well controlled.

PART XII

CARDIOVASCULAR AGENTS AND DIURETICS

THE CARDIOVASCULAR SYSTEM provides a constant supply of oxygen and nutrients to the cells and removes excess fluids and waste products. The heart propels the blood, and the blood vessels transport the blood through the pulmonary circulation from the heart's right side and the systemic circulation from the left side of the heart.

Cardiovascular disorders are the leading cause of death in the United States, as well as a primary cause of disability among adults. The drugs in this section increase the efficiency of the cardiovascular system. Digitalis preparations increase the force of the heart's contraction; antiarrhythmic agents correct disorders of heart rate and/or rhythm; diuretics control blood volume; and antihypertensive agents control excessive blood pressure.

Cardiac physiology The heart is divided into the right and left atria and ventricles. The coordinated contraction of the ventricles is called *systole,* and the period of relaxation is termed *diastole.* The quantity of blood expelled by each contraction of the left ventricle is termed the *stroke volume.* The amount of blood ejected is determined by the strength of the heart's muscle cells and the length of time the chambers take to fill. Factors that alter stroke volume include contractility, excessive blood volume, tachycardia and other arrhythmias, cardiac valve disorders (stenosis or regurgitation), excessive pressure (due to systemic or pulmonary hypertension), and muscular defects in the myocardium (myocardial infarction, pericarditis, myocarditis).

Coordination of the *heart rate*—the number of cardiac contractions per minute—is provided by the conduction system in the heart. Impulse formation occurs automatically. The myocardium is capable of initiating a contraction without external stimuli; the heart's pacemaker is termed the *SA node.* The impulse spreads through the atria, enters the *AV node,* and descends through the *bundle of His* and the left and right *bundle branches* to the *Purkinje fibers* in the ventricular muscles. A recording of the electrical impulses that pass through the heart is called an electrocardiogram. Factors that affect the speed of contraction are said to have a *dromotropic effect* on the heart; a *chronotropic effect* is an alteration in heart rate, and an *inotropic effect* is a change in the rate of speed at which an impulse is conducted through the heart. Cardiac and vascular disorders can result in dromotropic, chronotropic, or inotropic effects.

Congestive heart failure Congestive heart failure occurs when the heart is unable to respond adequately to the demands of the peripheral tissues for oxygen. The cardiac output can fail to keep pace with the body's demands either because of an abnormality in the heart muscle (myocardial infarction) or because eventually the work load becomes greater than the strength of the myocardium (hypertension). Although hypertension is the most common preexisting condition, arrhythmias, pneumonia, pulmonary emboli, and other disorders may precipitate pump failure.

Initially, the body attempts to compensate for the decrease in cardiac output by stimulating the sympathetic nervous system and inducing an increase in the heart rate (rapid, weak pulse). As the quantity of blood flowing through the renal arteries decreases, the kidneys respond by increasing the reabsorption of sodium and water; as the volume of blood is expanded, the work load on the heart becomes greater. When the right ventricle fails to pump adequately, the venous circulation becomes excessive and the organs and peripheral tissues become edematous. When the left ventricle fails, the heart can no longer accept the blood coming from the pulmonary circulation and pulmonary edema develops. When left ventricular failure develops slowly, the gradual increase in pulmonary pressure eventually causes right ventricular failure as well.

Therapeutic objectives are (1) to increase the strength of myocardial contractions by giving digitalis glycosides, (2) to reduce the blood volume by administering diuretics, and (3) to decrease the cardiac workload. Cardiac glycosides have a positive inotropic effect (improved contractility) on the heart, a negative dromotropic effect (decreased conduction speed), and a negative chronotropic effect (slower heart rate). Diuretics reduce blood volume, decreasing the workload of the heart. Drugs that reduce the amount of blood coming to the heart are sometimes called *preload reducers,* and include some of the diuretics and vasodilators.

Hypertension Although the exact cause or causes of hypertension are unknown, the disease can be treated successfully. Drugs that decrease blood volume (diuretics) are often all that is necessary to control blood pressure. But when hypertension persists despite the consistent use of diuretics, other drugs are used to dilate the arterial bed and decrease the total peripheral resistance. Once the peripheral resistance is decreased, the force against which the heart must contract is reduced. Drugs that dilate the arterial bed are sometimes referred to as *afterload reducers*.

Angina and myocardial infarction Angina is probably caused by either a spasm in the coronary artery or an imbalance in the blood flow (oxygen supply) to the myocardium that results in a greater need for oxygen than the coronary arteries are able to supply. The nitrates are useful, since they decrease peripheral resistance and increase the diameter of the coronary arteries. Beta blockers are helpful in reducing the frequency of chest pain by decreasing the heart rate and cardiac contractility. If a coronary artery is completely blocked, a myocardial infarction results. Antiarrhythmic agents are used to prevent and treat the resulting arrhythmias, narcotics are used to control the pain, and tranquilizers are used to diminish anxiety, since anxiety can increase the oxygen requirements of the heart. Anticoagulants, particularly heparin, are helpful in preventing thrombophlebitis and subsequent pulmonary emboli.

Chapter 46

Digitalis and Cardiac Glycosides

CARDIAC GLYCOSIDES OF which digitalis is the most important, are said to be the fourth most frequently prescribed drug in the United States and are immensely important to the health care system. Plant extracts containing glycosides have been used medicinally throughout the world for centuries. Squill or sea onion (*Scilla maritima*), a plant containing digitaloid substances, was used as a medicine as early as 1500 B.C. by the Egyptians; the Romans used it as a diuretic, heart tonic, and emetic. However, it was not until about 200 years ago in 1785 that an English physician and botanist, William Withering, published a book entitled *An Account of the Foxglove and Some of Its Medicinal Uses: With Practical Remarks on Dropsy and Other Diseases.* Withering was aware of the effectiveness of digitalis preparations in certain forms of dropsy, but did not relate these findings to cardiac action. John Ferriar in 1799 first recognized the primary action of digitalis on the heart.

SOURCES OF CARDIAC GLYCOSIDES

Plants of the genera Digitalis (foxglove) and Strophanthus (oleander and periwinkle) contain pharmacologically active sugar derivatives of steroids that are known collectively as *cardiac glycosides.* Digitalis glycosides are conjugation products of sugars and an aglycone; an aglycone molecule contains a lactone attached to a steroid (sugar-steroid-lactone). On hydrolysis, these compounds yield a sugar and one or more additional substances. Plants containing digitalis are indigenous to all corners of the earth. In addition, digitalis-like substances are found in lawn weeds and the skin of toads. Although no synthetic alternatives to the naturally occurring agents have been found, semi-synthetic glycosides are being investigated experimentally.

PROPERTIES OF CARDIAC GLYCOSIDES

Pharmacodynamics

Digitalis preparations increase the force of myocardial contractions (positive inotropic effect), decrease the rate of conduction through the myocardium (negative dromotropic effect), and decrease the heart rate (negative chronotropic effect). As cardiac output increases, peripheral circulation improves, venous pressure drops, renal blood flow increases, and diuresis occurs primarily as a result of improved circulation and organ function. Another benefit of circulatory improvement is enhanced coronary circulation. Slowing of the heart rate is due in part to vagal stimulation, which results in diminished impulse conduction through the heart and therefore slowing of the ventricular rate. The electrocardiographic effects of digitalis preparations are as follows:

1. S-T segment—depressed
2. T wave—diminished or inverted
3. P-R interval—prolonged
4. Q-T interval—shortened (a reflection of the fact that the drug shortens ventricular systole)

Indications for Use

Digitalis compounds are used primarily to treat congestive heart failure. They are also of use in the treatment of heart diseases associated with hypertension and atherosclerosis. Furthermore, atrial flutter and fibrillation and other supraventricular arrhythmias may respond to treatment with digitalis compounds.

Parameters of Use

The degree of absorption of various glycosides varies from a minimal amount to almost complete absorption. The liver initially concentrates cardiac glycosides and excretes them in the bile. After intestinal reabsorption and hepatic detoxification, digitalis is excreted by the kidneys and a major portion of the glycoside is found in the urine as metabolites. Since most glycosides are eliminated over a period of several days, drug accumulation may occur and eventually result in toxicity.

Studies of placental transfer show that 1% of glycosides and less than 3.5% of metabolites occur in the fetus 1.7 to 5 hours after drug injection. In a near-term fetus, it has been demonstrated that there is hepatic excretion of digitoxin and its metabolites can be found in the liver, gall bladder, and small intestine.

TYPES OF DIGITALIS PREPARATIONS

Although the various digitalis compounds have a similar effect on the body, they do vary in their purity, stability, absorption, dosage, and onset and duration of action.

Digitalis leaf is a mixture of several glycosides. The glycoside digitoxin is responsible for most but not all of the action caused by this preparation. However, the use of a pure cardiac glycoside has replaced the use of digitalis leaf.

Digoxin is probably the most prescribed cardiac glycoside because it is well absorbed from the gastrointestinal tract and is eliminated fairly rapidly; thus it has a relatively wide margin of safety. When administered orally, digoxin reaches its peak concentration in 45 to 60 minutes and then levels fall for the next 4 to 6 hours. Intravenously administered digoxin or *deslanoside* are often used during life-threatening emergencies, such as acute pulmonary edema, because they act rapidly. Although deslanoside is considered less toxic than digoxin, it is poorly absorbed from the gastrointestinal tract and is therefore not available in oral drug form.

Digitoxin can be administered orally or parenterally even though it has a relatively slow onset of action. This preparation has a long duration of action and is often used to provide long-term therapeutic drug levels. However, because digitoxin is very slowly eliminated from the body (half-life of 4 to 9 days), excessive accumulation of the drug can occur and result in digitalis toxicity, which requires treatment over 24 to 36 hours.

G-strophanthin, an intravenous cardiac glycoside, has a rapid onset of action (15 minutes) followed by a rapid fall in serum drug levels.

Digitalis glycosides may be administered orally, intravenously, or intramuscularly. However, most authorities do not recommend the intramuscular route, since it is painful and skeletal muscles absorb these drug preparations poorly. The subcutaneous route is not used because of possible drug unreliability. The rectal route has been used when others are not feasible.

DIGITALIZATION

When treating heart failure, it is essential to give the digitalis compound of choice to achieve optimum effect and then to maintain this effect. The cumulative property of digitalis glycosides is of prime concern in the process called *digitalization.* Data obtained by radioimmunoassay can be correlated with the drug dosage and the client's clinical symptoms in order to determine the accuracy of optimal loading and maintenance dosages.

Digitalization may be accomplished in hours or in days and is highly individualized. Examples of average digitalizing dosages are: digitalis leaf 100 mg three times a day for five days; or digitoxin 0.4 mg every eight hours for three doses. A single full dose for rapid action is rarely, if ever, used. Body weight, age, and pathology determine the dosage in pediatrics.

Many clients require lifelong maintenance dosages of digitalis glycosides and since these are highly individualized, various biologic factors must always be considered. The objective of the maintenance dosage is to replace the quantity of drug eliminated daily.

Clients receiving digitalis therapy should be observed for any variations in their absorption and elimination of the drug. Unusual alterations in eating habits, urinary output, and bowel movements will undoubtedly affect the cumulative ratio of cardiac glycosides and therefore drug performance. Maintenance implies an even and sustained drug action, but frequently, due to physiologic changes, such as electrolyte imbalances, endocrine disturbances, or underlying heart and lung disease, the maintenance dosage may result in toxic drug levels.

DIGITALIS TOXICITY

All digitalis preparations cause similar signs and symptoms of intoxication, which is usually due to the cumulative effects of maintenance dosages taken over relatively long periods of time. There are three major areas of concern: gastrointestinal, neurologic, and cardiac.

Gastrointestinal disturbances include nausea, vomiting, and diarrhea. These are early significant warning signs and often lead to anorexia. Neurologic symptoms are vertigo, headache, drowsiness, restlessness, irritability, weakness, delusions, convulsions and stupor. Ophthalmologic disorders are part of the central nervous system response to toxicity and include symptoms such as photophobia, disturbed color vision, and flickering light sensations.

The toxic effects on the cardiac system comprise depressed conduction and arrhythmias. Partial or complete heart block must be always viewed as evidence of digitalis intoxication and should be suspected if the ventricular rate falls below 60 beats per minute. Since a client may have a pulse deficit, the apical heart rate should be counted for one full minute. The mechanism of the bradycardiac effect of digitalis on sinus rhythm is probably due to a number of factors, including vagal stimulation. However, some experts believe that this rate change is secondary to changes in calcium levels. All rates and rhythm changes must be checked as the arrhythmia may occasionally present as tachycardia. Ventricular fibrillation is undoubtedly the most common cause of death from digitalis poisoning and is a serious problem with intravenous medications.

Treatment

If digitalis-induced arrhythmias occur, the drug should be discontinued and propranolol, a beta-adrenergic blocking agent, administered. Phenytoin is used when ventricular tachycardia occurs.

Potassium IV can be administered for its positive effect on cardiac contractions. When cardiac glycosides are in the blood the level of potassium ions is critical. If the concentration of potassium ions is increased the effect of the drug is reduced.

Another specific antidote for digitalis glycosides involves the administration of steroid-binding resins (cholestyramine, colestipol). These resins bind to glycosides and prevent their reabsorption by carrying them through the gastrointestinal tract and into the feces.

Predisposing Factors

Hypokalemia caused by diuretics tends to increase the client's susceptibility to digitalis-induced arrhythmias; the potassium depletion increases the automaticity of the ectopic pacemaker. To counteract hypokalemia, potassium salts are administered and the diuretic changed to a potassium-sparing one (aldactone, spironolactone). Hyperkalemia, on the other hand, may lead to AV block or severe bradycardia.

Some endocrine diseases, such as hypothyroidism and hyperthyroidism, may also predispose clients to digitalis toxicity. Clients with myxedema show an increased sensitivity to small dosages of digitalis, and bradycardia may result; however, hyperthyroid clients are resistant to digitalis and ordinary dosages may not be adequate.

Many authorities consider that the following conditions merit special consideration before administering a cardiac glycoside: recent myocardial infarction, ventricular tachycardia, partial heart block, and concurrent administration of calcium.

Factors that predispose clients to digitalis toxicity can be summarized as follows:

- Electrolyte imbalances
  - Hypokalemia
  - Hyperkalemia
  - Hypomagnesemia
  - Hypercalcemia
- Endocrine diseases
  - Hypothyroidism (myxedema)
  - Hyperthyroidism
- Heart and lung diseases
  - Hypoxia
  - Hypercapnea
  - Structural deformities (aortic stenosis, mitral stenosis, fibrotic conditions)
  - Infectious myocarditis
  - Myocardial infarction
- Elderly clients
- Impaired renal function

In addition to the above factors, it should be noted that epinephrine and related catecholamines have long been known to precipitate arrhythmias, especially in the digitalized heart.

NURSING MANAGEMENT

Pertinent factors that should be considered when caring for clients receiving a digitalis glycoside are as follows:

1. Always take the client's pulse for one full minute prior to administration. Take the apical heart beat and note rate and rhythm. If the rate is 60 beats per minute or lower, is excessively rapid, or the rhythm is altered, the drug should be withheld and the physician notified. It is essential to become familiar with pulse rate and rhythm so that deviations can be easily identified.

2. If a client is receiving a diuretic, the diet should be checked so that effective measures can be initiated to maintain electrolyte balance—for example, citrus fruits or bananas daily to provide potassium.

3. As vomiting, diarrhea, or surgical procedures (colostomy) may result in fluid and electrolyte imbalances that will alter drug effectiveness; thus dosage adjustments may have to be made.

4. Elderly clients tolerate cardiac glycosides poorly; therefore frequent blood level checks should be made and dosages adjusted accordingly.

5. When clients are on maintenance dosages, the drug should be administered at the same time daily, thereby decreasing the possibility of altered drug levels. This point should be explained in detail to clients.

6. Client teaching should include an understanding of the signs of toxicity and instruction in taking pulse rate. If the client is unable to measure pulse rate, then a family member should be taught how to count the pulse and to note the quality of the pulse and rhythm. This instruction should be done several days prior to discharge so that there is time for adequate practice.

7. The client should be instructed to store drug in airtight, light-resistant containers.

8. Clients should be aware of the fact that they must not miss or stop taking the drug and that they cannot "catch up" by taking extra medication. If a dosage is missed, the physician should be consulted.

CARDIAC GLYCOSIDES

GENERIC NAME Digoxin (RX)

TRADE NAMES Digoxin, Lanoxin, SK-Digoxin

CLASSIFICATION Cardiac glycoside

Source Glycoside often obtained from the leaves of *Digitalis lanata*.

Action Although the exact mechanism of action is unknown, digoxin is thought to inhibit the enzyme sodium, potassium-adenosinetriphosphatase ($Na^+ - K^+ -$ ATPase). This inhibition results in a reduction of energy available for the sodium pump and leads to an increase in intracellular sodium ions with a corresponding loss of potassium ions; calcium levels may also be affected. The major effect of the drug is an increase in the force of myocardial contractions. In addition, stroke volume and therefore cardiac output increase, circulation improves, and central venous pressure decreases. Although improved cardiac output will result in a decrease in heart rate, digoxin directly effects cardiac electrophysiology by slowing conduction velocity through the heart, particularly the AV node, thus resulting in prolongation of the P-R interval as shown on an EKG. As the vagus nerve is stimulated the ventricular rate decreases. The drug is therefore useful in treating supraventricular tachycardias and counteracting vagal blockade induced by quinidine and procainamide.

Indications for Use Congestive heart failure, atrial fibrillation and flutter, paroxysmal atrial tachycardia.

Contraindications Any signs of digitalis toxicity (hypokalemia), ventricular tachycardia not associated with digitalis toxicity, ventricular fibrillation, recent myocardial infarction.

Warnings and Precautions Use with caution in clients with inflammatory conditions of the heart, such as myocarditis, since digitalis-induced arrhythmias may occur; in neonates and premature infants, since metabolism and excretion of the drug is delayed; in clients with "high output" heart failure caused by a noncardiac disorder, such as severe anemia, infection, or hyperthyroidism; and in clients with incomplete heart block, pericarditis, or heart failure due to mechanical causes, such as cardiac tamponade. Use with extreme caution in clients with electrolyte imbalances, particularly hypokalemia, hypomagnesemia, and hypercalcemia, since arrhythmias may develop; and in clients with heart failure in the presence of glomerulonephritis, since digitalis toxicity may occur. Elderly clients and clients with myxedema (hypothyroidism) or renal insufficiency require smaller than average dosages. The differences in bioavailability between parenterally and orally administered drug must be considered before dosage form is changed.

Untoward Reactions Ventricular fibrillation, usually preceded by ventricular tachycardia, is the most common cause of death as a result of digitalis toxicity. Toxicity in adults often produces GI or CNS disturbances prior to the development of arrhythmias. GI disturbances include anorexia, nausea, vomiting, and occasionally diarrhea. CNS disturbances include disturbed color vision (yellow), photophobia, flickering light sensations, weakness, vertigo, headache, drowsiness, restlessness, irritability, delusions, convulsions, and stupor. Unifocal or multifocal premature ventricular contractions, particularly in bigeminy or trigeminy, are the most common arrhythmias in adults with cardiac disease. Other common arrhythmias include AV dissociation, atrial tachycardia with block, and an accelerated nodal rhythm. Depressed cardiac conduction, including partial or complete heart block and bradycardia, may occur. A Wenckebach AV block may progress to complete heart block. Toxicity in infants is rarely manifested initially by GI or CNS disturbances. Cardiac arrhythmias are more common. Sinus bradycardia with or without block is a sign of impending toxicity. Toxicity in children may induce any arrhythmia. AV block, atrial tachycardia with or without block, and nodal tachycardia are common. Prolonged drug therapy may induce gynecomastia in male clients. Irritation and pain occur at intramuscular injection sites; when possible, this route should be avoided.

Parameters of Use

Absorption Rapid, uniform, and relatively complete from parenteral sites and GI tract. About 50 to 80% of tablets and 70 to 90% of elixir is absorbed. Rate of absorption is decreased if taken after meals. The absolute bioavailability of Lanoxin is: 60 to 80% (tablet); 70 to 85% (elixir); 70 to 85% (IM); 100% (IV). Therapeutic serum drug levels: 0.5 to 2.5 mg/ml. Onset of action is: 30 to 60 minutes (po); 30 minutes (IM); 10 minutes (IV). Peak action occurs in: 5 to 6 hours (po); 2 to 6 hours (IM); 1 to 2 hours (IV). Half-life is 34 to 51 hours. About 20 to 25% bound to plasma proteins. Crosses placenta and enters breast milk. There appears to be little or no harm to the fetus or infant; however, caution is recommended. Crosses blood-brain barrier.

Distribution Widely to lean tissue; little to fatty tissue. Distribution phase takes 6 to 8 hours. Little accumulated drug is removed from the body by hemodialysis, since most of the drug is distributed in tissues rather than circulating blood.

Metabolism In the liver. Some metabolites excreted in bile or reabsorbed for GI tract.

Excretion First-order kinetics: About 50% of the total amount in the body will be excreted within 24 hours with 27% in the urine as unchanged drug and 15% in feces. About 80% is excreted in 48 hours. Clients with renal impairment may take 4 to 6 days to excrete the drug.

Drug Interactions GI absorption of digoxin is inhibited by meals high in bran fiber and the drugs neomycin, antacids, sulfasalazine, cholestyramine, colestipol, metoclopramide, kaolin-pectin, and propantheline. Hypokalemia and the potential for digitalis toxicity may be induced by amphotericin B, carbenicillin, ticarcillin, furosemide, depleting diuretics, and corticosteroids. Concurrent administration of quinidine will increase serum concentrations of digoxin. Concomitant parenteral administration of calcium may induce digitalis toxicity and arrhythmias. Succinylcholine potentiates the cardiac effects of digoxin and may result in arrhythmias.

Administration Highly individualized according to client's age, lean body weight, and cardiac status. Adults: Digitalizing dosage: 0.5 to 1.5 mg po, IM, or IV bolus in divided doses over 24 hours; Maintenance dosage: 0.25 to 0.75 mg po daily. Children: Ages 2 to 10 years: Digitalizing dosage: 0.01 to 0.02 mg/lb po in divided doses over 24 hours; Maintenance dosage: 25 to 30% of digitalizing dosage daily. Ages 2 weeks to 2 years: Digitalizing dosage: 0.03 to 0.04 mg/lb po or 0.02 to 0.03 mg/lb IV bolus in divided doses over 24 hours; Maintenance dosage: 25 to 35% of digitalizing dosage daily. Newborns: Digitalizing dosage: 0.02 to 0.03 mg/lb po or 0.01 to 0.02 mg/lb IV bolus in divided doses over 24 hours; Maintenance dosage: 20 to 30% of digitalizing dosage daily.

Available Drug Forms Pediatric elixir containing 50 mcg (0.05 mg/ml) in bottles containing 2 fl oz with a calibrated dropper; scored tablets containing 0.125 mg (yellow), 0.25 mg (white), or 0.5 mg (green); ampules containing 0.1 or 0.25 mg/ml.

Nursing Management

Planning factors

1. Obtain history of cardiac, renal, hepatic, and endocrine function.
2. Obtain baseline data on vital signs, blood pressure, electrolytes, and complete blood cell count before administering drug.
3. Obtain drug history. Determine whether client has received digitalis preparations within the last 2 weeks, since this may affect therapeutic effectiveness.
4. Cardiac monitoring is required during digitalization.

Administration factors

1. Divide digitalizing dosage into 2 or 3 doses given over 24 hours.
2. Obtain apical pulse for 1 full minute before administering drug.
3. Give oral drug preparations on an empty stomach. If GI disturbances occur, give drug with meals.
4. Administer drug at the same time every day, since its action is cumulative.
5. When administering IM, inject deep into large muscle mass.
6. Administer IV bolus slowly over 1 to 2 minutes. It may be diluted in normal saline or 5% D/W.

Evaluation factors

1. Withhold drug and report findings to physician immediately if pulse falls below 60 beats/min. or suddenly rises over 100 beats/min. or if a pulse deficit or premature beats suddenly occur.
2. Obtain serum electrolytes periodically. If abnormalities occur, notify physician.
3. Cardiac monitoring is highly recommended during digitalization and dosage adjustments. A prolonged P-R interval, a depressed S-T segment, and a shortened Q-T segment should be expected. If any of these intervals are excessively prolonged, shortened, or depressed, notify physician.
4. Serum levels of digoxin assist in determining dosage and should be taken at least 6 to 8 hours after the last dose; they are usually obtained just before the next scheduled dose. Serum drug levels will be 10 to 25% lower if sample is drawn 24 hours, rather than 8 hours, after last drug administration.
5. Observe for signs and symptoms of toxicity. The average toxic dose is 7 mg. Toxicity may last from a few hours to 1 to 2 days.

Client teaching factors

1. Instruct client and/or family members how to take a pulse.
2. Explain digitalis toxicity and the symptoms that should be reported to the physician before taking an additional dose.
3. Explain the necessity of taking the drug at the same time daily.

4. Inform clients receiving potassium-depleting drugs to eat foods high in potassium daily.
5. Emphasize the need for regular medical checkups and laboratory evaluations.

GENERIC NAME Acetyldigitoxin (RX)

TRADE NAME Acylanid

CLASSIFICATION Cardiac glycoside

See digoxin for Contraindications, Warnings and precautions, and Untoward reactions.

Source Prepared by enzymatic degradation of lanatoside A, a glycoside obtained from the leaves of *Digitalis lanata.*

Action Cardiotonic agent that is similar to digitoxin. It increases the force of cardiac contractions and thus increases cardiac output. Heart rate is decreased by direct action on the heart and by stimulation of the vagus nerve. Acetyldigitoxin is thought to have a wider margin of safety, since it is eliminated twice as fast as digitoxin.

Indications for Use Congestive heart failure, atrial fibrillation and flutter.

Parameters of Use

Absorption Slow but fairly complete from GI tract. About two-thirds of oral dose is absorbed. Onset of action is 2 to 4 hours. Peak action occurs in 12 to 24 hours and duration of action is 1 to 3 days.
Metabolism In the liver; metabolites reabsorbed by GI tract.
Excretion By the kidneys; some found in feces (about 9%). About 21% is excreted by the kidneys within 6 days. Complete elimination takes about 9 to 12 days.

Drug Interactions Cholestyramine and colestipol may bind with acetyldigitoxin in the GI tract and thereby prevent absorption. Concurrent use of diuretics may result in potassium and magnesium imbalances. (See digoxin.)

Administration Adults: Digitalizing dosage: Rapid: 1.6 to 2.2 mg po in divided doses over 24 hours; Slow: 1.8 to 3.2 mg po in divided doses over 2 to 6 days; Maintenance dosage: 0.1 to 0.2 mg daily.

Available Drug Forms Tablets containing 0.1 mg (orchid-pink) or 0.2 mg (white).

Nursing Mangement The average toxic dose is 5.5 mg. Toxicity may last for 3 to 7 days. (See digoxin.)

GENERIC NAME Deslanoside (RX)

TRADE NAME Cedilanid-D

CLASSIFICATION Cardiac glycoside

See digoxin for Contraindications, Untoward reactions, and Drug interactions.

Source Prepared by alkaline hydrolysis of lanatoside C, a glycoside obtained from *Digitalis lanata.*

Action Deslanoside is a rapid-acting cardiotonic agent similar to digoxin. It increases the force of myocardial contractions and thus increases cardiac output. Heart rate is decreased by direct action on the heart and by stimulation of the vagus nerve. Being more water soluble than most cardiac glycosides, deslanoside is often administered intravenously for rapid digitalization in the acute phase of congestive heart failure.

Indications for Use Acute pulmonary edema, congestive heart failure, atrial fibrillation and flutter, paroxysmal atrial tachycardia.

Warnings and Precautions Not recommended for children. (See digoxin.)

Parameters of Use

Absorption Poor and irregular from GI tract. Onset of action is 5 to 30 minutes. Peak action occurs in 2 to 4 hours and duration of action is 2 to 5 days. Half-life is 33 hours. Weakly bound to serum proteins.
Metabolism Rapidly in the liver.
Excretion Primarily by the kidneys; about 20% daily.

Administration Digitalization should be performed within 12 hours by giving 1.6 mg IM or IV in 2 divided doses; Maintenance therapy: With oral preparations, such as Acylanid, instituted within 12 hours of digitalization.

Available Drug Forms Ampules of 2 ml containing 0.2 mg/ml.

Nursing Management (See digoxin.)

1. Protect ampules from light.
2. When administering IM, inject deep into gluteal muscle and massage site after injection. Only inject 2 ml in each site.

GENERIC NAME Digitalis (powdered leaf and tincture)

TRADE NAMES Digifortis, Pil-Digis (RX)

CLASSIFICATION Cardiac (digitalis) glycoside

See digoxin for Contraindications, Untoward reactions, Drug interactions, and Nursing management.

Source Obtained from *Digitalis purpurea.* The leaves are dried and then pulverized. Main constituents are digitoxin, gitalin, and gitoxin.

Action Digitalis leaf is the oldest cardiotonic. The amount of activity varies according to the percent of each glycoside found in a preparation. The drug increases the force of cardiac contractions and thereby increases cardiac output. Heart rate is decreased by direct action on the heart and by stimulation of the vagus nerve.

Indications for Use Congestive heart failure, atrial fibrillation and flutter.

Warnings and Precautions Not recommended for children. (See digoxin.)

Parameters of Use (See digoxin.)

Absorption Onset of action is 2 to 4 hours. Peak action occurs in 12 to 24 hours and duration of action is 2 to 3 days. Some reversible binding to serum proteins occurs.

Administration Digitalizing dosage: 1.2 to 1.8 g po in divided doses over 24 hours; Maintenance dosage: 100 mg daily.

Available Drug Forms Tablets containing 100 mg; bottles of digitalis tincture.

GENERIC NAME Digitoxin (RX)

TRADE NAMES Crystodigin, Digitaline Nativelle, Purodigin

CLASSIFICATION Cardiac glycoside

See digoxin for Contraindications, and Warnings and precautions.

Source Crystalline glycoside obtained from *Digitalis purpurea*.

Action Digitoxin increases the force of cardiac contractions and thus increases cardiac output. Heart rate is decreased by direct action on the heart and by stimulation of the vagus nerve. Digitoxin has a slower rate of elimination than digoxin and is therefore useful for long-term maintenance therapy. Toxicity is difficult to treat because of the drug's cumulative characteristics.

Indications for Use Congestive heart failure, atrial fibrillation and flutter.

Untoward Reactions Cardiovascular toxicity may continue to develop after the drug has been withdrawn. Prolonged treatment may be required as the toxic effects disappear gradually. (See digoxin.)

Parameters of Use

Absorption Slow but complete from GI tract. Onset of action is 1 to 2 hours. Peak action occurs in 4 to 12 hours. Half-life is 4 to 6 days. About 97% bound to proteins in a loose and reversible bond.

Distribution Low affinity for heart. High concentrations are found in the liver, gall bladder, kidneys, and GI tract.

Metabolism In the liver; enters enterohepatic recirculation.

Excretion By the kidneys; some found in feces. About 11.4% is lost in the first 24 hours (4% via kidneys and 7% via intestines). After 3 weeks, about 60 to 70% is excreted by the kidneys and 17% in feces. About 30 days are required for nearly complete elimination.

Drug Interactions Cholestyramine may bind with digitoxin in the GI tract and thereby prevent absorption. Phenobarbital, phenylbutazone, and phenytoin may enhance the metabolism of digitoxin as a result of enzyme induction. (See digoxin.)

Administration Adults: Oral: Digitalizing dosage: 0.6 mg followed by 0.4 mg; then 0.2 mg at intervals of 4 to 6 hours; Maintenance dosage: 0.05 to 0.3 mg daily; Average dosage: 0.1 to 0.15 mg daily. Intravenous: Digitalizing dosage: 0.6 mg followed by 0.4 mg 4 to 6 hours later; then 0.2 mg every 4 to 6 hours; Maintenance dosage: As for oral administration. Children: Digitalizing dosage: Over 2 years: 0.03 mg/kg; Ages 1 to 2 years: 0.04 mg/kg; Under 1 year: 0.045 mg/kg; Newborns: 0.022 mg/kg. Give in 3 to 4 or more divided doses every 6 hours. Maintenance dosage: $\frac{1}{10}$ of digitalizing dosage.

Available Drug Forms Tablets containing 0.05 mg (orange), 0.1 mg (pink), 0.15 mg (yellow), or 0.2 mg (white); ampules containing 0.2 mg/ml.

Nursing Management (See digoxin.)

1. It is very important that the client has not had any digitalis preparations in the 3 weeks prior to therapy with digitoxin.
2. Check and double check that the correct drug is being administered; digitoxin can be mistaken for digoxin and vice versa.
3. Apical pulse should be at least 60 beats/min.
4. Special precautions and dosage adjustments are required for elderly clients and clients with impaired renal function.
5. Digitoxin is insoluble in water. Parenteral administration should be used only when the drug cannot be taken orally.
6. If IM injection is used, it should be given deep in the gluteal muscle and massaged after administration. Never give more than 2 ml in one site.
7. It should be remembered that this drug has a slow onset of action and is highly cumulative, taking as long as 3 weeks to be eliminated. The signs and symptoms of toxicity are persistent and require long-term treatment.

GENERIC NAME Gitalin (RX)

TRADE NAME Gitaligin

CLASSIFICATION Cardiac glycoside

See digoxin for Contraindications, Untoward reactions, and Drug interactions.

Source Water-soluble glycoside mixture obtained from *Digitalis purpurea*.

Action Gitalin contains some digitoxin and gitalin glycosides. It increases the force of cardiac contractions and thus increases the cardiac output. Heart rate is decreased by direct action on the heart and by stimulation of the vagus nerve. Although well absorbed, gitalin tends to cause local GI irritation and nausea.

Indications for Use Congestive heart failure, atrial fibrillation and flutter.

Warnings and Precautions Not recommended for children. (See digoxin.)

Parameters of Use

Absorption Well absorbed from GI tract. Onset of action is within 1 hour. Peak action occurs in 24 to 48 hours and duration of action is 10 to 12 days.

Metabolism In the liver.

Excretion About 20 to 30% daily in urine.

Administration Digitalizing dosage: 6 mg po in divided doses over 24 hours (every 6 to 8 hours); Maintenance dosage: About 0.5 mg daily.

Available Drug Forms Green tablets containing 0.5 mg.

Nursing Management Give with meals if nausea develops. (See digoxin.)

GENERIC NAME G-strophanthin (RX)

TRADE NAME Ouabain

CLASSIFICATION Cardiac glycoside

See digoxin for Contraindications, Warnings and precautions, Untoward reactions, and Drug interactions.

Source Crystalline glycosides obtained from *Strophanthus gratus* plant seeds.

Action This drug increases the force of cardiac contractions and thus increases cardiac output. Heart rate is decreased by direct action on the heart and by stimulation of the vagus nerve. Because the drug is so poorly absorbed from the GI tract, it is used only parenterally in emergency situations.

Indications for Use Acute pulmonary edema, congestive heart failure, atrial fibrillation and flutter.

Parameters of Use

Absorption Oral dosage forms are not available because the drug is poorly and irregularly absorbed from GI tract. Onset of action is 3 to 10 minutes. Peak action occurs in 90 minutes and duration of action is 8 to 12 hours. Half-life is 24 hours.

Distribution Cardiac tissue preferentially takes up drug so that it contains 5 to 10 times the plasma concentration 30 to 90 minutes after administration. Distribution is completed in 7 hours.

Metabolism None known.

Excretion About 37% is excreted in urine daily.

Administration Initial dosage: 0.25 mg IV bolus; Emergency dosage: 0.5 mg IV: then 0.1 mg hourly until desired effect, or a total of 1 mg/24 hours.

Available Drug Forms Ampules containing 0.5 mg/2 ml.

Nursing Management (See digoxin.)

1. Because the drug is poorly absorbed from the GI tract and is inactivated by gastric juices, it should be administered only via IV route.
2. Full digitalis effect occurs within 2 hours.
3. Since G-strophanthin is very potent and rapid acting, close observation of the client is essential.
4. Inject drug slowly.
5. G-strophanthin acts more rapidly than any other cardiac glycoside and cumulative effects are less likely. Onset of toxic symptoms is rapid.
6. Care must be taken when administering the drug to clients who have received any digitalis preparations during the preceding 3 weeks.

GENERIC NAME Lanatoside C (RX)

GENERIC NAME Cedilanid

CLASSIFICATION Cardiac glycoside

See digoxin for Contraindications, Untoward reactions, and Drug interactions.

Source Glycoside obtained from the leaves of *Digitalis lanata*.

Action Lanatoside C is similar to digoxin. The drug increases the force of cardiac contractions and thus increases cardiac output. Heart rate is decreased by direct action on the heart and by stimulation of the vagus nerve. Lanatoside C has a shorter duration of action and is less cumulative than digitoxin. This preparation is seldom used because it is poorly absorbed from the GI tract.

Indications for Use Congestive heart failure, atrial fibrillation and flutter.

Warnings and Precautions Not recommended for children. (See digoxin.)

Parameters of Use

Absorption Poorly absorbed from GI tract; about 10% of administered dose reaches bloodstream. Onset of action is 1 to 2 hours. Peak action occurs in 4 to 6 hours and duration of action is 24 to 36 hours.

Distribution Widely distributed.

Excretion Nearly 20% is excreted in urine daily.

Administration Digitalizing dosage: 7.5 to 10.0 mg po over 3 days; Maintenance dosage: 0.5 to 1.5 mg daily.

Nursing Management (See digoxin.)

Chapter 47

Antiarrhythmic Agents

ANTIARRHYTHMIC AGENTS CAME into common use as identification of arrhythmias became possible with technologic advances, particularly the cardiac monitor. An *arrhythmia* is a disturbance in the rate and/or rhythm of the heart that arises from physiologic or pathologic alterations in cardiac impulse formation or conduction and may ultimately result in a lethal decrease in cardiac output. Antiarrhythmic agents are drugs that are used to restore or maintain normal electrophysiologic function of the heart.

CARDIAC ELECTROPHYSIOLOGY

The heart contracts in response to coordinated electrical impulses that originate in the sinoatrial node (SA node), spread through the atria to the atrio-ventricular node (AV node), pass down the right and left branches of the bundle of His to the Purkinje fibers, and finally cross the ventricular myocardium. Conductive cells of the heart possess the property of *automaticity;* that is, the ability to contract spontaneously without neurologic intervention or other outside stimulus. Since automaticity in the SA node is faster than in the rest of the myocardial cells, the SA node initiates normal cardiac impulses and is often called the *pacemaker node*.

The rate at which an electrical impulse spreads through cardiac tissue is termed *conduction velocity*. Whereas the conduction velocity through the Purkinje fibers is very fast, about 4000 mm/second, the rate of conduction through the AV node is only about 400 mm/second. This slower AV conduction velocity enables the atria to contract before the ventricle contracts and advances impulses. Like skeletal muscle cells, cardiac cells are unresponsive, or *refractory*, to further stimulation until they have recovered from a previous excitation. The length of time before the cells can respond to another stimulus is termed the *refractory period*.

Sodium, potassium, calcium, and magnesium ions all affect the action of the heart. A sodium-potassium pump is responsible for the formation and conduction of electrical impulses through the heart. This pump creates an electrical gradient across the membrane of cardiac cells by influencing the flux of ions into and out of the cells. The inside of a resting heart cell has a negative charge because positive ions, including some potassium ions, have been shifted to the outside of the membrane. This resting gradient is aptly called the *resting potential*. However, as the *threshold potential* is reached, a rapid influx of sodium ions occurs and cell excitation results. As a consequence of this influx, the cell membrane loses its resting electrical balance and becomes rapidly *depolarized*. This depolarization eventually results in contraction. *Repolarization* is the phase in which the membrane reestablishes its resting polarity. The depolarization and repolarization phases are together termed the *action potential*. To differentiate the various phases of the action potential, the phases have been numbered as follows:

- Phase 0—depolarization
- Phase 1—early rapid depolarization
- Phase 2—slow repolarization
- Phase 3—late rapid repolarization
- Phase 4—resting potential

ELECTROCARDIOGRAM

The tiny electrical impulses emitted from the heart can be picked up and recorded by an *electrocardiograph* machine. A recording of these impulses on paper is termed an *electrocardiogram* (EKG). Positive (upward) and negative (downward) deflections from the baseline occur as an electrical impulse spreads through the heart and are differentiated as follows:

- P wave—spread of impulse through the atria
- QRS complex—spread of impulse through the ventricles
- T wave—repolarization
- P-R interval—distance (fraction of a second) between the onset of the P wave and the peak of the R wave
- Q-T interval—distance (fraction of a second) between the peak of the Q wave and the end of the T wave

Monitoring the electrical impulses of the heart is essential when antiarrhythmic drugs are given. However, as it is impractical to take a continuous

EKG, the client is attached to a *cardiac monitor* and one section of the EKG (usually using a lead II or a modified lead II) is displayed on the screen of the monitor, which is watched continuously by a certified coronary care nurse or another trained professional. If arrhythmias appear, a recording, or *tracing*, is taken and analyzed. If the arrhythmia proves to be life threatening, the certified coronary care nurse treats the arrhythmia according to agency standing orders and then notifies the physician. Drug therapy is the primary method for treating these abnormalities.

ARRHYTHMIAS

Arrhythmias frequently occur in clients with heart and lung disorders. Atrial arrhythmias are disturbing in many clients with pulmonary disorders, particularly chronic obstructive pulmonary disease, but are seldom life threatening. Although clients are often able to survive an initial myocardial infarction but not the arrhythmias that follow, the ability to accurately identify and treat arrhythmias immediately has dramatically reduced the mortality rate of clients with infarctions.

Arrhythmias are often divided into sinus, atrial, and ventricular and conduction pathway disturbances. Heart rates above 100 beats per minute are termed *tachycardia,* whereas rates below 60 beats per minute are termed *bradycardia;* the normal heart rate is between 60 and 100 beats/minute. *Ectopic beats* occur when a tiny section of the myocardium begins to generate impulses faster than the SA node and therefore usurps the SA node's pacing of the heart. Ectopic beats that originate in the atria or ventricles are termed *premature atrial* or *ventricular contractions* (PAC or PVC), respectively. Although PACs are seldom, if ever, life threatening, frequent PVCs (6 or more per minute) are considered dangerous because they may lead to ventricular tachycardia or fibrillation. These arrhythmias are lethal and death will occur in minutes if treatment with electrical countershock (defibrillation) and rapid-acting drugs, such as lidocaine, is not instituted immediately to decrease the automaticity of the abnormal pacing section of the heart, thereby allowing the SA node to resume its pacing of the heart.

Although more common, atrial flutter and fibrillation are not lethal in themselves, since it is the ventricles and not the atria that possess the strength and power to pump blood to the lungs for oxygenation and then out to the body. These arrhythmias are thought to occur as a result of a "circus-type movement" in the atria in which an impulse spreads in a circular route around and around the atria. Although the AV node often blocks some of these impulses, they can be transmitted to the ventricles, which then beat too fast. By stimulating the vagus nerve and inducing other changes, digitalis is effective in prolonging AV node conduction and thus reducing heart rate.

TYPES OF ANTIARRHYTHMIC AGENTS

Drugs used to treat arrhythmias are obtained from a variety of chemical sources and each drug affects the heart in a different way. Quinidine and other Type I antiarrhythmic agents act as cardiac depressants by decreasing myocardial automaticity and conduction velocity while increasing the refractory period. Cardiac contractility is also decreased and may result in a decrease in cardiac output, which is a potentially dangerous secondary effect of these drugs.

Lidocaine and phenytoin are sometimes classified as Type II antiarrhythmic agents as they depress heart action but by a different mechanism than quinidine. These agents decrease myocardial automaticity as well as the refractory period; but lidocaine has little or no effect on conduction velocity or cardiac contractility.

Adrenergic blocking agents are effective for certain tachyarrhythmias because they decrease the excitation induced by catecholamines and adrenergic neurons to the heart. Calcium channel blockers, which are a relatively new type of antiarrhythmic agent, block the entry of calcium via tiny channels in the membrane of conductive heart cells. Consequently, AV conduction velocity is decreased and the refractory period of the AV node is prolonged. These drugs exert their action without inducing untoward effects, including peripheral arterial spasms and bronchoconstriction, characteristic of traditional antiarrhythmic agents.

Bradycardia and disturbances of the conduction system that result in complete heart block are usually treated by the insertion of an electrical pacemaker, rather than by drugs. However, atropine and isoproterenol, which increase heart rate, can be used for the temporary treatment of severe bradycardia until a pacemaker can be inserted.

NURSING MANAGEMENT

In the acute stage following a myocardial infarction or other possible causes of arrhythmias, such as organic heart diseases, pulmonary diseases, and electrolyte disorders of drugs, the client will usually be treated in a coronary or intensive care unit, where continuous cardiac monitoring is required to promptly identify and treat the arrhythmia before it becomes lethal. Nurses in these situations function in an expanded role, because they are often the identifiers of the arrhythmia and must administer the appropriate drug immediately, which requires special training and an in-depth knowledge of the medications. It is therefore important for every nurse to understand the action of antiarrhythmic drugs and to be alert to possible side effects because of the hazards of toxicity. The nurse should check the client's heart rate prior to administering antiarrhythmic drugs and apical-radial rates and blood pressure when appropriate.

TYPE I ANTIARRHYTHMIC AGENTS

GENERIC NAME Quinidine sulfate (RX)

TRADE NAMES Cin-Quin, Quinidex, Quinidinium Sulfate, Quinora

CLASSIFICATION Antiarrhythmic, cardiac depressant

Source Dextrorotatory alkaloid of Cinchona and isomer of quinine.

Action This salt of quinidine contains more than 80% of anhydrous quinidine. Quinidine is considered a cardiac depressant because it depresses myocardial excitability, conduction velocity, and contractility. In addition, the refractory period of the myocardium is prolonged. These direct actions on the heart are thought to be due to the drug's ability to decrease sodium ion influx during depolarization, retard the shift of potassium ions during repolarization, and reduce the movement of calcium ions across the cell membrane. Therapeutic dosages of quinidine not only depress the automaticity of the SA node, but also ectopic pacemaker sites, thus decreasing heart rate and the occurrence of ectopic beats. Unfortunately, the decrease in conduction velocity increases the potential of heart block in clients with conduction defects. The anticholinergic properties of quinidine may cause an increase in heart rate by blocking vagal stimulation of the AV node. Large dosages may cause hypotension and a reflex increase in heart rate by inducing peripheral vasodilation. Some of the antimalarial, antipyretic, and oxytocic properties of quinine are also exhibited by quinidine.

Indications for Use Atrial fibrillation and flutter, paroxysmal atrial or ventricular tachycardia, atrial or ventricular premature contractions, paroxysmal AV or junctional tachycardia, maintenance of normal cardiac rhythm following cardioversion.

Contraindications Hypersensitivity to quinidine or quinine; history of thrombocytopenia purpura or cinchonism (quininism); tachycardia due to severe infections; digitalis intoxication manifested by AV conduction disorders; complete AV block with an AV nodal or idioventricular pacemaker; protective ectopic impulses or rhythms due to escape mechanisms.

Warnings and Precautions Since quinidine suppresses vagal stimulation and thereby increases AV conduction, the drug should not be used in clients with atrial flutter or fibrillation and a rapid ventricular response; prior digitalization will minimize this effect. Use with extreme caution in clients with incomplete AV block, since complete block or asystole may occur, and in clients with congestive heart failure in hypotensive states. Benefits must outweigh risks in pregnant women.

Untoward Reactions Cardiotoxicity: Excessive widening of QRS complex (greater than 0.12) or frequent premature ventricular contractions. Ventricular fibrillation, tachycardia, SA or AV block, or asystole may occur. The drug also widens the Q-T interval, induces depression of the S-T segment, and causes peaked P waves. Cinchonism: Ringing in the ears, headache, nausea, or disturbed vision may occur after a single dose in hypersensitive clients. Severe hypotension and precipitation of congestive heart failure have occurred in susceptible clients. Nausea, vomiting, and diarrhea are common; abdominal pain and anorexia may occur. Blood dyscrasias, including hemolytic anemia, thrombocytopenia, and agranulocytosis, are relatively common after prolonged use. Petechial hemorrhage of buccal mucosa may occur. Headache, low-grade fever, vertigo, and light headaches are common. Apprehension, confusion, delirium, syncope, disturbed color perception, photophobia, diplopia, night blindness, and optic neuritis may occur. Other hypersensitivity reactions include cutaneous flushing with intense pruritus, angioedema, and asthmatic episodes.

Parameters of Use

Absorption Readily absorbed from upper GI tract. Peak action occurs in 1 to 3 hours and duration of action is 6 to 8 hours. Plasma half-life is 4 to 6 hours. Therapeutic serum drug levels are less than 8 mcg/ml. Rapidly bound to plasma albumin (about 60%).

Distribution Widely distributed in body tissues.

Metabolism Primarily in the liver.

Excretion By the kidneys as unchanged drug and metabolites. Excretion rate is decreased by alkaline urine and increased by acidic urine.

Drug Interactions Antacids, sodium bicarbonate, acetazolamide, and other drugs that alkalize the urine will decrease the rate of quinidine excretion. Barbiturates and phenytoin may antagonize the effects of quinidine. Potassium enhances the effects of quinidine whereas hypokalemia reduces them. Excessive depression of vagal stimulation may occur when anticholinergic agents are used concurrently. Hypotensive agents may have an additive vascular effect with quinidine. May displace protein-bound drugs such as digoxin and other cardiac glycosides, thus increasing their serum levels and the potential for toxic reactions induced by the latter drugs.

Administration Maintenance dosage: 200 to 300 mg po itd or qid; Maximum dosage: 4 g/day. Initially, clients may require around-the-clock doses every 4 to 6 hours.

- *Paroxysmal atrial tachycardia:* 400 to 600 mg po every 2 to 3 hours until conversion.
- *Atrial fibrillation:* 200 mg po every 2 to 3 hours for 5 to 8 doses; then increase daily until conversion occurs.

Available Drug Forms Tablets containing 100, 200, or 300 mg; capsules containing 200 or 300 mg.

Nursing Management:

Planning factors

1. Obtain a complete cardiovascular history of drug hypersensitivity.
2. Obtain baseline EKG, serum electrolytes, and complete blood cell count before initiating therapy.
3. Obtain vital signs. Cardiac monitoring is recommended until stabilization occurs.
4. Digitalization should be accomplished before initiating quinidine therapy.

Administration factors

1. Give between meals with a full glass of water.
2. If nausea or diarrhea occur, administer drug 30 to 60 minutes after meals.

Evaluation factors

1. Watch cardiac monitor for the following:
   (a) Drug effect: peaking P waves, elongation of QRS complex and Q-T interval
   (b) Signs of drug toxicity: QRS complex wider than 0.12 seconds
   (c) Development of complete heart block or tachycardia
   Notify physician if toxicity, heart block, or tachycardia occur.
2. Lidocaine may be effective in treating certain quinidine-induced arrhythmias.
3. Diarrhea is a sign of drug toxicity and the dosage should be reduced or an alternative drug used. If symptoms occur, notify physician.
4. Monitor vital signs frequently (once a shift). If fever or hypotension develop, notify physician.
5. Observe client for congestive heart failure frequently (once a shift). If rales develop in the lung bases, notify physician.
6. Obtain complete blood cell count and hepatic function tests periodically (every 1 to 6 months).
7. As conversion from atrial flutter or fibrillation to normal sinus rhythm occurs, observe client frequently (qlh) for signs of thromboembolism, since a mural clot may be dislodged from the atria. Preventive heparin injections may be prescribed when therapy is initiated.
8. Monitor intake and output. If oliguria occurs, notify physician.
9. Monitor serum electrolytes periodically and notify physician of any abnormalities immediately, particularly in serum calcium and potassium levels.

Client teaching factors

1. Explain the purpose and the necessity of maintaining drug levels to client and family.
2. Instruct client and family in the toxic and other untoward reactions. Emphasize the necessity of notifying the physician immediately if shortness of breath, oral bleeding, syncope, or a sudden change in heart rate occur. Have client return demonstration of how to count a pulse and what to look for.
3. Emphasize the need to maintain regularly scheduled checkups and laboratory appointments.
4. Instruct client to store drug in tightly sealed containers in a dark area (cupboard) away from excessive heat.

GENERIC NAME Quinidine gluconate (injection)

TRADE NAME Quinidinium Gluconate (RX)

CLASSIFICATION Antiarrhythmic, cardiac depressant

See quinidine sulfate for Indications for use, Contraindications, Warnings and precautions, Untoward reactions, Parameters of use, and Drug interactions.

Action Unlike the sulfate salt, this salt is freely soluble in water and can therefore be used parenterally. Little or no local irritation occurs. (See quinidine sulfate.)

Administration

- *Paroxysmal atrial tachycardia:* Adults: 400 to 600 mg IM every 2 to 3 hours, as needed.
- *Other arrhythmias:* Adults: Initial dosage: 600 mg IM; then 200 to 400 mg, as needed, or 700 mg via dilute IV bolus.

Available Drug Forms Multidose vials of 70 ml containing 80 mg/ml (50 mg of anhydrous quinidine); contains approximately 62% of anhydrous quinidine.

Nursing Management (See quinidine sulfate.)

1. Intravenous use can be hazardous; observe client's response continuously for toxicity.
2. Dilute IV bolus in 50 ml or more of 5% D/W and infuse slowly.
3. Do not exceed 1 mg/min. IV bolus.

GENERIC NAME Quinidine gluconate (oral) RX

TRADE NAMES Duraquin, Quinaglute Dura-Tabs, Quinate

CLASSIFICATION Antiarrhythmic, cardiac depressant

See quinidine sulfate for Indications for use, Contraindications, Warnings and precautions, Untoward reactions, Parameters of use, and Drug interactions.

Action Well tolerated orally with little or no drug-induced GI disturbances. (See quinidine sulfate.)

Administration Adults: 1 to 2 tablets po every 8 to 12 hours.

Available Drug Forms Sustained-release tablets containing 324 mg of the glucose salt; sustained-release tablets containing 330 mg (206 mg of anhydrous quinidine); contains approximately 62% of anhydrous quinidine.

Nursing Management May be given with food if GI disturbances occur. (See quinidine sulfate.)

GENERIC NAME Quinidine polygalacturonate

TRADE NAME Cardioquin RX

CLASSIFICATION Antiarrhythmic, cardiac depressant

See quinidine sulfate for Indications for use, Contraindications, Warnings and precautions, Untoward reactions, Parameters of use, Drug interactions, and Nursing management.

Action Slightly ionized and slightly soluble in water. Little or no drug-induced GI disturbances occur. (See quinidine sulfate.)

Administration Adults: 1 to 2 tablets po every 8 to 12 hours.

Available Drug Forms Uncoated scored tablets containing 275 mg (166 mg of anhydrous quinidine); contains approximately 60.5% of anhydrous quinidine.

GENERIC NAME Quinidine bisulfate RX

TRADE NAME Biquin Durule

CLASSIFICATION Antiarrhythmic, cardiac depressant

See quinidine sulfate for Indications for use, Contraindications, Warnings and precautions, Untoward reactions, Parameters of use, Drug interactions, and Nursing management.

Action May be better tolerated than quinidine sulfate. (See quinidine sulfate.)

Administration Adults: 1 to 2 capsules po every 8 to 12 hours.

Available Drug Forms Contains approximately 66% of anhydrous quinidine.

GENERIC NAME Procainamide hydrochloride (injection)

TRADE NAME Pronestyl Injection RX

CLASSIFICATION Antiarrhythmic

Action Similar to quinidine, but less effective in treating atrial arrhythmias. The drug decreases cardiac automaticity, conduction velocity, cardiac contractility, blocks vagal stimulation, and increases the refractory period. Drug induces some anticholinergic effects that result in untoward reactions.

Indications for Use Premature ventricular contractions, ventricular tachycardia, refractory atrial arrhythmias unresponsive to quinidine, paroxysmal atrial tachycardia, atrial fibrillation.

Contraindications Hypersensitivity to procaine and related substances; clients with second-degree or greater heart block; myasthenia gravis.

Warnings and Precautions Use with caution in clients with hepatic or renal impairment. Parenteral administration may cause severe hypotension due to peripheral vasodilation.

Untoward Reactions Toxicity induces ventricular tachycardia, extrasystoles, fibrillation, or cardiac standstill. A reaction similar to systemic lupus erythematosus manifested by polyarthralgia, arthritis, pleuritic pain, myalgia, pleural effusion, pericarditis, rashes, fever, and chills may occur, particularly after prolonged use. Hypersensitivity reactions include angioneurotic edema and maculopapular rash. Agranulocytosis has occurred and may result in death. Thrombocytopenia and hemolytic anemia have been reported after prolonged use. Other reactions include nausea, vomiting, loss of appetite, diarrhea, and flushing. Hallucinations may occur, particularly in the elderly.

Parameters of Use

Absorption Onset of action is: less than 15 minutes (IM); in 30 minutes (IV). Peak action occurs in: 15 to 60 minutes (IM). Plasma half-life is $3\frac{1}{2}$ hours. Therapeutic serum drug levels: 3 to 10 mcg/ml.

Metabolism In the liver to active metabolite N-acetyl procainamide and inactive metabolites.

Excretion By the kidneys as unchanged drug (60%) and metabolites (10%).

Drug Interactions May increase the neuromuscular blockade induced by skeletal muscle relaxants such as tubocurarine and succinylcholine.

Administration Adults: Initial dosage: 100 mg via slow IV bolus at a rate not exceeding 50 mg/min. repeated every 2 to 5 minutes, as needed; then 2 to 6 mg via continuous IV infusion. Do not exceed 1 g at any one time. Anesthesia-induced arrhythmias: 100 to 500 mg IM every 4 to 8 hours until oral therapy can be started.

Available Drug Forms Vials of 10 ml containing 100 mg/ml; vials of 2 ml containing 500 mg/ml.

Nursing Management (See quinidine sulfate.)

1. Cardiac monitoring is essential. Drug will widen QRS complex and prolong P-R and Q-T intervals. Voltage of QRS and T wave may decrease.
2. Dilute IV bolus and infusion in 5% D/W.
3. Give IV bolus slowly; do not exceed 50 mg/min. Can be given as an intermittent IV drip of 500 to 1000 mg in 100 ml of 5% D/W over 30 minutes or until arrhythmias subside; then start a dilute continuous IV drip.
4. Add 1000 mg to 500 ml of 5% D/W to yield 2 mg/ml for continuous IV drip; an IV pump is highly recommended.
5. Monitor blood pressure and pulse continuously. If blood pressure drops 15 mm Hg or more, slow the rate of administration and notify physician.

GENERIC NAME Procainamide hydrochloride (oral)

TRADE NAMES Procan-SR, Pronestyl (RX)

Classification Antiarrhythmic

See procainamide hydrochloride (injection) for Action, Contraindications, Warnings and precautions, and Drug interactions.

Indications for Use Often used to prevent recurrence of arrhythmias. [See procainamide hydrochloride (injection).]

Untoward Reactions Large dosages may cause anorexia, nausea, urticaria, or pruritus. Allergic reactions, including bronchial asthma, to FD&C No. 5 yellow may occur in susceptible clients. [See procainamide hydrochloride (injection).]

Parameters of Use

[See procainamide hydrochloride (injection).]

Absorption Onset of action is 30 minutes. Peak action occurs in 60 minutes.

Administration

- *Ventricular arrhythmias:* 50 mg/Kg/day po in divided doses q3h (regular form) or q6h (sustained-release tablet).
- *Atrial fibrillation and paroxysmal atrial tachycardia:* 500 to 1000 mg po every 4 to 6 hours; 1000 mg sustained-release tablet po q6h.

Available Drug Forms Capsules containing 250 or 500 mg; tablets containing 250, 375, or 500 mg; sustained-release tablets (Procan-SR) containing 250 or 500 mg.

Nursing Management (See quinidine sulfate.)

1. Reduced dosages are required for clients with impaired renal or hepatic function.
2. Perform complete blood cell count, Coombs' test, and antinuclear antibody titers periodically to detect the development of blood dyscrasias and systemic lupus erythematosus syndrome.

GENERIC NAME Disopyramide; disopyramide phosphate

TRADE NAMES Rythmoden; Norpace (RX)

CLASSIFICATION Antiarrhythmic

Action Similar to quinidine and procainamide. Disopyramide decreases automaticity, conduction velocity, and contractility of the myocardium. Cardiac output may decrease as much as 10%. Increases the refractory time. Although the drug has an anticholinergic effect, it does not affect alpha- or beta-adrenergic receptors.

Indications for Use Unifocal and multifocal premature beats, couplets (paired premature ventricular contractions), mild to moderate ventricular tachycardia.

Contraindications Cardiogenic shock, second-degree or greater heart block, myasthenia gravis, glaucoma, urinary retention.

Warnings and Precautions Use with caution in clients with hepatic or renal impairment. Clients with organic heart disease or congestive heart failure may develop hypotension and other untoward reactions. Electrolyte imbalances, particularly hypokalemia, should be corrected before initiating therapy. Safe use in children and during pregnancy has not been established. Lactating mothers should bottle-feed their babies.

Untoward Reactions Anticholinergic side effects, including dry mouth, urinary hesitancy, and constipation, are common. Blurred vision, dryness of eyes, nasal, and oral mucosa, nausea, abdominal distension, and excessive flatulence may occur. Hypotension may occur. Hypoglycemia may occur, particularly in clients with congestive heart failure, malnutrition, hepatic or renal impairment. Cholestatic jaundice has been reported after prolonged use. Blood urea nitrogen, liver enzymes, and creatinine may be elevated. CNS disturbances include dizziness, fatigue, syncope, muscular weakness, insomnia, depression, and nervousness. Generalized skin rashes may occur.

Parameters of Use

Absorption Well absorbed from GI tract. Peak action occurs in 2 hours. Therapeutic serum drug levels (base drugs): 2 to 4 mcg/ml. About 50 to 65% bound to proteins. Plasma half-life is about 6.7 hours; but may be considerably longer (8 to 18 hours) in clients with severe renal impairment.

Metabolism Primarily in the liver.

Excretion Primarily as unchanged drug (50%) and metabolites by the kidneys.

Administration Adults: Over 50 kg: 150 to 200 mg po q6h; Under 50 kg: 100 mg po q6h. In clients with renal insufficiency, the dosage depends on creatinine clearance: 15 to 40 ml/min.: 100 mg po q10h; 5 to 15 ml/min.: 100 mg po q20h; 1 to 5 ml/min.: 100 mg po q30h.

Available Drug Forms Hard gelatin capsules containing 100 or 150 mg.

Nursing Management (See quinidine sulfate.)

1. Cardiac monitoring is essential initially and should be continued until stabilization occurs or drug is discontinued.
2. Check apical pulse before administration.
3. Monitor intake and output. Check serum electrolytes periodically.

TYPE II ANTIARRHYTHMIC AGENTS

GENERIC NAME Lidocaine hydrochloride (RX)

TRADE NAMES Auto-Injector, Lidocaine, Lido-Pen, Lignocaine, Xylocaine

CLASSIFICATION Antiarrhythmic

Action This aminoacyl amide is resistant to hydrolysis and has been used as a local anesthetic for decades because it is stable; it has twice the potency of procaine and has a more rapid onset of action. Lidocaine was also found to have antiarrhythmic properties and is now widely used for emergency treatment of ventricular arrhythmias, particularly those associated with myocardial infarction and heart surgery. Lidocaine is thought to increase the threshold of ventricles during diastole, thus decreasing excitability and the emergence of ectopic beats. Unlike quinidine, lidocaine has no effect on cardiac conduction velocity, myocardial contractility, or systolic blood pressure.

Indications for Use Particularly effective in preventing and treating premature ventricular contractions and ventricular tachycardia; digitalis-induced ventricular arrhythmias.

Contraindications Hypersensitivity to amine local anesthetics, Adams-Stokes disease, complete heart block, second- or third-degree heart block, sinus bradycardia.

Warnings and Precautions Use with caution in the elderly and in clients with severe hepatic or renal impairment or a history of congestive heart failure. Safe use in children (under 50 kg) has not been established.

Untoward Reactions Toxicity and other untoward reactions rarely occur. Toxicity effects include dizziness, bradycardia, syncope, and hypotension due to poor cardiac output. Convulsions, coma, or cardiac arrest may also occur. CNS disturbances include lightheadedness, drowsiness, apprehension, euphoria, tinnitus, blurred or double vision, vomiting, and sensations of heat, cold, or numbness. Respiratory depression, which eventually leads to respiratory arrest, has been reported. Irritation at intramuscular injection sites has been reported.

Parameters of Use

Absorption Onset of action is: 5 to 15 minutes (IM); 30 seconds to 2 minutes (IV). Duration of action is: 60 to 90 minutes (IM); about 20 minutes (IV). Plasma half-life is about 2 hours (elimination) and distribution half-life is only 8 to 10 minutes. Between 50 to 75% bound to plasma proteins.

Crosses blood-brain barrier and placenta. Drug rapidly metabolized by fetus.

Metabolism About 90% in the liver.

Excretion Primarily as metabolites by the kidneys; about 10% excreted as unchanged drug.

Drug Interactions Concurrent use of propranolol, quinidine, or phenytoin may have an additive cardiac depressant effect. Concurrent use of procainamide may augment CNS untoward reactions to lidocaine. Barbiturates may decrease the antiarrhythmic effect of lidocaine. Large dosages of lidocaine will increase the neuromuscular blocking action of succinylcholine; use with caution concurrently.

Administration

- *Emergency treatment of ventricular arrhythmias:* Initial dosage: 50 mg IV bolus followed by another 50 mg in 10 to 15 minutes (up to 300 mg may be given in divided doses); then 1 to 4 mg/min. via continuous IV drip. Toxicity usually occurs with rates greater than 5 mg/min. Continuous IV drip must be started within 20 minutes of IV bolus to maintain therapeutic serum drug levels. One-half of the drug dosage is used in elderly clients with renal insufficiency.
- *Short-term prevention of ventricular arrhythmias:* 200 to 300 mg IM or 2 mg/min. continuous IV drip.

Available Drug Forms (Without preservatives or additives.) Prefilled syringes containing 100 mg with 20 mg/ml (IV bolus); vials containing solutions of 1 or 2 g for adding to 500 ml of 5% D/W IV solution (continuous IV drip); injection syringes containing undiluted solutions of 1 or 2 g for adding to 500 ml of 5% D/W IV solution (continuous IV drip or IV bolus); ampules containing 100 mg/ml (IM injection).

Nursing Management

Planning factors

1. Obtain history of cardiovascular disturbances, when possible. Six or more premature ventricular contractions (PVCs) per minute and multifocal PVCs are usually treated immediately to prevent further deterioration of arrhythmias.
2. Cardiac monitoring is essential.
3. IV therapy is the preferred route of administration. Start 5% D/W or normal saline with 20- or 18-gauge indwelling catheter into a large blood vessel KVO. Drug solution is given as a secondary line.
4. Avoid administering other medications or blood products into drug IV administration line.
5. Check that the concentration of lidocaine (without preservatives) is correct.
6. Obtain baseline serum electrolytes. Abnormalities should be corrected before or concurrently with lidocaine therapy, when necessary.
7. When accurate creatine phosphokinase levels are important for diagnosis of myocardial infarction, drug should be administered IV instead of IM.

Administration factors

1. When administering IM,
   - (a) Although seldom used, IM administration is sometimes used by ambulance personnel to prevent arrhythmias in clients with myocardial infarctions during transport to hospital.
   - (b) Inject into deltoid muscle mass; this site provides higher serum peak drug levels than the gluteus muscles.
   - (c) Avoid giving more than 3 ml into the same muscle mass.
2. When administering IV bolus,
   - (a) Check patency of IV before administering drug.
   - (b) Can be given as a direct IV puncture or into the Y port of a continuous IV drip. Clamp distal section of IV tubing during injection.
   - (c) Administer at a rate of 25 to 50 mg/min. If administered too slowly, therapeutic drug levels will not be reached as the drug is rapidly destroyed by the liver and distribution to protein-binding sites occurs.
3. When administering via continuous IV drip,
   - (a) Add 2 g of lidocaine to 500 ml of 5% D/W. (1 g of lidocaine can be used.)
   - (b) Start continuous IV drip as soon as possible after IV bolus has been given (less than 20 minutes).
   - (c) Check patency of IV site before adding drug solution IV piggyback.
   - (d) An IV pump is recommended but a 60 gtt/ml IV administration set can be used.
   - (e) If the rate is not prescribed, a rate of 2 mg/min. is recommended. (This is equal to 30 gtt/min. or 0.5 ml/min. when 2 g is added to 500 ml of 5% D/W.)
   - (f) Never add a lidocaine drip to a blood transfusion line.
   - (g) Change IV drug solution at least once every 24 hours.

Evaluation factors

1. Constant cardiac monitoring is essential. Observe client for the following:
   - (a) Drug's effectiveness—cessation of ventricular arrhythmia. "Breakthrough" PVCs should not exceed 5/min. P-R interval may increase and Q-T interval may decrease with large dosages or prolonged use.
   - (b) Bradycardia and/or aggravation of arrhythmia—stop drug administration and notify physician.
2. Monitor intake and output, blood pressure, and respirations frequently. Initial dosage is usually maintained for 24 to 48 hours and then gradually decreased before discontinuing drug in order to prevent the resurgence of arrhythmia.
3. Observe client for initial CNS toxicity (usually seen when serum drug levels are between 5 to 8 mcg/ml). Serum drug levels above 9 mcg/ml will induce convulsions and respiratory arrest. If symptoms occur, decrease IV rate. When indicated, stop drug infusion until toxic reaction disappears.
4. Obtain serum electrolytes periodically (daily) and notify physician if abnormalities occur so that they can be corrected promptly.

GENERIC NAME Phenytoin sodium (RX)

TRADE NAME Dilantin, Dantoin

CLASSIFICATION Antiarrhythmic

Action Phenytoin sodium is a hydantoin derivative. It is an effective anticonvulsant that was found to decrease cardiac automaticity and the refractory time without increasing contractility (inotropic effect). The drug also increases conduction velocity and the threshold of atrial and ventricular fibers against the formation of premature beats.

Indications for Use Digitalis-induced extrasystoles, such as paroxysmal atrial tachycardia; refractory ventricular arrhythmias unresponsive to lidocaine.

Contraindications Hypersensitivity to hydantoin derivatives, sinus bradycardia, SA block, second- or third-degree heart block, Adams-Stokes disease.

Warnings and Precautions Use with caution in the elderly and clients with hypotension, severe myocardial insufficiency, acute heart failure, or impaired hepatic or renal function. May alter serum glucose levels in diabetic clients.

Safe use during pregnancy has not been established. Drug use has been associated with birth defects.

Untoward Reactions Rapid intravenous administration may cause severe hypotension and vascular collapse or life-threatening arrhythmias, including ventricular fibrillation and depressed AV conduction. Toxic CNS disturbances include ataxia, drowsiness, nystagmus, and diplopia. Respiratory depression, which may progress to apnea, has occurred. Toxic hepatitis may occur in the elderly and critically ill clients. Allergic reactions and blood dyscrasias may occur. Gingival hyperplasia, nausea, and vomiting are common. The gum overgrowth is irreversible and occurs most frequently in children. Although the gum condition may be annoying, the drug is usually continued. Meticulous oral hygiene may prevent further gum overgrowth. Local irritation and pain may occur at injection sites.

Parameters of Use

Absorption Onset of action is 3 to 5 minutes after IV administration. Plasma half-life is 22 hours, but varies widely depending on hepatic function. About 70 to 95% bound to plasma proteins. Slowly absorbed from GI tract; absorption may vary with drug dosage, form, and manufacturer. Peak plasma levels occur in 3 to 12 hours. Crosses blood-brain barrier.

Crosses placenta and enters breast milk. May cause birth defects.

Metabolism By saturable liver enzyme system; hypermetabolizers may have low serum drug levels. Excessive serum drug levels may be induced by liver disorders, congenital enzyme deficiency, or drug interaction.

Excretion Inactive metabolites are excreted into the bile and then reabsorbed and excreted by the kidneys. About 5% is excreted as unchanged drug. Severe kidney impairment may cause retention of drugs or metabolites.

Drug Interactions There are numerous drug interactions reported for phenytoin, primarily because of the drug's high plasma protein binding and its method of metabolism and excretion. Phenytoin is displaced from its plasma binding sites by salicylates, sulfonamides, phenothiazines, phenylbutazone, and phenyramidol. Drugs that inhibit the liver metabolism of phenytoin include oral anticoagulants, oral contraceptives, aminosalicylic acid, chloramphenicol, disulfiram, and isoniazid. Phenytoin decreases the body's supply of folic acid, and the two substances are antagonistic. Supplemental use of folic acid may decrease the anti-convulsant effect. The ingestion of alcohol increases the hepatic metabolism of phenytoin and may cause loss of drug's effect. Phenytoin and lidocaine have additive cardiac depressant effects; however, phenytoin may decrease the action of lidocaine through enzyme induction.

Administration Adults: 250 mg IV bolus over 5 minutes at a rate not exceeding 50 mg/min.; or 100 mg IV bolus repeated in 15 to 30 minutes as needed; or 1000 mg po in divided doses over 24 hours; then 300 to 500 mg po daily. Children: 3 to 8 mg/kg via IV bolus or infusion; may be given in 2 divided doses.

Available Drug Forms Ampules containing 50 mg/ml; prefilled syringes containing 50 mcg/ml.

Nursing Management (See quinidine sulfate.)

1. Often given as divided IV bolus. First bolus is a loading dose; second bolus often elicits a marked cardiac effect.
2. Continuous cardiac monitoring is essential.
3. Do not administer in 5% D/W IV line. Flush IV line with normal saline before and after drug administration. Administer intermittent IV infusion in saline over 1 hour or less.
4. Monitor blood pressure and pulse frequently.

ADRENERGIC BLOCKERS

GENERIC NAME Propranolol hydrochloride (RX)

TRADE NAME Inderal

CLASSIFICATION Antiarrhythmic

Action Propranolol is a beta-blocking agent that induces a marked reduction in heart rate. Propranolol competitively antagonizes the effects of catecholamines. It decreases cardiac automaticity, conduction velocity, refractory period, cardiac contractility, and cardiac output (slight). The drug is effective in treating tachyarrhythmias due to hyperthyroidism and catecholamines.

Indications for Use Tachyarrhythmias; atrial, supraventricular, and ventricular arrhythmias; angina. Primarily used for tachyarrhythmias caused by adrenergic response.

Contraindications Bronchial asthma, allergic rhinitis, sinus bradycardia, heart block greater than first degree, cardiogenic shock, right ventricular failure, clients taking adrenergic-augmenting psychotropic agents (such as MAO inhibitors).

Warnings and Precautions Abrupt withdrawal may precipitate myocardial infarction, thyrotoxicosis, angina, or pheochromocytoma. When surgery is indicated, notify anesthesiologist that client is taking propranolol. May cause bronchospasm in clients with asthma. May precipitate cardiac failure in the elderly and clients with a history of cardiac failure. Clients with Wolff-Parkinson-White syndrome may develop severe bradycardia when drug is initiated; insertion of a demand pacemaker may be required. The signs and symptoms of hypoglycemia may be masked in diabetic clients.

Untoward Reactions Bradycardia, hypotension, and congestive heart failure are common. Cardiac standstill may occur. Agranulocytosis, purpura, and other blood dyscrasias have been reported. May cause bronchoconstriction and GI disturbances, including nausea, vomiting, and diarrhea. Hypotension and hypoglycemia without tachycardia may occur in diabetic clients. CNS disturbances, including lightheadedness, depression, insomnia, visual disturbances, hallucinations, disorientation, and short-term memory loss, have occurred.

Parameters of Use

Absorption Well absorbed from GI tract. Onset of action is about 30 minutes (po); about 2 minutes (IV). Peak plasma levels occur in 60 to 90 minutes (po); 15 minutes (IV). Duration of action is about 6 hours (po); 3 to 6 hours (IV)). Plasma half-life varies from 3.4 to 6 hours; some clients metabolize the drug faster than others. About 90% bound to plasma proteins. Crosses blood-brain barrier and may cause CNS disturbances.

Crosses placenta and enters breast milk.

Distribution Widely distributed in body tissues.

Metabolism In the liver.

Excretion By the kidneys as unchanged drug and metabolites. Less than 5% excreted in feces.

Drug Interactions The cardiac depressant action of phenytoin and quinidine may be enhanced. Bradycardia may occur in digitalized clients. Propranolol is antagonized by aminophylline and other theophylline-containing drugs. Also antagonized by isoproterenol, norepinephrine, and glucagon; can be used as an antidote. May alter the requirements for insulin and other hypoglycemic agents in diabetes. Action of neuromuscular blocking agents, such as tubocurarine, may be prolonged; watch client for respiratory depression. Anesthetic agents that depress the myocardium (ether, cyclopropane, trichloroethylene) may cause severe hypotension, bradycardia, and cardiovascular collapse; discontinue beta blockers 48 hours prior to surgery.

Administration Adults: Initial dosage: 1 to 3 mg dilute IV bolus or infusion at a rate not exceeding 1 mg/min.; may be repeated in 2 to 5 minutes; do not repeat for 4 hours. Transfer to oral therapy as soon as possible. Maintenance dosage: 10 to 30 mg po tid or qid before meals and at bedtime (for arrythmias).

Available Drug Forms Ampules containing 1 mg/ml; tablets containing 10, 20, 40, 60, 80 or 90 mg; capsules (long-acting) containing 80, 120, or 160 mg.

Nursing Management

Planning factors

1. Obtain baseline data about the arrhythmia.
2. Assess cardiovascular and respiratory status for possible contraindications. Record baseline vital signs.
3. Assess hepatic and renal function. If blood urea nitrogen (BUN) or serum creatinine are elevated, notify physician. If oliguria exists, notify physician.
4. Keep drug on units where clients may need it for life-threatening arrhythmias (emergency room, intensive care unit, coronary care unit, extended coronary care unit).
5. Store drug in a dark area (closet).
6. Keep appropriate drugs readily available for use in the event of toxicity: atropine for bradycardia, isoproterenol for cardiac failure, epinephrine for hypotension, and aminophylline or isoproterenol for bronchospasm.
7. Withdraw drug temporarily 48 hours prior to surgery that requires general anesthetic agents, with the exception of clients with pheochromocytoma.

Administration factors

1. Check blood pressure and pulse before therapy is initiated or dosage adjusted. If severe bradycardia or hypotension exist, notify physician before administering drug. Initially, cardiac monitoring is essential.
2. Give drug before meals and at bedtime on an empty stomach. Follow with a full glass of water.
3. When administering IV,
   - (a) IV bolus given over 1 to 3 minutes is often used to treat life-threatening arrhythmias; diluted IV drug solution (50 or 100 ml) every 4 hours is then used to maintain serum levels.
   - (b) Desired dose can be diluted in 50 to 100 ml of normal saline or 5% D/W.
   - (c) Do not administer at a rate faster than 1 mg/min.
   - (d) Continuous cardiac monitoring is essential.
   - (e) Monitor blood pressure and pulse continuously.
   - (f) A second dose may be required.

Evaluation factors

1. When IV therapy is used, monitor blood pressure and pulse every 2 minutes until stable. Cardiac monitoring is essential to determine type of arrhythmia. If no response occurs after 2 doses, another antiarrhythmic agent or cardioversion may be required.
2. Initially, check blood pressure and pulse before each dosage; then check periodically.
3. Obtain complete blood cell count, blood urea nitrogen, and serum creatinine levels periodically.
4. Record intake and output.
5. Dosage must be reduced gradually before discontinuing drug.

Client teaching factors

1. Inform client of potential untoward reactions and to notify physician immediately if low pulse rate (below 60 beats/min.), shortness of breath, or hypoglycemia occur.
2. Advise client (particularly if normotensive) to change positions slowly to avoid lightheadedness.
3. Advise client to avoid excessive use of CNS depressants and stimulants (alcohol or caffeinated drinks such as coffee, cola, or tea), since untoward reactions may occur.
4. Inform client that adaptation to stressful situations will be altered and to avoid stress if possible.
5. Advise client that untoward reactions may occur if the drug is discontinued abruptly.

GENERIC NAME Bretylium tosylate (RX)

TRADE NAME Bretylol

CLASSIFICATION Antiarrhythmic

Action Bretylium tosylate, a bromobenzyl quaternary ammonium compound, inhibits the release of norepinephrine by depressing the excitability of adrenergic nerve endings. It increases the automaticity and refractory period of the heart, and may increase conduction velocity. The drug has little or no effect on cardiac contractility. The exact mechanism by which bretylium tosylate suppresses ventricular fibrillation and arrhythmias has not been established.

Indications for Use Ventricular arrhythmias. Has been used to prevent and treat ventricular fibrillation.

Contraindications Digitalis toxicity.

Warnings and Precautions Hypotension occurs in 50% of clients with continued use. Initial release of norepinephrine may cause transient hypertension and premature ventricular contractions. Use with caution in clients with a fixed cardiac output, such as those with aortic stenosis or severe pulmonary hypertension, since severe hypotension may occur due to a fall in peripheral resistance without a compensatory rise in cardiac output. Safe use in children and during pregnancy has not been established.

Untoward Reactions Hypotension and postural hypotension are common. Vertigo, dizziness, lightheadedness, and syncope may occur. Bradycardia, angina, and substernal discomfort may occur. Rapid infusion may induce nausea and vomiting. Renal dysfunction, hyperthermia, flushing, diarrhea, abdominal cramps, diaphoresis, and mild conjunctivitis have been reported. Confusion, paranoia, emotional lability, anxiety, lethargy, and shortness of breath have also been reported.

Parameters of Use

Absorption Onset of action is: in minutes after IV administration for ventricular fibrillation; 20 minutes to 2 hours for suppressing other ventricular arrhythmias. Half-life is about 7.8 hours in normal clients and about 16 hours in clients with a creatinine clearance of 21 ml/min.

Excretion By the kidneys as unchanged drug; rapidly eliminated during hemodialysis.

Drug Interactions Antihypertensive agents may potentiate the hypotensive effects of bretylium.

Administration

- *Life-threatening arrhythmias:* Initial dosage: 5 to 10 mg/kg via IV bolus or intermittent infusion; repeat every 1 to 2 hours, as needed; then continuous IV drip at 1 to 2 mg/min.
- *Other arrhythmias:* 5 to 10 mg/kg IV bolus over 8 minutes or more q6h, as needed.

Available Drug Forms Ampules containing 500 mg/10 ml.

Nursing Management (See propranolol hydrochloride.)

1. Dopamine or norepinephrine should be available for immediate use to treat hypotension (blood pressure of 75 mm Hg or less).
2. Cardiac monitoring is essential.
3. IV bolus and infusion must be diluted in at least 4 parts of 5% D/W or sodium chloride injection to each part of drug volume.
4. Continuous IV drip is prepared by adding 500 mg (10 ml) to 50 or 100 ml of 5% D/W or normal saline. Infuse at a rate of 1 to 2 mg/min.
5. Slow the rate of IV administration if blood pressure drops excessively or nausea occurs.
6. Continuous monitoring of blood pressure and pulse is highly recommended until stabilizaiton occurs.
7. Drug is given IM as undiluted solution.
8. Keep client in a supine position, whenever possible, to avoid hypotension. Elevation of the legs may be helpful.
9. Reduced dosages are required in clients with renal impairment.

CALCIUM CHANNEL BLOCKERS

GENERIC NAME Verapamil hydrochloride (RX)

TRADE NAMES Calan, Isoptin

CLASSIFICATION Antiarrhythmic

Action Verapamil inhibits slow-channel movement of calcium (and sodium) ions into conductive and contractile myocardial cells and vascular smooth cells; serum calcium levels are not altered. It slows AV conduction and prolongs the refractory period of AV nodes, thus decreasing ventricular rate in clients with supraventricular arrhythmias. Normal sinus rhythm is restored in clients with paroxysmal atrial tachycardia by interrupting reentry in the AV node. Afterload and myocardial contractility are reduced by verapamil.

Indications for Use Supraventricular arrhythmias; rapid conversion of paroxysmal atrial tachycardia to sinus rhythm, including Wolff-Parkinson-White, Lown-Ganong-Levine, and other syndromes; short-term control of rapid ventricular rate in atrial flutter or fibrillation.

Contraindications Severe hypotension, cardiogenic shock, second- or third-degree heart block, sick sinus syndrome, severe primary congestive heart failure, concurrently or within a few hours of propranolol IV or other beta-adrenergic blockers, since both drugs depress cardiac contractility and AV conduction.

Warnings and Precautions A rapid ventricular response may occur in clients with atrial flutter or fibrillation due to an aberrant conduction pathway that bypasses the AV node. Excessive bradycardia or asystole may occur in elderly clients and clients with sick sinus syndrome. May increase heart failure (pulmonary wedge pressure above 20 mm Hg) when the cause is not related to rate; concurrent digitalization may be helpful.

Untoward Reactions Hypotension, bradycardia, or severe tachycardia may occur. Dizziness and headache may also occur. Nausea and abdominal discomfort have been reported.

Parameters of Use

Absorption Peak action occurs in 3 to 5 minutes after IV bolus. Biphasic half-life: 4 minutes (distribution phase); 2 to 5 hours (elimination phase).

Metabolism Rapidly in the liver to several metabolites.

Excretion Primarily in urine (70%); some in feces (16%).

Drug Interactions Do not administer disopyramide within 48 hours before or 24 hours after verapamil because of potential interaction. Avoid concurrent use with beta-adrenergic blockers since excessive cardiac depression may occur, particularly when the beta blocker has been administered intravenously.

Administration Adults: Initial dosage: 5 to 10 mg (0.075 to 0.15 mg/kg) IV bolus over 2 minutes or more; then 10 mg in 30 minutes, if necessary. Maintenance dose: 240 to 480 mg/day. Children: Ages 1 to 15 years: Initial dosage: 0.1 to 0.3 mg/kg IV bolus over 2 minutes or more; do not exceed 5 mg; repeat in 30 minutes, if necessary; do not exceed 10 mg. Infants: 0.1 to 0.2 mg/kg IV bolus over 2 minutes or more; repeat in 30 minutes, if necessary.

Available Drug Forms Ampules containing 2.5 mg/ml. Tablets containing 80 or 120 mg.

Nursing Management

1. Vasopressor agents and isoproterenol should be available for immediate use in the event of severe hypotension or bradycardia.
2. For IV use, administer slowly as initial but transient hypotension is common.
3. Inspect solution for particulate matter or discoloration before using. Discard solution if changes occur.
4. It may take 10 minutes for normal sinus rhythm to be restored in paroxysmal atrial tachycardia.
5. Ventricular response is usually reduced by 20% in clients with atrial flutter or fibrillation. Conversion seldom occurs.
6. Continuous cardiac monitoring is essential.
7. Monitor blood pressure and pulse. If systolic pressure drops below 100 mg Hg, notify physician.
8. Dosages must be individualized by titration.

GENERIC NAME Nifedipine hydrochloride (RX)

TRADE NAME Procardia

CLASSIFICATION Antiarrhythmic

Action Nifedipine is a calcium channel blocker similar to verapamil hydrochloride. Although serum calcium levels are not altered, the slow-channel movement of calcium ions into conductile and contractile myocardial cells and vascular smooth cells is inhibited. However, nifedipine induces more relaxation of vascular smooth muscle than verapamil, thereby reducing blood pressure, but has less effect on SA and AV node conduction; therefore, verapamil is often preferred for emergency treatment of arrhythmias.

Indications for Use Supraventricular arrhythmias.

Contraindications Acute episodes of congestive heart failure, severe hypotension, cardiogenic shock, second- or third-degree heart block, sick sinus syndrome.

Warnings and Precautions Use with extreme caution in clients with aortic stenosis. Peripheral edema in the legs (pedal edema) may result from the drug-induced decrease in peripheral resistance; diuretics are effective in relieving the edema. Safe use in clients with hepatic or renal impairment and during pregnancy has not been established. A rapid ventricular response may occur in clients with atrial flutter or fibrillation due to an aberrant conduction pathway that bypasses the AV node. Excessive bradycardia or asystole may occur in elderly clients and clients with sick sinus syndrome.

Untoward Reactions Dose-related transient hypotension may occur, but is usually mild and well tolerated. Dizziness, lightheadedness, giddiness, flushing, a sensation of warmth, and headache are common. Syncope is rare and is dose related. GI disturbances include nausea and gastric distress. Diarrhea, cramps, and constipation have been reported. Weakness, muscle cramps, and nervousness have occurred. Peripheral edema, palpitations, dyspnea, wheezing, nasal congestion, and sore throat have been reported. Cholestasis has been reported after prolonged therapy, but rarely.

Parameters of Use

Absorption Rapid and complete, from GI tract. Onset of action is 10 minutes. Peak action occurs in 30 minutes. Half-life is 2 hours.

Excretion About 80% by the kidneys as unchanged drug and metabolites.

Drug Interactions Concurrent therapy with beta-adrenergic blockers is usually well tolerated, but the development of acute congestive heart failure, severe hypotension, and angina have been reported. Nifedipine may increase serum levels of digitalis glycosides as much as 50%; when used concurrently, observe client for digitalis toxicity.

Administration Adults: Initial dosage: 10 mg po every 8 hours for 1 to 2 weeks; then adjust dosage according to client's response; Dosage range: 10 to 30 mg every 6 to 8 hours; Maximum dosage: 180 mg po daily.

Available Drug Forms Capsules (orange) containing 10 mg.

Nursing Management

Planning factors

1. Obtain history of arrhythmia and other cardiovascular disorders.

2. Obtain baseline vital signs. If hypotension or pulmonary edema are present, notify physician before initiating therapy.
3. Obtain baseline EKG, serum transaminase levels, and hepatic function tests. If abnormalities exist, notify physician.

Administration factors

1. Give with 4 to 6 fl oz of water.
2. Drug can be administered tid, but the preferred schedule is every 8 hours.

Evaluation factors

1. Continuous cardiac monitoring of arrhythmia is essential.
2. Check blood pressure and pulse frequently (every 4 to 8 hours) for the first 2 to 3 days following institution of therapy and when dosage is adjusted. If hypotension or bradycardia occur, notify physician.
3. Observe legs for pedal edema and notify physician if edema occurs.

Client teaching factors

1. Warn client that abrupt withdrawal of drug may precipitate angina, arrhythmias, and other disorders.
2. Warn client about the expected secondary reactions to the drug, such as dizziness and headache. If symptoms are annoying and persistent, the physician should be notified.
3. When prescribed, instruct client in the proper use of antiembolic stockings.
4. Emphasize the need for regular medical checkups.

ANTIBRADYCARDIAC AGENTS

GENERIC NAME Atropine sulfate (RX)

TRADE NAME Atropine

CLASSIFICATION Antibradycardiac agent

Action In large dosages, this antimuscarinic agent blocks inhibitory vagal impulses to the heart and results in increased AV conduction (shortened P-R interval) and heart rate. It also blocks the effects of acetylcholine on the myocardium. The drug has little or no effect on blood pressure, but may cause flushing of head and neck due to vasodilation.

Indications for Use Bradycardia, bradyarrhythmias, such as junctional or escape rhythms. May be used until pacemaker can be inserted.

Contraindications Narrow-angle glaucoma, urinary retention, obstruction of GI or genitourinary tract.

Warnings and Precautions Use with caution in clients with hyperthyroidism, hypertension, congestive heart failure, or severe coronary artery disease; and in debilitated clients with chronic obstructive pulmonary disease, since mucus plugs may occur. Small dosages (less than 0.5 mg) may cause a decrease in heart rate. Children under 6 years of age may have an exaggerated response to the drug's action.

Untoward Reactions Extreme tachycardia and angina may occur with large dosages (over 2 mg). Common secondary effects include dry mouth, blurred vision, photophobia, urinary retention, and constipation. CNS disturbances, including headache, dizziness, restlessness, and tremors, may occur, particularly when dosages greater than 5 mg are administered.

Parameters of Use

Absorption Crosses placenta and is found in breast milk. Use with caution during pregnancy.

Distribution Rapidly disappears from blood into tissues.

Metabolism Hydrolyzed by enzymes in the liver and in tissues.

Excretion Primarily by the kidneys, as unchanged drug and metabolites. Small quantities found in body secretions.

Drug Interactions Physostigmine salicylate is an effective antidote for extreme tachycardia. Drugs that have some anticholinergic activity, such as the tricyclic antidepressants, meperidine, certain antihistamines, and phenothiazines may have additive or potentiating effects when given concurrently. MAO inhibitors may potentiate atropine. Administer atropine sulfate with extreme caution to clients who have taken MAO inhibitors within the last 2 weeks.

Administration Adults: 0.5 to 1.0 mg IV push; repeat every 5 to 15 minutes, as needed; do not exceed 2 mg. Children: 0.01 mg/kg IV push; repeat as needed; do not exceed 0.4 mg.

Available Drug Forms Prefilled syringes containing 0.5 mg/5 ml or 1 mg/10 ml; multidose vials containing 0.4, 1.0, or 1.2 mg/ml.

Nursing Management

1. Cardiac monitoring is essential.
2. Administer via rapid IV bolus. Avoid mixing with other IV medications.
3. Monitor blood pressure and pulse frequently.
4. Protect client's face from direct light.
5. Monitor intake and output.

GENERIC NAME Isoproterenol hydrochloride

TRADE NAME Isuprel (RX)

CLASSIFICATION Antibradycardiac agent

Action Isoproterenol is a potent stimulator of beta-adrenergic receptors. It induces an increase in heart rate, conduction velocity through the AV node, and contractility.

Indications for Use Heart block prior to insertion of a pacemaker, Adams-Stokes disease, AV block.

Contraindications Digitalis-induced tachycardia, pre-existing tachyarrhythmias, recent myocardial infarction.

Warnings and Precautions Use with caution in clients with coronary insufficiency, diabetes, or hyperthyroidism. A drug-induced heart rate of 130 beats/min. may precipitate a ventricular arrhythmia.

Untoward Reactions Tachycardia, ventricular arrhythmias, and hypotension may occur and lead to shock or pulmonary edema. Blood pressure may be elevated initially and then drop. Headache, dizziness, nervousness, and mild tremors are relatively common. Nausea, vomiting, anginal or precordial pain, and hyperglycemia may occur. Weakness, flushing, and sweating have been reported.

Parameters of Use

Absorption Readily absorbed from parenteral sites; sublingual absorption is unreliable.
Distribution Widely distributed, particularly to liver, kidneys, and brain.
Metabolism Rapid
Excretion Primarily by the kidneys as unchanged drug and metabolites.

Drug Interactions Propranolol and other beta blockers antagonize the action of isoproterenol. Do not give concurrently with epinephrine, since both are direct cardiac stimulants.

Administration

- *Heart block:* Adults: Initial dosage: 0.02 to 0.06 mg IV bolus; then 0.01 to 0.02 mg IV bolus, as needed, or 5 mcg/min. via continous IV drip. 0.2 mg IM can be used and followed by 0.2 to 0.1 mg IM, as needed. Children: $\frac{1}{2}$ of adult dosage.
- *Prevention of AV block and acute episodes of Adams-Stokes disease:* Adults: 30 to 180 mg po daily (sustained-release preparation).
- *shock:* 0.5 to 5.0 mcg/min. via continuous IV drip.

Available Drug Forms Ampules containing 0.2 mg/1 ml (1:5000 solution) or 1.0 mg/5 ml (1:5000 solution); tablets containing 10 or 15 mg.

Nursing Management

1. Dilute IV bolus and infusions in 5% D/W or sodium chloride.
2. Drug can be given undiluted intracardiac (shock), intramuscular, or subcutaneously. Usual dosage is 0.2 mg (1 ml).
3. IV bolus is prepared by adding 0.2 mg (1 ml) to 10 ml of diluent.
4. IV infusion is prepared by adding 2 mg (10 ml) to 500 ml of diluent to yield 4 mcg/ml.
   (a) Initial infusion rate is 5 mcg/ml or 1.25 ml/min.
   (b) An infusion pump is highly recommended.
5. Cardiac monitoring is essential.
6. Continuous monitoring of blood pressure and pulse is necessary.
7. Hypovolemia should be corrected before instituting therapy.
8. If anginal or precordial pain occur, discontinue the drug immediately.

Chapter 48

Antianginal Agents

ANGINA PECTORIS IS a coronary artery disease that is characterized by acute substernal chest pain, which may or may not radiate. Pain radiation usually occurs in the inner aspect of the left arm, but may also be radiated to the left shoulder or the right side of the neck. Although actual injury to the heart does not occur, frequent or severe anginal pain may interfere with the client's ability to work and perform other activities of daily living.

CAUSES OF ANGINA

In the 18th century, angina was postulated to be caused by spasms of the coronary arteries. However, in the middle of the 20th century, the cause of anginal pain was thought to be atherosclerosis of the coronary arteries, which caused a fluid blockage of the vessels. Indeed, most clients with angina experience pain upon exercising or performing other activities that increase the myocardial demand for oxygen above the coronary arteries' ability to supply oxygen. Anxiety, extreme cold weather, and heavy meals can also precipitate anginal pain.

During the 1970s, it was documented that spasms of the coronary arteries occur in clients with Prinzmetal's angina, a form of angina in which pain occurs at rest. It has now been determined that there are two primary causes of myocardial ischemia associated with acute anginal pain: (1) A *fixed obstruction* is produced in atherosclerosis that decreases the oxygen supply to the heart during exertion; and (2) a *variable obstruction* occurs when the coronary arteries go into spasm, which can cause pain at rest. Although the cause of coronary artery spasm is unknown, it seems to be related to an electrolyte disturbance within the smooth muscles of the arteries, since agents that block calcium channels are helpful in preventing it. Generally, fluid obstruction is more common, but many clients may have various degrees of both fixed and variable obstruction. Drugs used to prevent and treat acute angina include the nitrates, beta-adrenergic blocking agents, and calcium channel blocking agents.

DRUGS USED TO TREAT ANGINAL ATTACKS

129Anginal pain can be relieved in minutes by short-acting nitrate and nitrite vasodilators such as nitroglycerin and amyl nitrite, which are rapid-acting smooth muscle relaxants. Nitrates were originally thought to allay pain of angina by causing coronary artery dilation, but this is a secondary effect. Their primary action results in dilation of the postcapillary bed, which reduces the venous return of blood, or *preload*, to the heart. Some arterial dilation also occurs and the heart has less arterial pressure, or *afterload*, to pump against. Anginal pain is relieved when the work load of the heart is decreased by a reduction in the afterload and preload—reduction of the preload is of primary importance. There is some evidence to indicate that nitroglycerin directly affects the heart's ability to deliver blood to ischemic myocardial tissue by causing dilation of collateral coronary arteries, thereby increasing the blood supply to ischemic tissue.

As short-acting nitrates are effective within minutes for most clients with angina, clients must have these drugs readily available for use. Amyl nitrate is a vapor for inhalation and is inconvenient to carry, but nitroglycerin is available in small tablets that can be placed under the tongue for quick relief. Unfortunately, these tablets lose their potency rapidly and remain effective for only five months, even when they are carefully stored in airtight, light-resistant containers. Prevention of angina is preferred to treatment of acute angina.

DRUGS USED TO PREVENT ANGINA

Nitrates Long-acting nitrates, such as erythrityl tetranitrate, that have been used for decades with some success cause gradual vasodilation that is mild and prolonged. Unfortunately, these early preparations are only effective for a few hours and have to be taken several times a day. Preparations are now available that provide the slow release of nitroglycerin or the sustained release of longer-acting nitrates, thus requiring infrequent drug administration.

Beta-adrenergic blocking agents Although nitrates are effective in preventing angina in most clients, some clients are granted no pain relief whereas others experience a reduction, not elimination, in the number of acute anginal attacks. The drug propranolol, a beta-adrenergic blocker, was released for use in angina during the 1970s. Beta blockers are used in selected clients who have little or no relief with conventional measures. Propranolol and nadolol antagonize the heart's response to sympathetic stimulation. They decrease heart rate, cardiac output, and blood pressure. Although the blood supply through the coronary arteries is often reduced, the oxygen requirements of the myocardial tissue are reduced as well.

Abrupt withdrawal of these agents can precipitate the return of angina and possibly myocardial infarction, particularly in clients with severe coronary artery disease. Beta blockers are often administered concomitantly with nitrates, since these drugs complement each other's effects on the heart.

Calcium channel blocking agents Clients with severe coronary artery spasms may have little or no relief with any of the beta blockers and large, even toxic, dosages of nitrates are required to relieve their symptoms. The calcium channel blockers nifedipine and verapamil have been released for the treatment of vasospastic and classical fixed obstruction angina. Calcium blockers inhibit the transmembrane influx of extracellular calcium into cardiac and vascular smooth muscle and produce vasodilation as well as a decrease in heart rate. In addition, the afterload of the heart is decreased, the spasms of the coronary arteries are decreased or eliminated, and the coronary arteries are dilated. Arrhythmias associated with ischemic heart disease may be decreased and sometimes eliminated with these agents.

Combination therapy Nitrates, beta-adrenergic blockers, and calcium channel blockers all relieve angina by different mechanisms. Each class of agents can assist in either fixed obstruction or variable obstruction angina by decreasing the work load of the heart. Calcium channel blockers are specific for the type of angina that is caused by variable obstruction of the coronary arteries and is associated with pain at rest. Since many clients have various degrees of fixed and variable obstruction, they often benefit from a combination of therapeutic agents. The dosage of each drug is reduced in combination therapy and this also decreases the chance of toxicity from any one agent.

Some clients do not tolerate combination therapy as well as others. Clients with aortic stenosis may actually develop heart failure when beta blockers and calcium blockers are used concurrently because the reduction in afterload is limited by the stenosis. However, the concomitant use of nitrates with either the beta blockers or the calcium blockers seems to be complementary in most adults.

NURSING MANAGEMENT

When assessing the client with angina, the nurse needs to obtain a complete description of the pain, including type, location, radiation, duration, precipitating factors, and factors that relieve the pain. The effects the pain has on the client's ability to work and perform other activities of daily living are also important.

The client should be instructed to have the prescribed short-acting nitrate within reach at all times and should be asked to notify the nurse when angina occurs. If the pain is not relieved after taking three tablets 5 to 10 minutes apart, the physician should be notified. The frequency and duration of pain should be recorded on a chart.

Blood pressure and the frequency of pain are the primary factors by which the dosage of antianginal agents is regulated. The objective of therapy is to decrease or eliminate the frequency of acute pain by maintaining the lowest possible serum drug level. Although the client is cautioned to change position slowly, orthostatic hypotension or other symptoms of toxicity may occur and necessitate a dosage reduction. Dizziness is a low-level toxicity symptom and usually precedes orthostatic hypotension. Frequent and careful measurement of blood pressure is helpful in determining the hemodynamic effects of antianginal agents.

OTHER USES OF NITRATES

The use of nitroglycerin and other nitrates has been expanded in recent years. Although the effectiveness of nitrates has not been determined for some disorders, these agents are now being used for acute bronchial asthma, biliary colic, coronary vasospasm, congestive heart failure, mitral regurgitation, acute myocardial infarction, diffuse esophageal spasm, open-angle glaucoma, and for the control of blood pressure during surgical procedures.

SHORT-ACTING NITRATE AND NITRITE VASODILATORS

GENERIC NAME Amyl nitrite (RX)

TRADE NAME Amyl Nitrate Pearls

CLASSIFICATION Vasodilator

Source Mixture of isomeric amyl nitrates produced from amyl alcohol and nitrous acid. It is volatile at room temperature and the vapor forms an explosive mixture with oxygen.

Action Amyl nitrite is a potent smooth muscle relaxant. Although it is similar to nitroglycerin, amyl nitrite is faster acting, has a shorter duration of action, causes more pronounced tachycardia, and produces a greater increase in cardiac output. However, amyl nitrite causes less venous dilation than nitroglycerin. It is also less convenient to carry and use than nitroglycerin tablets. As amyl nitrite induces the formation of methemoglobin by oxidizing the ferrous ion of hemoglobin to the ferric form, it can be used to treat cyanide poisoning, since cyanide has a greater affinity for methemoglobin. Amyl nitrite is less effective as an antidote for cyanide than other preparations, but it does not require IV administration. (See nitroglycerin.)

Indications for Use Treatment of angina pectoris due to coronary artery disease. Has been used to treat acute bronchospasm, such as asthma, and biliary colic, such as cholelithiasis. Has also been used as an antidote for cyanide poisoning.

Contraindications Hypersensitivity to nitrates or nitrites, severe anemia, closed-angle glaucoma, increased intracranial pressure, cerebral hemorrhage, head injury.

Warnings and Precautions Use with caution in clients with acute or recent myocardial infarction; in clients with a history of postural hypotension; and in clients with glaucoma, since intraocular pressure may be increased. Tolerance to amyl nitrite and other organic nitrates may occur after prolonged use.

Untoward Reactions Toxicity can occur and includes syncope, tachycardia, arrhythmias, pronounced hypotension, nausea, and vomiting. (Syncope caused by an abrupt drop in blood pressure may occur after excessively deep inhalations.) Hypersensitivity to usual dosages of nitrates can occur and includes nausea, vomiting, restlessness, pallor, diaphoresis, and prolonged hypotension. Secondary effects, such as tachycardia, pounding of the heart, headache, dizziness, and flushing, may occur but the symptoms usually subside in less than 30 minutes.

Parameters of Use

Absorption Rapidly absorbed through mucous membranes of respiratory tract. Onset of action is 10 to 30 seconds and duration of action is 4 to 8 minutes.

Distribution Widely distributed.

Metabolism Rapidly in the liver.

Excretion By the kidneys as unchanged drug and metabolites.

Drug Interactions Concurrent use of alcohol may increase the effects of amyl nitrite. Cross-tolerance with long-acting nitrates can occur.

Administration Dosage is determined by the length of exposure and depth of inhalation (surface area).

- *Treatment of angina pectoris, acute biliary colic, and bronchospasm (asthma attack):* 0.2 to 0.3 ml inhaled as needed.
- *Antidote for cyanide poisoning:* 0.2 to 0.3 ml inhaled for 30 to 60 seconds every 5 minutes until consciousness returns.

Available Drug Forms Pearls (fragile, thin-glassed ampules enclosed in woven cloth) containing 0.2 to 0.3 ml of solution.

Nursing Management

Planning factors

1. Place client in a sitting or lying down position before administering drug.
2. Store drug in a place that is easy to locate.

Administration factors

1. Ampul is wrapped in cotton, gauze, or cloth and crushed between the fingers. The fabric protects the fingers from being lacerated.
2. Place drug near client's nose and mouth and instruct client to inhale normally once or twice. A second inhalation may be required if angina persists after 1 to 2 minutes.
3. Hold wrapped ampul in hand until it can be disposed of safely.

Evaluation factors

1. Check vital signs frequently. Do not administer a second inhalation if adverse reactions occur.
2. If angina is not relieved within 10 minutes after a second inhalation, notify physician.

Client teaching factors

1. Instruct client to sit or lie down before using drug.
2. Teach client and family how to break and use ampuls.

A cotton handkerchief or other thin cloth can be used.
3. Family should know where ampuls are stored.
4. Instruct client and family that drug is volatile and highly inflammable and should not be used near sparks or flames. All cigarettes should be extinguished before breaking ampul.
5. Instruct client to carry 2 or 3 ampuls in a protective container at all times. A small metal container such as a large pillbox lined with cotton can be used.
6. Instruct client to remain in a resting position for at least 15 minutes after drug administration.
7. Instruct family in the care of syncope: Place the client's head lower than the trunk; for example, between the knees if sitting or raising the legs if lying. Client should then deep breathe and do isometric exercises of the extremities.
8. Caution client to avoid excessively deep or several repeated inhalations, since toxicity may occur.
9. Inform client that the drug smells fruity and slightly pungent.

GENERIC NAME Nitroglycerin glyceryl trinitrate (sublingual)

TRADE NAMES GTN, Nitrostat, NTG (RX)

CLASSIFICATION Vasodilator

Source Organic nitrate produced from an explosive and volatile liquid. Made nonexplosive by the addition of the carbohydrate lactose.

Action Nitroglycerin relaxes all smooth muscles. The work load of the heart is decreased by the following drug-induced actions:

1. Dilates of numerous postcapillary blood vessels, thus reducing the venous blood return to the heart (reduces preload).
2. Dilates of peripheral arterioles, thus reducing the peripheral resistance against which the heart pumps (reduces afterload).
3. Increases the efficiency of left ventricular pumping by enhancing myocardial oxygen consumption. This action is thought to be caused by a drug-induced reduction in ventricular wall tension.

Precise mechanism of action is unknown, but sublingual administration of nitroglycerin relieves anginal attacks within minutes and prevents the occurrence of exertional angina for about 30 minutes. Although tachycardia and an increase in cardiac output occur initially, the reduction in preload decreases cardiac output. Renal blood flow decreases as blood pressure is reduced. Dilation of meningeal vessels may cause a transient pulsating headache. As retinal vessels dilate, intraocular pressure increases and can cause difficulty in clients with glaucoma. Coronary arteries are dilated but the oxygen content of coronary blood flow decreases as blood pressure decreases. However, there seems to be an increase in blood flow to inadequately perfused myocardial tissue, thus increasing cardiac output from an ischemic and incompetent heart. Smooth muscle of the bronchial tree, biliary tract, GI system, and uterus is also relaxed, but to a lesser degree.

Indications for Use Prevention and treatment of angina pectoris due to coronary artery disease, coronary insufficiency. Has been used to treat certain types of acute migraine headache.

Contraindications Hypersensitivity to nitrates or nitrites, severe anemia, closed-angle glaucoma, increased intracranial pressure, cerebral hemorrhage, head injury.

Warnings and Precautions Use with caution in clients with acute or recent myocardial infarction; in clients with a history of postural hypotension; and in clients with glaucoma, since intraocular pressure may be increased. Tolerance to nitroglycerin and other organic nitrates may occur after prolonged use; only a few day's withdrawal from the drug is needed to restore the drug's effectiveness.

Untoward Reactions Transient headache is common. The headache may be pulsating, but usually disappears within 5 to 20 minutes. Toxicity may result in marked tachycardia and severe hypotension. Hypersensitivity to the drug's hypotensive effect can occur. Usual drug dosages may induce the following symptoms: nausea, vomiting, restlessness, pallor, diaphoresis, apprehension, and collapse.

Parameters of Use

Absorption Rapidly absorbed through oral mucous membranes. Onset of action is 3 to 5 minutes and duration of action is 30 minutes.

Metabolism Rapidly metabolized in the liver by the enzyme glutathione and organic nitrate reductase. Inactive metabolites are formed.

Drug Characteristics Drug is rapidly inactivated by heat, light, air, and moisture. Store in light-resistant glass containers with metal caps; absorbed by plastic. Remains stable for about 5 months.

Drug Interactions Concurrent ingestion of alcohol enhances the action of nitroglycerin and the client may develop nausea, vomiting, cramps, and other unpleasant effects; avoid concurrent use. Physiologic antagonists of nitroglycerin are norepinephrine, acetylcholine, and histamine. Cross-tolerance with long-acting nitrates may occur.

Administration

- *Anginal attack:* Usual dosage: gr $\frac{1}{150}$ sublingual every 5 minutes times 3 doses, as necessary; Dosage range: gr $\frac{1}{400}$ to $\frac{1}{100}$.
- *Prevention of angina:* Usual dosage: gr $\frac{1}{150}$ sublingual just prior to exertional activity; Dosage range: gr $\frac{1}{400}$ to $\frac{1}{100}$.

Available Drug Forms Sublingual tablets containing gr $\frac{1}{400}$, gr $\frac{1}{200}$, gr $\frac{1}{150}$, or gr $\frac{1}{100}$.

Nursing Management

Planning factors

1. Place client in a sitting or lying down position before administering drug.
2. If taken as a preventive measure, intended activity can usually be performed safely after 5 minutes.
3. Date tablets and replace after 5 months; dispose of old tablets.
4. Leave tablets at bedside within easy reach of client.
5. All clients should receive their first drug dose under supervision in case of severe untoward reactions.

Administration factors

1. For best results, tablet should be placed under the tongue near sublingual vessels; but may be held anywhere under the tongue in contact with mucous membranes.
2. A second dose may be given after 5 minutes if no relief is obtained. A third dose is occasionally required.
3. If the tablet does not cause a slight burning sensation, it lacks potency. A fresh supply of tablets should be obtained.

Evaluation factors

1. Check blood pressure and pulse frequently. If hypotension occurs, place the client in a lying down position and elevate the legs. Notify physician; a reduced dosage may be required.
2. If severe hypotension occurs, phenylephrine hydrochloride or norepinephrine may be required.
3. If pain is not relieved after 3 doses, notify physician.
4. Duration of preventive effect is usually about 30 minutes.

Client teaching factors

1. Instruct client to keep a fresh supply of drug within reach at all times and to use drug at the first sign of an anginal attack.
2. Inform client to discard tablets every 4 to 5 months and obtain a new supply. Tablets must be kept tightly sealed in glass containers away from light.
3. Family should know where tablets are stored. Keep out of the reach of children.
4. Instruct client and family in method of administration.
5. Instruct family to seek medical assistance (call physician, take client to emergency room) if relief does not occur after 3 doses.
6. Warn client against chewing or swallowing tablets.
7. Instruct client to remain in a resting position for 15 to 30 minutes after drug administration.
8. Warn client to change position slowly to avoid dizziness, which will progress to orthostatic hypotension.
9. Warn client against the concurrent use of alcohol.

GENERIC NAME Nitroglycerin (injection) (RX)

TRADE NAMES Nitrostat IV, Tridil

CLASSIFICATION Vasodilator

Action Nitroglycerin is a smooth muscle relaxant that (1) promotes the peripheral pooling of blood, thus decreasing the venous blood return to the heart (reduces preload); (2) causes relaxation of arterioles (reduces afterload); and (3) enhances the oxygen supply-demand ratio of the heart. Therapeutic drug levels decrease systolic, diastolic, and mean arterial blood pressures. Although heart rate is usually increased, an excessive drop in blood pressure can cause inadequate perfusion of the coronary arteries. [See nitroglycerin glyceryl trinitrate (sublingual).]

Indications for Use Control of hypertension associated with surgical procedures, including cardiac bypass and sternotomy; congestive heart failure associated with acute myocardial infarction; treatment of angina pectoris in clients who are unresponsive to traditional therapies; induction of controlled hypotension during surgery, thus reducing the surgical risk in clients with severe hypertension.

Contraindications None known.

Warnings and Precautions Use with caution in clients with severe renal or hepatic impairment. Excessive hypotension must be avoided since poor organ perfusion may occur and cause deleterious effects to the brain, heart, liver, and kidneys. Long-term studies of the drug's cardiogenic potential have not been completed. Safe use in children and during pregnancy has not been established.

Untoward Reactions Headaches, which are sometimes throbbing, are the most common reaction. Toxicity by accidental overdose may result in severe hypotension and reflex tachycardia. Paradoxic bradycardia and an increase in anginal pain associated with drug-induced hypotension may occur in susceptible clients, particularly those with normal or low pulmonary wedge pressure. Other reactions include tachycardia, arrhythmias, nausea, vomiting, apprehension, restlessness, muscle twitching, chest discomfort, dizziness, and abdominal cramps. Cutaneous flushing, weakness, and exfoliative dermatitis have occurred with oral and topical nitroglycerin preparations.

Parameters of Use

Absorption Half-life is 1 to 4 minutes. About 60% bound to plasma proteins; some metabolites are also bound to plasma proteins. The dinitrates may be somewhat active, but the mononitrates are inactive.

Distribution Widely distributed in the body.

Metabolism In the liver to mononitrates and dinitrates.

Excretion Rapidly by the kidneys; primarily as metabolites.

Drug Interactions Although seldom needed, antagonists of nitroglycerin are the alpha-adrenergic agonists, such as methoxamine and phenylephrine. Cross-tolerance with long-acting nitrates can occur.

Administration Dosage depends on the client's blood pressure and clinical response. Initial titration rate: 5 mcg/min. IV; increase by 5 mcg/min. every 3 to 5 minutes, as necessary. If no response is seen at 10 mcg/min., increments of 20 mcg/min. may be tried. When blood pressure begins to drop, dosage increments should be 5 mcg/min. or less and the time interval between dosage increments should be lengthened (every 10 to 15 minutes) until desired effect.

Available Drug Forms Ampules containing 50 mg/10 ml (5 mg/ml) and 8 mg/10 ml (0.8 mg/ml). Ampules containing other concentrations may be available in the near future. Diluted solution remains stable for 48 hours at room temperature or 7 days under refrigeration.

Nursing Management

Planning factors

1. Baseline vital signs, blood pressure, and EKG are essential. Central venous pressure and pulmonary wedge pressure readings are recommended. Other cardiovascular parameters may be helpful.
2. Note whether the client has or is thought to have a normal or low left ventricular filling pressure (or pulmonary wedge pressure), since these clients may be very sensitive to nitroglycerin IV.
3. Obtain hepatic and renal function tests (blood urea nitrogen, creatinine) prior to initiating therapy.
4. Record intake and output.
5. An automatic blood pressure machine can be helpful when frequent blood pressure readings are required.
6. Obtain the desired IV solutions in glass bottles and specialized, nonabsorbent IV tubing, such as Tridiset. Do not use standard PVC tubing. Notify physician concerning the type of tubing available.
7. An IV pump is highly recommended.

Administration factors

1. Add concentrated drug solution to 500 ml of 5% D/W or 0.9% sodium chloride IV solution in glass bottles.
2. Do not exceed an IV dilution of 400 mcg/ml (200 mg in 500 ml of IV solution).
3. Check IV site for patency before adding medicated solution, since extravasation may cause tissue irritation.
4. Start IV rate at 5 mcg/min. and increase slowly according to client's blood pressure and other clinical responses.
5. Clients with normal or low left ventricular filling pressure may require only 5 mcg/min. or less.
6. The following table correlates dosage with flow rate when 50 mg of drug is added to 500 ml of IV solution.

	IV Flow Rates	
Dosage (mcg/min.)	IV Pump (ml/hr)	60 gtt/ml IV set (micro gtt/min.)
5	3	3
10	6	6
20	12	12
40	24	24
80	48	48
120	72	72
160	96	96

7. The following table correlates dosage with flow rate when 100 mg of drug is added to 500 ml of IV solution.

	IV Flow Rates	
Dosage (mcg/min.)	IV Pump (ml/hr)	60 gtt/ml IV set (micro gtt/min.)
5	1.5	1.5
10	3	3
20	6	6
40	12	12
80	24	24
160	48	48
240	72	72
320	96	96

8. The following table correlates dosage with flow rate when 200 mg of drug is added to 500 ml of IV solution.

	IV Flow Rates	
Dosage (mcg/min.)	IV Pump (ml/hr)	60 gtt/ml IV set (micro gtt/min.)
20	3	3
40	6	6
80	12	12
160	24	24
320	48	48
480	72	72
640	96	96

9. Since IV tubing has a capacity of 15 ml, it should be changed when the IV drug concentration is adjusted.
10. The time interval between dosage increments should be lengthened as the dosage exceeds 20 mcg/min.
11. The client's fluid requirements must be considered during maintenance drug therapy.

Evaluation factors

1. Continuously monitor blood pressure and pulse and adjust IV rate accordingly. Change dosage increments slowly.

2. If hypotension occurs, slow the IV rate to KVO (or discontinue if necessary) and elevate legs. Notify physician immediately.
3. Check IV site frequently (q1h) for extravasation or signs of irritation. Restart if necessary.
4. Monitor intake and output.
5. Monitor pulmonary wedge pressure frequently (every 5 to 10 minutes), if available. Arterial hypotension is preceded by a drop in pulmonary wedge pressure.
6. Cardiac monitoring is essential. If marked tachycardia or life-threatening arrhythmias occur, slow the IV rate to KVO (or discontinue if necessary) and notify physician immediately.

LONG-ACTING NITRATE VASODILATORS

GENERIC NAME Erythrityl tetranitrate (RX)

TRADE NAMES Anginar, Cardilate

CLASSIFICATION Vasodilator

See nitroglycerin glyceryl trinitrate (sublingual) for Contraindications, Warnings and precautions, Untoward reactions, and Drug interactions.

Action Explosive tetranitrate ester that is similar to nitroglycerin in action. Lactose is added to permit safe handling of the drug. Causes gradual vasodilation that is mild and prolonged.

Indications for Use Anginal pain, reduction of blood pressure. May be used at bedtime to prevent nocturnal angina.

Parameters of Use

Absorption Onset of action is: 30 minutes (oral tablet); 5 minutes (chewable tablet); 5 minutes (sublingual). Peak action occurs in: 1 to $1\frac{1}{2}$ hours (oral tablet); 30 to 45 minutes (chewable tablet); 30 to 45 minutes (sublingual). Duration of action is: 2 to 4 hours (oral tablet); 2 to 4 hours (chewable tablet); 2 hours (sublingual).

Administration Oral or chewable tablet: Initial dosage: 10 mg tid 30 minutes before meals. Sublingual or buccal tablet: Initial dosage: 5 mg tid; may be increased every 2 to 3 days until desired effect.

Available Drug Forms Sublingual and oral tablets containing 5, 10, or 15 mg; chewable tablets containing 10 mg.

Nursing Management If sublingual burning annoys client, buccal administration is recommended. [See nitroglycerin glyceryl trinitrate (sublingual).]

GENERIC NAME Isosorbide dinitrate (RX)

TRADE NAMES Dilatrate-SR, Isordil, Isosorbide Dinitrate, Isosorbide Dinitrate T.D., Isotrate, Sorate-2.5, Sorate-5, Sorate 10, Sorate 40, Sorbide T.D., Sorbitrate

CLASSIFICATION Vasodilator

See nitroglycerin glyceryl trinitrate (sublingual) for Contraindications, Untoward reactions, and Drug interactions.

Indications for Use Acute angina; prevention of anginal pain; reduction of preload in chronic coronary insufficiency; as an adjunct in congestive heart failure.

Warnings and Precautions Sublingual and chewable forms have been classified as probably effective; oral and sustained-release forms have been classified as possibly effective. Safe use in clients with a recent myocardial infarction has not been established. Hypersensitivity reactions (severe hypotension) may occur with dosages greater than 5 mg.

Parameters of Use

Absorption Onset of action is: 15 to 30 minutes (oral tablet); 2 to 5 minutes (chewable tablet); 2 to 5 minutes (sublingual); 15 to 30 minutes (sustained-release capsule). Duration of action is: 4 to 6 hours (oral tablet); 1 to 3 hours (chewable tablet); 1 to 3 hours (sublingual); 6 to 12 hours (sustained-release capsule).

Administration Oral or chewable tablet: Prophylaxis: 2 to 5 mg every 4 to 6 hours on an empty stomach (30 minutes before meals and at bedtime). Sublingual: Acute attack: 2.5 to 10.0 mg prn; Prophylaxis: 5 to 20 mg every 3 to 6 hours on an empty stomach (30 minutes before meals and at bedtime). Sustained-release capsule: Prophylaxis: 40 mg every 6 to 12 hours.

Available Drug Forms Oral tablets containing 5, 10, or 20 mg; chewable tablets containing 5 or 10 mg; sublingual tablets containing 2.5 mg; sustained-release capsules containing 40 mg.

Nursing Management [See nitroglycerin glyceryl trinitrate (sublingual).]

1. Dosage may be repeated every 10 to 15 minutes times 3 doses.
2. If pain persists, physician should be notified.

GENERIC NAME Mannitol hexanitrate (RX)

TRADE NAMES Mannex, Mannitol Nitrate, Nitranitol, Vascunitol

CLASSIFICATION Vasodilator

See nitroglycerin glyceryl trinitrate (sublingual) for Contraindications, Warnings and precautions, Untoward reactions, Drug interactions, and Nursing management.

Action Explosive compound that is combined with carbohydrates to permit safe handling. Similar actions to nitroglycerin.

Indications for Use Prevention of angina pectoris; reduction of blood pressure.

Parameters of Use

Absorption Onset of action is 15 minutes. Peak action occurs in 1 hour and duration of action is 5 hours.

Administration Dosage range: 16 to 64 mg every 4 to 6 hours.

Available Drug Forms Scored tablets containing 32 mg.

GENERIC NAME Pentaerythritol tetranitrate (RX)

TRADE NAMES Duotrate, Duotrate 45, P.E.T.N., P.E.T.N. S.R., Pentritol, Peritrate, Peritrate S.A., S.K.-P.E.T.N.

CLASSIFICATION Vasodilator

See nitroglycerin glyceryl trinitrate (sublingual) for Contraindications, Untoward reactions, Drug interactions, and Nursing management.

Action Powerful explosive that is combined with lactose, mannitol, or other carbohydrates to permit safe handling. Similar actions to nitroglycerin.

Indications for Use Prevention of angina.

Warnings and Precautions Has been classified as possibly effective. Often given combined with phenobarbital or an antianxiety agent (Cartrax). Sustained-release capsule may not be reliable.

Parameters of Use

Absorption Onset of action is: 20 minutes (oral tablet); 1 to 2 hours (sustained release capsule). Peak action occurs in: 1 hour (oral tablet). Duration of action is: 5 to 6 hours (oral tablet); 12 hours (sustained-release capsule).

Administration Oral tablet: 10 mg tid or qid on an empty stomach; Dosage range: 10 to 20 mg. Sustained-release capsule: 30 to 45 mg q12h on an empty stomach; Dosage range: 30 to 80 mg.

Available Drug Forms Tablets containing 10 or 20 mg; sustained-release capsules containing 30, 45, or 80 mg.

GENERIC NAME Nitroglycerin (oral and topical)

TRADE NAMES Nitro-Bid, Nitrodisc, Nitroglyn, Nitrol, Nitrong, Nitrospan, Transderm-Nitro

CLASSIFICATION Vasodilator (RX)

Action Although nitroglycerin is an effective smooth muscle relaxant for acute anginal attacks, sublingual tablets have a very short duration of action and are therefore ineffective for preventing angina. Oral and topical preparations provide a slow continuous release of nitroglycerin and are used to maintain therapeutic serum drug levels. Topical preparations are thought to maintain a more consistent serum drug level than oral controlled-release preparations. Although topical microseal and transderm drug delivery methods are more expensive, they are more convenient to apply than 2% nitroglycerin ointments. [See nitroglycerin glyceryl trinitrate (sublingual).]

Indications for Use Prevention and treatment of angina pectoris due to coronary artery disease; myocardial insufficiency.

Contraindications Hypersensitivity to nitrates or nitrites, severe anemia, increased intracranial pressure, cerebral hemorrhage, head injury.

Warnings and Precautions Use with caution in clients with acute myocardial infarction, congestive heart failure, glaucoma, or a history of postural hypertension. Tolerance to nitroglycerin and other organic nitrates may occur after prolonged use. Oral controlled-release preparations are not intended to relieve acute anginal attacks. The benefit of oral controlled-release preparations has not been proven and these drugs have been classified as possibly effective.

Untoward Reactions Transient headache is a common side effect. Hypotension, particularly orthostatic hypotension, is a symptom of toxicity. Other signs and symptoms of toxicity include tachycardia, syncope, dizziness, flushing, and nausea. Exfoliative dermatitis and other drug rashes have occurred, particularly when large dosages are used. Topical preparations may cause contact dermatitis after prolonged use. Oral controlled-release preparations may cause blurred vision and dry mouth.

Parameters of Use

Absorption Topical preparations are well absorbed from thin-layered skin surfaces, such as the inner surface of the forearm and nonhairy areas of the chest. The absorption rate for oral controlled-release preparations has not been established. Onset of action is: 1 hour (oral); 30 to 60 minutes (ointment); 30 minutes (skin pads). Peak action occurs in: 3 to 4 hours (oral). Duration of action is: 6 to 12 hours (oral); 3 to 4 hours (ointment); 24 hours (skin pads). Residual effect after removal is 30 minutes for topical preparations.

Metabolism In the liver to inactive metabolites.

Excretion By the kidneys.

Drug Interactions Concurrent ingestion of alcohol increases the absorption of oral controlled-release nitroglycerin preparations, thus increasing the effects of nitroglycerin and the potential for toxicity. Physiologic antagonists of nitroglycerin include norepinephrine, acetylcholine, and histamine. Cross-tolerance with long-acting nitrates may occur.

Administration Oral controlled-release capsule: 2.5 to 6.5 mg every 8 to 12 hours; Dosage range: 1.3 to 9.0 mg; the smallest effective dosage should be used. Topical: Skin pad (skin surface covered determines the dosage): 1 daily; each square centimeter of skin covered absorbs 0.5 mg every 24 hours in vivo. Ointment: Apply 1 to 2 inches of 2% ointment spread under applicator q8h; Dosage range: $\frac{1}{2}$ to 5 inches every 4 to 8 hours.

Available Drug Forms Oral controlled-release capsules containing 1.3, 2.5, 6.5, or 9.0 mg. Nitroglycerin ointment (2%) containing lactose, lanolin, and a petroleum base; each inch contains 15 mg of nitroglycerin. Stick-on skin pads containing 16 or 32 mg that cover 8 or 16 cm^2 of skin area, respectively (Nitrodisc). Stick-on skin pads containing 25 or 50 mg that cover 10 or 20 cm^2 of skin area, respectively (Transderm).

Nursing Management

Planning factors

1. Plan drug administration and application of topical preparations so that it does not interfere with sleep.
2. Store capsules and topical preparations in a cool, dry place, but do not refrigerate.
3. Obtain baseline blood pressure, pulse, and EKG.
4. Obtain plastic wrap when ointment is to be used.

Administration factors

1. Give oral capsules with water 1 hour before meals or 2 hours after meals.
2. When applying topical preparations,
   a. Check skin surfaces. Locate thin-layered skin surfaces without scars or other lesions. Avoid hairy areas and skin over moveable body parts.
   b. Application to the chest wall is effective, but hair in the immediate area must be shaved for best results. Consult client for preferences.
   c. Application to the left chest may have an additional physiologic benefit; but avoid the sternum area (the ointment would have to be removed before cardiopulmonary resuscitation could be instituted).
   d. Rotate skin sites.
   e. Remove previous skin pad or ointment before applying fresh medication. Wipe area thoroughly with a dry tissue.
3. When applying skin pads,
   a. Remove the backing from the pad and place firmly over the desired area.
   b. Although the pads generally adhere well, a pad that comes off prematurely should be replaced with a fresh one.
4. When applying ointment,
   a. Squeeze prescribed amount evenly on to a calibrated applicator (thin paper); be careful to avoid touching ointment.
   b. Place applicator with ointment on the skin.
   c. Gently press down on applicator to spread ointment over the skin. Ointment should be spread uniformly under applicator (2 × 3 in. area).
   d. Cover applicator and surrounding tissue with plastic wrap and secure with tape (preferably nonallergic tape).
   e. Avoid applying ointment to moveable body parts or areas where the covering may be accidentally pulled off.

Evaluation factors

1. The decrease in systolic pressure is a good indicator of hemodynamic response.
2. Check blood pressure and pulse frequently (every 2 to 4 hours) for the first 2 to 3 days following institution of therapy and when dosage is adjusted. If hypotension occurs, notify physician.
3. Cardiac monitoring is recommended for the first 2 to 3 days following initiation of therapy and when dosage is adjusted. If tachycardia or arrhythmias develop, notify physician.
4. Headaches are expected and can be effectively controlled with mild analgesics, such as acetaminophen. If symptoms occur, notify physician; severe and persistent headaches may require a reduction in dosage.
5. Orthostatic hypotension and dizziness are signs of low-level toxicity. If these or other signs of toxicity occur, notify physician; dosage reduction may be required if symptoms persist.
6. Notify physician if anginal pain continues to recur.
7. Topical corticosteroids may be required to treat dermatitis.
8. If blurred vision and dry mouth persist, the drug should be discontinued.

Client teaching factors

1. Instruct client to store drug in a cool, dry place, but not in a refrigerator.
2. Instruct client and family in the application of topical preparations.
3. Caution client and family to avoid skin contact with ointment.
4. Instruct client to schedule baths and showers around the time at which a new pad or ointment is to be applied, so that therapy is not interrupted.
5. Ointment should be removed before swimming. Inform client that swimming, if permitted by physician, should not last longer than 30 minutes, since the residual drug effects last only 30 minutes. Client should reapply ointment when out of the water.
6. Skin pads may remain in place during swimming. If the pad falls off, a fresh one should be applied.

BETA-ADRENERGIC BLOCKERS

GENERIC NAME Propranolol hydrochloride (RX)

TRADE NAME Inderal

CLASSIFICATION Beta-adrenergic blocker

Action Propranolol is a nonselective beta-adrenergic blocker that has no other autonomic nervous system activity. The drug competes with the body's catecholamines (epinephrine and norepinephrine) for beta-adrenergic sites, thus blocking the stimulation of beta receptors. Propranolol affects the heart (beta$_1$ receptors) by decreasing rate, output, and conduction velocity. Beta$_2$ blockade prevents relaxation of bronchial, GI, and uterine smooth muscle. Blood pressure is decreased probably as a result of decreased cardiac output, inhibition of renin secretion (decreases reabsorption of sodium by the kidneys), and depression of sympathetic innervation from the brain's vasomotor centers. The oxygen requirements of the heart are decreased. (See Chapter 42.)

Indications for Use Prevention of angina; hypertension, often in conjunction with thiazide diuretics; tachyarrhythmias.

Contraindications Bronchial asthma, allergic rhinitis, sinus bradycardia, overt congestive heart failure, diabetes mellitus, heart block greater than first degree.

Warnings and Precautions Use with caution in the elderly and in clients with Wolff-Parkinson-White syndrome, respiratory, hepatic, or renal disorders, or a history of heart failure. Safe use during pregnancy and lactation has not been established.

Untoward Reactions Bradycardia, congestive heart failure, and excessive hypotension have occurred and may be life threatening. Bronchospasm can occur in susceptible clients and may be life threatening. GI disturbances, including nausea, vomiting, and diarrhea, may occur. Hypoglycemia or thyrotoxicosis may occur without tachycardia. CNS disturbances, including lightheadedness, insomnia, weakness, and visual disturbances, may occur.

Parameters of Use

Absorption Onset of action is about 30 minutes. Peak action occurs in 60 to 90 minutes and duration of action is about 6 hours. Plasma half-life varies from 3.4 to 6 hours due to individual variations in metabolism. About 90% bound to plasma proteins.

Metabolism In the liver.

Excretion By the kidneys as unchanged drug and metabolites.

Drug Interactions Propranolol enhances bradycardia in digitalized clients. It may alter insulin requirements in diabetics. Isoproterenol, glucagon, aminophylline, and norepinephrine antagonize the effects of propranolol.

Administration Initial dosage: 10 to 20 mg po tid or qid before meals and at bedtime; then gradually increase every 3 to 7 days until desired effect; Maintenance dosage: About 160 mg daily in 3 or 4 divided doses; Maximum dosage: 320 mg/day.

Available Drug Forms Tablets containing 10, 20, 40, and 80 mg.

Nursing Management

Planning factors

1. Obtain baseline data about the type of angina.
2. Assess cardiovascular and respiratory status for possible contraindications. Record baseline vital signs.
3. Assess hepatic and renal function. If blood urea nitrogen (BUN) or serum creatinine are elevated, notify physician. If oliguria exists, notify physician.
4. Keep drug on units where clients may need it for life-threatening arrhythmias (emergency room, intensive care unit, coronary care unit, extended coronary care unit).
5. Store drug in a dark area (closet).
6. Keep appropriate drugs readily available for use in the event of toxicity: atropine for bradycardia, isoproterenol for cardiac failure, epinephrine for hypotension, and aminophylline or isoproterenol for bronchospasm.
7. Withdraw drug temporarily 48 hours prior to surgery that requires general anesthetic agents, with the exception of clients with pheochromocytoma.

Administration factors

1. Check blood pressure and pulse before therapy is initiated or dosage adjusted. If severe bradycardia (pulse below 56 beats/min.) or hypotension exist, notify physician before administering drug. Initially, cardiac monitoring is recommended.
2. Give drug before meals and at bedtime on an empty stomach. Follow with a full glass of water.

Evaluation factors

1. Initially, check blood pressure and pulse before each dosage; then check periodically.
2. Record frequency of angina to determine the drug's effectiveness. It may take 1 or 2 weeks of drug therapy before client is free of angina.
3. Obtain complete blood cell count, blood urea nitrogen, and serum creatinine levels periodically.
4. Record intake and output.
5. Dosage must be reduced gradually before discontinuing drug.

Client teaching factors

1. Inform client of potential untoward reactions and to notify physician immediately if low pulse rate (below 60 beats/min.), shortness of breath, or hypoglycemia occur.
2. Advise client (particularly if normotensive) to change positions slowly to avoid lightheadedness.
3. Advise client to avoid excessive use of CNS depressants and stimulants (alcohol or caffeinated drinks such as coffee, cola, or tea), since untoward reactions may occur.
4. Inform client that adaptation to stressful situations will be altered and to avoid stress if possible.
5. Warn client that abrupt withdrawal of drug may precipitate anginal pain or a myocardial infarction.

GENERIC NAME Nadolol (RX)

TRADE NAME Corgard

CLASSIFICATION Beta-adrenergic blocker

See propranolol hydrochloride for Warnings and precautions and Drug interactions.

Action Nadolol is similar to propranolol. Both drugs are nonselective beta-adrenergic blockers that reduce heart rate and cardiac output, systolic and diastolic blood pressure, and reflex orthostatic tachycardia, and inhibit isoproterenol-induced tachycardia. Whereas the duration of action of propranolol is only 6 hours, the effects of nadolol last 24 hours. Client compliance with drug therapy is theoretically better with nadolol because it needs to be taken only once per day compared with 4 times a day for propranolol. Toxic and other untoward reactions seem to be milder than with propranolol.

Indications for Use Prevention of angina pectoris; treatment of hypertension, usually with a thiazide diuretic.

Contraindications Bronchial asthma, sinus bradycardia, heart block greater than first-degree, cardiogenic shock, acute heart failure.

Untoward Reactions Although the reported incidence of untoward reactions to nadolol is less than propranolol, the same type of reactions occur. (See propranolol hydrochloride.)

Parameters of Use

Absorption Well absorbed from GI tract; food may increase absorption. Onset of action is about 30 to 60 minutes and duration of action is about 24 hours.
Crosses placenta and enters breast milk.
Metabolism In the liver.
Excretion By the kidneys.

Administration Highly individualized. Initial dosage: 40 mg po daily; then increase by 40 to 80 mg every 3 to 7 days until desired effect; Maintenance dosage: 80 to 240 mg daily.

Available Drug Forms Tablets containing 40, 80, 120, or 160 mg.

Nursing Management (See propranolol hydrochloride.)

1. Monitor vital signs frequently during dosage adjustments. Withhold drug and notify physician if pulse is below 56 beats/min.
2. May be administered without regard for meals; but should be given consistently with or without meals.
3. Warn client that abrupt withdrawal of drug may precipitate anginal pain or a myocardial infarction.

GENERIC NAME Timolol maleate (RX)

TRADE NAME Blocadren

CLASSIFICATION Beta-adrenergic blocker

See propranolol hydrochloride for Warnings and precautions and Drug interactions.

Action Timolol is the only beta blocker presently recommended for increasing the longevity of clients following an acute myocardial infarction. Like other beta blockers, timolol reduces heart rate, cardiac output, systolic and diastolic blood pressure, and reflex orthostatic tachycardia, and inhibits isoproterenol-induced tachycardia. Timolol tends to decrease myocardial contractility less than propranolol and other beta blockers.

Indications for Use Prevention of reinfarction following myocardial infarction; mild to moderate hypertension.

Contraindications Bronchospasm (including bronchial asthma and chronic obstructive pulmonary disease), sinus bradycardia, second- and third-degree heart block, overt heart failure, cardiogenic shock.

Untoward Reactions Although the reported incidence of untoward reactions to timolol is less than propranolol, the same type of reactions occur. (See propranolol hydrochloride.)

Parameters of Use

Absorption Rapidly absorbed from GI tract. Peak plasma levels occur in 1–2 hours. Half-life is 4 hours. Not significantly protein-bound.
Metabolism Partially in the liver.
Excretion Mainly by the kidneys.

Administration Highly individualized.

- *Post–myocardial infarction:* 10 mg po bid; usually instituted 1 to 3 weeks following myocardial infarction.
- *Hypertension:* Initial dosage: 10 mg po bid; then increase by 10 mg every 3 to 7 days until desired effect; Maintenance dosage: 10 to 20 mg bid; Maximum dosage: 60 mg/day.

Nursing Management (See propranolol hydrochloride.)

1. Monitor vital signs frequently during dosage adjustments. Withhold drug and notify physician if pulse is below 56 beats/min.
2. Warn client that abrupt withdrawal of drug may precipitate anginal pain or a myocardial infarction.

CALCIUM CHANNEL BLOCKERS

GENERIC NAME Nifedipine (RX)

TRADE NAME Procardia

CLASSIFICATION Calcium channel blocker

Action Although the exact antianginal mechanism of action is unknown, nifedipine is known to inhibit the influx of calcium ions into cardiac and vascular smooth muscle cells. (The contractile process of both cardiac and vascular smooth muscle depends on this movement of calcium ions.) Serum calcium levels are not altered, however. Coronary arteries and arterioles are relaxed, thereby preventing arterial spasms. Nifedipine also dilates peripheral arterioles, thus reducing blood pressure. As the total peripheral resistance decreases (afterload is decreased), the energy consumption and oxygen requirements of the heart are decreased and chronic stable angina is relieved and prevented from recurring. Myocardial contractility is also decreased. Nifedipine induces more relaxation of vascular smooth muscle than verapamil, thereby reducing blood pressure, but has less effect on SA and AV node conduction; therefore, nifedipine is often preferred for the treatment of angina.

Indications for Use Vasospastic angina; as an adjunct in chronic stable angina (exertional angina). May prove to be useful in treating hypertension.

Contraindications Acute episode of congestive heart failure; severe hypotension; cardiogenic shock.

Warnings and Precautions Use with extreme caution in clients with aortic stenosis. Nifedipine will not prevent the development of angina when beta blockers are withdrawn; beta blockers must be tapered before discontinuing. Peripheral edema in the legs (pedal edema) may occur from the drug-induced decrease in peripheral resistance; diuretics are effective in relieving the edema. Safe use in clients with hepatic or renal impairment, in conjunction with long-acting nitrates, and during pregnancy has not been established.

Untoward Reactions Dose-related transient hypotension may occur, but is usually mild and well tolerated; systolic and diastolic pressure are generally reduced by 5 to 10 mm Hg. Dizziness, lightheadedness, giddiness, flushing and a sensation of warmth, and headaches are common. Syncope is rare and is dose related. GI disturbances, including nausea and gastric distress, have occurred. Diarrhea, cramps, and constipation have been reported. Weakness, muscle cramps, and nervousness have occurred. Peripheral edema, palpitations, dyspnea, wheezing, nasal congestion, and a sore throat have been reported. Cholestasis has been reported after prolonged therapy, but rarely.

Laboratory Interactions Prolonged therapy may cause a mild to moderate increase in serum alkaline phosphatase, lactic dehydrogenase, serum glutamic-oxaloacetic transaminase, serum glutamic-pyruvic transaminase, and creatinine phosphokinase.

Parameters of Use

Absorption Rapid and complete from GI tract. Onset of action is 10 minutes. Peak action occurs in 30 minutes. Half-life is 2 hours. Highly bound to serum proteins.

Excretion About 80% by the kidneys as unchanged drug and metabolites.

Drug Interactions Concurrent therapy with beta-adrenergic blockers is usually well tolerated, but the development of acute congestive heart failure, severe hypotension, and recurrence of angina have been reported. Nifedipine may increase serum levels of digitalis glycosides as much as 50%; when used concurrently, observe client for digitalis toxicity.

Administration Initial dosage: 10 mg po q8h for 1 to 2 weeks; then adjust dosage according to client's response; Dosage range: 10 to 30 mg every 6 to 8 hours; Maximum dosage: 180 mg day.

Available Drug Forms Capsules (orange) containing 10 mg.

Nursing Management

Planning factors

1. Obtain history of cardiovascular disorders.
2. Obtain baseline vital signs. If hypotension or pulmonary edema are present, notify physician before initiating therapy.
3. Obtain baseline EKG, serum transaminase levels, and hepatic function tests. If abnormalities exist, notify physician.

Administration factors

1. Give with 4 to 6 fl oz of water.
2. Drug can be administered tid, but the preferred schedule is q8h.

Evaluation factors

1. Check blood pressure and pulse frequently (every 4 to 8 hours) for the first 2 to 3 days following institution of therapy and when dosage is adjusted. If hypotension or bradycardia occur, notify physician.
2. Cardiac monitoring is recommended for the first 2 to 3 days following initiation of therapy and when dosage is adjusted. If arrhythmias develop, notify physician.
3. Notify physician if anginal pain continues to recur.
4. Observe legs for pedal edema and notify physician if edema occurs.

Client teaching factors

1. Warn client that abrupt withdrawal of drug may precipitate angina or other disorders.
2. When prescribed, instruct client in the proper use of antiembolic stockings.
3. Warn client about the expected secondary reactions to the drug, such as dizziness and headache. If symptoms are annoying and persistent, the physician should be notified.
4. Emphasize the need for regular medical checkups.

GENERIC NAME Verapamil hydrochloride (RX)

TRADE NAMES Calan, Isoptin

CLASSIFICATION Calcium channel blocker

Action Although the exact antianginal mechanism of action is unknown, verapamil is known to inhibit the transmembrane influx of calcium ions into cardiac and vascular smooth muscle cells. Serum calcium levels are not altered, however. Both conductive and contractile myocardial cells are affected. SA node function and AV conduction are also inhibited, thus inducing a decrease in heart rate. Unlike nifedipine, verapamil induces little vasodilation. Myocardial contractility is decreased and there is some reduction in afterload. Verapamil is primarily used as an antiarrhythmic agent.

Indications for Use Vasospastic angina; chronic stable angina (exertional angina).

Contraindications Severe hypotension, cardiogenic shock, second- or third-degree heart block, sick sinus syndrome, severe primary congestive heart failure, within a few hours of propranolol IV or other beta-adrenergic blockers, since both drugs depress cardiac contractility and AV conduction.

Warnings and Precautions A rapid ventricular response may occur in clients with atrial flutter or fibrillation due to an aberrant conduction pathway that bypasses the AV node. Excessive bradycardia or asystole may occur in elderly clients and clients with sick sinus syndrome. May increase heart failure (pulmonary wedge pressure above 20 mm Hg) when the cause is not related to rate; concurrent digitalization may be helpful. Hepatic or renal failure do not alter the effects of a single dose, but duration of action may be prolonged with continued drug use. Safe use during pregnancy and lactation has not been established. Safe use in children is under investigation; present experience indicates that children respond to drug therapy equally as well as adults.

Untoward Reactions Initial but transient hypotension is common. Bradycardia, particularly in the elderly, asystole, and severe tachycardia may occur. Dizziness, headache, nausea, and abdominal discomfort may occur. Constipation is common. Emotional depression, rotary nystagmus, sleepiness, vertigo, muscle fatigue, and diaphoresis have been reported, but rarely. Prolonged use may cause hepatocellular damage with elevation in transaminase levels; symptoms are reversible when drug is discontinued.

Parameters of Use

Absorption Onset of action is 2 hours. Peak action occurs in 5 hours. Biphasic half-life is 4 minutes (distribution phase); 2 to 5 hours (elimination phase).

Metabolism Rapidly in the liver to several metabolites.

Excretion Primarily in urine (70%); some in feces (16%).

Drug Interactions Do not administer disopyramide within 48 hours before or 24 hours after verapamil because of potential interaction. Avoid concurrent use with beta-adrenergic blockers since excessive cardiac depression may occur, particularly when the beta blocker has been administered intravenously.

Administration Initial dosage: 60 mg po q8h for 7 to 14 days; then increase as needed; Dosage range: 60 to 120 mg.

Available Drug Forms Capsules containing 60 or 80 mg.

Nursing Management (See nifedipine.)

1. Monitor blood pressure and pulse. If hypotension occurs, notify physician immediately.
2. Obtain hepatic function tests periodically when prolonged therapy is required.
3. Stool softeners are helpful in preventing constipation.
4. Isoproterenol, atropine, lidocaine, and procainamide should be available for immediate use in the event of untoward reactions, such as bradycardia, asystole, or tachycardia. Cardiac pacing and cardioversion may also be required.

GENERIC NAME Diltiazem (RX)

TRADE NAME Cardizem

CLASSIFICATION Calcium channel blocker

See verapamil hydrochloride for Contraindications, Warnings and precautions, and Untoward reactions.

Action Although the exact antianginal mechanism of action is unknown, diltiazem is known to inhibit the transmembrane influx of calcium ions into cardiac and vascular smooth muscle cells. Serum calcium levels are not altered, however. Like verapamil, diltiazem affects both conductive and contractile myocardial cells. SA node function and AV conduction are also inhibited, thus inducing a decrease in heart rate. Myocardial contractility is decreased and there is some reduction in afterload. Diltiazem is used to treat supraventricular arrhythmias and angina.

Indications for Use Vasospastic angina; chronic stable angina (exertional angina).

Parameters of Use (See verapamil hydrochloride.)

Absorption Onset of action is about 15 minutes. Peak action occurs in about 30 minutes.

Drug Interactions Concurrent therapy with beta-adrenergic blockers is usually well tolerated, but the development of acute congestive heart failure, severe hypotension, and recurrence of angina have been reported.

Administration Initial dosage: 60 mg po q8h for 1 to 2 weeks; then adjust dosage according to client's response; Dosage range: 60 to 90 mg.

Available Drug Forms Capsules containing 30 mg.

Nursing Management Monitor blood pressure and pulse. If hypotension, bradycardia, or congestive heart failure develop, notify physician immediately. (See nifedipine and verapamil hydrochloride.)

Chapter 49

Anticoagulants

TYPES OF ANTICOAGULANTS

INDICATIONS FOR USE

TREATMENT OF OVERDOSE

FACTORS KNOWN TO ALTER PROTHROMBIN TIME

DETERMINATION OF DOSAGE

NATURAL ANTICOAGULANTS

- Heparin sodium
- Heparin lock flush
- Protamine sulfate

WARFARIN AND DERIVATIVES

- Warfarin sodium
- Warfarin potassium
- Dicumarol
- Ethyl biscoumacetate
- Acenocoumarol
- Phenprocoumon

INDANDIONE DERIVATIVES

- Phenindione
- Anisindione
- Bromindione
- Diphenadione

WHEN BLEEDING OCCURS, a series of complex events are initiated that culminate in the formation of a clot and the cessation of bleeding. This process is called *hemostasis*. Although the process is not completely understood, scientists have discovered a number of factors, most of which are blood proteins, involved in the complex process of coagulation. (See Table 49-1.) The basic stages of the clotting mechanism are (1) the formation and activation of Factor X; (2) the conversion of prothrombin to thrombin; and (3) the conversion of fibrinogen to fibrin; the agglutination of platelets is another essential factor. Anticoagulants are drugs that antagonize blood clotting factors in one or more stages of coagulation.

TYPES OF ANTICOAGULANTS

The first anticoagulant used therapeutically was heparin. This *natural anticoagulant* is found in the liver and other tissues of several animals, including humans. Heparin is a potent substance that is measured in units of activity rather than weight. It inhibits all three stages of coagulation, but it does not affect bleeding time. Heparin is active in vivo and in vitro. The drug is administered parenterally and is effective within minutes. Protamine sulfate, another natural anticoagulant, exhibits weak anticoagulant activity, but is very effective in neutralizing heparin.

After observing a temporary hemorrhagic disorder in cattle who had eaten spoiled sweet clover, Link and Campbell, in 1934, isolated and identified the toxic substance as dicumarol, which is an active principle of *warfarin*. Warfarin preparations are effective anticoagulants when administered orally and are therefore cheaper to use therapeutically than parenteral drugs. As warfarin was originally considered unsafe for humans, dicumarol was the first available oral anticoagulant. Warfarin preparations antagonize both the intrinsic and extrinsic mechanisms for the formation of prothrombin and its conversion to thrombin. Thus, these drugs are potent hypoprothrombin agents.

Indandione derivatives are very similar to those of warfarin; but they affect the prothrombin time by functioning as an antimetabolite for vitamin K, which is used by the liver to form prothrombin.

Several drugs, such as *aspirin*, are known to antagonize the agglutination of platelets. These substances have been used prophylactically to provide a mild anticoagulant effect. The use of antiagglutination drugs is no longer as popular as it was in the last decade.

INDICATIONS FOR USE

Anticoagulants are used to prevent or treat thromboembolic disorders. Intravenously administered heparin is used for situations in which an immediate anticoagulant effect is desired and the oral anticoagulants, warfarin and indandione derivatives, which are inexpensive, are used when a more prolonged action is required. Clients who need both immediate and long-term drug therapy are often given heparin and an oral anticoagulant concurrently. However, heparin is discontinued as soon as the oral anticoagulant has decreased the client's prothrombin time adequately.

TREATMENT OF OVERDOSE

Bleeding is the primary toxic reaction to anticoagulants. Heparin tends to cause gastrointestinal bleeding, hematuria, and hematomas at injection sites. Protamine sulfate (a basic compound) effectively neutralizes heparin (an acidic compound) by combining with it to form a stable salt. This salt has no anticoagulant activity and is eliminated from the body. Since protamine is also an anticoagulant, the quantity of protamine must be just enough to neutralize the activity level of heparin. The longer the time lapse between heparin and protamine administration, the smaller the dosage of protamine required because heparin is rapidly excreted. Administration of whole blood also assists in reversing heparin-induced hemorrhaging by diluting serum drug levels.

The administration of vitamin K, particularly vitamin K_1 (phytonadione), is usually effective in reversing the toxic effects of warfarin and indandione derivatives. However, whole blood may also be required, particularly when toxicity is due to very-long-acting oral anticoagulants.

TABLE 49-1 Blood Clotting Factors

Factor Number	Commonly Accepted Names	Other Names	Remarks
I	Fibrinogen		Plasma protein that is synthesized by the liver in relatively large quantities (100 to 700 mg per 100 ml of blood).
II	Prothrombin		Chemical substance found in serum that is converted to thrombin.
III	Tissue thromboplastin	Platelet factor 3	Found in plasma and intracellularly.
IV	Calcium (ions)		Acts as a catalyst in most reactions of the coagulation process.
V	Labile factor	Proaccelerin, accelerator globulin (Ac-G)	Plasma protein that is easily destroyed by heat (labile).
VI	(Accelerin)		No longer considered to have a clotting function.
VII	Stable factor	Proconvertin, serum prothrombin conversion accelerator (SPCA), autoprothrombin	Plasma protein that requires vitamin K for its synthesis in the liver.
VIII	Antihemophilic factor (AHF)	Antihemophilic globulin	Plasma protein. Genetic deficiency results in hemophilia.
IX	Christmas factor	Plasma thromboplastin, autoprothrombin II	Plasma protein that requires vitamin K for its synthesis in the liver. Genetic deficiency results in hemophilia.
X	Stuart-Prower factor		Plasma protein of major importance in the coagulation process. Vitamin K is required for its synthesis in the liver.
XI	Plasma thromboplastin antecedent (PTA)		Plasma protein that accelerates blood coagulation.
XII	Hageman factor		Plasma protein.
XIII	Fibrin-stabilizing factor	Thrombokinase, complete thromboplastin	Stabilizes clot during formation.

The early detection of excessive hypoprothrombinemia is advisable. Clients should be observed for asymptomatic hematuria (use appropriate dipsticks to determine the presence of blood in the urine), bleeding of the gums, nosebleeds, and petechiae. Unfortunately, prothrombin levels can also be altered by many other factors.

FACTORS KNOWN TO ALTER PROTHROMBIN TIME

Hundreds of drugs, travel, dietary changes, and states of health can increase or decrease the prothrombin time. Clients should be warned against the self-administration of over-the-counter drugs and altering their dietary habits. If alterations occur or are anticipated, the physician should be notified. States of health that can increase the prothrombin time include carcinoma, collagen disease, congestive heart failure, diarrhea, fever, hepatic disorders, hyperthyroidism, malnutrition, and steatorrhea (vitamin K deficiency). Factors known to decrease the prothrombin time include edema, hyperlipemia, and hypothyroidism.

DETERMINATION OF DOSAGE

The dosage of an anticoagulant is determined by appropriate coagulation tests. The clotting time (Lee-White) is used for heparin and the prothrombin time is used for oral anticoagulants. The test for heparin is performed about 1 hour before each therapeutic dose. When heparin is given prophylactically in small doses, tests need only be done intermittently after dosage stabilization. Determination of the prothrombin time is done prior to the administration of each dose until stabilization occurs; then once or twice a week. If at any point the prothrombin time decreases or increases abruptly, tests should be reinstituted on a daily basis until stabilization is apparent again. As these tests are of the utmost importance in determining drug effectiveness, the need for regular laboratory evaluations should be stressed to the client. Furthermore, the margin of safety is very narrow for anticoagulants.

NATURAL ANTICOAGULANTS

GENERIC NAME Heparin sodium (RX)

TRADE NAMES Depo-Heparin, Heprinar, Lipo-Hepin, Liquaemin, Panheprin, Panheprin SDS

CLASSIFICATION Anticoagulant

Source Highly acidic mucopolysaccharide prepared commercially from porcine intestinal mucosa or bovine lung.

Action Heparin inhibits several reactions that lead to the clotting of blood both in vitro and in vivo. Although heparin does not inhibit the formation of prothrombin per se, it does antagonize the intrinsic formation of thromboplastin and Factor X, thereby inhibiting the conversion of prothrombin to thrombin. The thrombin-catalyzed conversion of fibrinogen to fibrin is also antagonized and the agglutination, or clumping, of platelets is inhibited. Although heparin can prolong the clotting time, the bleeding time is often unaffected. Therapeutic doses of heparin have an antilipemic effect. The activation of Factor XIII is reported to be inhibited, thus preventing the formation of a stable clot. Although little or no heparin can be detected in blood, heparin, or a heparinlike substance, does occur naturally in the lungs, liver, and platelets of humans. Heparin has no fibrinolytic activity but does prevent the extension of a preexisting thrombus, and therefore reduces the possibility of embolism.

Indications for Use Situations in which an immediate anticoagulant effect is desired; treatment and prevention of thromboembolic disorders, including primary embolism, cerebral thrombosis, coronary occlusion, and phlebitis; prevention of thromboembolic disorders that may occur during or following cardiac, arterial, and other forms of major abdominothoracic surgery; atrial fibrillation with embolization and prevention of a mural clot following myocardial infarction; prophylaxis during dialysis and extracorporeal circulation procedures; as an anticoagulant in blood transfusions and laboratory blood samples, including arterial blood gases.

Contraindications Hypersensitivity to heparin; situations in which there is active or a potential for active bleeding, including intracranial hemorrhage, arterial sclerosis, subacute bacterial endocarditis, inaccessible ulcerative lesions (peptic ulcer), continuous tube drainage of the stomach or small intestines, threatened abortion, and shock; situations in which there is a bleeding tendency, including hemophilia, purpura (thrombocytopenia), severe deficiency of ascorbic acid, and severe hepatic and renal disorders; following certain invasive procedures (spinal tap, spinal anesthesia) and certain types of major surgery, including brain, spinal cord, or eye surgery.

Warnings and Precautions Use with caution in clients with hypertension, hepatic or renal disorders, alcoholism, indwelling catheters, and during menstruation. Also use with caution in pregnant women during the last trimester and in the immediate postpartum period. Effects on human fertility and teratogenic potential have not been established. A higher incidence of bleeding has been reported in women over 60 years. Transfusions with ACD-converted blood may contain heparin and therefore can affect the coagulation system.

Untoward Reactions Hemorrhage or bleeding, particularly from the GI tract (diarrhea that progresses to melena and then frank bleeding, hematemesis) and the urinary tract (hematuria), is the primary untoward reaction. Surgical clients may develop a wound hematoma. Adrenal hemorrhage with resultant acute adrenal insufficiency (hypotension, decreased cardiac output, electrolyte imbalances, shock) has occurred and requires prompt therapy with corticosteroids IV. Acute reversible thrombocytopenia has occurred following heparin IV. Mild pain, local irritation, and hematoma formation may occur if heparin is injected intramuscularly. Common hypersensitivity reactions include chills, fever, and urticaria. Anaphylaxis, asthma, rhinitis, and excessive tearing have occurred, but infrequently. Vasospasms in an extremity can occur and may be due to hypersensitivity; but also occur in a recently catheterized lung. The onset may occur 6 to 10 days following initiation of therapy and may last for 4 to 6 hours. The extremity becomes ischemic, cyanotic, and painful. An itching and burning sensation on the plantar surface of the extremity may precede the condition. If the disorder goes unrecognized and heparin therapy is continued, generalized venospasms will occur and the client will become cyanotic, develop tachypnea, and complain of headache and a feeling of oppression. Chest pain, hypertension, joint pains, and headache have been reported without signs of venospasm. Osteoporosis with resulting fractures, suppression of renal function, and suppression of aldosterone synthesis may occur, particularly following long-term therapy at high dosages. Rare reactions include delayed transient alopecia and priapism. Rebounding hyperlipemia may occur following withdrawal of therapy.

Parameters of Use

Absorption Well absorbed but slowly after subcutaneous injection. Not effective after oral administration. Well absorbed after intramuscular injection. Peak action occurs in: 1 hour (subc); 5 to 10 minutes (IV). Duration of action is: 12 to 16 hours (subc); 2 to 6 hours (IV). Bound to plasma proteins; may displace certain drugs from binding sites.

Does not cross placenta or enter breast milk.

Distribution Evenly distributed in the blood; small quantities absorbed and stored in most cells.

Metabolism In the liver by heparinase and other enzymes. The metabolite uroheparin weakly inhibits the formation of thrombin.

Excretion About 50% is excreted slowly by the kidneys as unchanged drug and uroheparin. Other metabolites are excreted in urine.

Drug Interactions Although it is a weak anticoagulant, protamine sulfate is effective as a heparin antidote. The following drugs interfere with the agglutination of platelets, the primary hemostatic defense of heparinized clients: aspirin, dextran, phenylbutazone, ibuprofen, indomethacin, dipyridamole, hydroxychloroquine, guaifenesin; concurrent use should be avoided. Antineoplastic agents increase the possibility of hemorrhage in heparinized clients; do not give concomitantly. Digitalis preparations inhibit the action of heparin and should not be administered concurrently. Tetracyclines, nicotine, ascorbic acid, antihistamines (including chlorpheniramine, cyclizine, and diphenhydramine), phenothiazines (including perphenazine, promazine, and promethazine), and hydroxyzine antagonize the anticoagulant action of heparin; concurrent therapy should be avoided. Penicillin inhibits the action of heparin and hemorrhage may occur when penicillin IV is discontinued in a heparinized client. Heparin increases the anticoagulant effect of oral anticoagulants. When the drugs are administered concurrently, a period of at least 5 hours after heparin IV or 24 hours after subcutaneous heparin must elapse in order to obtain a valid prothrombin level.

Laboratory Interactions Heparinized blood should not be used to determine isoagglutinins, complement platelet counts, or erythrocyte fragility tests.

Administration Dosage is determined and adjusted according to the partial thromboplastin time. The following therapeutic dosages are those for a 150-lb adult with normal clotting tests. Subcutaneous: Initial dosage: 10,000 to 20,000 units; then 8000 to 10,000 units q8h or 15,000 to 20,000 units q12h. Intravenous (IV bolus): Initial dosage: 10,000 units; then 5000 to 10,000 units every 4 to 6 hours. Intravenous (IV infusion): Initial dosage: 5000 units IV bolus; then 20,000 to 40,000 units in 1000 ml of normal saline over 24 hours. For clients undergoing total body perfusion (cardiac or arterial surgery) the usual dosage is 150 to 400 units/kg IV; the dosage varies with the length of perfusion required. Prophylactic dosage: 5000 units subc every 8 to 12 hours. When used for extracorporeal dialysis, the manufacturer's instructions should be followed. A typical priming dosage is 2000 units injected into the arterial blood line; then 1000 to 2000 units q1h during dialysis.

Available Drug Forms Multidose vials containing 1000, 5000, 10,000, or 20,000 units/ml; single-dose vials containing 10,000, 20,000, or 40,000 units/ml; 1-ml single-dose disposable cartridges containing 5000, 10,000, or 20,000 units/ml (Panheprin SDS); 1-ml single-dose Tubex cartridges containing 1000, 2500, 5000, 7500, 10,000, 15,000, or 20,000 units/ml and 5000 units/0.5 ml; 5-ml ampules containing 1000 units/ml (heparin without preservatives).

Nursing Management

Planning factors

1. A test dose (1000 units) should be given to clients with a history of multiple allergies. Observe the client for chills, fever, urticaria, and other hypersensitivity reactions for 1 hour or more.
2. Client should be hospitalized for heparin therapy, so that untoward reactions can be managed quickly and effectively.
3. Clotting time and other coagulation tests must be obtained in order to determine the correct dosage of heparin. The "two syringe technique" should be

used to prevent contamination of the blood sample in the second syringe by tissue fluids. The tests used may include whole blood clotting time, recalcified clotting time, prothrombin time (PT), or partial thromboplastin time (PTT). Notify physician as soon as the results are known.

4. Obtain complete blood cell count, including leukocyte and platelet count, prior to initiating therapy. Notify physician of any abnormalities before administering drug.
5. Protamine sulfate should be readily available.
6. If client is receiving other drugs intramuscularly, the drug order should be changed to a different route of administration by the physician, since hematoma and other untoward reactions may occur at the injection site, particularly in the elderly and debilitated clients.
7. Notify laboratory personnel when the client is heparinized and again before each venipuncture.
8. Keep venipunctures to a minimum.
9. Schedule all essential invasive procedures, including venipunctures, enemas, catheterization, and injections, prior to heparin administration.

Administration factors

1. Check the heparin container several times, since heparin comes in many strengths and forms.
2. Obtain clotting time and/or PTT prior to each injection. PTT should be about double control levels.
3. Measure dosage carefully in a disposable 100-unit insulin syringe or disposable TB syringe (25- or 26-gauge needle, $\frac{5}{8}$ in. long).
4. Avoid IM injections if at all possible.
5. When administering subcutaneously,
   a. Inject deep into fatty tissue. Large fat pads are located just above the iliac crests and in the abdominal wall.
   b. Avoid scar tissue and tissue within 2 inches of the umbilicus.
   c. Explain to client that these are the best sites for heparin administration and that there are relatively few pain nerve endings in the area.
   d. Wipe selected area gently with an alcohol swab and allow site to dry. Do not rub vigorously.
   e. Inject straight into fat at 90° angle. (Fat tissue can be gently gathered prior to insertion.)
   f. Do not aspirate, since trauma may occur to tissue.
   g. Inject heparin slowly but steadily into the tissue.
   h. Withdraw needle in the same direction as introduced.
   i. Apply gentle but even pressure to the injection site for 15 seconds or longer; do not rub.
   j. Rotate sites; the same site should not be used twice in any one week.
6. When administering via IV bolus,
   a. Notify physician of clotting time or PTT prior to each drug administration.
   b. The Y port of an infusion line or a heparin lock can be used. Check the patency of the IV before injecting drug.
   c. Inject slowly over several minutes depending on the dosage (2 minutes per 5000 units). The rate of injection should be prescribed by the physician.
7. When administering via intermittent IV infusion,
   a. Notify physician of clotting time or PTT prior to each drug administration.
   b. Add to 50 or 100 ml of normal saline.
   c. Run IV over 30 minutes. An IV infusion pump is recommended.
8. When administering via continuous IV infusion,
   a. Obtain clotting time or PTT every 4 hours and adjust the IV rate accordingly.
   b. An IV infusion pump is highly recommended.
9. Record all data on a flowchart (date, time, dosage, injection sites, laboratory tests).

Evaluation factors

1. Obtain coagulation studies periodically. Platelet count usually decreases after 2 days of therapy, but may not occur for as long as 2 weeks.
2. Check all skin openings (previous injections, wounds) for hematoma each shift. Check extremities and sacral area for bruising or other signs of bleeding.
3. Examine urine, feces, and vomitus for signs of bleeding.
4. Monitor all signs frequently for the first 2 hours following drug administration. If hypotension or tachycardia occur, notify physician immediately. Vital signs should be monitored at least once a shift.
5. Report all untoward reactions to a physician.
6. Male clients can shave safely with a safety razor when the platelet count is normal.
7. Heparin overdose can be treated with protamine sulfate or whole blood transfusions.

GENERIC NAME Heparin lock flush (RX)

TRADE NAMES Heparin Lock Flush Solution, Hep-Lock, Panheprin Lock

CLASSIFICATION Anticoagulant

Action Heparin lock flush solution contains a low dose of heparin sodium within an intermittently used indwelling venipuncture device called a heparin lock. The device is used to administer intermittent medications or for withdrawing venous blood samples. The lumen of a heparin lock holds less than 0.5 ml and the heparin lock flush solution will maintain the lock's patency for about 4 hours. (See heparin sodium.)

Administration

1. Flush lock with 1 ml of sterile water or normal saline for injection.
2. Administer medication or withdraw blood sample.
3. Flush lock with 1 ml of sterile water or normal saline for injection.
4. Inject 1 ml of heparin lock flush solution.

Available Drug Forms Disposable cartridges of 1 ml with 25-gauge, $\frac{5}{8}$-in. needle containing 100 units/ml of heparin in normal saline.

GENERIC NAME Protamine sulfate (RX)

CLASSIFICATIONS Anticoagulant, Heparin antagonist

Source Purified proteins obtained from the sperm of salmon and certain other species of fish.

Action Protamine is a weak anticoagulant that interferes with the production of thromboplastin. In large dosages, protamine is able to inhibit the activation of fibrinogen by thrombin. Since protamine is highly basic, it will combine with heparin, a highly acidic anticoagulant, to form a stable salt, which has no anticoagulant activity. Therefore, protamine is highly effective as an antidote for heparin toxicity.

Indications for Use Antidote for heparin toxicity; used to treat accidental heparin overdoses and to counteract heparin activity following certain surgical procedures, such as cardiac bypass surgery.

Contraindications None known.

Warnings and Precautions Use with caution in clients with severe cardiovascular disease and those known to have a hypersensitivity to fish. Safe use during pregnancy has not been established.

Untoward Reactions Bleeding will occur if excessive amounts of protamine are given for heparin toxicity, particularly in clients who are hypoprothrombinemic. Abrupt hypotension, bradycardia, and dyspnea may occur, particularly when the drug is administered too fast or when large dosages (100 mg or more) are given. A transient flushing and a feeling of warmth can occur.

Parameters of Use

Absorption Onset of action as an antidote to heparin is within 5 minutes.

Administration Dosage depends on residual heparin activity and should be guided by coagulation studies, such as plasma thrombin time and the heparin titration test. Usual dosage: 50 mg IV; repeat as necessary; do not give more than 100 mg at any one time.

Available Drug Forms Ampules containing 5 ml of solution with 50 mg of drug activity (1 ml contains 10 mg of drug activity); multidose vials containing 25 ml of solution with 250 mg of drug activity (1 ml contains 10 mg of drug activity).

Nursing Management

Planning factors

1. Keep drug under refrigeration, but do not freeze. All nurses should be informed of the drug's exact location in the refrigerator and the location should be noted on the "crash cart."
2. Clients who undergo cardiac bypass and other forms of surgery that require the use of heparin may develop hyperheparinemia 30 minutes to 18 hours after surgery, despite complete neutralization of heparin with protamine at the time of surgery. Protamine should be kept in the unit's refrigerator (recovery room and intensive care unit). Watch these clients closely for bleeding.
3. Perform baseline coagulation studies (plasma thrombin time, heparin titration test) prior to protamine administration and periodically thereafter.

Administration factors

1. Each milligram of protamine neutralizes 90 USP units of heparin from lung tissue or 115 USP units of heparin from intestinal mucosa. Administer protamine as soon as possible. A 30-minute delay following heparin administration requires only half of the usual protamine dose.
2. Do not administer more than 50 mg of protamine in any 10-minute period.
3. Check patency of IV before administering drug.
4. IV bolus is the preferred method of administration. The recommended rate of administration is 10 mg/min. (1 ml/min.). Administer over 3 minutes or more to prevent untoward reactions.
5. Drug can be further diluted with 5% D/W or normal saline.
6. Do not mix with any other drugs. Protamine is known to be incompatible with several antibiotics, including cephalosporins and penicillins.

Evaluation factors

1. Check vital signs every 15 to 30 minutes for at least 3 hours following every administration of protamine. If any bleeding occurs, notify physician immediately.
2. Obtain blood coagulation studies hourly until all danger of bleeding has passed (4 to 24 hours) and then periodically, as necessary.

WARFARIN AND DERIVATIVES

GENERIC NAME Warfarin sodium (RX)

TRADE NAMES Coumadin, Panwarfin

CLASSIFICATION Anticoagulant

Source Originally obtained from spoiled sweet clover.

Action Warfarin inhibits the synthesis of prothrombin (Factor II) by depressing the formation of Factors VII, IX, and X in vivo. It competes with vitamin K in the clotting mechanism and thereby decreases the amount of circulating prothrombin. Warfarin is believed to interfere with the utilization of vitamin K by the liver to form prothrombin. Phytonadione (vitamin K_1) is an effective antidote for warfarin. As warfarin is so effective in blocking the clotting mechanism, only small dosages are required. Unlike heparin, warfarin does not affect coagulation immediately; the effects may take several days. However, warfarin has the advantage of being effective orally. Warfarin has no fibrinolytic activity but does prevent extension of a preexisting thrombus, and therefore reduces the possibility of embolism.

Indications for Use Treatment and prevention of venous thrombosis and its extension; atrial fibrillation with embolization; treatment and prevention of pulmonary embolism; as an adjunct in the treatment of coronary occlusion. May be effective as an adjunct in the treatment of transient cerebral ischemic attacks. Also used as a rodenticide.

Contraindications Hypersensitivity to warfarin or its derivatives; situations in which there is active bleeding or a potential for active bleeding, including ulcerations (or potential ulcerations) of the GI, genitourinary, or respiratory tracts, continuous tube drainage of the stomach or small intestines, cerebrovascular hemorrhage, aneurysms, pericarditis, pericardial effusions, subacute bacterial endocarditis, and threatened abortion; situations in which there is a bleeding tendency, including hemophilia, purpura (thrombocytopenia), other forms of blood dyscrasias, and severe hepatic or renal disorders; prior to or following surgery and certain invasive procedures, including brain, spinal cord, or eye surgery, traumatic surgery that results in large open surfaces, spinal tap, and spinal anesthesia; malignant hypertension; pregnancy, since the drug crosses the placental barrier and may cause fetal hemorrhage.

Warnings and Precautions Use with caution in clients with severe or moderately severe hepatic or renal insufficiency; in clients with indwelling catheters, since bleeding may occur; in clients with severe or moderately severe hypertension, polycythemia vera, vasculitis, or severe diabetes; during lactation, since the drug enters breast milk and can cause thrombocytopenia in the nursing infant; and in clients receiving antibiotics for an infection or those with sprue or other disorders that alter the intestinal flora, since bleeding may occur. Any form of trauma may result in internal bleeding. External traumas and surgery may result in severe bleeding or hemorrhage. Clients with congestive heart failure may be sensitive to warfarin and may require lower dosages. Abrupt cessation of warfarin is not recommended; dosage should be gradually tapered over 3 to 4 weeks. Numerous factors may influence the client's response to warfarin, including travel, changes in diet, environment, state of health, and medications.

Untoward Reactions Overdose will cause excessive thrombocytopenia and may result in bleeding. Thrombocytopenia frequently causes bleeding of the gums (particularly after brushing teeth), nosebleeds, petechiae, and excessive menstrual bleeding; oozing from shaving nicks can also occur. GI disturbances, including anorexia, nausea, hemoptysis, diarrhea, and tarry stools, may occur and are usually caused by a bleeding lesion (ulcer or tumor). Genitourinary bleeding (hematuria) can also occur. Asymptomatic hematuria occurs frequently. Cerebral and hepatic hemorrhages have occurred in susceptible clients (the elderly, those with an abnormality of the vasculature), but rarely. Hypersensitivity reactions include urticaria, dermatitis, and fever, but these occur rarely. Vasomotor spasms of the extremities that can result in necrotic toes (called "purple toes") have occurred, but rarely; this condition may be a hypersensitivity reaction. Other rare reactions include blood dyscrasias (incidence increases with the length of therapy), alopecia, priapism, nausea, vomiting, diarrhea, and abdominal cramps.

Parameters of Use

Absorption Fairly well absorbed from GI tract and intramuscular sites. Peak plasma concentration occurs in 1 to 9 hours after oral administration. Blood concentration is not related to therapeutic effect. Onset of hypoprothrombinemia is 36 to 72 hours and duration is 4 to 5 days depending on the length of time the drug remains in the liver. Half-life is $2\frac{1}{2}$ days. About 97% bound to plasma albumin as a result of numerous drug interactions.

Crosses placenta and enters breast milk; lactating mothers must bottle-feed their babies.

Distribution Mainly in liver, lungs, spleen, and kidneys.

Metabolism In the liver to inactive metabolites. Rate of metabolism varies widely from client to client.

Excretion Most is excreted by the kidneys as metabolites.

Drug Interactions There are literally hundreds of drugs that interact with warfarin. Some drug interactions cause lengthening of the prothrombin time, whereas others shorten the prothrombin time significantly. Only the most common interactions are listed here. Consult a pharmacist for other drug interactions. Commonly used drugs that potentiate warfarin by lengthening the prothrombin time are: salicylates (including aspirin), anabolic steroids, numerous antibiotics, chymotrypsin, dextran, ethacrynic acid, glucagon, MAO inhibitors, phenytoin, narcotics (if used for a prolonged period of time), quinidine, quinine, sulfonamides, thyroid hormones. Any enzyme inhibitor, such as allopurinol, has the potential for potentiating warfarin. Commonly used drugs that inhibit warfarin by shortening the prothrombin time are adrenocorticosteroids, antacids, antihistamines, barbiturates, meprobamate, oral contraceptives, paraldehyde. Any enzyme inducer, such as cimetidine, has the potential for inhibiting warfarin. Commonly used drugs that may either potentiate or inhibit warfarin are: alcohol, chloral hydrate, and diuretics. Warfarin anticoagulants potentiate the action of sulfonylurea antidiabetic agents (chlorpropamide, tolbutamide) by inhibiting their metabolism and excretion. These agents may displace warfarin from protein-binding sites. Warfarin anticoagulants also potentiate anticonvulsants (phenytoin, phenobarbital) by inhibiting their metabolism and excretion. Phytonadione (vitamin K_1) is an effective antidote for warfarin. Concurrent use of anticoagulants containing streptokinase or urokinase is not recommended and can be hazardous. Heparin increases the anticoagulant effect of warfarin. When the drugs are administered concurrently, a period of at least 5 hours after heparin IV or 24 hours after subcutaneous heparin must elapse in order to obtain a valid prothrombin level. Dietary deficiencies of vitamin C, K, and other substances needed for the clotting mechanism may cause bleeding. Prolonged hot weather may increase the prothrombin time. Diets high in vitamin K may decrease the prothrombin time.

Administration Dosage individualized according to the prothrombin time, which should be twice the control level. Initial dosage (average adult): 40 to 60 mg po, IM, or IV; Maintenance dosage: 2 to 10 mg po daily. Reduced dosages are required for the elderly, debilitated clients, and clients with severe renal or hepatic impairment. Initial dosage: 20 to 30 mg po, IM, or IV; Maintenance dosage: 2 to 10 mg po daily or every other day.

Available Drug Forms Scored tablets containing 2 mg (lavender), 2.5 mg (orange), 5 mg (peach), 7.5 mg (yellow), or 10 mg (white). Single injection units (amorphous warfarin sodium lyophilized) containing a vial of 50 mg warfarin and a 2-ml ampule of sterile water for injection; diluent can be used for intramuscular injections only. Consult a pharmacist if IV injection is desired.

Nursing Management

Planning factors

1. Obtain complete history and include information regarding (1) any unusual bleeding that has occurred; (2) whether there is a tendency to bruise easily; (3) drugs taken in the last month; (4) OTC preparations normally taken for common ailments; (5) usual diet; and (6) plans for travel in the near future. Since so many factors alter the client's response to warfarin, update the history frequently (weekly or biweekly).
2. Obtain prothrombin time (PT), other coagulation tests, and complete blood cell count (including platelet count) prior to instituting therapy. Notify physician of any abnormalities before administering drug.
3. Adequate laboratory facilities must be accessible for outpatients, who must be willing to keep their laboratory appointments.
4. Withdraw drug 2 days prior to surgery and take PT daily.
5. The antidote, vitamin K_1 (2.5 to 25.0 mg po or parenterally), should be readily available.
6. Keep venipuncture and IM injections to a minimum.
7. Dosage and duration of therapy highly individualized. Therapy is maintained until the danger of thrombosis or embolism has passed.

Administration factors

1. Obtain a PT test or one-stage PT test prior to each drug administration. Report test results to physician and reconfirm the drug and dosage before administering.
2. Check the type of warfarin drug and the dosage several times before administering.
3. When administering IM,
   a. Reconstitute warfarin with diluent provided.
   b. Use freshly prepared solution.
   c. Inject deep into muscle mass; the Z-track method is recommended.
   d. Rotate injection sites.
   e. Observe previous injection sites for signs of bleeding.
4. When warfarin IV is prescribed, consult the pharmacist for details on dilution and administration; however, this route is rarely used.
5. Record all data on a flowchart (date, time, dosage, injection sites, laboratory tests).

Evaluation factors

1. Obtain PT tests daily until stabilization occurs at $1\frac{1}{2}$ to $2\frac{1}{2}$ times the control level (at least 3 to 7 days). PT tests can be done weekly on outpatients.
2. If the PT is altered dramatically (either up or down), the PT test should be reinstituted on a daily basis until restabilization occurs.
3. Examine for signs and symptoms of external and internal bleeding once a shift. (Outpatients should be examined at each appointment.) Examine the mouth for signs of bleeding or petechiae and test the urine daily for hematuria (dipsticks are available). If symptoms occur, including asymptomatic hematuria, notify physician immediately.
4. Obtain complete blood cell count (including platelet count) and more complete coagulation studies periodically.

Client teaching factors

1. Instruct male client to shave with an electric razor.
2. Instruct client to use a soft bristle toothbrush.
3. Warn client to report any signs or symptoms of bleeding to physician immediately. Instruct client that the early signs of hypoprothrombinemia include bleeding of the gums and petechiae. Client should also be taught how to use dipsticks to detect asymptomatic hematuria.
4. Renal clients may be given a dose of vitamin K to carry at all times in case of accidental injury. Explain to the client when the dose should be used.
5. Instruct client to carry a card, tag, identification band, or some form of alert to indicate the anticoagulant being used.
6. Inform client of the factors that may alter the PT.
7. Caution client against poor dietary habits and the indiscriminate use of OTC drugs, since prothrombin levels may be altered. The client should be warned against (a) consuming large quantities of vitamin K-rich foods (green leafy vegetables, eggs, tomatoes) and (b) self-treating common ailments. The physician should be consulted before taking OTC drugs.
8. Caution client against drinking alcoholic beverages. (The physician may allow small amounts infrequently.)
9. Impress upon client the necessity of keeping laboratory and medical (physician) appointments.
10. Instruct client to store drug in tightly sealed containers away from moisture (not in the kitchen or bathroom). Explore possible locations with client. The drug must be kept out of the reach of children.
11. Instruct client to take medication at the same time each day (breakfast). Forgetful clients should "X-out" a calendar when they take the drug.

GENERIC NAME Warfarin potassium (RX)

TRADE NAME Athrombin-K

CLASSIFICATION Anticoagulant

See warfarin sodium for Indications for use, Contraindications, Warnings and precautions, Untoward reactions, Drug interactions, and Nursing management.

Action Potassium warfarin can be used interchangeably with sodium warfarin to inhibit the synthesis of prothrombin. As potassium warfarin is absorbed somewhat more readily from the GI tract, slightly lower dosages are required to produce the same anticoagulant effect as sodium warfarin.

Parameters of Use

Absorption Readily absorbed from GI tract. Onset of hypoprothrombinemia is 12 to 24 hours and duration is 4 to 5 days. Half-life is $2\frac{1}{2}$ days. About 97% bound to plasma albumin as a result of numerous drug interactions.

Crosses placenta and enters breast milk; lactating mothers must bottle-feed their babies.

Distribution Mainly in liver, lungs, spleen, and kidneys.

Metabolism In the liver to inactive metabolites. Rate of metabolism varies widely from client to client.

Excretion Most is excreted by the kidneys as metabolites.

Administration Dosage individualized according to the prothrombin time., which should be $1\frac{1}{2}$ to $2\frac{1}{2}$ times the control level. Initial dosage (average adult): 25 to 50 mg po; Maintenance dosage: 2.5 to 10.0 mg daily. Elderly and debilitated clients require reduced dosages.

Available Drug Forms Scored tablets containing 5 or 10 mg.

GENERIC NAME Dicumarol (RX)

TRADE NAMES Dicumarol

CLASSIFICATION Anticoagulant

See warfarin sodium for Indications for use, Contraindications, Warnings and precautions, Drug interactions, and Nursing management.

Action Dicumarol was the first oral anticoagulant available commercially. It inhibits the synthesis of prothrombin by depressing the formation of Factors VII, IX, and X in vivo. Dicumarol is similar to warfarin sodium, but is less potent and is slightly longer acting. (See warfarin sodium.)

Untoward Reactions GI disturbances, including nausea, vomiting, abdominal cramps, and diarrhea, are common. (See warfarin sodium.)

Parameters of Use (See warfarin sodium.)

Absorption Irregular and incomplete. Onset of hypoprothrombinemia is 12 to 72 hours and duration is 5 to 6 days, but may last as long as 2 weeks. About 98% bound to plasma albumin. Extensive protein binding may cause numerous drug interactions.

Administration Dosage individualized according to the prothrombin time, which should be $1\frac{1}{2}$ to $2\frac{1}{2}$ times the control level. Initial dosage (average adult): 200 to 300 mg po; Maintenance dosage: 50 to 100 mg daily. Elderly and debilitated clients require reduced dosages.

Available Drug Forms Tablets containing 25 mg (white), 50 mg (pink), or 100 mg (white).

GENERIC NAME Ethyl biscoumacetate (RX)

TRADE NAME Tromexan

CLASSIFICATION Anticoagulant

See warfarin sodium for Contraindications, Warnings and precautions, Drug interactions, and Nursing management.

Action Similar to dicumarol, but thought to be more rapidly absorbed, metabolized, and excreted; thus cumulative effect is less. (See dicumarol.)

Indications for Use Initiation of anticoagulant therapy.

Untoward Reactions May cause GI disturbances and hypersensitivity reactions (rash, urticaria, alopecia). (See warfarin sodium.)

Parameters of Use (See warfarin sodium.)

Absorption Onset of action is about 18 hours and duration of action is 2 to 3 days.

Administration Initial dosage: 1200 to 1800 mg po; Maintenance dosage: 150 to 900 mg daily.

Available Drug Forms Tablets containing 150 or 300 mg.

GENERIC NAME Acenocoumarol (RX)

TRADE NAME Sintrom

CLASSIFICATION Anticoagulant

See warfarin sodium for Indications for use, Contraindications, Warnings and precautions, Drug interactions, and Nursing management.

Action Similar to warfarin sodium, but thought to be more potent than other warfarin derivatives. (See warfarin sodium.)

Untoward Reactions May cause GI disturbances, including oral ulcerations. (See warfarin sodium.)

Parameters of Use (See warfarin sodium.)

Absorption Onset of action is about 12 hours and duration of action is $1\frac{1}{2}$ to 2 days.

Administration Initial dosage: 16 to 28 mg po; Second day: 8 to 16 mg po; Maintenance dosage: 2 to 12 mg daily.

Available Drug Forms Tablets containing 4 mg.

GENERIC NAME Phenprocoumon (RX)

TRADE NAME Liquamar

CLASSIFICATION Anticoagulant

See warfarin sodium for Indications for use, Contraindications, Warnings and precautions, Drug interactions, and Nursing management.

Action Similar to warfarin, but is very potent and has a prolonged duration of action. (See warfarin sodium.)

Untoward Reactions May cause diarrhea upon withdrawal and hypersensitivity reactions (rashes). (See warfarin sodium.)

Parameters of Use (See warfarin sodium.)

Absorption Onset of action is 24 to 36 hours and duration of action is 7 to 14 days.

Administration Initial dosage: 20 to 24 mg po; Maintenance dosage: 1 to 4 mg daily.

Available Drug Forms Tablets containing 3 mg.

INDANDIONE DERIVATIVES

GENERIC NAME Phenindione (RX)

TRADE NAME Hedulin

CLASSIFICATION Anticoagulant

See warfarin sodium for Contraindications, Warnings and precautions, and Drug interactions.

Action Phenindione functions like a vitamin K antimetabolite and therefore inhibits the synthesis of prothrombin by the liver. Although its action is similar to warfarin derivatives, the long-term use of phenindione causes a relatively high incidence of hepatitis, agranulocytosis, and other untoward reactions. Consequently, its use is usually restricted to clients who are unable to tolerate warfarin derivatives.

Indications for Use Prevention and treatment of thromboembolic disorders in clients who do not tolerate warfarin derivatives. (See warfarin sodium for further details.)

Untoward Reactions Hypersensitivity reactions include fever, malaise, headache, and rashes; exfoliative dermatitis has also occurred. Side effects that affect the blood and the hepatic and renal system are thought to be the result of hypersensitivity. Blood dyscrasias, including agranulocytosis, leukopenia, and eosinophilia, have occurred with long-term therapy. Hepatic disorders include hepatitis and jaundice. Renal disorders include albuminuria, generalized edema, and tubular necrosis. Other reactions include diarrhea, paralysis of eye accommodation, and blurred vision. Hemorrhagic reactions that occur with warfarin derivatives are also problematic. (See warfarin sodium for further details.)

Parameters of Use

Absorption Fairly well absorbed from GI tract. Marked variations occur from client to client. Onset of hypoprothrombinemia is 2 to 8 hours and duration is 1 to 4 days. Highly bound to serum proteins as a result of numerous drug interactions.

Crosses placenta and enters breast milk; lactating mothers must bottle-feed their babies.

Metabolism In the liver to inactive metabolites.

Excretion In urine, which turns red-orange. Difficult to distinguish from hematuria unless urine is tested.

Administration Dosage individualized according to the prothrombin time, which should be $1\frac{1}{2}$ to $2\frac{1}{2}$ times the control level. Initial dosage: 200 to 300 mg po in 2 divided doses q12h; Maintenance dosage: 25 to 100 mg daily; may be given in 2 divided doses q12h.

Available Drug Forms Tablets containing 20 or 50 mg.

Nursing Management (See warfarin sodium.)

1. Perform hepatic and renal function tests before instituting therapy. If abnormalities are present, an alternative anticoagulant should be used.
2. Warn client about harmless urine color change.
3. Instruct client to notify physician immediately if fever, infection, cloudy urine, or jaundice occurs.
4. Perform complete blood cell count (including platelet count), urinalysis for albumin, clotting time, and prothrombin time daily until stabilization occurs; then weekly or biweekly.

GENERIC NAME Anisindione (RX)

TRADE NAME Miradon

CLASSIFICATION Anticoagulant

See warfarin sodium for Contraindications, Warnings and precautions, and Drug interactions. See phenindione for Indications for use, Untoward reactions, and Nursing management.

Action Anisindione inhibits the synthesis of prothrombin by the liver. Well absorbed from GI tract.

Parameters of Use (See phenindione.)

Absorption Onset of action is 8 hours and duration of action is $1\frac{1}{2}$ to 3 days.

Administration Initial dosage: 300 mg po; Second day: 200 mg po; Maintenance dosage: 25 to 100 mg daily.

Available Drug Forms Tablets containing 50 mg.

GENERIC NAME Bromindione (RX)

TRADE NAME Halinone

CLASSIFICATION Anticoagulant

See warfarin sodium for Contraindications, Warnings and precautions, and Drug interactions. See phenindione for Indications for use, Untoward reactions, and Nursing management.

Action Bromindione is more potent and has a longer duration of action than phenindione. May be given once daily instead of q12h.

Parameters of Use (See phenindione.)

Absorption Onset of action is within 24 hours and duration of action is more than 4 days.

Administration Initial dosage: 12 to 18 mg po; Second day: 12 to 18 mg po; Maintenance dosage: 2 to 5 mg daily.

Available Drug Forms Scored tablets containing 2, 5, or 10 mg.

GENERIC NAME Diphenadione (RX)

TRADE NAME Dipaxin

CLASSIFICATION Anticoagulant

See warfarin sodium for Contraindications, Warnings and precautions, and Drug interactions. See phenindione for Indications for use, Untoward reactions, and Nursing management.

Action Similar to phenindione but less toxic and considerably longer acting. Nausea is a common side effect.

Parameters of Use (See phenindione.)

Absorption Onset of action is within 24 hours and duration of action is 15 to 20 days.

Administration Initial dosage: 20 to 30 mg po; Second day: 10 to 15 mg po; Maintenance dosage: 2.5 to 5 mg daily.

Available Drug Forms Scored tablets containing 5 mg.

Chapter 50

Antihypertensive Agents

PHYSIOLOGIC CONTROL OF BLOOD PRESSURE
TYPES OF ANTIHYPERTENSIVE AGENTS
CLASSIFICATION OF HYPERTENSION
CENTRAL-ACTING AGENTS
- Clonidine hydrochloride
- Methyldopa
- Methyldopate hydrochloride
- Pargyline hydrochloride
- Alkaverir
- Veratrum viride
- Cryptenamine acetates
- Cryptenamine tannates
- Protoveratrine A and B maleates
- Protoveratrine A

GANGLIONIC BLOCKING AGENTS
- Mecamylamine hydrochloride
- Trimethaphan camsylate

ALPHA- AND BETA-ADRENERGIC BLOCKERS
- Metoprolol tartrate
- Nadolol
- Oxprenolol
- Pindolol
- Propranolol hydrochloride
- Timolol maleate
- Phenoxybenzamine hydrochloride
- Phentolamine hydrochloride

NOREPINEPHRINE DEPLETORS
- Reserpine
- Rauwolfia serpentina
- Alseroxylon
- Deserpidine
- Rescinnamine
- Syrosingepine
- Guanethidine sulfate

TYROSINE HYDROXYLASE INHIBITORS
- Metyrosine

SELECTIVE ALPHA-ADRENERGIC BLOCKERS AND VASODILATORS
- Prazosin hydrochloride

DIRECT VASODILATORS
- Hydralazine hydrochloride
- Diazoxide (injection)
- Sodium nitroprusside
- Minoxidil

COMBINATION PREPARATIONS

- Aldoclor
- Aldoril
- Apresazide
- Apresoline-Esidrix
- Diupres
- Diutensen
- Diutensen-R
- Enduronyl, Enduronyl Forte
- Esimil
- Eutron
- Exna-R
- Hydropres, Hydrotensin
- Inderide
- Metatensin
- Minizide
- Naquival
- Oreticyl
- Rauzide
- Rease-R
- Salutensin, Salutensin Demi
- Ser-Ap-Es

HYPERTENSION IS A major health problem that affects nearly 15% of the white and 27% of the black population in the United States. Although most hypertensive clients can be well controlled by medication, clients with hypertension are often asymptomatic and remain untreated until one or more of their body organs becomes affected. Chronic severe hypertension may lead to angina, myocardial infarction, congestive heart failure, cerebral vascular accident (stroke), and impaired renal function. Antihypertensive agents are unable to correct the cause of hypertension, but they are effective in controlling the elevation in blood pressure, thereby preventing the resultant organ damage and prolonging the client's life span.

PHYSIOLOGIC CONTROL OF BLOOD PRESSURE

Just as daily activities cause normal fluctuations in heart rate, so does blood pressure experience normal elevations and depressions. However, a consistently elevated diastolic (resting) pressure above 90 or 95 mm Hg is considered pathologic. Although an abrupt increase in cardiac output, which is equal to stroke volume times heart rate, will cause a corresponding elevation in blood pressure, increases in blood pressure are usually due to an increase in total peripheral resistance. The normal state of vascular smooth muscle is mild constriction, but when any one of several physiologic mechanisms that control blood pressure are activated in response to the needs of body tissues, vasoconstriction (elevation of blood pressure) or vasodilation (lowering of blood pressure) is induced. Catecholamines and the autonomic nervous system, baroreceptor reflexes, and the renin-angiotensin system all have a role in the maintenance of total peripheral resistance. Clients with hypertension often have excessive constriction of arterioles and a resulting increase in peripheral vascular resistance.

Catecholamines, epinephrine and norepinephrine, increase heart rate and produce vasoconstriction of several blood vessels, thereby elevating blood pressure. Clients with pheochromocytoma release excessive quantities of catecholamines and therefore have a markedly elevated blood pressure. As stimulation of the adrenergic nervous system causes the release of catecholamines, excessive excitation of this system will result in an elevation of blood pressure.

Baroreceptors are sensory nerve endings located in the carotid sinus and arteries, aortic arch, and vena cava. These receptors are stimulated when the vessel walls are stretched and cause a decrease in arterial blood pressure and heart rate by inhibiting the vasomotor center in the medulla oblongata and stimulating the vagus nerve, respectively. For reasons yet unexplained, these baroreceptors maintain the blood pressure of hypertensive clients at a higher than normal level.

The enzyme *renin* is secreted by the kidneys in response to lowered renal arterial blood pressure and serum sodium levels. As a result of the release of renin into the bloodstream, angiotensin I is formed which is rapidly converted to *angiotensin II,* a potent vasopressor. Angiotensin

II also promotes the reabsorption of sodium and water by the kidneys by stimulating the release of aldosterone. (Aldosterone is a mineralocorticoid that induces sodium retention and the urinary loss of potassium.) It has been found that some hypertensive clients have a high serum renin level whereas others have low renin levels. Since catecholamines stimulate the secretion of renin by interaction with beta-adrenergic receptors, clients with high levels of renin respond to beta-adrenergic blockers, such as propranolol. Research in this area is continuing and the long-term results may take several years.

Other areas of hypertension research include the role of sodium and calcium in arteriole smooth muscle. It is believed that there is an excess of these electrolytes in muscle fibers and therefore excessive vasoconstriction. cAMP (adenosine 3′:5′-cyclic phosphate), an endogenous substance that plays a role in bronchodilation-constriction, may also affect arteriole smooth muscle. However, it is known that sodium-restricted diets, suppression of renin and aldosterone, and the use of diuretics that induce the excretion of sodium are effective in lowering an elevated blood pressure.

TYPES OF ANTIHYPERTENSIVE AGENTS

Antihypertensive agents lower elevated blood pressure by several different mechanisms. *Central-acting* agents affect the vasomotor center in the medulla and some also have an antianxiety effect. *Ganglionic blockers* are effective in decreasing arteriole vasoconstriction by interfering with autonomic nerve impulses at sympathetic ganglion. *Adrenergic blocking agents* block the nerve impulses that induce vasoconstriction and increase heart rate. Reserpine and related drugs *deplete norepinephrine* levels at adrenergic nerve endings, thus preventing excessive vasoconstriction. Other drugs, such as hydralazine and sodium nitroprusside, cause *direct vasodilation* and are effective in reducing blood pressure rapidly. Although *diuretics* have no direct antihypertensive effects, they have been found to lower blood pressure by their action on plasma volume (see Chapter 53 for a more detailed discussion of diuretics).

CLASSIFICATION OF HYPERTENSION

When hypertension is a symptom of an underlying primary pathology, such as pheochromocytoma, toxemia of pregnancy, coarctation of the aorta, or renal or hormonal disorders, it is termed *secondary hypertension.* Drugs and other substances, such as excessive licorice intake, hypersensitivity to sympathomimetics, and birth control pills, may cause secondary hypertension. Once the primary etiology is identified and corrected, blood pressure returns to normal.

Unfortunately, the etiology of hypertension is unknown in nearly 90% of the clients. An elevated blood pressure of unknown origin is called *primary* or *essential hypertension* and is characterized by constriction of arterioles, which increases the peripheral vascular resistance and results in a persistent diastolic pressure of 90 mm Hg or higher. When hypertension develops gradually over several years it is termed *benign,* but when the onset is abrupt and the diastolic pressure is markedly elevated it is termed *malignant hypertension,* since it will eventually lead to organ damage.

As the selection of appropriate treatment depends on the severity of the elevation in diastolic pressure, hypertension may be classified as mild, moderate, severe, or hypertensive crisis. *Mild* or *labile* hypertension is manifested by an asymptomatic and/or periodic elevation of diastolic pressure (90 to 105 mm Hg). No medication is required, but the client should avoid predisposing factors, such as excessive sodium intake, obesity, or smoking. If blood pressure remains elevated after conservative therapy, reserpine or a thiazide diuretic may be prescribed.

Moderate hypertension is manifested by a consistently elevated diastolic pressure between 105 and 120 mm Hg. The client may or may not be symptomatic and some organ damage will occur if the hypertensive state remains untreated. An adrenergic blocking agent, reserpine, or a central-acting antihypertensive agent is usually effective and is often prescribed concurrently with a thiazide diuretic.

A diastolic pressure between 120 and 140 mm Hg is termed *severe* hypertension, since it is symptomatic and will result in damage to the heart, kidneys, retina, or other organs. Clients with severe hypertension require a potent antihypertensive agent, such as guanethidine sulfate, or a ganglionic blocking agent, such as mecamylamine hydrochloride, and may even require two different types of antihypertensive agents. Thiazide diuretics are also helpful.

Hypertensive crisis is manifested by a diastolic pressure above 140 mm Hg and is considered a medical emergency, since severe organ damage such as retinopathy, pump failure, oliguria, and encephalopathy may occur. The client may experience severe headaches and visual and gastrointestinal disturbances. This condition is treated aggressively with parenterally administered short-acting vasodilators, such as sodium nitroprusside or diazoxide, to maintain the diastolic pressure at 100 mm Hg or less. The client is gradually titrated off the parenteral medication to oral antihypertensive agents.

CENTRAL-ACTING AGENTS

GENERIC NAME Clonidine hydrochloride (RX)

TRADE NAME Catapres

CLASSIFICATION Antihypertensive

Action Although the precise mechanism of action is unknown, clonidine (an imidazoline derivative) is thought to act by stimulating inhibitory alpha-adrenergic neurons in the CNS, which results in inhibition of the cardioaccelerator and vasoconstrictor centers in the brain stem. Consequently, blood pressure is reduced and pulse rate is slowed. Some transient vasoconstriction also occurs due to peripheral stimulation of alpha-adrenergic receptors. There is some reduction in cardiac output and peripheral resistance. Renal blood flow and glomerular filtration remain essentially unchanged. Plasma renin activity and excretion of aldosterone and catecholamines may be reduced with continued drug therapy. The concurrent use of clonidine with diuretics enhances the antihypertensive effect.

Indications for Use Mild to moderate hypertension. Has been used for essential, renal, and malignant hypertension.

Contraindications None known.

Warnings and Precautions Use with caution in clients with severe coronary insufficiency, recent myocardial infarction, cerebrovascular diseases, or chronic renal failure. Abrupt withdrawal of drug may cause a rapid increase in blood pressure, nervousness, agitation, and headache. Hypertensive encephalopathy and death have occurred, but rarely. A sedative effect may occur during the initial therapy with clonidine, but tolerance develops after continued use.

Safe use in children and during pregnancy has not been established.

Untoward Reactions Common untoward reactions include dry mouth, drowsiness, and sedation. Dizziness, constipation, headache, and fatigue occur frequently. These effects diminish with continued use of drug. Cardiovascular disturbances include bradycardia, which occurs frequently. Orthostatic hypotension has been reported, but less frequently than with most antihypertensive agents. Wenckebach and trigeminy arrhythmias have been reported. Congestive heart failure and Raynaud's phenomenon have also been reported, but rarely. GI disturbances include nausea, anorexia, vomiting, and parotid pain. Drug-induced hepatitis, jaundice, hyperbilirubinemia, and malaise have been reported. CNS disturbances, including insomnia, vivid dreams, nightmares, nervousness, restlessness, anxiety, and mental depression, may occur. Urinary retention and impotence have been reported. Rashes, angioneurotic edema, hives, urticaria, and pruritus have been reported and are associated with drug hypersensitivity. Dryness, itching and burning of the eyes, pallor, weight gain, transient elevation in blood glucose or serum creatinine phosphokinase, and gynecomastia have been reported. Accidental overdose may cause profound hypotension, weakness, somnolence, vomiting, and diminished reflexes. Retinal degeneration has been reported in animal toxicology studies.

Parameters of Use

Absorption Rapid from GI tract; oral administration may cause GI disturbances. Onset of action is 30 to 60 minutes. Peak action occurs in 2 to 4 hours and duration of action is 6 to 8 hours. Plasma half-life is 12 to 16 hours.

Metabolism Primarily in the liver.

Excretion By the kidneys as metabolites; about 20% excreted in feces.

Drug Interactions May potentiate CNS depression when given concurrently with alcohol, barbiturates, and other CNS depressants. Antihypertensive effect may be decreased by tricyclic antidepressants and MAO inhibitors. Drug-induced bradycardia may be enhanced by guanethidine, propranolol, and digitalis glycosides.

Administration Highly individualized. Initial dosage: 0.1 mg po bid; then increase by 0.1 to 0.2 mg daily until desired effect; Maintenance dosage: 0.2 to 0.8 mg daily in divided doses; Maximum effective dosage: 2.4 mg/day.

Available Drug Forms Scored tablets containing 0.1, 0.2, or 0.3 mg.

Nursing Management

Planning factors

1. Obtain the following baseline data: blood pressure in standing, sitting, and supine position; other vital signs; EKG tracing.
2. If any arrhythmias exist, notify physician before instituting therapy.
3. An eye examination should be done to detect actual or potential degeneration of the retina.

Administration factors Give between meals with a full glass of water.

Evaluation factors

1. Monitor blood pressure and pulse during peak plasma drug levels and before administering each dose when drug therapy is first instituted or dosage adjusted. If hypotension or arrhythmias occur, notify physician.
2. Dry mouth can be relieved by cool drinks, sugarless gum, and, if allowed, ice chips.
3. Since orthostatic hypotension and drowsiness may occur, assist client with ambulation, as indicated.
4. Stool softeners usually prevent drug-induced constipation.
5. Obtain periodic hepatic function tests and eye examinations (every 1 to 6 months depending on dosage).
6. When discontinued, taper drug dosage over 2 to 4 days to avoid a rapid rise in blood pressure.

Client teaching factors

1. Explain the necessity of maintaining drug schedule. Emphasize the reason for avoiding abrupt withdrawal.
2. Instruct client to avoid driving a car or engaging in other hazardous activity until drowsiness subsides (about 1 to 4 weeks).
3. Instruct client in methods to avoid orthostatic hypotension, dry mouth, and constipation.
4. Inform client that vivid dreams may occur and they are a reaction to the drug.
5. Instruct client to report untoward reactions to a physician.

GENERIC NAME Methyldopa (RX)

TRADE NAMES Aldomet, Dopamet

CLASSIFICATION Antihypertensive

Action Alpha-methylnorepinephrine, a metabolite of methyldopa, is thought to cause the stimulation of inhibitory alpha-adrenergic neurons in the CNS, thus resulting in lowered arterial blood pressure. Unlike clonidine, there is little or no effect on cardiac output or heart rate. False neurotransmission in the CNS may also be involved. Plasma renin activity and tissue concentrations of serotonin, dopamine, norepinephrine, and epinephrine are also reduced.

Indications for Use Moderate to severe hypertension.

Contraindications Hypersensitivity to drug; acute hepatitis cirrhosis, or other hepatic disorders.

Warnings and Precautions Use with caution in clients with renal impairment or a history of hepatic disease or dysfunction. Fatalities have been reported due to hemolytic anemia or hepatic dysfunction. Positive Coombs' test and other symptoms are reversed when drug is discontinued. Tolerance occasionally develops after 2 to 3 months of therapy; the dosage may be increased or a diuretic added. Avoid use during pregnancy and lactation unless benefits outweigh risks.

Untoward Reactions Transient sedation, headache, weakness, and dizziness are common when therapy is first initiated or dosage increased. Symptoms usually subside after a few weeks. Drug-induced fever associated with muscle pains, nausea, vomiting, and diarrhea frequently occurs during the first 2 to 3 weeks of therapy; eosinophilia, skin rashes, and abnormal hepatic function tests (serum alkaline phosphatase, serum glutamic-oxaloacetic transaminase, serum glutamic-pyruvic transaminase, bilirubin, cephalin cholesterol flocculation, prothrombin time, retention of Bromsulphalein) have also occurred; these reactions are thought to be due to hypersensitivity and the drug should be discontinued. CNS disturbances include symptoms of cerebrovascular insufficiency, paresthesia, decreased mental acuity, parkinsonism, Bell's palsy, and involuntary choreoathetotic movements. Nightmares, depression, and psychotic disturbances may also occur. Cardiovascular disturbances, including bradycardia and precipitation of anginal pain, may occur. If orthostatic hypotension occurs, the dosage should be reduced. Edema and weight gain are usually treated with the addition of diuretics; but if congestive heart failure is developing, the drug is discontinued. Myocarditis has been reported. GI disturbances, including dry mouth, nausea, vomiting, constipation, excessive flatulence, and diarrhea, may occur. Soreness of the tongue, pancreatitis, and sialadenitis have been reported. Hemolytic anemia, leukopenia, granulocytopenia, thrombocytopenia, and positive Coombs', antinuclear antibodies, lupus erythematosus cells, and rheumatoid factor tests have been reported. Lupuslike syndrome, eczema, and other rashes have been reported. Other reactions include nasal stuffiness, breast enlargement, gynecomastia, unexpected lactation, impotence, decreased libido, elevated blood urea nitrogen, and arthralgia.

Parameters of Use

Absorption Well absorbed from GI tract. Onset of action is 6 to 12 hours. Peak action occurs in 3 to 6 hours and duration of action is 8 to 12 hours. Biphasic elimination with half life of $1\frac{1}{2}$ hours; then 5 to 8 hours if renal function test is normal; severe renal impairment doubles the half-life.

Crosses placenta and enters breast milk.

Metabolism Primarily in the liver.

Excretion Primarily in urine. Renal dialysis causes loss of drug.

Drug Interactions Drugs that increase the antihypertensive effect of methyldopa include amphetamines, diuretics, levodopa, norepinephrine, phenothiazines, propranolol, procainamide, quinidine, and tricyclic antidepressants.

Laboratory Interactions May produce false-positive urine glucose with Clinitest; but does not affect Tes-Tape or Diastix. Interferes with the measurement of urinary uric acid by phosphotungstate method, serum creatinine by alkaline picrate, and serum glutamic-oxaloacetic transaminase by colorimetric methods. Causes fluorescence in urine and may cause false determination of urine catecholamines, thus interfering with the diagnosis of pheochromocytoma. However, drug does not alter vanilmandelic acid test for pheochromocytoma.

Administration Adults: Initial dosage: 250 mg po tid for 48 hours; then increase every 2 to 3 days until desired effect; may be given in divided doses; Maximum dosage: 3000 mg/day. Children: Initial dosage: 10 mg/kg po daily in 2 to 4 divided doses; then increase every 2 to 3 days until desired effect; Maximum dosage: 65 mg/kg or 3000 mg daily, whichever is lower.

Available Drug Forms Tablets containing 125, 250, or 500 mg; oral suspension containing 250 mg/ml.

Nursing Management (See clonidine hydrochloride.)

1. Obtain body temperature q4h of awake client when therapy is first initiated.
2. Obtain hepatic function tests frequently.
3. Elderly clients are prone to develop cerebral ischemia, which results in syncope. Lower dosages are usually required. If symptoms occur, notify physician.
4. Shake suspension well before measuring dose.
5. Cardiac monitoring is recommended when treating severe hypertension.

GENERIC NAME Methyldopate hydrochloride

TRADE NAME Aldomet (RX)

CLASSIFICATION Antihypertensive

See methyldopa for Contraindications, Warnings and precautions, Untoward reactions, and Drug interactions.

Action Unlike methyldopa, methyldopate hydrochloride is soluble in water and can be used for parenteral injection. Additional ingredients buffer the solution and protect it with antioxidants and chelating agents. (See methyldopa.)

Indications for Use Hypertension in clients who require parenteral injections. Has been used for initial treatment of severe hypotension. (Not the drug of choice for hypertensive crisis.)

Parameters of Use (See methyldopa.)

Absorption Onset of action is 4 to 6 hours and duration of action is 10 to 16 hours.

Administration Adults: Initial dosage: 250 to 500 mg q6h via intermittent IV drip; then change to oral drug as soon as possible; Maximum dosage: 1000 mg in 6 hours. Children: Initial dosage: 20 to 40 mg/kg daily in divided doses q6h via intermittent IV drip; then change to oral drug as soon as possible.

Available Drug Forms Vials of 5 ml containing 50 mg/ml. Generic contents in 5 ml of solution: Methyldopate HCl: 250 mg; citric acid anhydrous: 25 mg; sodium bisulfite: 16 mg; disodium edetate: 2.5 mg; monothioglycerol: 10 mg; sodium hydroxide and water qs.

Nursing Management (See clonidine hydrochloride.)

1. Add desired dose to 100 ml of 5% D/W and infuse over 30 to 60 minutes.
2. Do not mix with other drugs, since numerous incompatibilities exist.
3. Monitor vital signs and obtain hepatic function tests frequently.
4. Cardiac monitoring is recommended when treating severe hypertension.
5. Obtain body temperature q4h of awake client following administration.
6. Elderly clients are prone to develop cerebral ischemia, which results in syncope. Lower dosages are usually required. If symptoms occur, notify physician.

GENERIC NAME Pargyline hydrochloride (RX)

TRADE NAME Eutonyl

CLASSIFICATION Antihypertensive

Action Nonhydrazine MAO inhibitor with hypotensive action and little antidepressant activity. Mechanism of hypotensive activity is unknown, but is thought to be due to alterations in central or ganglionic neurotransmission.

Indications for Use Moderate to severe hypertension.

Contraindications Pheochromocytoma, paranoid schizophrenia, hyperthyroidism, severe renal failure, malignant hypertension, children under 12 years, clients taking central- or peripheral-acting sympathomimetic amines or other substances containing pressor amines such as tyramine (aged or processed cheese, beer, wine).

Warnings and Precautions Elderly clients and clients who have had a sympathectomy are particularly sensitive to the drug's antihypertensive effect; lower dosages are required. Not recommended for clients with mild or labile hypertension. Antihistamines, hypnotics, sedatives, narcotics, and tranquilizers must be used in reduced dosages if concurrent drug therapy is essential. Discontinue drug at least two weeks prior to surgery whenever possible. Use with caution in clients with renal insufficiency, diabetes, or parkinsonism. Use with caution in clients with impaired hepatic function. Drug-induced hypotension may precipitate coronary or cerebral thrombosis in clients with impaired cardiovascular function. Febrile disorders may accentuate drug-induced hypotension. The drug may have to be discontinued until fever subsides. Use with caution in clients with preexisting psychosis accompanied by hyperactivity or hyperexcitability.

Safe use in children and during pregnancy and lactation has not been established.

Untoward Reactions Orthostatic hypotension occurs frequently. Dizziness, weakness, palpitations, and syncope may also occur. CNS disturbances include tremors, hyperexcitability, muscle twitching and other extrapyramidal symptoms, nightmares, insomnia, and sweating. Weight gain may be due to fluid retention and edema or increased appetite. GI disturbances are common and include nausea, vomiting, constipation, and dry mouth. Other reactions include impotence, delayed ejaculation, rashes, purpura, and arthralgia. Toxicity may cause agitation, hallucinations, hyperreflexia, convulsions, hyperpyrexia, and hypotension or hypertension.

Parameters of Use

Excretion In urine as unchanged drug and metabolites.

Drug Interactions Concurrent use with tricyclic antidepressants may result in severe toxicity and convulsions. MAO inhibitors potentiate the CNS depression induced by barbiturates and meperidine. Pargyline blocks the metabolism of many adrenergic agents and may result in convulsions, hypertension, and fever. Pargyline impairs the metabolism of tyramine, a substance found in several foods and beverages (cheddar cheese, pickled herring, beans, bananas, beer, and Chianti wines). Concurrent ingestion of tyramine-rich foods may result in severe untoward reactions, including headaches, palpitations, and hypertension. Deaths have been reported. Transitory elevation in blood pressure may result from concurrent therapy with levodopa. Hypoglycemia may occur in diabetic clients who require insulin or oral hypoglycemic agents.

Administration Adults: Initial dosage: 25 mg po daily; then increase by 10 mg every 1 to 2 weeks until desired effect; Maximum dosage: 200 mg/day. Clients over 65 years and those who have had a sympathectomy should be initiated with 10 to 25 mg po daily.

Available Drug Forms Tablets containing 10, 25, or 50 mg.

Nursing Management (See clonidine hydrochloride.)

1. Administer one dose each day, usually early in A.M.
2. Monitor vital signs periodically for 2 to 3 weeks after therapy is first initiated or dosage adjusted.
3. Monitor intake and output. If fluid retention occurs, notify physician.
4. Stabilization of blood pressure may not occur for 1 to 3 weeks.
5. As drug causes orthostatic hypotension, obtain blood pressure in standing position when evaluating antihypertensive effect. If symptoms of orthostatic hypotension occur, notify physician; dosage reduction may be required.
6. Instruct client to avoid eating tyramine-rich foods and to seek medical advice before taking over-the-counter drugs, particularly decongestants.

GENERIC NAME Alkaverir (RX)

TRADE NAME Veriloid

CLASSIFICATION Antihypertensive

Source Mixture of alkaloids from *Veratrum viride*.

Action Alkaverir indirectly causes inhibition of the vasomotor center in the brain stem by sensitizing baroreceptors in the carotid sinus and aortic arch, thus reducing heart rate and arterial blood pressure. The drug has a narrow margin of safety.

Indications for Use Essential renal or malignant hypertension, toxemia of pregnancy.

Contraindications Hypersensitivity to veratrum alkaloids, pheochromocytoma.

Warnings and Precautions Use with caution in clients with angina, cardiovascular disease, or a history of bronchial asthma.

Safe use during pregnancy and lactation has not been established.

Untoward Reactions Nausea is a frequent untoward reaction. Other GI disturbances include vomiting, hiccups, and epigastric discomfort. Bronchial constriction, bronchospasm, and respiratory depression may occur. Orthostatic hypotension is common. Bradycardia and arrhythmias may occur. CNS disturbances, including confusion, disorientation, and blurred vision, have occurred. Pain may occur at injection sites and abscesses have been reported at intramuscular injection sites.

Parameters of Use

Absorption Onset of action is: about 4 hours (po); 60 to 90 minutes (IM); within minutes (IV). Duration of action is: 4 to 6 hours (po); 3 to 6 hours (IM); 1 to 3 hours (IV).

Drug Interactions Hypotension may occur when general anesthetics are administered concurrently. Antihypertensive effect may be reversed by tricyclic antidepressants.

Administration Adults: Oral: 3 to 5 mg daily in divided doses after meals; Intramuscular, intravenous: 0.1 to 0.5 mg daily.

Available Drug Forms Tablets containing 3 or 5 mg; vials containing 0.1 mg/ml.

Nursing Management (See clonidine hydrochloride.)

1. Give with a full glass of water immediately after meals.
2. When given by parenteral route, inject deep into muscle. Procainamide hydrochloride 1% may be added to decrease pain.
3. Monitor vital signs in standing and recumbent position.
4. Atropine can be effective for reversing excessive bradycardia.
5. Ephedrine is effective for reversing excessive hypotension.

GENERIC NAME Veratrum viride (RX)

TRADE NAME Vertavis

CLASSIFICATION Antihypertensive

See alkaverir for Contraindications, Warnings and precautions, and Drug interactions.

Source Standardized powdered preparation of crude Veratrum alkaloids.

Action Veratrum indirectly causes inhibition of vasomotor baroreceptors in the carotid sinus and aortic arch, thereby reducing heart rate and arterial blood pressure. The drug is seldom used today due to frequent nausea and other untoward reactions.

Indications for Use Mild to moderate hypertension.

Untoward Reactions Nausea occurs frequently.

Parameters of Use

Absorption Onset of action is about 2 hours and duration of action is 4 to 6 hours.

Administration Adults: 20 to 80 units po daily in divided doses after meals and at bedtime with a snack.

Available Drug Forms Tablets containing 5 or 10 Craw units.

Nursing Management Give with food in order to decrease nausea. (See clonidine hydrochloride.)

GENERIC NAME Cryptenamine acetates (RX)

TRADE NAME Unitensen

CLASSIFICATION Antihypertensive

See alkaverir for Contraindications, Warnings and precautions, Untoward reactions, and Drug interactions.

Source Mixture of alkaloids from *Veratrum viride* prepared as an acetate salt for solubility.

Action Cryptenamine indirectly causes inhibition of the vasomotor center in the brain stem by sensitizing baroreceptors in the carotid sinus and aortic arch, thus reducing heart rate and arterial blood pressure.

Indications for Use Short-term treatment of hypertensive crisis.

Parameters of Use

Absorption Onset of action is within minutes and duration of action is 1 to 3 hours.

Administration 0.5 ml of drug solution diluted in 20 ml or more of 5% D/W via slow IV bolus or intermittent drip at a rate not exceeding 1 ml/min.

Available Drug Forms Vials containing 2 ml of sterile solution; 1 mg is equal to 130 Carotid Sinus Reflex (CSR) units.

Nursing Management (See clonidine hydrochloride and alkaverir.)

1. Do not mix with other drugs, since numerous incompatibilities exist.
2. May be given by intermittent drip in 100 ml of 5% D/W.
3. A syringe or infusion pump is recommended.
4. Monitor blood pressure continuously when administering via IV bolus.

GENERIC NAME Cryptenamine tannates (RX)

TRADE NAMES Unitensen, Unitensyl

CLASSIFICATION Antihypertensive

See alkaverir for Contraindications, Warnings and precautions, Untoward reactions, and Drug interactions.

Source Mixture of alkaloids from *Veratrum viride* prepared as a tannate salt.

Action Cryptenamine indirectly causes inhibition of the vasomotor center in the brain stem by sensitizing baroreceptors in the carotid sinus and aortic arch, thus reducing heart rate and arterial blood pressure.

Indications for Use Mild to moderate hypertension, toxemia of pregnancy.

Parameters of Use

Absorption Onset of action is about 2 hours and duration of action is 4 to 6 hours.

Administration Adults: Initial dosage: 2 mg po bid; then increase dosage weekly until desired effect; Maximum dosage: 12 mg/day.

Available Drug Forms Tablets containing 2 mg; 1 mg is equal to 130 Carotid Sinus Reflex (CSR) units.

Nursing Management Give with a full glass of water after meals or with a snack. (See clonidine hydrochloride and alkaverir.)

GENERIC NAME Protoveratrine A and B maleates

TRADE NAME Provell Maleate (RX)

CLASSIFICATION Antihypertensive

See alkaverir for Indications for Use, Contraindications, Warnings and precautions, Untoward reactions, and Drug interactions. See clonidine hydrochloride and alkaverir for Nursing management.

Source Alkaloids obtained from *Veratrum album.*

Action Similar to other veratrums. (See alkaverir.)

Administration 1.0 to 2.5 mg po daily in divided doses after meals and at bedtime with a snack.

GENERIC NAME Protoveratrine A (RX)

TRADE NAME Protalba

CLASSIFICATION Antihypertensive

See alkaverir for Indications for Use, Contraindications, Warnings and precautions, Untoward reactions, and Drug interactions. See clonidine hydrochloride and alkaverir for Nursing management.

Source Purified alkaloid from rhizomes of *Veratum album.*

Action Similar to other veratrums. The A alkaloid is more potent than the B alkaloid and can be given parenterally. (See alkaverir.)

Administration 200 mcg po qid after meals and at bedtime with a snack.

GANGLIONIC BLOCKING AGENTS

GENERIC NAME Mecamylamine hydrochloride

TRADE NAME Inversine (RX)

CLASSIFICATION Antihypertensive

Action Mecamylamine, a potent secondary amine, induces a competitive and noncompetitive blockade of acetylcholine at nicotinic receptor sites. The drug reduces blood pressure in normotensive and hypertensive clients.

Indications for Use Moderate to severe essential hypertension, uncomplicated malignant hypertension.

Contraindications Severe cardiac disease, recent myocardial infarction, chronic pyelonephritis, uremia, severe renal insufficiency.

Warnings and Precautions Use with caution in clients with prostatic hypertrophy, glaucoma, pyloric stenosis, or renal, coronary, or cerebrovascular insufficiency. Fever, excessive environmental temperatures, and stress may increase the antihypertensive effect. Abrupt withdrawal may cause rebound hypertension.

Untoward Reactions Orthostatic hypotension, nausea, vomiting, constipation, dry mouth, paresthesias, blurred vision, fatigue, and tremors are common. Choreiform movements and weakness may lead to convulsions when high dosages are used. Headache, sedation, dizziness, and psychotic disturbances may occur. Urinary retention, impotence, and decreased libido may occur.

Parameters of Use

Absorption Readily absorbed from GI tract. Onset of action is 1 to 2 hours and duration of action is 6 to 12 hours. Crosses blood-brain barrier.

Distribution High concentrations found in liver and kidneys.

Excretion By the kidneys as unchanged drug; rate of excretion is increased by acidic urine, but decreased by alkaline urine.

Drug Interactions Toxicity may occur when sodium bicarbonate and other alkaline substances are administered concurrently. Antihypertensive effect may be potentiated by alcohol, antihypertensive agents, sympathomimetics, and thiazide diuretics.

Administration Adults: Initial dosage: 2.5 mg po bid; then increased by 2.5 mg every 2 days until desired effect.

Available Drug Forms Scored tablets containing 2.5 or 10 mg.

Nursing Management

1. Give with meals.
2. Sodium-restricted diets are not necessary.
3. Constipation can usually be relieved with diet changes, milk of magnesia, and an increase in fluid intake. Instruct client to notify physician before using an OTC laxative.
4. Instruct client to avoid excessive heat (showers) and to notify physician if fever occurs.
5. Warn client about orthostatic hypotension.

GENERIC NAME Trimethaphan camsylate (RX)

TRADE NAME Arfonad

CLASSIFICATION Antihypertensive

Action Trimethaphan competitively blocks acetylcholine by occupying nicotinic receptor sites and stabilizing the postsynaptic membrane. It does not prevent the release of acetylcholine; but it induces the release of histamine. It is an ultra-short-acting drug that induces vasodilation, which ultimately results in a lowering of blood pressure. Trimethaphan is ineffective when administered orally.

Indications for Use Hypertensive crisis; control of hypotension during surgery; emergency treatment of pulmonary hypertension (pulmonary edema) associated with systemic hypertension.

Contraindications Pregnancy, hypovolemia, shock, asphyxia, uncorrected respiratory insufficiency.

Warnings and Precautions Use with caution in clients with a history of allergic disorders. Use with extreme caution in children, the elderly, debilitated clients, in clients with arteriosclerosis, cardiac, hepatic, or renal disease, Addison's disease, or diabetes, and those receiving adrenocorticosteroids.

Untoward Reactions Tachycardia and severe orthostatic hypotension are common. Extreme weakness and respiratory depression may occur. Respiratory arrests have been reported. Urinary retention may occur.

Administration Adults: Initial dosage: 1 to 2 mg/min. via continuous IV drip; then adjust for desired effect; Dosage range: 0.2 to 6.0 mg/min.

Available Drug Forms Ampules containing 500 mg (50 mg/ml).

Nursing Management

1. Always use freshly prepared solution.
2. Add 500 mg (10 ml) to 50 ml of 5% D/W to yield 1 mg/ml (0.1%) solution strength.
3. Add as a secondary line to IV.
4. An IV pump is highly recommended. Adjust IV rate according to blood pressure response.
5. Continuous monitoring of blood pressure, cardiac monitoring, and maintenance of a recumbent position are essential.
6. Supplemental oxygen therapy is required.
7. Administered only by specially trained health professionals, usually physicians.
8. An indwelling urinary catheter is recommended.
9. If excessive hypotension occurs, administration should be discontinued. Blood pressure is usually restored in 10 minutes. Phenylephrine hydrochloride or mephentermine sulfate can be used to restore blood pressure, when necessary.
10. Pupillary dilation does not necessarily indicate anoxia or depth of anesthesia, since trimethaphan induces dilation of pupils.

ALPHA- AND BETA-ADRENERGIC BLOCKERS

GENERIC NAME Metoprolol tartrate (RX)

TRADE NAMES Lopressor, Lopressor Betaloc

CLASSIFICATION Antihypertensive

Action Metoprolol is a synthetic beta-adrenergic blocking agent that selectively affects $beta_1$-receptor sites (heart). Its action reduces heart rate, cardiac output, and blood pressure. High dosages will stimulate $beta_2$-receptor sites (bronchial and vascular smooth muscle).

Indications for Use Hypertension. Often used with other antihypertensive agents.

Contraindications Sinus bradycardia, heart block greater than first degree, cardiogenic shock, acute heart failure.

Warnings and Precautions Use with caution in the elderly; in clients with a history of cardiac failure, since the drug has the potential of depressing myocardial contractility and thereby precipitating cardiac failure; in clients with hyperthyroidism, since the signs and symptoms of thyrotoxicosis may be masked; in clients susceptible to bronchospasm (chronic bronchitis, emphysema); in clients with impaired hepatic or renal function; and in diabetic clients, since the signs and symptoms of hypoglycemia may be masked. Abrupt withdrawal of drug may precipitate angina pectoris, myocardial infarction, thyroid storm, and other disorders.

Safe use during pregnancy and lactation has not been established.

Untoward Reactions Bradycardia, congestive heart failure, and excessive hypotension have occurred and may be life-threatening. Arterial insufficiency with paresthesia of the hands may occur. Bronchospasm can occur in susceptible clients and may be life-threatening. GI disturbances, including nausea, vomiting, epigastric distress, abdominal cramps, diarrhea, and constipation, may occur. Mesenteric arterial thrombosis and ischemic colitis have been reported. Hypoglycemia without tachycardia and hypotension may occur in diabetic clients. Thyrotoxicosis without tachycardia may occur in clients with hyperthyroidism; thyroid function tests are unaffected. Blood dyscrasias, including agranulocytosis, nonthrombocytopenic purpura, and thrombocytopenic purpura, have been reported. CNS reactions, including lightheadedness, depression, insomnia, weakness, visual disturbances, hallucinations, disorientation, and short-term memory loss, have occurred. Allergic reactions include pharyngitis, agranulocytosis, rashes, fever, sore throat, and laryngospasm. Rare reactions include reversible alopecia and dry skin, mucous membranes, and conjunctiva.

Parameters of Use

Absorption Rapid and complete. Duration of effect on blood pressure is not dose related; repeated oral doses of 100 mg reduce blood pressure for about 12 hours. Half-life is 3 to 4 hours. About 12% bound to albumin.

Metabolism About 50% of serum level metabolized in the liver during the first pass. Causes highly variable serum drug levels.

Drug Interactions May alter insulin requirements of clients previously stabilized on oral hypoglycemic agents; watch clients for hypoglycemia. Isoproterenol and norepinephrine antagonize the effects of metoprolol and can be used as antidotes. May enhance the cardiac depressant action of phenytoin and quinidine. Drugs that deplete catecholamines, such as the antihypertensive agent reserpine, may have an additive effect when given concurrently with beta blockers; observe client closely for hypotension and marked bradycardia, since vertigo, syncope, or postural hypotension may occur. When clonidine is given concurrently with beta blockers, the latter should be discontinued several days before the gradual withdrawal of clonidine.

Administration Adults: Initial dosage: 50 mg po bid; then increase as needed; Dosage range: 200 to 400 mg daily in divided doses.

Available Drug Forms Tablets containing 50 or 100 mg.

Nursing Management

Planning factors

1. Obtain baseline blood pressure and pulse before initiating therapy.
2. Assess cardiovascular and respiratory status for potential contraindications.
3. Assess hepatic and renal function. If blood urea nitrogen (BUN) or serum creatinine are elevated, notify physician.

Administration factors

1. Check blood pressure and pulse before administering drug when therapy is first initiated or dosage adjusted. If severe bradycardia or hypotension occur, notify physician before administering drug.
2. Give drug before breakfast and at bedtime on an empty stomach. Follow with a full glass of water.

Evaluation factors

1. Initially and when dosage adjustments are required, maintain a vital sign flowchart. Check and record blood pressure and pulse of awake client q4h. Also record blood pressure 2 hours before administering drug and when drug is given. If blood pressure returns to untreated hypertensive state after 1 week of therapy, notify physician, since a dosage adjustment is required.
2. Obtain complete blood cell count, BUN, and serum creatinine periodically.
3. Record intake and output.
4. Reduce dosage gradually before discontinuing drug.

Client teaching factors

1. Inform client of untoward reactions and to notify physician immediately if symptoms occur, particularly low pulse rate (below 60 beats/min.), diarrhea, dizziness, or depression.
2. Advise client to change position slowly to avoid lightheadedness.
3. Advise client to avoid excessive use of CNS depressants and stimulants (coffee, cola, tea, alcohol), since untoward reactions may occur.
4. Inform client that adaptation to stressful situations will be altered and to avoid stress if possible.
5. Advise client that untoward reactions may occur if the drug is discontinued abruptly.
6. Inform client to store medication in tightly covered containers away from moisture (not in bathroom or kitchen).

GENERIC NAME Nadolol (RX)

TRADE NAME Corgard

CLASSIFICATION Antihypertensive

See metoprolol tartrate for Warnings and precautions.

Action Nadolol is a synthetic nonselective beta-adrenergic blocker. It reduces systolic and diastolic blood pressure, heart rate, cardiac output, and reflex orthostatic tachycardia. (See metoprolol tartrate.)

Indications for Use Hypertension. Often used with thiazide diuretics and other antihypertensive agents.

Contraindications Bronchial asthma, sinus bradycardia, heart block greater than first-degree, cardiogenic shock, acute heart failure.

Untoward Reactions Bradycardia, heart failure, hypotension, bronchospasm. (See metoprolol tartrate.)

Parameters of Use

Absorption Well absorbed from GI tract; food may increase absorption. Onset of action is about 30 to 60 minutes. Duration of action is about 24 hours. Crosses placenta and enters breast milk.

Metabolism In the liver.

Excretion By the kidneys.

Drug Interactions May alter requirements for insulin and other hypoglycemic agents. Excessive bradycardia may occur if used concurrently with digitalis glycosides.

Administration Adults: Initial dosage: 40 mg po daily; then increase gradually every 3 to 7 days by increments of 40 or 80 mg until desired effect; Maintenance dosage: 80 to 320 mg daily. Lower dosages are required for clients with impaired renal function; dosage is usually administered every other day.

Available Drug Forms Tablets containing 40, 80, 120, or 160 mg; 1-ml ampules containing 1 mg/ml.

Nursing Management

Planning factors

1. Obtain baseline data relevant to the purpose for which the drug is to be administered.
2. Assess cardiovascular and respiratory status for potential contraindications. Record baseline vital signs.
3. Assess hepatic and renal function. If blood urea nitrogen (BUN) or serum creatinine is elevated, notify physician. If oliguria exists, notify physician.
4. Appropriate antidote should be readily available: atropine for bradycardia, epinephrine for hypotension, isoproterenol for cardiac failure, and aminophylline for bronchospasm.

Administration factors

1. Check blood pressure and pulse before administering drug when therapy is first initiated or dosage adjusted. If severe bradycardia or hypotension exist, notify physician before administering drug.
2. Give drug with meals or a snack.

Evaluation factors

1. Initially, record blood pressure and pulse before each dose; then periodically.
2. Obtain complete blood cell count, BUN, and serum creatinine levels periodically.
3. Record intake and output.
4. Reduce dosage gradually before discontinuing drug.

Client teaching factors

1. Inform client of untoward reactions and to notify physician immediately if symptoms occur, particularly low pulse rate (below 60 beats/min.).
2. Advise client (particularly normotensive client) to change position slowly to avoid lightheadedness, since hypotension may occur.
3. Advise client to avoid excessive use of CNS depressants and stimulants (coffee, cola, tea, alcohol), since untoward reactions may occur.
4. Inform client that adaptation to stressful situations will be altered and to avoid stress if possible.
5. Advise client that untoward reactions may occur if the drug is discontinued abruptly.

GENERIC NAME Oxprenolol (RX)

TRADE NAMES ISET, Trasicor

CLASSIFICATION Antihypertensive

See metoprolol tartrate for Warnings and precautions, Drug interactions, and Nursing management. See pindolol for Contraindications and Untoward reactions.

Action Oxprenolol is a nonselective beta-adrenergic blocker with intrinsic sympathomimetic activity. Like pindolol, oxprenolol is theoretically less likely to precipitate congestive heart failure, bradycardia, bronchospasm, and peripheral vasoconstriction than other beta blockers. A disadvantage of the drug's sympathomimetic activity is its potential for increasing myocardial oxygen needs, which would make the drug less effective for treating angina than other beta blockers. Because the drug is rapidly metabolized by the liver to inactive metabolites, oxprenolol can probably be safely used in the elderly. Delayed-release formulations are required to maintain serum levels.

Indications for Use Exertional angina, hypertension, some ventricular arrhythmias.

Parameters of Use

Absorption Well absorbed from the GI tract. Crosses blood-brain barrier. Half-life is 2 to 4 hours.

Metabolism Rapidly metabolized in the liver.

Excretion By the kidneys; some is excreted in bile and eliminated in feces.

Administration Highly individualized. Initial dosage: 40 mg po tid; then increase gradually every 1 to 2 weeks until desired response occurs. Maximum daily dosage: 160 mg po tid.

Available Drug Forms Tablets containing 40 mg; Slow-release tablets containing 160 or 320 mg.

GENERIC NAME Pindolol (RX)

TRADE NAME Visken

CLASSIFICATION Beta-adrenergic blocker

See metoprolol tartrate for Warnings and precautions, Drug interactions, and Nursing management.

Action Pindolol is a nonselective beta-adrenergic blocker with intrinsic sympathomimetic activity. It reduces blood pressure but, unlike propranolol, it reduces total peripheral resistance and slightly increases cardiac output. Theoretically it is less likely to precipitate congestive heart failure, bradycardia, bronchospasm, and peripheral vasoconstriction than other beta blockers. However, it may increase myocardial oxygen needs, making the drug ineffective for treating angina.

Indications for Use Treatment of hypertension, either alone or in conjunction with thiazide diuretics.

Contraindications Bronchial asthma, overt cardiac failure, cardiogenic shock, second- and third-degree heart block, severe bradycardia.

Parameters of Use

Absorption Rapid and complete from the GI tract. Peak effects occur in about 1 hour. About 40% is bound to plasma proteins. Half-life is about 3 to 4 hours, but may be about 7 hours in the elderly and as long as 15 hours in clients with renal impairment.

Excretion Primarily by the kidneys as metabolites; some is excreted in bile and eliminated in feces. Slowed excretion may occur in clients with cirrhosis of the liver.

Untoward Reactions Similar to the other beta blockers, but milder. (See metoprolol tartrate.) Other untoward reactions include the following: CNS disturbances include reversible mental depression (catatonia), disorientation to time and place, and short-term memory loss. May intensify AV block. Agranulocytosis and purpura (particularly thrombocytopenic purpura) may occur. Allergic reactions include erythemic rash, fever accompanied by aching and a sore throat, laryngospasm, and respiratory distress. Mesenteric arterial thrombosis and ischemic colitis have been reported. Reversible alopecia and Peyronie's disease have been reported.

Administration Highly individualized. Initial dosage: 10 mg po bid for 2 to 3 weeks. Increase by 10 mg daily every 2 to 3 weeks until desired response occurs. Maximum daily dose: 60 mg.

Available Drug Forms Scored tablets containing 5 or 10 mg.

GENERIC NAME Propranolol hydrochloride (RX)

TRADE NAME Inderal

CLASSIFICATION Antihypertensive

See metoprolol tartrate for Contraindications, Warnings and precautions, Untoward reactions, and Drug interactions. See metoprolol tartrate and nadolol for Nursing management.

Action Propranolol competes for beta-adrenergic receptor sites, thus decreasing heart rate and cardiac output. It inhibits the release of renin, decreases tonic adrenergic outflow from vasomotor centers, and results in a lowered blood pressure.

Indications for Use Hypertension. Often used with thiazide diuretics and other antihypertensive agents.

Parameters of Use

Absorption Well absorbed from the GI tract. Plasma half-life is variable (3.4 to 6 hours).

Distribution Widely distributed. About 90% bound to plasma proteins. Onset of action occurs in about 30 minutes (po) or about 2 minutes (IV); peak plasma level occurs in 60 to 90 minutes (po) or 15 minutes (IV); duration is about 6 hours (po) or 3 to 6 hours (IV).

Metabolism In the liver; impaired hepatic function may cause prolonged drug action.

Excretion Via the kidneys as unchanged drug and metabolites; impaired kidney function may prolong drug action. Crosses blood-brain barrier. Crosses placenta and enters breast milk.

Administration Adults: Initial dosage: 40 mg po bid for 3 to 7 days; then increase dosage until desired effect; Maintenance dosage: 160 to 480 mg daily. Full antihypertensive effect may take several weeks.

Available Drug Forms Tablets containing 10, 20, 40, or 80 mg; vials containing 1 mg/ml for parenteral use.

GENERIC NAME Timolol maleate (RX)

TRADE NAME Blocadren

CLASSIFICATION Antihypertensive

See metoprolol tartrate for Contraindications, Warnings and precautions, Untoward reactions, Drug interactions, and Nursing management.

Action Timolol maleate is a beta-adrenergic blocker similar to propranolol hydrochloride. It reduces systolic and diastolic blood pressure, heart rate, cardiac output, and reflex orthostatic tachycardia.

Indications for Use Hypertension; used alone or combined with other antihypertensive agents, particularly the thiazide diuretics.

Parameters of Use

Absorption Well absorbed from the GI tract.
Metabolism Some metabolism occurs in the liver.
Excretion Primarily by the kidneys.

Administration 10 mg po bid.

Available Drug Forms Tablets or capsules containing 10 mg.

GENERIC NAME Phenoxybenzamine hydrochloride

TRADE NAME Dibenzyline (RX)

CLASSIFICATION Antihypertensive

Action Phenoxybenzamine is a long-acting blocker of alpha-adrenergic receptor sites. It induces chemical sympathectomy, lowers blood pressure, and increases blood flow to skin and abdominal organs. Propranolol may be used to control phenoxybenzamine-induced tachycardia. The drug is effective in controlling hypertensive episodes and sweating associated with pheochromocytoma.

Indications for Use Hypertensive episodes due to pheochromocytoma, vasospastic peripheral vascular disorders.

Contraindications Any disorder in which a drop in blood pressure is undesirable.

Warnings and Precautions Use with caution in clients with restricted circulation to the brain, heart, or kidneys. Use with caution in the elderly. May aggravate the symptoms of respiratory infection.

Untoward Reactions Nasal congestion, postural hypotension, and tachycardia are common. Inhibition of ejaculation has been reported. Symptoms tend to subside with continued drug therapy. GI disturbances have been reported. May cause exacerbation of a preexisting peptic ulcer. Toxicity may occur; symptoms include postural hypotension, dizziness, fainting, tachycardia, vomiting, lethargy, and shock.

Parameters of Use

Absorption Poorly absorbed from the GI tract; about one-third enters bloodstream. Half-life is about 24 hours. Onset of action occurs in about 2 hours. Complete blockade takes about 2 weeks.

Metabolism In the liver.

Excretion By the kidneys; some is excreted in bile and eliminated in feces.

Drug Interactions Excessive hypotension and tachycardia may occur if given concurrently with alpha- or beta-adrenergic stimulants. Epinephrine is ineffective in counteracting toxicity. Propranolol and other beta-adrenergic blockers may be used to control tachycardia and other untoward reactions.

Administration Adults: Initial dosage: 10 mg po daily for 4 days; then increase by increments of 10 mg until desired effect; Maintenance dosage: 20 to 60 mg daily. Children: Initial dosage: 0.2 mg/kg po daily; then increase dosage until desired effect.

Available Drug Forms Capsules containing 10 mg.

Nursing Management

Planning factors

1. Monitor baseline vital signs and blood pressure for several days.
2. Obtain a complete history, including symptoms of cerebral insufficiency, cardiac disorders, and renal impairment. If oliguria or other abnormalities exist, notify physician.
3. Creatinine clearance test is recommended.

Administration factors

1. Give on an empty stomach and follow with a full glass of water.
2. Can be taken with milk if GI disturbances occur.

Evaluation factors

1. Monitor blood pressure and pulse before giving drug and periodically (every 4 hours while awake) until blood pressure is stabilized, then daily as needed.
2. If tachycardia or hypotension occur, notify physician.

Client teaching factors

1. Instruct client to notify health professional if GI distress occurs. Milk or an antacid is usually effective.
2. Instruct client to consult physician before ingesting alcohol or OTC drugs for colds.
3. Instruct client in measures to avoid orthostatic hypotension.
4. Instruct client to avoid abrupt cessation of drug.

GENERIC NAME Phentolamine hydrochloride

TRADE NAME Regitine (RX)

CLASSIFICATION Antihypertensive

See phenoxybenzamine hydrochloride for Untoward reactions, Drug interactions, and Nursing management.

Action Phentolamine is a competitive blocker of alpha-adrenergic receptor sites and circulating epinephrine. It produces vasodilation and increases gastric secretions, which may cause nausea, vomiting, and diarrhea.

Indications for Use Hypertension before and after pheochromocytomectomy.

Contraindications Hypersensitivity to drug, myocardial infarction, coronary artery disease.

Warnings and Precautions Use with caution in clients with a peptic ulcer.

Parameters of Use

Absorption Fairly well absorbed from the GI tract. Onset of action occurs in 30 to 60 minutes; duration of action is about 4 to 6 hours.

Metabolism Unknown.

Excretion About 10% as unchanged drug in urine.

Administration Adults: 50 mg po qid; Children: 5 mg/kg po daily in divided doses.

Available Drug Forms Tablets containing 50 mg. Also available in vials for parenteral use.

NOREPINEPHRINE DEPLETORS

GENERIC NAME Reserpine (RX)

TRADE NAMES Alkarau, Broserpine, De Serpa, Elserpine, Hiserpia, Hyperine, Lemiserp, Raurine, Rau-Sed, Rauseroid, Sandril, Serpalan, Serpate, Serpasil, Sermina, T-Serp, Vio-Serpine, Zepine

CLASSIFICATION Antihypertensive

Source Main alkaloid obtained from Indian snakeroot *Rauwolfia serpentina*.

Action Reserpine lowers blood pressure by depleting norepinephrine and other catecholamines at postganglionic adrenergic nerve endings. The reuptake of norepinephrine into storage vesicles at these nerve endings is decreased, thus allowing the destruction of the neurotransmitter. After a few days of therapy there is a considerable decrease in the amount of norepinephrine in the storage vesicles and so there is less neurotransmitter available to induce vasoconstriction of arterioles upon stimulation; thus there is a decrease in peripheral resistance and blood pressure gradually drops. Bradycardia and a decrease in cardiac output also occur. There is little or no drug-induced orthostatic hypotension. Reserpine crosses the blood-brain barrier and produces a marked tranquilizing effect on the CNS. It is believed that the drug causes a depletion of norepinephrine and serotonin from the brain. Reserpine was originally used to control agitated psychotic states, but it has been replaced by phenothiazines and other tranquilizers. Effects resulting from a lack of adrenergic stimulation include an increase in gastric motility and secretions.

Indications for Use Mild to moderate essential hypertension; as an adjunct in severe hypertension; as an adjunct in hypertensive crisis when administered parenterally.

Contraindications Hypersensitivity to any *Rauwolfia serpentina* alkaloid, mental depression, suicidal tendencies, acute peptic ulcer, ulcerative colitis, clients receiving electroconvulsive therapy.

Warnings and Precautions Use with caution in the elderly, debilitated clients; in clients with a history of mental depression; in clients with a history of peptic ulcer or gall stones, since biliary colic may be precipitated; and in clients with bronchial asthma, renal insufficiency, bradycardia, or severe cardiac or cerebrovascular disorders. Safe use during pregnancy and lactation has not been established. Congestion due to an increase in respiratory secretions, hypoxia, and anoxia may occur in breast-fed babies. Preoperative withdrawal of drug may cause circulatory instability during and following surgery.

Untoward Reactions GI disturbances, including hypersecretion, nausea, vomiting, anorexia, and diarrhea, are common; peptic ulcers and GI bleeding have been reported. Nasal congestion is a common reaction. Epitaxis has occurred. Dyspnea may occur. Cardiovascular disturbances, including bradycardia, angina, arrhythmias, and syncope, may occur. CNS disturbances include drowsiness, mental depression, nervousness, paradoxic anxiety, nightmares, and dizziness. Parkinsonism has been reported. Early symptoms of CNS toxicity include despondency, early morning insomnia, loss of appetite, impotence, and self-depreciation. Toxicity also induces altered level of consciousness, which progresses to coma, hypotension, marked bradycardia, hypothermia, central respiratory depression, and diarrhea. Water retention and weight gain may occur. Hypersensitivity reactions include pruritus, rashes, and purpura.

Parameters of Use

Absorption Slowly absorbed from GI tract. Onset of action is: 1 to 3 days (po); up to 4 hours (IM). Duration of action is: 10 to 12 hours (IM). Effects of drug may persist for weeks after discontinuation of therapy.

Crosses placenta and enters breast milk.

Distribution Widely distributed in body.

Excretion By the kidneys as metabolites.

Drug Interactions Hypotensive effects are potentiated by diuretics, phenothiazines, procainamide, quinidine, thiothixene, and methotrimeprazine. MAO inhibitors and tricyclic antidepressants may alter the antihypertensive effect of reserpine; excitability may occur; use with extreme caution concurrently. Clients taking quinidine or digitalis glycosides concomitantly may develop arrhythmias. Concurrent therapy with other antihypertensive agents, including guanethidine, veratrum, hydralazine, methyldopa, and chlorthalidone, may cause excessive hypotension.

Administration Highly individualized. Adults: Oral: Initial dosage: 0.5 mg daily for 1 to 2 weeks; then 0.1 to 0.25 mg daily. Intramuscular: Initial dosage: 0.5 to 1.0 mg; then 2 to 4 mg every 2 to 3 hours, as needed; Maximum dosage: 4 mg; if 4 mg is ineffective, use of another agent is recommended. Children: 0.7 mg/kg every 12 to 24 hours. Often given with hydralazine.

Available Drug Forms Tablets containing 0.1 or 0.25 mg; ampules containing 2.5 mg/ml.

Nursing Management

Planning factors

1. Obtain history of mental, cardiovascular, cerebral, and GI diseases.
2. Obtain baseline blood pressure in standing, sitting, and recumbent position.
3. EKG tracing is recommended.
4. Obtain serum electrolytes. Imbalances should be corrected before instituting therapy.
5. A sodium-restricted diet should be prescribed concurrently.
6. Check expiration date and discard drug when indicated. Color change is not an indication of decomposition.

Administration factors

1. Give after meals or with a snack with a full glass of water to avoid gastric irritation.
2. When administering IM, inject deep into well-vascularized muscle.
3. Discontinue drug therapy 2 weeks before surgery or electroconvulsive therapy.
4. Drug is rapidly decomposed by light and oxidation, particularly when in solutions. Protect from light.

Evaluation factors

1. Monitor blood pressure and pulse frequently for at least 2 weeks when drug therapy is first initiated; then daily for 2 or more weeks.

2. If hypotension occurs, notify physician. Treat with catecholamines (not the indirect sympathomimetics).
3. If bradycardia or arrhythmias occur, notify physician. Cardiac monitoring or an EKG can be used to determine the type of arrhythmia. Treat accordingly.
4. If excessive sedation or dependency occur, notify physician. Institute suicide precautions. Drug dose is either reduced or discontinued.
5. GI disturbances are treated symptomatically.
6. Monitor intake and output. Weigh daily. If water retention occurs, notify physician. A thiazide diuretic may be required.

Client teaching factors

1. Instruct client to take tablets with food to avoid gastric irritation.
2. Instruct client and family about untoward reactions. Explain the early symptoms of depression and the danger of suicide if mental depression occurs. (May not occur for 6 months.) Prompt reporting is essential.
3. Instruct client to check and record weight frequently and to notify physician if weight gain or edema occur.
4. Emphasize the need for regular medical checkups.
5. Instruct client to store drug in tightly sealed containers away from light.

GENERIC NAME Rauwolfia serpentina (RX)

TRADE NAMES Hiwolfia, Hyper-Rauw, Hywolfia, Raudixin, Rauja, Rauserpa, Rauserpin, Rauwoldin, Raufola, Serfia, Serfolia, Wolfina

CLASSIFICATION Antihypertensive

See reserpine for Contraindications, Warnings and precautions, Untoward reactions, Parameters of use, Drug interactions, and Nursing management.

Source Powdered whole root of *Rauwolfia serpentina.*

Action This drug depletes norepinephrine at postganglionic adrenergic nerve endings, thus inducing vasodilation. Antihypertensive activity is due to reserpine alkaloid (50%) and other alkaloids. Not recommended for children. About 200 to 300 mg of this drug is equal to 500 mcg of reserpine.

Indications for Use Mild to moderate hypertension.

Administration Adults: Initial dosage: 200 to 400 mg po daily for 2 to 3 weeks; can be given in divided doses; then 50 to 300 mg daily.

Available Drug Forms Coated tablets containing 50 or 100 mg.

GENERIC NAME Alseroxylon (RX)

TRADE NAME Rauwiloid

CLASSIFICATION Antihypertensive

See reserpine for Contraindications, Warnings and precautions, Untoward reactions, Parameters of use, Drug interactions, and Nursing management.

Source Fat-soluble fraction of *Rauwolfia serpentina.*

Action Alseroxylon is the primary antihypertensive alkaloid. Not recommended for children.

Indications for Use Mild to moderate hypertension.

Administration Adults: 2 to 4 mg po daily.

Available Drug Forms Tablets containing 2 mg.

GENERIC NAME Deserpidine (RX)

TRADE NAME Harmonyl

CLASSIFICATION Antihypertensive

See reserpine for Contraindications, Warnings and precautions, Untoward reactions, Parameters of use, Drug interactions, and Nursing management.

Source Chemically similar to reserpine, but lacks a methoxyl group.

Action May act faster than reserpine, but is less potent. Less mental depression occurs. The 100-mcg tablet (yellow) contains FD&C No. 5 yellow (tartrazine) and allergic reactions, such as bronchial asthma, may occur.

Indications for Use Mild essential hypertension; as an adjunct in severe states of hypertension.

Administration Adults: Initial dosage: 250 mcg po tid for 10 to 14 days; then 250 mcg daily.

Available Drug Forms Tablets containing 100 mcg (0.1 mg) or 250 mcg (0.25 mg).

GENERIC NAME Rescinnamine (RX)

TRADE NAMES Anaprel, Cinnasil, Moderil

CLASSIFICATION Antihypertensive

See reserpine for Contraindications, Warnings and precautions, Untoward reactions, Parameters of use, and Drug interactions.

Source Prepared from Rauwolfia alkaloids.

Action Rescinnamine depletes norepinephrine at postganglionic adrenergic nerve endings, thus inducing vasodilation.

Indications for Use Mild to moderate hypertension.

Administration Adults: Initial dosage: 500 mcg po daily for 1 to 2 weeks, then 250 to 500 mcg daily; Dosage range: 250 to 500 mcg daily.

Available Drug Forms Tablets containing 250 or 500 mcg.

Nursing Management Administer with meals. (See reserpine.)

GENERIC NAME Syrosingopine (RX)

TRADE NAME Singoserp

CLASSIFICATION Antihypertensive

See reserpine for Contraindications, Warnings and precautions, Untoward reactions, Parameters of use, Drug interactions, and Nursing management.

Source Chemically similar to reserpine, from which it is produced.

Action Said to be less toxic and less potent than reserpine. Frequently used in combination with diuretics.

Indications for Use Mild to moderate hypertension.

Administration Adults: Initial dosage: 1 mg po bid for 1 to 2 weeks; then 0.5 to 3 mg daily.

Available Drug Forms Tablets containing 1 mg; often used in combination with hydrochlorothiazide (a diuretic).

GENERIC NAME Guanethidine sulfate (RX)

TRADE NAME Ismelin

CLASSIFICATION Antihypertensive

Action Guanethidine is a potent and long-acting adrenergic blocking agent. Like reserpine, it depletes norepinephrine from peripheral storage sites by preventing reuptake of the neurotransmitter at postganglionic adrenergic nerve endings, but at a slower rate. In addition, guanethidine prevents the release of norepinephrine in response to impulses along these adrenergic neurons, thus preventing sympathetic vasoconstriction. These drug actions produce a gradual drop in blood pressure due to vasodilation, a decrease in blood pressure, a decrease in venous return, and a subsequent decrease in cardiac output. Although there may be some decrease in the activity of plasma renin, fluid retention may occur due to a lack of cardiac output and the subsequent increase in reabsorption of sodium and water by the kidneys. Consequently, the drug is often given with a thiazide diuretic (Esimil). The lack of adrenergic inhibition of cholinergic impulses results in bradycardia and GI disturbances. Guanethidine is sometimes given with hydralazine and other antihypertensive agents.

Indications for Use Moderate to severe hypertension, renal hypertension associated with pyelonephritis, renal amyloidoisis, and renal artery stenosis.

Contraindications Known or suspected pheochromocytoma, acute congestive heart failure, clients who have received MAO inhibitors in the last 2 weeks.

Warnings and Precautions Use with caution in clients with bronchial asthma, renal disorders associated with elevated blood urea nitrogen (BUN) levels, severe coronary artery disease, recent myocardial infarction, cerebrovascular disease, peptic ulcer, or ulcerative colitis. Safe use during pregnancy has not been established.

Untoward Reactions Orthostatic and exertional hypotension, dizziness, weakness, and syncope are common. Common reactions resulting from cholinergic stimulation include bradycardia and diarrhea. Arrhythmias, dyspnea due to bronchoconstriction, nausea, vomiting, nocturia, urinary incontinence, and blurred vision may also occur. Fluid retention, which may progress to congestive heart failure, may occur. Edema and weight gain are common. A rise in BUN levels may occur. Inhibition of ejaculation is common. Other reactions include dermatitis, loss of scalp hair, dry mouth, parotid tenderness, ptosis of the eyelids, myalgia, muscle tremors, mental depression, angina, chest pains, and paresthesia. Anemia, thrombocytopenia, and leukopenia have been reported, but no causal relationship has been established.

Parameters of Use

Absorption Partially absorbed from GI tract. Absorption rate varies from client to client, but tends to remain at the same rate in each client. Absorption may be increased if given with meals.

Small amount enters breast milk. Can be used by lactating mothers, but not advised since the drug is potent. Unable to cross blood-brain barrier.

Distribution High concentrations found in liver, kidneys, and lung tissues.

Metabolism Probably in the liver.

Excretion By the kidneys as unchanged drug and metabolites; unabsorbed drug excreted in feces.

Drug Interactions Drugs that antagonize the antihypertensive effect include amphetamines, cocaine, ephedrine, MAO inhibitors, methylphenidate, norepinephrine, phenylephrine, phenothiazines, and tricyclic antidepressants. Drugs that may increase the antihypertensive effect include alcohol, levodopa, and thiazide diuretics. Excessive bradycardia may occur when used concurrently with digitalis glycosides. Excessive orthostatic hypotension and bradycardia may occur when used concomitantly with rauwolfia derivatives; use together with caution.

Administration Highly individualized. Adults: Initial dosage: 10 mg po daily for at least 5 to 7 days; then increase by 10 mg until desired effect; Maintenance dosage: 25 to 50 mg daily; Maximum dosage: 300 mg/day. Children: Initial dosage: 200 mcg/kg po daily for 1 to 3 weeks; then increase dosage until desired effect; Maximum dosage: 8 times initial dosage or 300 mg daily.

Available Drug Forms Tablets containing 10 or 25 mg.

Nursing Management

Planning factors

1. Obtain baseline blood pressure when client is recumbent, sitting, and after standing 10 minutes.
2. Obtain history of arrhythmias and cardiac diseases, renal disorders, and cerebral insufficiency. If orthostatic hypotension occurs normally, notify physician before initiating therapy.
3. Obtain baseline BUN level. If elevated, notify physician before instituting therapy.
4. Schedule drug to be given at mealtime.
5. Withhold drug 2 weeks prior to surgery to avoid cardiac arrest or severe hypotension during anesthesia.

Administration factors

1. Obtain blood pressure before administering drug, when therapy is first initiated, dosage adjusted, and other antihypertensive agents added. Standing blood pressure is used to determine whether a dosage increase is required.
2. Give with a full glass of water at mealtime.

Evaluation factors

1. Obtain blood pressure 10 minutes after standing, at least daily, and when client is sitting and recumbent periodically. A lack of standing blood pressure response will require an increase in dosage as long as dizziness, weakness, and syncope do not occur.
2. If orthostatic hypotension occurs, have client lie down with feet elevated.
3. Obtain temperature frequently. If fever occurs, notify physician.
4. Monitor intake and output. If fluid retention occurs, drug should be discontinued.
5. Monitor bowel movements. If severe diarrhea occurs, drug should be discontinued.
6. Dosage may be increased weekly or monthly to ensure that stabilizing drug effect is present; stabilizing drug effect occurs in 5 to 7 days.

Client teaching factors

1. Inform client of the potential of orthostatic and exertional hypotension. Assist client with ambulation when drug dosage is adjusted. Instruct client to sit or lie down immediately when dizziness or weakness occur.
2. Warn client to avoid strenuous activity.
3. Warn client that noncompliance with a sodium-restricted diet may result in excessive fluid retention and edema.
4. Emphasize the need for maintaining regular medical checkups.
5. Instruct client to notify physician if fever occurs, since dosage reduction is required.
6. Emphasize the need to consult physician before taking OTC drugs. Hypertensive crisis may occur if certain sympathomimetics are taken concurrently (decongestants).
7. Instruct client to store drug in tightly closed containers.

TYROSINE HYDROXYLASE INHIBITORS

GENERIC NAME Metyrosine (RX)

TRADE NAME Demser

CLASSIFICATION Antihypertensive

Action The enzyme tyrosine hydroxylase catalyzes the first step in the biosynthesis of catecholamines. Clients with pheochromocytoma, a tumor of the adrenal medulla, produce excessive quantities of norepinephrine and epinephrine. Therapeutic doses of metyrosine inhibit tyrosine hydroxylase, thus decreasing the biosynthesis of endogenous norepinephrine and epinephrine by 35 to 80% in clients with pheochromocytoma. The reduction in catecholamines is determined by measuring the urinary excretion of catecholamines and their metabolites (metanephrine and vanilmandelic acid). Alpha-adrenergic blockers may also be required, particularly during surgical manipulation of the tumor, to prevent hypertensive crisis and arrhythmias.

Indications for Use Treatment of clients with pheochromocytoma prior to surgery and when surgery is contraindicated.

Contraindications Hypersensitivity to drug.

Warnings and Precautions High fluid intake is required to prevent metyrosine crystalluria and urolithiasis. Large volumes of fluid and plasma may be required to prevent hypotension postoperatively, particularly when alpha-adrenergic blockers and metyrosine were given concurrently preoperatively to control hypertension. Hypertensive crisis and arrhythmias may occur during surgical manipulation of the tumor; alpha-adrenergic blockers, such as phentolamine, are recommended. Safe use during pregnancy has not been established.

Untoward Reactions Moderate to severe sedation occurs in all clients within 24 hours of instituting therapy. Maximum sedation occurs after 2 to 3 days of therapy and then gradually subsides over the next week unless dosage is increased. Residual sedative effects persist when dosages of 2000 mg daily are used. Temporary insomnia and other sleep disturbances usually occur when the drug is discontinued. Psychic stimulation may occur in clients who did not experience the sedative effect during therapy. Extrapyramidal reactions, including drooling, speech impairment, and tremors, have occurred in approximately 10% of clients. Trismus and parkinsonism reactions have occurred in some clients. Anxiety, depression, hallucinations, disorientation, confusion, and other mental disturbances may occur, particularly when high dosages are used; symptoms subside when dosage is reduced. Diarrhea occurs in nearly 10% of clients. Nausea, vomiting, and abdominal pain may also occur. Crystalluria, transient dysuria, and hematuria may occur if urine output drops below 2000 ml daily. Hypersensitivity reactions, including urticaria, pharyngeal edema, and eosinophilia, may occur, but rarely. Other reported reactions include slight swelling of the breast, galactorrhea, nasal stuffiness, decreased salivation with dry mouth, headache, impotence, and an elevated serum glutamic-oxaloacetic transaminase level.

Parameters of Use

Absorption Well absorbed from GI tract.

Enters breast milk; lactating mothers should bottle-feed their babies.

Excretion Nearly 70% as unchanged drug in urine. Some drug excreted as catechol metabolites (alpha-methyldopa, alpha-methyldopamine, alpha-methylnorepinephrine).

Drug Characteristics Subject to oxidative degradation in alkaline aqueous solutions. Give with water or acidic juices. Do not give with other drugs.

Drug Interactions Metyrosine may potentiate the extrapyramidal effects of phenothiazines and butyrophenones; use with caution concurrently. Additive effects may occur with alcohol and other CNS depressants.

Laboratory Interactions May produce a false increase in urinary excretion of catecholamines due to drug metablites in urine.

Administration Adults and children over 12 years: Initial dosage: 250 mg po qid; then increase by 250 mg daily until desired effect; Dosage range: 2000 to 3000 mg daily; Maximum dosage: 4000 mg/day. When given as a preoperative medication, maintain dosage that produces desired effect for 5 to 7 days prior to pheochromocytoma surgery.

Available Drug Forms Capsules containing 250 mg.

Nursing Management

Planning factors

1. Obtain baseline vital signs and EKG. Start blood pressure and pulse flowchart.
2. Obtain baseline laboratory work, including determination of urinary catecholamines.
3. Schedule medications to prevent drug interactions. Sedative drug effect may be better tolerated if drug is administered q6h instead of qid.
4. Determine baseline intake and output.

Administration factors

1. Obtain blood pressure and pulse before administering drug. If severe hypotension occurs, notify physician before administration.
2. Give drug alone on an empty stomach to prevent degradation and drug interactions.
3. Follow drug with a full glass of water or acidic juice; drug is subject to oxidative degradation in alkaline aqueous solutions.
4. Encourage client to drink between 2000 to 3000 ml of fluid a day (1 glassful every hour for 12 hours when awake).
5. When drug is administered at bedtime, encourage client to follow drug with 2 glassfuls of water.

Evaluation factors

1. Sedative effect is expected initially. Assist client with meals and adequate fluid intake, as necessary.
2. Maintain intake and output. Give adequate quantities of fluid to maintain 2000 ml or more of urine.
3. Maintain blood pressure and pulse flowchart when therapy is first initiated or dosage adjusted.
4. Measure urinary catecholamines daily until optimal response (50% reduction) occurs.
5. Observe client for extra pyramidal and other reactions frequently. If symptoms occur, notify physician.

Client teaching factors

1. Emphasize the need of maintaining 2000 ml or more of urine daily. Instruct client in methods of increasing fluid intake.
2. Warn client about sedative effects and caution client against performing activities that require constant attention (driving a car).
3. Inform client to notify physician immediately if diarrhea, tremors, difficulty with speech, drooling, dysuria, or crystals in urine occur.

SELECTIVE ALPHA-ADRENERGIC BLOCKERS AND VASODILATORS

GENERIC NAME Prazosin hydrochloride (RX)

TRADE NAME Minipress

CLASSIFICATION Antihypertensive

Action Prazosin, a quinazoline derivative, was previously thought to reduce blood pressure by direct relaxation of arteriole smooth muscle, which then decreases peripheral resistance. Further animal studies revealed that the decrease in total peripheral resistance is also related to blockade of postsynaptic alpha-adrenergic receptors but without the usual reflex tachycardia. The precise mechanism of action is still unknown. Prazosin controls hypertension with little or no increase in serum renin levels, cardiac output, renal blood flow, or glomerular filtration rate. It may be used concurrently with thiazide diuretics.

Indications for Use Mild to moderate hypertension. Also used to decrease afterload in severe congestive heart failure.

Contraindications None known.

Warnings and Precautions May cause syncope and sudden loss of consciousness in 1% of clients initially. This is probably due to excessive postural hypotension, and may be preceded by an episode of severe tachycardia. May be prevented by small initial dosages and a gradual increase in dosage. Safe use in children and during pregnancy has not been established.

Untoward Reactions Syncope usually occurs within 30 to 90 minutes after an initial dosage of 2 mg or more. Dizziness, headache, drowsiness, lethargy, weakness, palpitations, and nausea are common reactions; however, symptoms usually disappear after continued therapy. Cardiovascular disturbances include edema, dyspnea, and tachycardia. GI disturbances include dry mouth, vomiting, diarrhea, constipation, and abdominal discomfort or pain. CNS disturbances include nervousness, vertigo, depression, and paresthesia. Skin reactions include rashes, pruritus, alopecia, and lichen planus. Blurred vision, reddened sclera, epitaxis, nasal congestion, tinnitus, and diaphoresis may occur.

Parameters of Use

Absorption Well absorbed from GI tract. Onset of action is about 30 minutes. Peak action occurs in about 3 hours. Plasma half-life is 2 to 3 hours. Highly bound to proteins. May cause displacement of other protein-bound drugs.

Metabolism Primarily in the liver by demethylation and conjugation.

Excretion Primarily via bile and feces.

Drug Interactions Syncope may occur when other antihypertensive agents or thiazide diuretics are added. Hypotension may develop with concomitant use of beta-adrenergic blockers, such as propranolol; use with caution concurrently.

Administration Adults: Initial dosage: 1 mg po bid or tid; then gradually increase to 6 to 15 mg daily in 2 divided doses. Maximum effective dosage for most clients is 20 mg day.

Available Drug Forms Capsules containing 1, 2, or 5 mg.

Nursing Management

Planning factors

1. Obtain history of cardiovascular disturbances.
2. Obtain baseline blood pressure in standing, sitting, and recumbent position.
3. A test dose of 1 mg should be given at bedtime to avoid syncope.

Administration factors Give with a full glass of water between meals.

Evaluation factors

1. Check blood pressure and pulse every 15 to 30 minutes for at least 2 hours after initial dosage. Assist client with ambulation.
2. Check blood pressure and pulse 2 to 3 hours after each dose when therapy is first initiated, dosage adjusted, and other antihypertensive agents added.
3. Monitor output daily and check for the presence of edema.
4. Check for other untoward reactions periodically.
5. If syncope occurs, have client lie down with feet elevated. Although the episode is self-limiting, supportive measures should be used, as indicated.

Client teaching factors

1. Inform client of the possibility of initial syncope and to notify physician if dizziness occurs. Instruct client to rise from a recumbent position slowly.
2. Explain the reason for taking medication regularly. Emphasize avoidance of abrupt withdrawal.
3. Instruct client to inform physician if untoward reactions occur.

DIRECT VASODILATORS

GENERIC NAME Hydralazine hydrochloride (RX)

TRADE NAMES Apresoline, Dralzine

CLASSIFICATION Antihypertensive

Action Hydralazine, a phthalazine derivative, lowers blood pressure by direct action on arteriole smooth muscle, causing vasodilation with a resultant decrease in peripheral resistance. There is usually a greater diastolic response than systolic. Since blood flow through renal and cerebral vessels is increased, hydralazine can be used in clients with renal insufficiency. Unlike other antihypertensive agents (ganglionic blocking agents), postural hypotension seldom occurs. Unfortunately, a compensatory sympathetic reflex is stimulated and results in an increase in heart rate (tachycardia) and cardiac output.

Indications for Use Moderate to severe hypertension, hypertensive crisis (parenteral administration).

Contraindications Hypersensitivity to drug, coronary artery disease (including myocardial infarction and ischemia), severe mitral valvular rheumatic heart disease (may increase pulmonary artery pressure), lupus erythematosus.

Warnings and Precautions Use with caution during pregnancy, since teratogenic effects (cleft palate and malformed facial and cranial bones) have occurred in animal studies; in clients with suspected coronary artery disease (the elderly), since myocardial ischemia (angina) and myocardial infarction may occur; in clients with severe renal damage (lack of adequate number of functioning nephrons); in clients with disorders of the valve on the left-hand side of the heart, since an increase in pulmonary artery pressure and pulmonary edema may occur; in clients with cerebral vascular accidents, since drug may precipitate cerebral ischemia if a preexisting increase in intracranial pressure, particularly after parenteral administration; and in clients receiving MAO inhibitors.

Untoward Reactions Tachycardia, headache, palpitations, and angina pectoris occur frequently, particularly when large dosages are given. Other common reactions include nausea, vomiting, anorexia, and diarrhea; these reactions usually subside when the dosage is reduced. A reaction characteristic of lupus erythematosus (LE) with the presence of LE cells can occur; watch for joint pains, fever, chest pains, persistent malaise, and other unexplained symptoms. Hypersensitivity reactions include rashes, urticaria, fever, chills, joint pains, eosinophilia, and hepatitis. Toxic reactions include hypotension (which can progress to shock), tachycardia, arrhythmias, myocardial ischemia, and a generalized flushing of the skin. Blood dyscrasias include reduction in hemoglobin and red blood cell count, leukopenia, agranulocytosis, and purpura. Psychotic reactions characterized by depression, disorientation, or anxiety have occurred, but rarely. Peripheral neuritis (paresthesia, numbness, tingling) may occur and is probably due to an antipyridoxine effect. Rare reactions include nasal congestion, lacrimation, conjunctivitis, dizziness, tremors, paradoxic pressor response, muscle cramps, difficulty in micturition, constipation, paralytic ileus, and dyspnea.

Parameters of Use

Absorption Readily absorbed from GI tract. Onset of action is: about 1 hour (po); within 15 minutes (IM); 1 to 2 minutes (IV). Peak action occurs in: 3 to 4 hours (po); 10 to 80 minutes (IV). Duration of action is: up to 24 hours (po); about 3 to 4 hours (IM); about 2 hours (IV). Peak levels and duration of action may vary from client to client. Half life varies according to rate of acetylation; Range: 2 to 8 hours.

Metabolism Primarily in the liver by acetylation; some conjugation occurs. The rate of acetylation is genetically determined.

Excretion By the kidneys as metabolites. Rate of excretion may vary considerably; Range: 2 to 4 hours.

Drug Interactions Often used concurrently with other antihypertensive agents (reserpine) or thiazide diuretics (hydrochlorothiazide) and potentiation occurs. Since profound hypotension may result when combination therapy is initiated, client should be closely monitored. The pressor response to epinephrine, levarterenol, and other vasopressors may be inhibited, thus requiring larger dosages of vasopressors, which increases the risk of untoward reactions (arrhythmias) when the client is in shock. Concurrent therapy with MAO inhibitors may result in potentiation of vasodilatory effect. Other drugs that may antagonize the hypotensive effect of hydralazine include amphetamines and sympathomimetics. The oral antidiabetic agent tolbutamide may inhibit the hypotensive effect of hydralazine. Other drugs that may potentiate the hypotensive effect of hydralazine include anesthetics, ethacrynic acid, guanethidine, spironolactone, and triamterene.

Administration Highly individualized. Oral: Initial dosage: 10 mg qid for 2 to 4 days; then increase to 25 mg qid for remainder of week; increase to 50 mg qid for second week; Maintenance: Adjust dosage to lowest effective level. If the client requires 300 mg or more daily, the incidence of untoward reactions increases, thus combination drug therapy (reserpine, hydrochlorothiazide) is often tried. Intramuscular, intravenous: 20 to 40 mg every 4 to 8 hours for 24 to 48 hours, as necessary; oral drug form is started as soon as possible.

Available Drug Forms Tablets containing 10, 25, or 50 mg; 1-ml ampules containing 20 mg/ml.

Nursing Management

Planning factors

1. Obtain the following baseline data: blood pressure in standing, sitting, and supine position; other vital signs; an EKG tracing; LE cell preparation, complete blood cell count, and antinuclear antibody titer.
2. If any arrhythmias exist or the LE preparation and Coombs' test are positive, notify physician before therapy is initiated.
3. When IV administration is required,
   a. Start continuous infusion at a KVO rate or faster, so that plasma expanders (not vasopressors) and appropriate drugs can be given readily in the event of drug-induced shock.
   b. Insert an indwelling urinary catheter to determine adequacy of output.
   c. Cardiac monitoring is required to detect the development of arrhythmias.
4. Oral administration is the preferred route.

Administration factors

1. Give oral drug forms between meals with a full glass of water.
2. When administering IM, inject into large muscle mass with good circulation.
3. When administering IV,
   a. Check patency of IV.
   b. Check blood pressure and pulse before administering drug.
   c. Give via IV bolus over 2 to 5 minutes.
   d. Check blood pressure, pulse, and EKG tracings every 5 minutes for the first 30 minutes; then every 15 minutes until blood pressure stabilizes (about 2 hours).

Evaluation factors

1. Monitor blood pressure and pulse during peak plasma levels. Remember that peak plasma levels vary widely from client to client.

2. EKG monitoring is recommended during the first week of therapy. Arrhythmias are most apt to occur during peak plasma levels (3 to 4 hours after oral administration). If arrhythmias develop, notify physician.
3. Headache, tachycardia, premature ventricular contractions, anginal pain, and other common untoward reactions usually occur during peak plasma levels. If symptoms develop, notify physician before the next dose is administered, since a reduction in dosage or the concurrent administration of a beta-blocker (propranolol) may be required.
4. Record intake and output, particularly in clients with hypertensive crisis or renal impairment. Urinary output is usually increased. If output decreases, notify physician.
5. Too rapid a reduction in blood pressure may cause cerebral ischemia (sensory disturbances, anxiety, slowing of mental process) and impair renal blood flow (decrease in urinary output). If symptoms occur, keep client supine with legs elevated and notify physician immediately.
6. As with other antihypertensive agents, postural hypotension may occur. Caution client to change position slowly (lying to sitting) and lie down if faintness occurs.
7. When long-term therapy is required,
   a. Obtain LE preparation, complete blood cell count, and antinuclear antibody titer periodically. If lupus erythematosus develops, notify physician. Drug may be discontinued and long-term steroid therapy may be required.
   b. Assess client for antipyridoxine effect, drug tolerance, and other untoward reactions monthly Pyridoxine (vitamin B_6) may be required.
8. When discontinued, reduce dosage gradually so that a sudden increase in blood pressure does not occur.

GENERIC NAME Diazoxide (injection) (RX)

TRADE NAME Hyperstat I.V.

CLASSIFICATION Antihypertensive

Action Diazoxide, a nondiuretic benzethiadiazine (thiazide) derivative, is a potent vasodilator that acts directly on the smooth muscle of peripheral arterioles, thus reducing peripheral resistance. As arterial blood pressure decreases, cardiac output increases. Since coronary and cerebral blood flow is maintained, diazoxide can be administered to clients with a decreased myocardial reserve, and since renal blood flow is increased, the drug can safely be given to clients with renal insufficiency. Unlike other thiazide derivatives, diazoxide is devoid of diuretic activity. In fact, diazoxide increases extracellular fluid volume by promoting the retention of sodium and water. This untoward reaction can be controlled by concurrent use of diuretics. (It should be remembered that thiazide diuretics potentiate the antihypertensive action of diazoxide.) Like thiazide diuretics, diazoxide inhibits insulin release and catecholamine-induced glycogenesis, which results in hyperglycemia. Additional insulin may be required for clients with diabetes mellitus and those receiving multiple injections of diazoxide.

Indications for Use Hypertensive crisis, particularly when associated with malignant hypertension.

Contraindications Hypersensitivity to thiazides or sulfonamides unless benefits outweigh risks, compensatory hypertension associated with aortic coarctation or arteriovenous shunt, ineffective for hypertension due to pheochromocytoma.

Warnings and Precautions Use with caution in clients with diabetes mellitus, a family history of diabetes, uremia, or severe renal impairment; and in clients with impaired cerebral or coronary circulation, since cerebral, myocardial, and optic nerve infarctions have been caused by a rapid decrease in blood pressure. Use with extreme caution during pregnancy, since fetal or neonatal hyperbilirubinemia, thrombocytopenia, and altered carbohydrate metabolism have occurred. Subendocardial necrosis and necrosis of the papillary muscles of the heart have occurred in animals due to hypoxia associated with reflex tachycardia and a rapid decrease in blood pressure. Safe use in children has not been established.

Untoward Reactions Common reactions include hyperglycemia, fluid retention (which may result in edema), and congestive heart failure, particularly after multiple injections. Transient myocardial ischemia may result in angina, arrhythmias, and other EKG changes. Cerebral ischemia or infarction manifested by unconsciousness, convulsions, paralysis, confusion, or focal neurologic deficit may occur. Repeated injections may cause optic nerve infarction and persistent retention of nitrogenous wastes. Hypersensitivity reactions include rashes, leukopenia, and fever. CNS disturbances include papilledema, feeling of warmth, headache, dizziness, euphoria, drowsiness, and ringing in the ears. Cardiovascular disturbances include orthostatic hypotension, flushing, and tightness in the chest. GI disturbances include nausea, vomiting, anorexia, abdominal discomfort, dry mouth, constipation, and diarrhea. Pancreatitis has been reported. Dyspnea and a choking sensation have been reported. Pain, inflammation, and phlebitis may occur at the injection site. Painful cellulitis without sloughing frequently occurs after extravasation.

Parameters of Use

Absorption Onset of action is about 30 seconds after rapid IV administration. Peak action occurs in about 5 minutes and duration of action is up to 12 hours. Plasma half-life is about 28 hours. About 90% bound to plasma proteins.

Crosses placenta and enters breast milk; lactating mothers should bottle-feed their babies.

Excretion By the kidneys; removal by renal dialysis.

Drug Interactions Concurrent use of hydralazine potentiates the antihypertensive effect and may result in excessive hypotension. The effects of diazoxide may be potentiated by thiazide diuretics and excessive hypotension, hyperglycemia, and hyperuricemia may occur. Concomitant use of coumarin derivatives may cause excessive anticoagulant activity. Potentiation of antihypertensive effect may occur when methyldopa, reserpine, hydralazine, nitrates, papaverine compounds, or other direct peripheral vasodilators are used concurrently.

Administration Adults: Initial dosage: 1 to 3 mg/kg via rapid IV bolus over 30 seconds or less (Maximum: 150 mg); then repeat every 5 to 15 minutes until desired effect, as necessary; then repeat every 4 to 24 hours, as needed. *Elderly clients with a decrease in cerebral or myocardial blood flow* require a minibolus for a more gradual decrease in blood pressure. Treatment is limited to a few days; then change to an oral antihypertensive agent.

Available Drug Forms Ampules of 20 ml containing 15 mg/ml.

Nursing Management

Planning factors

1. Obtain the following baseline data: blood pressure in standing, sitting, and supine position; other vital signs; an EKG tracing; blood sugar and complete blood cell count.
2. If arrhythmias or hyperglycemia exist, notify physician before therapy is instituted.
3. Start continuous infusion at a KVO rate or faster, so that plasma expanders and appropriate drugs can be given readily in the event of drug-induced shock. An 18- or 20-in. gauge angiocath in a large peripheral vessel is recommended.
4. An indwelling urinary catheter may be required to monitor output and urinary sugar content in diabetic clients.
5. Cardiac monitoring is required to detect the development of arrhythmias.

Administration factors

1. Never inject into muscle or subcutaneous tissue.
2. Check patency of IV.
3. Give rapid IV bolus over 30 seconds unless otherwise directed by physician.
4. Obtain blood pressure and pulse (and monitor tracings) continuously for the first 30 minutes; then every 15 minutes for about 2 hours; then as indicated.

Evaluation factors

1. If blood pressure continues to drop for more than 30 minutes after rapid IV bolus, the drop is probably not drug induced. Assess client for other causes of reduction.
2. Instruct client to remain in a low Fowler's position for at least 30 minutes after each injection to avoid cerebral insufficiency.
3. If cerebral ischemia occurs, keep client supine with legs elevated and notify physician. Start nasal oxygen.
4. Cardiac monitoring is recommended during therapy. If arrhythmias occur, notify physician.
5. Monitor intake and output hourly. If oliguria occurs notify physician immediately.
6. Monitor and record urinary glucose levels frequently in all clients. Obtain serum blood glucose periodically. Insulin coverage may be required in nondiabetic clients after repeated injections of diazoxide.
7. Assess client for other untoward reactions frequently. If observed, notify physician immediately.

GENERIC NAME Sodium nitroprusside (RX)

TRADE NAMES Nipride, Nitropress

CLASSIFICATION Antihypertensive

Action Sodium nitroprusside is a potent rapid-acting vasodilator that acts directly on vascular smooth muscle, thus reducing peripheral resistance and lowering blood pressure. It is chemically similar to nitrites.

Indicators for Use Short-term management of hypertensive crisis; control of hypotension during anesthesia to reduce bleeding; reduces preload and afterload in clients with pump failure.

Contraindications Compensatory hypertension, emergency surgery in moribund clients, surgical procedures in clients with cerebral ischemia.

Warnings and Precautions Use with caution in clients with hepatic or renal insufficiency or hyperthyroidism. Preexisting anemia and hypovolemia should be corrected before starting drug therapy.

Safe use during pregnancy and lactation has not been established.

Untoward Reactions Severe hypotension can result from too rapid administration. Too rapid reduction in blood pressure may cause nausea, retching, diaphoresis, apprehension, headache, restlessness, muscular twitching, chest pain, palpitations, dizziness, and abdominal discomfort. Metabolic acidosis and an increased tolerance to drug is a sign of toxicity. Cyanide poisoning may occur and result in coma, weak pulse, absence of reflexes, dilated pupils, pink coloring, distant heart sounds, and shallow breathing. Extravasation will cause sloughing and necrosis. Irritation may occur at the injection site.

Parameters of Use

Absorption Onset of action is about 2 minutes and effects persist 1 to 5 minutes after infusion is stopped.

Metabolism Rapidly metabolized to cyanide in erythrocytes and tissues. Subsequently converted to thiocyanate in the liver with the assistance of the hepatic enzyme rhodanase. Rate of conversion depends on availability of sulfur (thiosulfate).

Excretion In urine primarily as thiocyanate metabolites.

Drug Interactions Concurrent therapy with other antihypertensive agents will result in increased sensitivity to the effects of sodium nitroprusside.

Administration Adults: Continuous IV infusion at 0.5 to 10 mcg/kg/min.; Usual dosage: 3 mcg/kg/min.; Maximum dosage: 10 mcg/kg/min.

Available Drug Forms Vials containing 50 mg of powder for reconstitution.

Nursing Management

1. Calculate mcg/kg of body weight, as shown in the following table.

RECOMMENDED DOSAGE (mcg) BASED ON BODY WEIGHT

Body Weight (kg)	0.5 mcg/kg	1.0 mcg/kg	3.0 mcg/kg	5.0 mcg/kg	10.0 mcg/kg
50	25	50	150	250	500
60	30	60	180	300	600
70	35	70	210	350	700
80	40	80	240	400	800
90	45	90	270	450	900
100	50	100	300	500	1000
110	55	110	330	550	1100
120	60	120	360	600	1200

2. Reconstitute powder with 5% D/W; use only freshly prepared solution.
3. Add 1 vial (50 mg) to 250 ml (200 mcg/ml) or 500 ml (100 mcg/ml) of 5% D/W. Date and time solution.
4. Cover bottle of medicated IV solution with aluminum foil to keep light out (special bags are available).
5. Check patency of IV before administering. Add medicated solution as a piggyback IV line. An infusion pump is recommended.
6. Start with a slow IV rate (0.5 to 1.0 mcg/kg/min.) and titrate according to blood pressure response every 5 minutes.
7. Check blood pressure every 5 minutes until stable; then every 15 minutes. If hypotension occurs, turn medicated IV off, start primary IV solution, and notify physician.
8. If extravasation occurs, turn IV off and quickly restart IV with primary solution before restarting medicated solution. Notify physician.
9. Watch for cyanide poisoning (monitor serum thiocyanate levels daily) and other untoward reactions. Overdosage is treated with nitrates to induce methemoglobin formation, thereby promoting the formation of nontoxic complexes.

Desired mcg/min.	Flow Rate: ml/min. with 100 mcg/ml solution	ml/min. with 200 mcg/ml solution
50	0.5	0.25
100	1.0	0.50
150	1.5	0.75
200	2.0	1.00
250	2.5	1.25
300	3.0	1.50
350	3.5	1.75
400	4.0	2.00
450	4.5	2.25
500	5.0	2.50
600	6.0	3.00
700	7.0	3.50
800	8.0	4.00
900	9.0	4.50
1000	10.0	5.00

GENERIC NAME Minoxidil (RX)

TRADE NAME Loniten

CLASSIFICATION Antihypertensive

See hydralazine hydrochloride for Contraindications and Warnings and precautions.

Action Minoxidil has properties similar to hydralazine. It acts directly on smooth muscle of arterioles to induce vasodilation. The resultant decrease in peripheral vascular resistance leads to a drop in systolic and diastolic blood pressure, inhibition of vagal stimulation (which results in tachycardia), and an increase in renin secretion, which accelerates heart rate and output and causes the retention of sodium and water. Minoxidil is often given with a beta-adrenergic blocker to control tachycardia and a diuretic to promote diuresis of retained fluid and sodium.

Indications for Use Refractory severe symptomatic hypertension that is unresponsive to other drugs.

Untoward Reactions Tachycardia and edema are common, and may precipitate congestive heart failure and myocardial lesions, including pericardial effusion followed by tamponade. EKG changes, particularly alterations in the T wave, frequently occur. Hypertrichosis (elongation, thickening, and enhanced pigmentation of fine body hair) frequently occurs within 3 to 6 weeks, but disappears within 6 months after discontinuation of drug.

Allergic rashes are rare. Thrombocytopenia and leukopenia occur, but rarely. Breast tenderness has been reported.

Parameters of Use

Absorption 90% absorbed from the GI tract; peak drug level occurs in one hour, then declines rapidly. Plasma half-life is about 4 hours. Drug effect on blood pressure does not correlate with drug plasma levels. Onset of action is about one hour; duration of drug effect is approximately 75 hours.

Metabolism Rapid, by the liver; conjugation with glucuronic acid and conversion to more polar metabolites occurs. Some metabolites are active, but not as active as the drug.

Excretion By the kidneys.

Drug Interactions Severe orthostatic hypotension and a rapid decrease in blood pressure may occur if given concurrently with guanethidine; use with extreme caution concomitantly.

Administration Adults and children over 12 years: Initial dosage: 5 mg po daily for 2 days; then increase to 10 mg as needed; then 20 mg, then 40 mg in divided doses daily; Dosage range: 10 to 40 mg daily; Maximum dosage: 50 mg/day. Children: Under 12 years: Initial dosage: 0.2 mg/kg po daily for 3 days; then increase by 1.0 to 0.2 mg/kg daily until desired effect; Dosage range: 0.25 to 1.0 mg/kg/day.

Available Drug Forms Tablets containing 2.5 or 10 mg.

Nursing Management

1. Give at the same time daily.
2. If supine diastolic pressure is decreased more than 30 mm Hg, dosage should be divided and given bid.
3. Give client the available information insert. Answer client's questions.
4. Store drug at room temperature.

COMBINATION PREPARATIONS

See monographs of individual constituents of combination preparations for further details.

TRADE NAME Aldoclor (RX)

CLASSIFICATION Combination antihypertensive and diuretic agent

Indications for Use Treatment of hypertension after drug dosage has been determined.

Contraindications Hypersensitivity to methyldopa or sulfonamides; active hepatic disease, including hepatitis and cirrhosis.

Warnings and Precautions Tolerance may develop after 2 to 3 months.

Administration 1 tablet po bid or tid; maximum dosage: 3000 mg methyldopa/24 hours.

Available Drug Forms Generic contents in each beige Aldoclor 150 tablet: methyldopa: 250 mg; chlorothiazide: 150 mg. Generic contents in each green Aldoclor 250 tablet: methyldopa: 250 mg; chlorothiazide: 250 mg.

Nursing Management Dosage increases should begin with the evening dose to minimize the sedative effect of methyldopa.

TRADE NAME Aldoril (RX)

CLASSIFICATION Combination antihypertensive and diuretic agent

Indications for Use Treatment of hypertension after drug dosage has been determined.

Contraindications Hypersensitivity to methyldopa or sulfonamides; active hepatic disease, including hepatitis and cirrhosis.

Warnings and Precautions Tolerance may develop after 2 to 3 months. Syncope may occur in the elderly.

Administration 1 tablet po bid or tid; Maximum dosage: 3000 mg methyldopa/24 hours.

Available Drug Forms Generic contents in each salmon Aldoril 15 tablet: methyldopa: 250 mg; hydrochlorothiazide: 15 mg. Generic contents in each white Aldoril 25 tablet: methyldopa: 250 mg; hydrochlorothiazide: 25 mg. Generic contents in each salmon Aldoril D30 tablet: methyldopa: 500 mg; hydrochlorothiazide: 30 mg. Generic contents in each white Aldoril D50 tablet: methyldopa: 500 mg; hydrochlorothiazide: 50 mg.

Nursing Management Dosage increases should begin with the evening dose to minimize the sedative effect of methyldopa.

TRADE NAME Apresazide (RX)

CLASSIFICATION Combination antihypertensive and diuretic agent

Indications for Use Treatment of hypertension after drug dosage has been determined.

Contraindications Hypersensitivity to hydralazine or sulfonamides, coronary artery disease, mitral valvular rheumatic heart disease, anuria.

Administration 1 capsule po bid adjusted to lowest effective dosage; Maximum dosage: 300 mg hydralazine/24 hours.

Available Drug Forms Generic contents in each blue and white Apresazide 25/25 capsule: hydralazine hydrochloride: 25 mg; hydrochlorothiazide: 25 mg. Generic contents in each pink and white Apresazide 50/50 capsule: hydralazine hydrochloride: 50 mg; hydrochlorothiazide: 50 mg. Generic contents in each pink flesh and white Apresazide 100/50 capsule: hydralazine hydrochloride: 100 mg; hydrochlorothiazide: 50 mg.

TRADE NAME Apresoline-Esidrix (RX)

CLASSIFICATION Combination antihypertensive and diuretic agent

Indications for Use Treatment of hypertension after drug dosage has been determined.

Contraindications Hypersensitivity to hydralazine or sulfonamides, coronary artery disease, mitral valvular rheumatic heart disease, anuria.

Administration 1 tablet po tid; Maximum dosage: 2 tablets tid.

Available Drug Forms Generic contents in each orange tablet: hydralazine hydrochloride: 25 mg; hydrochlorothiazide: 15 mg.

TRADE NAME Diupres (RX)

CLASSIFICATION Combination antihypertensive and diuretic agent

Indications for Use Treatment of hypertension after drug dosage has been determined.

Contraindications Hypersensitivity to chlorothiazide, sulfonamides, or reserpine; anuria; active peptic ulcer or ulcerative colitis; mental depression; clients receiving electroconvulsive therapy.

Administration 1 to 2 tablets po daily or bid.

Available Drug Forms Generic contents in each pink Diupres 250 tablet: chlorothiazide: 250 mg; reserpine: 0.125 mg Generic contents in each pink Diupres 500 tablet: chlorothiazide: 500 mg; reserpine: 0.125 mg.

TRADE NAME Diutensen (RX)

CLASSIFICATION Combination antihypertensive and diuretic agent

Indications for Use Treatment of hypertension after drug dosage has been determined.

Contraindications Hypersensitivity to thiazides, sulfonamides, or *Veratrum viride;* recent myocardial infarction; recent cerebral thrombosis; severe renal or hepatic failure.

Warnings and Precautions Potentiates the action of ganglionic blocking agents and may cause bradycardia.

Administration 1 to 4 tablets po daily.

Available Drug Forms Generic contents in each white and blue tablet: cryptenamine (tannate salts): 2 mg; methyclothiazide: 2.5 mg.

TRADE NAME Diutensen-R (RX)

CLASSIFICATION Combination antihypertensive and diuretic agent

Indications for Use Treatment of hypertension after drug dosage has been determined.

Contraindications Hypersensitivity to thiazides, sulfonamides, or reserpine; anuria; active peptic ulcer or ulcerative colitis; mental depression; severe renal or hepatic failure; clients receiving electroconvulsive therapy.

Warnings and Precautions Use with caution in clients with a history of bronchial asthma. Potentiates the action of ganglionic or peripheral adrenergic blocking agents.

Administration 1 to 4 tablets po daily.

Available Drug Forms Generic contents in each white and pink tablet: methyclothiazide: 2.5 mg; reserpine: 0.1 mg.

TRADE NAMES Enduronyl, Enduronyl Forte (RX)

CLASSIFICATION Combination antihypertensive and diuretic agent

Indications for Use Treatment of hypertension after drug dosage has been determined.

Contraindications Hypersensitivity to thiazides, sulfonamides, or deserpidine; anuria; active peptic ulcer or ulcerative colitis; mental depression; renal failure; clients receiving electroconvulsive therapy.

Warnings and Precautions Potentiates the action of ganglionic blocking agents. May cause bradycardia or hypokalemia.

Administration 1 tablet po daily in early A.M.

Available Drug Forms Generic contents in each yellow Enduronyl tablet: methyclothiazide: 5 mg; deserpidine: 0.25 mg. Generic contents in each gray Enduronyl Forte tablet: methyclothiazide: 5 mg; deserpidine: 0.5 mg.

TRADE NAME Esimil (RX)

CLASSIFICATION Combination antihypertensive and diuretic agent

Indications for Use Treatment of hypertension after drug dosage has been determined.

Contraindications Hypersensitivity to guanethidine or sulfonamides, anuria, known or suspected pheochromocytoma, acute congestive heart failure, concurrent therapy with MAO inhibitors.

Warnings and Precautions Frequently causes orthostatic hypotension.

Administration Initial dosage: 1 tablet po daily in A.M.; then 2 tablets daily in A.M.

Available Drug Forms Generic contents in each white tablet: guanethidine monosulfate: 10 mg (equivalent to 8.4 mg guanethidine sulfate); hydrochlorothiazide: 25 mg.

Nursing Management Dosage adjustments are made after a minimum of 1 week of therapy, when necessary.

TRADE NAME Eutron (RX)

CLASSIFICATION Combination antihypertensive and diuretic agent

Indications for Use Treatment of hypertension after drug dosage has been determined.

Contraindications Hypersensitivity to sulfonamides, pheochromocytoma, paranoid schizophrenia, hyperthyroidism, severe renal failure, malignant hypertension, children under 12 years.

Warnings and Precautions Clients must avoid tyramine and high pressor amine foods.

Administration 1 tablet po daily in early A.M.

Available Drug Forms Generic contents in each tablet: pargyline hydrochloride: 25 mg; methyclothiazide: 5 mg.

TRADE NAME Exna-R (RX)

CLASSIFICATION Combination antihypertensive and diuretic agent

Indications for Use Treatment of hypertension after drug dosage has been determined.

Contraindications Hypersensitivity to thiazides, sulfonamides, or reserpine; anuria; active peptic ulcer or ulcerative colitis; mental depression; severe renal or hepatic failure; clients receiving electroconvulsive therapy.

Warnings and Precautions Use with caution in clients with a history of bronchial asthma. May cause bradycardia or hypokalemia.

Administration 1 tablet po daily in early A.M.

Available Drug Forms Generic contents in each white tablet: benzthiazide: 50 mg; reserpine: 0.125 mg.

TRADE NAMES Hydropres, Hydrotensin (RX)

CLASSIFICATION Combination antihypertensive and diuretic agent

Indications for Use Treatment of hypertension after drug dosage has been determined.

Contraindications Hypersensitivity to sulfonamides, rauwolfia derivatives, or reserpine; anuria; active peptic ulcer or ulcerative colitis; mental depression; clients receiving electroconvulsive therapy.

Warnings and Precautions May cause bradycardia.

Administration 1 tablet po daily, bid, tid, or qid.

Available Drug Forms Generic contents in each green Hydropres 25 and Hydrotensin 25 tablet: hydrochlorothiazide: 25 mg; reserpine: 0.125 mg. Generic contents in each green Hydropres 50 and Hydrotensin 50 tablet: hydrochlorothiazide: 50 mg; reserpine: 0.125 mg.

TRADE NAME Inderide (RX)

CLASSIFICATION Combination antihypertensive and diuretic agent

Indications for Use Treatment of hypertension after drug dosage has been determined.

Contraindications Hypersensitivity to any ingredient or sulfonamides, bronchial asthma, allergic rhinitis, sinus bradycardia or heart block greater than first degree, cardiogenic shock, right ventricular failure due to pulmonary hypertension, congestive heart failure, anuria.

Warnings and Precautions Use with caution in clients with hyperthyroidism, Wolff-Parkinson-White syndrome, diabetes, susceptibility to bronchospasm, history of bronchial asthma, or severe renal disorder.

Administration 1 to 2 tablets po bid in early A.M.

Available Drug Forms Generic contents in each Inderide-40/25 tablet: propranolol hydrochloride: 40 mg; hydrochlorothiazide: 25 mg. Generic contents in each Inderide-80/25 tablet: propranolol hydrochloride: 80 mg; hydrochlorothiazide: 25 mg.

TRADE NAME Metatensin (RX)

CLASSIFICATION Combination antihypertensive and diuretic agent

Indications for Use Treatment of hypertension after drug dosage has been determined.

Contraindications Hypersensitivity to thiazides, sulfonamides, or reserpine; anuria; active peptic ulcer or ulcerative colitis; mental depression; severe renal or hepatic failure; clients receiving electroconvulsive therapy.

Administration 1 to 2 tablets po daily; Maximum dosage: 8 mg trichlormethiazide daily.

Available Drug Forms Generic contents in each tablet: trichlormethiazide: 2 or 4 mg; reserpine: 0.1 mg.

TRADE NAME Minizide (RX)

CLASSIFICATION Combination antihypertensive and diuretic agent

Indications for Use Treatment of hypertension after drug dosage has been determined.

Contraindications Hypersensitivity to thiazides or sulfonamides, anuria.

Warnings and Precautions Use with caution in clients with renal disorders and elderly or debilitated clients. May cause syncope or severe tachycardia.

Administration Highly individualized. 1 tablet po bid or tid.

Available Drug Forms Generic contents in each blue-green Minizide 1 tablet: prazosin hydrochloride: 1 mg; polythiazide: 0.5 mg. Generic contents in each blue-green/pink Minizide 2 tablet: prazosin hydrochloride: 2 mg; polythiazide: 0.5 mg. Generic contents in each blue-green/blue Minizide 3 tablet: prazosin hydrochloride: 5 mg; polythiazide: 0.5 mg.

TRADE NAME Naquival (RX)

CLASSIFICATION Combination antihypertensive and diuretic agent

Indications for Use Treatment of hypertension after drug dosage has been determined.

Contraindications Hypersensitivity to thiazides, sulfonamides, or reserpine; anuria; active peptic ulcer or ulcerative colitis; mental depression; severe renal or hepatic failure; clients receiving electroconvulsive therapy.

Administration 1 tablet po daily in early A.M.

Available Drug Forms Generic contents in each tablet: trichlormethiazide: 4 mg; reserpine: 0.1 mg.

TRADE NAME Oreticyl (RX)

CLASSIFICATION Combination antihypertensive and diuretic agent

Indications for Use Treatment of hypertension after drug dosage has been determined.

Contraindications Hypersensitivity to thiazides, sulfonamides, or deserpidine; anuria; active peptic ulcer or ulcerative colitis; mental depression; severe renal or hepatic failure; clients receiving electroconvulsive therapy.

Administration 1 tablet po bid in early A.M.

Available Drug Forms Generic contents in each rose-colored Oreticyl 25 tablet: hydrochlorothiazide: 25 mg; deserpidine: 0.125 mg. Generic contents in each rose-colored Oreticyl 50 tablet: hydrochlorothiazide: 50 mg; deserpidine: 0.125 mg. Generic contents in each gray-colored Oreticyl Forte tablet: hydrochlorothiazide: 25 mg; deserpidine: 0.25 mg.

TRADE NAME Rauzide (RX)

CLASSIFICATION Combination antihypertensive and diuretic agent

Indications for Use Treatment of hypertension after drug dosage has been determined.

Contraindications Hypersensitivity to thiazides, sulfonamides, or rauwolfia derivatives; anuria; active peptic ulcer or ulcerative colitis; mental depression; clients receiving electroconvulsive therapy.

Warnings and Precautions May cause mental depression.

Administration 1 to 4 tablets po daily.

Available Drug Forms Generic contents in each tablet: powdered rauwolfia serpentina: 50 mg; bendroflumethiazide: 4 mg.

TRADE NAME Rease-R (RX)

CLASSIFICATION Combination antihypertensive and diuretic agent

---

Indications for Use Treatment of hypertension after drug dosage has been determined.

Contraindications Hypersensitivity to thiazides, sulfonamides, or reserpine; anuria; active peptic ulcer or ulcerative colitis; mental depression; severe renal or hepatic failure; clients receiving electroconvulsive therapy.

Warnings and Precautions Use with caution in clients with a history of bronchial asthma. May cause bradycardia or hypokalemia.

Administration $\frac{1}{2}$ to 2 tablets po daily.

Available Drug Forms Generic contents in each scored tablet: polythiazide: 2 mg; reserpine: 0.25 mg.

TRADE NAMES Salutensin, Salutensin Demi (RX)

CLASSIFICATION Combination antihypertensive and diuretic agent

---

Indications for Use Treatment of hypertension after drug dosage has been determined.

Contraindications Hypersensitivity to sulfonamides, rauwolfia derivatives, or reserpine; anuria; active peptic ulcer or ulcerative colitis; mental depression; clients receiving electroconvulsive therapy.

Warnings and Precautions Use with caution in clients with a history of bronchial asthma. May cause bradycardia or hypokalemia.

Administration 1 tablet po daily or bid; Maximum dosage: 3 to 4 tablets daily in divided doses.

Available Drug Forms Generic contents in each Salutensin tablet: hydroflumethiazide: 50 mg; reserpine: 0.125 mg. Generic contents in each Salutensin-Demi tablet: hydroflumethiazide: 25 mg; reserpine: 0.125 mg.

TRADE NAME Ser-Ap-Es (RX)

CLASSIFICATION Combination antihypertensive and diuretic agent

---

Indications for Use Treatment of hypertension after drug dosage has been determined.

Contraindications Hypersensitivity to hydralazine, sulfonamides, rauwolfia derivatives, or reserpine; anuria; active peptic ulcer or ulcerative colitis; mental depression; coronary artery disease; mitral valvular rheumatic heart disease; clients receiving electroconvulsive therapy.

Administration 1 to 2 tablets po tid.

Available Drug Forms Generic contents in each salmon pink tablet: hydralazine hydrochloride: 25 mg; hydrochlorothiazide: 15 mg; reserpine: 0.1 mg.

Nursing Management Maximum reduction in blood pressure may take as long as 2 weeks.

Chapter 51

Antilipemic Agents

HYPERLIPEMIA AND THE ROLE OF ANTILIPEMIC AGENTS

Although the relationship between serum lipid levels and atherosclerosis is controversial, it is established that individuals with higher than normal lipid levels are at increased risk of developing atherosclerosis. Hyperlipemia is a condition characterized by increased serum levels of cholesterol, triglycerides and phospholipids, which are transported in the circulation in combination with proteins called *lipoproteins*. Low-density lipoproteins contain most of the total cholesterol in the body and are therefore potentially the most harmful. High-density lipoproteins, on the other hand, contain about 20% cholesterol. These lipoproteins also transport cholesterol from body cells to the liver where it is then excreted in bile. Individuals with high concentrations of high-density lipoproteins have a lower risk factor for cardiovascular disease.

Antilipemic agents currently available show no evidence of reversing atherosclerosis once the process is begun. Use of these drugs for long-term lowering of serum lipid levels is still controversial, but those who prescribe these agents feel that lower lipid levels may retard the atherosclerotic process. In any case, drug therapy with antilipemic agents is always used as an adjunct to a low-cholesterol (saturated fat) diet. The available drugs act in one of three ways: (1) some (clofibrate, dextrothyroxine) enhance the metabolism of lipoproteins; (2) some (cholestyramine, colestipol, probucol) bind with and thereby remove lipoproteins from the circulation; (3) some (nicotinic acid) interfere with the production of cholesterol and triglycerides.

ANTILIPEMIC AGENTS

GENERIC NAME Cholestyramine resin (RX)

TRADE NAMES Cuemid, Questran

CLASSIFICATION Antilipemic

Action Cholestyramine is a chloride salt of a quaternary ammonium anion-exchange resin. It releases chloride ions and adsorbs intestinal bile salts to form an insoluble product that is excreted in feces. As a consequence of the increased fecal loss of bile acids, increased amounts of cholesterol are oxidized to bile acids, thereby lowering plasma cholesterol levels. Cholestyramine also binds digitoxin in the GI tract.

Indications for Use As an adjunct to diet therapy for reduction of low-density lipoprotein levels; treatment of pruritus associated with biliary stasis; acute digitoxin toxicity.

Contraindications Hypersensitivity, biliary obstruction.

Warnings and Precautions Use with caution in clients with steatorrhea or impaired renal function. Safe use during pregnancy and lactation has not been established.

Untoward Reactions Severe constipation, fecal impaction, abdominal distention, flatulence, nausea, vomiting, anorexia, steatorrhea, skin rashes, ecchymoses, anemia. May interfere with calcium and fat absorption and lead to deficiencies of vitamins A, D, E, K, and calcium. Hyperchloremic acidosis has been reported.

Parameters of Use

Absorption Is not absorbed from GI tract.
Excretion In feces.

Drug Interactions Cholestyramine may bind other drugs (organic acids) given concurrently, thereby impeding their absorption. It interferes with the absorption of oral anticoagulants, digitalis, glycosides, iron, thiazide diuretics, phenylbutazone, thyroid hormones, tetracycline, and phenobarbital.

Administration *Cholestyramine:* Adults: 4 g po tid or qid; Children: Over 6 years: 80 mg/kg po tid.

Available Drug Forms Packets of dry powder containing 4 g of active ingredient.

Nursing Management

Planning factors High-bulk, high-fluid diet is essential to avoid severe constipation.

Administration factors

1. Give before meals.
2. Never give powder in dry form, since it is irritating to mucous membranes.
3. Place contents of packet on surface of beverage. Allow to stand for 2 minutes before stirring. Can also be mixed with soups or pureed fruits. Rinse glass after ingestion and have client drink remainder.
4. Any other oral drugs must be taken at least 1 hour prior to or 4 to 6 hours after cholestyramine to avoid binding.
5. Stool softeners are often prescribed concurrently.

Evaluation factors Long-term therapy requires parenteral treatment with fat-soluble vitamins.

Client teaching factors

1. Teach client signs of hypoprothrombinemia, since drug can cause increased bleeding tendency.
2. Warn client to avoid taking any other drugs with cholestyramine and to take drug at least 1 hour after meals and snacks.

GENERIC NAME Clofibrate (RX)

TRADE NAME Atromid-S

CLASSIFICATION Antilipemic

Action Exact mechanism of action is unknown, but may block cholesterol synthesis and enhance the catabolism of low-density lipoproteins. Serum phospholipids and triglycerides are reduced. Excretion of neutral sterols is increased.

Indications for Use As an adjunct to diet therapy for reduction of serum cholesterol and triglyceride levels.

Contraindications Pregnancy, lactation, hepatic or renal dysfunction, biliary cirrhosis.

Warnings and Precautions Use with caution in clients with diabetes. Not recommended for children.

Untoward Reactions Nausea and diarrhea are common. Drowsiness, weakness, and giddiness may occur. An acute syndrome of severe muscle cramps, stiffness, weakness, and muscle tenderness has been reported occasionally. Other untoward reactions include flatulence, headache, dry skin, alopecia, leukopenia, agranulocytosis, and dermatologic reactions.

Parameters of Use

Absorption Well absorbed from the GI tract; found in plasma as chlorophenoxyisobutyric acid. Plasma acid is highly bound to plasma albumin receptor sites for fatty acids and thyroxine. Onset of drug action is 3 to 24 hours. Half-life is about 12 hours.

Excretion In urine as the metabolite glucuronide.

Drug Interactions Clofibrate enhances the action of anticoagulants.

Laboratory Interactions Increases serum glutamic-oxaloacetic transaminase, serum glutamicpyruvic transaminase, Bromsulphalein retention, thymol turbidity, creatinine, phosphatase, and proteinuria.

Administration 500 mg po qid.

Available Drug Forms Capsules containing 500 mg.

Nursing Management

Planning factors

1. Obtain baseline routine hepatic studies, including prothrombin levels. If abnormal, notify physician.
2. Obtain baseline studies on serum cholesterol and triglyceride levels.

Administration factors

1. Give drug between meals, with a full glass of water.
2. If GI disturbances occur, give drug 1 hour after meals.

Evaluation factors

1. In clients on concomitant anticoagulant therapy, obtain prothrombin levels daily until stabilized. Anticoagulant dosage is usually reduced by one-half.
2. Obtain periodic serum cholesterol and triglyceride levels (weekly, then monthly).
3. Obtain periodic hepatic studies, since abnormalities usually occur. Notify physician, since drug may have to be discontinued if studies are significantly abnormal.
4. Drug must be taken for 1 to 3 months before lipid levels reach normal levels.
5. Long-term effects of clofibrate are unknown.

Client teaching factors

1. Instruct client to report any GI disturbances, since times of drug administration may need to be changed.
2. Instruct client to report symptoms of cold to physician, since they may indicate the onset of drug-induced acute syndrome.
3. Emphasize the importance of regular checkups and blood work.

GENERIC NAME Colestipol hydrochloride (RX)

TRADE NAME Colestid

CLASSIFICATION Antilipemic

See cholestyramine resin for Warnings and precautions, Drug interactions, and Nursing management.

Action Colestipol hydrochloride is similar to cholestyramine resin, but colestipol is a high-molecular-weight anion-exchange copolymer of diethylenetriamine and an epoxypropane. Like cholestyramine, colestipol binds bile acids in the GI tract to form complexes that are eliminated in the feces. Although hydrophilic, colestipol is virtually insoluble in water, is not hydrolyzed by digestive enzymes, and very little, if any, is absorbed into the systemic circulation. (See cholestyramine resin.)

Indications for Use As an adjunct to diet therapy for reduction of low-density lipoprotein levels.

Contraindications Hypersensitivity to any ingredient.

Parameters of Use

Absorption Virtually not absorbed from the GI tract.

Excretion In feces, complexed with bile salts; if

absorbed, the drug is excreted as unchanged drug in the urine. Up to 0.05% may be excreted in urine.

Administration Adults: 5 g po tid or qid. Maximum daily dose: 30 g daily.

Available Drug Forms Packets of granules containing 5 g; bottles of granules containing 500 g, with one level scoop containing 5 g.

GENERIC NAME Niacin (nicotinic acid)

TRADE NAMES Nicobid, Nicolar, Nico-Span, SK-Niacin

CLASSIFICATION Antilipemic (OTC) (RX)

Action Besides its function as a vitamin, large dosages of niacin are known to reduce serum lipids. Although the exact mechanism of action is unknown, niacin is thought to interfere with the production of cholesterol and triglycerides.

Contraindications Clients with hepatic dysfunction or an active peptic ulcer.

Indications for Use As an adjunct to diet in the treatment of hypercholesterolemia and hyperbetalipoproteinemia.

Warnings and Precautions Use with caution in clients with a history of peptic ulcer, jaundice, or liver dysfunction. Use with caution in clients with diabetes, since adjustments in diet or hypoglycemic therapy may be required. Since elevated uric acid levels have occurred, use with caution in clients predisposed to gout.

Safe use during pregnancy and lactation has not been established.

Untoward Reactions Severe flushing and an alteration in glucose tolerance are common. GI disturbances, including epigastric distress, bleeding of a previous ulcer, and other disorders, may occur. Hyperuricemia, abnormal liver function tests, jaundice, toxic amblyopia, hypotension, and transient headache may occur. Skin disorders include dry skin, keratosis nigricans, and pruritus.

Drug Interactions Adrenergic blocking agents used for treating hypertension may have an additive vasodilating effect and should not be given concurrently.

Administration 1 to 2 g po daily; may be increased to a maximum dosage of 6 g/day after several weeks.

Available Drug Forms Long-acting capsules containing 400 mg; tablets containing 500 mg.

Nursing Management

1. For maximum response to niacin therapy, tablets may be chewed and followed with a large glass of water.
2. Nicotinic acid therapy has been used in clients for up to 5 years to maintain reduced serum lipid levels. When drug is discontinued, lipid levels return to pretreatment levels within 6 weeks.
3. Resistance to niacin occurs in 25% of clients.

GENERIC NAME Probucol (RX)

TRADE NAME Lorelco

CLASSIFICATION Antilipemic

See cholestyramine resin for Drug interactions

Action Mechanism of action is unknown, but may inhibit the transport of cholesterol from the intestine, thereby lowering serum lipoproteins.

Indications for Use As an adjunct to diet therapy for reduction of serum cholesterol levels.

Contraindications Hypersensitivity, pregnancy, lactation, children.

Untoward Reactions Generally mild and of short duration. Untoward reactions include diarrhea, flatulence, nausea, vomiting, headache, dizziness, palpitations, chest pain, angioneurotic edema, dermatologic reactions, and blurred vision.

Parameters of Use

Absorption Limited and variable from GI tract. Up to 90% is unabsorbed.

Excretion Via biliary tract.

Administration 500 mg po bid.

Available Drug Forms Coated tablets containing 250 mg.

Nursing Management (See cholestyramine resin.)

1. Give with meals. When administered with food, peak blood levels are less variable than when given on an empty stomach.
2. Store in dry, light-resistant containers. Avoid excessive heat.

GENERIC NAME Sitosterols (RX)

TRADE NAME Cytellin

CLASSIFICATION Antilipemic

Action Mechanism of action is unknown, but may interfere with intestinal absorption of cholesterol.

Indications for Use As an adjunct to diet therapy for reduction of serum lipids.

Untoward Reactions Anorexia, diarrhea, and abdominal cramps may occur, but rarely.

Parameters of Use

Absorption Almost none is absorbed.
Excretion Unchanged in feces.

Drug Interactions None known, but may interfere with absorption of other drugs taken concurrently.

Administration 12 to 24 g po daily in divided doses; Maximum dosage: 36 g/day.

Available Drug Forms Suspension in 16-oz bottles; do not freeze.

Nursing Management

1. Mix with liquid and give immediately before meals. Dosage may be increased when large or high-fat meals are eaten.
2. For optimum response to drug, any foods eaten between meals should be preceded by a fractional dose.
3. Maximum therapeutic effect usually occurs after 2 or 3 months. When drug is discontinued, lipid levels return to pretreatment levels in 3 weeks.
4. Inform client that drug may produce bulky, light-colored stools.

GENERIC NAME Sodium dextrothyroxine (RX)

TRADE NAMES Choloxin, *D*-Thyroxine

CLASSIFICATION Antilipemic

Action Dextrothyroxine sodium is the sodium salt of an isomer of thyroxine. Although it does not decrease the production of cholesterol, dextrothyroxine does stimulate the liver to increase the catabolism and excretion of cholesterol (and its by-products) into bile, which enters the GI tract and is then eventually eliminated in feces.

Indications for Use As an adjunct to diet therapy in the treatment of hyperlipidemia.

Contraindications Euthyroid clients with known organic heart disease, moderate to severe hypertension, marked liver or kidney dysfunction, or a history of iodism; pregnancy and lactation.

Warnings and Precautions Use with caution in clients with coronary artery insufficiency or diabetes and in clients with impaired hepatic or renal function. May increase serum thyroxine levels; this should not be interpreted as hypermetabolism. Safe use in children has not been established.

Untoward Reactions Secondary effects due to hypermetabolism include angina, extrasystoles, ectopic beats, supraventricular tachycardia, cardiac hypertrophy, insomnia, nervousness, tremors, weight loss, sweating, flushing, hyperthermia, hair loss, diuresis, menstrual irregularities, nausea, vomiting, constipation, diarrhea, and anorexia. Other reactions include headache, alterations in libido, hoarseness, tinnitus, dizziness, peripheral edema, malaise, visual disturbances, psychic changes, paresthesia, muscle pain, skin rashes, and itching. Iodism may occur. Gallstones have been reported.

Drug Interactions Dextrothyroxine may enhance the action of anticoagulants on prothrombin time. The dosage of anticoagulant may have to be reduced by as much as one-half. Additive effect may occur if given concurrently with thyroid preparations.

Administration Adults: Initial dosage: 1 to 2 mg po daily for 1 month, then increase by 1 to 2 mg daily, at monthly intervals. Maximum daily dosage: 4 to 8 mg daily. Children: Initial dosage: 50 mcg/kg daily for 1 month, then increase by 50 mcg daily, at monthly intervals. Maximum daily dosage: 4 mg daily.

Available Drug Forms Scored tablets containing 1 2, 4, or 6 mg.

Nursing Management

Planning factors

1. Obtain baseline thyroid studies, hepatic studies including prothrombin levels, cholesterol and triglyceride levels, and glucose levels.
2. Obtain a history of thyroid dysfunction.

Administration factors

1. Give drug with a full glass of water.
2. Avoid giving drug late at night, since insomnia may occur.
3. If GI disturbances occur, give drug one-half hour before meals.

Evaluation factors

1. In clients on concomitant anticoagulant therapy, obtain prothrombin levels daily until stabilization. Anticoagulant dosage is usually reduced by one-third to one-half.
2. Obtain periodic serum cholesterol and triglyceride levels (weekly, then monthly).
3. Thyroid studies may be required periodically (every 3 to 6 months).
4. Obtain periodic hepatic studies, since abnormalities sometimes occur.

Client teaching factors

1. Instruct client to take drug with a full glass of water.
2. Inform client of the secondary effects of drug and to report symptoms to physician if the effects are bothersome.
3. Emphasize the importance of regular checkups and blood work.

Chapter 52

Antianemic Agents

Icron-FA	Zentinic
I.L.X. B_{12} Elixir	Zentron
I.L.X. B_{12} Tablets	Zentron Chewable
Stuartinic	

THE ERYTHROPOIETIC SYSTEM

The aspect of the hematologic system concerned with the formation and function of erythrocytes, or red blood cells (RBCs), is termed the *erythropoietic system.* The importance of erythrocytes lies in their ability to carry oxygen from the lungs to the tissues. *Hemoglobin* (hgb) is the substance in erythrocytes that combines with oxygen. *Anemia* occurs when the number of circulating erythrocytes or the amount of hemoglobin falls below normal levels and can be the results of inadequate production of healthy erythrocytes or excessive loss of cells, due either to bleeding or premature cell destruction.

Although erythrocytes are formed by almost all the bones in children, in adults the cells are produced by the bone marrow of the sternum, vertebrae, ribs, and a few other bones. Even these bones produce fewer and fewer cells after humans reach the age of 30. Consequently, mild anemia is common in the elderly.

The primitive bone marrow cell, called a hemocytoblast, will develop into either a platelet, a leukocyte, or an erythrocyte. Gradually these cells lose their nucleus and hemoglobin forms within the cell. These cells are first called erythroblasts, then normoblasts, and eventually reticulocytes, the term used for young erythrocytes. Within 2 to 4 days, reticulocytes lose their remaining reticulum and stop producing hemoglobin. When the entire process is complete, the cells are mature erythrocytes. Substances required for the proper formation of erythrocytes include certain proteins, iron, and most of the B-complex vitamins, particularly cyanocobalamin (B_{12}), folic acid (B_9), pyridoxine (B_6), thiamine (B_1), riboflavin (B_2), and niacinamide (B_3). (For a complete explanation of the B-complex vitamins' role, see Chapter 18.) Normally only 0.5% of the circulating red blood cells are reticulocytes; the remainder are mature erythrocytes. The average adult male's blood has 4.5 to 6.5 million RBC/mm^3, whereas adult females usually have a total of only 4.0 to 5.6 million RBC/mm^3.

Hemoglobin is a conjugated protein that contains 4 *heme* molecules, the iron-containing substance, and a simple protein, *globin.* The average adult male has 14.0 to 18.0 gm/100 ml of hemoglobin in his blood, whereas the normal adult female averages 12 to 16 gm/100 ml. Hemoglobin combines loosely with oxygen in the lungs to form *oxyhemoglobin* and then readily releases the oxygen in exchange for carbon dioxide in the capillaries of tissues. Not only are amino acids and iron important for the formation of hemoglobin, but small quantities of copper, pyridoxine, and cobalt are necessary as catalysts or enzymes. Long-term deficiencies of any one of these substances can eventually result in anemia.

The body tends to conserve iron and some of the other components of hemoglobin and red blood cells. When a worn-out erythrocyte finally breaks apart after about 120 days of work, the hemoglobin is released into the plasma and the remaining cell fragments are taken up by the reticuloendothelial cells of the spleen, liver, bone marrow, and other tissues. Eventually the freed hemoglobin lodges in the reticuloendothelial cells, where it is separated into heme and globin molecules. Most of the iron is transported by a glycoprotein, transferrin, to the bone marrow and other storage sites such as the liver. The remainder of the heme molecule is reduced to *bilirubin* and is gradually released into the bloodstream, finally ending up in the liver to be used to form bile. Anemia develops if the equilibrium between cell destruction and production of new erythrocytes is disturbed.

TYPES OF ANEMIA

The most common type of anemia is *iron-deficiency anemia.* Initial symptoms include mild weakness, fatigability, periodic dizziness, anorexia, and slight pallor of the skin. Because of the lack of hemoglobin, the red blood cells tend to be small and pale, thus the term hypochromic microcytic anemia.

A deficiency of iron can result from several causes, including:

1. inadequate dietary intake of iron;
2. inadequate absorption of iron, due to:
   a. lack of hydrochloric acid to free iron from foodstuffs:
   b. defective absorbing surface (duodenal ulcers);
   c. the presence of interfering substances such as phosphates, antacids, and dietary products;
3. Excessive blood loss due to chronic or acute bleeding.

Pregnancy, growth spurts, and heavy menstruation cause an increased need for iron. If the iron intake is inadequate, anemia eventually occurs. However, the most common cause of iron-deficiency anemia is chronic blood loss, particularly from the gastrointestinal or genitourinary tract. Until the cause of bleeding is identified and treated, the client is given iron supplements.

Pernicious anemia, or Addison's anemia, is caused by a lack of vitamin B_{12}. For reasons not fully understood, the glandular mucosa of the stomach fundus atrophies, and the stomach fails to secrete adequate quantities of hydrochloric acid to free the iron ingested in food and intrinsic factor to ensure intestinal absorption of vitamin B_{12}. Signs and symptoms include weakness, sore tongue, paresthesia (tingling and numbness) of the extremities, gastrointestinal disturbances including diarrhea, nausea, and vomiting, and eventually cardiac failure. Clients with pernicious anemia will produce normal red blood cells if they receive vitamin B_{12} in adequate quantities; but since the vitamin is not absorbed when taken orally, these clients must receive vitamin B_{12} injections at least once each month.

ANTIANEMIC AGENTS

Drugs used to treat anemia are selected according to the cause of the anemia. Iron supplements are the most frequently used drug and are usually administered orally. Since the absorption of orally administered iron is enhanced by the presence of vitamin C in the intestines, many iron preparations contain vitamin C. If the iron is poorly absorbed when given orally, it may be administered parenterally. Unfortunately, iron tends to stain the skin when administered intramuscularly and must be given by the Z-track method in order to trap the medication in the muscle. When skin staining does occur, it can take months or even years for the discoloration to disappear.

Other substances used to treat anemia include vitamin B_{12}, vitamin B complex, copper sulfate, liver extract, liver injection, folic acid, and glutamic acid. Since the vitamins are explained in Chapter 18, they have been excluded from this chapter. Copper sulfate is used to treat iron-deficiency anemias, since copper is also necessary for the formation of hemoglobin and may be involved in the absorption and transport of iron in the body. Liver extracts and injections have been used for decades, but since the isolation of specific vitamin substances, the liver preparations are seldom used today. Glutamic acid hydrochloride is a chemical combination of an amino acid and hydrochloric acid. This drug is used to treat the hydrochloric acid deficiency that is often associated with pernicious anemia.

ORAL IRON PREPARATIONS

GENERIC NAME Ferrous sulfate (RX)

TRADE NAMES Feosol (Dried), Fer-In-Sol (Dried), Fero-Gradumet, Mol-Iron

CLASSIFICATION Hematopoietic

Action Iron is essential for the normal formation of hemoglobin, myoglobin, and numerous enzymes (cytochromes, cytochrome oxidase) necessary for cellular oxidation. Iron is transferred from its storage sites as the need arises. As the storage sites become depleted, the intestinal mucosa absorbs greater quantities of dietary iron. However, if there is a lack of dietary iron, an iron deficiency occurs which results in hypochromic and often microcytic anemia and alterations in the gastric and esophageal mucosa. Only about 10 to 20% of dietary iron is absorbed in the normal client. A well-balanced diet provides about 10 to 15 mg of iron daily. It is doubtful whether adequate quantities of iron for adolescents, females of childbearing age, pregnancy, and lactation can be met by diet alone; supplemental iron is usually required.

Foods rich in iron include organ meats, particularly liver. Small quantities of iron present in whole wheat bread and cereals, green leafy vegetables, nuts, and legumes are absorbed.

Indications for Use Treatment and prevention of iron-deficiency anemia: hypochromic anemia, malnutrition, chlorosis (iron-deficiency anemia of adolescents). Conditions that may cause malabsorption of iron: lack of gastric hydrochloric acid (gastrectomy), extensive resection of the small intestines (ileostomy), severe or chronic diarrhea, advanced age. Conditions that may cause excessive loss of iron through bleeding: menstruation, lesions of the GI tract (malignancy), advanced age. Chronic blood loss is the most common cause of iron-deficiency anemia (menstruation, slow genitourinary or GI bleeding). States of increased requirement: pregnancy, lactation, infancy (particularly bottle-fed babies), adolescence.

Contraindications Conditions in which there is an excessive accumulation of iron: hemosiderosis, repeated blood transfusions, hemochromatosis (bronzed diabetes), hemolytic anemia.

Warnings and Precautions Use with caution in clients with a preexisting GI disorder that may be aggravated by supplemental oral iron preparations: peptic ulcer, ulcerative colitis, regional enteritis.

Untoward Reactions Although an overdose of oral iron preparations is relatively nontoxic to adults, the accidental ingestion of 1 g or more may cause acute toxicity in infants and young children. The signs and symptoms of GI irritation occur within 30 minutes (nausea, vomiting, hematemesis, diarrhea of green stools). The progressive necrosis of the stomach and small intestines results in acidosis and shock due to cardiovascular collapse (pallor, lethargy, drowsiness, tarry stools). Death usually occurs within 48 hours. Survivors will have severe gastric scarring and may develop pyloric stenosis. Severe rickets due to interference of phosphorus assimilation may occur in infants who ingest large dosages over a long period of time. GI disturbances due to irritation are common and include diarrhea, abdominal cramps, epigastric distress, and constipation. Staining of the teeth may occur with liquid oral preparations. Stools turn a harmless black color. Secondary hemosiderosis (iron overload) can occur, but rarely.

Parameters of Use

Absorption Primarily from the duodenum, jejunum, stomach, and proximal portion of the ileum. As the severity of the iron deficiency increases, the absorption of iron increases. Ascorbic acid increases the absorption of iron by inhibiting the formation of the less soluble ferric form. Normal serum iron levels: 70 to 170 mcg/100 ml; Normal iron-binding capacity: 275 to 380 mcg/100 ml.

Distribution About 75% in hemoglobin (70% in red blood cells and 5% in myoglobin). About 20% stored in liver, spleen, and bone marrow as ferritin or hemosiderin and about 5% in various other tissues. Iron is carried by transferrin (a beta-globulin) to the bone marrow and other distribution sites (free ionized iron is toxic). Normally, one-third of transferrin is in use at any one time. Transferrin levels may vary with changes in tissue oxygenation and protein synthesis. When red blood cells are destroyed, most of the iron is transported back to hematopoietic centers for reuse in hemoglobin synthesis. A single blood transfusion may contain as much as 200 to 250 mg of iron; this iron is also recycled by the body. Excessive storage of iron can occur with multiple blood transfusions and may cause hemosiderin deposits in body organs (secondary hemochromatosis).

Excretion Minimal amounts excreted (0.5 to 1.0 mg daily); primarily by ferritin being sloughed off with epithelial cells of the GI tract or skin. Trace amounts excreted in urine, sweat, and nails.

Drug Interactions Antacids and pancreatic extracts inhibit the absorption of iron by forcing insoluble complexes. Tetracycline inhibits iron absorption and vice versa. Multivitamin preparations containing vitamin E may inhibit iron absorption, particularly in children; do not give concurrently. Ascorbic acid (vitamin C) enhances the absorption of oral iron preparations; between 50 to 100 mg may be given concomitantly. The chelating agent dimercaprol forms a toxic iron-chelating complex and should not be used. The chelating agent deferoxamine mesylate has a high affinity for ferric ions and is used as an antidote for iron poisoning. Oral contraceptives may increase the amount of iron bound to serum proteins. Dairy products, particularly milk and eggs, interfere with the absorption of oral iron preparations. The phytic acid content of cereals interferes with the absorption of oral iron preparations by forming nonabsorbable chelating complexes. Large quantities of fruit juices containing vitamin C may enhance the absorption of oral iron preparations.

Laboratory Interactions Large dosages of iron may cause false-positive results for occult blood in the stools with *o*-toluidine and guaiac reagent; but the benzidine test is unaffected.

Administration Highly individualized. Adults: 300 mg po daily is commonly used in mild deficiency states; 600 to 1200 mg po daily is commonly used in severe deficiency states. Children: 120 to 600 mg po daily in divided doses.

Available Drug Forms Film-coated tablets containing 300 mg; enteric-coated tablets containing 300 mg; liquid containing 125 mg/ml or 300 mg/5 ml; timed-release capsules containing 250 mg; Graduments containing 525 mg. Also an ingredient in several multivitamin preparations. Preparations contain 65 mg of elemental iron in 300 mg of ferrous sulfate or 365 mg of dried ferrous sulfate.

Nursing Management

Planning factors

1. Obtain complete history to determine potential causes of blood loss and the normal dietary intake of iron before instituting therapy. Consult a dietitian and physician, as needed.
2. Obtain baseline data, including complete blood cell count (CBC), serum iron, and iron-binding capacity, prior to instituting therapy. A serum bilirubin and bone marrow test are also helpful in determining the type of anemia.
3. Schedule drug therapy between meals, since food

inhibits absorption. In addition, drug administration in early morning and late evening should be avoided because GI irritation may result.

4. Divided doses are required in children to prevent GI irritation.
5. Avoid giving iron preparations with interacting drugs (antacids).
6. Store drug in a dry area away from children.
7. The recommended daily allowance varies with body size, rate of growth, and the presence of menstruation. The average allowances are: Males: 10 mg; Females: 18 mg (during childbearing years); Infants: 6 to 15 mg; Adolescents: 18 mg; Children: 10 mg; pregnancy: 18 mg; Lactation: 18 mg.

Administration factors

1. When administering liquid iron preparations,
   a. Use a straw placed as far back in the mouth as is comfortable to avoid staining of the teeth. Client should rinse the mouth with plain water after ingestion.
   b. Give with a large quantity of water (8 fl oz), since some liquid preparations are incompatible with fruit juices or milk (Feosol Elixir). Most of the pediatric drops (Fer-In-Sol) are compatible with water or fruit juices.
2. When administering tablets,
   a. Give with a full glass of orange juice or water.
   b. Client should avoid milk or dairy products for 1 hour before and after drug administration.
   c. If client has difficulty swallowing the tablet, a liquid preparation can be given. Consult physician, as needed.

Evaluation factors

1. If client develops gastric distress, notify physician. Reducing the dosage, using an enteric-coated tablet or sustained-release capsule, or changing to a better tolerated iron preparation (ferrous gluconate) may be required.
2. Sustained-release capsules may not provide a satisfactory response, since the iron in these capsules may be released in the lower intestines and therefore be poorly absorbed.
3. The signs and symptoms of iron deficiency usually respond to some degree within 2 days of therapeutic dosages, particularly in children. The appetite increases, the client feels more energetic and less irritable, and dysphagia may disappear. CBC begins to improve within 5 days and usually returns to normal in 2 to 3 weeks.
4. Monitor the blood picture (CBC) weekly.
5. If an appreciable improvement does not occur within 3 weeks, the cause of anemia may still be present, the client may have developed an infection, inadequate absorption may be occurring, or the client may not be complying with drug therapy on a regular basis. Long-term therapy is required (3 to 6 months).
6. Iron and vitamin C drug preparations may be required for inadequate absorption.
7. Treatment of an overdose consists of inducing vomiting quickly, giving dairy products (milk), gastric lavage within the first hour (sodium bicarbonate solution), and instilling iron-chelating drugs (deferoxamine).

Client teaching factors

1. Warn client that drug may cause black or tarry stools.
2. Emphasize the importance of keeping the drug away from children, since deaths in children have occurred from accidental overdose.
3. Instruct client to store tablets and capsules in a dry area (not the kitchen or bathroom).
4. Demonstrate how liquid preparations should be taken.
5. Inform client that mild irritation can be avoided by taking the drug between meals and not in early morning or late evening. If a light breakfast is normally eaten, client should take the drug in the middle of the afternoon. If irritation persists, client should notify physician.
6. Explain to client the necessity of maintaining laboratory appointments to monitor the drug's effectiveness.
7. Diet education of client and family may assist in avoiding iron-deficiency anemias in the future.

GENERIC NAME Ferrous fumarate (OTC) (RX)

TRADE NAMES Feostat, Ferranol, Fumerin, Hemocyte, Ircon, Laud-Iron, Palmiron, Span-FF, Toleron

CLASSIFICATION Hematopoietic

See ferrous sulfate for Indications for use, Contraindications, Warnings and precautions, Untoward reactions, Parameters of use, Drug interactions, and Nursing management.

Action Ferrous fumarate is an iron preparation similar to ferrous sulfate. Although it is more expensive, ferrous fumarate does not deteriorate as rapidly as ferrous sulfate and does not need to be protected against oxidation. (See ferrous sulfate.)

Administration Highly individualized. Adults and older children: 200 mg po daily or bid; Dosage range: 200 to 800 mg daily. Children: Under 6 years: 100 to 300 mg po daily in divided doses.

Available Drug Forms Tablets containing 200 or 325 mg; chocolate-flavored chewable tablets containing 100 mg; capsules containing 325 mg; suspension containing 100 mg/5 ml; pediatric drops containing 45 mg/0.6 ml. Preparations contain 33 mg of elemental iron in 100 mg of ferrous fumarate.

GENERIC NAME Ferrous gluconate (OTC) (RX)

TRADE NAMES Fergon, Ferralet

CLASSIFICATION Hematopoietic

See ferrous sulfate for Indications for use, Contraindications, Warnings and precautions, Untoward reactions, Parameters of use, Drug interactions, and Nursing management.

Action Ferrous gluconate is an iron preparation similar to ferrous sulfate. Although it is considerably more expensive than ferrous sulfate, ferrous gluconate appears to be better tolerated and results in fewer GI disturbances. (See ferrous sulfate.)

Administration Highly individualized. Adults: 200 to 600 mg po daily; Children: Ages 6 to 12 years: 100 to 300 mg po tid; Under 6 years: 100 to 300 mg po tid in divided doses; Infants: 30 gtt po daily.

Available Drug Forms Tablets containing 300 or 434 mg; elixir containing 320 mg/5 ml; pediatric drops containing 64 mg/ml. Preparations contain about 37 mg of elemental iron in 320 mg of ferrous gluconate.

GENERIC NAME Ferrocholinate (RX)

TRADE NAMES Chel-Iron, Ferrolip

CLASSIFICATION Hematopoietic

See ferrous sulfate for Indications for use, Contraindications, Warnings and precautions, Untoward reactions, Parameters of use, Drug interactions, and Nursing management.

Action Since ferrocholinate is a chelated compound, it is not absorbed as well as ferrous sulfate and causes fewer untoward reactions. (See ferrous sulfate.)

Administration Adults: 330 mg po tid; Infants and children under 6 years: 104 mg po daily in divided doses.

Available Drug Forms Tablets containing 330 mg. Also available as syrup or solution. Preparations contain 40 mg in 1 tablet or 10 mg/ml of solution of elemental iron in 330 mg of ferrocholinate.

GENERIC NAME Ferrous carbonate (RX)

CLASSIFICATION Hematopoietic

See ferrous sulfate for Indications for use, Contraindications, Warnings and precautions, Untoward reactions, Parameters of use, Drug interactions, and Nursing management.

Action Similar to ferrous sulfate, but not recommended for children. (See ferrous sulfate.)

Administration Adults: 1 tablet po tid.

Available Drug Forms An ingredient of some multivitamin and mineral preparations. Preparations contain 66.7 mg of elemental iron.

GENERIC NAME Ferric pyrophosphate (RX)

CLASSIFICATION Hematopoietic

See ferrous sulfate for Indications for use, Contraindications, Warnings and precautions, Untoward reactions, Parameters of use, Drug interactions, and Nursing management.

Action Similar to ferrous sulfate, but not recommended for children. (See ferrous sulfate.)

Administration Adults: 30 ml po daily.

Available Drug Forms An ingredient of some multivitamin and mineral preparations, including Rouite Tonic. Preparations contain 20 mg elemental iron in 30 ml.

IRON AND VITAMIN C PREPARATIONS

Since it increases the absorption of iron, vitamin C is added to several iron preparations. (See ferrous sulfate and vitamin C.)

TRADE NAME Fe-O.D. (RX)

CLASSIFICATION Hematopoietic

Administration 1 tablet po daily or bid.

Available Drug Forms Generic contents in each yellow tablet: ferrous fumarate: 300 mg; ascorbic acid: 500 mg. Time release base. Contains 100 mg of elemental iron in 300 mg of ferrous fumarate.

TRADE NAME Ferancee (OTC) (RX)

CLASSIFICATION Hematopoietic

Untoward Reactions Hypersensitivity reactions (bronchoconstriction) to FD&C No. 5 yellow may occur.

Administration 1 tablet po daily or bid.

Available Drug Forms Generic contents in each brown and yellow tablet: ferrous fumarate: 200 mg; ascorbic acid: 49 mg; sodium ascorbate: 114 mg. Also contains FD&C No. 5 yellow (tartrazine) as a color additive. Contains 67 mg of elemental iron in 200 mg of ferrous fumarate.

TRADE NAME Ferancee-HP (OTC) (RX)

CLASSIFICATION Hematopoietic

Untoward Reactions Hypersensitivity reaction (bronchoconstriction) to FD&C No. 5 yellow may occur.

Administration Adults over 12 years: 1 tablet po daily, bid, or tid.

Available Drug Forms Generic contents in each red tablet: ferrous fumarate: 330 mg; ascorbic acid: 350 mg; sodium ascorbate: 281 mg. Also contains FD&C No. 5 yellow. Contains 110 mg of elemental iron in 330 mg of ferrous fumarate.

TRADE NAME Fero-Grad-500 (RX)

CLASSIFICATION Hematopoietic

Administration 1 Gradument po daily or bid.

Available Drug Forms Generic contents in each red tablet: ferrous sulfate: 525 mg; sodium ascorbate: 500 mg. Controlled-release drug form. Contains 105 mg of elemental iron in 525 mg of ferrous sulfate.

TRADE NAME Mol-Iron Chronosule with Vitamin C

CLASSIFICATION Hematopoietic (OTC)

Untoward Reactions Hypersensitivity reaction (bronchoconstriction) to FD&C No. 5 yellow may occur.

Administration 1 capsule po daily or bid.

Available Drug Forms Generic contents in each capsule: ferrous sulfate: 390 mg; ascorbic acid: 150 mg. Sustained-release drug form. Also contains FD&C No. 5 yellow. Contains 75 mg of elemental iron in 390 mg of ferrous sulfate.

IRON PLUS OTHER ADDITIVE PREPARATIONS

TRADE NAME Fermalox (OTC)

CLASSIFICATION Hematopoietic

Action May be better tolerated by some clients. Less iron absorption occurs than when pure ferrous sulfate is administered.

Administration 1 to 2 tablets po daily.

Available Drug Forms Generic contents in each tablet: ferrous sulfate: 200 mg; magnesium and aluminum hydroxide (Maalox): 200 mg. Contains 43 mg of elemental iron in 200 mg of ferrous sulfate.

TRADE NAME Ferro-Sequels (OTC)

CLASSIFICATION Hematopoietic

Administration 1 capsule po daily or bid.

Available Drug Forms Generic contents in each green capsule: ferrous fumarate: 100 mg. Sustained-release drug form (5 to 6 hours). Also contains docusate sodium 100 mg to counteract constipation. Contains 50 mg of elemental iron in 100 mg of ferrous fumarate.

TRADE NAME Simron (OTC)

CLASSIFICATION Hematopoietic

Administration 1 capsule po tid.

Available Drug Forms Generic contents in each maroon, soft-gelatin capsule: ferrous gluconate: 86 mg. Also contains polysorbate 20 (Sacagen) 400 mg to enhance iron absorption and counteract constipation. Contains 10 mg of elemental iron in 86 mg of ferrous gluconate.

TRADE NAME Simron Plus (OTC)

CLASSIFICATION Hematopoietic

Administration 1 capsule po tid.

Available Drug Forms Generic contents in each maroon, soft-gelatin capsule: ferrous gluconate: 86 mg. Also contains: polysorbate 20: 400 mg; vitamin C (sodium ascorbate): 50 mg; pyridoxine HCl (B_6): 1 mg; folic acid: 0.1 mg; cyanocobalamin (B_{12}): 3.33 mcg. Contains 10 mg of elemental iron in 86 mg of ferrous gluconate.

INJECTABLE IRON PREPARATIONS

GENERIC NAME Iron dextran (RX)

TRADE NAMES Dextraron-50, Hematran, Imferon, K-FeRon, Proferdex

CLASSIFICATION Hematopoietic

Action Iron complexed with dextran is a sterile colloidal solution of ferric hydroxide that can be administered parenterally. Since oral iron preparations are inexpensive, usually effective in iron-deficiency anemia, and produce relatively few untoward reactions, the use of injectable iron is restricted to clients who are either unresponsive to iron salts or are unable to take them. Iron is essential for the normal function of hemoglobin, myoglobin, and numerous enzymes necessary for cellular oxidation. Iron deficiency results in hypochromic and often microcytic anemia and alterations in the gastric and esophageal mucosa.

Indications for Use Used only when oral iron salts are ineffective or impractical, such as GI disorders, inability to absorb adequate quantities of oral iron, intolerance to oral salts, and noncompliance. Treatment and prevention of iron-deficiency anemia: hypochromic anemia, malnutrition, excessive loss of iron through bleeding, states of increased requirement. (See ferrous sulfate.)

Contraindications Hypersensitivity to iron dextran; conditions in which there is an excessive accumulation of iron: hemosiderosis, repeated blood transfusions, hemochromatosis (bronzed diabetes), hemolytic anemia; all anemias other than iron-deficiency anemia; severe hepatic impairment.

Warnings and Precautions Use with caution in clients known to have multiple allergies or asthma; during pregnancy, since an increase in the number of stillbirths and fatal anomalies has occurred in test animals (benefits should outweigh risks in pregnancy and women of childbearing potential); and in clients with rheumatoid arthritis, since an acute swelling and pain may occur, particularly following intravenous drug therapy. Unnecessary parenteral iron therapy will cause excessive iron storage and will eventually cause hemosiderosis. Large dosages have been shown to be carcinogenic in test animals (sarcomas in rats, mice, and rabbits).

Untoward Reactions Hypersensitivity reactions, including anaphylaxis (which may be fatal), bronchospasm, dyspnea, and urticaria, have occurred within 30 minutes of injection. Rashes, pruritus, arthralgia, myalgia, fever, and sweating have also occurred. Irritation at the injection site occurs frequently. Pain, inflammation, and soreness may persist. Intramuscular sites may develop sterile abscesses and a brown discoloration of the skin due to drug leakage into subcutaneous tissue, which may persist for 1 or 2 years. Local phlebitis may occur following intravenous injection. Secondary hemochromatosis, the excessive storage of iron (hemosiderin deposits) in tissue, can occur. Intravenous administration may result in peripheral vascular flushing, particularly if the rate of administration is too rapid. Cardiovascular reactions, including hypotension, chest pain, tachycardia, arrhythmias, and transient paresthesia, have occurred, particularly following intravenous administration. Neurologic reactions, including dizziness and convulsions, have occurred. Leukocytosis (with or without fever) and regional lymphadenopathy have been reported. Exacerbation of rheumatoid arthritis has occurred in susceptible clients, particularly after intravenous administration. Other reactions include headache, nausea, vomiting, and shivering.

Parameters of Use

Absorption Slowly absorbed from intramuscular sites (over 50% in the first 3 days and almost 90% within 3 weeks); residual deposits may not be completely absorbed for several months. Drug is removed from these sites by the lymphatic system. Iron dextran complex is dissociated by the reticuloendothelial system, particularly the liver. Normal serum iron levels: 70 to 170 mcg/100 ml; Normal iron-binding capacity: 275 to 380 mcg/100 ml.

Distribution About 75% in hemoglobin (70% in red blood cells and 5% in myoglobin). About 20% stored in liver, spleen, and bone marrow as ferritin or hemosiderin and about 5% in various other tissues. Iron is carried by transferrin (a beta-globulin) to the bone marrow and other distribution sites (free ionized iron is toxic). Normally, one-third of transferrin is in use at any one time. Transferrin levels may vary with changes in tissue oxygenation and protein synthesis. When red blood cells are destroyed, most of the iron is transported back to hematopoietic centers for reuse in hemoglobin synthesis. A single blood transfusion may contain as much as 200 to 250 mg of iron; this iron is also recycled by the body. Excessive storage of iron can occur with multiple blood transfusions and may cause hemosiderin deposits in body organs (secondary hemochromatosis).

Excretion Minimal amounts excreted (0.5 to 1.0 mg daily); primarily by ferritin being sloughed off with epithelial cells of the GI tract or skin. Trace amounts excreted in urine, sweat, and nails. Excretion cannot be enhanced when toxicity occurs.

Drug Interactions The chelating agent deferoxamine mesylate has a high affinity for ferric ions and is used as an antidote for iron poisoning. The chelating agent dimercaprol forms a toxic iron-chelating complex and should not be used. Oral contraceptives may increase the amount of iron bound to serum proteins.

Laboratory Interactions Large dosages of iron may cause false-positive results from occult blood in the stools with *o*-toluidine and guaiac reagent; but the benzidine test is unaffected.

Administration Dosage varies according to the client's body weight and amount of iron depletion in hemoglobin (Hgb) and iron stores. Bone marrow biopsy can give an estimate of total iron store depletion. Serum iron provides an estimate of iron depletion. Formula for estimating total dosage (mg) required to restore Hgb and replenish iron stores is: $0.3 \times$ body weight in lb $\times$ (100 − Hgb in g/dl $\times$ 100)/14.8. Factors to be considered in the formula are: blood volume—8.5% of body weight; normal Hgb—14.8 g/dl; iron content of Hgb—0.34%; Hgb deficit and weight. Substitute 12.0 g/dl for normal Hgb in children under 30 lb. The dosage is divided and given over several days. A test dose of 25 mg (0.5 ml) IM or IV should be given. Adults: 250 mg (5 ml) IM or 100 mg (2 ml) IV daily or every other day; adults under 110 lb require smaller daily dosages. Infants and children: Under 10 lb: 25 mg IM daily or every other day; 10 to 20 lb: 50 mg IM daily or every other day; 20 to 110 lb: Up to 100 mg IM daily or every other day.

Available Drug Forms Ampules of 2 or 5 ml containing 50 mg iron/ml; 10-ml multidose vials containing 50 mg iron/ml for IM use only (contains 0.5% phenol as a preservative).

Nursing Management

Planning factors

1. Obtain complete history to determine potential causes of blood loss and the normal dietary intake of iron before instituting therapy. Consult a dietitian and physician, as needed.
2. Obtain baseline data, including complete blood cell count (CBC), serum bilirubin, bone marrow, and other laboratory procedures, to determine the type of anemia and the iron requirements.
3. Administration of oral iron salts should be attempted before considering parenteral administration.
4. Discontinue oral iron salts before starting parenteral iron.
5. Calculate the iron requirements and record total needs on medication record or Cardex.

Administration factors

1. A test dose of 25 mg (0.5 ml) must be given on the first day. If no hypersensitivity reactions occur, drug therapy may begin the next day or several hours later.
2. When administering IM,
   a. Use a 2- or 3-in., 19- or 20-gauge needle.
   b. Place client in supine position before administering injection.
   c. Inject deep into muscle mass of the upper outer quadrant of the buttocks. Since drug may cause staining of skin, never use the arm or an exposed area for injection.
   d. Inject using the Z-track method to avoid infiltration into subcutaneous tissue and eventual staining of the skin. Add a small air bubble into syringe (0.5 ml). Displace the skin laterally and inject needle. Be sure to aspirate to prevent accidental IV administration. Inject medication away from the needle.
   e. Rotate injection sites and record.
   f. Do not inject more than 5 ml in one injection site.
   g. IV administration may be required for clients with small muscle masses.
3. When administering IV,
   a. Be sure to withdraw dose from an ampule for IV use.
   b. Place client in supine position before administering drug.
   c. Check patency of IV site.
   d. Inject medication slowly over 5 minutes or more. Do not exceed 50 mg/min. A syringe pump is recommended.
   e. Instruct client to remain in bed for 1 hour to prevent untoward reactions.

Evaluation factors

1. Observe client for at least 1 hour following test dose. Hypersensitivity reactions usually occur within 10 to 60 minutes. If a hypersensitivity reaction occurs, notify physician immediately and follow agency protocol.
2. If the drug is initiated in an outpatient facility, retain client for at least 1 hour. Examine client before discharging.
3. The signs and symptoms of iron deficiency usually improve to some degree within 2 days. The appetite increases, the client feels more energetic and less irritable, and dysphagia may disappear. CBC begins to improve within 5 days and usually returns to normal in 2 to 3 weeks.
4. Monitor the blood picture (CBC) weekly or biweekly.
5. If an appreciable improvement does not occur within 3 weeks, the cause of anemia may still be present, the client may have developed an infection, inadequate absorption may be occurring, or the client may not be complying with drug therapy on a regular basis.
6. The use of iron salts should replace parenteral administration as soon as possible.

Client teaching factors

1. Warn client that skin may remain discolored at injection sites for 1 to 2 years.
2. Inform client to report any unusual signs and symptoms immediately, particularly those that occur within 24 hours of drug administration.
3. Explain to client the necessity of frequent laboratory examinations to monitor the drug's effectiveness.
4. Diet education of client and family may assist in avoiding iron-deficiency anemias in the future.

GENERIC NAME Iron sorbitex (RX)

TRADE NAME Jectofer

CLASSIFICATION Hematopoietic

See ferrous sulfate for Indications for use. See iron dextran for Drug interactions.

Action Iron complexed with sorbitol and citric acid is a sterile aqueous solution that can be administered intramuscularly. Iron sorbitex is similar to iron dextran and contains 50 mg of elemental iron per millimeter.

Contraindications Severe renal impairment. (See iron dextran.)

Warnings and Precautions Use with caution in clients with active urinary tract infections. Use in children is not recommended until further testing is completed. (See iron dextran.)

Untoward Reactions Urinary tract reactions, including urinary frequency, hematuria, and albuminuria, have been reported. Secondary organ reactions, including a transient alteration in taste, blurred vision, and hearing impairment, have been reported. (See iron dextran.)

Parameters of Use

Absorption Rapidly absorbed into the bloodstream. Although injections are painful, there is little residual accumulation at injection site. Peak serum levels occur within 2 hours. Distribution to bone marrow and other sites occurs within 3 days.

Distribution (See iron dextran.)

Excretion Primarily by the kidneys within 24 hours. Some excreted in feces and saliva. Urinary excretion may cause damage to the kidneys.

Administration Total dosage is determined by using formula (see iron dextran). 1.5 mg/kg IM daily (100 to 200 mg daily); do not exceed 250 mg (5 ml) daily.

Available Drug Forms Multidose vials of 10 ml containing 50 mg iron/ml.

Nursing Management (See iron dextran.)

1. Cannot be administered intravenously.
2. Warn client about harmless brown discoloration of urine.
3. Frequent oral hygiene may be required due to excretion in saliva.

GENERIC NAME Dextriferron (RX)

TRADE NAME Astrafer

CLASSIFICATION Hematopoietic

See ferrous sulfate and iron dextran for Indications for use, Contraindications, Warnings and precautions, Untoward reactions, Parameters of use, and Drug interactions.

Action Iron complexed with dextrin is a sterile collodial solution of ferric hydroxide that can be administered intravenously. Dextriferron is similar to iron dextran, but this preparation contains only 20 mg of elemental iron per milliliter.

Administration Total dosage is determined by using formula (see iron dextran). Therapy is started 2 to 3 days after test dose (30 mg, or 1.5 ml, IV). Dosage is increased in increments of 20 to 30 mg until a maximum daily dosage of 100 mg (5 ml) is attained.

Available Drug Forms Ampules of 5 ml containing 20 mg iron/ml.

Nursing Management (See iron dextran.)

1. Administer slowly by IV injection. A rate of 20 mg/min. is recommended to prevent untoward reactions.
2. Hypersensitivity reactions usually occur within 10 to 60 minutes of test dose, but may take several hours.
3. Delayed hypersensitivity and other untoward reactions may occur if dosage is increased too rapidly.

ANTIDOTES—IRON POISONING

GENERIC NAME Deferoxamine mesylate (RX)

TRADE NAME Desferal

CLASSIFICATION Iron poisoning antidote

Source Trihydroxamic acid, a compound isolated from *Streptomyces pilosus*.

Action This compound is a chelating agent with an affinity for ferric ions. It forms a water-soluble chelate that is excreted by the kidneys. Although excessive tissue iron (ferritin and hemosiderin) is removed, the drug does not displace appreciable quantities of iron from transferrin, hemoglobin, and other essential proteins. Deferoxamine does not disrupt or chelate other metals, such as calcium and copper, theoretically. Approximately 8.5 mg of iron can be chelated by 100 mg of deferoxamine. There is little or no increase in the excretion of electrolytes and trace metals.

Indications for Use As an adjunct to standard measures in treating acute iron intoxication. Also used in secondary hemosiderosis due to multiple blood transfusions, hemolytic anemia, accidental overdose, and other causes of chronic iron overload.

Contraindications Hypersensitivity to drug, severe renal impairment, anuria, children under 3 years.

Warnings and Precautions Use with caution in clients with impaired renal function; exacerbation has been reported in clients with chronic renal infections. Not indicated for the treatment of primary hemochromatosis. Benefits should outweigh the risks in women of childbearing age, since animal studies have indicated that fetal skeletal anomalies can occur.

Untoward Reactions Urticaria, hypotension, generalized erythema, and shock may occur due to a release of histamine, particularly after rapid intravenous infusion. Hypersensitivity reactions, including generalized itching, rashes (cutaneous wheals), and anaphylaxis, have occurred. Localized pain may occur at injection sites. Localized pruritus, erythema, inflammation, and other signs of skin irritation may occur after subcutaneous injection. Cataracts may develop with prolonged drug therapy. Other reactions include blurred vision, dysuria, abdominal discomfort, diarrhea, leg cramps, tachycardia, and fever.

Parameters of Use

Absorption Fairly well absorbed from intramuscular and subcutaneous sites. Less than 15% absorbed from GI tract; an unabsorbable iron complex is produced within the lumen of the GI tract.

Metabolism By plasma enzymes; but mechanism is unknown.

Excretion Rapidly by the kidneys; some excreted via bile and eliminated in feces.

Administration Highly individualized. Maximum dosage: 6 g/day.

- *Acute iron toxicity:* Initial dosage: 1 g IM or IV followed by 0.5 g IM q4h times 2 doses; then 0.5 g IM every 4 to 12 hours, as needed.
- *Acute iron toxicity with cardiovascular collapse:* Initial dosage: 1 g IV followed by 0.5 g IV q4h times 2 doses (but do not exceed 15 mg/kg/hour); then 0.5 g IV every 4 to 12 hours, as needed.
- *Chronic iron overload:* 0.5 to 1 g IM daily. If blood transfusions are required, an additional 2 g should be given IV for each unit of blood or 1 to 2 g (20 to 40 mg/kg) daily over 8 to 24 hours.

Available Drug Forms Vials containing 500 mg of dried powder for reconstitution with 2 ml of sterile water to yield 250 mg/ml.

Nursing Management

Planning factors

1. Obtain baseline data, including complete blood cell count, serum iron, iron-binding capacity, serum bilirubin, and renal function tests, before instituting therapy.
2. Protect reconstituted solution from light; discard after 7 days.
3. Obtain baseline vital signs.
4. Each unit of blood contains 200 to 250 mg of iron.

Administration factors

1. Deferoxamine does not dissolve quickly. Be sure all powder is dissolved before withdrawing desired dose. Label vial with concentration and date of reconstitution.
2. When administering IM,
   a. Inject deep into large muscle mass.
   b. Rotate sites.
   c. Monitor vital signs every 15 to 30 minutes.
3. When administering by IV infusion,
   a. Reserved for clients in shock.
   b. Do not give as IV bolus unless carefully calibrated syringe pump is available.
   c. Dilute reconstituted solution in 50 or 100 ml (or more) of normal saline, glucose in water, or Ringer's lactate.
   d. Check patency of IV before administering drug.
   e. Rate of administration is prescribed by physician; do not exceed 15 mg/kg/hour.
   f. Monitor vital signs every 5 to 15 minutes. If hypersensitivity reaction occurs, turn medication off but keep IV open with nonmedicated IV solution and notify physician immediately.
   g. An infusion pump is highly recommended.
   h. Discontinue IV administration as soon as client's condition permits.
4. When administering subcutaneously,
   a. Reserved for the administration of frequent small dosages to clients with chronic iron overload.
   b. A small portable pump capable of providing continuous minidoses is recommended.
   c. Administer over 8 to 12 hours daily for best results.

Evaluation factors

1. Carefully observe client for hypersensitivity reaction during the first 24 hours following initiation of therapy.
2. Monitor vital signs at least once a shift after client's condition has stabilized.
3. Record intake and output. If an imbalance occurs, notify physician.
4. Obtain hematopoietic (serum iron) and renal function tests frequently (daily) when therapy is initiated. Periodic examinations (weekly or biweekly) are adequate when prolonged therapy is required.
5. Perform split-lamp eye examinations weekly or biweekly when prolonged therapy is required.

Client teaching factors

1. Warn client about harmless red discoloration of urine.
2. Emphasize the necessity of frequent laboratory examinations.
3. Inform client to report any unusual signs and symptoms immediately.

OTHER HEMATOPOIETIC SUBSTANCES

GENERIC NAMES Copper sulfate; cupric oxide

CLASSIFICATION Hematopoietic (OTC) (RX)

Action Copper and iron are interrelated and function together in several metabolic activities. Like iron, copper is essential for the formation of hemoglobin and enzymes required for cellular oxygenation. Copper may assist in the absorption of iron from the GI tract and the transport of iron from the tissues into blood. Although an actual copper-deficiency state is unknown in humans, hypocupremia (or low serum copper levels) may occur in malnutrition, malabsorption disorders, such as sprue and celiac disease, and in nephrosis. The latter disorder can induce the excretion of ceruloplasmin, which is a copper-bound serum protein. Once the underlying condition and iron deficiency are treated, serum levels return to normal. Copper is widely distributed in nature and an adequate caloric intake of food supplies more than ample quantities of copper. There is no evidence to indicate the need for prophylactic or therapeutic copper supplements.

Indications for Use Treatment and prevention of hypocupremia and iron-deficiency anemias.

Parameters of Use

Absorption Well absorbed from the proximal end of the small intestines. Mechanism of absorption has not been established. Serum copper levels: Men: 70 to 140 mcg/100 ml; Women: 85 to 155 mcg/100 ml. Normal values are considerably lower in neonates and somewhat lower in young children.

Distribution Liver, red blood cells, muscles, bone, kidneys, and CNS. Ceruloplasmin is thought to be synthesized in the liver. Transported from intestines to liver bound to serum proteins. About 90% of serum copper is bound to the alpha-globulin ceruloplasmin. Some serum copper is unbound and may diffuse across the glomerular membrane and be excreted in urine.

Excretion In feces, urine, and sweat.

Drug Interactions Estrogen therapy may elevate serum copper levels.

Administration Small quantities (1 to 3 mg) added to some multivitamin and mineral preparations.

Available Drug Forms An ingredient of several multivitamin and mineral preparations, including Hemo-Vite, Optilets-M-500, Vio-Bec Forte, and Berocca Plus (cupric oxide).

Nursing Management

1. Daily requirements have not been established.
2. The average diet contains 2 to 5 mg daily.

GENERIC NAME Liver extract (RX)

CLASSIFICATION Hematopoietic

Source Purified liver extract from mammals (calf liver).

Action Liver extract is no longer an official preparation, but is present in some multivitamin preparations. Besides being an expensive product, liver extract is poorly tolerated orally.

Warnings and Precautions Unreliable for treating pernicious anemia.

Parameters of Use

Absorption Irregular and incomplete.

Distribution By the blood to the liver and other sites.

Untoward Reactions GI disturbances include nausea, vomiting, and diarrhea.

Available Drug Forms An ingredient of some hematopoietic agents, including Hep-Forte.

GENERIC NAME Liver injection (RX)

TRADE NAME Pernaemon

CLASSIFICATION Hematopoietic

Source Purified liver fraction from mammals (calf liver).

Action Before the specific causes of anemia were identified, liver injections were used to treat anemia. Liver extract contains vitamin B_{12}, folic acid, folinic acid, and other substances. Its potency is measured by its vitamin B_{12} activity (1 to 2 mcg of cyanocobalamin per milliliter of extract). Liver injections are seldom used today. (See vitamin B_{12} in Chapter 18.)

Indications for Use Pernicious anemia and other forms of anemia. Has been used in anemia associated with alcoholism and malnutrition.

Contraindications Hypersensitivity to liver extract or any constituents.

Administration Adults: 1 mcg IM daily (7 to 15 mcg weekly); 1 mcg is equal to 1 U.S.P. unit.

Available Drug Forms Ampules containing 10 or 20 mcg/ml; multidose vials containing 10 or 20 mcg/ml. An ingredient in some hematopoietic agents, including Albaforte and Hemocyte.

GENERIC NAME Glutamic acid hydrochloride

TRADE NAME Acidulin (OTC)

CLASSIFICATION Hematopoietic–gastric acidifier

Source Produced synthetically by chemical combination of the amino acid and hydrochloric acid.

Action Glutamic acid not only acidifies the stomach, but is a necessary component for the biosynthesis of folic acid. This compound quickly dissociates upon contact with water in the stomach. Glutamic acid counteracts a deficiency of hydrochloric acid in the gastric juices. A deficiency of hydrochloric acid is often associated with pernicious anemia. Glutamic acid is tasteless, safe to carry, and does not discolor the teeth or injure mucous membranes.

Indications for Use Achlorhydria due to pernicious anemia.

Contraindications Gastric hyperacidity, gastric or peptic ulcer.

Untoward Reactions Systemic acidosis may occur, particularly when excessive quantities are ingested.

Administration 1 to 3 capsules or Pulvules po tid (600 to 1800 mg daily).

Available Drug Forms Capsules containing 200 mg; Pulvules containing 340 mg. Also an ingredient of several digestion aids.

Nursing Management

1. Give immediately before or during meals.
2. 340 mg of glutamic acid is equal to about 10 minims of diluted hydrochloric acid.

THERAPEUTIC ORAL HEMATOPOIETIC PREPARATIONS

TRADE NAME Chromagen (RX)

CLASSIFICATION Hematopoietic

Administration Adults: 1 capsule po daily.

Available Drug Forms Generic contents in each capsule: Vitamins: C (ascorbic acid): 250 mg; B_{12} (cyanocobalamin): 10 mcg. Minerals: ferrous fumarate: 200 mg. Contains 66 mg of elemental iron in 200 mg of ferrous fumarate. Also contains dessicated stomach substance 100 mg.

TRADE NAME Fergon Plus (RX)

CLASSIFICATION Hematopoietic

Indications for Use Sometimes used to supplement parenteral drug therapy for pernicious anemia.

Administration 1 Caplet po daily or bid.

Available Drug Forms Generic contents in each caplet: Vitamins: C (ascorbic acid): 75 mg; B_{12} (cyanocobalamin) with intrinsic factor: $\frac{1}{2}$ NF unit. Minerals: ferrous fumarate: 500 mg. Contains 58 mg of elemental iron in 500 mg of ferrous fumarate.

TRADE NAME Fero-Folic-500 (RX)

CLASSIFICATION Hematopoietic

Administration 1 tablet po daily.

Available Drug Forms Generic contents in each controlled-release gradumet: Vitamins: C (sodium ascorbate): 500 mcg; folic acid: 800 mcg. Minerals: ferrous sulfate: 525 mg. Contains 105 mg of elemental iron in 525 mg of ferrous sulfate.

TRADE NAME Fetrin (RX)

CLASSIFICATION Hematopoietic

Administration 1 capsule po daily or bid.

Available Drug Forms Generic contents in each sustained-release capsule: Vitamins: C (ascorbic acid): 60 mg; B_{12} (cyanocobalamin): 5 mcg. Minerals: ferrous fumarate: 200 mg. Contains 66 mg of elemental iron in 200 mg of ferrous fumarate. Also contains intrinsic factor.

TRADE NAME Folvron (RX)

CLASSIFICATION Hematopoietic

Administration 1 capsule po daily or bid.

Available Drug Forms Generic contents in each capsule: Vitamins: folic acid: 0.33 mg. Minerals: ferrous sulfate (dried): 182 mg. Contains 57 mg of elemental iron in 182 mg of ferrous sulfate.

TRADE NAME Glytinic (RX)

CLASSIFICATION Hematopoietic

Action Glycine may increase the client's tolerance for iron salts.

Administration Adults: 1 tablet or tbsp po bid; Children: Ages 6 to 12 years: 1 tsp po tid; Ages 2 to 6 years: 1 tsp po bid.

Available Drug Forms Generic contents in each tablet and tablespoon: Vitamins: B_1 (thiamine): 7.5 mg; B_3 (niacinamide): 45 mg; B_5 (pantothenate): 6.5 mg; B_6 (pyridoxine): 2.25 mg; B_{12} (cyanocobalamin): 10 mcg. Minerals: ferrous fumarate: 865 mg; aminoacetic acid (glycine): 1.3 g; liver: 5 gr. Contains 100 mg of elemental iron in 865 mg of ferrous fumarate.

TRADE NAME Hemocyte-F (RX)

CLASSIFICATION Hematopoietic

Administration 1 tablet po daily or bid.

Available Drug Forms Generic contents in each tablet: Vitamins: folic acid: 1 mg. Minerals: ferrous fumarate: 324 mg. Contains 106 mg of elemental iron in 324 mg of ferrous fumarate.

TRADE NAME Hemocyte Plus (RX)

CLASSIFICATION Hematopoietic

Administration 1 tablet po daily.

Available Drug Forms Generic contents in each tablet: Vitamins: C (sodium ascorbate): 200 mg; B_1 (thiamine mononitrate): 10 mg; B_2 (riboflavin): 6 mg; B_3 (niacinamide): 30 mg; B_5 (calcium pantothenate): 10 mg; B_6 (pyridoxine HCl): 5 mg; B_{12} (cyanocobalamin): 15 mcg; folic acid: 1 mg. Minerals: ferrous fumarate: 324 mg; zinc sulfate: 80 mg; magnesium sulfate: 70 mg; manganese sulfate: 4 mg; copper sulfate: 2 mg. Contains 106 mg of elemental iron in 324 mg of ferrous fumarate.

TRADE NAME Hemo-Vite (RX)

CLASSIFICATION Hematopoietic

Administration 1 tablet po daily.

Available Drug Forms Generic contents in each tablet: Vitamins: C (ascorbic acid): 150 mg; B_1 (thiamine HCl): 5 mg; B_2 (riboflavin): 5 mg; B_3 (niacinamide): 50 mg; B_5 (calcium pantothenate): 10 mg; B_6 (pyridoxine HCl): 1 mg; B_{12} (cyanocobalamin) with intrinsic factor: $\frac{1}{2}$ NF unit; folic acid: 0.2 mg. Minerals: ferrous fumarate: 240 mg; copper sulfate: 1 mg. Contains 79 mg of elemental iron in 240 mg of ferrous fumarate.

TRADE NAME Iberet-500 (RX)

CLASSIFICATION Hematopoietic

Administration 1 tablet po daily.

Available Drug Forms Generic contents in each controlled-release gradument: Vitamins: C (sodium ascorbate): 500 mg; B_1 (thiamine mononitrate): 6 mg; B_2 (riboflavin): 6 mg; B_3 (niacinamide): 30 mg; B_5 (calcium pantothenate): 10 mg; B_6 (pyridoxine HCl): 5 mg; B_{12} (cyanocobalamin): 25 mcg. Minerals: ferrous sulfate: 525 mg. Contains 105 mg of elemental iron in 525 mg of ferrous sulfate.

TRADE NAME Iberet-500 Liquid (RX)

CLASSIFICATION Hematopoietic

Administration Adults: 2 tsp po bid; Children: Ages 1 to 3 years: 1 tsp po bid.

Available Drug Forms Generic contents in each teaspoon (5 ml): Vitamins: C (ascorbic acid): 125 mg; B_1 (thiamine mononitrate): 1.5 mg; B_2 (riboflavin): 1.5 mg; B_3 (niacinamide): 7.5 mg; B_5 (dexpanthenol): 2.5 mg; B_6 (pyridoxine HCl): 1.25 mg; B_{12} (cyanocobalamin): 6.25 mg. Minerals: elemental iron (ferrous sulfate): 26.25 mg. Fruit flavor for infants and children. May be added to water or fruit juice.

TRADE NAME Iberet-Folic-500 (RX)

CLASSIFICATION Hematopoietic

Administration 1 tablet po daily.

Available Drug Forms Generic contents in each controlled-release gradument: Vitamins: C (sodium ascorbate): 500 mg; B_1 (thiamine mononitrate): 6 mg; B_2 (riboflavin): 6 mg; B_3 (niacinamide): 30 mg; B_5 (calcium pantothenate): 10 mg; B_6 (pyridoxine HCl): 5 mg; B_{12} (cyanocobalamin): 25 mcg; folic acid: 800 mcg. Minerals: ferrous sulfate: 525 mg. Contains 105 mg of elemental iron in 525 mg of ferrous gluconate.

TRADE NAME Icron-FA (RX)

CLASSIFICATION Hematopoietic

Indications for Use Often used as a prenatal supplement to prevent anemia during second and third trimester.

Administration 1 tablet po daily.

Available Drug Forms Generic contents in each tablet: Vitamins: folic acid: 1.0 mg. Minerals: ferrous fumarate: 200 mg. Contains 82 mg of elemental iron in 200 mg of ferrous fumarate.

TRADE NAME I.L.X. B_{12} Elixir (RX)

CLASSIFICATION Hematopoietic

Administration 1 tsp po tid.

Available Drug Forms Generic contents in each tablespoon (15 ml): Vitamins: B_1 (thiamine HCl): 5 mg; B_2 (riboflavin): 2 mg; B_3 (nicotinamide): 10 mg; B_{12} (cyanocobalamin): 10 mcg. Minerals: iron ammonium citrate; liver fraction 1: 98 mg. Contains 102 mg of elemental iron in 15 ml. Also contains 8% alcohol.

TRADE NAME I.L.X. B_{12} Tablets (RX)

CLASSIFICATION Hematopoietic

Indications for Use Has been used for anemia in geriatrics and other adults.

Administration 1 tablet po tid.

Available Drug Forms Generic contents in each tablet: Vitamins: C: 60 mg; B_1 (thiamine HCl): 2 mg; B_2 (riboflavin): 2 mg; B_3 (niacinamide): 20 mg; B_{12} (cyanocobalamin): 10 mcg. Minerals: ferrous gluconate: 380 mg; dessicated liver: 2 gr. Contains 38 mg of elemental iron in each tablet.

TRADE NAME Stuartinic (RX)

CLASSIFICATION Hematopoietic

Untoward Reactions Hypersensitivity reaction (bronchoconstriction) to FD&C No. 5 yellow may occur.

Administration 1 tablet po daily.

Available Drug Forms Generic contents in each tablet: Vitamins: C (ascorbic acid): 300 mg; (sodium ascorbate): 225 mg; B_1 (thiamine mononitrate): 6 mg; B_3 (niacinamide): 20 mg; B_5 (calcium pantothenate): 10 mg; B_6 (pyridoxine HCl): 1 mg; B_{12} (cyanocobalamin): 25 mcg. Minerals: ferrous fumarate: 300 mg. Contains 100 mg of elemental iron in 300 mg of ferrous fumarate. Also contains FD&C No. 5 yellow.

TRADE NAME Zentinic (RX)

CLASSIFICATION Hematopoietic

Administration 1 to 2 Pulvules po daily.

Available Drug Forms Generic contents in each pulvule: Vitamins: C(ascorbic acid): 200 mg; B_1 (thiamine mononitrate): 7.5 mg; B_2 (riboflavin): 7.5 mg; B_3 (niacinamide): 30 mg; B_5 (calcium pantothenate): 15 mg; B_6 (pyridoxine HCl): 7.5 mg; B_{12} (cyanocobalamin): 50 mcg; folic acid: 0.05 mg. Minerals: ferrous fumarate: 300 mg. Contains 100 mg of elemental iron in 300 mg of ferrous fumarate.

TRADE NAME Zentron (RX)

CLASSIFICATION Hematopoietic

Administration Adults: 1 to 2 tsp po tid; Infants and children: $\frac{1}{2}$ to 1 tsp po daily, bid, or tid.

Available Drug Forms Generic contents in each teaspoon (5 ml): Vitamins: C (ascorbic acid): 100 mg; B_1 (thiamine HCl): 1 mg; B_2 (riboflavin): 1 mg; B_3 (niacinamide): 5 mg; B_5 (pantothenate): 1 mg; B_6 (pyridoxine HCl): 1 mg; B_{12} (cyanocobalamin): 5 mcg. Minerals: ferrous sulfate: 92 mg. Contains 20 mg of elemental iron in 92 mg of ferrous sulfate. Also contains 2% alcohol.

TRADE NAME Zentron Chewable (RX)

CLASSIFICATION Hematopoietic

Administration Adults: 1 to 2 tablets po tid; Children: Over 2 years 1 tablet po daily, bid, or tid.

Available Drug Forms Generic contents in each tablet: Vitamins: C (ascorbic acid): 100 mg; B_1 (thiamine HCl): 1 mg; B_2 (riboflavin): 1 mg: B_3 (niacinamide): 5 mg; B_5 (pantothenate): 1 mg; B_6 (pyridoxine HCl): 1 mg; B_{12} (cyanocobalamin): 5 mcg. Minerals: ferrous fumarate: 60 mg. Contains 20 mg of elemental iron in 60 mg of ferrous fumarate.

Chapter 53

Diuretics

TYPES OF DIURETICS

MERCURIAL DIURETICS

- Meralluride
- Mercaptomerin sodium
- Merethoxylline procaine
- Chlormerodin
- Mercurophyllin
- Mercumatilin sodium
- Mersalyl
- Mersalyl with theophylline

CARBONIC ANHYDRASE INHIBITORS

- Acetazolamide
- Methazolamide
- Ethoxzolamide
- Dichlorphenamide

THIAZIDE DIURETICS

- Chlorothiazide
- Hydrochlorothiazide
- Benzthiazide
- Bendroflumethiazide
- Cyclothiazide
- Hydroflumethiazide
- Methyclothiazide
- Polythiazide
- Trichlormethiazide

THIAZIDE-LIKE DIURETICS

- Chlorthalidone
- Metolazone
- Quinethazone

LOOP DIURETICS

- Furosemide
- Ethacrynic acid, sodium ethacrynate

POTASSIUM-SPARING DIURETICS

- Spironolactone
- Triamterene

OSMOTIC DIURETICS

- Mannitol
- Urea
- Glucose (50%)

XANTHINE DIURETICS

- Aminophylline
- Caffeine
- Theobromine
- Theophylline

ANY DRUG THAT increases diuresis and therefore promotes the loss of water from the body is called a *diuretic*. For example, caffeine increases glomerular filtration and thus promotes diuresis by increasing cardiac output and blood flow to the renal arteries. However, the diuretic effect of caffeine is mild compared to some drugs that can cause the loss of as much as 2000 ml from one dose. These potent diuretics are termed *saluretics* and they promote diuresis by increasing the loss of sodium, chloride, and water from the body. Saluretics, such as the thiazides, are emphasized in this chapter, since they are the most commonly used diuretics.

TYPES OF DIURETICS

Mercurial diuretics are among the oldest diuretic agents used for medicinal purposes. From the 16th century, when Paracelsus first used one of them medicinally, until the late 1940s, mercurial diuretics were the only effective agents for promoting diuresis in various states of edema. These drugs exert their action by interfering with the active reabsorption of sodium and chloride ions from the proximal renal tubule into the blood, thus causing an increase in water excretion. Since the mercurials are poorly absorbed from the gastrointestinal tract, they must be injected. Unfortunately, clients may stop responding to mercurials after repeated doses and they can cause some serious untoward reactions, particularly hypochloremia. The cheaper oral diuretics are used more frequently today for mild edema.

Carbonic anhydrase inhibitors are sulfonamide derivatives that inhibit the enzyme carbonic anhydrase and ultimately promote diuresis by decreasing the reabsorption of both bicarbonate and sodium ions. These agents are effective for the treatment of mild edema. They also are useful as an adjunct to miotics in the treatment of chronic open-angle glaucoma because they inhibit the formation of aqueous humor. Since these agents alkalize the urine, they interfere with the normal excretion process of numerous drugs.

Benzothiadiazine diuretics, which are more commonly referred to as *thiazide diuretics*, are inexpensive and orally effective for mild and moderate edema. They act by inhibiting the reabsorption of sodium and chloride ions from the distal renal tubule. Although thiazide diuretics do not affect the blood pressure of normotensive clients, they are effective in treating hypertension. Unfortunately, thiazides can cause hypokalemia (lack of potassium) and hyperuricemia (gout) and can suppress the release of insulin in clients with diabetes mellitus and potential diabetics.

Loop diuretics (ethacrynic acid and furosemide) are very potent saluretics that are effective for refractory edema and are useful in emergency situations, such as pulmonary edema. They act by inhibiting the reabsorption of sodium and chloride ions in the ascending limb of the loop of Henle. Unlike thiazides, loop diuretics can be safely used in diabetes, since they cause little or no alteration in carbohydrate metabolism. However, these diuretics are so potent that they can cause severe electrolyte imbalances and even reduce the blood volume so markedly that cardiovascular collapse occurs.

Potassium-sparing diuretics act by different mechanisms, but they all promote the retention of potassium in the body. Spironolactone is an aldosterone antagonist that acts on the distal renal tubule and causes sodium to be lost while potassium is retained. Although triamterene is not an aldosterone antagonist, it also acts directly on the distal tubule to cause the retention of potassium and the loss of sodium. Since the quantity of sodium that reaches the distal tubule is small, the excretion of sodium and water is limited. Potassium-sparing diuretics are often used concurrently with more proximal-acting diuretics, such as thiazides, since the combination increases diuresis while preventing hypokalemia.

Although *osmotic diuretics* cause little or no saluretic effect, they do promote water excretion by increasing the osmotic pressure of the tubular filtrate. These hypertonic solutions are excreted by the kidneys, but once in the tubular fluid they are not absorbed by the body, thus promoting water excretion. When infused into the blood, osmotic diuretics increase the blood's osmolality and thus promote the diffusion of fluid into the blood. Therefore, they are useful in the emergency treatment of elevated cerebrospinal fluid and intraocular pressure. However, osmotic diuretics can cause circulatory overload and induce pulmonary edema.

Xanthine diuretics are seldom used only for their diuretic effect. Their primary actions include bronchial dilation, stimulation of the heart, and relaxation of smooth muscles. They promote water excretion by increasing cardiac output and dilating afferent arterioles, thereby increasing glomerular filtration.

MERCURIAL DIURETICS

GENERIC NAME Meralluride (RX)

TRADE NAME Mercuhydrin

CLASSIFICATION Mercurial diuretic

Action This divalent organic mercurial compound combines with the sulfhydryl groups attached to certain renal enzymes. The affected enzymes are inactivated, thus inhibiting the reabsorption of several substances. There is a marked interference with the active reabsorption of sodium and chloride ions from the proximal tubule into the blood. The retention of osmotically active sodium in the filtrate causes an increase in water excretion. Potassium is normally secreted into the fluid in the distal tubule and collecting duct. Since the drug depresses tubular secretion of potassium, there is no significant loss of this electrolyte.

Indications for Use Congestive heart failure, ascites due to portal obstruction or cirrhosis of the liver, chronic nephrosis.

Contraindications Hypersensitivity to mercury ion, dehydration, renal insufficiency (may cause mercury poisoning due to inadequate drug excretion), hypochloremia.

Untoward Reactions Systemic mercury poisoning may occur after prolonged use. The first signs and symptoms include saliva with a strong metallic taste, followed by stomatitis, gingivitis, anorexia, colitis, hypertension, peripheral neuritis, anemia, and oliguria. Hyperchloremic acidosis, due to excessive loss of chloride ion, may occur after prolonged therapy. Arrhythmias can occur following administration of a large dosage or if excessive accumulation of drug occurs. Hypersensitivity reactions, including flushing, nausea, vomiting, fever with chills, itching and urticaria, agranulocytosis, thrombocytopenia, and neutropenia, have been reported. Renal damage may occur with prolonged use. Local irritation around injection sites, ecchymoses, induration, or necrosis may occur. Hyperuricemia is rare. Intravenous injection may cause cardiac toxicity and result in ventricular fibrillation.

Parameters of Use

Absorption Well absorbed from parenteral sites; slowly and incompletely absorbed from intestines. Onset of diuresis is 1 to 2 hours. Peak action occurs in 6 to 8 hours and duration of action is 12 to 24 hours.

Distribution Mainly to the kidneys; binds to renal tubules.

Excretion Rapidly excreted by the kidneys; about 95% in 24 hours. Some may be excreted via the GI tract.

Drug Interactions Ammonium chloride and other urinary acidifiers, chlorides, and theophylline derivatives increase the diuretic effect of meralluride, whereas alkalizing agents, such as sodium bicarbonate, decrease the diuretic effect.

Administration Intramuscular, subcutaneous: 65 to 260 mg as needed; Intravenous: 65 to 130 mg via IV bolus over 5 minutes or more as needed.

Available Drug Forms Ampules of 1 or 2 ml containing 130 mg/ml; also contains a small quantity of theophylline (39 mg) to increase the absorption rate; 1 ml contains approximately 39 mg of mercury. (Due to popularity of other less expensive and less toxic drugs, meralluride may not be available in some areas.)

Nursing Management

Planning factors

1. A test dose (65 mg IM) is recommended, since toxic and hypersensitivity reactions can be severe and difficult to treat. Test dose should be given 24 hours before administering the first therapeutic dose.
2. Administer in early morning so that sleep will not be disturbed by diuresis.
3. Dietary content should include chloride and some sodium (4 g sodium diet). Excessive low salt intake or excessive loss of salt (hot weather, vomiting) may precipitate hypochloremic alkalosis and prevent diuresis.
4. Some potassium-rich foods, such as citrus fruits and bananas, should be ingested daily. Although potassium loss is minimal with meralluride, some loss of potassium can occur.

Administration factors

1. Inject deep into large muscle mass with good circulation (upper outer quadrant of gluteus maximus).
2. Avoid edematous sites and other sites with poor circulation, since tissue necrosis and sloughing may occur.
3. Rotate sites to decrease tissue irritation.
4. The Z-track method is recommended when given intramuscularly, since this minimizes tissue irritation.
5. Administer IV bolus over 5 minutes or more and monitor heart rate continuously.

Evaluation factors

1. Monitor heart rate and rhythm periodically during the first 3 to 6 hours following administration. If arrhythmias develop, notify physician.
2. Monitor blood pressure periodically. Excessive diuresis may cause dehydration and hypovolemia, thus causing hypotension in the elderly and clients with severe cardiac disease. If blood pressure falls dramatically (lightheadedness, dizziness, syncope), notify physician immediately.

3. Weigh client daily to determine quantity of water loss. A weight loss of 1 to 2 kg (2.2 to 4.4 lb) is common.
4. Record intake and output. If diuresis does not begin within 6 hours, notify physician.
5. Determine serum electrolyte levels (sodium, potassium, chloride, carbon dioxide-combining capacity, magnesium) and blood urea nitrogen daily. If abnormal, notify physician before administering the next dose.
6. Perform urinalysis at least biweekly in clients receiving repeated doses. If albumin, red blood cells, or casts appear, notify physician before administering the next dose.
7. Measure abdominal girth each morning in clients with ascites.
8. Assess lung rales and rhonchi at least q2h in clients with congestive heart failure.

GENERIC NAME Mercaptomerin sodium (RX)

TRADE NAME Thiomerin

CLASSIFICATION Mercurial diuretic

See meralluride for Indications for use, Contraindications, Untoward reactions, and Drug interactions.

Action This mercurial diuretic is complexed with thioglycolate. As with meralluride, diuresis is produced by inhibition of tubular reabsorption of sodium and chloride ions. Thioglycolate causes this compound to release mercury ions at a slower rate from the injection site, thus reducing local irritation and the potential of cardiac toxicity that occurs with meralluride.

Parameters of Use

Absorption Well absorbed from subcutaneous tissue and muscles. Onset of diuresis is 2 to 3 hours. Peak action occurs in 5 to 9 hours and duration of action is 12 to 24 hours. Bound to plasma proteins.
Distribution Distributed to kidneys and liver; localizes in renal tubules.
Excretion Rapidly excreted by the kidneys; some bowel excretion.

Administration 25 to 250 mg IM or subc daily.

Available Drug Forms Vials containing 125 mg/ml; Tubex containing 2 ml with 125 mg/ml; 1 ml contains approximately 40 mg of mercury.

Nursing Management (See meralluride.)

1. Keep drug refrigerated, as it is unstable to heat and light.
2. Discard drug if it becomes turbid.
3. Test dose (62.5 mg IM) should be given 24 hours before administering the first therapeutic dose.

GENERIC NAME Merethoxylline procaine (RX)

TRADE NAME Dicurin Procaine

CLASSIFICATION Mercurial diuretic

See meralluride for Indications for use and Untoward reactions.

Action This organic mercurial diuretic contains procaine and theophylline. As with other mercurials, diuresis is produced by inhibition of tubular reabsorption of sodium and chloride ions and other electrolytes. Procaine is added to decrease the discomfort at the injection site. Theophylline (xanthine diuretic) is added to stabilize the solution; it improves absorption and decreases irritation.

Contraindications Hypersensitivity to procaine or theophylline. (See meralluride.)

Parameters of Use (See meralluride.)

Excretion Approximately 75% is excreted in 24 hours.

Drug Interactions Cross-sensitization may occur with drugs containing the *p*-aminobenzoic acid group (benzocaine, tetracaine, butacaine). (See meralluride.)

Administration 0.5 to 2.0 ml IM or subc daily, or as needed.

Available Drug Forms Ampules and vials containing 2 or 10 ml; 1 ml contains 39.3 mg of mercury, 100 mg of the procaine salt, and 50 mg of theophylline.

Nursing Management (See meralluride.)

1. Keep drug refrigerated as it is unstable to heat and direct sunlight.
2. Test dose (0.5 ml IM) should be given 24 hours before administering the first therapeutic dose.

GENERIC NAME Chlormerodin (RX)

TRADE NAME Neohydrin

CLASSIFICATION Mercurial diuretic

See meralluride for Indications for use, Contraindications, Untoward reactions, Parameters of use, Drug interactions, and Nursing management.

Action Radioactive chlormerodin (^{197}Hg) has been used to diagnose kidney and brain disorders.

Administration 1 to 6 tablets (18 to 110 mg) po daily.

Available Drug Forms Tablets containing 18.3 mg of chlormerodin (10 mg of mercury).

GENERIC NAME Mercurophyllin (RX)

TRADE NAME Mercupurin

CLASSIFICATION Mercurial diuretic

See meralluride for Indications for use, Contraindications, Untoward reactions, Parameters of use, Drug interactions, and Nursing management.

Action Peak diuresis from oral form is in 48 hours.

Administration Oral: 200 mg daily; intramuscular: 68 to 270 mg (0.5 to 2.0 ml) daily.

Available Drug Forms One milliliter contains 135 mg of mercurophyllin (38 mg of mercury).

GENERIC NAME Mercumatilin sodium (RX)

TRADE NAME Cumertilin Sodium

CLASSIFICATION Mercurial diuretic

See meralluride for Action, Indications for use, Contraindications, Untoward reactions, Parameters of use, Drug interactions, and Nursing management.

Administration 50 to 200 mg (0.5 to 2.0 ml) IM as needed.

Available Drug Forms One milliliter contains 132 mg of mercumatilin, 50 mg of theophylline, and 30 mg of mercury.

GENERIC NAME Mersalyl (RX)

TRADE NAME Salyrgan

CLASSIFICATION Mercurial diuretic

See meralluride for Action, Indications for use, Contraindications, Untoward reactions, Parameters of use, Drug interactions, and Nursing management.

Administration 0.5 to 2.0 ml IM initially; then 100 to 200 mg weekly or twice weekly. Has been given IV.

Available Drug Forms One milliliter contains 39.6 mg of mercury.

GENERIC NAME Mersalyl with theophylline (RX)

TRADE NAME Mersalyn, Salyrgan-Theophyllin

CLASSIFICATION Mercurial diuretic

See meralluride for Action, Indications for use, Contraindications, Untoward reactions, Parameters of use, Drug interactions, and Nursing management.

Administration 1 to 2 ml IM weekly or twice weekly.

Available Drug Forms One milliliter contains 50 mg of theophylline and 39.6 mg of mercury.

CARBONIC ANHYDRASE INHIBITORS

GENERIC NAME Acetazolamide (RX)

TRADE NAMES Diamox, Diamox Sequels

CLASSIFICATION Diuretic, carbonic anhydrase inhibitor

Action Acetazolamide, a sulfonamide derivative with no bacteriostatic action, inhibits the action of the enzyme carbonic anhydrase. This enzyme catalyzes the hydration of carbon dioxide to carbonic acid, which rapidly dissociates into hydrogen and bicarbonate ions. The hydrogen ions are then exchanged in the renal tubule for sodium and, to some degree, potassium ions. When the enzyme is inhibited by acetazolamide, hydrogen ions are not secreted by the tubular cells. Thus, many sodium and carbonate ions cannot be reabsorbed from the tubular fluid back into the blood. Retention of these osmotically active substances in the tubular fluid causes diuresis of alkaline urine. Metabolic acidosis may eventually develop due to the excretion of bicarbonate ions and the retention of hydrogen ions. Since acidosis can reduce and even prevent seizure activity, this drug is effective as an adjunct to anticonvulsants in the treatment of epilepsy. In addition, inhibition of carbonic anhydrase decreases the rate at which aqueous humor is produced. Therefore, acetazolamide is an effective adjunct to miotics in the treatment of glaucoma. Since some potassium is lost due to enhanced secretion in the distal tubule, hypokalemia can occur if there is an adequate intake of dietary potassium. A decrease in ammonia and chloride ion excretion also occurs in many clients.

Indications for Use Mild or moderate states of edema, including drug-induced edema, premenstrual edema, and cardiac edema; chronic open-angle glaucoma; preoperatively for acute angle-closure glaucoma (to reduce intraocular pressure); drug-induced glaucoma; petit mal epilepsy and certain other seizure disorders; correction of metabolic acidosis caused by mercurial diuretics.

Contraindications Hypersensitivity to sulfonamides, hyponatremia, hypokalemia, hyperchloremic acidosis, dehydration, renal failure, severe hepatic disease, nephritis, Addison's disease, prolonged use in clients with chronic noncongestive angle-closure glaucoma (since the symptoms of worsening glaucoma will be masked).

Warnings and Precautions Diuresis is not dose-related and excessive dosage may induce severe untoward reactions. Teratogenic effects have been demonstrated in rats. Use with great caution during pregnancy. Use with caution in clients with diabetes, chronic obstructive pulmonary disease, and other lung disorders.

Untoward Reactions Fever accompanied by headache, chills, malaise, pruritus, or a skin rash may develop as a result of hypersensitivity to sulfonamides. Toxic nephrosis, tubular necrosis with or without hematuria, and blood dyscrasias, including acute hemolytic anemia, agranulocytosis, aplastic anemia, thrombocytopenia, and eosinophilia, may also occur. Common side effects, particularly when large dosages are used, include drowsiness and mild or transient paresthesia of the head, face, and extremities. Confusion can occur, particularly in the elderly. Urinary calculi formation and renal colic may be caused by the drug-induced decrease in urinary citrate. Electrolyte disturbances may occur due to excessive loss of sodium (hyponatremia) or potassium (hypokalemia) or the excessive retention of chloride (hyperchloremia). Disorientation has been reported in clients with hepatic dysfunction, such as cirrhosis. Rare reactions include transient myopia, glycosuria, flaccid paralysis, and convulsions.

Parameters of Use

Absorption Readily absorbed from GI tract. Onset of diuresis is: 30 minutes (po); 5 to 10 minutes (IV). Peak plasma levels occur in: 2 to 4 hours (regular tablet); 8 to 12 hours (sustained-release capsule). Duration of action is: 8 to 12 hours (regular tablet); 18 to 24 hours (sustained-release capsule); 2 hours (IV).

Crosses placenta.

Excretion By the kidneys as unchanged drug within 24 hours.

Drug Interactions When acetazolamide alkalizes the urine, weak acidic drugs will be excreted at a slower rate. Consequently, the effects of weak acidic drugs, including amphetamines, tricyclic antidepressants, catecholamines, ganglionic blocking agents, the beta-adrenergic blocker dichloroisoproterenol, the anticonvulsant gallamine, procainamide, and quinidine, are potentiated due to excessive renal absorption. When acetazolamide alkalizes the urine, weak basic drugs will be excreted at a faster rate. Consequently, the effects of weak basic drugs, including lithium carbonate, salicylates, phenobarbital, and methenamine, are decreased due to rapid excretion. Since acetazolamide causes the renal excretion of some potassium, the incidence of hypokalemia will increase markedly if another drug that causes potassium loss, including corticosteroids and certain other diuretics, is given concomitantly. Digitalis toxicity may occur if acetazolamide is given concurrently with digitalis glycosides. Acetazolamide tends to increase the blood glucose level of diabetics receiving oral antidiabetic agents.

Administration

- *Mild or moderate edema:* 5 mg/kg; Dosage range: 250 to 375 mg po daily or every other day.
- *Glaucoma:* 250 to 1000 mg po daily in divided doses every 8 to 12 hours; 250 to 500 mg IM or IV in acute cases.
- *Seizure disorders:* 8 to 30 mg/kg po in divided doses q8h; Initial dosage: 250 mg.

Available Drug Forms Tablets containing 125 or 250 mg; sustained-release capsules containing 500 mg; vials containing 500 mg of yellowish white crystalline powder for reconstitution with 5 ml of sterile water.

Nursing Management

Planning factors

1. When diuresis is desired, administer in early morning so that sleep is not disturbed.
2. Best diuretic effect occurs when kidneys are allowed to "rest" every other day or once every 3 days since drug's effectiveness diminishes with continuous use. If ordered on alternate days, confusion can be avoided by remembering if the drug is administered on even or odd days of the calendar.
3. If a potassium supplement is not ordered some potassium-rich foods (citrus fruits, bananas) should be ingested daily.

Administration factors

1. Tablets can be crushed and added to warm water, when necessary. Add $\frac{1}{2}$ teaspoon of honey or 1 teaspoon of syrup to mask the bitter taste.
2. Sustained-release capsules should not be crushed. Use tablets if dosage must be administered in liquid form.
3. Reconstituted parenteral solution has an alkaline pH (approximately 9.2). The IV route is recommended because IM administration causes severe pain. Administer IV bolus slowly.
4. When administering IM, inject deep into large muscle mass and rotate sites to decrease tissue irritation.
5. Use parenteral solution within 24 hours of reconstitution.

Evaluation factors

1. Common side effects tend to occur during the drug's peak plasma levels. If symptoms occur, assist with ambulation.
2. When administering drug for diuretic effect, complete the following:
   a. Record intake and output.
   b. If diuresis does not begin by the end of the drug's peak plasma level, notify physician.
   c. Weigh client daily to determine quantity of water loss.
3. Determine serum electrolyte levels, particularly potassium, periodically. It has been recommended that potassium levels be determined at least once or twice a week in clients receiving concomitant therapy with digitalis, corticosteroids, or other diuretics.

4. Assess client daily, prior to morning dosage, for hypokalemia and marked acidosis (disorientation, rapid and deep respirations, weakness). If symptoms occur, notify physician before administering drug.
5. When drug is administered for 2 weeks or longer, obtain complete blood cell counts periodically to detect developing blood dyscrasias.
6. Observe diabetic clients and potential diabetics for hyperglycemia.

GENERIC NAME Methazolamide (RX)

TRADE NAME Neptazane

CLASSIFICATION Diuretic, carbonic anhydrase inhibitor

See acetazolamide for Contraindications, Warnings and precautions, Drug interactions, and Nursing management.

Action This nonbacteriostatic sulfonamide derivative has similar actions to acetazolamide, but is more active in inhibiting carbonic anhydrase. May be used safely with miotics, osmotic diuretics, and epinephrine for the treatment of acute open-angle glaucoma. (See acetazolamide.)

Indications for Use Chronic open-angle glaucoma, preoperatively for acute angle-closure glaucoma, drug-induced glaucoma, petit mal epilepsy and certain other seizure disorders.

Untoward Reactions May cause profound CNS disturbances (paresthesia, drowsiness, confusion). (See acetazolamide).

Parameters of Use

Absorption Readily absorbed from GI tract; may cause GI disturbances. Onset of diuresis is 2 to 4 hours and duration of action is 10 to 12 hours.

Crosses placenta.

Distribution Widely distributed. High concentrations found in plasma (erythrocytes), aqueous humor, cerebrospinal fluid, and kidneys. Reported to penetrate into brain and eye more than acetazolamide.

Metabolism Some metabolized in the liver.

Excretion About 20 to 30% excreted by the kidneys as unchanged drug. Causes less diuresis than acetazolamide.

Administration 50 to 100 mg po bid or tid.

Available Drug Forms Tablets containing 50 mg.

GENERIC NAME Ethoxzolamide (RX)

TRADE NAMES Cardrase, Ethamide

CLASSIFICATION Diuretic, carbonic anhydrase inhibitor

See acetazolamide for Contraindications, Warnings and precautions, Untoward reactions, Drug interactions, and Nursing management.

Action This nonbacteriostatic sulfonamide derivative is almost twice as active as a carbonic anhydrase inhibitor as acetazolamide. Ethoxzolamide is primarily used for its diuretic effect and for lowering intraocular pressure. It causes less GI disturbances than methazolamide. (See acetazolamide.)

Indications for Use Mild or moderate states of edema, including drug-induced edema, premenstrual edema, and cardiac edema; chronic open-angle glaucoma; secondary glaucoma; petit mal epilepsy and certain other seizure disorders; correction of metabolic acidosis caused by mercurial diuretics.

Parameters of Use

Absorption Readily absorbed from GI tract. Onset of diuresis is 30 minutes. Peak plasma levels occur in 2 to 4 hours and duration of effect is 8 to 12 hours.

Crosses placenta.

Distribution Widely distributed. High concentrations in plasma (erythrocytes), aqueous humor, cerebrospinal fluid, and kidneys. Some also found in muscles, liver, and lungs.

Excretion About 40% excreted by the kidneys as unchanged drug. Causes more diuresis than acetazolamide.

Administration

- *Mild or moderate edema:* 62.5 to 125 mg po daily times 3 days or every other day.
- *Glaucoma:* 62.5 to 250 mg po bid, tid, or qid; dosage is regulated by tonometric measurements.

Available Drug Forms Scored tablets containing 125 mg.

GENERIC NAME Dichlorphenamide (RX)

TRADE NAMES Daranide, Oratrol

CLASSIFICATION Diuretic, carbonic anhydrase inhibitor

See acetazolamide for Contraindications, Warnings and precautions, Untoward reactions, Drug interactions, and Nursing management.

Action This nonbacteriostatic sulfonamide derivative inhibits carbonic anhydrase. Although it has some diuretic effect and prevents the reabsorption of sodium and bicarbonate ions, dichlorphenamide is primarily recommended as an adjunct for the treatment of glaucoma. It reduces intraocular pressure by inhibiting the rate at which aqueous humor is formed. It also causes metabolic acidosis. Much of the enzyme activity must be suppressed before a physiologic response is observed.

Indications for Use Chronic open-angle glaucoma, drug-induced glaucoma, preoperatively for acute angle-closure glaucoma. May be effective for glaucoma when other therapies fail or are poorly tolerated. Normally used concurrently with miotic agents (pilocarpine, physostigmine).

Parameters of Use

Absorption Rapidly absorbed from GI tract. Onset of diuresis is 30 to 60 minutes. Peak plasma levels occur in 2 to 4 hours and duration of action is 6 to 12 hours.

Crosses placenta.

Administration 25 to 50 mg po daily, bid, or tid. As much as 300 mg daily (150 mg g12h) may be given initially to decrease intraocular pressure.

Available Drug Forms Scored tablets containing 50 mg.

Nursing Management See Chapter 79 for further details about glaucoma.

THIAZIDE DIURETICS

GENERIC NAME Chlorothiazide (RX)

TRADE NAMES Diuril, Ro-Chlorozide

CLASSIFICATION Thiazide diuretic, antihypertensive

Action Chlorothiazide is a synthetic diuretic chemically related to sulfonamides. It inhibits the reabsorption of sodium and chloride ions from the tubular fluid into the blood at the distal tubule. It also increases the excretion of potassium and bicarbonate ions. Retention of these osmotically active substances in the tubular fluid causes an increase in water excretion. Initially, hypertensive clients are helped by the diuresis and the resulting decrease in plasma volume. Further antihypertensive action occurs, but is not completely understood. Alterations in sodium metabolism, which cause a decrease in peripheral resistance, are thought to occur. The blood pressure of normotensive patients is unaffected. There is also a decrease in the excretion of calcium and uric acid. Resulting hyperuricemia may precipitate an attack of gout. Chlorothiazide may suppress the release of insulin in clients with diabetes mellitus and potential diabetes; but clients with diabetes insipidus will experience a reduction in fluid loss.

Indications for Use Mild or moderate states of edema associated with chronic congestive heart failure, chronic hepatic disease, nephrosis, chronic renal failure, nephrotic syndrome, acute glomerulonephritis, and corticosteroid and estrogen therapy; mild hypertension with or without other antihypertensive agents; polyuria of diabetes insipidus; hypercalcemia.

Contraindications Hypersensitivity to thiazides or sulfonamides; anuria or pronounced oliguria; electrolyte imbalances, including hyponatremia, hypochloremic alkalosis, and hypokalemia; intravenous use in infants and young children.

Warnings and Precautions Use with caution in clients with gout. Clients with a history of bronchial asthma and other allergic conditions may develop a hypersensitivity reaction. May precipitate hepatic coma in clients with severe hepatic impairment and azotemia in clients with renal impairment. Cumulative effects may also develop in clients with impaired renal function. May exacerbate systemic lupus erythematosus. May be hazardous during pregnancy and lactation. May increase insulin requirements in clients with diabetes mellitus or latent diabetes. Clients who have had a sympathectomy may become hypotensive.

Untoward Reactions Toxicity to thiazides includes lethargy that progresses to coma within a few hours after drug administration. There may be little or no effect on respiratory or cardiovascular functioning and the electrolytes may be normal. Vomiting and diarrhea may precede lethargy. Hypersensitivity reactions include anaphylactic reactions, purpura, photosensitivity, dermatitis, urticaria, vasculitis, fever, and respiratory distress. GI disorders, including nausea, vomiting, diarrhea, abdominal cramps, anorexia, and constipation, may occur. Intrahepatic cholestatic jaundice, elevated serum ammonia, mental confusion, disorientation, and hepatic coma have been reported, particularly in clients with impaired hepatic function. Hyperglycemia and accompanying glycosuria may occur in diabetics and latent diabetics. Acute attacks of gout may be precipitated by hyperuricemia. Common side effects include headache, restlessness, orthostatic hypotension, and transient dizziness, vertigo, and paresthesia; the elderly are particularly susceptible to these effects. Hypokalemia (progressive muscular weakness, paresthesia, hyporeflexes, anorexia, vomiting) occurs frequently. Other electrolyte disturbances may arise as a result of excessive loss of sodium (hyponatremia) or chloride (hypochloremia). Retention of calcium may cause hypercalcemia and pathologic changes of the parathyroid in clients on prolonged thiazide therapy. Blood dyscrasias, including leukopenia, agranulocytosis, thrombocytopenia, and aplastic anemia, occur, but rarely. Rare reactions include transient blurred vision, xanthopsia (objects appear yellow), pancreatitis, and hematuria. Lupus erythematosus may be precipitated in susceptible clients.

Parameters of Use

Absorption Relatively rapid; effective when given orally. Onset of diuresis is: 2 hours (po); 15 minutes (IV). Peak action occurs in: 4 hours (po); 30 minutes (IV). Duration of action is: 6 to 12 hours (po); 2 to 4 hours (IV).

Crosses placenta and appears in breast milk; lactating mothers should not breast-feed their babies.

Distribution Distributed throughout extracellular fluid, but concentrated in the kidneys.

Excretion By the kidneys, as unchanged drug within 6 hours.

Drug Interactions

Since thiazide diuretics cause renal excretion of potassium, the severity of hypokalemia will increase if other drugs that cause potassium loss, including corticosteroids, ACTH, and certain other diuretics, are given concurrently. Digitalis toxicity may be precipitated by the hypokalemia produced by thiazide diuretics if digitalis glycosides are given concomitantly. Orthostatic hypotension, which can progress to general hypotension, may occur when alcohol, other antihypertensive agents, barbiturates, or narcotics are given concomitantly. Absorption of chlorothiazide is inhibited by the ion-exchange resin cholestyramine. Insulin requirements and dosages of oral antidiabetic agents may need to be increased in diabetics. Thiazide diuretics may increase the responsiveness to norepinephrine. Renal excretion of amphetamines and lithium may be decreased by thiazides and toxicity may result.

Laboratory Interactions

Serum levels of protein-bound iodine may be decreased in the absence of thyroid disorders. Thiazides should be discontinued at least one day prior to parathyroid function tests. A false increase in the Bromsulphalein test for hepatic function may occur.

Administration

- *Mild edema:* 0.5 to 1.0 g po daily or bid; may be given every other day after initial diuresis.
- *Hypertension:* 0.5 to 1.0 g po daily usually in divided doses; dosage is adjusted according to blood pressure response; up to 2 g may be required daily in divided doses.
- *Pediatric:* 10 mg/lb/day (22 mg/kg/day) in divided doses.
- *Acute congestive heart failure:* 0.5 to 1.0 g IV daily or bid.

Available Drug Forms

White scored tablets containing 250 or 500 mg; oral suspension containing 250 mg/5 ml; vials containing 0.5 g of dry powder for reconstitution with at least 18 ml of sterile water for injection.

Nursing Management

Planning factors

1. When diuresis is desired, administer after breakfast (and immediately after supper if bid) so that gastric irritation and nocturnal diuresis is prevented. Do not administer after 6 P.M. so that sleep is not interrupted.
2. If a potassium supplement is not ordered, some potassium-rich foods (citrus fruits, bananas, dates, dried apricots) should be ingested daily.
3. Discontinue thiazide therapy 48 hours prior to surgery if possible, thus preventing interaction with tubocurarine or pressor amines (norepinephrine).
4. Obtain the following baseline data: blood pressure in sitting, standing, and supine position; serum electrolytes, blood urea nitrogen (BUN), serum glucose, and uric acid; body weight.

Administration factors

1. Oral suspension can be used if client is unable to swallow the tablets; consult physician.
2. Do not administer intramuscular or subcutaneous.
3. Intravenous chlorothiazide is used in emergencies and clients unable to take oral medication (postsurgical clients).
   a. Reconstitute in at least 18 ml of sterile water.
   b. Label multidose vial with date, time, strength, and initials.
   c. Solution may be stored at room temperature, but must be discarded after 24 hours.
   d. May be administered slowly with a syringe pump or given over 30 minutes in 50 ml of 5% D/W.
   e. Check patency of IV before administering. Extravasation can cause extreme irritation.

Evaluation factors

1. When therapy is initiated, monitor blood pressure every 15 to 30 minutes from the time of drug onset through peak plasma levels. If hypertension occurs, notify physician immediately. Once the maintenance dosage has been determined, check blood pressure before administration and once during peak plasma levels.
2. When administering drug for diuretic effect, complete the following:
   a. Record intake and output.
   b. Weigh client daily to determine quantity of water loss.
3. Test urine of diabetics and potential diabetics for sugar and acetone at least 4 times each day, since hyperglycemia may occur.
4. Assess client prior to morning drug dose for hypokalemia and other electrolyte imbalances. If symptoms occur, notify physician before administering drug.
5. Determine serum electrolytes, BUN, uric acid, and glucose levels periodically. Determine potassium levels at least once or twice a week in clients receiving concomitant therapy with digitalis glycosides, corticosteroids, or other diuretics.
6. When drug is administered for 2 weeks or longer, diuretic action may subside although hypotensive effect will continue. Assess blood pressure at least once a week.

Client teaching factors

1. Instruct client to avoid using table salt and highly salted foods (bacon, processed meats).
2. Instruct client to avoid the use of salt substitutes unless the physician is consulted first.
3. Instruct client to eat potassium-rich foods daily.
4. Advise client to take drug immediately after meals or with food.
5. Warn client to avoid alcoholic beverages during therapy.
6. Instruct client to avoid very hot showers or baths, sunbathing, strenuous exercise, or rapid position changes, since hypotension can occur.
7. Instruct client in the signs and symptoms of hypokalemia and other untoward reactions and to notify physician if symptoms occur.

8. Instruct client to avoid caffeinated drinks (coffee, tea, cola).
9. Instruct diabetic clients to report any consistent appearance of urinary sugar to physician.

GENERIC NAME Hydrochlorothiazide (RX)

TRADE NAMES Esidrix, HydroDIURIL, Hydro-Z, Lexor, Oretic, Ro-Hydrazide, Thiuretic

CLASSIFICATION Thiazide diuretic, antihypertensive

See chlorothiazide for Indications for use, Contraindications, Warnings and precautions, and Untoward reactions.

Action Hydrochlorothiazide is a synthetic diuretic chemically related to sulfonamides. It is similar to the parent drug chlorothiazide, but is approximately 10 times more potent and produces fewer toxic and other side effects. (See chlorothiazide.)

Parameters of Use

Absorption Relatively rapid; effective when given orally. Onset of diuresis is 2 hours. Peak action occurs in 4 hours and duration of action is 6 to 12 hours. Half-life is 3 hours.

Crosses placenta and appears in breast milk; lactating mothers should not breast-feed their babies.

Distribution Distributed throughout extracellular fluid but concentrated in the kidneys.

Excretion By the kidneys as unchanged drug within 24 hours.

Drug Interactions Clients who develop photosensitivity reactions to the diuretic and antihypertensive agent quinethazone may develop the same untoward effect when given hydrochlorothiazide. Hyperglycemia is enhanced if hydrochlorothiazide is given concomitantly with the antihypertensive agent diazoxide. (See chlorothiazide.)

Administration

- *Edema:* Initial dosage: 50 to 200 mg po daily (may be given in divided doses); Maintenance dosage: 25 to 100 mg daily (may be given in divided doses daily or every other day).
- *Hypertension:* Initial dosage: 50 to 100 mg po daily; occasionally 200 mg in divided doses is required. Maintenance dosage is determined by blood pressure response; Dosage range: 50 to 100 mg daily. Some clients respond better when dosage is given twice a day (25 to 50 mg bid).
- *Pediatric:* Ages 6 months and under: 1.0 to 1.5 mg/lb/day in divided doses; Over 6 months: 1.0 mg/lb/day in divided doses.

Available Drug Forms Scored tablets containing 25, 50, or 100 mg. Also available in single-dose packages.

Nursing Management (See chlorothiazide.)

1. Tablets can be softened in 30 ml of warm water and mixed with formula for infants.
2. Monitor infants, children, the elderly, and debilitated clients frequently for the first week, since they are more susceptible to toxicity and electrolyte imbalances.
3. Desired blood pressure should be obtained within a week.

GENERIC NAME Benzthiazide (RX)

TRADE NAMES Aquastat, Aquatag, Exna, Hydrex

CLASSIFICATION Thiazide diuretic, antihypertensive

See chlorothiazide for Indications for use, Contraindications, Warnings and precautions, Untoward reactions, and Drug interactions.

Action Benzthiazide is a synthetic diuretic chemically related to sulfonamides. It is about 85% more potent than hydrochlorothiazide and prolonged use can cause hypokalemia and other electrolyte imbalances. (See chlorothiazide.)

Parameters of Use Onset of diuresis occurs in 2 hours. Peak action occurs in 4 to 6 hours; duration of action is 12 to 8 hours. (See chlorothiazide.)

Administration

- *Edema:* Initial dosage: 50 to 200 mg po daily in 2 divided doses; Maintenance dosage: 50 to 150 mg daily in 2 divided doses.
- *Hypertension:* Dosage depends on blood pressure. Dosage range: 25 to 50 mg po bid. Dosage is adjusted over a 1-week trial period before stabilization occurs. Maximum dosage: 50 mg tid.

Available Drug Forms Scored tablets containing 25 or 50 mg.

Nursing Management Give immediately after breakfast and supper. (See chlorothiazide.)

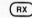

GENERIC NAME Bendroflumethiazide (RX)

TRADE NAME Benuran, Naturetin

CLASSIFICATION Long-acting thiazide diuretic

See chlorothiazide for Indications for use, Contraindications, Warnings and precautions, Untoward reactions, Drug interactions, and Nursing management.

Action Bendroflumethiazide, an analog of hydrochlorothiazide, is one of the most potent thiazides.

Less potassium and bicarbonate is lost than with hydrochlorothiazide. Prolonged use may require potassium supplementation.

Parameters of Use

Absorption Onset of action is 1 to 2 hours. Peak action occurs in 6 to 12 hours and duration of action is 18 hours.

Administration Initial dosage: 5 to 20 mg po daily; Maintenance dosage: 2.5 to 15.0 mg daily.

Available Drug Forms Tablets containing 0.5, 5, or 10 mg.

GENERIC NAME Cyclothiazide (RX)

TRADE NAME Anhydron

CLASSIFICATION Long-acting thiazide diuretic

See chlorothiazide for Indications for use, Contraindications, Warnings and precautions, Untoward reactions, Drug interactions, and Nursing management.

Action Cyclothiazide, an analog of hydrochlorothiazide,is a potent antihypertensive. Severe hypertensives may require a daily maintenance dosage.

Parameters of Use

Absorption Onset of action is 6 hours. Peak action occurs in 7 to 12 hours and duration of action is 18 to 24 hours.

Administration Initial dosage: 1 to 2 mg po daily; Maintenance dosage: 1 to 2 mg every other day.

Available Drug Forms Scored tablets containing 2 mg.

GENERIC NAME Hydroflumethiazide (RX)

TRADE NAMES Diucardin, Na Clex, Saluron

CLASSIFICATION Long-acting thiazide diuretic

Action Hydroflumethiazide, an analog of hydrochlorothiazide, has a potency similar to hydrochlorothiazide.

Parameters of Use

Absorption Onset of action is 1 to 2 hours. Peak action occurs in 4 hours and duration of action is 18 to 24 hours.

Administration

- *Edema:* 25 to 200 mg po daily.
- *Hypertension:* 50 to 100 mg po daily.

Available Drug Forms Scored tablets containing 50 mg.

GENERIC NAME Methyclothiazide (RX)

TRADE NAMES Aquatensen, Enduron

CLASSIFICATION Long-acting thiazide diuretic

See chlorothiazide for Indications for use, Contraindications, Warnings and precautions, Untoward reactions, Drug interactions, and Nursing management.

Action Methyclothiazide is an analog of hydrochlorothiazide. It is well absorbed and well tolerated. The drug has little effect on serum potassium levels. Only one daily dose is necessary.

Parameters of Use

Absorption Absorption Onset of action is 2 hours. Peak action occurs in 6 hours and duration of action is 24 hours.

Administration 2.5 to 10.0 mg po daily.

Available Drug Forms Tablets containing 2.5 and 5 mg.

GENERIC NAME Polythiazide (RX)

TRADE NAME Renese

CLASSIFICATION Long-acting thiazide diuretic

See chlorothiazide for Indications for use, Contraindications, Warnings and precautions, Untoward reactions, Drug interactions, and Nursing management.

Action Polythiazide, an analog of hydrochlorothiazide, has approximately 10 times the diuretic effect of hydrochlorothiazide. Only one daily dose is necessary.

Parameters of Use

Absorption Onset of action is 2 hours. Peak action occurs in 6 hours and duration of action is 24 to 48 hours (can last up to 72 hours). Binds to plasma proteins.

Administration 1 to 4 mg po daily.

Available Drug Forms Tablets containing 1, 2, and 4 mg.

GENERIC NAME Trichlormethiazide (RX)

TRADE NAMES Aquazide, Metahydrin, Methydrin, Naqua

CLASSIFICATION Long-acting thiazide diuretic

See chlorothiazide for Indications for use, Contraindications, Warnings and precautions, Untoward reactions, Drug interactions, and Nursing management.

Action Trichlormethiazide, an analog of hydrochlorothiazide, has approximately 10 times the diuretic effect of hydrochlorothiazide. It is excreted slower than the parent drug chlorthiazide.

Parameters of Use

Absorption Onset of action is 2 hours. Peak action occurs in 6 hours and duration of action is 24 hours.

Administration Initial dosage: 2 to 4 mg po bid; Maintenance dosage: 2 to 4 mg daily.

Available Drug Forms Tablets containing 2 and 4 mg.

THIAZIDE-LIKE DIURETICS

GENERIC NAME Chlorthalidone (RX)

TRADE NAME Hygroton

CLASSIFICATION Thiazide-like diuretic

See chlorothiazide for Indications for use, Contraindications, Warnings and precautions, Untoward reactions, and Drug interactions.

Action Chlorthalidone (phthalimidine sulfonamide) is chemically different but physiologic action is similar to chlorothiazide. It has a saluretic effect with minimal loss of potassium and bicarbonate. (See chlorothiazide for further details.)

Parameters of Use

Absorption Slower than chlorothiazide. Onset of action is 2 hours. Peak action occurs in 6 to 18 hours and duration of action is 60 hours (48 to 72 hours).

Excretion By the kidneys as unchanged drug; some in bile (often reabsorbed).

Administration Adults: 50 to 200 mg po daily or every other day immediately after breakfast; Children: 3 mg/kg 3 times per week.

Available Drug Forms Tablets containing 25, 50, or 100 mg.

Nursing Management Give with a full glass of water. (See chlorothiazide.)

GENERIC NAME Metolazone (RX)

TRADE NAMES Diulo, Zaroxolyn

CLASSIFICATION Thiazide-like diuretic

See chlorothiazide for Indications for use, Contraindications, Warnings and precautions, Untoward reactions, Drug interactions, and Nursing management.

Action Metolazone (quinazoline sulfonamide) is chemically different but physiologic action is similar to chlorothiazide. (See chlorothiazide.) Marked diuresis occurs when given with furosemide. The drug may produce diuresis in severe oliguria. Antihypertensive effect may occur after 3 to 4 days. (See chlorothiazide.)

Parameters of Use

Absorption Onset of action is 1 hour. Peak action occurs in 2 hours and duration of action is 12 to 24 hours. Highly bound to proteins.

Administration

- *Edema:* 5 to 20 mg po daily in early A.M.
- *Hypertension:* 2.5 to 5.0 mg po daily.

Available Drug Forms Tablets containing 2.5, 5, or 10 mg.

GENERIC NAME Quinethazone (RX)

TRADE NAME Hydromox

CLASSIFICATION Thiazide-like diuretic

See chlorothiazide for Indications for use, Contraindications, Warnings and precautions, Untoward reactions, Drug interactions, and Nursing management.

Action Quinethazone (quinazoline sulfonamide) has the same potency as hydrochlorothiazide, but a longer duration of action.

Parameters of Use

Absorption Rapid. Onset of action is 2 hours. Peak action occurs in 6 hours and duration of action is 12 to 24 hours.

Excretion By the kidneys as unchanged drug.

Administration 50 to 100 mg po daily; Dosage range: 50 to 200 mg daily.

Available Drug Forms Scored tablets containing 50 mg.

Nursing Management Give as one dose early in A.M. (See chlorothiazide.)

LOOP DIURETICS

GENERIC NAME Furosemide (RX)

TRADE NAME Lasix

CLASSIFICATION Loop diuretic

Action Furosemide, a sulfonamide derivative (anthranilic acid), is a potent diuretic that inhibits the reabsorption of sodium and chloride ions in the ascending limb of the loop of Henle as well as in the proximal and distal tubules. It reduces renal vascular resistance. The renal excretion of potassium is increased, but the excretion of bicarbonate is essentially unchanged. Low dosages cause retention of uric acid, but high dosages increase the excretion of uric acid. Thus, hyperuricemia is less problematic than with other diuretics. Unlike thiazide diuretics, furosemide has little effect on carbohydrate metabolism.

Indications for Use Refractory edema; acute and chronic edema; pulmonary edema; edema associated with congestive heart failure, cirrhosis of the liver, nephrotic syndrome, and other renal diseases; hypertension (particularly when associated with blood volume overload or edema) with or without other antihypertensive agents.

Contraindications Hypersensitivity to furosemide or sulfonamides, anuria, hyponatremia, hypokalemia, hypochloremic alkalosis, women of childbearing age unless the situation is life threatening.

Warnings and Precautions Use with caution in clients with gout or diabetes mellitus. Excessive diuresis may result in severe reduction of blood volume, circulatory collapse, and/or thrombosis, particularly in the elderly and debilitated clients. May precipitate hepatic coma in clients with severe hepatic impairment or azotemia in clients with renal impairment. May exacerbate systemic lupus erythematosus.

Untoward Reactions Hypersensitivity reactions include purpura, photosensitivity, rash, urticaria, vasculitis, exfoliative dermatitis, and erythema multiforme. Hypokalemia (arrhythmias, flattened T waves, progressive muscular weakness, paresthesia, hyporeflexes, anorexia, vomiting) occurs relatively frequently. Other electrolyte disturbances may arise as a result of excessive loss of sodium (hyponatremia), chloride (hypochloremia), or calcium (hypocalcemia), but tetany is rare. Hypovolemia and dehydration may also occur. Hypotension, circulatory collapse, and thromboembolic episodes may occur, particularly in the elderly and debilitated clients. GI disorders (nausea, vomiting, diarrhea, abdominal cramps, anorexia, constipation) are relatively common with long-term administration. Intrahepatic cholestatic jaundice, elevated serum ammonia levels, elevated blood urea nitrogen, mental confusion, disorientation, and hepatic coma have been reported, particularly in clients with impaired hepatic function. Common side effects include orthostatic hypotension and transient dizziness; the elderly are particularly susceptible to these effects. Tinnitus and temporary or permanent hearing loss can occur, particularly when the drug is injected rapidly intravenous, there is some renal impairment, or the client is receiving certain antibiotics concomitantly; it is sometimes preceded by a feeling of fullness in the ears. Blood dyscrasias include anemia, leukopenia, agranulocytosis, thrombocytopenia, and aplastic anemia. Lupus erythematosus may occur in susceptible clients. Hyperuricemia may occur with long-term therapy and acute attacks of gout may be precipitated, but rarely. Rare reactions include paresthesia, headache, xanthopsia, blurred vision, urinary bladder spasm, pancreatitis, and hematuria.

Parameters of Use

Absorption Rapidly absorbed from GI tract. Biphasic diuresis. Onset of action is: 30 to 60 minutes (po); 20 to 60 minutes (IM); 5 minutes (IV). Peak action occurs in: 1 to 2 hours (po); 1 to 2 hours (IM); 15 to 60 minutes (IV). Duration of action is: 6 to 8 hours (po); 6 to 8 hours (IM); 2 hours (IV). About 95% bound to plasma proteins.

Crosses placenta and appears in breast milk; lactating mothers should bottle-feed their babies.

Distribution Distributed throughout the extracellular fluid, but concentrated in the kidneys and liver.

Metabolism Small amount metabolized by the liver; may cause temporary elevation of blood urea nitrogen.

Excretion Rapidly excreted by the kidneys as unchanged drug and metabolites; some excreted in feces.

Drug Interactions Since furosemide causes renal excretion of potassium, the severity of hypokalemia will increase if other drugs that cause potassium loss, including corticosteroids, ACTH, and certain other diuretics, are given concurrently. Digitalis toxicity may be precipitated by the hypokalemia produced by furosemide if digitalis glycosides are given concomitantly. Ototoxicity (tinnitus and hearing impairment) can occur when aminoglycoside antibiotics, such as gentamicin and kanamycin, are given concomitantly. Orthostatic hypotension, which can progress to general hypotension, may occur when alcohol, other antihypertensive agents, barbiturates, or narcotics are given concurrently. Insulin requirements and the dosage of oral antidiabetic agents may need to be increased in diabetics, but rarely. Renal excretion of salicylates and lithium may be decreased by furosemide resulting in salicylate or lithium toxicity. Furosemide may increase the responsiveness to norepinephrine and other pressor amines. Nephrotoxicity may be enhanced if cephaloridine or other cephalosporin antibiotics are given concomitantly. Hypertension and tachycardia can occur if chloral hydrate is given within the same 24-hour period as furosemide.

Administration Highly individualized.

- *Edema:* Oral: 40 to 80 mg daily; Dosage range: 40 to 600 mg daily; may be given in divided doses. Intramuscular, intravenous: 20 to 40 mg; Dosage range: 20 to 80 mg as a single dose. A second dose may be given in 1 hour if no response occurs.
- *Hypertension:* 40 mg po bid; Dosage range: 20 to 100 mg bid.

- *Pediatric:* Oral: 2 mg/kg daily; do not exceed 6 mg/kg/day. A second dose of 1 to 2 mg/kg can be given in 6 to 8 hours if no response occurs. Intramuscular, intravenous: 1 mg/kg; do not exceed 6 mg/kg/day. A second dose of 1 mg/kg may be given in 2 to 4 hours if no response occurs. Do not administer IV bolus faster than 1 mg/min.

Available Drug Forms Scored tablets containing 20, 40, or 80 mg; orange-flavored oral solution containing 10 mg/ml (droppers are available for infants); sterile injectable solution in ampules of 2 or 10 ml containing 10 mg/ml; 2-ml prefilled syringes containing 10 mg/ml.

Nursing Management

Planning factors

1. When diuresis is desired, administer early in A.M. so that nocturnal diuresis is prevented. If the drug is administered twice a day, the first dose should be given as early as possible (8 A.M.) and the second dose 6 to 8 hours later (2 P.M. or 4 P.M.). When possible, do not administer after 6 P.M. so that sleep is not interrupted.
2. If a potassium supplement is not ordered, some potassium-rich foods (citrus fruits, bananas, dates, dried apricots) should be ingested daily.
3. Hypokalemia may be avoided by administering the drug for the first 4 days of each week. However, potassium-rich foods should be ingested all week long.
4. A 4-g or more sodium diet is usually required to prevent hyponatremia.
5. Discontinue drug at least 1 week (if po) or 2 days (if parenteral) prior to surgery.
6. Obtain the following baseline data prior to initiating therapy: blood pressure in sitting, standing, and supine position; serum electrolytes, blood urea nitrogen (BUN), serum glucose, and uric acid; body weight.
7. Store drug in dark area. Discard parenteral solution if it has a yellow discoloration.
8. Store oral suspension in refrigerator (36 to 46 F).

Administration factors

1. Oral solution can be used if client is unable to swallow tablets.
2. When administering IM,
   a. Inject deep into muscle mass with good circulation (upper outer quadrant of buttock into gluteus maximus), since drug is irritating.
   b. Avoid edematous sites and sites with poor circulation.
   c. Rotate sites to decrease tissue irritation.
3. When administering IV,
   a. Instruct client to report any feelings of faintness, tinnitus, or "fullness in the ears." If any of these symptoms occur, discontinue medication and notify physician.
   b. Check patency of IV before administering drug.
   c. Small dosages (20 to 40 mg) can be administered rapidly (1 to 2 minutes), but large dosages should not be administered faster than 4 mg/min. If the client is elderly or has severe cardiac or renal disease, the drug should always be administered at 4 mg/min. or less. Never exceed 10 mg/min.
   d. An IV syringe pump is highly recommended.

Evaluation factors

1. Monitor heart rate, rhythm, and blood pressure frequently from the time of drug onset through peak plasma levels. If arrhythmia develops (premature ventricular contractions) or blood pressure falls dramatically (20 mm Hg or more), notify physician immediately.
2. Record intake and output. If diuresis does not begin in 1 hour following parenteral administration or 2 hours following oral administration, notify physician.
3. Weigh client daily to determine quantity of water loss. A weight loss of 1 to 2 kg is common.
4. Determine serum electrolyte levels (sodium, potassium, chloride, carbon dioxide binding capacity, calcium) and BUN daily. If abnormal, notify physician before administering drug.
5. Measure abdominal girth each morning in clients with ascites.
6. Assess lung rales and rhonchi at least q2h in clients with pulmonary edema and congestive heart failure.
7. Test urine of diabetics and potential diabetics for sugar at least 4 times daily.
8. Assess client daily, prior to morning dose, for hypokalemia and other electrolyte disturbances. If symptoms occur, notify physician before administering drug.

Client teaching factors

1. Instruct client about the appropriate times to take medication.
2. Inform client to eat foods high in potassium at least once daily.
3. Advise client to seek medical advice if any untoward reactions occur.

GENERIC NAMES Ethacrynic acid; sodium ethacrynate

TRADE NAMES Edecrin; Sodium Edecrin (RX)

CLASSIFICATION Loop diuretic

See furosemide for Warnings and precautions.

Action This potent synthetic diuretic is an unsaturated ketone derivative of phenoxyacetic acid. It inhibits the reabsorption of sodium and chloride ions in the ascending limb of the loop of Henle as well as in the proximal and distal tubules. There is also some loss of potassium, calcium, and hydrogen ions. Although uric acid is retained when low dosages are administered, high dosages cause its excretion. Unlike thiazide diuretics, ethacrynic acid has little effect on carbohydrate metabolism. Calcium excretion is increased in hypercalcemia and diabetes insipidus. Hypoproteinemia may reduce the diuretic effect of ethacrynic acid and should be corrected with salt-poor albumin before administering drug.

Indications for Use Refractory edema; acute and chronic edema; pulmonary edema; edema associated with congestive heart failure, cirrhosis of the liver, nephrotic syndrome and other renal diseases, and ascites (lymphedema); hypercalcemia; diabetes insipidus.

Contraindications Hypersensitivity to ethacrynic acid (or mannitol if IV), anuria, hypokalemia, hypochloremic alkalosis, women of childbearing age unless the situation is life threatening, hepatic coma, pregnancy.

Untoward Reactions Severe watery diarrhea with sudden onset may occur; this may be an allergic reaction. Tinnitus vertigo and a feeling of "fullness in the ears" can progress to temporary or permanent hearing loss, particularly when the drug is injected rapidly intravenous, there is severe renal impairment, or the client is receiving ototoxic drugs, such as certain antibiotics, concomitantly. Hypokalemia occurs relatively frequently and may lead to fatal arrhythmias, particularly in elderly cardiac clients receiving digitalis glycosides concurrently. Other electrolyte disturbances may arise as a result of excessive loss of sodium (hyponatremia), chloride (hypochloremia, hypochloremic alkalosis), or calcium (hypocalcemia). These disturbances may have fatal consequences in clients with ascites and severely decompensated cirrhosis of the liver. Hypovolemia and dehydration may occur, particularly in infants, children, the elderly, and debilitated clients. Hypotension, circulatory collapse, and thromboembolic episodes may also occur, particularly in the elderly and debilitated clients. GI disorders (anorexia, nausea, vomiting, dysphagia, abdominal cramps, diarrhea) may occur with large dosages and long-term therapy. Blood dyscrasias include agranulocytosis, severe neutropenia, and thrombocytopenia. Hyperuricemia may occur and acute attacks of gout may be precipitated, but rarely. Hyperglycemia and glucosuria may occur in diabetics and latent diabetics, but rarely. Schönlein-Henoch purpura has been reported in clients with rheumatic disease. Rare reactions include jaundice, pancreatitis, elevated blood urea nitrogen, fatigue, and malaise.

Parameters of Use

Absorption Relatively rapid. Onset of diuresis is: 30 minutes (po); 5 minutes (IV). Peak action occurs in: 2 hours (po); 30 minutes (IV). Duration of action is: 6 to 8 hours (po); 2 hours (IV). Half-life is 30 to 70 minutes. Bound to proteins; may displace other drugs from protein-binding sites.

Probably crosses placenta and appears in breast milk; lactating mothers should bottle-feed their babies.

Distribution Distributed throughout extracellular fluid, but concentrated in the kidneys and liver.

Metabolism Metabolized to cysteine conjugate.

Excretion Approximately two-thirds in urine and one-third in bile.

Drug Interactions Since ethacrynic acid causes renal excretion of potassium, the severity of hypokalemia will increase if other drugs that cause potassium loss, including corticosteroids, ACTH, and certain other diuretics, are given concurrently. Digitalis toxicity may be precipitated by the hypokalemia produced by ethacrynic acid if digitalis glycosides are given concomitantly. Ototoxicity and hearing loss can occur with concurrent use of aminoglycoside antibiotics, such as gentamicin, kanamycin, neomycin, and streptomycin. Renal excretion of lithium may be decreased by ethacrynic acid resulting in lithium toxicity. Ethacrynic acid may displace warfarin and oral antidiabetic agents from protein-binding sites, thus potentiating their effects. The drug may also potentiate the effects of alcohol. Ethacrynic acid increases the responsiveness to tubocurarine and other curare derivatives.

Administration Highly individualized. Adults: Oral: 50 mg bid; Dosage range: 50 to 400 mg daily. Intravenous: 0.5 to 1.0 mg/kg (50 mg for average adult); do not exceed 100 mg in a single dose. Children: 25 mg po; then increase gradually by 25 mg until desired effect.

Available Drug Forms Scored tablets containing 25 or 50 mg; 50-ml vials containing 50 mg of powder (contains 62.5 mg mannitol).

Nursing Management

Planning factors

1. Administer early in A.M. with breakfast so that nocturnal diuresis is prevented. If the drug is administered twice a day, the second dose should be given with food during midafternoon or early evening.
2. A 4-g or more sodium diet is usually required to prevent hyponatremia.
3. Obtain the following baseline data prior to initiating therapy: blood pressure in sitting, standing, and supine position; complete blood cell count, serum electrolytes, blood urea nitrogen, and uric acid; body weight. Hepatic function tests should be done periodically if long-term therapy is required.

Administration factors

1. Give tablets with milk or meals to prevent GI irritation.
2. Reconstitute sterile ethacrynate powder with 50 ml of sodium chloride. Give as slow IV bolus or add solution to 50 ml of 5% D/W. Use solution within 24 hours.
3. Discard solution if it becomes hazy.
4. When administering IV,
   a. Do not use IV route in children.
   b. Check patency of IV before administering
   c. Instruct client to report any feelings of faintness, tinnitus, or "fullness in the ears." If any of these symptoms occur, discontinue medication and notify physician.
   d. An IV syringe or infusion pump is highly recommended.
   e. Check IV site frequently, since extravasation can cause severe tissue irritation.

Evaluation factors

1. Monitor heart rate, rhythm, and blood pressure frequently from the time of drug onset through peak plasma levels.
2. Observe client frequently for hyponatremia and other untoward reactions.
3. Record intake and output.
4. Weigh client daily to determine quantity of water loss.

5. Measure abdominal girth each morning in clients with ascites.
6. Assess rales and rhonchi frequently in clients with cardiac or pulmonary disorders.

Client teaching factors

1. Instruct client about appropriate time to take drug.
2. Inform client to eat foods high in potassium at least once daily.
3. Advise client to seek medical advise if any untoward reactions occur.

POTASSIUM-SPARING DIURETICS

GENERIC NAME Spironolactone (RX)

TRADE NAME Aldactone

CLASSIFICATION Potassium-sparing diuretic (aldosterone antagonist)

Action Spironolactone, which is synthetically produced, inhibits the effects of aldosterone by competing for its receptor sites. This action results in inhibition of the aldosterone-mediated exchange of sodium for potassium in the distal renal tubule and sodium ions remain in the tubule instead of being exchanged for potassium ions in the bloodstream. Although the mechanism of action is unknown, spironolactone can lower blood pressure in hypertensive clients. Unlike other diuretics, reports indicate that this drug does not precipitate gout (hyperuricemia) or hyperglycemia. Spironolactone may be administered with thiazide or loop diuretics. It exhibits a supplemental diuretic effect and reduces the loss of potassium induced by other diuretics.

Indications for Use Primary hyperaldosteronism (aldosterone-producing adrenal adenomas, nodular adrenal hyperplasia); used alone or as an adjunct to other diuretics for congestive heart failure, ascites, cirrhosis of the liver, nephrotic syndrome, and other renal disorders; as an adjunct to antihypertensive agents for essential hypertension or hypokalemia; hypokalemia secondary to therapy with digitalis glycosides.

Contraindications Anuria, acute renal insufficiency or impairment, hyperkalemia.

Warnings and Precautions Use with caution in clients with blood urea nitrogen greater than 40 mg%. Use may be hazardous during pregnancy and lactation and is restricted to life-threatening situations. Has been found to be carcinogenic in rats after long-term administration of toxic doses. Hyperkalemia may occur if potassium supplements or potassium-rich foods are ingested concomitantly or if renal function is severely impaired.

Untoward Reactions Hyperkalemia (irritability, nausea, diarrhea, weakness, arrhythmias including ventricular fibrillation or cardiac standstill, peaked T waves) can occur and should be treated promptly with intravenous injections of glucose and insulin. Gynecomastia (abnormally enlarged mammary glands in males or females), decreased libido in males, menstrual irregularities, hirsutism, voice deepening, and other symptoms of hormonal imbalance can occur due to the drug's structural similarities to steroids; symptoms usually disappear when drug is discontinued. Other electrolyte imbalances may arise as a result of excessive loss of sodium (hyponatremia) and water (dehydration, lethargy); mild acidosis can also occur. Hypersensitivity reactions include maculopapular or erythematous rash, urticaria, and fever. CNS disturbances (mental confusion, ataxia, headache, lethargy, drowsiness) have occurred. Common GI symptoms include anorexia and diarrhea and abdominal cramps with long-term therapy, particularly in the elderly and debilitated clients.

Parameters of Use

Absorption Rapidly absorbed. Biphasic diuresis. Although peak serum levels of the metabolite canrenone occur in 2 to 4 hours, maximum diuresis usually takes 3 to 5 days. Activity persists for about 3 days after discontinuing the drug. Half-life is: 10 minutes (spironolactone); 13 to 24 hours (canrenone). About 90% bound to proteins.

Spironolactone may cross placenta and canrenone appears in breast milk; lactating mothers should bottle-feed their babies.

Metabolism Rapidly metabolized to canrenone (active) and inactive metabolites. Canrenone produces most of the drug effect.

Excretion As metabolites in urine and bile.

Drug Interactions Hyperkalemia can occur if spironolactone is given concomitantly with potassium. Spironolactone potentiates the effects of antihypertensive agents, particularly ganglionic blocking agents; the dosage of the latter drugs should be reduced by 50% when administered with spironolactone. Spironolactone may decrease the effect of cardiac glycosides. Systemic acidosis can occur if ammonium chloride is administered concurrently. Large doses of salicylates may antagonize the effects of spironolactone.

Administration

- *Test for hyperaldosteronism:* Short method: 400 mg po daily for 4 days; Long method: 400 mg po daily for 3 to 4 weeks. If serum potassium decreases sharply after drug is discontinued, test is considered positive.
- *Edema:* 25 mg po bid, tid, or qid; Dosage range: 25 to 200 mg daily. Administer for at least 5 days; then adjust dosage until desired effect.
- *Hypertension:* 25 mg po bid; Dosage range: 50 to 100 mg daily. Administer for at least 2 weeks; then adjust dosage until desired effect.
- *Hypokalemia:* 25 to 100 mg daily. (Use only when traditional therapy is considered inappropriate.)
- *Pediatric:* 3.3 mg/kg/day (1.5 mg/lb/day) in divided doses.

Available Drug Forms Scored tablets containing 25 mg.

Nursing Management

Planning factors

1. If client is unable to swallow tablets, notify pharmacist who can prepare an appropriate suspension. Suspensions are usually stable for 1 month.
2. If client is taking a potassium supplement or ingesting potassium-rich foods daily, notify physician before administering drug. Consult physician, dietitian, and client if diet adjustments are required to prevent hyperkalemia and hyponatremia.
3. Obtain the following baseline data prior to initiating therapy: blood pressure in standing, sitting, and supine position; serum electrolytes; body weight; status of breasts (size, shape, nodules) in males and females.
4. Store drug in a dark area.

Administration factors

1. Tablets can be crushed and added to applesauce or custard if client is unable to swallow tablets. (Add to a flavored syrup to facilitate administration to children.)
2. Check client daily, prior to administering drug, for electrolyte imbalances. If symptoms occur, notify physician before administering drug.
3. Administer drug in early morning to avoid nocturnal diuresis.

Evaluation factors

1. Check blood pressure daily for the first 2 weeks of therapy; then periodically.
2. Record intake and output.
3. Determine serum electrolytes daily for the first week; then periodically. Measure potassium levels frequently (weekly).
4. Weigh client daily to determine quantity of water loss.
5. Measure abdominal girth daily in clients with ascites.
6. Assess hepatic clients for CNS disturbances prior to each drug administration. If lethargy, confusion, or other symptoms occur, notify physician.
7. Assess breasts for gynecomastia at least biweekly. (Teach client breast self-examination.)

GENERIC NAME Triamterene (RX)

TRADE NAME Dyrenium

CLASSIFICATION Potassium-sparing diuretic

Action This weak diuretic is a synthetic pteridine derivative. It increases urinary excretion of sodium ions in exchange for potassium and hydrogen ions in the distal tubule. Although triamterene does not inhibit aldosterone, it does act directly on the section of the distal tubule influenced by the hormone. Since relatively small quantities of sodium reach this distal site, excretion of sodium and water is limited; however, concurrent use of more proximal-acting diuretics will increase the degree of diuresis. Carbonate and some chloride are also excreted. Uric acid excretion is not affected except in susceptible clients (gouty arthritis). Since glomerular filtration is reduced, blood urea nitrogen may increase; thus, triamterene should not be used in severe renal or hepatic diseases. Elevation of blood urea nitrogen can be minimized by administering the drug every other day.

Indications for Use Used alone or as an adjunct to other diuretics for congestive heart failure, cirrhosis of the liver, nephrotic syndrome and other renal disorders, or steroid-induced edema; edema of secondary hyperaldosteronism.

Contraindications Hypernsensitivity to triamterene, anuria, severe or progressive renal impairment (except nephrosis), severe hepatic impairment, hyperkalemia.

Warnings and Precautions Use with caution in clients with impaired renal or hepatic function, gouty arthritis, or diabetes mellitus. Use may be hazardous during pregnancy and lactation. Do not use if blood urea nitrogen is elevated. Hyperkalemia may occur if potassium supplements or potassium-rich foods are ingested concomitantly.

Untoward Reactions Hypersensitivity reactions include anaphylaxis, photosensitivity, and rashes. Hyperkalemia (irritability, nausea, diarrhea, weakness, arrhythmias including ventricular fibrillation or cardiac standstill, peaked T waves) can occur and should be treated promptly. Diabetics, clients with renal insufficiency, the elderly, and clients on long-term therapy may be particularly susceptible to hyperkalemia. GI disturbances, including nausea, vomiting, and diarrhea, are relatively common. Other electrolyte imbalances may arise as a result of excessive loss of sodium (hyponatremia) and water (dehydration); metabolic acidosis can also occur. Megaloblastic anemia can occur (since triamterene is a weak folic acid antagonist), particularly in clients with splenomegaly and cirrhosis of the liver. Granulocytopenia and eosinophilia may also occur. Nitrogen retention can occur, particularly in clients with renal or hepatic impairment. Hypotension has occurred with large dosages and long-term drug administration. Hyperuricemia has been reported in clients with a history of gouty arthritis.

Parameters of Use

Absorption Rapid and irregular absorption. Onset of diuresis is 2 to 4 hours and duration of action is 7 to 9 hours. Maximum therapeutic effect may not occur for several days. Half-life is 2 to 3 hours. Approximately 66% bound to proteins; may be displaced from binding sites by other drugs.

May cross placenta and appear in breast milk; lactating mothers should bottle-feed their babies.

Excretion By the kidneys, but the rate of elimination is variable.

Drug Interactions Hypotension may occur if triamterene is given concomitantly with antihypertensive agents. Hyperkalemia can occur if triamterene is given concurrently with potassium supplements. Triamterene may decrease the effect of cardiac glycosides.

Laboratory Interactions Triamterene interferes with fluorometric measurement of quinidine and lactate dehydrogenase.

Administration Highly individualized. Initial dosage: 100 mg po bid for 3 or 4 days; Maintenance dosage: 100 mg daily or every other day; Dosage range: 100 to 300 mg daily. When administered with other diuretics the usual dosage is 100 mg daily or every other day.

Available Drug Forms Capsules containing 50 or 100 mg.

Nursing Management

Planning factors

1. Administer early in A.M. with breakfast so that nocturnal diuresis is prevented. If the drug is administered twice a day, the second dose should be given with food during midafternoon or early evening.
2. A 4-g sodium diet or more is usually required to prevent hyponatremia.
3. If client is taking potassium supplements or ingesting potassium-rich foods daily, notify physician before administering drug. Consult physician, dietitian, and client if diet adjustments are required to prevent hyperkalemia and hyponatremia.
4. Obtain the following baseline data prior to initiating therapy: blood pressure; body weight; serum electrolytes, blood urea nitrogen (BUN), and uric acid.

Administration factors

1. Check client daily, prior to administering drug, for electrolyte imbalances. If symptoms occur, notify physician before administering drug.
2. Give with food or meals to prevent GI irritation.

Evaluation factors

1. Check blood pressure daily for the first week of therapy; then periodically.
2. Record intake and output.
3. Determine serum electrolytes and BUN daily for the first week; then weekly.
4. Weigh client daily to determine quantity of water loss.
5. Measure abdominal girth daily in clients with ascites.

OSMOTIC DIURETICS

GENERIC NAME Mannitol (RX)

TRADE NAMES D-Mannitol, Osmitrol

CLASSIFICATION Osmotic diuretic

Source Sugar alcohol that occurs in fruits and vegetables; commercially prepared by reducing dextrose.

Action Mannitol increases the osmolarity of the glomerular filtrate and thereby decreases the tubular reabsorption of water, thus causing diuresis. Average dosages of mannitol will increase the loss of sodium and chloride. Additional electrolytes (potassium, calcium) may be lost when large dosages are administered. As mannitol is a hypertonic solution that remains in extracellular fluid after intravenous injection, it increases the osmolarity of blood and promotes the diffusion of fluid into blood, thereby decreasing elevated cerebrospinal fluid and intraocular pressures.

Indications for Use Emergency treatment of elevated cerebrospinal fluid pressure (head injuries) and elevated intraocular pressure unresponsive to other therapies; oliguria following cardiovascular surgery, severe trauma, hemolytic transfusion reaction, and other causes of acute renal failure; toxic overdose of some substances; diagnostic kidney test (measuring the rate of glomerular filtration).

Contraindications Anuria, severe renal failure, pulmonary edema, severe congestive heart failure, active intracranial bleeding, severe dehydration.

Warnings and Precautions Safe use in pregnancy and children under 12 years has not been established. Electrolyte-free mannitol should not be given when blood is being administered.

Untoward Reactions Circulatory overload, pulmonary edema, or congestive heart failure may occur in susceptible clients or if mannitol is administered too rapidly. Electrolyte imbalances include alterations in sodium and potassium. Dehydration may occur with brisk diuresis. Acidosis has occurred in some clients. Osmotic nephrosis may occur and progress to severe irreversible nephrosis. Hypersensitivity reactions include urticaria and fever. Thrombophlebitis can occur in susceptible clients, particularly the elderly. Extravasation will cause local edema and tissue necrosis. Other reactions include urinary retention, headache, blurred vision, convulsions, nausea, vomiting, rhinitis, anginalike pain, hypotension, hypertension, and tachycardia.

Parameters of Use

Absorption Cerebrospinal fluid pressure begins to drop in 15 minutes and persists for 3 to 8 hours. Intraocular pressure begins to drop in 30 to 60 minutes and persists for 4 to 6 hours. Diuresis occurs in 1 to 3 hours. Half-life is approximately 100 minutes. Does not cross blood-brain barrier unless client has severe acidosis, active bleeding, or excessive drug concentrations in blood.

Distribution Essentially remains in extracellular fluid.

Metabolism In the liver to glycogen, but very little metabolized.

Excretion Rapidly excreted by the kidneys; about 80% eliminated within 3 hours.

Drug Interactions Mannitol increases the urinary excretion of lithium and may decrease the client's response to lithium.

Administration Total dosage, concentration, and rate of administration is determined by nature of injury, client's food requirements, and urinary output.

- *Test Dose:* 0.2 g/kg infused over 5 minutes; Usual adult dosage: 75 to 100 ml. If no diuresis occurs, a second test dose may be tried.
- *Oliguria:* 50 to 100 g/24 hours; Dosage range: 50 to 200 g/24 hours; do not exceed 200 g daily.
- *Reduction of intracranial pressure and brain mass:* 1.5 to 2.0 g/kg (0.75 to 1.0 g/lb) infused over 30 to 60 minutes. A continuous mannitol drip may be required. Titrate IV rate to maintain urine output between 30 to 50 ml/hour.
- *Reduction of intraocular pressure:* 1.5 to 2.0 g/kg (0.75 to 1.0 g/lb). If given as a prophylactic preoperatively, administer 1 to $1\frac{1}{2}$ hours prior to surgery.
- *Diagnostic test:* Dilute 100 ml of 20% solution (10 g) with 180 ml of injectable sodium chloride solution (yields 280 ml of a 7% solution) and infuse at 20 ml/min. Normal clearance rates: Males: 125 ml/min.; Women: 116 ml/min. Collect all urine over a specified time interval and analyze for drug excretion/min. When test is finished, take blood samples and determine the drug concentration in mg/ml of plasma.

Available Drug Forms Ampules containing 12.5 g in 50 ml of solution; IV bottles containing 20% solution in 500 ml, 15% solution in 500 ml, 10% solution in 1000 ml, or 5% solution in 1000 ml.

Nursing Management

Planning factors

1. Insert an indwelling urinary catheter and attach to a drainage bag so that hourly urinary output can be determined.
2. Obtain the following baseline data prior to initiating therapy: blood pressure and pulse; serum electrolytes; urinary output over the last hour; blood pH (presence of acidosis).
3. Attach cardiac clients and the elderly to an EKG monitor.
4. Insert central venous pressure (CVP) line and measure pressure prior to instituting therapy.
5. Administer drug through an angiocath.
6. Measure intraocular pressure, particularly if drug therapy has been instituted for an elevation in this pressure.
7. Do not use drug if crystals are present. The crystals will disappear if the container is heated in warm water and shaken well. Cool to body temperature before administering.

Administration factors

1. Give test dose to clients with oliguria prior to initiation of therapy. If diuresis is less than 30 ml, notify physician.
2. Check patency of IV line before administering. Restart IV if it appears infiltrated.
3. Do not administer through a CVP line.
4. When administering via IV bolus,
   a. Give at a rate of 10 ml/min. or less in order to prevent untoward reactions.
   b. Check CVP line before administering each bolus and 15 minutes after bolus is completed. If postbolus CVP is elevated 20 mm Hg or more above prebolus CVP, observe client for potential cardiovascular overload and notify physician.
5. When administering via IV intermittent infusion,
   a. Use a IV pump to control the rate of infusion, if available.
   b. If pump is unavailable, use a minidrip IV administration set. (Infusion rate is prescribed by physician.) Do not administer faster than 100 ml/hour unless specifically prescribed.
   c. Monitor CVP, blood pressure, and pulse every 10 minutes during administration and every 15 to 30 minutes following until diuresis is complete (about 3 hours).
   d. Check urinary output hourly.
6. When administering via continuous IV drip,
   a. Use an IV pump to control the rate of infusion, if available.
   b. Infusion rate may be prescribed by physician as "a rate sufficient to maintain output between 30 to 50 ml/hour." Adjust IV rate up or down according to the previous hour's urinary output.
   c. Do not exceed 100 ml/hour unless specifically prescribed.
   d. Monitor CVP, blood pressure, and pulse every 15 to 30 minutes during therapy. If CVP rises rapidly, slow IV rate to KVO and notify physician immediately.
   e. If urinary output remains below 30 ml/hour for 2 consecutive hours, notify physician.
   f. Check IV site for extravasation every 30 minutes.

Evaluation factors

1. Record intake and output.
2. Determine serum electrolytes periodically during therapy.
3. Observe for progressive oliguria. If it occurs, slow IV rate to KVO and notify physician immediately.
4. Observe for circulatory overload (elevated CVP, rales in the lungs). If symptoms occur, slow IV rate to KVO and notify physician immediately.
5. If diuresis does not begin within 2 hours, notify physician.

GENERIC NAME Urea (RX)

TRADE NAMES Carbamide, Urephil, Urevert

CLASSIFICATION Osmotic diuretic

Source Synthetically produced diamide salt of carbonic acid.

Action Intravenous administration of hypertonic urea solution increases the concentration of urea so that it is greater in the blood than in extracellular body fluids. Consequently, cerebrospinal and intraocular fluid will move into the blood. As the concentration of urea increases in the glomerular filtrate, the reabsorption of water is decreased in the proximal tubule and diuresis occurs.

Sodium, chloride, and some potassium are also excreted. Topical administration promotes skin hydration and is useful for removing keratin.

Indications for Use Treatment of elevated intracranial pressure (control of edema) and elevated intraocular pressure; removal of keratin in hyperkeratotic disorders.

Contraindications Anuria, severe renal failure, active intracranial bleeding, marked dehydration, severe hepatic failure.

Warnings and Precautions Use with caution in infants, children, during pregnancy, in clients with impaired hepatic function (since there may be a significant rise in serum ammonia levels), and in clients with impaired renal function. Blood urea nitrogen below 40 mg/100 ml does not preclude the use of urea in most cases, but frequent laboratory studies should be done to determine renal function.

Untoward Reactions Hemolysis and adverse effects on the cerebral vasomotor centers (causing increased capillary bleeding) may occur if urea is infused rapidly. Minor arterial oozing can occur following intracranial surgery. Venous thrombosis and hemoglobinuria may occur, particularly if hypothermia therapy is used concurrently. Common reaction include headache, nausea, vomiting, syncope, and disorientation. Transient confusion and agitation can occur, particularly when urea is infused too fast or there is marked impairment of renal function. Electrolyte imbalances include alterations in sodium and potassium. Dehydration may occur with brisk diuresis. Intraocular hemorrhage has been reported following rapid intravenous infusion in clients with glaucoma. Chemical phlebitis and thrombosis at or near the injection site has been reported, but infrequently. Extravasation will cause local irritation and pain and sloughing may occur.

Parameters of Use

Absorption Poorly absorbed from GI tract; oral administration is seldom used because very large dosages are required. Cerebrospinal fluid and intraocular pressures begin to decrease in 1 to 2 hours and persist for 3 to 10 hours. Diuresis occurs in 6 to 12 hours.

Distribution Distributed throughout extracellular fluid; also found in intracellular fluid.

Excretion By the kidneys as unchanged drug.

Drug Interactions Urea increases the urinary excretion of lithium and may decrease the client's response to lithium. Urea may counteract elevations in intraocular pressure induced by the skeletal muscle relaxant succinylcholine. Due to its fibrinolytic activity, urea may potentiate the effects of anticoagulants.

Administration Total dosage and rate of administration are determined by nature of injury and urinary output. Adults: 1.0 to 1.5 g/kg daily via IV infusion (30% solution) at a rate not exceeding 4 ml/min. Infants: 0.1 g/kg.

Available Drug Forms Sterile 150-ml vials containing 40 g for reconstitution with 5% D/W, 10% D/W, or 10% invert sugar. Topical preparations: 2 to 25% in cream or lotion form.

Nursing Management

Planning factors

1. Insert an indwelling urinary catheter and attach to a drainage bag so that hourly urinary output can be determined.
2. Obtain the following baseline data prior to initiating therapy: vital signs, including temperature; serum electrolytes, ammonia levels, and blood urea nitrogen (BUN); urinary output over the last hour.
3. If not already inserted, insert an angiocath into a large blood vessel. Do not use a CVP line.
4. Measure intraocular pressure, particularly if drug therapy has being instituted for an elevation in this pressure.

Administration factors

1. Always use freshly prepared solution, since ammonia is produced with storage.
2. Reconstitute with 105 ml of the appropriate diluent to yield 135 ml of 30% solution; 1 ml of solution contains 300 mg of urea.
3. If the whole vial is not required, remove undesired portion before hanging IV container (run through IV administration set into sink).
4. Discard all unused preparation immediately.
5. Check patency and adequacy of IV site before administering drug.
6. Infusion rate is prescribed by physician. Do not exceed 4 ml/min. An IV rate of 65 to 135 ml/hour is common for an adult.
7. Use an IV pump to maintain the desired flow rate, if available.

Evaluation factors

1. Monitor vital signs every 30 minutes until diuresis; then every 1 to 2 hours.
2. Measure urinary output hourly.
3. Record intake and output. If diuresis does not begin within 6 hours, notify physician immediately.
4. Check IV site for infiltration and irritation every 30 minutes.
5. Observe for signs and symptoms of CNS irritation (disorientation, confusion, agitation, nausea, vomiting, headache). If symptoms occur during drug administration, slow IV rate to KVO and notify physician immediately. If symptoms occur after drug administration, notify physician.
6. Determine BUN, serum ammonia levels, and serum electrolytes periodically (q12h). Elevation of BUN is common, but does not require discontinuation of therapy unless levels are markedly elevated.
7. Observe client for indications of bleeding frequently, particularly postoperative clients.

GENERIC NAME Glucose (50%) (RX)

CLASSIFICATION Osmotic diuretic

See mannitol for Contraindications, Warnings and precautions, Untoward reactions, Parameters of use, Drug interactions, and Nursing management.

Action Similar to mannitol in action. (See mannitol.)

Administration 50 ml of 50% glucose via slow IV bolus or intermittent infusion.

Available Drug Forms Ampules or vials containing 50 ml of 50% glucose.

XANTHINE DIURETICS

Xanthine diuretics are used to treat a variety of disorders. Complete monographs for these drugs are located in the chapters that deal with the drug's most frequent use. For example, the complete monograph for aminophylline, a potent bronchodilator, will be found in Chapter 54.

GENERIC NAME Aminophylline (RX)

TRADE NAMES Lixaminol, Mini-Lix, Somophyllin

CLASSIFICATION Xanthine diuretic

Action Aminophylline dilates the afferent arterioles and therefore increases glomerular filtration and urinary output.

Indications for Use Bronchodilator, peripheral vasodilator, myocardial stimulant, antiasthmatic.

Administration 200 to 500 mg po or rectal suppository daily.

GENERIC NAME Caffeine (RX)

CLASSIFICATION Xanthine diuretic

Action Caffeine dilates the afferent arterioles and therefore increases glomerular filtration and urinary output.

Indications for Use CNS stimulant in respiratory depression and other disorders.

Administration Oral: 65 to 250 mg daily; Intravenous: 250 to 600 mg q4h as needed (administer slowly).

GENERIC NAME Theobromine (RX)

CLASSIFICATION Xanthine diuretic

Action Theobromine dilates the afferent arterioles and therefore increases glomerular filtration and urinary output.

Indications for Use Bronchodilator and smooth muscle relaxant; often combined with other diuretics.

Administration 300 to 500 mg po daily.

GENERIC NAME Theophylline (RX)

TRADE NAMES Elixophyllin, Slo-Phyllin, Theobid, Theocin

CLASSIFICATION Xanthine diuretic

Action Most active diuretic of the xanthine alkaloids. Theophylline is seldom used alone, but combined with other diuretics (mercurials) to reduce irritation and improve absorption.

Indications for Use Bronchodilator and smooth muscle relaxant.

Administration 100 to 200 mg po daily.

PART XIII

RESPIRATORY SYSTEM AGENTS

RESPIRATION IS THE exchange of gases (air) between body cells and the atmosphere and involves the nose, pharynx, larynx, trachea, bronchi, bronchioles, and lungs. Abnormal breathing may be due to a disease or disorder of the respiratory organs or a systemic abnormality, such as anemia, acidosis, or infection. Respiration can also be affected directly or indirectly by many drugs, including central nervous system depressants and stimulants, adrenergic agents, cholinergic agents, autonomic blocking agents, diuretics, and certain antiinfective agents. However, this part only describes those drugs used to treat disorders of the external respiratory organs, namely bronchodilators, decongestants, mucolytics, and expectorants.

Breathing, or the act of inhaling and exhaling air through the external respiratory organs, is under the control of the *respiratory center* in the medulla oblongata. This center controls the rate and depth of inspiration and expiration and responds rapidly to changing body needs for oxygen. *Chemoreceptors,* which are located in the aortic arch, carotid body, and other large arteries, are sensitive to changes in arterial blood gases (pO_2, pCO_2) and hydrogen ion concentrations (pH) and send nervous impulses to the respiratory center that induce an increase or decrease in respirations. Emotions, body temperature, vasomotor activity, and other forms of stimuli can also affect the respiratory center.

Bronchial smooth muscle and respiratory secretions from the mucous membranes are influenced by the autonomic nervous system. Cholinergic neurons assist in maintaining normal bronchoconstriction and mucoid secretions. Alpha-adrenergic neurons also assist in the maintenance of bronchoconstriction, but suppress mucoid secretions. On the other hand, $beta_2$-adrenergic neurons mediate the relaxation of bronchial smooth muscle and thus induce bronchodilation. The mechanics that induce bronchoconstriction and bronchodilation are explained in detail in Chapter 54.

The body also has several other respiratory reflex mechanisms, such as sneezing and coughing. *Sneezing* is stimulated by the presence of certain irritants in the nasal cavities. These substances cause a buildup of air pressure in the pharynx. When the pressure is suddenly released by depression of the uvula, air is rapidly expelled through the nasal cavities, clearing them. The *cough reflex* is the sudden expulsion of air from the lungs. This reflex clears the respiratory passages of excessive secretions and foreign matter. Incomplete expulsion of infected mucous and debris may cause the infection to spread to other parts of the lungs. As prolonged or violent coughing may eventually lead to emphysema or pneumothorax, the defensive cough reflex must be suppressed.

Cough suppressants act via the central nervous system (CNS depressants). When these agents are administered, excessive mucus, infection, and other cough stimuli should be treated concurrently. Cough suppressants most commonly used, such as codeine and terpin hydrate, also decrease the flow of bronchial secretions. *Expectorants,* such as guaifenesin and potassium iodide, facilitate the removal of excessive mucus and debris. By increasing bronchial secretions, the secretions become watery and more easily expelled. *Mucolytics,* such as acetylcysteine, are a type of expectorant that literally "breaks" the mucus secretions apart, thus facilitating drainage and removal. Although inhaled mucolytics have lost popularity due to untoward reactions, these substances can be effective and desirable in selected clinical situations.

Decongestants are alpha-adrenergic agents that prevent the formation of nasal secretions by inducing vasoconstriction. These agents are frequently applied topically and some may be given concurrently with other respiratory drugs.

Many *bronchodilators* are stimulants of adrenergic receptors. The ideal bronchodilator would selectively stimulate $beta_2$-receptor sites without affecting the $beta_1$-receptor sites in the heart and other areas of the body. As a result of recent developments in pharmacotherapeutics, terbutaline and albuterol, two $beta_2$-adrenergic agents, are now available; others will probably follow. Theophylline and theophylline-containing agents have been used for a decade. Unlike adrenergic agents, these substances induce bronchodilation by inhibiting phosphediesterase and may be used concurrently with an adrenergic agent, such as ephedrine.

Multiple ingredient prescription and over-the-counter preparations are also available for treating respiratory disorders, but their benefit is questionable. The action of one ingredient may counteract another, augment the untoward reactions of another, or even be ineffective in combination. Research is being conducted to determine the effectiveness of these preparations. At the present time, many physicians are prescribing one or more single ingredient prescriptions to be administered at different times. When appropriate, nurses should be cautioned when administering multiple ingredient preparations and instructed to evaluate the therapeutic and untoward reactions of clients frequently.

Chapter 54

Bronchodilators

Mudrane GG Elixir
Quadrinal
Quibron Plus
Tedral, Tedral Suspension
Tedral-25
Tedral Expectorant
Tedral Elixir
Tedral SA

COMBINATION PREPARATIONS CONTAINING THEOPHYLLINE-CONTAINING SUBSTANCES AND AN EXPECTORANT

Asbron G
Elixophyllin-KI
Isufil T.D.
Quibron
Quibron-300
Slo-Phyllin GG
Synophylate-GG
Theolair-Plus 125
Theolair-Plus 250
Theolair-Plus Liquid
Theo-Organidin
Dilor-G
Emfaseem
Lufyllin-GG
Neothylline-GG
Brondecon

MULTIPLE INGREDIENT PREPARATIONS

KIE Syrup
Lufyllin-EPG
Mudrane
Mudrane GG Tablets
PBZ with Ephedrine
Quelidrine
Rynatuss Tablets
Rynatuss Pediatric Suspension
Duo-Medihaler
Mucomyst with Isoproterenol
Norisodrine with Calcium Iodide

BRONCHOCONSTRICTION CAN BE caused by several respiratory diseases, including bronchial asthma, bronchitis, emphysema, and other disorders that lead to chronic obstructive lung disease. All these disorders have one common manifestation; that is, an increase in airway resistance. Bronchodilators act by different mechanisms to assist in the relief of wheezing dyspnea and other symptoms of these disorders. They exert their action by affecting the sympathetic (adrenergic) or parasympathetic (cholinergic) nervous systems or other chemical substances that influence the diameter of the bronchi and bronchioles.

BRONCHOCONSTRICTION AND BRONCHODILATION

The normal state of bronchial smooth muscle is mild constriction. This normal muscular tone is balanced by (1) the bronchodilating influence mediated by beta-adrenergic neurons; and (2) the bronchoconstricting influence mediated by alpha-adrenergic and cholinergic neurons. Catecholamines released from adrenergic receptor sites alter the activity of adenosine 3^1:5^1-cyclic phosphate (cAMP). Elevations in the concentration of cAMP cause relaxation of bronchial smooth muscle and result in bronchodilation. Stimulation of *beta$_2$-adrenergic* receptor sites increases the activity of adenylate cyclase. This enzyme increases the conversion of adenosine triphosphate (ATP) to cAMP, thus increasing the concentration of cAMP and producing bronchodilation. cAMP is inactivated by the enzyme phosphodiesterase. When the degradation of cAMP is inhibited, the concentration of cAMP increases and bronchodilation results.

Cyclic guanosine monophosphate (cGMP) is the antagonist of cAMP. Whereas stimulation of *alpha-adrenergic* receptor sites results in a decrease in the concentration of cAMP, stimulation of *cholenergic* receptor sites increases the concentration of cGMP. Thus, stimulation of either alpha-adrenergic or cholinergic receptor sites in the bronchial smooth muscle induces bronchoconstriction.

In extrinsic (atopic or allergic) asthma, exposure to an allergen results in the production of the immunoglobulin IgE and its ultimate fixation to mast cells in the respiratory tract. Mast cells have granules that contain histamine, serotonin, and other chemical mediators. Upon subsequent exposure to the allergen, an antibody-antigen reaction occurs on the membranes of mast cells that ultimately results in a decrease of cAMP and the release of histamine, serototin, slow-reacting substances of anaphylaxis (SRS-A), and other chemical mediators. Histamine induces smooth muscle constriction, an increase in capillary permeability, and an excessive secretion of mucus in the upper respiratory tract. Serotonin may also induce constriction of smooth muscle and an increase in capillary permeability. Thus, immediate bronchoconstriction and an increase in airway resistance occur. SRS-A production is induced by the antibody-antigen reaction and SRS-A release induces bronchoconstriction and an increase in capillary permeability 6 to 12 hours after exposure to the allergen. Whereas histamine is the primary chemical mediator involved in anaphylaxis, SRS-A is thought to be the major mediator in bronchial asthma.

TYPES OF BRONCHODILATORS

Most bronchodilators act by altering the concentration of cAMP. Sympathomimetic bronchodilators induce relaxation of bronchial smooth muscle by stimulation of beta$_2$-adrenergic receptor sites. These agents may stimulate alpha, beta$_1$-, or beta$_2$-receptor sites. Although stimulation of alpha-receptor sites may induce bronchoconstriction, vasoconstriction of bronchial mucosal blood vessels with subsequent reduction in mucosal inflammation and congestion also occurs. Thus, alpha-adrenergic agents may aid in the reduction of respiratory secretions, but may induce the development of thick, tenacious mucus, mucus plugs, and bronchoconstriction.

Adrenergic agents Although these agents stimulate alpha-receptor sites, epinephrine and ephedrine are of benefit because they also stimulate beta-receptor sites. Epinephrine is the drug of choice in anaphylaxis and acute asthmatic attacks. This adrenergic agent has a rapid onset of action when inhaled or administered parenterally. However, as its duration of action is short and tolerance to the drug's bronchodilating effect can develop, epinephrine is usually reserved for aborting acute episodes. Ephedrine is useful in preventing excessive bronchoconstriction and aborting mild to moderately severe acute episodes.

Beta-adrenergic agents Isoproterenol is a sympathomimetic amine that stimulates beta-adrenergic receptor sites. It is the most potent beta-adrenergic agent known. This agent is particularly effective in relaxing bronchial smooth muscle when excessive muscle tone is present. Unfortunately, isoproterenol induces tachycardia, arrhythmias, and other untoward reactions by stimulating beta$_1$-adrenergic receptor sites. To restrict the drug's effects to the respiratory tract, isoproterenol is often administered via oral inhalation. Thus, the quantity of drug absorbed from the bronchi into the bloodstream is limited and fewer systemic effects on the heart and other tissues occur. Several beta-adrenergic agents are also effective in preventing excessive bronchoconstriction.

Beta$_2$-adrenergic agents Drugs that stimulate beta$_2$-adrenergic receptor sites have been the subject of intense investigation in the last few years. Terbutaline was the first to be released and metaproterenol soon followed. Other agents are presently under investigation and may be released in the near future.

Phosphodiesterase inhibitors Theophylline and theophylline-containing agents induce bronchodilation by inhibiting the enzyme phosphodiesterase, which degrades cAMP. Theophylline-containing drugs not only induce dilation of bronchial smooth muscle, but they also cause vasodilation of the coronary arteries, reduce vascular resistance, and stimulate the myocardium, skeletal muscles, and central nervous system. A transitory increase in cardiac output causes diuresis. Toxic effects can occur as a result of secondary actions of theophylline. Stimulation of the central nervous system may cause insomnia, nervousness, convulsions, and eventually coma. Tachycardia, hypotension, and arrhythmias may also occur. Therapeutic dosages range from 10 to 20 mcg/ml; toxic effects occur when serum drug levels exceed 20 mcg/ml.

ANTIASTHMATIC AGENTS

Although cromolyn sodium is not a bronchodilator, the drug is effective in decreasing the body's requirements for bronchodilators and antiinflammatory agents in extrinsic asthma. Mast cells are inhibited from releasing chemical mediators that induce bronchoconstriction after 3 to 4 weeks of therapy. Although the drug is ineffective in aborting acute episodes of bronchospasm, it is effective in decreasing the frequency and severity of asthmatic attacks.

CORTICOSTEROIDS

When bronchospasm cannot be relieved by bronchodilators, the antiinflammatory effect of corticosteroids may be required. Intravenous administration of hydrocortisone sodium succinate (Solu-Cortif) may be life saving in anaphylaxis, status asthmaticus, and other acute episodes. The continued use of oral corticosteroids may be required in order to prevent acute episodes of bronchospasm. Cromolyn is particularly effective in clients who require corticosteroids, since the dosage of the latter may be reduced or eliminated as the prophylactic effect of cromolyn increases.

EXPECTORANTS AND OTHER AGENTS

Excessive respiratory secretions and the production of thick, tenacious mucus accompanies many respiratory diseases. Consequently, preparations that contain bronchodilators, expectorants, and/or mucolytics are frequently required. Ephedrine and theophylline are frequently used to prevent excessive bronchoconstriction in chronic respiratory disorders. However, as both these bronchodilators cause central nervous system stimulation, phenobarbital and other barbiturates are used to counteract this drug-induced stimulation.

NURSING MANAGEMENT

Since bronchodilators cause severe untoward reactions when administered orally or parenterally, many of these agents are given by inhalation. Hand-held nebulizers that emit a specific amount of drug are referred to as *metered-dose inhalers*. Other nebulizers require the careful measurement and instillation of medicated solution. Nurses need to familiarize themselves with the proper use of these nebulizers and should show the client how to operate and clean them. Medicated solutions may be diluted and administered via oxygen aerosolization or IPPB (see Chapter 16 for details). At least three parts normal saline should be used to dilute one part medicated solution.

As excessive use of a bronchodilator may result in tolerance or paradoxic bronchospasm, the client must be warned against excessive use of the drug, particularly when administered by inhalation. In addition, as clients with respiratory diseases are prone to infections of the respiratory tract, inhalers and medicated solutions should be kept as clean as possible, so that inhalation of pathogens is avoided.

SYMPATHOMIMETIC BRONCHODILATORS

Adrenergic Agents

GENERIC NAME Epinephrine hydrochloride (RX)

TRADE NAMES Adrenalin, Asmolin, Sus-Phrine

CLASSIFICATION Bronchodilator, adrenergic agent

Action This drug provides both rapid (20% drug in solution) and sustained (80% in suspension) epinephrine action. It stimulates alpha- and beta-adrenergic receptors, thus inducing bronchial dilation and increasing vital capacity by relieving congestion in the bronchial mucosa and constricting pulmonary vessels.

Indications for Use Acute bronchospasm, bronchial asthma, reversible bronchospasm associated with chronic bronchitis and emphysema.

Contraindications Hypersensitivity to any ingredient; clients with narrow-angle glaucoma, shock, cerebral arteriosclerosis, and organic heart disease; during labor; during general anesthesia with halogenated hydrocarbons or cyclopropane.

Untoward Reactions Anxiety, headache, fear, tremor, weakness, dizziness, palpitations, pallor, and urinary retention are common secondary effects. Toxic effects include a sharp rise in blood pressure, which may cause cerebral hemorrhage (pressor effect can be counteracted with nitrates or rapid-acting alpha-adrenergic blockers), severe, throbbing headache, and ventricular arrhythmias. Arrhythmias, including tachycardia that may progress to ventricular fibrillation, may occur. Altered perception and thought processes can occur and progress to frank psychosis. Tissue necrosis at the injection site, due to vasoconstriction, can occur.

Warnings and Precautions Use with caution in the elderly, in clients with cardiovascular disorders, diabetes, hypertension, hyperthyroidism, or psychoneurosis, and during pregnancy. Use with extreme caution in clients with prostatic hypertrophy.

Parameters of Use

Absorption Onset of action is 3 to 5 minutes and peak action occurs in about 20 minutes.

Crosses placenta and enters breast milk. Does not cross blood-brain barrier.

Metabolism Metabolized by sympathetic nerve endings, liver, and other tissues.

Excretion In urine.

Drug Interactions Tricyclic antidepressants potentiate the effects of epinephrine on the cardiovascular system and increase the risk of severe alterations in blood pressure, arrhythmias, convulsions, and other untoward effects. Digitalis preparations and mercurial diuretics potentiate the effects of epinephrine on the myocardium and increase the risk of ventricular tachycardia, fibrillation, and other arrhythmias. Some of the anthihistamines potentiate the effects of epinephrine by inhibiting tissue storage, thereby increasing the amount of epinephrine available at the receptor sites. Propranolol potentiates the pressor effects of epinephrine and may cause severe reflex bradycardia and AV block. Concurrent administration with thyroid preparations may precipitate an acute episode of coronary insufficiency. Epinephrine action may be potentiated by thyroxine. Oral hypoglycemic agents are antagonized by epinephrine. Measure blood sugar levels frequently and take appropriate measures. Insulin requirements are increased. Alcohol may decrease the client's response to epinephrine by increasing the rate of excretion.

Administration Adults: 0.1 to 0.3 ml subc; may be repeated in 6 hours, if necessary. Children: 0.005 ml/kg; Maximum dosage: 0.15 ml (under 30 kg).

Available Drug Forms Ampules of 0.5 ml containing 2.5 mg; 5-ml multidose vials containing 5 mg/ml.

Nursing Management

Planning factors

1. Promptness is essential when administering drug during emergency situations. Know where the drug is located and the strengths available.
2. Store drug in closed containers away from light.
3. Check drug supply monthly. Replace all drug packages that have expired.
4. Discard drug if solution becomes discolored or forms a precipitate.
5. Have rapid-acting nitrates available for treating toxic pressor effects and propanolol for treating arrhythmias.
6. When possible, obtain baseline pulse, respiration, and blood pressure.
7. Date multidose vials when opened and discard vial after time period indicated by the manufacturers.

Administration factors

1. Triple-check drug form and concentration, since fatalities have occurred from using improper dosage and route of administration.
2. Suspensions are only for IM or subc use; do not inject suspension intravenously. Rotate suspension well but gently; inject deep into well-vascularized tissue. Initial drug absorption can be enhanced by rubbing the injection site gently for one minute.
3. Rotate injection sites to prevent tissue necrosis from drug's pressor effect; check injection site for signs of necrosis (blanching of skin or cool to touch).

Evaluation factors

1. Monitor client's blood pressure and pulse frequently (every 1 to 3 minutes) until blood pressure stabilizes.
2. Assess the drug's effect on the client's breathing.
3. Notify physician immediately if hypertension or arrhythmias develop. Nitrates may be required to treat toxicity.
4. Acidosis may develop. Be prepared to administer sodium bicarbonate IV as needed.

GENERIC NAME Epinephrine bitartrate (RX)

TRADE NAME Medihaler-Epi

CLASSIFICATION Bronchodilator, adrenergic agent

See epinephrine hydrochloride for Contraindications, Warnings and precautions, and Drug interactions.

Action Potent bronchodilator. (See epinephrine hydrochloride.)

Indications for Use Acute bronchospasm associated with bronchial asthma.

Untoward Reactions Repeated use may cause bronchial irritation and edema.

Parameters of Use (See epinephrine hydrochloride.)

Absorption Slowly absorbed into bloodstream from bronchi. Onset of action is immediate. Low serum drug levels.

Administration 1 inhalation; if no relief in 1 to 2 minutes, repeat inhalation.

Available Drug Forms Metered-dose inhaler that delivers 0.3 mg (equal to 0.16 mg of epinephrine base per inhalation).

Nursing Management

1. After forced expiration, instruct client to inhale deeply while depressing inhaler.
2. If no relief occurs after 2 inhalations, notify physician.

GENERIC NAME Racepinephrine (OTC)

TRADE NAME Vaponefrin

CLASSIFICATION Bronchodilator, adrenergic agent

See epinephrine hydrochloride for Warnings and precautions and Drug interactions. See epinephrine hydrochloride and epinephrine bitartrate for Parameters of use.

Action Racepinephrine induces bronchodilation.

Indications for Use Bronchospasm associated with bronchial asthma.

Contraindications Do not use in children under 4 years. (See epinephrine hydrochloride.)

Untoward Reactions Repeated use may cause bronchial irritation and edema.

Administration Place 10 to 15 gtt into nebulizer and instruct client to inhale spray normally 2 to 3 times. Repeat 2 to 3 inhalations after 5 minutes, as necessary. May be used 4 to 6 times daily; smallest effective dosage should be used.

Available Drug Forms Bottles with measured dropper and metered dose inhaler. Solution of racemic epinephrine as the hydrochloride; equivalent to 2.25% of epinephrine base.

Nursing Management

1. Instruct client to rinse mouth and throat after each use.
2. Do not use solution if it has a brown color or a precipitate has formed.
3. If no relief occurs, notify physician.

GENERIC NAME Ephedrine sulfate (RX)

TRADE NAME Ephedsol, Estasule Minus III

CLASSIFICATION Bronchodilator, adrenergic agent

See epinephrine hydrochloride for Untoward reactions.

Action Ephedrine stimulates alpha- and beta-adrenergic receptors. It also stimulates the release of stored norepinephrine and reduces engorgement and edema of the respiratory tract. Similar to epinephrine, but has slower onset and longer duration of action. Produces less bronchodilation than epinephrine. Ephedrine is ineffective in aborting acute bronchospasm due to its slow onset of action.

Indications for Use Bronchospasm and congestion.

Contraindications Hypersensitivity to ephedrine, narrow-angle glaucoma, arrhythmias, porphyria, psychosis or marked neurosis, concurrent therapy with MAO inhibitors.

Warnings and Precautions Use with caution in the eldery and clients with cardiovascular disorders, hypertension, hyperthyroidism, and prostatic hypertrophy. Tolerance develops within 2 to 3 weeks.

Parameters of Use

Absorption Well absorbed from GI tract. Peak bronchodilation occurs in about 1 hour and persists for 3 to 4 hours. Crosses blood-brain barrier.

Excretion Primarily by the kidneys as unchanged drug (60 to 70%).

Drug Interactions Concurrent use of MAO inhibitors and tricyclic antidepressants may precipitate hypertensive crisis. (See epinephrine hydrochloride.)

Administration Adults: 12.5 to 50 mg po bid, tid, or qid; Recommended dosage: 400 mg/day. Children: 2 to 3 mg/kg po in divided doses every 4 to 6 hours; Maximum dosage: 3 mg/kg/day.

Available Drug Forms Tablets and capsules containing 25 or 50 mg; syrup containing 16 mg/4 ml.

Nursing Management (See epinephrine hydrochloride.)

1. Hypoxia, acidosis, and elevated arterial carbon dioxide levels may reduce drug's effectiveness and increase untoward reactions. Prompt correction of these disorders is essential.
2. Store drug at room temperature.
3. Avoid administering at bedtime, since insomnia may occur.

GENERIC NAME Ephedrine hydrochloride (RX)

CLASSIFICATION Bronchodilator, adrenergic agent

See ephedrine sulfate for Contraindications, Warnings and precautions, Parameters of use, Drug interactions, and Nursing management.

Action Same action and effects as ephedrine sulfate. This drug is seldom used because it causes more GI irritation than ephedrine sulfate.

Indications for Use Bronchospasm and congestion.

Administration Adults: 25 mg po q4h.

Available Drug Forms Tablets and capsules containing 25 mg. Found in several multiple ingredient preparations.

Beta-Adrenergic Agents

GENERIC NAME Isoproterenol hydrochloride (inhalation) RX

TRADE NAMES Aerolone, Aerotrol, Isuprel, Norisodrine, Vapo-N-Iso

CLASSIFICATION Bronchodilator, beta-adrenergic agent

Action Isoproterenol, a synthetic sympathomimetic amine chemically related to epinephrine, is a potent beta-adrenergic agent that has little or no effect on alpha-receptor sites. The primary effect of inhaled isoproterenol is relaxation of bronchial smooth muscle by stimulation of $beta_2$-receptor sites. Marked bronchodilation occurs in acute episodes of bronchospasm and therefore drug inhalation is effective in acute asthmatic attacks. The drug is well absorbed into blood after inhalation and causes some cardiac excitation, relaxation of GI smooth muscle, and a decrease in peripheral resistance of skeletal muscle vasculature. Excessive inhalation can cause systemic toxicity, particularly tachycardia and palpitations. However, fewer secondary effects occur after inhalation than after sublingual administration.

Indications for Use Bronchospasm associated with acute and chronic bronchial asthma, pulmonary emphysema, bronchitis, and bronchiectasis.

Contraindications Hypersensitivity to sympathomimetic amines, tachycardia, arrhythmias.

Warnings and Precautions Use with caution in clients with cardiac disease, hypertension, or hyperthyroidism. Safe use during pregnancy has not been established.

Untoward Reactions Toxic effects include tachycardia, palpitations, nervousness, vertigo, and insomnia. Irritation of the respiratory tract may occur and result in inflammation and edema. Cardiac disturbances include tachycardia, aggravation of preexisting arrhythmia, EKG evidence of coronary insufficiency, and precordial ache or anginal pain. Changes in blood pressure and flushing may occur. CNS disturbances, including headache, mild tremors, nervousness, insomnia, tinnitus, dizziness, and restlessness, may occur. Nausea, weakness, and sweating may occur. Cardiac arrest and paradoxic airway resistance have occurred after excessive use, but the reason is unclear.

Parameters of Use

Absorption Well absorbed. Onset of action is in minutes and duration of action is 1 to 2 hours.

Drug Interactions Concurrent administration of epinephrine or other sympathomimetic amines may cause systemic toxic effects.

Administration

- *Acute attack:* Smallest number of inhalations that will provide relief.
- *Hand-held nebulizer:* 5 to 15 inhalations 1:200 solution every 3 to 4 hours, as needed; 3 to 7 inhalations 1:100 solution every 3 to 4 hours, as needed; 6 to 12 inhalations Aerolone; can be repeated twice at 15-minute intervals; 1 inhalation Norisodrine (Mistometer); can be repeated twice at 5- to 10-minute intervals; Maximum dosage: 8 treatments daily; 1 inhalation equals 5 to 7 of a 1:100 solution.
- *Oxygen aerosolization or IPPB (chronic obstructive pulmonary disease):* Adults: 0.3 to 0.5 ml 1:200 solution diluted in 2.0 to 2.5 ml of normal saline over 10 to 20 minutes 3 to 5 times daily; Maximum dosage: 0.5 ml 1:800, 1:1000, or 1:1200 solution. Children: 0.25 ml 1:200 solution diluted in 1.5 to 2.0 ml of normal saline over 10 to 15 minutes 3 to 5 times daily.

Available Drug Forms Nonisotonic solution (Aerolone) containing 2.5 mg/ml; also contains 80% propylene glycol, ascorbic acid, coloring, and sodium hydroxide. Isotonic solution (Isuprel, Vapo-N-Iso) 1:200 (0.5%) or 1:100 (1.0%) with dropper; also contains citric acid, sodium chloride, chlorobutanol, and sodium bisulfate. Metered-dose nebulizers that deliver 131 mcg/inhalation (Mistometer) or 120 mcg/inhalation (Norisodrine); also contain 33% alcohol and ascorbic acid.

Nursing Management

Planning factors

1. Obtain history of pulmonary and cardiovascular disorders. If angina, arrhythmias, or other disturbances are noted, notify physician.
2. Perform baseline pulmonary function tests, particularly forced expiratory volume.
3. Instruct client in the use of hand-held nebulizers before an acute episode occurs.
4. Practice the use of oxygen aerosolization and IPPB equipment with plain normal saline before preparing equipment for client's use.
5. Obtain baseline EKG, particularly in clients over 40 years.
6. Obtain baseline blood pressure and vital signs.
7. Schedule inhalations between meals so that drug-induced nausea does not interfere with meals.
8. Store drug in refrigerator.

Administration factors

1. Prepare equipment for use with sterile technique to prevent contamination.
2. Discard solution if it has a brown color or has formed a precipitate.
3. Use undiluted solutions for nebulization. Dilute solutions for oxygen aerosolization and IPPB with at least 3 times the amount of water or saline.
4. When using oxygen aerosolization,
   a. Set oxygen flow rate at 4 to 6 l/min. before giving client the equipment.

   b. Administer over 10 to 20 minutes.
   c. Wash equipment at least once every 24 hours.
5. When using IPPB,
   a. Know the capacity of the nebulizer unit when preparing dilution; most units hold 3 to 5 ml.
   b. Usual settings are 15 l/min. for inspiratory flow rate and 15 cm of water for cycling pressure.
   c. Administer over 10 to 20 minutes.
   d. Wash equipment at least once every 24 hours.
6. Long-term therapy with oxygen aerosolization and IPPB are used to progressively reach deep bronchitis.
7. Do not leave client alone during first treatment as untoward reactions may occur. Assist in proper use of equipment, when necessary.
8. Administer oxygen after an acute asthmatic episode.
9. Instruct client to rinse mouth with water after treatment to avoid dryness of the oropharynx.

Evaluation factors

1. Check client for tachycardia, arrhythmias, and other untoward reactions 15 to 30 minutes after treatment. If reactions occur, notify physician.
2. Check client's breathing pattern for relief. Reassure client and assist client to relax.
3. Tolerance to drug may develop after prolonged use.
4. Perform pulmonary function tests periodically.

Client teaching factors

1. Instruct client in use of equipment.
   a. Use normal saline when assisting client in proper use of equipment.
   b. Check manufacturer's instructions for use of hand-held nebulizers and demonstrate the use of the equipment.
   c. Demonstrate how to fill and clean equipment.
2. Instruct client to clear nasal and oral passages before beginning treatment.
3. Inform client that metered-dose nebulizers usually recommend deep inhalation after forced expiration, whereas other equipment requires normal inhalation.
4. Instruct client to rinse mouth with water after treatment, since dry mouth, sore throat, tooth decay, and parotiditis may occur.
5. Warn client against excessive use, since toxicity may occur.
6. Warn client that solution turns pink with use and that they should not be alarmed if saliva and sputum turn pink.
7. Instruct client not to use solutions with a brown discoloration or precipitate.
8. Instruct client to notify physician if arrhythmias or lack of relief occur.

GENERIC NAME Isoproterenol hydrochloride (systemic)

TRADE NAME Isuprel Glossets (RX)

CLASSIFICATION Bronchodilator, beta-adrenergic agent

Action Isoproterenol is a potent beta-adrenergic agent (synthetic catecholamine), which has little or no effect on alpha receptors. Primary actions are on the heart ($beta_1$), inducing acceleration of heart rate and increased conduction velocity and contractility, and on bronchial smooth muscle ($beta_1$), causing bronchodilation.

Indications for Use Bronchoconstriction associated with bronchopulmonary diseases.

Contraindications Preexisting tachyarrhythmias, recent myocardial infarction.

Warnings and Precautions Clients with status asthmaticus and abnormal blood gas tensions may not have an improvement in vital capacity and blood gases although bronchospasm is relieved; oxygen should be given. Use with caution in clients with coronary insufficiency, diabetes, or hyperthyroidism. Hypovolemia and acid-base imbalances should be corrected before initiating drug therapy. Use with caution in clients who are hypersensitive to sympathomimetic amines. Drug-induced tachycardia of 130 beats/minute may induce ventricular arrhythmias. Discontinue drug immediately if precordial or anginal pain occurs.

Untoward Reactions Tachycardia, palpitations, nervousness, mild tremors, sweating, and flushing of the face are common secondary reactions. Arrhythmias may occur, particularly if client has a preexisting arrhythmia or if toxicity occurs. Nausea, vomiting, and hyperglycemia may occur.

Parameters of Use

Absorption Erratic. Onset of action is in minutes and duration of action is 1 to 4 hours.

Metabolism Conjugated in liver, lungs, and other tissues.

Excretion Primarily by the kidneys as inactive metabolites.

Drug Interactions Propranolol and other beta blockers will antagonize isoproterenol's action. Excessive cardiac stimulation will occur if given concurrently with epinephrine.

Administration Adults: 10 to 20 mg sublingual q4h, as needed; Maximum dosage: 60 mg/day. Children: 5 to 10 mg sublingual q4h, as needed; Maximum dosage: 30 mg/day.

Available Drug Forms Sublingual tablets containing 10 or 15 mg.

Nursing Management

Planning factors

1. Obtain a complete history of respiratory and cardiovascular disorders.
2. Correct hypovolemia and acid-base balance before instituting drug therapy.
3. Not recommended for children under 6 years.

Administration factors Instruct client to hold tablet under tongue until completely dissolved. Warn client to avoid swallowing tablet or saliva, since GI disturbances may occur. (See isoproterenol hydrochloride in Chapter 38.)

Evaluation factors

1. Monitor blood pressure and pulse rate frequently.
2. If anginal or precordial pain occurs, notify physician immediately.
3. If pulse rate is above 100 beats/minute, notify physician before giving drug.

Client teaching factors

1. Instruct client to protect tablets from heat and light. Store drug in a dark area.
2. Instruct client in the appropriate placement of tablet in the mouth.
3. Instruct client and family members to seek medical assistance immediately if bronchospasm persists or if fainting occurs.
4. Inform client about the drug's common secondary effects.

GENERIC NAME Isoproterenol sulfate (RX)

TRADE NAMES Medihaler-Iso, Norisodrine Sulfate

CLASSIFICATION Bronchodilator, beta-adrenergic agents

See isoproterenol hydrochloride (inhalation) for Contraindications, Warnings and precautions, Untoward reactions, and Nursing management.

Action This bronchodilator is similar to isoproterenol hydrochloride (systemic). (See isoproterenol hydrochloride.)

Indications for Use Bronchoconstriction associated with bronchopulmonary diseases.

Parameters of Use

Absorption Erratic. Onset of action is in minutes and duration of action is 1 to 4 hours.

Administration

- *Acute episode:* 1 inhalation; if no relief in 2 to 5 minutes, give a second inhalation per treatment; Maximum dosage: 6 inhalations hourly.
- *Maintenance therapy:* 1 to 2 inhalations 4 to 6 times daily.

Available Drug Forms Metered-dose oral inhaler. Inhaled solution 10 or 25% (Norisodrine) with lactose as a diluent. Medihaler-Iso delivers 0.08 mg of isoproterenol/inhalation suspension in an inert propellent.

GENERIC NAME Ethylnorepinephrine hydrochloride

TRADE NAME Bronkephrine (RX)

CLASSIFICATION Bronchodilator, beta-adrenergic agent

See isoproterenol hydrochloride (systemic) for Contraindications.

Action Ethylnorepinephrine is a relatively mild beta-adrenergic agent with actions similar to isoproterenol; but as it is less potent it causes fewer systemic effects (similar to isoetharine). Since it has little or no pressor effect, it can be used in hyperactive clients. In addition, it causes little or no CNS stimulation and can therefore be used in children and debilitated clients.

Indications for Use Acute bronchospasm.

Warnings and Precautions Use with caution in clients with cardiovascular disease or a history of stroke or coronary artery disease. [See isoproterenol hydrochloride (systemic).]

Untoward Reactions An elevation in pulse rate, palpitations, headache, dizziness, nausea, and alterations in blood pressure may occur. [See isoproterenol hydrochloride (systemic).]

Parameters of Use Unknown.

Administration Adults: 1 to 2 mg IM or subc depending on severity of episode; Children: 0.2 to 1.0 mg IM or subc depending on severity of episode.

Available Drug Forms Ampules containing 2 mg/ml.

Nursing Management Protect ampules from light. [See isoproterenol hydrochloride (systemic).]

GENERIC NAME Isoetharine mesylate (RX)

TRADE NAME Bronkometer

CLASSIFICATION Bronchodilator, beta-adrenergic agent

See isoproterenol hydrochloride (inhalation) for Contraindications and Nursing management.

Action Isoetharine is a synthetic beta-adrenergic agent with preferential affinity for $beta_2$-receptor sites of bronchial and certain vascular smooth muscles. It has little affinity for $beta_1$-receptor sites.

Warnings and Precautions Tolerance may develop after prolonged use. Benefits should outweigh risks during pregnancy and lactation.

Untoward Reactions Cardiac arrest and paradoxic airway resistance have been reported with excessive use. Toxicity may result in tachycardia, palpitations, nausea, headache, and epinephrine-like effects.

Parameters of Use Similar to isoproterenol but with a shorter duration of action.

Administration Adults: 1 to 2 inhalations q4h, as needed; severe episodes may require an additional inhalation after 2 to 5 minutes.

Available Drug Forms Vials with oral 0.61% nebulizer containing saccharin, menthol, 30% alcohol, fluorochlorohydrocarbons, and 0.1% ascorbic acid. Refill vials containing 10 or 20 ml.

GENERIC NAME Isoetharine hydrochloride (RX)

TRADE NAME Bronkosol

CLASSIFICATION Bronchodilator, beta-adrenergic agent

See isoproterenol hydrochloride (inhalation) for details.

Action Solutions of isoetharine for use in conventional nebulizers, by oxygen aerosolization, and in IPPB machines.

Administration

- *Hand-held nebulizer:* 4 inhalations of undiluted solution q4h; Dosage range: 3 to 7 inhalations.
- *Oxygen aerosolization:* 0.5 ml diluted with 1.5 ml of saline over 15 to 20 minutes q4h; Dosage range: 0.25 to 1.0 ml. Unit dose per nebulization q4h.

Available Drug Forms 1.0% aqueous glycerin solution with sodium chloride, citric acid, sodium hydroxide, methylparaben, and acetone bisulfate. Unit dose contains 0.25% aqueous glycerin solution with same ingredients.

Nursing Management [See isoproterenol hydrochloride (inhalation).]

1. Screw plunger into rubber stopper at rear of barrel.
2. Carefully remove cap from front of barrel. Avoid contamination of open end.
3. Insert open end into nebulizer cup of medication port and depress plunger until barrel is empty.
4. Follow usual procedures for treatment.
5. When using oxygen aerosolization,
   a. Set oxygen flow rate at 4 to 6 l/min.
   b. Dilute with 3 times the amount of saline.
6. When using IPPB,
   a. Dilute with 2 times the amount of saline.
   b. Usual settings are 15 l/min. for inspiratory flow rate and 15 cm of water for cycling pressure.

GENERIC NAME Metaproterenol sulfate (systemic)

TRADE NAMES Alupent, Metaprel (RX)

CLASSIFICATION Bronchodilator, beta-adrenergic agent

See isoproterenol hydrochloride (systemic) for details.

Action Metaproterenol is a potent beta-adrenergic agent similar to isoproterenol, but with greater selectivity for $beta_2$-receptor sites. Although isoproterenol has a more rapid onset, metaproterenol has a longer duration of action and causes fewer untoward reactions.

Indications for Use Asthma and reversible bronchospasm associated with bronchitis and emphysema.

Contraindications Tachycardia, tachyarrhythmias.

Warnings and Precautions Use with caution in clients with hypertension, coronary artery disease, congestive heart failure, hyperthyroidism, or diabetes. Adequate time should elapse before using another sympathomimetic. Not recommended for children under 6 years. Safe use during pregnancy and lactation has not been established.

Untoward Reactions Nervousness, tachycardia, tremors, and nausea are common.

Parameters of Use

Absorption About 40% absorbed from GI tract. Duration of action is about 4 hours.

Excretion In urine as glucuronic acid conjugates.

Administration Adults and children over 9 years (27 kg or more): 20 mg (or 10 ml) po tid or qid; Children: Ages 6 to 9 years (under 27 kg): 10 mg (or 5 ml) po tid or qid.

Available Drug Forms Tablets containing 10 or 20 mg; syrup containing 10 mg/5 ml.

GENERIC NAME Metaproterenol sulfate (inhalation)

TRADE NAMES Alupent, Metaprel (RX)

CLASSIFICATION Bronchodilator, beta-adrenergic agent

See metaproterenol sulfate (systemic) for Action. See isoproterenol (inhalation) for further details.

Indications for Use Acute reversible bronchospasm.

Warnings and Precautions Not recommended for children under 12 years.

Parameters of Use

Absorption Duration of action after 1 dose from hand-held nebulizer is 1 to 5 hours; duration after repeated doses is 1 to 2½ hours. Onset of action is 5 to 30 minutes after IPPB and duration of action is 2 to 6 hours.

Administration

- *Metered dose:* 1 to 3 inhalations every 3 to 4 hours, as needed; Maximum dosage: 12 inhalations daily.
- *Hand-held nebulizer:* 10 inhalations of undiluted solution; Dosage range: 5 to 15 inhalations.
- *IPPB:* 0.3 ml diluted in 2.5 ml of normal saline; Dosage range: 0.2 to 0.3 ml.

Available Drug Forms Metered-dose (0.65 mg) aerosol unit for oral nebulization; 5% solution for nebulization with calibrated dropper.

Nursing Management Store at room temperature and protect from light.

GENERIC NAME Methoxyphenamine (RX)

TRADE NAME Orthoxine

CLASSIFICATION Bronchodilator, beta-adrenergic agent

See isoproterenol hydrochloride (systemic) for details.

Action Sympathomimetic amine similar to ephedrine, but has more selectivity for beta-receptor sites. Primarily causes bronchodilation and relaxation of smooth muscle. Causes a mild vasopressor effect.

Indications for Use Bronchial asthma, allergic rhinitis, urticaria, allergic GI and headache reactions.

Warnings and Precautions Tolerance develops after 2 to 3 weeks.

Untoward Reactions Palpitations, tachycardia, hypertension, nausea, vomiting, insomnia, nervousness, anxiety, dizziness, sweating.

Parameters of Use Similar to ephedrine but slightly longer duration of action.

Administration Adults: 100 mg po every 4 to 6 hours; Maximum dosage: 600 mg/day. Children: 25 to 50 mg po every 4 to 6 hours.

Nursing Management Avoid administering drug within 1 to 2 hours of bedtime.

Beta$_2$-Adrenergic Agents

GENERIC NAME Albuterol (RX)

TRADE NAMES Proventil, Ventolin

CLASSIFICATION Bronchodilator, beta$_2$-adrenergic agent

See terbutaline sulfate for Drug interactions.

Action Albuterol (salbutamol) induces bronchodilation by stimulating beta$_2$-receptor sites in bronchial smooth muscle. It relaxes smooth muscle of the bronchi, uterus, and vascular supply to skeletal muscles. The drug is similar to terbutaline, but has only been released for oral inhalation in the United States to date. This method of administration causes fewer systemic untoward reactions because the drug is gradually absorbed into the bloodstream from the bronchi. Albuterol is longer acting than isoproterenol and produces less severe secondary cardiovascular effects (less than half the effect).

Indications for Use Reversible bronchospasm associated with obstructive pulmonary diseases.

Warnings and Precautions Safe use in children under 12 years and during pregnancy and lactation has not been established. Do not use other sympathomimetic aerosols concurrently.

Untoward Reactions Paradoxic bronchospasm and other fatalities may occur after excessive use. (See terbutaline sulfate.)

Parameters of Use

Absorption Gradual from bronchi. Low serum drug levels when recommended dosages inhaled. Peak plasma levels occur in 2 to 4 hours. Peak pulmonary effects occur in 60 to 90 minutes and persist for 3 to 4 hours. Half-life is 3.8 hours.

Excretion About 72% by the kidneys in 24 hours as unchanged drug (28%) and metabolites (44%).

Administration Adults and children 12 years and older: 1 to 2 inhalations every 4 to 6 hours, as needed.

Available Drug Forms Metered-dose (90 mcg) aerosol unit for oral inhalation.

Nursing Management

Planning factors

1. Obtain history of pulmonary and cardiovascular disorders. If angina, arrhythmias, or other disturbances are noted, notify physician.
2. Perform baseline pulmonary function tests, particularly forced expiratory volume.

3. Instruct client in the use of hand-held nebulizers before an acute episode occurs.
4. Obtain baseline EKG, particularly in clients over 40 years.
5. Obtain baseline blood pressure and vital signs.
6. Store drug at room temperature between 15 and 30 C (59 to 86° F); canister may explode if exposed to temperatures above 120 F.

Administration factors

1. Prepare equipment for use with sterile technique to prevent contamination.
2. Do not leave client alone during first treatment, as untoward reactions may occur. Assist client in proper use of equipment, when necessary.
3. Instruct client to rinse mouth with water after treatment to avoid dryness of the oropharynx.

Evaluation factors

1. Check client for tachycardia, hypertension, arrhythmias, and other untoward reactions 15 to 30 minutes after treatment. If reactions occur, notify physician.
2. Check client's breathing pattern for relief. Reassure client and assist client to relax.
3. Perform pulmonary function tests periodically.

Client teaching factors

1. Check manufacturer's instructions for use of equipment and demonstrate use to client.
2. Instruct client to clear nasal and oral passages before beginning treatment.
3. Instruct client to take a deep inhalation after a forced expiration.
4. Instruct client to rinse mouth with water after treatment, since dry mouth, sore throat, tooth decay, and parotiditis may occur.
5. Warn client against excessive use, since toxicity may occur.
6. Instruct client to notify physician if arrhythmias or lack of relief occur.

GENERIC NAME Terbutaline sulfate (RX)

TRADE NAMES Brethine, Bricanyl

CLASSIFICATION Bronchodilator, $beta_2$-adrenergic agent

Action Terbutaline, a synthetic sympathomimetic amine, induces bronchodilation by stimulating $beta_2$-receptor sites in the bronchial musculature to release adenylate cyclase, the enzyme that catalyzes the conversion of ATP to AMP. AMP induces relaxation of bronchial smooth muscle. Terbutaline is relatively selective in its stimulation of $beta_2$-receptor sites. Untoward reactions are minimal. The drug has a relatively long duration of action, but is poorly absorbed from the GI tract. Only oral and subcutaneous administration (deltoid area) have been approved to date, but studies indicate that inhalation is also effective.

Indications for Use Bronchial asthma, reversible bronchospasm associated with bronchitis and emphysema.

Contraindications Hypersensitivity to sympathomimetic amines, labor and delivery (injectable form only).

Warnings and Precautions Use with caution in clients with diabetes, hypertension, hyperthyroidism, or a history of seizures. Use with caution in cardiac clients, particularly those with preexisting arrhythmias. Safe use during pregnancy has not been established, but animal reproductive studies have not demonstrated any adverse effects to date. Safe use in children under 12 years has not been established. Concurrent use with other systemic sympathomimetics is not recommended, since untoward cardiovascular reactions may occur. Inhaled sympathomimetics can be used concurrently with caution. Injectable terbutaline has caused transitory hypokalemia, pulmonary edema, and hypoglycemia (mother and neonate) when used during labor.

Untoward Reactions Secondary reactions typical of other sympathomimetics are common, but the frequency and severity of these reactions tend to decrease with continued therapy. CNS disturbances, including nervousness and tremors, are common. Headache and dizziness are common after injection. Drowsiness, anxiety, and sweating may also occur. Cardiovascular disturbances, including palpitations and increased heart rate, are common after injection in excess of 0.25 mg, but tend to be transitory after oral administration. Transitory nausea, vomiting, and muscular cramps have been reported.

Parameters of Use

Absorption About 40% absorbed from GI tract; well absorbed from injection sites. Dosage and safety have not been determined for other routes to date. Onset of action is: 30 minutes (po); 5 minutes (subc). Peak action occurs in: 2 to 3 hours (po); 30 to 60 minutes (subc). Duration of action is: 4 to 8 hours (po); 1½ to 4 hours (subc). Effects are measured by a 15% or greater increase in forced expiratory volume and results from other pulmonary function studies. Half-life is about 3½ hours.

Crosses placenta.

Drug Interactions Not recommended for use with MAO inhibitors, since concurrent use with sympathomimetic amines may cause severe hypertension. Beta blockers will block the effects of terbutaline.

Administration Oral: Adults: 2.5 mg q6h while awake; maximum dosage: 7.5 mg/day. Subcutaneous: Adults: 0.25 mg; can be repeated in 15 to 30 minutes; do not exceed 0.5 mg in 4 hours.

Available Drug Forms Scored tablets containing 2.5 or 5.0 mg; 1-ml ampules containing 1.0 mg/ml.

Nursing Management

Planning factors

1. Obtain history of pulmonary and cardiovascular disorders.

2. Perform baseline pulmonary function tests, particularly forced expiratory volume.
3. Obtain baseline vital signs.
4. Store drug in dark area at room temperature. Check expiration date periodically (monthly) and replace as necessary.

Administration factors

1. Give tablets with a full glass of water.
2. Check clarity of parenteral solution before using and discard if discolored.
3. Inject deep into subcutaneous tissue of lateral deltoid area (other injection sites have not been approved to date)
4. Rotate injection sites.

Evaluation factors

1. Monitor vital signs. If tachycardia or arrhythmias occur, notify physician.
2. Observe and record the presence of resting tremors periodically. Tremors usually subside with continued use.
3. Perform pulmonary function tests periodically, since tolerance to drug may develop with prolonged use.

Client teaching factors

1. Explain reason for drug use (prevention of bronchoconstriction) and emphasize the need for maintaining the prescribed schedule.
2. Instruct client to keep drug in dark area away from excessive heat and light.
3. Instruct client to inform physician if tachycardia or palpitations occur.
4. Warn client about common secondary effects and explain that symptoms subside with continued use.

PHOSPHODIESTERASE INHIBITORS

GENERIC NAME Theophylline (RX)

TRADE NAMES Accurbron, Aerolate, Aquaphyllin, Bronkodyl, Constant-T, Elixicon, Elixophyllin, LaBID, Physpan, Pulm, Quibron-T, Quibron-T/SR, Respbid, Slo-Phyllin, Somophyllin-T, Somophyllin-CRT, Sustaire, Theobid, Theoclear, Theo-Dur, Theolair, Theon, Theophyl, Theospan SR, Theostat, Theovent

CLASSIFICATION Bronchodilator, phosphodiesterase inhibitor

Action Theophylline relaxes smooth muscles of the respiratory tract and relieves bronchospasm by inhibiting phosphodiesterase, the enzyme that degrades intracellular AMP. Bronchodilation is minimal in the absence of bronchospasm. Vital capacity is increased by bronchodilation and the medullary respiratory center is stimulated. The coronary arteries are dilated and the myocardium is stimulated directly, thus resulting in an increase in cardiac output. Preexisting arrhythmias may be precipitated but tachycardia is avoided, except in large dosages when theophylline causes some stimulation of the vagus nerve. The renal arteries are dilated and theophylline inhibits sodium and chloride reabsorption at the proximal tubules, but the resulting diuresis is of short duration. The smooth muscles of the GI and biliary tract are also relaxed, but to a lesser degree than the bronchial tract. The CNS is stimulated and excitation may occur, particularly when high dosages are given. Stimulation of skeletal muscles also occurs. Since little or no tolerance to the drug develops, theophylline can be used for long periods of time.

Indications for use Prophylaxis and relief of bronchial asthma; reversible bronchospasm associated with obstructive pulmonary disease, such as chronic bronchitis and emphysema.

Contraindications Hypersensitivity to xanthines, peptic ulcer, active gastritis.

Warnings and Precautions Use with caution in clients with cardiovascular, hepatic, or renal disorders. Use with caution in young children and the elderly. Safe use of sustained-release preparations in children under 6 years has not been established. Safe use during pregnancy has not been established. Should not be given concurrently with xanthine-containing drugs, since xanthine toxicity may occur. Toxicity may occur with conventional therapeutic dosages in clients (1) over 55 years, particularly males; (2) with hepatic disorders, including alcoholism; (3) with chronic obstructive pulmonary disease; and (4) with low body clearances, including transient cardiac decompensation.

Untoward Reactions The early signs of toxicity, nausea and restlessness, occur in about 50% of the clients prior to the onset of convulsions. Ventricular arrhythmias and seizures are often the first sign of toxicity. Tachycardia may occur and a preexisting arrhythmia may worsen before seizures develop. Coma often follows seizure activity. GI disturbances, including nausea, vomiting, and epigastric distress, are common. Hematemesis and diarrhea have been reported. CNS disturbances, including headache and insomnia, are common. Irritability, restlessness, hyperexcitability, and muscular twitching (toxicity) may lead to clonic-tonic generalized convulsions. Cardiovascular disturbances, including tachycardia, extrasystoles, and flushing, may occur. Hypotension and ventricular arrhythmias may lead to circulatory collapse. Diuresis is a common secondary effect. Albuminuria and excretion of red blood cells and renal tubular cells may also occur. Hyperglycemia and inappropriate ADH syndrome may occur. Tachypnea and respiratory arrest have been reported.

Parameters of Use

Absorption Complete from GI tract; but poor solubility makes rate of absorption erratic. Absorption of elixir is relatively rapid. Rate of absorption is decreased when given with food. Plasma half-life varies widely because of variable rates of metabolism and excretion: Average: About 4 hours; Range in adults: 2 to 16 hours; Nonsmokers: 7 to 9 hours; Smokers: 4 to 5 hours; Range in children: 2 to 10 hours; Ages 0 to 3 months: Up to 24 hours; Ages 4 to 6 months; Approaches range in older children; Over 6 years: 3 to 5 hours. Half-life is shortened by cigarette smoking, but prolonged by as much as 24 hours in clients with alcoholism, hepatic and renal disorders, or chronic obstructive pulmonary disease. Steady-state serum levels occur in about 3 days. Therapeutic serum drug levels: 10 to 20 mcg/ml. Nearly 20% bound to plasma proteins. Crosses placenta and enters breast milk. Crosses blood-brain barrier and causes CNS stimulation.

Distribution Demethylated and oxidized in the liver and other tissues. Enzymatic degradation occurs.

Excretion By the kidneys as unchanged drug (about 10%) and metabolites (methyduric acids and methylxanthines). Some excreted in feces, saliva, and other secretions.

Drug Interactions Theophylline increases the excretion of lithium carbonate and may precipitate digitalis toxicity and toxicity to sympathomimetic amines. Tachycardia may occur if administered concurrently with reserpine. High dosages of theophylline may increase the anticoagulant effect of oral anticoagulants. Concurrent therapy with erythromycin, clindamycin, lincomycin, troleandomycin, and cimetidine may elevate theophylline serum levels and increase the chance of toxicity. Concurrent therapy with furosemide causes marked diuresis; with chlordiazepoxide may cause drug-induced fatty acid metabolism; and with hexamethonium decreases the chronotropic effect.

Laboratory Interactions Colorimetric methods of determining serum uric acid levels are affected. May increase test results for urinary catecholamines, plasma free fatty acids, bilirubin, and sedimentation rate. May decrease thyroid test results of ^{131}I uptake.

Administration Highly individualized. A loading dose of 0.5 mg/kg produces serum drug levels of 1 mcg/ml. Theophyllinization (higher initial dosages) is recommended for clients who have not been receiving theophylline-containing preparations. Adults: Initial dosage: 100 to 200 mg po q6h or every 8 to 12 hours (sustained-release preparation); then adjust dosage according to serum drug levels. Children: 4 mg/kg po q6h for 3 days or every 8 to 12 hours (sustained-release preparation); Under 9 years: 4 to 5 mg/kg po q6h or every 8 to 12 hours (sustained-release preparation); do not exceed 100 mg.

Available Drug Forms Elixir containing 10 mg/ml, 50 mg/5 ml, or 80 mg/15 ml; alcohol-free liquid (Aerolate) containing 160 mg/15 ml, syrup (Aquaphyllin, Slo-Phyllin, Theostat) containing 80 mg/15 ml, and liquid (Theolair) containing 80 mg/15 ml; syrup containing 80 mg/15 ml; suspension (Elixicon) containing 100 mg/5 ml; chewable tablets containing 25 mg; tablets containing 100, 125, 200, 225, 250, or 300 mg; capsules containing 50, 100, 200 or 250 mg; sustained-release capsules (Aerolate, Bronkodyl S-R, Elixophyllin SR, Physpan, Pulm, Quibron-T/SR, Respbid, Slo-Phyllin Gyrocaps, Somophyllin-CRT, Sustaire, Theobid, Theoclear L.A., Theo-Dur, Theolair-SR, Theophyl-SR, Theospan SR, Theovent) and tablets (Constant-T, LaBID) containing 100, 200, 250, 300, or 500 mg.

Nursing Management

Planning factors

1. Perform baseline pulmonary function tests, when possible.
2. Obtain history of cigarette smoking, alcohol consumption, and pulmonary, cardiovascular, hepatic, and renal disorders.
3. Obtain baseline vital signs.
4. Avoid administering within 2 hours of bedtime, when possible.

Administration factors

1. Shake suspension well before measuring dosage.
2. Give all preparations with a full glass of water.
3. Do not crush or chew sustained-release tablets or capsules.
4. Give after meals or with food if GI disturbances occur. If symptoms persist, dosage reduction may be required.
5. If client is unable to swallow tablets or capsules, notify physician so that a liquid preparation can be prescribed.
6. Sustained-release preparations can be given at bedtime.

Evaluation factors

1. Observe for initial signs and symptoms of toxicity when drug is first initiated or dosage adjusted. If symptoms occur, notify physician.
2. Monitor vital signs frequently when drug is first initiated or dosage adjusted.
3. Monitor elderly clients for arrhythmias.
4. Monitor intake and output.
5. If seizure activity (toxicity) occurs, diazepam IV (0.1 to 0.3 mg/kg; up to 10 mg) can be given. Coma may follow seizure activity and is treated with supportive therapy.
6. Obtain serum drug levels frequently until optimal response is obtained; then periodically (every 1 to 3 months).
7. Obtain serum drug levels periodically when high dosages or prolonged therapy are required. Monitor dosages above 16 mg/kg/day or 400 mg/day by serum drug levels.

Client teaching factors

1. Explain how to take and when to take drug preparation prescribed. Emphasize the importance of taking the drug on schedule.
2. Instruct client to avoid contact with infectious diseases and irritants (smoke, hairspray, insecticide sprays).
3. Inform client that humidification of room air may be helpful in expectorating respiratory secretions.
4. Instruct client to consult physician before taking any OTC drugs, since several of these preparations contain ephedrine and other sympathomimetic amines.
5. Instruct elderly and debilitated clients to change position slowly to avoid dizziness, particularly when therapy is initiated.
6. Instruct client to store drug in airtight containers at room temperature.

GENERIC NAME Aminophylline (RX)

TRADE NAMES Aminodur, Aminophyl, Aminophyllin, Lixaminol, Phyllocontin, Somophyllin, Somophyllin-DF

CLASSIFICATION Bronchodilator, phosphodiesterase inhibitor

See theophylline for Indications for use, Contraindications, Warnings and precautions, and Untoward reactions.

Action Aminophylline (theophylline ethylenediamine) is the principle purine salt of theophylline and contains approximately 85% anhydrous theophylline and 15% ethylenediamine, an inactive ingredient. The drug's action is due to its theophylline content. As it is more soluble in water than its parent compound, aminophylline can be administered parenterally and rectally. (See theophylline.)

Parameters of Use (See theophylline.)

Absorption Rate of metabolism and excretion is variable, thus serum levels achieved and sustained will vary from client to client. Therapeutic serum drug levels: 10 to 20 mcg/ml. Usual time required to achieve therapeutic serum levels: Tablet: 60 to 90 minutes; Sustained-release capsule: 3 to 7 hours; Rectal suppository: 2 to 4 hours; Retention enema; 30 to 60 minutes; intermittent IV infusion: 15 to 60 minutes. Rectal enema and intermittent IV infusion achieve similar therapeutic blood levels. Oral doses and rectal suppositories are more erratic in absorption. Duration of effect is variable, but usually sustained for 6 to 12 hours. Neonates may maintain therapeutic serum levels for 24 hours.

Drug Interactions Aminophylline is an alkaline solution; do not mix with drugs that interact with alkaline solutions. Aminophylline antagonizes the effects of propranolol and nadolol; use with caution concurrently. (See theophylline.)

Administration Highly individualized. Adults: Loading dose: 6 to 7 mg/kg (or 500 mg) po, IV, or via rectal enema; then in 6 hours: 2.4 to 3.5 mg/kg (or 250 to 500 mg) po, IV, or rectally every 6 to 8 hours. IV is usually given by intermittent IV infusion, but may be given by continuous IV infusion: Adults: 0.6 to 0.9 mg/kg/hour. Children: Ages: 9 to 16 years: Loading dose: 6.0 to 7.5 mg/kg po or IV; then 3.5 to 3.8 mg/kg po or IV q6h or 3 to 6 mg/kg po or IV every 6 to 8 hours. Continuous IV infusion: 0.8 to 1.0 mg/kg/hour. Ages 6 months to 9 years: Loading dose: 6 to 7 mg/kg po or IV; then 4 to 6 mg/kg po or IV q6h. Intermittent or continuous IV infusions are often preferred: 1.0 to 1.2 mg/kg/hour.

Available Drug Forms Flavored oral liquid containing 105 mg/ml; dye-free oral colorless liquid (Somophyllin-DF) containing 105 mg/5 ml; Rectal solution for enema containing 300 mg/5 ml; rectal suppositories containing 150 or 300 mg; capsules containing 100, 200, or 250 mg; sustained-release capsules containing 50, 100, or 250 mg; ampules containing 10 or 20 mg with 25 mg/ml.

Nursing Management

Planning factors

1. Perform baseline pulmonary function tests.
2. Obtain history of cigarette smoking, alcohol consumption, pulmonary, cardiovascular, hepatic, and renal disorders.
3. Obtain baseline vital signs.
4. Avoid administering within 2 hours of bedtime when possible.

Administration factors

1. When administering oral preparations,
   a. Give all oral preparations with a full glass of water.
   b. Do not crush or chew sustained-release capsules.
   c. Give after meals or with food if GI disturbances occur. If symptoms persist, dosage reduction may be required.
   d. Sustained-release preparations can be given at bedtime.
2. When administering rectal preparations,
   a. Rectal enemas are not recommended for children.
   b. Administer after bowel movements, whenever possible.
   c. Retention of suppositories or enema fluid may be better between meals, since food ingestion stimulates GI motility, particularly in children.
   d. Insert rectal suppository well beyond internal sphincter.
   e. Rectal solutions may be instilled with a rectal syringe.
   f. Retention of drug may be increased if client remains recumbent for 30 minutes.
3. When administering IV,
   a. Do not use solution if a precipitate has formed.
   b. Can be given via slow IV bolus at a rate of 25 mg/min. or less, but this method is not recommended.
   c. Add drug to 50 or 100 ml of 5% D/W or 5% D/S and administer over 30 to 60 minutes.
   e. Continuous IV solution can be given in 250 to 500 ml of 5% D/W or 5% D/S.
   f. If an infusion pump is not available, use a microdrip IV administration set.

Evaluation factors

1. Observe for initial signs and symptoms of toxicity when drug is first initiated or dosage adjusted. If symptoms occur, notify physician.
2. Monitor vital signs frequently when drug is first initiated, dosage adjusted, or administered intravenously.
3. Monitor elderly clients for arrhythmias.
4. Monitor intake and output.
5. If seizure activity (toxicity) occurs, diazepam IV (0.1 to 0.3 mg/kg; up to 10 mg) can be given. Coma may follow seizure activity and is treated with supportive therapy.

6. Obtain serum drug levels frequently until optimal response is obtained; then periodically (every 1 to 3 months).
7. Check for premature expulsion of rectal preparations.

Client teaching factors

1. Explain how to take and when to take drug preparation prescribed. Emphasize the importance of taking drug on schedule.
2. Instruct client to avoid contact with infectious diseases and irritants (smoke, hairspray, insecticide sprays).
3. Inform client that humidification of room air may be helpful in expectorating respiratory secretions.
4. Instruct client to consult physician before taking any OTC drugs, since several of these preparations contain ephedrine and other sympathomimetic amines.
5. Instruct elderly and debilitated clients to change positions slowly to avoid dizziness, particularly when therapy is initiated.
6. Instruct client to store drug in airtight containers at room temperature.

GENERIC NAME Theophylline sodium glycinate

TRADE NAMES Glynazan, Glytheonate, Synophylate

CLASSIFICATION Bronchodilator, phosphodiesterase inhibitor (RX)

See theophylline for Contraindications, Warnings and precautions, Untoward reactions, Parameters of use, Drug interactions, and Nursing management.

Action This drug is a mixture of sodium theophylline and glycine. It is more soluble than theophylline. (See theophylline.)

Administration Adults: 1 to 2 tablets or 15 to 30 ml po every 6 to 8 hours; Children: Ages 6 to 12 years: 1 tablet or 10 to 15 ml po every 6 to 8 hours; Ages 3 to 6 years: 5.0 to 7.5 ml po every 6 to 8 hours; Ages 1 to 3 years: 2.5 to 5.0 ml po every 6 to 8 hours.

Available Drug Forms Tablets containing 300 mg; elixir containing 300 mg/15 ml. Theophylline equivalency per dose: 165 mg per tablet or 15 ml (50%).

GENERIC NAME Theophylline sodium acetate

TRADE NAME Soluble Theocin (RX)

CLASSIFICATION Bronchodilator, phosphodiesterase inhibitor

See theophylline for Contraindications, Warnings and precautions, Untoward reactions, Parameters of use, Drug interactions, and Nursing management.

Action This drug is seldom used today except in combination preparations. (See theophylline.)

Administration Adults: 200 to 300 mg po daily.

Available Drug Forms Tablets containing 200 or 300 mg.

GENERIC NAME Theophylline calcium salicylate

TRADE NAME Phyllicin, Theophyl-225 (RX)

CLASSIFICATION Bronchodilator, phosphodiesterase inhibitor

See theophylline for Action, Contraindications, Warnings and precautions, Untoward reactions, Parameters of use, Drug interactions, and Nursing management.

Administration Adults: 16 mg/kg/day (or 450 mg/day) in 3 to 4 divided doses every 6 to 8 hours; Children: Over 9 kg: 4 to 6 mg/kg/day in 3 to 4 divided doses every 6 to 8 hours.

Available Drug Forms Tablets containing 500 mg; elixir containing 500 mg/30 ml and 5% alcohol. Theophylline equivalency per dose: 225 mg per tablet or 30 ml (about 50%). Also contains 225 mg of calcium salicylate as a solubilizing agent.

GENERIC NAME Theophylline (retention enema)

TRADE NAME Fleet-Brand Theophylline (RX)

CLASSIFICATION Bronchodilator, phosphodiesterase inhibitor

See theophylline for Contraindications, Warnings and precautions, Untoward reactions, Parameters of use, Drug interactions, and Nursing Management.

Action This drug is administered only by retention enema. It is erratically absorbed, but is useful in clients who cannot tolerate theophylline orally. (See theophylline.)

Administration 250 to 500 mg rectally.

Available Drug Forms Retention enema containing theophylline equivalency per dose: 75%.

GENERIC NAME Theophylline dihydroxypropyl

TRADE NAMES Asminyl, Dilor, Lufyllin, Neothylline

CLASSIFICATION Bronchodilator, phosphodiesterase inhibitor (RX)

See theophylline for Indications for use, Contraindications, and Drug interactions.

Action Theophylline dihydroxypropyl (dyphylline) is not a theophylline salt, but is chemically related to theophylline. (See theophylline.)

Warnings and Precautions Use with extreme caution in clients with congestive heart failure.

Untoward Reactions High dosages (500 to 1000 mg) may cause GI irritation. (See theophylline.)

Parameters of Use

Absorption More consistent and less irritating to GI tract than theophylline salts.

Administration Adults: Oral: 15 mg/kg (or 300 mg) q6h, as needed. Intramuscular: 250 to 500 mg q6h, as needed.

Available Drug Forms Elixir containing 100 or 160 mg/15 ml; tablets containing 200 or 400 mg; vials containing 250 mg/ml. Theophylline equivalency per dose: 70%.

Nursing Management Do not use injectable drug form if a precipitate has developed. (See theophylline.)

GENERIC NAME Theophylline cholinate (RX)

TRADE NAME Choledyl

CLASSIFICATION Bronchodilator, phosphodiesterase inhibitor

See theophylline for Indications for use, Contraindications, Warnings and precautions, Untoward reactions, Parameters of use, Drug interactions, and Nursing management.

Action This choline salt (oxtriphylline) of theophylline is well tolerated and absorbed. It produces little or no GI irritation in therapeutic dosages.

Administration Adults: 200 mg po q6h; Children: Ages 2 to 12 years: 100 mg/50 lb po q6h. Pediatric syrup: Initial dosage: 25 mg/kg/day (or 625 mg/day) in 3 to 4 divided doses every 6 to 8 hours; then 13 to 375 mg/kg/day, as tolerated.

Available Drug Forms Enteric-coated tablets containing 100 or 200 mg; elixir containing 100 mg/5 ml and 20% alcohol; pediatric syrup containing 50 mg/5 ml. Theophylline equivalency per dose: 32 mg/50 mg of oxtriphylline (64%).

ANTIASTHMATIC AGENTS

GENERIC NAME Cromolyn sodium (RX)

TRADE NAMES Intal, Rynacrom

CLASSIFICATION Antiasthmatic agent

Action Although the exact mechanism of action is unknown, cromolyn acts on mast cells to inhibit the release of histamine, slow-reacting substances of anaphylaxis (SRS-A), serotonin, and other chemical mediators that induce bronchoconstriction. Hypersensitivity reactions cause mast cells to release these mediators that induce smooth muscle contraction and increase capillary permeability and respiratory airway resistance. As cromolyn is neither a bronchodilator nor an antiinflammatory agent, it is ineffective in aborting acute asthmatic attacks or other hypersensitivity reactions. However, the drug is effective in preventing these hypersensitivity reactions and reduces the amount of bronchodilators and corticosteroids needed to treat subsequent reactions. Cromolyn is effective in decreasing asthmatic episodes in clients with reversible airway obstruction.

Indications for Use As an adjunct in the treatment of severe bronchial asthma, particularly perennial asthma. It is ineffective in the treatment of acute episodes of bronchial asthma, particularly status asthmaticus.

Contraindications Hypersensitivity to cromolyn.

Warnings and Precautions Use with caution in clients with impaired hepatic or renal function. Animal studies (monkey) have indicated the possibility of arterial kidney lesions with prolonged therapy. Safe use during pregnancy has not been established. Not recommended for children under 5 years. Symptoms of asthma may recur if drug dosage is reduced or discontinued.

Untoward Reactions Relatively few severe untoward reactions occur. Cough and bronchospasm may occur following inhalation. Nasal congestion, sore throat, and wheezing are relatively common following inhalation. Laryngeal edema has been reported. Hypersensitivity reactions include angioedema, rash, urticaria, and painful swollen joints. Eosinophilic pneumonia (pulmonary infiltration with eosinophilia), exfoliative dermatitis, periarteritic vasculitis, and photodermatitis have been reported. Dysuria and urinary frequency may occur. Nephrosis has been reported. Nausea, headache, swollen parotid glands, and dizziness may occur. Hemoptysis and hoarseness have been reported. Anemia has occurred, but rarely.

Parameters of Use

Absorption Not absorbed from GI tract; rapidly absorbed from lung tissue and blood. Ineffective if swallowed and may cause GI irritation. About 10 to 20% of drug actually reaches lung tissue. Most of the drug enters GI tract after inhalation. Therapeutic results occur in 3 to 4 weeks.

Crosses placenta and may enter breast milk.

Excretion Primarily by the kidneys; enters GI tract via bile; excreted as unchanged drug.

Drug Interactions None known.

Administration Adults and children over 5 years: Initial dosage: 20 mg of powder inhaled qid; then dosage may be reduced in 2 to 4 weeks to 20 mg of powder inhaled tid. If asthmatic symptoms become worse, dosage is returned to qid administration.

Available Drug Forms Capsules containing 20 mg of micronized drug with lactose powder to improve delivery properties. Capsules are used with the Spinhaler turbo-inhaler.

Nursing Management

Planning factors

1. Obtain history of respiratory disorders. Record symptoms of asthma and their severity.
2. Perform baseline pulmonary function tests.
3. Store capsules in airtight container away from moisture and heat above 40 C (104 F).

Administration factors

1. Place whole capsule in inhaler. Powder is released as capsule is pierced by inhaler.
2. Instruct client to exhale deeply, place the mouthpiece between the lips and inhale steadily and deeply, remove the inhaler from the mouth before exhaling, and repeat until all the powder is gone.
3. Instruct client to rinse mouth with water after inhalation and then eat or drink an alkaline nutrient.

Evaluation factors

1. Assess client's asthmatic symptoms weekly. A flowchart may be helpful in recording the frequency and severity of symptoms.
2. Obtain pulmonary function tests periodically.
3. Spinhaler may cause accidental inhalation of gelatin particles or pieces of mouthpiece or propeller. Observe client for dyspnea after use.

Client teaching factors

1. Instruct client in the proper use of inhaler. (Demonstrate use of equipment without capsule.) Instruct client in proper cleansing of inhaler.
2. Caution client against swallowing capsule.
3. Encourage client to follow dosage schedule and inform client that therapeutic results may not occur for 3 to 4 weeks.
4. Inform client that dosage reduction or discontinuation of corticosteroids and bronchodilators may be possible, depending on client's response to cromolyn therapy.
5. Caution client against using a cracked or worn inhaler. (Inhaler should be replaced periodically.)
6. Instruct client to rinse mouth with water after each treatment to decrease oropharyngeal irritation. (Milk may decrease GI irritation.)
7. Instruct client in the proper storage of capsules.

COMBINATION PREPARATIONS CONTAINING EPHEDRINE AND THEOPHYLLINE

TRADE NAME Bronkolixir (OTC) (RX)

CLASSIFICATION Bronchodilator/expectorant

Action Provides bronchodilation, decongestion, and expectorant actions. Phenobarbital provides sedation to relieve anxiety.

Indications for Use Asthma, bronchitis.

Warnings and Precautions Phenobarbital may be habit forming. Use with caution in clients with hypertension, heart disease, diabetes, or hyperthyroidism.

Untoward Reactions Frequent or prolonged use may cause nervousness, restlessness, or insomnia. May cause drowsiness and urinary retention.

Administration Adults: 10 ml po qid; Children over 6 years: 5 ml po qid.

Available Drug Forms Cherry-flavored elixir. Generic contents in 5 ml: ephedrine sulfate: 12 mg; guaifenesin: 50 mg; theophylline: 15 mg, phenobarbital: 4 mg; alcohol: 19%.

TRADE NAME Bronkotabs (OTC) (RX)

CLASSIFICATION Bronchodilator/expectorant

Action Provides bronchodilation and decongestion and promotes expectoration. Phenobarbital counteracts drug-induced CNS stimulation and provides mild sedation.

Indications for Use Bronchial asthma, asthmatic bronchitis, chronic bronchitis with emphysema.

Warnings and Precautions Phenobarbital may be habit forming. Use with caution in clients with hypertension, heart disease, diabetes, or hyperthyroidism.

Untoward Reactions Frequent or prolonged use may cause nervousness, restlessness, or insomnia. May cause drowsiness and urinary retention.

Administration Adults: 1 tablet po 4 to 5 times daily; Children over 6 years: $\frac{1}{2}$ tablet po 4 to 5 times daily.

Available Drug Forms Generic contents in each tablet: ephedrine sulfate: 24 mg; guaifenesin: 100 mg; theophylline: 100 mg; phenobarbital: 8 mg.

TRADE NAME Co-Xan (Improved) (RX)

CLASSIFICATION Bronchodilator/expectorant

Action Provides bronchodilation, thins respiratory secretions, and relieves pain or discomfort.

Indications for Use Acute episodes of asthma and other respiratory disorders characterized by bronchospasm, inflamed mucous membranes, and adherent secretions.

Contraindications Hypersensitivity to any ingredient.

Warnings and Precautions Use with caution in clients with hypertension, heart disease, diabetes, or hyperthyroidism.

Untoward Reactions May cause drowsiness and urinary retention.

Administration Adults: 15 ml po q6h; Children: over 12 years: 10 to 15 ml po q6h; Ages 6 to 12 years: 5 to 10 ml po q6h; Ages 3 to 6 years: 5 ml po q6h; Ages 1 to 3 years: 2.5 ml po q6h.

Available Drug Forms Syrup. Generic contents in 15 ml: theophylline: 165 mg; codeine phosphate: 15 mg; ephedrine hydrochloride: 25 mg; guaifenesin: 100 mg; alcohol: 10%.

Nursing Management

1. Do not administer within 12 hours of theophylline or aminophylline suppositories.
2. Caution client against driving a car or operating heavy equipment.

TRADE NAME Isuprel (RX)

CLASSIFICATION Bronchodilator/expectorant

Action Combination preparation with three bronchial dilators that have different mechanisms of action.

Indications for Use Bronchial asthma, allergic coughs, bronchitis. Severe bronchospasms may require other therapies.

Contraindications Hypersensitivity to any ingredient.

Warnings and Precautions Phenobarbital may be habit forming. Use with caution in clients with glaucoma or prostatic hypertrophy and in those with hyperthyroidism, hypertension, or heart disease, since tachycardia, ventricular arrhythmias, nausea, or headache may occur. Not recommended during pregnancy.

Untoward Reactions May elevate serum protein-bound iodine.

Administration Adults: 30 ml po tid or qid, as needed; Children: Ages 6 to 12 years: 5 to 30 ml po tid, as needed; Ages 3 to 6 years: 10 to 15 ml po tid, as needed; Ages 1 to 3 years: 5 to 10 ml po tid, as needed.

Available Drug Forms Vanilla-flavored elixir. Generic contents in 15 ml: phenobarbital: 6 mg; isoproterenol hydrochloride: 2.5 mg; ephedrine sulfate: 12 mg; theophylline: 45 mg; potassium iodide: 150 mg; alcohol: 19%.

Nursing Management Do not use if crystals or precipitate have formed.

TRADE NAME Marax (RX)

CLASSIFICATION Bronchodilator

Action Provides bronchodilation. Hydroxyzine modifies the CNS stimulation of ephedrine. Syrup has an expectorant effect.

Indications for Use Possibly effective for the relief of bronchospasm and bronchial asthma.

Contraindications Hypersensitivity to any ingredient, hypertension, heart disease, hyperthyroidism, early pregnancy.

Warnings and Precautions Use with caution in clients with prostatic hypertrophy.

Untoward Reactions May cause drowsiness and may potentiate CNS depressants, such as alcohol.

Administration Adults: $\frac{1}{2}$ to 1 tablet po bid, tid, or qid; Children: Over 5 years: $\frac{1}{4}$ to $\frac{1}{2}$ tablet po bid, tid, or qid or 5 ml po tid or qid; Ages 2 to 5 years: 2.5 to 5.0 ml po tid or qid.

Available Drug Forms Scored tablets and colorless syrup. Generic contents in each tablet or 20 ml: ephedrine sulfate: 25 mg; theophylline: 130 mg; hydroxyzine hydrochloride: 10 mg. Syrup also contains 5% alcohol.

Nursing Management

1. Protect syrup from light.
2. Caution client against driving a car or operating heavy equipment.

TRADE NAME Mudrane GG Elixir (RX)

CLASSIFICATION Bronchodilator/expectorant

Action Sugar-free bronchodilator-mucolytic for children. Provides bronchodilation and thins respiratory secretions.

Indications for Use Asthma, asthmatic bronchitis.

Contraindications Hypersensitivity to any ingredient.

Warnings and Precautions Use with caution in clients with heart disease, diabetes, or hyperthyroidism.

Untoward Reactions May cause drowsiness and urinary retention.

Administration Adults: 1 tbsp po every 6 to 8 hours. Children: 1 ml/10 lb po every 6 to 8 hours.

Available Drug Forms Red-colored elixir. Generic contents in 5 ml: theophylline: 20 mg; ephedrine hydrochloride: 4 mg; phenobarbital: 2.5 mg; guaifenesin: 26 mg; alcohol: 20%. Also contains paraben as a preservative.

Nursing Management Follow with a glass of water.

TRADE NAME Quadrinal (RX)

CLASSIFICATION Bronchodilator/expectorant

Action Provides bronchodilation and expectorant-mucolytic effects. Phenobarbital counteracts drug-induced CNS stimulation and provides mild sedation.

Indications for Use Chronic respiratory disease in which tenacious mucus and bronchospasm are dominant symptoms, such as bronchial asthma, chronic bronchitis, and pulmonary emphysema.

Contraindications Hypersensitivity to any ingredient, enlarged thyroid, pregnancy, lactation, neonates.

Warnings and Precautions Phenobarbital may be habit forming. Use with caution in the elderly. Use as short-term therapy only in children.

Administration Adults: 1 tablet or 10 ml po every 6 to 8 hours; severe episodes may require $1\frac{1}{2}$ tablets or 15 ml q8h. Children: Ages 6 to 12 years: $\frac{1}{2}$ tablet or 5 ml po q8h; Under 6 years: Proportionately less.

Available Drug Forms Scored tablets and fruit-flavored suspension. Generic contents in each tablet or 10 ml: potassium iodide: 320 mg; theophylline (calcium salicylate): 65 mg; ephedrine hydrochloride: 24 mg; phenobarbital: 24 mg.

Nursing Management

1. Store between 59 and 86 F (15 to 30 C).
2. Shake suspension well before measuring dosage.
3. Discontinue drug if client develops skin rash, swelling of eyelids, or severe frontal headache (iodism).

TRADE NAME Quibron Plus (RX)

CLASSIFICATION Bronchodilator/expectorant

Action Provides bronchodilation and thins respiratory secretions. Butabarbital counteracts drug-induced CNS stimulation.

Indications for Use Possibly effective for the relief of bronchial asthma, bronchitis, bronchiectasis, and emphysema.

Contraindications Hypersensitivity to any ingredient, within 14 days of therapy with MAO inhibitors.

Warnings and Precautions Butabarbital may be habit forming. Use with caution in the elderly, in clients with disorders of the cardiovascular, hepatic, or endocrine system, and those with right-sided heart failure, hyperthyroidism, history of peptic ulcers, porphyria, urinary retention, or angle-closure glaucoma.

Untoward Reactions Severe toxic reactions, such as seizures and ventricular arrhythmias, are not necessarily preceded by less severe symptoms.

Administration Adults: 1 to 2 capsules or 15 to 30 ml po bid or tid; Children: Ages 8 to 12 years: 1 capsule or 15 ml po bid or tid; Under 8 years: 2 to 5 ml/10 lb po bid or tid.

Available Drug Forms Soft gelatin capsules and flavored elixir. Generic contents in each capsule or 15 ml: theophylline: 150 mg; guaifenesin: 100 mg; ephedrine hydrochloride: 25 mg; butabarbital: 20 mg. Elixir also contains 15% alcohol.

TRADE NAMES Tedral; Tedral Suspension (OTC)

CLASSIFICATION Bronchodilator

Action Provides bronchodilation. Phenobarbital counteracts drug-induced CNS stimulation and provides mild sedation.

Indications for Use Symptomatic relief of bronchial asthma, asthmatic bronchitis, and other bronchospastic disorders; prevention and treatment of acute asthmatic episodes. Suspension is useful for children and adults unable to swallow tablets.

Contraindications Hypersensitivity to any ingredient, porphyria, children under 2 years.

Warnings and Precautions Phenobarbital may be habit forming.

Untoward Reactions Epigastric distress, palpitations, insomnia, tremulousness, CNS stimulation, difficult micturition.

Warnings and Precautions Use with caution in clients with hypertension, heart disease, diabetes, or hyperthyroidism.

Administration Adults: 1 to 2 tablets or 10 to 20 ml po q4h; Children: Over 60 lb: $\frac{1}{2}$ tablet or 5 to 10 ml po every 4 to 6 hours.

Available Drug Forms Scored tablets and licorice-flavored suspension. Generic contents in each tablet or 10 ml: theophylline: 130 mg; ephedrine hydrochloride: 24 mg; phenobarbital: 8 mg.

Nursing Management Shake suspension well before measuring dosage.

TRADE NAME Tedral-25H (RX)

CLASSIFICATION Bronchodilator

See Tedral for Contraindications and Untoward reactions.

Action Same as Tedral but contains 25 mg of barbiturate.

Indications for Use Used for clients who are unduly sensitive to the effects of ephedrine. (See Tedral.)

Warnings and Precautions Butabarbital may be habit forming.

Administration Adults: 1 tablet po q4h; Children: $\frac{1}{2}$ tablet po q4h.

Available Drug Forms Generic contents in each scored tablet: theophylline: 130 mg; ephedrine hydrochloride: 24 mg; butabarbital: 25 mg.

TRADE NAME Tedral Expectorant (RX)

CLASSIFICATION Bronchodilator/expectorant

See Tedral for Contraindications, Warnings and Precautions, and Untoward reactions.

Action Similar to Tedral, but also contains guaifenesin to increase the volume and decrease the viscosity of respiratory secretions.

Indications for Use Used only when bronchospasm is accompanied by thick, viscous secretions. (See Tedral.)

Administration Adults: 1 to 2 tablets po q6h; Children: Under 12 years: Dosage not established.

Available Drug Forms Generic contents in each scored tablet: theophylline: 130 mg; ephedrine hydrochloride: 24 mg; phenobarbital: 8 mg; guaifenesin 100 mg.

TRADE NAME Tedral Elixir (OTC)

CLASSIFICATION Bronchodilator

See Tedral for Contraindications, Warnings and precautions, and Untoward reactions.

Action Same as Tedral but half the strength.

Indications for Use Elixir is useful for clients who have difficulty swallowing tablets. (See Tedral.)

Administration Adults: 15 to 30 ml po q4h; Children: 5 ml/30 lb po every 4 to 6 hours.

Available Drug Forms Cherry-flavored elixir. Generic contents in 5 ml: theophylline: 32.5 mg; ephedrine hydrochloride: 6 mg; phenobarbital: 2 mg; alcohol: 15%.

TRADE NAME Tedral SA (RX)

CLASSIFICATION Bronchodilator

See Tedral for Contraindications, Warnings and precautions, and Untoward reactions.

Action Provides immediate and sustained bronchodilation. Similar to Tedral but has convenience of twice-a-day dosage.

Indications for Use May be useful in clients who are sensitive to ephedrine. (See Tedral.)

Administration Adults: 1 tablet po q12h; Children: Under 12 years: Dosage not established.

Available Drug Forms Generic contents in each double-layered tablet: Immediate release layer: theophylline: 90 mg; ephedrine hydrochloride: 16 mg; phenobarbital: 25 mg; Sustained-release layer: theophylline: 90 mg; ephedrine hydrochloride: 32 mg.

Nursing Management

1. Instruct client not to chew tablets.
2. Give first dose immediately on awakening in the morning.

COMBINATION PREPARATIONS CONTAINING THEOPHYLLINE-CONTAINING SUBSTANCES AND AN EXPECTORANT

TRADE NAME Asbron G (RX)

CLASSIFICATION Bronchodilator/expectorant

Action Provides bronchodilation and thins respiratory secretions.

Contraindications Hypersensitivity to xanthines, peptic ulcer, active gastritis.

Warnings and Precautions Use with caution in clients with cardiovascular, hepatic, or renal disorders. Safe use during pregnancy and in children under 6 years has not been established.

Untoward Reactions The early signs of theophylline toxicity are nausea and restlessness. Convulsions may follow. Tachycardia may occur and a preexisting arrhythmia may worsen before seizures develop. GI disturbances include nausea, vomiting, and epigastric distress. Headache and insomnia are common. Diuresis is common. Hyperglycemia and tachypnea may occur.

Administration Adults: 1 to 2 tablets or 15 to 30 ml po every 6 to 8 hours; Children: Ages 6 to 12 years: 10 to 15 ml po every 6 to 8 hours; Ages 3 to 6 years: 5.0 to 7.5 ml po every 6 to 8 hours; Ages 1 to 3 years: 2.5 to 5.0 ml po every 6 to 8 hours.

Available Drug Forms Inlay tablets and elixir. Generic contents in each tablet or 15 ml: theophylline sodium glycinate: 300 mg; guaifenesin: 100 mg. Elixir also contains 15% alcohol.

TRADE NAME Elixophyllin-KI (RX)

CLASSIFICATION Bronchodilator/expectorant

See Asbron G for Action, Contraindications, and Untoward reactions.

Warnings and Precautions Use with caution in clients with cardiovascular, hepatic, renal, or thyroid disorders. Not recommended during pregnancy and lactation; safe use during pregnancy and in children under 6 years has not been established.

Administration Adults: 30 ml po tid upon arising, at 3 P.M., and hs; Children: 0.2 ml/lb po tid as for adults.

Available Drug Forms Elixir. Generic contents in 15 ml: theophylline: 80 mg; potassium iodide: 130 mg; alcohol: 10%.

Nursing Management Store at room temperature.

TRADE NAME Isufil T.D. (RX)

CLASSIFICATION Bronchodilator/expectorant

See Asbron G for Action and Contraindications.

Warnings and Precautions Use with caution in the elderly and debilitated clients. (See Asbron G.)

Untoward Reactions Some drowsiness may occur. (See Asbron G.)

Administration 1 tablet po every 6 to 8 hours.

Available Drug Forms Generic contents in each tablet: theophylline: 200 mg; noscapine: 30 mg.

TRADE NAME Quibron (RX)

CLASSIFICATION Bronchodilator/expectorant

See Asbron G for Action, Contraindications, Warnings and precautions, and Untoward reactions.

Administration Adults: 1 to 2 capsules or 15 to 30 ml po every 6 to 8 hours; Children: Ages 9 to 12 years: 4 to 5 mg/kg po every 6 to 8 hours; Under 9 years: 4 to 6 mg/kg po every 6 to 8 hours.

Available Drug Forms Generic contents in each soft gelatin capsule or 15 ml: theophylline: 150 mg; guaifenesin: 90 mg. (Both preparations have a bitter taste.)

TRADE NAME Quibron-300 (RX)

CLASSIFICATION Bronchodilator/expectorant

See Asbron G for Action, Contraindications, Warnings and precautions, and Untoward reactions.

Indications for Use Used for adults who need higher dosages.

Administration 1 capsule po every 6 to 8 hours.

Available Drug Forms Generic contents in each soft gelatin capsule: theophylline: 300 mg; guaifenesin: 180 mg.

TRADE NAME Slo-phyllin GG (RX)

CLASSIFICATION Bronchodilator/expectorant

See Asbron G for Action, Contraindications, Warnings and precautions, and Untoward reactions.

Administration Adults: 1 to 2 capsules or 15 to 30 ml po every 6 to 8 hours; Children: Ages 9 to 12 years: 4 to 5 mg/kg po every 6 to 8 hours; Under 9 years: 4 to 6 mg/kg po every 6 to 8 hours.

Available Drug Forms White, soft gelatin capsules and lemon-vanilla flavored syrup. Generic contents in each capsule or 15 ml: theophylline: 150 mg; guaifenesin: 90 mg. Syrup also contains sugar.

TRADE NAME Synophylate-GG (RX)

CLASSIFICATION Bronchodilator/expectorant

See Asbron G for Contraindications, Warnings and precautions, and Untoward reactions.

Action Large dosages are less irritating to the GI tract than theophylline. (See Asbron G.)

Administration Adults: 1 to 2 tablets or 15 to 30 ml po every 6 to 8 hours; Children: Ages 6 to 12 years: 1 tablet or 10 to 15 ml po every 6 to 8 hours; Ages 3 to 6 years: 5.0 to 7.5 ml po every 6 to 8 hours; Ages 1 to 3 years: 2.5 to 5.0 ml po every 6 to 8 hours.

Available Drug Forms Generic contents in each tablet or 15 ml: theophylline sodium glycinate: 300 mg; guaifenesin: 100 mg. Syrup also contains 10% alcohol.

TRADE NAME Theolair-Plus 125 (RX)

CLASSIFICATION Bronchodilator/expectorant

See Asbron G for Action, Contraindications, Warnings and precautions, and Untoward reactions.

Administration Adults: 1 to 2 capsules or 15 to 30 ml po every 6 to 8 hours; Children: Ages 9 to 12 years: 4 to 5 mg/kg po every 6 to 8 hours; Under 9 years: 4 to 6 mg/kg po every 6 to 8 hours.

Available Drug Forms Generic contents in each tablet: theophylline: 125 mg; guaifenesin: 100 mg.

TRADE NAME Theolair-Plus 250 (RX)

CLASSIFICATION Bronchodilator/expectorant

See Asbron G for Action, Contraindications, Warnings and precautions, and Untoward reactions.

Administration Adults: 1 to 2 tablets po every 6 to 8 hours.

Available Drug Forms Generic contents in each tablet: theophylline: 250 mg; guaifenesin: 200 mg.

TRADE NAME Theolair-Plus Liquid (RX)

CLASSIFICATION Bronchodilator/expectorant

See Asbron G for Action, Contraindications, Warnings and precautions, and Untoward reactions.

Indications for Use Liquid is often used for children, the elderly, and debilitated clients.

Administration Adults: 1 to 2 capsules or 15 to 30 ml po every 6 to 8 hours; Children: Ages 9 to 12 years: 4 to 5 mg/kg po every 6 to 8 hours; Under 9 years: 4 to 6 mg/kg po every 6 to 8 hours.

Available Drug Forms Generic contents in 15 ml: theophylline: 125 mg; guaifenesin: 100 mg.

TRADE NAME Theo-Organidin (RX)

CLASSIFICATION Bronchodilator/expectorant

See Asbron G for Action, Warnings and precautions, and Untoward reactions.

Contraindications Hypersensitivity to inorganic iodides or xanthines, pregnancy, lactation, neonates. Peptic ulcer, active gastritis.

Administration Adults: 15 to 30 ml po every 6 to 8 hours; Children: 5 ml/9 kg po bid or tid.

Available Drug Forms Elixir. Generic contents in 15 ml: theophylline: 120 mg; iodinated glycerol: 30 mg; alcohol: 15%.

Nursing Management Store at room temperature in airtight containers.

TRADE NAME Dilor-G (RX)

CLASSIFICATION Bronchodilator/expectorant

See Asbron G for Contraindications and Warnings and precautions.

Action Usually better tolerated than theophylline. (See Asbron G.)

Untoward Reactions May cause drowsiness. (See Asbron G.)

Administration Adults: 1 to 2 tablets or 10 to 20 ml po every 6 to 8 hours; Children: Ages 6 to 12 years: 10 to 15 ml po every 6 to 8 hours; Ages 3 to 6 years: 5.0 to 7.5 ml po every 6 to 8 hours; Ages 1 to 3 years: 2.5 to 5.0 ml po every 6 to 8 hours.

Available Drug Forms Generic contents in each pink scored tablet or 10 ml: dyphylline: 200 mg; guaifenesin: 200 mg.

TRADE NAME Emfaseem (RX)

CLASSIFICATION Bronchodilator/expectorant

See Asbron G for Action, Contraindications, Warnings and precautions, and Untoward reactions.

Administration Adults: 1 to 2 tablets po every 6 to 8 hours; Children: Ages 9 to 16 years: 1 tablet po every 6 to 8 hours.

Available Drug Forms Generic contents in each blue and white capsule: dyphylline: 200 mg; guaifenesin: 100 mg.

TRADE NAME Lufyllin-GG (RX)

CLASSIFICATION Bronchodilator/expectorant

See Asbron G for Action, Contraindications, and Warnings and precautions.

Untoward Reactions May cause drowsiness. (See Asbron G.)

Administration Adults: 1 to 2 tablets or 15 to 30 ml po every 6 to 8 hours; Children: Ages 6 to 12 years: 1 tablet or 10 to 15 ml po every 6 to 8 hours; Ages 3 to 6 years: 5 to 7 ml po every 6 to 8 hours; Ages 1 to 3 years: 2.5 to 5.0 po every 6 to 8 hours.

Available Drug Forms Light yellow, monogrammed tablets and clear yellow-orange elixir with a fruity odor and taste. Generic contents in each tablet or 30 ml: dyphylline: 200 mg; guaifenesin: 200 mg. Elixir also contains 17% alcohol.

TRADE NAME Neothylline-GG (RX)

CLASSIFICATION Bronchodilator/expectorant

See Asbron G for Action, Contraindications, and Warnings and precautions.

Untoward Reactions May cause drowsiness. (See Asbron G.)

Administration Adults: 1 to 2 tablets or 15 to 30 ml po every 6 to 8 hours; Children: Ages 6 to 12 years: 1 tablet or 10 to 15 ml po every 6 to 8 hours; Ages 3 to 6 years: 5 to 7 ml po every 6 to 8 hours; Ages 1 to 3 years: 2.5 to 5.0 ml po every 6 to 8 hours.

Available Drug Forms Generic contents in each white tablet or 30 ml: dyphylline: 200 mg; guaifenesin: 200 mg. Elixir also contains 10% alcohol.

TRADE NAME Brondecon (RX)

CLASSIFICATION Bronchodilator/expectorant

See Asbron G for Action, Contraindications, Warnings and precautions, and Untoward reactions.

Administration Adults and children over 12 years: 1 tablet or 10 ml po q6h; Children: Ages 2 to 12 years: 5 ml/60 lb po q6h.

Available Drug Forms Salmon-pink tablets and dark red, cherry-flavored elixir. Generic contents in each tablet or 10 ml: oxtriphylline: 200 mg; guaifenesin: 100 mg. Elixir also contains 20% alcohol.

Nursing Management Store at room temperature.

MULTIPLE INGREDIENT PREPARATIONS

TRADE NAME KIE Syrup (RX)

CLASSIFICATION Bronchodilator/expectorant

Action Provides bronchodilation and mucolytic effects.

Indications for Use Symptomatic relief of bronchial asthma, emphysema, and asthmatic bronchitis.

Contraindications Hypersensitivity to any ingredient, severe heart disease, arrhythmias, pregnancy, tuberculosis, acne.

Warnings and Precautions Discontinue if client develops skin rash, swelling of eyelids, or severe frontal headache (iodism).

Administration Adults 5 ml po every 6 to 8 hours with a full glass of water.

Available Drug Forms Green syrup. Generic contents in 5 ml: potassium iodide: 150 mg; ephedrine hydrochloride: 8 mg.

TRADE NAME Lufyllin-EPG (RX)

CLASSIFICATION Bronchodilator/expectorant

Action Provides bronchodilation, expectorant effects, and sedation to counteract drug-induced CNS stimulation.

Indications for Use Acute bronchial asthma, reversible bronchospasm associated with bronchitis and emphysema.

Warnings and Precautions Phenobarbital may be habit forming. Use with caution in clients with severe heart disease, renal or hepatic dysfunction, or glaucoma. Do not administer to children under 6 years.

Untoward Reactions May cause nausea, headache, arrhythmias, or CNS stimulation.

Administration Adults: 1 tablet or 10 ml po q6h; larger dosages are required in acute asthma. Children: Over 6 years: Start on low dosages po every 6 to 8 hours; then gradually increase to lowest effective dosage; Maximum dosage: 5 mg/kg/day.

Available Drug Forms Pink monogrammed tablets and clear red elixir with a fruity odor and taste. Generic contents in each tablet or 10 ml: dyphylline: 100 mg; guaifenesin: 200 mg; ephedrine hydrochloride: 16 mg; phenobarbital: 16 mg. Elixir also contains 5.5% alcohol.

TRADE NAME Mudrane (RX)

CLASSIFICATION Bronchodilator/expectorant

Action Provides bronchodilation, mucolytic effects, and sedation to counteract drug-induced CNS stimulation.

Indications for Use Symptomatic relief of bronchial asthma, emphysema, and asthmatic bronchitis.

Contraindications Hypersensitivity to any ingredient, arrhythmias, heart disease, hypertension, hyperthyroidism, porphyria, pregnancy, tuberculosis, acne.

Warnings and Precautions Phenobarbital may be habit forming. Discontinue if client develops skin rash, swelling of eyelids, or severe frontal headache (iodism).

Administration Adults: 1 tablet po every 6 to 8 hours with a full glass of water; Older children: $\frac{1}{2}$ tablet po every 6 to 8 hours with a full glass of water.

Available Drug Forms Generic contents in each yellow scored tablet: potassium iodide: 195 mg; aminophylline: 130 mg; phenobarbital: 8 mg; ephedrine hydrochloride: 16 mg.

TRADE NAME Mudrane GG Tablets (RX)

CLASSIFICATION Bronchodilator/expectorant

See Mudrane for Indications for Use, Contraindications, and Warnings and precautions.

Action Same as Mudrane, but guaifenesin replaces potassium iodide as mucolytic-expectorant. This drug is prescribed for clients with acne and tuberculosis, during pregnancy, or when client is intolerant to iodides. It may be substituted every fourth week for Mudrane to reduce the incidence of iodide sensitivity.

Administration Adults: 1 tablet po every 6 to 8 hours with a full glass of water.

Available Drug Forms Generic contents in each yellow tablet: aminophylline: 130 mg; guaifenesin: 100 mg; ephedrine hydrochloride: 16 mg; phenobarbital: 8 mg.

TRADE NAME PBZ with Ephedrine (RX)

CLASSIFICATION Bronchodilator/expectorant

Action Provides antihistamine effects, bronchodilation, and drying of respiratory secretions.

Indications for Use Persistent, unproductive cough associated with allergies and bronchitis; as an adjunct in the treatment of asthma and allergic respiratory disorders.

Contraindications Neonates, lactation.

Untoward Reactions Causes CNS depression and may cause dizziness and hypotension in the elderly.

Administration Adults: 4 to 8 ml po every 3 to 4 hours with a full glass of water; Older children: 2 to 4 ml po every 3 to 4 hours with a full glass of water.

Available Drug Forms Yellow liquid. Generic contents in 4 ml: tripelennamine citrate: 30 mg; ephedrine sulfate: 10 mg; ammonium chloride: 80 mg.

Nursing Management Protect from light.

TRADE NAME Quelidrine (OTC)

CLASSIFICATION Bronchodilator/decongestant

Action Provides bronchodilation. Nonnarcotic antihistaminic cough suppressant. Safe for clients of all ages.

Indications for Use Symptomatic relief of cough associated with acute or subacute simple respiratory infections.

Warnings and Precautions Use with caution in clients with hypertension, heart disease, angina, diabetes, thyroid disorders, or those receiving digitalis. Reevaluation of underlying cause is required if cough persists or high fever ocurs.

Untoward Reactions Infrequent.

Administration Adults: 5 ml po daily, bid, tid, or qid; Children: Over 6 years: 2.5 ml po daily, bid, tid, or qid; Ages 2 to 6 years: 1.25 ml po daily, bid, tid, or qid. May be diluted with syrup to facilitate administration to children.

Available Drug Forms Generic contents in 5 ml: dextromethorphan hydrobromide: 10 mg; chlorpheniramine maleate: 2 mg; ephedrine hydrochloride: 5 mg; phenylephrine hydrochloride: 5 mg; ammonium chloride: 40 mg; ipecac fluid extract: 0.005 ml; alcohol: 2%.

TRADE NAME Rynatuss Tablets (RX)

CLASSIFICATION Bronchodilator/decongestant

Action Provides bronchodilation, decongestion, antihistamine, and antitussive effects.

Indications for Use Relief of cough associated with the common cold, bronchial asthma, and acute or chronic bronchitis.

Contraindications Hypersensitivity to any ingredient, neonates, lactation.

Warnings and Precautions Use with caution in clients with hypertension, cardiovascular disease, hyperthyroidism, diabetes, narrow-angle glaucoma, or prostatic hypertrophy. May have additive CNS effects with CNS depressants and alcohol.

Untoward Reactions Drowsiness, sedation, dryness of mucous membranes, GI disturbances.

Administration 1 to 2 tablets po q12h.

Available Drug Forms Generic contents in each lavender-rose tablet: carabetapentane tannate: 60 mg; chlorpheniramine tannate: 5 mg; ephedrine tannate: 10 mg; phenylephrine tannate: 10 mg.

TRADE NAME Rynatuss Pediatric Suspension (RX)

CLASSIFICATION Bronchodilator/decongestant

See Rynatuss Tablets for Action, Indications for use, Contraindications, and Warnings and precautions.

Untoward Reactions An allergic reaction (bronchial asthma) may occur to FD&C No. 5 yellow. (See Rynatuss Tablets.)

Administration Children: Over 6 years: 5 to 10 ml po q12h; Ages 2 to 6 years: 2.5 to 5.0 ml po q12h.

Available Drug Forms Strawberry-currant flavored suspension. Generic contents in 5 ml: carbetapentane tannate: 30 mg; chlorpheniramine tannate: 4 mg; ephedrine tannate: 5 mg; phenylephrine tannate: 5 mg. Also contains FD&C No. 5 yellow.

Nursing Management

1. Store at room temperature.
2. Shake suspension well before measuring dosage.

TRADE NAME Duo-Medihaler (RX)

CLASSIFICATION Bronchodilator/decongestant

Action Provides bronchodilation and vasoconstruction to reduce edema and congestion of bronchial vascular beds.

Indications for Use Dyspnea associated with bronchospasm and excessive respiratory secretions in acute and chronic bronchial asthma, emphysema, bronchitis, and bronchiectasis.

Contraindications Hypersensitivity to any ingredient, arrhythmias, tachycardia.

Untoward Reactions Excessive use may cause paradoxic airway resistance or cardiac arrest.

Administration

- *Acute episode:* 1 to 2 inhalations.
- *Maintenance:* 1 to 2 inhalations 4 to 6 times daily.

Available Drug Forms Metered-dose inhaler and refills. Generic contents in each inhalation: isoproterenol hydrochloride: 0.16 mg; phenylephrine bitartrate: 0.24 mg.

TRADE NAME Mucomyst with Isoproterenol (RX)

CLASSIFICATION Bronchodilator/mucolytic

Action Provides bronchodilation and mucolytic effects.

Indications for Use Adjunct therapy for clients with viscid or inspissated mucous secretions associated with chronic obstructive pulmonary disease, cystic fibrosis, posttrauma conditions, and atelectasis.

Contraindications Hypersensitivity to any ingredient, arrhythmias, tachycardia.

Warnings and Precautions Use with caution in children under 6 years.

Administration Oxygen aerosolization or IPPB: 4 ml qid.

Available Drug Forms Solution 10 or 20%. Generic contents: acetylcysteine: 10%; isoproterenol hydrochloride: 0.05%.

Nursing Management Mechanical suctioning may be required after treatment.

TRADE NAME Norisodrine with Calcium Iodide

CLASSIFICATION Bronchodilator/expectorant (RX)

Action Provides bronchodilation and expectorant effects.

Indications for Use Hypersensitivity to any ingredient, arrhythmias, tachycardia.

Contraindications Hypersensitivity to any ingredients, arrythmias, tachycardia.

Administration 5 to 10 ml po qid.

Available Drug Forms Syrup. Generic contents in 5 ml: isoproterenol sulfate: 3 mg; calcium iodide: 150 mg; alcohol: 6%.

Chapter 55

Decongestants

4-Way Tablets
Histabid Duracap
Sinulin
Sine-Aid
Triaminic Tablets
Triaminic Juvelets
Triaminic-12 Tablets
Triaminic Infant Drops
Triaminic Syrup

TOPICAL DECONGESTANTS

Phenylephedrine hydrochloride
Cyclopentamine hydrochloride
Methylhexaneamine carbonate
Naphazoline hydrochloride
Oxymethazoline hydrochloride
Propylhexedrine
Tetrahydrozoline hydrochloride
Tuaminoheptane sulfate
Xylometazoline hydrochloride

TEMPORARY INFLAMMATION AND congestion of the upper respiratory tract occurs in practically all individuals and may be due to an infection, an allergy, or a nonallergic vasomotor reaction. Millions of dollars are spent on over-the-counter and prescription decongestants annually by the public. Decongestant preparations may contain one or more ingredients. Unfortunately, combination preparations sometimes contain ingredients that the client may neither need nor want and the use of these preparations may cause unnecessary and adverse reactions. It is the responsibility of health professionals to assist the client in understanding the types of preparations available and the rationale for using each type of decongestant. The selection of an appropriate decongestant requires a knowledge of the anatomical structures involved, the etiology of the disorder, and the pharmacologic action of the ingredients in decongestant preparations.

STRUCTURES OF THE UPPER RESPIRATORY SYSTEM

The nose, sinuses, and nasopharynx are considered components of the upper respiratory tract. Inspired air is filtered, humidified, and warmed to near body temperature by the nose. The superior, middle, and inferior turbinates (or conchae) increase the surface area through which air passes and thereby facilitate the ability of the nose to perform its functions.

The perpetually moist and highly vascular mucous membrane lining the nasal cavities ensures that inspired air achieves a relatively constant temperature and humidity before entering the nasopharynx. The sinuses drain into the nasal cavities and are in danger of being inflamed whenever the nasal mucous membranes are congested, as is the membrane lining the eustachian tube and middle ear, which connects the nasopharynx with the middle ear.

INDICATIONS FOR USE

Rhinitis is the inflammation of the nasal mucous membrane and *Rhinorrhea* refers to the free discharge of watery nasal mucus. The etiologic classification of rhinitis is usually subdivided as follows:

1. Acute infections or simple rhinitis-coryza
2. Allergic rhinitis
   (a) Acute or seasonal
   (b) Chronic or perennial

Infectious rhinitis (common cold) is caused by one of several viruses and is characterized by a red, inflamed nasal membrane and excessive rhinorrhea that persists for six to seven days. Headache and sneezing may also be present. Some experts believe that the swelling of the nasal membrane is beneficial because it prevents the infection from spreading and therefore do not advocate the use of locally applied decongestants during the first two days. Instead, systemic decongestants, particularly pseudoephedrine hydrochloride, are recommended. When infectious rhinitis is accompanied by fever and aches and pains, a combination of a single decongestant and either aspirin or acetaminophen is usually used.

Allergic rhinitis occurs when a hypersensitive client is exposed to an allergen. Although removal of the allergen from the client's environment is the preferred method of treatment, this is not always possible. The allergic reaction results in inflammation of the nasal mucosa, but the mucosa has a pale and edematous appearance rather than a reddish appearance as in infectious rhinitis. Acute or seasonal allergic rhinitis usually lasts a few weeks; but chronic or perennial rhinitis is constantly present and the client experiences intermittent periods of nasal obstruction. Eventually, the nasal mucosa becomes thickened as connective tissue forms. Antihistamines are helpful in limiting the allergic reaction, although they do not prevent it, and decongestants are used to treat the congestion. Several antihistamine-decongestant preparations are also available, but their effectiveness is questionable. (Some of these multiple ingredient preparations have already been listed as only possibly effective.) Further research is required to determine the effectiveness of these preparations in acute and chronic allergic rhinitis. The judicious use of mild, topically applied decongestants is helpful in relieving nasal obstruction, but excessive or prolonged use may lead to rebounding congestion or nonallergic vasomotor rhinitis—a chronic disorder characterized by intermittent nasal obstruction with excessive rhinorrhea. Stress, hypothyroidism, and other disorders can also cause a neurovascular imbalance in the nasal cavity.

Sinusitis is the inflammation of the mucous membranes of the sinuses and may present as a complication of rhinitis. Headache in the area of the involved sinus frequently occurs; fever may also occur if the sinus passageway is completely blocked. Topically applied decongestants may be helpful in treating this condition and are administered by adjusting the position of the client's head so that the medication is directed toward the nasal opening of the sinus. As clients with sinusitis tend to misuse topical decongestants, rebounding congestion may eventually develop. Most forms of sinusitis are allergic in origin, not infectious; consequently, antihistamines and systemic decongestants are often prescribed. However, it should be remembered that treatment of chronic sinusitis requires the expertise of an otolaryngologist.

Acute *otitis media* (inflammation of the middle ear) is a frequent complication of acute rhinitis, particularly in children, since their eustachian tube is relatively short and broad. Systemic decongestants are used to treat this disorder as otic solutions are unable to reach the involved area. Although the accompanying earache quickly subsides after instilling decongestants in serious otitis media, the medication must be continued as prescribed in order to facilitate drainage of the accumulated fluid.

TYPES OF DECONGESTANTS

Agents used as decongestants stimulate the alpha-adrenergic systems and thus promote vasoconstriction of nasal arterioles, thereby relieving congestion and inflammation. Ephedrine is an effective decongestant, but as this drug causes other alpha and beta effects, it is seldom used. Ideally, a decongestant should induce nasal vasoconstriction similar to or greater than ephedrine without causing other adrenergic effects. Pseudoephedrine and phenylpropanolamine are frequently used because they cause little or no central nervous system disturbances. However, restlessness, arrhythmias, and other untoward reactions can result from the use of adrenergic agents (see Chapter 39). Although the onset of action of these drugs is not as immediate as when topical decongestants are used, their effects last longer and rebounding congestion does not occur.

The autonomic nervous system controls the engorgement of the nasal vasculature, but the normal reflex reaction can be disturbed by excessive or prolonged use of topical decongestants. Consequently, the client may eventually develop congestion soon after the effects of the topical agent subside; thus a cyclic drug-induced congestion results. Rebounding congestion is treated by the withdrawal of all decongestants until normal reflexes return. Normal saline nose drops can be used to clear the nasal membranes and promote nasal clearing.

Antihistamines can be beneficial in allergic rhinitis and sinusitis. Mild antihistamines are preferred because their anticholinergic effects will induce dryness of the nasal and other mucous membranes (dry mouth). As these substances can cause untoward reactions, such as drowsiness and central nervous system depression, alcohol, hypnotics, and other central nervous system depressants must be avoided. Urinary retention, blurred vision, and constipation can also occur as a result of anticholinergic properties. Young children may develop insomnia and irritability as a result of central nervous system stimulation. Decongestants containing antihistamines should not be used routinely for acute rhinitis unless an allergic reaction is suspected.

SYSTEMIC DECONGESTANTS

GENERIC NAME Pseudoephedrine hydrochloride

TRADE NAMES Besan, Cenafed, D-Feda, Ehor, Novafed, Sudabid, Sudafed, Sudafed S.A. (OTC)

CLASSIFICATION Systemic decongestant, adrenergic agent

Action Pseudoephedrine is an adrenergic agent similar to ephedrine, but it induces less intense pressor and CNS stimulation. The decongestant effect on the upper respiratory tract mucosa is the result of vasoconstriction. Tissue hyperemia and edema are decreased, thus the patency of the nasal airway increases. Some bronchodilation also occurs. There is little or no increase in the blood pressure of normotensive clients; but the drug should be used with caution in hypertensive clients. CNS stimulation may occur, particularly in young children. Unlike decongestants containing antihistamines, pseudoephedrine does not produce drowsiness and is therefore useful during the daytime. When indicated, the drug may be given concurrently with analgesics, antihistamines, expectorants, or antibiotics.

Indications for Use Upper respiratory tract congestion associated with the common cold or infections, sinusitis, or allergic rhinitis; eustachian tube congestion associated with acute eustachian salpingitis, aerotitis media, and serous otitis media.

Contraindications Hypersensitivity to sympathomimetic amines (manifested by insomnia, dizziness, weakness, tremors, or arrhythmias), severe hypertension, severe coronary artery disease, clients taking MAO inhibitors, lactation.

Warnings and Precautions Use with caution in clients with diabetes, hypertension, cardiovascular diseases, glaucoma, hyperthyroidism, or prostatic hypertrophy and in the elderly (60 years or older), since high dosages or prolonged therapy may cause hallucinations, convulsions, and CNS depression. Safe use during pregnancy has not been established.

Untoward Reactions Common hypersensitivity reactions include tachycardia, palpitations, headache, dizziness, and nausea. Although less common with pseudoephedrine, sympathomimetics may cause fear, anxiety, tenseness, restlessness, tremors, weakness, pallor, dyspnea, dysuria, insomnia, hallucinations, convulsions, CNS depression, arrhythmias, hypotension, and death.

Parameters of Use

Absorption Well absorbed from GI tract. Onset of action is about 15 to 30 minutes. Peak action occurs in about 1 hour and duration of action is about 4 hours. Long-acting preparations are released slowly and have a duration of action of about 10 to 12 hours. Serum half-life is about 4 to 6 hours.

Excretion By the kidneys; acidic urine (pH lower than 6) will increase drug excretion, whereas alkaline urine (pH above 8) will decrease drug excretion.

Drug Interactions Hypertensive crisis may occur in clients receiving MAO inhibitors concurrently. Beta-adrenergic blockers will increase the effects and therefore the untoward reactions of pseudoephedrine. May decrease the antihypertensive effects of methyldopa, mecamylamine, reserpine, and veratrum alkaloids. Urinary acidifiers will increase and urinary alkalizers will decrease the excretion of pseudoephedrine.

Administration Adults and children over 12 years: 60 mg po q4h (regular tablet); 60 to 120 mg po q12h (long-lasting drug form); Children: Ages 6 to 12 years: 30 mg po q4h; Maximum dosage: 120 mg/day; Ages 2 to 5 years: 15 mg po q4h; Maximum dosage: 60 mg/day.

Available Drug Forms Tablets containing 30 or 60 mg; syrup or liquid containing 30 mg/5 ml; long-acting tablets and capsules containing 60 or 120 mg.

Nursing Management

Planning factors

1. Obtain history of CNS and cardiovascular disorders.
2. Obtain baseline blood pressure and pulse. If hypertension, tachycardia, or arrhythmias are present, notify physician before initiating therapy.
3. Schedule therapy so that drug is not administered within 2 hours of bedtime.

Administration factors

1. Give with water.
2. If anorexia occurs, give at least 2 hours before meals or 1 hour after meals.
3. If nausea occurs, give after meals.

Evaluation factors

1. Obtain blood pressure and pulse of hypertensive and elderly clients 1 to 2 hours after administering drug. If hypertension, tachycardia, or an irregular pulse occur, notify physician.
2. Check urinary output of elderly clients. If urinary retention or incontinence occur, notify physician.
3. Observe the behavior of young children and the

elderly 1 to 2 hours after administration. If CNS stimulation occurs, notify physician.

Client teaching factors

1. Inform client to avoid OTC drugs containing ephedrine or other sympathomimetics.
2. Instruct client to avoid taking drug within 2 hours of bedtime, since insomnia may occur.
3. Warn elderly clients and the parents of children under 12 years to avoid excessive use of drug. Only 4 doses should be taken in 24 hours.
4. Caution client to notify medical personnel if tachycardia, dizziness, tremors, or other untoward reactions occur.
5. Instruct client to store drug at room temperature away from light, excessive heat, and moisture (long-acting drug form).

GENERIC NAME Pseudoephedrine sulfate

TRADE NAME Afrinol (OTC)

CLASSIFICATION Systemic decongestant, sympathomimetic

See pseudoephedrine hydrochloride for Indications for use, Contraindications, Warnings and precautions, Untoward reactions, Parameters of use, and Drug interactions.

Source Naturally occurring alkaloid of the plant *Ephedra*.

Action Similar to pseudoephedrine hydrochloride.

Administration Adults and children over 12 years: 1 tablet po q12h.

Available Drug Forms Long-acting drug form with an easily dissolved outer surface and a center that releases drug several hours after ingestion.

Nursing Management Instruct client not to chew tablets. (See pseudoephedrine hydrochloride.)

GENERIC NAME Phenylephrine hydrochloride

CLASSIFICATION Systemic decongestant, sympathomimetic (OTC) (RX)

See pseudoephedrine hydrochloride for Indications for use, Contraindications, Untoward reactions, Parameters of use, Drug interactions, and Nursing management.

Action Often marketed as a locally applied decongestant solution (Neo-Synephrine). May induce more intense pressor effect than pseudoephedrine. May increase intraocular pressure.

Warnings and Precautions Use with extreme caution in clients with hypertension, ischemic heart disease, or glaucoma.

Administration 15 mg po every 8 to 12 hours.

Available Drug Forms Found in several combination decongestant preparations, such as Broncon C.R., Dimetapp, Leder-BP, Neo-Synephrine, and Ru-Tuss.

GENERIC NAME Phenylephrine tannate (RX)

CLASSIFICATION Systemic decongestant, sympathomimetic

See pseudoephedrine hydrochloride for Indications for use, Contraindications, Untoward reactions, Parameters of use, Drug interactions, and Nursing management.

Action May induce more intense pressor effect than pseudoephedrine. May increase intraocular pressure.

Warnings and Precautions Use with extreme caution in clients with hypertension, ischemic heart disease, or glaucoma.

Administration 25 mg po q12h.

Available Drug Forms Found in several combination decongestant preparations.

GENERIC NAME Phenylpropanolamine hydrochloride (OTC)

TRADE NAMES Norephedrine, Propadrine, Propagest

CLASSIFICATION Systemic decongestant, sympathomimetic

See pseudoephedrine hydrochloride for Indications for use, Contraindications, Warnings and precautions, Untoward reactions, Parameters of use, Drug interactions, and Nursing management.

Action Primary amine similar to ephedrine, but less toxic and induces less CNS stimulation. Stable when administered orally. Frequently used for young children.

Untoward Reactions Prolonged or excessive use may result in hypertension, tachycardia, palpitations, nervousness, or insomnia, particularly in the elderly.

Administration Adults and children under 12 years: 25 mg po q4h; Maximum dosage: 150 mg/day; Children: Ages 6 to 12 years: 12.5 mg po q4h; Maximum dosage: 75 mg/day; Ages 2 to 5 years: 6.25 mg (2.5 ml) po q4h; Maximum dosage: 37.5 mg/day.

Available Drug Forms Scored tablets containing 25 mg; flavored syrup containing 12.5 mg/5 ml. Also found in several combination decongestant preparations, such as Comtrex, Congespirin, Coricidin D, CoTylenol, Ornade, and Triaminic.

DECONGESTANTS CONTAINING PSEUDOEPHEDRINE

TRADE NAMES Anamine; Ryna (OTC)

CLASSIFICATION Systemic decongestant

See pseudoephedrine hydrochloride for Untoward reactions.

Action Preparation with decongestant properties of pseudoephedrine and antihistaminic effects of chlorpheniramine. It has little sedative effect.

Indications for Use Upper respiratory tract congestion, perennial allergic rhinitis, acute rhinitis, rhinosinusitis, eustachian tube congestion.

Contraindications Hypersensitivity to any ingredient, severe hypertension, coronary artery disease, pregnancy, lactation, clients receiving MAO inhibitors.

Warnings and Precautions Use with caution in clients with hypertension, cardiovascular disease, glaucoma, prostatic hypertrophy, diabetes, or hyperthyroidism. Additive effects may occur with alcohol or CNS depressants.

Drug Interactions MAO inhibitors and beta-adrenergic blockers increase the effects of pseudoephedrine.

Administration Adults: 10 ml po every 4 to 6 hours; Children: Ages 6 to 12 years: 5 ml po every 4 to 6 hours; Ages 1 to 6 years: 2.5 to 5.0 ml po q6h; Infants: 1.25 to 2.5 ml po q6h.

Available Drug Forms Flavored syrup. Generic contents in 5 ml: pseudoephedrine hydrochloride: 30 mg; chlorpheniramine maleate: 2 mg.

Nursing Management Caution client against engaging in hazardous activities. (See pseudoephedrine hydrochloride.)

TRADE NAME Anamine T.D. (RX)

CLASSIFICATION Systemic decongestant

See pseudoephedrine hydrochloride for Untoward reactions. See pseudoephedrine hydrochloride and Anamine for Nursing management. See Anamine for Indications for use, Contraindications, and Drug interactions.

Action Prolonged-release drug form that hampers the release of antihistamine.

Warnings and Precautions Not recommended for children under 12 years. (See Anamine.)

Administration Adults and children over 12 years: 1 capsule po every 8 to 12 hours.

Available Drug Forms Generic contents in each capsule: pseudoephedrine hydrochloride: 120 mg; chlorpheniramine maleate: 8 mg.

TRADE NAME Brexin L.A. (RX)

CLASSIFICATION Systemic decongestant

See pseudoephedrine hydrochloride for Untoward reactions.

Indications for Use Symptomatic relief of the common cold, allergic rhinitis, and sinusitis.

Contraindications Hypersensitivity to any ingredient, diabetes, narrow-angle glaucoma, urinary retention, peptic ulcer, acute asthma.

Warnings and Precautions Use with caution in the elderly (over 60 years).

Administration Adults and children over 12 years: 1 capsule po q12h.

Available Drug Forms Generic contents in each red and clear colored capsule: pseudoephedrine hydrochloride: 120 mg; chlorpheniramine maleate: 8 mg.

Nursing Management Store in airtight containers between 59 and 86 F.

TRADE NAME Bromfed (RX)

CLASSIFICATION Systemic decongestant

See pseudoephedrine hydrochloride for Untoward reactions. See Brexin L.A. for Contraindications and Warnings and precautions.

Action Decongestant and alkylamine-type antihistamine. Similar to Brexin L.A.

Indications for Use Symptomatic relief of the common cold, allergic rhinitis, and sinusitis.

Administration Adults and children over 12 years: 1 capsule po q12h.

Available Drug Forms Generic contents in each capsule: pseudoephedrine hydrochloride: 120 mg; brompheniramine maleate: 12 mg.

TRADE NAME Bromfed-PD (RX)

CLASSIFICATION Systemic decongestant

See pseudoephedrine hydrochloride for Untoward reactions. See Brexin L.A. for Contraindications and Warnings and precautions.

Action Pediatric drug form with half the contents of Bromfed for adults.

Indications for Use Symptomatic relief of the common cold, allergic rhinitis, and sinusitis.

Administration Adults and children over 6 years: 1 capsule po q12h.

Available Drug Forms Generic contents in each capsule: pseudoephedrine hydrochloride: 60 mg; brompheniramine maleate: 6 mg.

TRADE NAME Deconamine Tablets (RX)

CLASSIFICATION Systemic decongestant

See pseudoephedrine hydrochloride for Untoward reactions.

Action Preparation with decongestant properties of pseudoephedrine and antihistaminic effects of chlorpheniramine.

Indications for Use Upper respiratory tract congestion associated with the common cold, allergic rhinitis, and sinusitis; eustachian tube congestion.

Warnings and Precautions Not recommended for children under 12 years.

Administration Adults and children over 12 years: 1 tablet po tid or qid.

Available Drug Forms Generic contents in each white scored tablet: *d*-pseudoephedrine hydrochloride: 60 mg; chlorpheniramine maleate: 4 mg.

TRADE NAME Deconamine-SR (RX)

CLASSIFICATION Systemic decongestant

See pseudoephedrine hydrochloride for Untoward reactions.

Action Similar to Deconamine Tablets.

Indications for Use Upper respiratory tract congestion associated with the common cold, allergic rhinitis, and sinusitis; eustachian tube congestion.

Administration Adults and children over 12 years: 1 capsule po every 12 hours.

Available Drug Forms Generic contents in each blue and yellow sustained-release capsule: *d*-pseudoephedrine hydrochloride: 120 mg; chlorpheniramine maleate: 8 mg.

TRADE NAME Deconamine Syrup (RX)

CLASSIFICATION Systemic decongestant

See pseudoephedrine hydrochloride for Untoward reactions.

Action Similar to Deconamine Tablets.

Indications for Use Upper respiratory tract congestion associated with the common cold, allergic rhinitis, and sinusitis; eustachian tube congestion.

Administration Adults and children over 12 years: 5 to 10 ml po tid or qid; Children: Ages 6 to 12 years: 2.5 to 5.0 ml po tid or qid; Maximum dosage: 20 ml/day; Ages 2 to 6 years: 2.5 ml po tid or qid; Maximum dosage: 10 ml/day.

Available Drug Forms Clear liquid in grape-flavored aromatic vehicle. Generic contents in 5 ml: *d*-pseudoephedrine hydrochloride: 30 mg; chlorpheniramine maleate: 2 mg.

TRADE NAME Deconamine Elixir (RX)

CLASSIFICATION Systemic decongestant

See pseudoephedrine hydrochloride for Untoward reactions.

Action Similar to Deconamine Tablets.

Indications for Use Upper respiratory tract congestion associated with the common cold, allergic rhinitis, and sinusitis; eustachian tube congestion.

Administration Adults and children over 12 years: 5 to 10 ml po tid or qid; Children: Ages 6 to 12 years: 2.5 to 5.0 ml po tid or qid; Maximum dosage: 20 ml/day; Ages 2 to 6 years: 2.5 ml po tid or qid; Maximum dosage: 10 ml/day.

Available Drug Forms Blue-colored liquid in pleasant tasting aromatic vehicle. Generic contents in 5 ml: *d*-pseudoephedrine hydrochloride: 30 mg; chlorpheniramine maleate: 2 mg; alcohol: 15%.

TRADE NAME Historal Capsules (RX)

CLASSIFICATION Systemic decongestant

See pseudoephedrine hydrochloride for Untoward reactions.

Action Combination preparation with decongestant, antihistaminic, and atropine-like effects (methscopolamine).

Indications for Use Upper respiratory tract congestion associated with the common cold, allergic rhinitis, and sinusitis; eustachian tube congestion.

Administration Adults and children over 12 years: 1 capsule po q12h.

Available Drug Forms Generic contents in each sustained-release capsule: pseudoephedrine hydrochloride: 60 mg; chlorpheniramine maleate: 12 mg; methscopolamine nitrate: 2.5 mg.

TRADE NAME Historal Liquid (RX)

CLASSIFICATION Systemic decongestant

See pseudoephedrine hydrochloride for Untoward reactions.

Action Similar to Historal Capsules.

Indications for Use Upper respiratory tract congestion associated with the common cold, allergic rhinitis, and sinusitis; eustachian tube congestion.

Administration Adults and children over 12 years: 5 to 10 ml po every 4 to 6 hours; Children: Ages 6 to 12 years: 5 ml po every 4 to 6 hours; Ages 3 to 6 years: 2.5 ml po every 4 to 6 hours.

Available Drug Forms Generic contents in 5 ml: pseudoephedrine hydrochloride: 30 mg; chlorpheniramine maleate: 2 mg; methscopolamine nitrate: 0.5 mg.

TRADE NAME Historal Pediatric Oral Drops (RX)

CLASSIFICATION Systemic decongestant

See pseudoephedrine hydrochloride for Untoward reactions and Nursing management.

Indications for Use Used prophylactically to promote drainage through the eustachian tube.

Administration Ages 10 to 18 months: 1.0 ml po qid; Ages 7 to 9 months: 0.75 ml po qid; Ages 4 to 6 months: 0.5 ml po qid; Ages 1 to 3 months: 0.25 ml po qid.

Available Drug Forms Bottles containing 30 ml with a calibrated dropper; 1 ml contains 30 mg of pseudoephedrine.

TRADE NAMES Novafed A Capsules; ND Clear T.D

CLASSIFICATION Systemic decongestant (RX)

See pseudoephedrine hydrochloride for Untoward reactions.

Action Controlled-release drug form containing pellets. About half of drug is released soon after ingestion.

Indications for Use Symptomatic relief of upper respiratory tract congestion associated with the common cold, allergic rhinitis, and sinusitis; eustachian tube congestion.

Administration Adults and children over 12 years: 1 capsule po q12h.

Available Drug Forms Novafed A is a red and orange, hard gelatin capsule. ND Clear T.D. is a clear capsule. Generic contents in each capsule: pseudoephedrine hydrochloride: 120 mg; chlorpheniramine maleate: 8 mg.

TRADE NAME Novafed A Liquid (OTC)

CLASSIFICATION Systemic decongestant

See pseudoephedrine hydrochloride for Untoward reactions.

Indications for Use Symptomatic relief of upper respiratory tract congestion associated with the common cold, allergic rhinitis, and sinusitis; eustachian tube congestion.

Administration Adults and children over 12 years: 10 ml po qid; Children: Ages 6 to 12 years: 5 ml po qid; Under 6 years: 2.5 ml po qid; do not exceed 4 doses in 24 hours.

Available Drug Forms Bottles containing 120 ml of green liquid. Generic contents in 5 ml: pseudoephedrine hydrochloride: 30 mg; chlorpheniramine maleate: 2 mg; alcohol: 5%.

TRADE NAME Pseudo-Bid (RX)

CLASSIFICATION Systemic decongestant

See pseudoephedrine hydrochloride for Untoward reactions.

Action Prolonged-release drug form. Guaifenesin liquefies viscid secretions and promotes drainage of the bronchials.

Indications for Use Symptomatic relief of bronchial and upper respiratory tract congestion.

Warnings and Precautions Not recommended for children under 12 years.

Administration Adults and children over 12 years: 1 capsule po q12h.

Available Drug Forms Generic contents in each clear capsule: pseudoephedrine hydrochloride: 120 mg; guaifenesin: 250 mg.

TRADE NAME Pseudo-Hist Capsules (RX)

CLASSIFICATION Systemic decongestant

See pseudoephedrine hydrochloride for Untoward reactions.

Action Timed-release drug form similar to Anamine.

Indications for Use Systomatic relief of upper respiratory tract and bronchial congestion associated with the common cold, allergic rhinitis, influenza, and sinusitis.

Administration Adults and children over 12 years: 1 capsule po q12h.

Available Drug Forms Generic contents in each capsule: pseudoephedrine hydrochloride: 65 mg; chlorpheniramine maleate: 10 mg.

TRADE NAME Pseudo-Hist Liquid (RX)

CLASSIFICATION Systemic decongestant

See pseudoephedrine hydrochloride for Untoward reactions.

Indications for Use Symptomatic relief of upper respiratory tract and bronchial congestion associated with the common cold, allergic rhinitis, influenza, and sinusitis.

Administration Children: Ages 6 to 12 years: 5 ml po every 3 to 4 hours; 40 to 50 lb: 2.5 ml po every 3 to 4 hours; 20 to 30 lb: 1.25 to 2.5 ml po every 3 to 4 hours; 15 to 20 lb: 0.25 to 1.25 ml po every 3 to 4 hours; do not exceed 4 doses in 24 hours.

Available Drug Forms Generic contents in 5 ml; pseudoephedrine hydrochloride: 15 mg; chlorpheniramine maleate: 2 mg. Also available with expectorant hydrocodone (2.5 mg) as Pseudo-Hist Expectorant.

TRADE NAMES Rondec Tablets; Rondec Syrup

CLASSIFICATION Systemic decongestant (RX)

See pseudoephedrine hydrochloride for Untoward reactions.

Action Contains a decongestant and an antihistamine with mild anticholinergic and sedative effects (carbinoxamine).

Indications for Use Symptomatic relief of allergic and vasomotor rhinitis.

Administration Adults and children over 6 years: 1 tablet or 5 ml po qid; Children: Ages 18 months to 6 years: 2.5 ml po qid.

Available Drug Forms Film-coated orange tablets and berry-flavored syrup. Generic contents in each tablet or 5 ml: pseudoephedrine hydrochloride: 60 mg; carbinoxamine maleate: 4 mg.

Nursing Management Protect drug from excessive heat.

TRADE NAME Rondec Drops (RX)

CLASSIFICATION Systemic decongestant

See pseudoephedrine hydrochloride for Untoward reactions.

Action Contains a decongestant and an antihistamine with mild anticholinergic and sedative effects (carbinoxamine).

Indications for Use Symptomatic relief of allergic and vasomotor rhinitis.

Administration Children: Ages 9 to 18 months: 1.0 ml po qid; Ages 6 to 9 months: 0.75 ml po qid; Ages 3 to 6 months: 0.5 ml po qid; Ages 1 to 3 months: 0.25 ml po qid.

Available Drug Forms Bottles containing 30 ml of berry-flavored syrup and calibrated dropper. One dropperful is equal to 1 ml. Generic contents in 1 ml: pseudoephedrine hydrochloride: 25 mg; carbinoxamine maleate: 2 mg.

Nursing Management Protect drug from excessive heat.

TRADE NAME Rondec-TR tablets (RX)

CLASSIFICATION Systemic decongestant

See pseudoephedrine hydrochloride for Untoward reactions.

Indications for Use Symptomatic relief of allergic and vasomotor rhinitis.

Administration Adults and children over 12 years: 1 tablet po bid.

Available Drug Forms Film-coated blue tablets; slow-release drug form. Generic contents in each tablet: pseudoephedrine hydrochloride: 120 mg; carbinoxamine maleate: 8 mg.

Nursing Management Protect drug from excessive heat.

TRADE NAME Ryna-C Liquid (Ci)

CLASSIFICATION Systemic decongestant

See pseudoephedrine hydrochloride for Untoward reactions.

Indications for Use Symptomatic relief of upper respiratory tract congestion and cough associated with the common cold and allergic rhinitis.

Warnings and Precautions Codeine may be habit forming.

Untoward Reactions May cause drowsiness.

Administration Adults and children over 12 years: 10 ml po q6h; Children: Ages 6 to 12 years: 5 ml po q6h; Ages 2 to 6 years: 2.5 ml po q6h; do not exceed 4 doses in 24 hours.

Available Drug Forms Cinnamon-flavored liquid. Generic contents in 5 ml: pseudoephedrine hydrochloride: 30 mg; chlorpheniramine maleate; 2 mg; codeine phosphate: 10 mg.

MULTIPLE INGREDIENT SYSTEMIC DECONGESTANTS

TRADE NAMES Leder-BP Sequels; Broncon C.R.; Dimetapp Extentabs (OTC) (RX)

CLASSIFICATION Multiple ingredient systemic decongestant

Action Contains an antihistamine (brompheniramine). Considered to be possibly effective for congestion.

Indications for Use Symptomatic relief of upper respiratory tract congestion associated with infections and allergies.

Administration Adults and children over 12 years: 1 tablet po q8h or bid.

Available Drug Forms Generic contents in each sustained-release tablet: phenylephrine hydrochloride: 15 mg; phenylpropanolamine hydrochloride: 15 mg; brompheniramine maleate: 12mg.

TRADE NAME Rynatan Tablets (RX)

CLASSIFICATION Multiple ingredient systemic decongestant

Action Contains two antihistamines and a decongestant (phenylephrine).

Indications for Use Particularly effective for allergic rhinitis.

Administration Adults and children over 12 years: 1 to 2 tablets po q12h.

Available Drug Forms Generic contents in each capsule-shaped tablet: phenylephrine tannate: 25 mg; chlorpheniramine tannate: 8 mg; pyrilamine tannate: 25 mg.

Nursing Management Store drug at room temperature.

TRADE NAME Rynatan Pediatric Suspension (RX)

CLASSIFICATION Multiple ingredient systemic decongestant

Action Contains two antihistamines and a decongestant (phenylephrine).

Indications for Use Particularly effective for allergic rhinitis.

Administration Children: Over 6 years: 5 to 10 ml po q12h; Ages 2 to 6 years: 2.5 to 5.0 ml po q12h.

Available Drug Forms Strawberry-currant flavored suspension. Generic contents in 5 ml: phenylephrine tannate: 5 mg; chlorpheniramine tannate: 2 mg; pyrilamine tannate: 12.5 mg.

Nursing Management

1. Shake suspension well before using.
2. Store drug at room temperature.

TRADE NAME Dimetapp Elixir (RX)

CLASSIFICATION Multiple ingredient systemic decongestant

Action Contains an antihistamine (brompheniramine). Considered probably effective.

Indications for Use Upper respiratory tract congestion, eustachian tube congestion.

Administration Adults and children over 12 years: 10 ml po tid or qid; Children: Ages 4 to 12 years: 5 ml po tid or qid; Ages 2 to 4 years: 3.75 ml po tid or qid; Ages 7 months to 2 years: 2.5 ml po tid or qid; Ages 1 to 6 months: 1.25 ml po tid or qid.

Available Drug Forms Grape-flavored elixir. Generic contents in 5 ml: phenylephrine hydrochloride: 5 mg; phenylpropanolamine hydrochloride: 5 mg; brompheniramine maleate: 5 mg; alcohol: 2.3%.

TRADE NAME Ru-Tuss Plain (OTC)

CLASSIFICATION Multiple ingredient systemic decongestant

Action Contains two decongestants and two antihistamines.

Indications for Use Temporary relief of congestion and symptoms associated with allergies and the common cold.

Untoward Reactions May cause drowsiness, blurred vision, viscous respiratory secretions, dysuria, and CNS disturbances.

Administration Adults and children over 12 years: 10 ml po every 4 to 6 hours; Children: Ages 6 to 12 years: 5 ml po every 4 to 6 hours; Ages 2 to 6 years: 2.5 to 5.0 ml every 4 to 6 hours.

Available Drug Forms Generic contents in 5 ml: phenylephrine hydrochloride: 6 mg; phenylpropanolamine hydrochloride: 4 mg; pheniramine maleate: 4 mg; pyrilamine maleate: 4 mg; alcohol: 5%.

TRADE NAME T-Dry (RX)

CLASSIFICATION Multiple ingredient systemic decongestant

Action Contains two decongestants and an antihistamine (chlorpheniramine). Duration of action is 6 to 10 hours.

Indications for Use Symptomatic relief of allergies, sinusitis, and the common cold.

Administration Adults: 1 capsule po bid.

Available Drug Forms Generic contents in each timed-release capsule: phenylpropanolamine hydrochloride: 50 mg; phenylephrine hydrochloride: 25 mg; chlorpheniramine maleate: 12 mg.

TRADE NAME Congespirin Chewable (OTC)

CLASSIFICATION Multiple ingredient systemic decongestant

Indications for Use Temporary relief of nasal congestion, fever, and aches and pains associated with the common cold.

Contraindications Hypertension, diabetes, hyperthyroidism, heart disease.

Administration Children: Ages 12 years and over: 8 tablets po q4h; Age 11 years: 6 tablets po q4h; Ages 9 to 10 years: 5 tablets po q4h; Ages 6 to 8 years: 4 tablets po q4h; Ages 4 to 5 years: 3 tablets po q4h; Ages 2 to 3 years: 2 tablets po q4h.

Available Drug Forms Generic contents in each chewable tablet: aspirin: 81 mg; phenylephrine hydrochloride: 1.25 mg.

Nursing Management

1. Give with a full glass of water.
2. If fever or other symptoms persist for more than 10 days, instruct client to notify physician.

TRADE NAME Congespirin Liquid (OTC)

CLASSIFICATION Multiple ingredient systemic decongestant

Indications for Use Temporary relief of nasal congestion, fever, and aches and pains associated with the common cold.

Administration Children: Ages 6 to 12 years: 10 ml po every 3 to 4 hours; Ages 3 to 5 years: 5 ml po every 3 to 4 hours; do not exceed 4 doses in 24 hours.

Available Drug Forms Generic contents in 5 ml: acetaminophen: 130 mg; phenylpropanolamine hydrochloride: 6.25 mg; alcohol: 10%.

TRADE NAME Headway (OTC)

CLASSIFICATION Multiple ingredient systemic decongestant

Action Acetaminophen is an analgesic and antipyretic. Chlorpheniramine is an antihistamine.

Indications for Use Temporary relief of nasal congestion, rhinitis, sneezing, itching nose, watery eyes, and aches and pains associated with allergies and the common cold.

Warnings and Precautions May cause drowsiness. Alcoholic beverages should be avoided.

Administration Adults and children over 12 years: 2 tablets or capsules po q4h. Children: Ages 6 to 12 years: 1 tablet or capsule po q4h; do not exceed 4 doses in 24 hours.

Available Drug Forms Generic contents in each tablet or capsule: acetaminophen: 325 mg; phenylpropanolamine hydrochloride: 18.75 mg; chlorpheniramine maleate: 2 mg.

TRADE NAME 4-Way Tablets (OTC)

CLASSIFICATION Multiple ingredient systemic decongestant

Action Similar to Headway.

Indications for Use Temporary relief of nasal congestion, rhinitis, sneezing, itching nose, watery eyes, and aches and pains associated with allergies and the common cold.

Warnings and Precautions May cause drowsiness.

Administration Adults: 2 tablets po q4h; do not exceed 6 tablets daily. Children: Ages 6 to 12 years: 1 tablet po q4h; do not exceed 4 tablets daily.

Available Drug Forms Generic contents in each pink and white tablet: aspirin: 324 mg; phenylpropanolamine hydrochloride: 12.5 mg; chlorpheniramine maleate: 2 mg.

TRADE NAME Histabid Duracap (RX)

CLASSIFICATION Multiple ingredient systemic decongestant

Indications for Use Symptomatic relief of allergies, sinusitis, and the common cold.

Administration Adults and children over 6 years: 1 capsule po q12h.

Available Drug Forms Generic contents in each timed-release capsule: phenylpropanolamine hydrochloride: 75 mg; chlorpheniramine maleate: 8 mg.

TRADE NAME Sinulin (OTC)

CLASSIFICATION Multiple ingredient systemic decongestant

Indications for Use Sinus congestion and headache.

Contraindications Hypertension, diabetes, heart or thyroid disease, glaucoma, elderly clients.

Warnings and Precautions May cause drowsiness. Drug should be discontinued if tachycardia, dizziness, or blurred vision occur.

Administration Adults: 1 tablet po q4h; do not exceed 4 doses in 24 hours.

Available Drug Forms Generic contents in each peach tablet: phenylpropanolamine hydrochloride: 37.5 mg; chlorpheniramine maleate: 2 mg; acetaminophen: 325 mg; salicylamide: 250 mg; homatropine methylbromide: 0.75 mg.

Nursing Management Caution client against engaging in hazardous activities.

TRADE NAME Sine-Aid (OTC)

CLASSIFICATION Multiple ingredient systemic decongestant

Action Contains an analgesic and a decongestant. Does not contain an antihistamine.

Indications for Use Sinus headache, sinusitis.

Administration Adults: 2 tablets po q4h; do not exceed 6 doses in 24 hours.

Available Drug Forms Generic contents in each tablet: acetaminophen: 325 mg; phenylpropanolamine hydrochloride: 25 mg.

Nursing Management Instruct client to consult physician if pain persists for more than 3 days.

TRADE NAME Triaminic Tablets (RX)

CLASSIFICATION Multiple ingredient systemic decongestant

Action Long-acting drug form containing a decongestant and two antihistamines.

Indications for Use Nasal congestion and postnasal drip associated with colds, allergies, sinusitis, rhinitis, and allergic reactions.

Untoward Reactions May cause drowsiness, dizziness, restlessness, and epigastric distress.

Administration Adults and children over 12 years: 1 tablet po every 6 to 8 hours when awake; do not exceed 3 doses in 24 hours.

Available Drug Forms Generic contents in each yellow film-coated tablet: phenylpropanolamine hydrochloride: 50 mg; pheniramine maleate: 25 mg; pyrilamine maleate: 25 mg.

Nursing Management Instruct client to avoid chewing tablet.

TRADE NAME Triaminic Juvelets (RX)

CLASSIFICATION Multiple ingredient systemic decongestant

Action Long-acting drug form similar to Triaminic Tablets, but contains half the ingredients.

Indications for Use Nasal congestion and postnasal drip associated with colds, allergies, sinusitis, rhinitis, and allergic reactions.

Untoward Reactions May cause drowsiness, dizziness, restlessness, and epigastric distress.

Administration Adults and children over 12 years: 2 tablets po every 6 to 8 hours when awake; Children: Ages 6 to 12 years: 1 tablet po every 6 to 8 hours when awake; do not exceed 3 doses in 24 hours.

Available Drug Forms Generic contents in each pink film-coated tablet: phenylpropanolamine hydrochloride: 25 mg; pheniramine maleate: 12.5 mg; pyrilamine maleate: 12.5 mg.

Nursing Management Instruct client to avoid chewing tablet.

TRADE NAME Triaminic-12 Tablets (OTC)

CLASSIFICATION Multiple ingredient systemic decongestant

Action Long-acting drug form containing a decongestant and an antihistamine.

Indications for Use Nasal congestion and postnasal drip associated with colds, allergies, sinusitis, rhinitis, and allergic reactions.

Warnings and Precautions May cause excitability in children.

Untoward Reactions May cause drowsiness, dizziness, restlessness, and epigastric distress.

Administration Adults and children over 12 years: 1 tablet po every 12 hours.

Available Drug Forms Generic contents in each pink film-coated tablet: phenylpropanolamine hydrochloride: 75 mg; chlorpheniramine maleate: 12 mg.

Nursing Management Instruct client to avoid chewing tablet.

TRADE NAME Triaminic Infant Drops (RX)

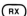

CLASSIFICATION Multiple ingredient systemic decongestant

Action Contains a decongestant and two antihistamines.

Indications for Use Nasal congestion and postnasal drip associated with colds, allergies, sinusitis, rhinitis, and allergic reactions.

Untoward Reactions May cause drowsiness.

Administration Infants: 1 gtt/2 lb po qid.

Available Drug Forms Squeeze bottle containing 15 ml with 24 gtt/ml. Generic contents in 1 ml: phenylpropanolamine hydrochloride: 20 mg; pheniramine maleate: 10 mg; pyrilamine maleate: 10 mg.

Nursing Management Store drug at room temperature.

TRADE NAME Triaminic Syrup (OTC)

CLASSIFICATION Multiple ingredient systemic decongestant

Action Contains a decongestant and an antihistamine.

Indications for Use Nasal congestion and postnasal drip associated with colds, allergies, sinusitis, rhinitis, and allergic reactions.

Warnings and Precautions May cause excitability in children.

Untoward Reactions May cause drowsiness, dizziness, restlessness, and epigastric distress.

Administration Adults: 10 ml po q4h; Children: Ages 6 to 12 years: 5 ml po q4h; Ages 2 to 6 years: 2.5 ml po q4h; Ages 3 months to 2 years: 4 to 5 gtt/kg po q4h.

Available Drug Forms Generic contents in 5 ml: phenylpropanolamine hydrochloride: 12.5 mg; chlorpheniramine maleate: 2 mg.

TOPICAL DECONGESTANTS

GENERIC NAME Phenylephedrine hydrochloride

TRADE NAMES Alconefrin, Coricidin Nasal Mist, Isophrin, Neo-Synephrine Nose Drops, Rhinall, Sinarest Nasal Spray, Synasal (OTC)

CLASSIFICATION Topical decongestant

Action Sympathomimetic with potent alpha-adrenergic and weak beta-adrenergic activity. Decongestant action has a longer duration than epinephrine. Little or no CNS stimulation occurs. Some systemic absorption can occur and cause untoward reactions.

Indications for Use Rhinitis.

Untoward Reactions Prolonged use may cause rebound congestion.

Administration Adults: 2 to 3 gtt 1.0% or 0.5% solution into each nostril every 3 to 4 hours, as needed; Adults and children: 2 to 3 gtt 0.25% solution into each nostril every 3 to 4 hours, as needed; Infants and young children: 2 to 3 gtt 0.125% solution into each nostril every 3 to 4 hours, as needed.

Available Drug Forms Solution 0.125, 0.25, 0.5, or 1.0%.

Nursing Management

1. Do not use if solution develops a precipitate or turns dark brown.
2. Protect drug from light and excessive heat.
3. Keep bottle tightly closed.
4. Instruct client in proper application.
5. Inform client to avoid excessive use and to notify physician if nasal congestion persists.

GENERIC NAME Cyclopentamine hydrochloride

TRADE NAME Clopane (OTC)

CLASSIFICATION Topical decongestant

Action Decongestant effect of cyclopentamine, an aliphatic adrenergic amine, is similar to ephedrine, but it induces little or no CNS stimulation. Absorbed drug may cause hypertension, dizziness, nervousness, and nausea.

Indications for Use Rhinitis.

Administration 1 to 2 gtt 0.5% to 1.0% solution every 3 to 4 hours.

Available Drug Forms Nasal solution with dropper.

GENERIC NAME Methylhexaneamine carbonate

TRADE NAME Forthane (OTC)

CLASSIFICATION Topical decongestant

Action Methylhexaneamine carbonate, a volatile aliphatic amine, is a more potent local vasoconstrictor than ephedrine. It has a short duration of action and an ammonialike odor.

Indications for Use Allergic rhinitis.

Administration 1 to 2 inhalations in each nostril, as needed; should not be used more often than every 30 minutes.

Available Drug Forms Nasal inhaler.

GENERIC NAME Naphazoline hydrochloride

TRADE NAME Privine (OTC)

CLASSIFICATION Topical decongestant

Action Potent alpha-adrenergic agent.

Indications for Use Rhinitis.

Contraindications Glaucoma.

Untoward Reactions May cause burning, stinging, or sneezing. May slow heart rate.

Administration Adults and children over 6 years: 2 gtt 0.05% solution every 3 to 4 hours, as needed.

Available Drug Forms Nasal solution with dropper (0.05%) and nasal spray (0.05%).

Nursing Management Instruct client to seek medical advice if no relief occurs after 3 days.

GENERIC NAME Oxymethazoline hydrochloride

TRADE NAMES Afrin, Duration (OTC)

CLASSIFICATION Topical decongestant

Action Oxymethazoline, an imidazoline derivative, is a long-acting vasoconstrictor.

Indications for use Rhinitis.

Administration Adults and children over 6 years: 2 to 3 gtt 0.05% solution bid; Children: Ages 2 to 5 years: 2 to 3 gtt 0.025% solution.

Available Drug Forms Nose drops, nasal spray, and menthol nasal spray 0.05% solution; pediatric nose drops 0.025% solution.

GENERIC NAME Prophylhexedrine (OTC)

TRADE NAME Benzedrex

CLASSIFICATION Topical decongestant

Action Propylhexedrine, a volatile aliphatic compound, is a less effective vasoconstrictor than ephedrine, but does not induce CNS stimulation. It has a short duration of action and a fishy odor.

Indications for Use Rhinitis.

Administration 1 to 2 inhalations in each nostril, as needed.

Available Drug Forms Nasal inhaler.

Nursing Management Store in tightly sealed containers, since drug absorbs carbon dioxide when exposed to the air.

GENERIC NAME Tetrahydrozoline Hydrochloride

TRADE NAME Tyzine (OTC)

CLASSIFICATION Topical decongestant

Action Tetrahydrozoline, an aliphatic adrenergic amine, has a greater vasoconstrictor effect than a similar solution of ephedrine. It also has a longer duration of action than ephedrine.

Indications for Use Rhinitis.

Administration 2 gtt 0.05% to 2% solution, as needed.

Available Drug Forms Nasal solution with dropper.

GENERIC NAME Tuaminoheptane sulfate

TRADE NAME Tuamine (OTC)

CLASSIFICATION Topical decongestant

Action Tuaminoheptane, an aliphatic adrenergic amine, has a greater vasoconstrictor effect than a similar solution of ephedrine. It also has a longer duration of action than ephedrine.

Indications for Use Rhinitis.

Administration 2 gtt 0.05% to 2% solution every 4 to 6 hours, as needed.

Available Drug Forms Nasal solution with dropper.

GENERIC NAME Xylometazoline hydrochloride

TRADE NAMES Otrivin, Sinex-LA, 4-Way LA Spray

CLASSIFICATION Topical decongestant (OTC)

Action Xylometazoline, an imidazoline derivative, is an effective nasal vasoconstrictor with a relatively long duration of action.

Indications for Use Rhinitis.

Administration Adults and children over 2 years: 2 to 3 gtt 0.05% to 0.1% solution every 8 to 10 hours.

Available Drug Forms Adult nasal drops and spray 0.1% solution; pediatric nasal drops 0.05% solution.

Chapter 56

Mucolytics and Expectorants

THE FLUID SECRETED by the glands and cells of the bronchial tree is normally sufficiently watery to cleanse the lungs of bacteria and other foreign particles. However, when the atmosphere of the respiratory tract becomes dry, respiratory secretions become highly viscous and may form plugs that are difficult to expectorate. Clients with respiratory disorders may require assistance in preventing the formation of viscous respiratory secretions. Theoretically, *mucolytic agents* reduce the viscosity and *expectorants* increase the volume of respiratory secretions, thereby permitting easier expulsion of thick secretions. However, the clinical value of these agents is in doubt. Adequate maintenance of the client's general state of hydration seems to be of greater benefit.

CHARACTERISTICS OF MUCOLYTIC AGENTS

These agents reduce the viscosity of respiratory secretions by breaking down the constituent protein molecules into smaller and more soluble particles that can be expectorated or drained from the bronchial tree. Mucolytics are most commonly used for clients with pulmonary disease as the normal ciliary cleansing mechanisms are impaired in these clients. Clients with chronic pulmonary disease also tend to be dehydrated, which further increases the viscosity of respiratory secretions. Water is often administered via vaporizer or nebulizer to help liquefy the secretions. Unless the client is on restricted fluid intake, adequate quantities of drinking fluids aid in liquefying the respiratory secretions so that they can be more easily expectorated.

The *nursing management* of clients receiving mucolytic agents includes the following factors:

1. Suctioning equipment should be kept at the client's bedside in the event that the client is unable to expectorate the increased secretions.
2. Postural drainage may be ordered to assist the client in expectoration.
3. Clients, particularly asthmatic clients, should be observed for the development of bronchospasm. If this condition develops, therapy should be discontinued and appropriate treatment instituted.
4. If symptoms are relieved and breath sounds improve, the client may be instructed in self-administration of the drug. Teaching should include possible side effects and procedure for discontinuing the drug when symptoms have abated.
5. Clients with chronic obstructive pulmonary disease may also benefit from breathing exercises, increased fluid intake (unless contraindicated), and special exercise programs.

CHARACTERISTICS OF EXPECTORANTS

These agents stimulate the production of respiratory secretions, thus reducing their viscosity and making expulsion easier. Some expectorants are thought to act by causing gastric irritation, which in turn stimulates bronchial glands innervated by the vagus nerve and causes increased secretion. There is much debate about the effectiveness of expectorants and many health professionals feel that these agents are no more effective than increased fluid intake and/or humidification. Therefore, a high fluid intake, unless contraindicated, and humidification of the environment will aid in increasing the effectiveness of these agents.

With the exception of potassium iodide, most expectorants are quite safe when taken as prescribed and rarely cause adverse effects. They are commonly used in combination with antitussive agents, since the increased lubrication of the respiratory tract may decrease the irritation caused by a dry, hacking cough.

TYPES OF COMBINATION PREPARATIONS

Expectorants are most commonly used in commercially prepared formulations in combination with one or more of the following:

- Analgesics—to ease fever and aches associated with colds and flu
- Anticholinergics—to combat rhinorrhea and congestion associated with colds
- Antihistamines—to combat congestion and to help relieve sneezing, itchy eyes, and other allergic reactions

- Bronchodilators—to ease bronchospasm associated with asthma and related conditions
- Decongestants—to relieve congestion by vasoconstriction.

The effectiveness of these ingredients in the strengths available in over-the-counter preparations is doubtful; moreover, some of the ingredients, such as antihistamines and decongestants, are contraindicated in certain disease states, such as hypertension. As over-the-counter cold preparations are very popular, clients should be carefully instructed in the side effects and contraindications of these commonly available preparations.

MUCOLYTICS

GENERIC NAME Acetylcysteine (RX)

TRADE NAMES Airbron, Mucomyst

CLASSIFICATION Mucolytic

Action Acetylcysteine is a derivative of L-cysteine, a naturally occurring amino acid. It decreases viscous pulmonary secretions. It is thought to act by breaking the disulfide bonds of mucoproteins in respiratory secretions.

Indications for Use Cystic fibrosis, bronchitis, chronic obstructive pulmonary disease and other respiratory disorders, as an adjunct in atelectasis.

Contraindications Hypersensitivity to acetylcysteine.

Warnings and Precautions Use with caution in the elderly and debilitated clients. Use with extreme caution in clients with a history of asthma or bronchoconstriction.

Untoward Reactions Nausea without vomiting often occurs as drug has a rotten-egg odor. Prolonged use may cause stomatitis. Bronchospasm and severe dyspnea may occur, particularly in clients with a history of asthma. Rhinorrhea frequently occurs. Hemoptysis has been reported.

Parameters of Use

Absorption Small amount absorbed by epithelium. Maximum effect occurs in 5 to 10 minutes.

Metabolism In the liver.

Drug Interactions No significant interactions.

Administration Nebulization: 3 to 5 ml 20% solution tid or qid or 6 to 10 ml 10% solution tid or qid.

Available Drug Forms Vials containing 10 or 30 ml of a 20% solution.

Nursing Management

Planning factors

1. Obtain history of pulmonary disorders, including asthma.
2. Obtain suction equipment and keep at bedside.
3. Store drug in tightly sealed containers in a refrigerator.

Administration factors

1. May be diluted with sterile water. Most effective when used as a 10 to 20% solution with a pH adjusted to between 7 and 9.
2. Equipment should not contain iron, copper, or rubber.
3. Label newly opened container with date and time. Use within 48 hours.

Evaluation factors

1. Monitor client during first few treatments and ensure that airway patency is maintained.
2. Observe clients with asthma for possible bronchospasm, which necessitates immediate discontinuation of drug.
3. Do not mix mucolytic agents with other drugs, unless specifically prescribed by physician and validated by pharmacist. (Known to be incompatible with tetracycline, erythromycin, and other antibiotics.)
4. Monitor vital signs before, during, and after the first few treatments.

Client teaching factors

1. Explain the purpose of the agent and the importance of expectorating liquefied secretions.
2. Instruct client in postural drainage, if indicated.

GENERIC NAME Tyloxapol (RX)

TRADE NAME Alevaire

CLASSIFICATION Mucolytic

Action Tyloxapol (alkyl phenol) has a local action on bronchial secretions. It lowers the surface tension of viscous pulmonary secretions. The drug is relatively stable and is nonirritating to the skin. Bronchodilators or vasoconstrictors may be added to the solution.

Indications for Use Cystic fibrosis, bronchitis, chronic obstructive pulmonary disease and other respiratory disorders, as an adjunct in atelectasis.

Contraindications None known.

Warnings and Precautions Use with caution in clients with a history of asthma or bronchospasm.

Untoward Reactions Seldom causes untoward reactions. May cause nausea. Prolonged use may cause a local skin irritation.

Drug Interactions No significant interactions.

Administration 10 to 20 ml 0.125% solution tid or qid or 500 ml over 12 to 24 hours via facial tent or other form of inhalation equipment.

Available Drug Forms Vials containing 5 ml.

Nursing Management (See acetylcysteine.)

1. Do not dilute.
2. When used as a vehicle, add bronchodilator before administering.
3. Discard unused solution after treatment.
4. Encourage client to deep breathe during treatment.

EXPECTORANTS

GENERIC NAME Guaifenesin (OTC) (RX)

TRADE NAMES Balminil, Colrex, Demo-Cined, Dilyn, Glycotuss, Glytuss, G-Tussin, Guaiatussin, Hytuss, Motussin, Resyl, Robitussin, Sedatuss, Tussanca

CLASSIFICATION Expectorant

Action Although it has been used for its sedative effects, guaifenesin (glyceryl guaiacolate) is the most frequently used expectorant. The exact mechanism of action is unknown, but guaifenesin is thought to increase the flow of respiratory secretions by stimulating a reflex action induced by gastric irritation. This drug is often used in combination with antihistamines, analgesics, and vasoconstrictors.

Indications for Use Combats productive and nonproductive coughs associated with the common cold, sinusitis, pharyngitis, and other respiratory disorders.

Contraindications None reported.

Warnings and Precautions Use with caution in clients with blood dyscrasias.

Untoward Reactions GI disturbances, including nausea and vomiting, have occurred, but rarely. Drowsiness has been reported, particularly with large dosages.

Drug Interactions May inhibit platelet function; therefore, can increase the risk of bleeding in clients on heparin therapy.

Laboratory Interactions May interfere with the determination of 5-hydroxyindoleacetic acid and vanilmandelic acid.

Administration Adults: 100 to 200 mg po every 3 to 4 hours; Children: 25 to 100 mg po every 3 to 4 hours.

Available Drug Forms Syrup containing 100 mg/5 ml (contains 3.5% alcohol).

Nursing Management

Planning factors Obtain history of respiratory disorder.

Administration factors Give after meals with a full glass of water.

Evaluation factors

1. Evaluate type, characteristics, and frequency of cough periodically.
2. Observe for bleeding of gums, excessive bruising, hematuria, or other signs of bleeding. If symptoms occur, withhold drug and notify physician.

Client teaching factors

1. Unless contraindicated, encourage client to drink 3000 ml or more of fluid daily.
2. Instruct client to deep breathe frequently.
3. Instruct client to seek medical assistance if cough persists for more than 5 to 7 days.

GENERIC NAME Ammonium chloride (OTC)

CLASSIFICATION Expectorant

Action Although the exact mechanism of action is unknown, ammonium chloride is thought to increase the flow of respiratory secretions by stimulating a reflex action induced by gastric irritation. Consequently, enteric-coated tablets should not be used for expectorant action.

Indications for Use Combats productive and nonproductive coughs associated with the common cold, sinusitis, pharyngitis, and other respiratory disorders.

Contraindications Hepatic or renal failure.

Untoward Reactions Acidosis may occur with prolonged therapy.

Parameters of Use

Absorption Complete absorption occurs in 3 to 6 hours.

Excretion By the kidneys.

Administration Adults: 300 mg po every 2 to 4 hours; Children: 75 to 150 mg po every 2 to 4 hours.

Available Drug Forms Powder, tablets, and enteric-coated tablets.

Nursing Management

1. Observe client for the onset of acidosis. If symptoms occur, withhold drug and notify physician.
2. Unless contraindicated, encourage client to drink 3000 ml or more of fluid daily.
3. Instruct client to deep breathe frequently.
4. Instruct client to seek medical assistance if cough persists for more than 5 to 7 days.

GENERIC NAME Hydroiodic acid (OTC) (RX)

CLASSIFICATION Expectorant

See potassium iodide for Untoward reactions.

Action Hydroiodic acid is thought both to have a direct effect on the secretory glands of the respiratory tract and to stimulate a reflex action induced by gastric irritation.

Indications for Use Chronic bronchitis, bronchial asthma.

Contraindications Tuberculosis.

Warnings and Precautions The acidic characteristics of the drug can be very destructive to teeth.

Administration Adults 17 to 70 mg po bid or tid; Children: 0.7 to 7.0 mg po daily, bid, or tid.

Available Drug Forms Bottles containing 17 mg/ml with a calibrated dropper.

Nursing Management

1. Dilute drug in water and administer with a straw to avoid damage to the client's tooth enamel.
2. Discard drug if it has a deep brown discoloration.
3. Give after meals to avoid GI disturbances.
4. Unless contraindicated, encourage client to drink 3000 ml or more of fluid daily.

GENERIC NAME Iodinated glycerol (RX)

TRADE NAME Organidin

CLASSIFICATION Expectorant

See potassium iodide for Untoward reactions and Nursing management.

Action Iodinated glycerol is thought to have both a direct effect on the secretory glands of the respiratory tract and to stimulate a reflex action induced by gastric irritation.

Indications for Use Chronic bronchitis, bronchial asthma, as an adjunct in the treatment of emphysema.

Contraindications Hypersensitivity to iodides, tuberculosis, hypothyroidism.

Administration Adults: 50 to 60 mg po qid; Children: 25 to 30 mg po qid.

Available Drug Forms Tablets containing 30 mg; 30-ml dropper bottle containing 3 mg/gtt; elixir containing 1.2% clear amber liquid.

GENERIC NAME Potassium iodide (OTC)

TRADE NAME SSKI

CLASSIFICATION Expectorant

Action Potassium iodide is thought both to have a direct effect on the secretory glands of the respiratory tract and to stimulate a reflex action induced by gastric irritation.

Indications for Use Chronic bronchitis, bronchial asthma.

Contraindications Hypersensitivity to iodides, tuberculosis, hyperthyroidism, hyperkalemia, acute bronchitis.

Warnings and Precautions Use with caution during pregnancy, since high dosages or prolonged use may cause untoward reactions in the fetus. Prolonged use of high dosages may cause hypothyroidism. Use with caution in clients with a history of peptic ulcer or other disorders associated with upper gastrointestinal irritation.

Untoward Reactions GI disturbances, including nausea and epigastric discomfort, are common. Vomiting and small bowel lesions have been reported with prolonged use. Various types of hypersensitivity rashes can occur. Iodism (chronic iodine poisoning) may occur with prolonged drug therapy. The symptoms include metallic taste, stomatitis, increased salivation, coryza, sneezing, periorbital edema, pulmonary edema, and circulatory collapse.

Parameters of Use

Absorption From small intestine as iodide; little free iodine is absorbed from the GI tract. Bound to plasma proteins as iodide and thyroxine.

Distribution Wide; about 30% to thyroid gland. Enters saliva and gastric juices.

Metabolism Thyroxine is metabolized by the liver and the iodine is then excreted in bile.

Excretion Primarily by the kidneys, in 2 to 3 days. Crosses placenta and enters breast milk.

Drug characteristics Unstable in moist air. Store in airtight containers located in a dry area.

Drug Interactions Concurrent use of oral thiazide diuretics may predispose the client to gastrointestinal ulcerations. Concurrent use of lithium may predispose the client to hypothyroidism. Concurrent use of antithyroid agents is not recommended.

Administration Adults: 300 mg every 4 to 6 hours; Children: 60 to 600 mg po daily in divided doses.

Available Drug Forms Syrup containing 300 mg in 5 ml; enteric-release tablets containing 120 mg and 300 mg; saturated oral solution (SSKI) containing 300 mg in 0.3 ml, provided with calibrated dropper marked at the 0.3-ml and 0.6-ml levels; oral solution containing 500 mg in 15 ml.

Nursing Management

1. Dilute drug in 3 to 4 fl oz of water or orange juice.
2. Adequate hydration of the client may prevent the need for expectorants.
3. Determine if there is an allergy to iodine or iodine compounds; if so, notify the physician.
4. Follow iodine solutions with a full glass of water.
5. Administer drug after meals to prevent GI irritation.
6. Observe client frequently for hypersensitivity reactions after the first dose (first 3 to 4 hours).
7. Warn client that vomitus will have a purple color if starch and iodine are vomited.

GENERIC NAME Terpin hydrate (RX)

TRADE NAMES Creoterp, Terp, Terpinol

CLASSIFICATION Expectorant

Action Although there is little scientific evidence of its value, terpin hydrate (volatile oil) has been used as an expectorant for decades. It is thought to have a direct stimulatory effect on the secretory glands of the respiratory tract, thus increasing fluid production and expectoration. The drug is often combined with an antitussive agent, such as codeine, to relieve coughing. Terpin hydrate elixir has a high alcoholic content (greater than 40%).

Indications for Use Combats productive and nonproductive coughs associated with the common cold, sinusitis, pharyngitis, and other respiratory disorders.

Contraindications Uncontrolled diabetes mellitus, active peptic ulcer or a history of peptic ulcer.

Warnings and Precautions Use with caution in clients known to have a history of alcohol or other substance abuse.

Administration 5 to 10 ml po every 3 to 4 hours, as needed.

Available Drug Forms Bottles of elixir (plain); bottles of elixir containing 10 mg/5 ml of codeine.

Nursing Management

1. Terpin hydrate with codeine is a controlled substance.
2. Give after meals as nausea frequently occurs when drug is administered on an empty stomach.
3. Maximize local soothing effect by administering drug undiluted. Do not follow with water.
4. Unless contraindicated, encourage client to drink 3000 ml or more of fluid daily.

COMBINATION EXPECTORANT PREPARATIONS

TRADE NAME Cheracol D Syrup (OTC)

CLASSIFICATION Combination expectorant preparation

Indications for Use Helps quiet dry, hacking cough and loosen phlegm.

Administration Adults: 10 ml po q4h prn; Children: Ages 6 to 11 years: 5 ml po q4h prn; Ages 2 to 6 years: 2.5 ml po q4h prn.

Available Drug Forms Generic contents in 5 ml: dextromethorphan hydrobromide: 10 mg; guaifenesin: 100 mg; alcohol: 4.75%.

TRADE NAME Coricidin Syrup (OTC)

CLASSIFICATION Combination expectorant preparation

Indications for Use Relief of cough and nasal congestion.

Contraindications Heart or thyroid disease, diabetes, hypertension, children under 2 years.

Warnings and Precautions Do not exceed recommended dosage. Do not give concurrently with MAO inhibitors.

Untoward Reactions May induce nervousness or dizziness.

Administration Adults: 10 ml po q4h prn; Children: Ages 6 to 11 years: 1 to 5 ml po q4h prn; Ages 2 to 5 years: 2.5 ml po q4h prn; do not exceed 6 doses daily.

Available Drug Forms Generic contents in 5 ml: dextromethorphan hydrobromide: 10 mg; phenylpropanolamine hydrochloride: 12.5 mg; guaifenesin: 100 mg; alcohol: less than 0.5%.

TRADE NAME Dorcol Pediatric Cough Syrup (OTC)

CLASSIFICATION Combination expectorant preparation

Indications for Use Common cold.

Warnings and Precautions Use with caution in clients with a history of chronic bronchitis, bronchial asthma, emphysema, hypertension, heart or thyroid disease, or diabetes. Do not give concurrently with MAO inhibitors.

Untoward Reactions May induce blurred vision, flushing, GI disturbances, dizziness, or sleeplessness.

Administration Children: Ages 6 to 12 years: 10 ml po q4h prn; Ages 2 to 6 years: 5 ml po q4h prn; Ages 3 months to 2 years: 3 gtt/kg po q4h prn.

Available Drug Forms Generic contents in 5 ml: phenylpropanolamine hydrochloride: 6.25 mg; guaifenesin: 50 mg; dextromethorphan hydrobromide: 5 mg; alcohol: 5%.

TRADE NAME Entex (RX)

CLASSIFICATION Combination expectorant preparation

Indications for Use Sinusitis, pharyngitis, bronchitis, and asthma complicated by tenacious mucus; as an adjunct in serous otitis media.

Contraindications Severe hypertension, lactation.

Warnings and Precautions Use with caution in clients with a history of heart or thyroid disease, diabetes, or prostatic hypertropy. Do not give concurrently with MAO inhibitors.

Untoward Reactions May induce nervousness, insomnia, GI disturbances, or headache.

Administration Adults and children over 12 years: 1 capsule or 10 ml po qid; Children: Ages 6 to 12 years: 7.5 ml po qid; Ages 4 to 6 years: 5 ml po qid; Ages 2 to 4 years: 2.5 ml po qid.

Available Drug Forms Generic contents in each orange and white capsule: phenylephrine hydrochloride: 5 mg; phenylpropanolamine hydrochloride: 45 mg; guaifenesin: 200 mg. Generic contents in 5 ml: phenylephrine hydrochloride: 5 mg; phenylpropanolamine hydrochloride: 20 mg; guaifenesin: 100 mg; alcohol: 5%.

TRADE NAME Iodo-Niacin (RX)

CLASSIFICATION Combination expectorant preparation

Indications for Use Used to thin mucus in the bronchial tubes.

Contraindications Acute bronchitis.

Warnings and Precautions Use with caution during pregnancy. Use with extreme caution in clients with tuberculosis. May induce nonspecific small bowel lesions; discontinue immediately if symptoms of abdominal pain, distention, nausea, vomiting, or GI bleeding appear.

Untoward Reactions May induce thyroid adenoma, goiter, myxedema, iodism, and GI disturbances.

Administration 2 tablets po tid after meals.

Available Drug Forms Generic contents in each controlled-action tablet: potassium iodide: 135 mg; niacinamide hydroiodide: 25 mg.

TRADE NAME Mudrane (RX)

CLASSIFICATION Combination expectorant preparation

Indications for Use Bronchial asthma, emphysema, asthmatic bronchitis.

Contraindications Severe heart disease, hypertension, hyperthyroidism, tuberculosis, porphyria, acne, pregnancy.

Warnings and Precautions Phenobarbital may be habit forming. Discontinue if client develops skin rash, eye irritation, swelling of eyelids, or severe frontal headache (iodism).

Untoward Reactions May induce headache, tachycardia, vomiting, dizziness, urinary retention, or skin rash.

Administration 1 tablet po tid or qid prn.

Available Drug Forms Generic contents in each yellow scored tablet: potassium iodide: 195 mg; aminophylline: 130 mg; phenobarbital: 8 mg; ephedrine hydrochloride: 16 mg.

TRADE NAME Novahistine (OTC)

CLASSIFICATION Combination expectorant preparation

Indications for Use Colds, influenza, pertussis.

Contraindications Emphysema, asthma, chronic cough accompanied by excessive secretions.

Warnings and Precautions Do not give concurrently with MAO inhibitors.

Untoward Reactions May induce GI disturbances or dizziness.

Administration Adults: 10 ml po q4h prn; Children: Ages 6 to 12 years: 5 ml po q4h prn; Ages 2 to 6 years: 2.5 ml po q4h prn; do not exceed 4 doses in 24 hours.

Available Drug Forms Generic contents in 5 ml: dextromethorphan hydrobromide: 10 mg; guaifenesin: 100 mg; alcohol: 7.5%

TRADE NAME Quadrinal (RX)

CLASSIFICATION Combination expectorant preparation

Action Contains bronchodilators and an expectorant.

Indications for Use Bronchial asthma, chronic bronchitis, pulmonary emphysema.

Contraindications Enlarged thyroid or goiter, pregnancy, lactation.

Warnings and Precautions Phenobarbital may be habit forming. Use with caution in clients with a history of severe heart disease or hypoxemia, hypertension, hyperthyroidism, hepatic disease, peptic ulcer, diabetes, prostatic hypertrophy, porphyria, or acne. Use with extreme caution in clients with a history of hepatic dysfunction or chronic obstructive lung disease. Do not give concurrently with other xanthine derivatives.

Untoward Reactions May induce GI disturbance, headache, iodism, dizziness, or skin rash.

Administration Adults: 1 tablet or 10 ml po tid or qid; Children: Ages 6 to 12 years: $\frac{1}{2}$ tablet or 5 ml po tid.

Available Drug Forms Scored tablets and fruit-flavored suspension. Generic contents in each tablet or 10 ml: ephedrine hydrochloride: 24 mg; phenobarbital: 24 mg; theophylline (calcium salicylate): 130 mg; potassium iodide: 320 mg.

TRADE NAME Ryna-CX (Ci)

CLASSIFICATION Combination expectorant preparation

Indications for Use Relief of dry, nonproductive cough and nasal congestion.

Contraindications Children under 2 years.

Warnings and Precautions Codeine may be habit forming. Use with caution in clients with a history of chronic pulmonary disease, hypertension, thyroid disease, or diabetes. Do not give concurrently with MAO inhibitors.

Untoward Reactions May induce excitability, drowsiness, or constipation.

Drug Interactions Additive effects occur with other CNS depressants, alcohol, and sedatives.

Administration Adults: 10 ml po q6h; Children: Ages 6 to 12 years: 5 ml po q6h ; Ages 2 to 6 years: 2.5 ml po q6h; do not exceed 4 doses in 24 hours.

Available Drug Forms Colorless, cherry-vanilla-menthol flavored liquid. Generic contents in 5 ml: codeine phosphate: 10 mg; pseudoephedrine hydrochloride: 30 mg; guaifenesin: 100 mg.

TRADE NAME Theo-Organidin (RX)

CLASSIFICATION Combination expectorant preparation

Action Contains a bronchodilator and an expectorant.

Indications for Use Bronchial asthma, bronchitis, pulmonary emphysema.

Contraindications Pregnancy, lactation, neonates.

Warnings and Precautions Use with extreme caution in clients with a history of thyroid disease. Discontinue if rash appears. Do not give concurrently with other xanthine derivatives or CNS stimulants.

Untoward Reactions May induce gastric irritation or iodism.

Drug Interactions Iodides may increase the hypothyroid effect of antithyroid preparations.

Administration Adults: 10 to 20 ml po every 6 to 8 hours; Children 5 ml/20 lb po every 8 to 12 hours.

Available Drug Forms Clear amber elixir. Generic contents in 15 ml: theophylline: 120 mg; iodinated glycerol: 30 mg; alcohol: 15%.

TRADE NAME Tussagesic (OTC)

CLASSIFICATION Combination expectorant preparation

Indications for Use Common cold.

Warnings and Precautions Use with caution in clients with a history of cardiovascular disease, diabetes, hyperthyroidism, or hypertension.

Untoward Reactions May induce drowsiness, blurred vision, flushing, dizziness, or GI disturbances.

Administration Adults: 1 tablet po q8h or 10 ml po q4h; Children: Ages 6 to 12 years: 5 ml po q4h; Ages 1 to 6 years: 2.5 ml po q4h.

Available Drug Forms Generic contents in each timed-release tablet: phenylpropanolamine hydrochloride: 25 mg; pheniramine maleate: 12.5 mg; pyrilamine maleate: 12.5 mg; dextromethorphan hydrobromide: 30 mg; terpin hydrate: 180 mg; acetaminophen: 325 mg. Generic contents in 5 ml: phenylpropanolamine hydrochloride: 12.5 mg; pheniramine maleate: 6.25 mg; pyrilamine maleate: 6.25 mg; dextromethorphan hydrobromide: 15 mg; terpin hydrate: 90 mg; acetaminophen: 120 mg.

Nursing Management Caution client that mental and/or physical abilities may be impaired.

TRADE NAME Tussi-Organidin (Ci)

CLASSIFICATION Combination expectorant preparation

Indications for Use Chronic bronchitis, bronchial asthma, common cold.

Contraindications Pregnancy, lactation, neonates.

Warnings and Precautions Codeine may be habit forming. Use with caution in clients with a history of thyroid disease or acne. Discontinue if rash appears. Do not give concurrently with MAO inhibitors.

Untoward Reactions May induce GI disturbances, constipation, drowsiness, sedation, or dry mouth.

Drug Interactions Additive effects occur with other CNS depressants, alcohol, and tranquilizers. Iodides may increase the hypothyroid effect of antithyroid preparations.

Administration Adults: 5 to 10 ml po q4h; Children: 2.5 to 5.0 ml po q4h.

Available Drug Forms Clear red elixir. Generic contents in 5 ml: iodinated glycerol: 30 mg; codeine phosphate: 10 mg; chlorpheniramine maleate: 2 mg; alcohol: 15%. Also available without codeine as Tussi-Organidin DM.

Nursing Management Caution client that mental and/or physical abilities may be impaired.

TRADE NAME Viro-Med (OTC)

CLASSIFICATION Combination expectorant preparation

Indications for Use Viral colds and flu.

Contraindications Children under 6 years.

Warnings and Precautions Use with caution in clients with a history of asthma, glaucoma, hypertension, diabetes, prostatic hypertrophy, or heart or thyroid disease.

Untoward Reactions May induce drowsiness or excitability.

Administration Adults: 2 tablets po q4h; Children: Ages 6 to 12 years: 1 tablet po q4h.

Available Drug Forms Generic contents in each tablet: aspirin: 325 mg; chlorpheniramine maleate: 1 mg; pseudoephedrine hydrochloride: 15 mg; dextromethorphan hydrobromide: 7.5 mg; guaifenesin: 50 mg.

Nursing Management Caution client that mental and/or physical abilities may be impaired.

PART XIV

ANTIINFECTIVE AGENTS

FOR COUNTLESS AGES, tremendous numbers and varieties of microorganisms have inhabited the earth. Many of these organisms cause human disease; exposure occurs through food, water, soil, air, and bodily contact. For every type of infection a corresponding antimicrobial agent is sought. Some have broad spectrums of use, being effective against many microorganisms, and others are specific in action, being effective against one or a few microorganisms.

Scientists first discovered that "germs" caused disease in the mid-1800s. However, it was not until the 1930s that the antibiotic era began. Discovery of the first sulfonamide, Prontosil, paved the way for extensive research in antiinfective agents. Since then many sulfonamides have been synthesized, and all in current use are synthetic compounds.

Meanwhile, Alexander Fleming, working with his microscope, discovered that a colony of microorganisms was partially destroyed by a blue-green mold that had contaminated it. This mold, which had reached his culture by air, was not unlike those found on bread, cheese, or other foods. Fleming gave the destructive material the name *penicillin* after the mold already known as *Penicillium.* It was not until the 1940s that the curative powers of this agent were recognized and techniques for mass production developed. Since that time millions of lives have been saved by penicillin, which is still the most widely used of all the antimicrobial agents.

When it became evident that penicillin would have to be produced for wide-scale use, individual cultures of the mold became impractical. Many pharmaceutical firms worked diligently to perfect a successful manufacturing process. Today many synthetic and semi-synthetic penicillins are available. The forms of penicillin existing today are soluble, diffusible, and readily absorbed. Their actions may be bacteriostatic or bactericidal, depending upon the concentration employed and the organism's susceptibility. Gram-negative bacteria are generally less sensitive than gram-positive bacteria. Young pathogens are more readily killed than mature ones. Despite its relatively narrow spectrum of antimicrobial activity, however, penicillin is effective against the causative organisms of the most common human microbial infections.

The success of penicillin and its derivatives provided the impetus for research into a variety of other antibiotic agents. Antibiotics in current use are either extracts of chemicals produced by microorganisms (natural), or are synthesized in the laboratory (synthetic). Regardless of the source, all antibiotics act by interfering with the metabolism of the infecting organism in one of four ways:

1. by weakening the cell wall structure, causing it to disintegrate;
2. by changing the permeability of the cell membrane so that chemical composition of the cell is altered;
3. by altering cell protein synthesis, causing cell death; or
4. by interfering with nucleic acid synthesis so that the cell cannot grow and divide.

Successful treatment depends on choosing the antiinfective agent that will be most likely to destroy the offending microorganism. This determination is often made with the assistance of *culture and sensitivity testing* in the laboratory. This allows the physician to select the drug that is most effective without causing unnecessary adverse effects in the client. In the case of commonly seen infections, the physician may choose to omit the expensive laboratory testing and treat the client with a broad-spectrum antibiotic that has little risk of causing adverse effects during short-term therapy.

Several principles should always be considered in treating with antiinfectives. First, these drugs should never be used indiscriminately because the microorganism can adapt to the presence of the drug. When this happens, the microbe becomes resistant to the drug and continues to grow despite drug therapy. Second, many antiinfectives, while highly effective in destroying microorganisms, may also be highly toxic to human cells, causing life-threatening adverse effects. Finally, prolonged indiscriminate use of antiinfectives causes changes in the normal microbial population of the host's body. In other words, some of the helpful microbes (such as *Escherichia coli,* which aids digestion, or *Staphylococcus epidermidis,* a normal component of skin flora) are destroyed along with the offending ones. As a result, the client may develop a *superinfection.* This new infection may be much more serious than the primary infection, because it is often caused by a microorganism that is resistant to most antiinfective drugs.

The more recent discovery of fungal and viral causes of disease has presented even greater challenges to modern pharmaceutical research. Currently, the antifungal and antiviral drugs are few in number. Most antiviral drugs are highly toxic. Because the body naturally produces a substance called *interferon* in defense against viral invasion, many researchers feel that natural or synthetic production of this substance on a large scale will open the door to treatment of viral infections. One needs only to read a daily newspaper to follow the strides being made in this area.

Chapter 57

Sulfonamides

CHARACTERISTICS OF SULFONAMIDES

SHORT-ACTING SULFONAMIDES

- Sulfadiazine, sulfadiazine sodium
- Sulfamethizole
- Sulfisoxazole

INTERMEDIATE-ACTING SULFONAMIDES

- Sulfamethoxazole

LONG-ACTING SULFONAMIDES

- Sulfamethoxypyridazine

TROPICAL SULFONAMIDES

- Mafenide acetate
- Silver sulfadiazine
- Sulfacetamide sodium

COMBINATION PREPARATIONS

- Azo Gantanol
- Azo Gantrisin
- Bactrim, Septra, Sulfatrim
- Sultrin, Trysul
- Thiosulfil-A
- Vagilia, Cantri

CHARACTERISTICS OF SULFONAMIDES

Sulfonamides were the first group of antiinfective agents available for therapeutic use and comprised the major therapy for bacterial infections until penicillins were introduced in the 1940s. Sulfonamides have a broad spectrum of action against both gram-negative and gram-positive bacteria; however, resistance has developed among many organisms, so the sulfonamides have been largely replaced with newer and more effective antiinfective agents. Although the clinical use of sulfonamides is now limited, these drugs are still useful in specific conditions; namely, the treatment of urinary tract infections and severe burns.

The only significant differences between the various sulfonamide drugs concern their rates of absorption, metabolism, and excretion. Short-acting sulfonamides are rapidly absorbed and are used primarily for urinary tract and some systemic infections. Intermediate-acting sulfonamides are excreted more slowly than the short-acting drugs and are useful for long-term treatment of chronic urinary tract infections. Long-acting sulfonamides are relatively rapidly absorbed, but as they are slowly excreted therapeutic blood levels may be maintained for several days. In the past, the long-acting drugs have been used for urinary tract infections; however, their potential for toxicity is high and they have been largely replaced with the short-acting drugs.

A number of sulfonamide preparations are also available for local, topical, and ophthalmic use. Local application is used for the treatment of vaginal infections due to susceptible organisms and ulcerative colitis—sulfonamides seem to exert an antiinflammatory action in the intestine.

Sulfonamides are effective against a wide range of gram-negative and gram-positive organisms, including beta-hemolytic streptococci, pneumococci, *Escherichia coli, haemophilus influenzae, Neisseria meningitidis, N. gonorrhea, Bacillus anthracis, Shigella, Nocardia, Chlamydia,* and *Actinomyces.*

SHORT-ACTING SULFONAMIDES

GENERIC NAMES Sulfadiazine; sulfadiazine sodium

CLASSIFICATION Synthetic antibacterial (sulfonamide) RX

Action Sulfadiazine is bacteriostatic in therapeutic doses. It disrupts the production of folic acid in bacterial cells by replacing the metabolite *p*-aminobenzoic acid (PABA), thereby preventing further growth of the bacteria. Sulfonamide action is inhibited by the presence of pus and necrotic tissue because PABA is present in these materials.

Indications for Use Acute, recurrent, and chronic urinary tract infections, chancroid, nocardiosis, toxoplasmosis, falciparum malaria, trachoma, conjunctivitis and superficial eye infections, lymphogranuloma venerium, ulcerative colitis, dermatitis herpetiformis. Also used for prophylaxis in recurrent rheumatic fever and sensitive strains of meningococcal meningitis. Topical uses include prevention of *Pseudomonas* infections in second- and third-degree burns and treatment of ophthalmic and vaginal infections. Often used in combination with other sulfonamides.

Contraindications Advanced renal disease, urinary obstruction, intestinal obstruction, porphyria, group A beta-hemolytic streptococcal infections, pregnancy near term, lactation, infants under 2 months, hypersensitivity to sulfonamides.

Untoward Reactions The most common side effects are GI distress and urinary tract disturbances (crystalluria, hematuria, urinary obstruction probably due to the insolubility of the drug in acid urine). Other significant adverse reactions include blood dyscrasias, allergic and hypersensitivity reactions (primarily dermatologic), and CNS disturbances (headache, vertigo, tinnitus, ataxia, depression, convulsions, hallucinations, peripheral neuritis, ototoxicity, psychosis).

Parameters of Use

Absorption Readily absorbed from GI tract. Peak action occurs in: 3 to 6 hours (po); 2 to 4 hours (subc). About 35 to 60% bound to plasma proteins.

Crosses placenta and appears in breast milk.

Distribution Distributed to most body tissues, including cerebrospinal fluid.

Metabolism Acetylated in the liver.

Excretion By the kidneys; some reabsorption of the drug may occur. Drug is insoluble in acid urine and precipitation can cause crystalluria and hematuria.

Drug Interactions May potentiate, or be potentiated by, other protein-bound drugs because of competition for protein-binding sites. Local anesthetics that are PABA derivatives inhibit the effects of sulfonamides. The risk of crystalluria is increased with concurrent use of paraldehyde, methenamine, or urinary acidifiers. Absorption of sulfonamides is impaired by antacids and mineral oil. Concurrent ingestion of alcohol increases the risk of toxicity because oxidation of acetaldehyde is inhibited. Hypoglycemic effect of insulin is potentiated by sulfonamides. Sulfonamides can displace bilirubin in premature infants and newborns and result in kernicterus.

Laboratory Interactions Sulfadiazine interferes with Bromsulphalein, phenolsulfonphthalein, and thyroid function tests. May produce false-positive readings for urinary glucose with Benedict's solution and Clinitest and urinary protein. May interfere with urine urobilinogen determinations with Ehrlich's reagent or Urobilistix. Any follow-up cultures performed after initiation of sulfonamide therapy must have PABA in the culture medium for the results to be reliable.

Administration Adults: Oral: 2 to 4 g daily; Subcutaneous, intravenous: Initial dosage: 50 mg/kg; then 100 mg/kg/day. Children: 150 mg/kg po daily in divided doses.

Available Drug Forms Tablets containing 500 mg; 10-ml vials containing 250 mg/ml.

Nursing Management

Administration factors

1. Fluid intake should be sufficient to maintain an output of at least 1500 ml/day to prevent crystalluria.
2. Urinary alkalization with sodium bicarbonate may be necessary.
3. When administering IV, give over 10 to 30 minutes.
4. Dilute solution for IV or subc administration with sterile water to yield 50 mg/ml.

Evaluation factors

1. Test acidity of urine daily.
2. Hypersensitivity reactions (serum sickness or hemolytic anemia) usually develop within 10 days after initiation of therapy and generally begin with sudden fever. Monitor temperature daily.
3. Obtain renal and hepatic function and blood tests frequently in clients taking sulfonamides for more than 2 weeks.
4. Observe diabetic clients on oral hypoglycemics for hypoglycemic reactions. Perform serum glucose tests early in sulfonamide therapy.

Client teaching factors

1. Instruct client to report immediately any early manifestations of blood dyscrasias or hypersensitivity reaction. Symptoms include sore throat, malaise, fatigue, joint pains, pallor, abnormal bleeding, rash, and jaundice. A high fever, severe headache, stomatitis, conjunctivitis, rhinitis, or urticaria may precede Stevens-Johnson syndrome and mandate termination of therapy.
2. Warn client to avoid excessive exposure to sunlight to prevent photosensitivity reactions.
3. Instruct client to consult physician before taking any OTC preparations.
4. Instruct client to store drug in light-resistant containers.

GENERIC NAME Sulfamethizole (RX)

TRADE NAMES Microsul, Proklar, Thiosulfil, Urifon

CLASSIFICATION Synthetic antibacterial (sulfonamide)

See sulfadiazine for Action, Contraindications, Untoward reactions, and Drug interactions.

Indications for Use Primarily in the treatment of acute and chronic urinary tract infections.

Parameters of Use (See sulfadiazine.)

Absorption Readily absorbed from GI tract. Peak action occurs in about 2 hours after oral administration. About 90% bound to plasma proteins.

Distribution Does not diffuse into cerebrospinal fluid.

Administration Adults: 0.5 to 1.0 g po tid or qid; Children: 30 to 45 mg/kg po daily in 4 divided doses.

Available Drug Forms Tablets containing 250, 500, or 1000 mg.

Nursing Management May cause an orange-yellow discoloration of skin and urine. (See sulfadiazine.)

GENERIC NAME Sulfisoxazole (RX)

TRADE NAMES Gantrisin, Koro-Sulf, Lipo-Gantrisin, SK-Soxazole, Sulfasox, Sulfizin

CLASSIFICATION Synthetic antibacterial (sulfonamide)

See sulfadiazine for Action, Indications for use, Contraindications, Untoward reactions, and Drug interactions.

Parameters of Use (See sulfadiazine.)

Absorption Readily absorbed from GI tract. Peak action occurs in 2 to 4 hours (po, IM); 30 minutes (IV). Half-life is 3 to 6 hours. About 85% bound to plasma proteins.

Distribution Distributed to all extracellular fluids.

Administration Adults: Oral: Initial dosage: 2 to 4 g; then 4 to 8 g daily in divided doses. Intramuscular, subcutaneous, intravenous: Initial dosage: 50 mg/kg; then 100 mg/kg/day in 2 to 4 divided doses. Children: 150 mg/kg po daily in 4 to 6 divided doses. Ophthalmic use: 1 to 3 gtt every 1 to 4 hours. Vaginal use: 2 to 4 applications daily. Elixir (long-acting form): Adults: 4 to 5 g q12h; Children: 60 to 75 mg/kg q12h.

Available Drug Forms Tablets containing 500 mg; syrup containing 500 mg/5 ml; emulsion containing 1 g/5 ml; solution for injection containing 400 mg/ml; ophthalmic drops 4%; vaginal ointment 4%; vaginal cream 10%.

Nursing Management (See sulfadiazine.)

1. When oral administration is impractical, the preferred parenteral route is intravenous.
2. Solutions are incompatible with silver preparations.
3. Topical drug preparations may be inactivated by pus or serum.
4. Instruct client to discontinue topical drug form immediately if irritation or other sensitivity reactions occur.

INTERMEDIATE-ACTING SULFONAMIDES

GENERIC NAME Sulfamethoxazole (RX)

TRADE NAME Gantanol

CLASSIFICATION Synthetic antibacterial (sulfonamide)

See sulfadiazine for Action, Contraindications, Untoward reactions, Drug interactions, and Nursing management.

Indications for Use Primarily in the treatment of urinary tract infections.

Parameters of use (See sulfadiazine.)

Absorption More slowly absorbed than sulfadiazine. Half-life is 9 to 12 hours. About 50 to 70% bound to plasma proteins.

Excretion More slowly excreted than sulfadiazine.

Administration Adults: Initial dosage: 2 g po; then 1 g bid or tid. Children: Initial dosage: 50 to 60 mg/kg po; then 25 to 30 mg/kg bid; Maximum dosage: 75 mg/kg/day.

Available Drug Forms Tablets containing 500 or 1000 mg; suspension containing 500 mg/ml.

LONG-ACTING SULFONAMIDES

GENERIC NAME Sulfamethoxypyridazine (RX)

TRADE NAMES Kynex, Midicel

CLASSIFICATION Synthetic antibacterial (sulfonamide)

See sulfadiazine for Action, Contraindications, Untoward reactions, Drug interactions, and Nursing management.

Indications for Use Urinary tract infections, upper respiratory tract infections, dysentery, tissue infections. Also used for acne, meningococcal meningitis, and for prophylaxis in clients with rheumatic fever.

Parameters of Use (See sulfadiazine.)

Absorption Readily absorbed from GI tract. Peak action occurs in 1 to 2 hours and duration of action is about 10 hours. About 85% bound to plasma proteins.

Distribution Distributed to all body fluids; enters cerebrospinal fluid only if meninges are inflamed.

Administration Adults: Initial dosage: 1 g po; then 0.5 g/day. Prophylaxis against streptococcal infection: 2 to 3 g po in a single weekly dose. Children: Initial dosage: 30 mg/kg po; then 15 mg/kg/day

Available Drug Forms Tablets containing 500 mg.

TOPICAL SULFONAMIDES

GENERIC NAME Mafenide acetate (RX)

TRADE NAME Sulfamylon

CLASSIFICATION Synthetic antibacterial (sulfonamide)

See sulfadiazine for Contraindications and Untoward reactions.

Action A topical preparation which is active in the presence of pus or serum. (See sulfadiazine.)

Indications for Use Second- and third-degree burns, to prevent infection.

Parameters of Use

Absorption Rapidly absorbed from skin surface. Peak plasma concentrations occur in 2 to 4 hours.
Excretion Rapidly by the kidneys.

Administration Apply to affected areas daily or bid.

Available Drug Forms Cream containing 85 mg/g.

Nursing Management (See sulfadiazine.)

1. Cleanse wound before each application.
2. Apply cream to burn area with sterile gloved hand.
3. Wound dressings are not required.
4. Client may need an analgesic, since drug causes local pain.
5. Drug may be continued until healing is established or site is ready for grafting (30 to 60 days).
6. Allergic reactions may occur in 10 to 14 days; drug may be discontinued.

GENERIC NAME Silver sulfadiazine (RX)

TRADE NAME Silvadene

CLASSIFICATION Synthetic antibacterial (sulfonamide)

See sulfadiazine for Contraindications, Untoward reactions, and Drug interactions.

Action This drug affects bacterial cell membranes and cell walls only. It is effective against many gram-negative and gram-positive organisms. It remains active in the presence of pus or serum and is not inhibited by PABA. Sulfadiazine is slowly released as the silver salt interacts with sodium chloride in body tissues, and may be systemically absorbed.

Indications for Use Second- and third-degree burns, to prevent infection.

Administration Apply to affected areas daily or bid.

Available Drug Forms Cream (white) 1%.

Nursing Management (See sulfadiazine and mafenide acetate.)

1. Drug interacts with heavy metals and produces a dark discoloration; do not use discolored cream.
2. Drug may inactivate topically applied proteolytic enzymes.

GENERIC NAME Sulfacetamide sodium (RX)

TRADE NAME Sulamyd

CLASSIFICATION Synthetic antibacterial (sulfonamide)

See sulfadiazine for Action, Contraindications, and Drug interactions.

Indications for use Conjunctivitis, corneal ulcer, superficial ocular infections; as an adjunct to systemic treatment of trachoma.

Warnings and Precautions May retard corneal healing. May result in proliferation of nonsusceptible organisms. Incompatible with silver preparations.

Untoward Reactions Local irritation, transient stinging or burning.

Administration Ophthalmic use: Solution: 1 gtt into conjunctival sac every 2 hours. Ointment: Apply into conjunctival sac qid; may be used as an adjunct to solution.

Available Drug Forms Ointment 10%; solution 10 or 30% in dropper bottles.

Nursing Management (See sulfadiazine.)

1. Sensitivity reactions are rare; however, some systemic absorption from the eye may occur.
2. Store ointment away from heat.
3. Do not use solutions with a dark discoloration.

COMBINATION PREPARATIONS

TRADE NAME Azo Gantanol (RX)

CLASSIFICATION Synthetic antibacterial (sulfonamide)

Indications for Use Acute painful phase of urinary tract infections due to susceptible organisms.

Contraindications Pregnancy at term, lactation, children under 12 years.

Warnings and Precautions Use with caution in clients with impaired renal or hepatic function, severe allergies or bronchial asthma.

Administration Initial dosage: 4 tablets po; then 2 tablets morning and evening for 3 days.

Available Drug Forms Generic contents in each red film-coated tablet: sulfamethoxazole: 0.5 g; phenazopyridine hydrochloride: 100 mg.

Nursing Management

1. Inform client of harmless discoloration of urine.
2. Adequate fluid intake (at least 3000 ml/day) must be maintained to prevent crystalluria and stone formation.

TRADE NAME Azo Gantrisin (RX)

CLASSIFICATION Synthetic antibacterial (sulfonamide)

Indications for Use Acute painful phase of urinary tract infections due to susceptible organisms.

Contraindications Pregnancy at term, lactation, children under 12 years.

Warnings and Precautions Use with caution in clients with impaired renal or hepatic function, severe allergies, or bronchial asthma.

Administration Initial dosage: 4 to 6 tablets po; then 2 tablets qid until pain subsides; then initiate therapy with sulfisoxazole.

Available Drug Forms Generic contents in each red film-coated tablet: sulfisoxazole: 0.5 g; phenazopyridine hydrochloride: 50 mg.

Nursing Management

1. Inform client of harmless discoloration of urine.
2. Adequate fluid intake (at least 3000 ml/day) must be maintained to prevent crystalluria and stone formation.

TRADE NAMES Bactrim; Septra; Sulfatrim (RX)

CLASSIFICATION Synthetic antibacterial (sulfonamide)

Indications for Use Urinary tract infections due to susceptible strains of the following organisms: *Escherichia coli, Klebsiella-Enterobacter, Proteus mirabilis, Proteus vulgaris, Proteus morganii,* acute otitis media due to susceptible strains of *Haemophilus influenzae* or *Streptococcus pneumoniae;* acute attacks of chronic bronchitis due to susceptible strains of *Haemophilus influenzae* or *Streptococcus pneumoniae;* enteritis caused by susceptible strains of *Shigella flexneri* and *Shigella sonnei; pneumocystis carinii* pneumonitis.

Contraindications Pregnancy at term, lactation, infants under 2 months, streptococcal pharyngitis, glucose-b-phosphate dehydrogenase deficiency.

Warnings and Precautions Use with caution in clients with impaired renal or hepatic function, folate deficiency, severe allergies, or bronchial asthma.

Drug interactions May prolong the prothrombin time of clients receiving warfarin.

Administration 1 double strength tablet, 2 regular tablets, or 20 ml q12h for 10 to 14 days.

Available Drug Forms Generic contents in each regular tablet: sulfamethoxazole: 400 mg; trimethoprim: 80 mg. Generic contents in each double strength tablet: sulfamethoxazole: 800 mg; trimethoprim: 160 mg. Generic contents in 5 ml: sulfamethoxazole: 200 mg; trimethoprim: 40 mg.

Nursing Management

1. Adequate fluid intake (at least 3000 ml/day) must be maintained to prevent crystalluria and stone formation.
2. Obtain blood counts frequently as blood dyscrasias may develop.

TRADE NAMES Sultrin; Trysul (RX)

CLASSIFICATION Synthetic antibacterial (sulfonamide)

Indications for Use *Haemophilus vaginalis* vaginitis. Trysul may also be used as a deodorant for saprophytic infection following radiation therapy.

Contraindications Hypersensitivity to sulfonamides, renal disease.

Administration Cream: 1 applicatorful intravaginally bid for 4 to 6 days; dosage may then be reduced by one-half or one-quarter. Tablet: 1 intravaginally bid for 10 days.

Available Drug Forms Generic contents in vaginal cream: sulfathiazole: 3.42%; sulfacetamide: 2.86%; sulfabenzamide: 3.7%; urea: 0.64%. Generic contents in each vaginal tablet (Sultrin only): sulfathiazole: 172.5 mg; sulfacetamide: 143.75 mg; sulfabenzamide: 184 mg.

TRADE NAME Thiosulfil-A (RX)

CLASSIFICATION Synthetic antibacterial (sulfonamide)

Indications for Use Acute painful phase of urinary tract infections due to susceptible organisms.

Contraindications Pregnancy at term, lactation, infants under 2 months, group A streptococcal infections, glucose-b-phosphate dehydrogenase deficiency.

Warnings and Precautions Use with caution in clients with impaired renal or hepatic function, severe allergies, or bronchial asthma.

Administration 1 to 2 tablets po tid or qid.

Available Drug Forms Generic contents in each tablet: sulfamethizole: 0.5 g; phenazopyridine hydrochloride: 50 mg.

Nursing Management

1. Inform client of harmless discoloration of urine.
2. Obtain microscopic urinalysis once a week when client is treated for more than 2 weeks.
3. Adequate fluid intake (at least 3000 ml/day) must be maintained to prevent crystalluria and stone formation.
4. Obtain blood counts frequently as blood dyscrasias may develop.

TRADE NAMES Vagilia; Cantri (RX)

CLASSIFICATION Synthetic antibacterial (sulfonamide)

Indications for Use *Haemophilus vaginalis* vaginitis.

Contraindications Sensitivity to sulfonamides.

Warnings and Precautions Vaginal applications should not be used after seventh month of pregnancy. Observe for signs of systemic toxicity or skin rash.

Administration 6 g or 1 vaginal suppository daily or bid. Continue through one complete menstrual cycle.

Available Drug Forms Generic contents in suppositories or cream: sulfisoxazole: 10%; aminacrine hydrochloride: 0.2%; allantoin: 2.0%.

Nursing Management

1. Douching before insertion of medication may be necessary for hygienic purposes.
2. If there is no response within 3 to 4 days, treatment should be discontinued and another attempt made to isolate the offending organism.

Chapter 58

Cephalosporins

CEPHALOSPORINS

- Cefazolin sodium
- Cephalothin sodium
- Cephaloridine
- Cephaloglycin dihydrate
- Cephalexin monohydrate
- Cephapirin sodium
- Cefadroxil monohydrate
- Cefaclor
- Cefoxitin sodium
- Cephradine
- Cefamandole nafate

CEPHALOSPORINS HAVE A slightly different chemical structure than penicillins but their mechanism of action is the same. Although these drugs have a number of therapeutic uses, there is no outstanding indication for their use over penicillins.

Cross-sensitivity of cephalosporins and penicillins has been documented and controversy exists over whether to administer cephalosporins to penicillin-sensitive clients. However, most authorities agree that severe hypersensitivity reactions may occur in penicillin-sensitive clients. Both gram-positive and gram-negative organisms respond to cephalosporin therapy. Culture and sensitivity tests will delineate clearly which drug is specific for the identified organism.

CEPHALOSPORINS

GENERIC NAME Cefazolin sodium (RX)

TRADE NAMES Ancef, Kefzol

CLASSIFICATION Semisynthetic antibiotic (cephalosporin)

Action Cefazolin is a semisynthetic derivative of cephalosporin C, a substance produced by the fungus *Cephalosporium acremonium*. It is effective against a broad spectrum of bacteria and has the same action as penicillin G.; that is, it inhibits bacterial cell wall synthesis.

Indications for Use Penicillin-sensitive and penicillin-resistant organisms; soft tissue, blood, bone, and upper respiratory and genitourinary tract infections susceptible to cephalosporia respond well.

Contraindications Hypersensitivity to cephalosporins or penicillins.

Warnings and Precautions Use with caution in clients with elevated serum sodium levels, renal or hepatic dysfunction, and a history of anaphylaxis, allergies, bronchial asthma, hay fever, and allergic reactions to other drugs. Safe use in infants (under 1 year) and during pregnancy and lactation has not been established.

Untoward Reactions Allergic reactions include drug fever, maculopapular rash, anaphylaxis, urticaria, ulceration of mucous membranes, serum sickness, and eosinophilia; rashes are the most common reaction. Hemolytic anemia, thrombocytopenia, neutropenia, leukopenia, and a positive Coombs' test have occurred. GI disturbances include nausea, vomiting, and diarrhea. A transient rise in serum glutamic-oxaloacetic transaminase, serum glutamic-pyruvic transaminase, alkaline phosphatase, and blood urea nitrogen has been reported. Other untoward reactions include pain and phlebitis at the injection site, superinfections, genital and anal pruritus, and vaginitis.

Parameters of Use

Absorption Peak blood levels occur in 3 hours after an intravenous dose of 350 mg. Half-life is about 1.4 hours. Highly bound to plasma proteins.

Crosses placenta and small amounts enter breast milk.

Distribution Widely distributed. Bile levels may exceed serum levels by as much as five times.

Excretion About 60% in urine as unchanged drug during first 6 hours; 70 to 80% in 24 hours.

Drug Interactions A synergistic effect occurs with ampicillin. Concurrent use of probenecid, ethacrynic acid, furosemide, polymyxin B, or sulfinpyrazone causes prolonged elevated blood levels of cephalosporins, thereby increasing risk of nephrotoxicity. Cephalosporin may increase effects of oral anticoagulants.

Laboratory Interactions May produce false-positive results for urinary glucose and protein with certain reagents. Clinistix, Tes-Tape, and Ames reagent are not affected.

Administration Adults: 3 to 4 g IM or IV daily; do not exceed 6 g/day.

Available Drug Forms Vials containing 250, 500, or 1000 mg; piggyback IV sets containing 0.5, 1.0, 5.0, or 10.0 g.

Nursing Management

Planning factors

1. Complete culture and sensitivity tests before instituting therapy.
2. Obtain complete blood cell count (CBC) and renal and hepatic function tests prior to initiation of therapy.
3. Check for hypersensitivity (allergy) before administering drug.
4. Clients with impaired renal function require reduced dosages.
5. Solutions reconstituted with sterile water or 0.9% normal saline in original container are stable for 12 weeks if frozen immediately.
6. Crystals may be redissolved by warming the vial. (Poor solubility may require the administration of larger volumes.)

Administration factors

1. When administering IM, inject deep into large muscle mass and rotate injection sites.
2. When administering IV,
   - (a) Reconstitute with intravenous fluids. Label vial with date, time, and concentration. IV solutions are stable for 24 hours at room temperature and 96 hours under refrigeration.
   - (b) Administer by injection or continuous or intermittent infusion in 50 to 100 ml of solution. If

given via IV push, inject over 3 to 5 minutes through tubing.
   (c) Check patency of IV before starting infusion.
3. Lidocaine (1 to 2%) may be prescribed concurrently to decrease pain at the injection site.

Evaluation factors

1. Observe client continuously for at least 30 minutes for hypersensitivity (allergic) reaction when therapy is first initiated. If a reaction occurs, notify physician and institute measures according to agency protocol.
2. If drug is administered on an outpatient basis, retain client for at least 30 minutes. Examine client before discharging.
3. Continue therapy for at least 2 days after client has become asymptomatic or cultures are negative. Therapy is usually maintained for 10 days.
4. Monitor CBC, creatinine, urine, blood urea nitrogen, and other tests indicative of hematologic, renal, and hepatic function frequently, particularly with prolonged therapy or high dosages. (Elevation of creatinine may indicate impending acute tubular necrosis.)
5. Examine client daily for superinfections. GI and vaginal infections are common.

GENERIC NAME Cephalothin sodium (RX)

TRADE NAME Keflin

CLASSIFICATION Semisynthetic antibiotic (cephalosporin)

See cefazolin sodium for Action, Indications for use, Contraindications, Warnings and precautions, and Untoward reactions.

Parameters of Use

Absorption Peak blood levels occur in: 30 minutes (500 mg IM); 15 minutes (1000 mg IV).

Excretion About 60 to 70% in urine in 5 to 6 hours. (See cefazolin sodium.)

Drug Interactions Calcium gluceptate and tetracycline will cause precipitation when mixed with cephalothin. Sodium bicarbonate and aminophylline will cause deterioration in minibottle but not in regular infusion. Diphenhydramine will precipitate in minibottle. Use of heparin and steroids to diminish the incidence of thrombophlebitis will inhibit antimicrobial activity in add-a-line IV. High dosages in combination with gentamicin may lead to acute tubular necrosis. (See cefazolin sodium.)

Administration Adults: 500 to 2000 mg IM or IV every 4 to 6 hours; Children: 100 mg/kg IM or IV daily. Intraperitoneal: 0.1 to 4% irrigating solution; up to 6 mg/100 ml of dialysis fluid instilled in peritoneal cavity.

Available Drug Forms Vials containing 1, 2, 4, or 20 g.

Nursing Management (See cefazolin sodium.)

1. Superinfection is possible with *Pseudomonas*.
2. May be given via IV push through tubing over 3 to 5 minutes (1 g/10 ml), but this greatly enhances the risk of thrombophlebitis.
3. May be given intermittently or in large volume parenteral solutions administered within 24 hours.
4. Slight discoloration will not alter potency. Reconstituted solutions used for IM injection should be used within 24 hours.

GENERIC NAME Cephaloridine (RX)

TRADE NAME Loridine

CLASSIFICATION Semisynthetic antibiotic (cephalosporin)

See cefazolin sodium for Action, Indications for use, Contraindications, Warnings and precautions, and Untoward reactions.

Parameters of Use

Absorption Peak blood levels occur in 30 minutes following intramuscular injection. Half-life is 40 to 108 minutes. (See cefazolin sodium.)

Drug Interactions Do not mix with antibiotics. Nephrotoxicity may be increased by aminoglycosides, colistin, and polymyxin B. Concomitant use of furosemide and sodium edecrin may lead to acute tubular necrosis. (See cefazolin sodium.)

Administration Highly individualized. Adults: Dosage range: 250 to 1000 g IM or IV qid; Children: 30 to 50 mg/kg IM or IV daily.

Available Drug Forms Ampules containing 500 or 1000 mg/10 ml of dry powder.

Nursing Management (See cefazolin sodium.)

1. There is no pain on IM injection.
2. Rarely given by IV route. If given IV, inject slowly 3 to 4 times a day through IV tubing.
3. Do not dilute with paraben-containing solutions.
4. Protect ampules from light.
5. Extremely nephrotoxic. Observe renal function test protocol.

GENERIC NAME Cephaloglycin dihydrate (RX)

TRADE NAME Kafocin

CLASSIFICATION Semisynthetic antibiotic (cephalosporin)

See cefazolin sodium for Action, Contraindications, Warnings and precautions, Untoward reactions, Drug interactions, and Nursing management.

Indications for Use Acute and chronic infections of the urinary tract (cystitis, pyelonephritis, pyelitis); asymptomatic bacteriuria.

Parameters of Use

Absorption Absorbed from GI tract; stable in gastric acid. Peak serum levels high enough for urinary tract infections only. Half-life is 90 minutes.

Excretion 25% in urine within 8 hours. Excreted as desacetyl derivative. (See cefazolin sodium.)

Administration Adults: 250 to 500 mg po qid for 10 days; Children: 25 to 50 mg/kg po daily.

Available Drug Forms Capsules containing 250 mg.

GENERIC NAME Cephalexin monohydrate (RX)

TRADE NAME Keflex

CLASSIFICATION Semisynthetic antibiotic (cephalosporin)

See cefazolin sodium for Action, Indications for use, Contraindications, Warnings and precautions, Untoward reactions, and Drug interactions.

Parameters of Use

Absorption Peak blood levels occur in 1 hour. Half-life about 1 hour. About 6 to 15% bound to plasma protein. (See cefazolin sodium.)

Excretion About 90% as unchanged drug in urine within 8 hours.

Administration Adults: 1 to 4 g po daily; Children: 25 to 50 mg/kg po daily.

Available Drug Forms Capsules containing 250 mg; powder containing 1.5, 2.5, or 5.0 g; pediatric suspension containing 1g.

Nursing Management Shake suspension well before using; stable for 14 days if refrigerated. (See cefazolin sodium.)

GENERIC NAME Cephapirin sodium (RX)

TRADE NAME Cefadyl

CLASSIFICATION Semisynthetic antibiotic (cephalosporin)

See cefazolin sodium for Action, Contraindications, Warnings and precautions, Untoward reactions, and Drug interactions.

Indications for Use Treatment of penicillin G-resistant infections; penicillinase and nonpenicillinase *Staphylococcus aureus* infections respond well; respiratory, urinary tract, skin, and soft tissue infections.

Parameters of Use

Absorption Peak blood levels occur in 30 minutes after intramuscular administration. About 44 to 55% bound to plasma proteins. Half-life is 36 minutes.

Excretion About 70% in urine within 6 hours. (See cefazolin sodium.)

Administration Adults: 500 to 1000 mg IM or IV every 4 to 6 hours; up to 12 g daily; Children: 40 to 80 mg/kg IM or IV daily.

Available Drug Forms Vials containing 1 or 2 g; piggyback IV sets containing 1, 2, or 4 g.

Nursing Management (See cefazolin sodium.)

1. IM injection is well tolerated.
2. Low level of irritation associated with IV injection.
3. When administering via intermittent IV infusion, dilute 1 to 2 g in 10 ml and give through an auxiliary unit.

GENERIC NAME Cefadroxil monohydrate (RX)

TRADE NAME Duricef

CLASSIFICATION Semisynthetic antibiotic (cephalosporin)

See cefazolin sodium for Action, Contraindications, Warnings and precautions, Untoward reactions, Drug interactions, and Nursing management.

Indications for Use Upper respiratory tract infections caused by *Escherichia coli, Proteus mirabilis,* and *Klebsiella;* infections of the skin and/or skin structure caused by *Staphylococcus* and/or *Streptococcus* respond well.

Parameters of Use

Absorption Absorbed from GI tract; stable in gastric acid.

Metabolism Not metabolized in body.

Excretion About 90% in urine within 8 hours. (See cefazolin sodium.)

Administration 1 g po daily.

Available Drug Forms Capsules containing 500 mg; tablets containing 1 g.

GENERIC NAME Cefaclor (RX)

TRADE NAME Ceclor

CLASSIFICATION Semisynthetic antibiotic (cephalosporin)

See cefazolin sodium for Action, Contraindications, Warnings and precautions, Untoward reactions, and Drug interactions.

Indications for Use Active against otitis media caused by *Haemophilus influenzae* strains resistant to amoxicillin and ampicillin; gram-negative infections; upper and lower respiratory tract infections.

Parameters of Use

Absorption Readily absorbed from GI tract after oral administration. Peak blood levels occur in 30 to 60 minutes when taken on an empty stomach; 60 to 120 minutes with food in stomach. (See cefazolin sodium.)

Administration Adults: 250 mg po every 8 hours; do not exceed 4 g/day. Children: 20 mg/kg po daily; do not exceed 1 g/day.

Available Drug Forms Capsules containing 250 or 500 mg; oral suspension containing 125 or 250 mg/5 ml.

Nursing Management Best given on an empty stomach, but food does not inhibit absorption. (See cefazolin sodium.)

GENERIC NAME Cefoxitin sodium (OTC) (RX)

TRADE NAME Mefoxin

CLASSIFICATION Semisynthetic antibiotic (cephalosporin)

See cefazolin sodium for Contraindications, Warnings and precautions, and Untoward reactions.

Action Cefoxitin is a semisynthetic derivative of cephamycin C, a substance produced by *Streptomyces lactamdurans.* It is effective against a broad spectrum of bacteria, especially anaerobes *(Bacteroides fragilis, Providencia).*

Indications for Use Useful against mixed aerobes and anaerobes.

Parameters of Use

Absorption Peak serum levels occur in 30 minutes, following intramuscular injection; 5 minutes following intravenous injection. Half-life is 40 to 65 minutes. (See cefazolin sodium.)

Drug Interactions Nephrotoxicity may occur with concurrent use of aminoglycosides. (See cefazolin sodium.)

Administration 1 to 2 g IM or IV every 6 to 8 hours.

Available Drug Forms Vials containing 1 or 2 g of powder.

Nursing Management May sustain local thrombophlebitis when given by IV route. (See cefazolin sodium.)

GENERIC NAME Cephradine (RX)

TRADE NAMES Anspor, Velosef

CLASSIFICATION Semisynthetic antibiotic (cephalosporin)

See cefazolin sodium for Action, Contraindications, Warnings and precautions, Untoward reactions, and Drug interactions.

Indications for Use Chiefly upper and lower respiratory and urinary tract infections.

Parameters of Use

Absorption Well absorbed from GI tract; stable in gastric acid. Peak blood levels occur in 49 minutes following intramuscular injection or 1 hour following oral administration. Half-life is 1 to 2 hours. 20% bound to plasma proteins.
Excretion About 57 to 80% in urine during first 6 hours. (See cefazolin sodium.)

Administration Adults: 2 to 4 g po, IM, or IV qid; do not exceed 8 g/day. Children: Over 1 year: 250 to 500 mg po qid; 50 to 100 mg/kg IM or IV qid; do not exceed 300 mg/kg/day.

Available Drug Forms Vials containing 250, 500, or 1000 g; infusion bottles containing 2 or 4 g; capsules containing 250 or 500 mg; tablets containing 1 g; suspension containing 125 mg or 250 mg/5 ml.

Nursing Management (See cefazolin sodium.)

1. Do not mix Velosef with Ringer's lactate as calcium ions and sodium carbonate deactivate the drug. Contains 136 mg of sodium or 6 mg/1 g.
2. Give IM injection deep into gluteal muscle.
3. Hypernatremia may contraindicate continued therapy.
4. Monitor serum electrolytes and observe client for signs of sodium retention.
5. Solution is stable for 24 hours at 5 C.

GENERIC NAME Cefamandole nafate (RX)

TRADE NAME Mandol

CLASSIFICATION Semisynthetic antibiotic (cephalosporin)

See cefazolin sodium for Action, Contraindications, Warnings and precautions, and Untoward reactions.

Indications for Use Most effective against gram-negative organisms (*Enterobacter*, indole-positive *Proteus*); effective against anaerobes; relatively resistant to deactivation by penicillinase and cephalosporinase.

Parameters of Use

Absorption Peak blood levels occur in 30 to 120 minutes following intramuscular injection; 10 minutes following intravenous injection. Half-life is 30 to 60 minutes.

Metabolism Not metabolized in body.

Excretion About 65 to 85% in urine. (See cefazolin sodium.)

Drug Interactions Do not mix with antibiotics, especially aminoglycosides. (See cefazolin sodium.)

Laboratory Interactions Produces false-positive results for proteinuria with acid and denaturization precipitation tests.

Administration Adults: 500 to 2000 g IM or IV every 4 to 8 hours; Children: 50 to 150 mg/kg IM or IV daily.

Available Drug Forms Vials containing 0.5, 1.0, or 2.0 g of dry white powder.

Nursing Management (See cefazolin sodium.)

1. Reconstitute 1 g with 3 ml of bacteriostatic water for IM injection.
2. Do not mix with other antibiotics in same infusion. Dilute 1 g with 10 ml of sterile water, 5% dextrose, or 0.9% Sodium Chloride Injection for direct intermittent administration. If sterile water is used as diluent, reconstitute with 20 ml/g for intermittent infusion to avoid hypotonicity.

Chapter 59

Aminoglycosides

AMINOGLYCOSIDES

- Streptomycin sulfate, dihydrostreptomycin sulfate, streptoduocin
- Neomycin sulfate
- Gentamicin sulfate
- Kanamycin sulfate
- Amikacin sulfate
- Paromomycin sulfate
- Tobramycin sulfate

THIS GROUP OF antiinfective agents interferes with microbial protein synthesis causing faulty bacterial protein production. The drugs exert a wide range of bactericidal activity against both gram-positive and gram-negative organisms; they also demonstrate a high incidence of cross-resistance.

Most aminoglycosides are poorly absorbed from the gastrointestinal tract, but they are well absorbed from muscle masses. Like penicillins, they cross the placenta and only penetrate the blood-brain barrier when the meninges are inflamed. These drugs are excreted by the kidneys through glomerular filtration.

Pronounced toxic effects have been demonstrated clinically. Nephrotoxicity, ototoxicity, and neuromuscular blockade have been reported. Damage to the eighth cranial nerve may cause irreversible deafness, coordination difficulties, and vertigo. Although vestibular damage may be partially reversed, there is some question as to whether the damage can be remedied with discontinuance of the drug. Nephrotoxicity is manifested as albuminuria and an elevated nonprotein nitrogen level.

Nursing care varies according to the drug administered, dosage, compatibility in solution and other factors. Monitoring of laboratory data is extremely critical. Indications of azotemia progressing to oliguria may first appear in urine tests. An elevated blood urea nitrogen level and poor creatinine clearance are examples of indicators of potential toxicity. Detailed recording of intake and output is essential. Neurologic and respiratory assessment are an important part of nursing care for the client on aminoglycoside therapy.

AMINOGLYCOSIDES

GENERIC NAMES Streptomycin sulfate; dihydrostreptomycin sulfate; streptoduocin

TRADE NAME Strycin (RX)

CLASSIFICATION Antibiotic (aminoglycoside)

Action Streptomycin is isolated from *Streptomyces griseus*. It is thought to bind soluble RNA with the wrong specificity, thus producing faulty and ineffective bacterial proteins.

Indications for Use Effective against acid-fast bacilli (tuberculosis, leprosy, tularemia, plague, brucellosis); effective in combination with penicillins against meningitis, urinary tract infections, acute gonorrhea, granuloma inguinale, bacteremia, and pneumonia.

Contraindications Hypersensitivity to aminoglycosides, myasthenia gravis, disorders of the inner ear, concurrent use of neurotoxic or nephrotoxic agents.

Warnings and Precautions Use with caution during pregnancy, in children and the elderly, and in clients with impaired renal function.

Untoward Reactions Streptomycin causes vestibular damage whereas dihydrostreptomycin causes damage to the cochlear apparatus. Circumoral or peripheral paresthesias, amblyopia, and pancytopenia may also occur. Hypersensitivity reactions include rashes, pruritus, angioedema, lymph node enlargement, fever, blood dyscrasias, stomatitis, and anaphylactic shock.

Parameters of Use

Absorption Well absorbed following intramuscular injection and enters all body tissues. Peak blood levels occur in 1 to 2 hours.

Crosses placenta and appears in breast milk.

Metabolism Not metabolized in body.

Excretion About 85% by the kidneys within 24 hours.

Drug Interactions A synergistic effect occurs with ethambutal, rifampin, isoniazid, and p-aminosalicyclic acid. Synergistic effects also occur with penicillin G in the treatment of subacute bacterial endocarditis caused by enterococci (bacteremia, meningitis, brain abscess, urinary tract infections). Avoid concurrent use of viomycin, kanamycin, loridine, polymyxin B, colistin, and diuretics (which may give rise to ototoxicity). Concomitant use with muscle relaxants (tubocurarine, succinylcholine) may precipitate neuromuscular blockade and respiratory paralysis.

Laboratory Interactions Blood urea nitrogen may be decreased. May cause false-positive results for urinary glucose with Benedict's solution or Clinitest. Use of sodium, potassium, ammonium, calcium, or magnesium salts may cause inaccurate culture and sensitivity test results.

Administration Adults: 1 to 4 g IM daily; Children: 20 to 40 mg/kg IM daily. Maintenance dosage: 1 g 1 to 3 times weekly.

Available Drug Forms Ampules containing 500 or 1000 mg; vials containing 1 or 5 g of dry powder.

Nursing Management

Planning factors

1. Complete culture and sensitivity tests before instituting therapy.
2. Perform audiometric tests prior to initiation of therapy.
3. Dosage is regulated by renal function and audiometry tests.

Administration factors

1. Dilute drug with 0.9% normal saline or bacteriostatic water for injection. May be refrigerated up to 14 days after reconstitution.
2. IM injections are usually painful; inject deep into large muscle mass.
3. When handling drug, avoid direct contact as sensitization can occur.
4. Keep client well hydrated to prevent drug accumulation and/or nephrotoxicity.

Evaluation factors

1. Depression is a common but transient symptom.
2. Periodic audiometric testing and renal and hepatic function tests are recommended for clients on long-term therapy.
3. Adverse neurologic effects may begin with headache, nausea, vomiting, vertigo, and ataxia. Although symptoms may abate, even with continued use, residual damage may be permanent in some clients.
4. Symptoms of ototoxicity include tinnitus, impaired hearing, roaring noises, and a sense of fullness in the ears. If testing indicates auditory nerve damage, drug should be discontinued to avoid permanent hearing loss.
5. Clients on long-term therapy should be referred to community health nursing services for continued evaluation.

Client teaching factors

1. Teach client signs and symptoms of neurotoxicity and ototoxicity. Instruct client to report such symptoms promptly to physician.
2. Encourage client to keep appointments for periodic renal and hepatic function tests and audiometric testing. Inform client that permanent auditory and neurologic damage can be avoided if symptoms are reported promptly.
3. Instruct client to maintain adequate fluid intake to avoid renal damage and to promptly report changes in the intake-output ratio.

GENERIC NAME Neomycin sulfate (RX)

TRADE NAMES Mycifradin, Myciguent, Neobiotic, Neocin

CLASSIFICATION Antibiotic (aminoglycoside)

See streptomycin sulfate for Contraindications and Warnings and precautions.

Action Neomycin is isolated from *Streptomyces fradiae* and has properties similar to streptomycin.

Indications for Use Topical therapy chiefly for infected skin lesions, burns, and ulcerations; hepatic coma to reduce blood ammonia levels via alteration of intestinal flora; bowel cleanser preparatory to colon surgery; very effective as a genitourinary irrigant and topical irrigant preparatory to closure of colostomy.

Untoward Reactions Malabsorption syndrome (increased fecal fat, decreased serum carotene, decreased xylose). (See streptomycin sulfate.)

Parameters of Use

Absorption Poorly absorbed from GI tract, but well absorbed from muscle. Peak levels are reached in 48 hours.

Excretion About 97% in feces and 3% in urine. If given by parenteral route, 50% excreted in urine.

Drug Interactions Inhibits the absorption of penicillin V. (See streptomycin sulfate.)

Administration Oral: Bowel cleanser: 40 mg/kg every 24 hours for 3 days; Hepatic coma: 100 mg/kg times 4 doses; then 50 mg/kg; do not exceed 3 g. Intramuscular: 15 mg/kg/day. Topical: Solution or ointment 1%: apply daily or bid.

Available Drug Forms Tablets containing 500 mg; oral solution 0.5%; ointment 0.5%; vials containing 0.5 g of sterile powder. Several combination preparations are also available.

Nursing Management Neomycin is the most toxic of the aminoglycosides and is rarely given by parenteral route. (See streptomycin sulfate.)

GENERIC NAME Gentamicin sulfate (RX)

TRADE NAME Garamycin

CLASSIFICATION Antibiotic (aminoglycoside)

See streptomycin sulfate for Contraindications and Warnings and precautions.

Action Gentamicin is isolated from *Micromonospora purpurea* and has properties similar to streptomycin.

Indications for Use Topical therapy for infected skin lesions; parenteral therapy for gram-negative organisms (*Pseudomonas aeruginosa, Proteus* (indole positive and negative), *Escherichia coli, Klebsiella, Enterobacter, Serratia*); not effective against topical viral or fungal infections.

Untoward Reactions Generalized burning, joint pain, fever, weight loss, pseudotumor cerebri, alopecia, hepatomegaly, splenomegaly. Eye drops may cause burning, stinging, and transient irritation (hypersensitivity reactions). (See streptomycin sulfate.)

Parameters of Use

Absorption Absorbed following intramuscular and topical (slight) administration. Peak levels occur in 30 to 60 minutes after intravenous administration. About 30% bound to serum proteins.

Excretion About 30 to 100% in urine within 24 hours.

Drug Interactions Concurrent administration with ethacrynic acid or furosemide increases the risk of ototoxicity. Antimicrobial activity is decreased by carbenicillin. Concomitant use with penicillin G produces a synergistic bactericidal effect against *Streptococcus faecalis, S. liquifaciens,* and *S. zymogenes.* There is an increased chance of toxicity when given with cephalothin. (See streptomycin sulfate.)

Administration Intramuscular, intravenous: 2 to 3 mg/kg daily for 7 to 10 days. Topical: Cream or ointment 0.1%: Apply bid or tid; Eye drops: 1 to 2 gtt/eye every 4 hours; Ophthalmic ointment: Apply bid or tid.

Available Drug Forms Vials containing 80 mg/2 ml; pediatric vials containing 20 mg/2 ml; disposable syringes containing 60 mg/1.5 ml or 80 mg/2 ml; cream and ointment 0.1% in tubes containing 15 g; plastic bottles containing 5 mg of eye drops with dropper; ophthalmic ointment in $\frac{1}{8}$-oz. tubes.

Nursing Management (See streptomycin sulfate.)

1. When using cream, apply a small amount 2 to 3 times daily; an occlusive dressing may be indicated. Store away from heat.
2. Dilute with 100 to 200 ml of normal saline or dextrose for IV administration.
3. Give IV infusion over 1 to 2 hours. Never administer by IV push.
4. Watch for erythema, pruritus, or photosensitization, which are indicative of a reaction to topical preparations.
5. Ophthalmic drug forms may retard corneal healing and increase the possibility of fungal infections.

GENERIC NAME Kanamycin sulfate (RX)

TRADE NAME Kantrex

CLASSIFICATION Antibiotic (aminoglycoside)

See streptomycin sulfate for Contraindications, Warnings and precautions, and Untoward reactions.

Action Kanamycin is isolated from *Streptomyces kanamyceticus* and has properties similar to Streptomycin.

Indications for Use Short-term treatment of *Escherichia coli, Enterobacter aerogenes, Klebsiella pneumoniae,* and *Serratia marcescens.* It has been used as a preparatory to bowel surgery (less toxic than neomycin).

Parameters of Use

Absorption Absorbed from muscle. Peak effect occurs in 1 hour.

Excretion About 100% in feces after oral administration and 50 to 80% in urine after intramuscular administration within 24 hours.

Drug Interactions A synergistic effect occurs in methicillin-resistant *Staphylococcus aureus* when given with cephalosporins. Do not mix with barbiturates. Concurrent administration with ethacrynic acid increases the risk of ototoxicity. (See streptomycin sulfate.)

Administration Oral: Bowel cleanser: 1 g every 4 to 6 hours for 72 hours. Intramuscular, intravenous: 15 mg/kg daily; do not exceed 1.5 g/day. Inhalation: Aerosol: 250 mg in normal saline bid, tid, or qid.

Available Drug Forms Vials containing 500 mg/1.5 ml or 1.0 g/3.0 ml; disposable syringes containing 500 mg/2 ml; capsules containing 500 mg; aerosol (powder added to nebulizer in normal saline); pediatric vials containing 25 or 75 mg/2 ml.

Nursing Management (See streptomycin sulfate.)

1. When administering IM, inject deep into large muscle mass. Rotate sites to avoid induration and sterile abscess formation.
2. When administering IV,
   (a) Dilute 1 g in 400 ml of normal saline or dextrose.
   (b) Give 60 to 80 gtt/min.
   (c) This route is only used when IM route is contraindicated.
3. May be given intraperitoneal to irrigate surgical wounds; dilute 500 mg in 20 ml of distilled water.
4. Solutions may darken, but potency is unaffected.

GENERIC NAME Amikacin sulfate (RX)

TRADE NAMES Amikacin, Amikin

CLASSIFICATION Antibiotic (aminoglycoside)

See streptomycin sulfate for Contraindications and Warnings and precautions. See streptomycin sulfate and gentamicin sulfate for Untoward reactions and Drug interactions.

Action Amikacin is a semisynthetic aminoglycoside derived from kanamycin.

Indications for Use Reserved for treatment of gentamicin-resistant infections.

Parameters of Use

Absorption Peak blood levels occur in: 1 hour (IM); 30 minutes (IV). About 11% bound to serum proteins. Half-life is greater than 2 hours.

Excretion About 94 to 98% within 24 hours.

Administration 15 mg/kg IM or IV daily for no more than 10 days.

Available Drug Forms Vials containing 100 or 500 mg/2 ml; disposable syringes containing 500 mg/2 ml or 1.0 g/4 ml.

Nursing Management (See streptomycin sulfate.)

1. Stable at room temperature for 2 years.

2. Solution may develop a yellow discoloration, but potency is not affected.
3. When administering IV,
   (a) Dilute 500 mg in 200 ml of normal saline or dextrose.
   (b) Infuse over 30 to 60 minutes in adults.
   (c) Infuse over 1 to 2 hours in infants.

Administration In hepatic coma, 4 g po daily in 3 divided doses for 5 to 6 days. 25 to 35 mg/kg daily in 3 divided doses for 5 to 10 days.

Available Drug Forms Capsules containing 250 mg; pediatric syrup containing 125 mg/5 ml.

GENERIC NAME Paromomycin sulfate (RX)

TRADE NAME Humatin

CLASSIFICATION Antibiotic (aminoglycoside)

See streptomycin sulfate for Nursing Management.

Action Paromomycin is isolated from *Streptomyces rimosus.* Direct antibacterial and antimicrobial action occurs in gastrointestinal tract.

Indications for Use Bacillary dysentery and amebiasis. (See neomycin sulfate.)

Contraindications Hypersensitivity, intestinal obstruction.

Warnings and Precautions Use with caution in presence of gastrointestinal ulceration.

Untoward Reactions Diarrhea, abdominal cramps, nausea, headache, dizziness, rash, pruritus ani, heartburn, superinfection.

Parameters of Use

Absorption Not absorbed. Acts directly on organisms in GI tract.

Excretion Almost 100% of drug is excreted unchanged in feces.

Drug Interactions None reported.

GENERIC NAME Tobramycin sulfate (RX)

TRADE NAME Nebcin

CLASSIFICATION Antibiotic (aminoglycoside)

See streptomycin sulfate for Indications for use, Contraindications, Warnings and precautions, Untoward reactions, and Drug interactions.

Action Tobramycin is isolated from *Streptomyces tenebrarius* and has properties similar to streptomycin.

Parameters of Use

Absorption Peak blood levels occur in 30 to 90 minutes after intramuscular or intravenous administration. Not bound to serum proteins. Half-life is 2 hours.

Excretion About 93% in urine within 24 hours.

Administration 3 to 5 mg/kg IM or IV daily in 3 divided doses; do not exceed 5 mg/kg/day.

Available Drug Forms Ampules containing 80 mg/2 ml; pediatric ampules containing 20 mg/2 ml; disposable syringes containing 60 mg/1.5 ml or 80 mg/2 ml.

Nursing Management (See streptomycin sulfate.)

1. Dilute dose in 50 to 100 ml of normal saline or dextrose for IV administration and infuse over 20 to 60 minutes.
2. Secondary apnea may occur in anesthetized clients.

Chapter 60

Penicillins

THE FIRST OF the antibiotics, the penicillins, are still the most widely used antiinfective agents. Their usefulness in treating gram-positive infections is well documented and their reported efficacy in the treatment of some gram-negative organisms and spirochete infections has also been clinically validated.

MECHANISM OF ACTION

Although the exact mechanism of action is not completely understood, penicillins are thought to interfere with the biosynthesis of cell wall mucopeptide; consequently, the structural composition of the cell wall is altered. Penicillins appear to be more effective against immature cells that are actively dividing than against mature cells. These drugs are selectively toxic to susceptible bacteria while sparing human cells from their biochemical activity. Thus, their relatively low toxicity to mammalian cells makes them useful and potent antiinfective agents.

TYPES OF PENICILLINS

Penicillin G is the parent drug of over 30 penicillins that have been discovered. Some penicillins occur naturally whereas others are biosynthesized (semisynthetic) in the laboratory. Naturally occurring penicillins deteriorate rapidly in the acidic environment of the stomach and this has spurred the development of acid-resistant penicillins. In addition, penicillins resistant to penicillinase, an enzyme found naturally in many organisms that inactivates penicillins, have also been developed. Many of the penicillinase-resistant penicillins are also acid-resistant. More recently, broad-spectrum penicillins, the first of which was ampicillin, have been developed.

Since naturally occurring penicillins are unstable in gastric acid, they are best administered parenterally. If oral therapy is indicated, the dosage must be three to five times the parenteral dosage to achieve therapeutic blood levels. Many of the orally administered penicillins will bind with food and form insoluble complexes. Therefore, oral penicillins should be given at least one hour before or two hours after meals.

After parenteral administration, penicillins are widely distributed throughout the body. However, concentrations of the drug in various body tissues and fluids differs considerably. Furthermore, some drug molecules bind to plasma proteins. Penicillins are found in sputum and breast milk. They are also found in somewhat higher concentrations in peritoneal fluid, whereas joint, ocular, pleural, and pericardial fluids have relatively low concentrations. The highest concentration is found in the kidneys, from which 60 to 90% of the drug is excreted. Penicillins cross the placental barrier, but do not readily enter cerebrospinal fluid unless the meninges are inflamed. Renal excretion may be delayed by concurrent administration of probenecid (Benemid) or phenylbutazone (Butazolidin), which effectively block tubular transport of penicillins.

INDICATIONS FOR USE

With the exception of the broad-spectrum penicillins, the penicillins have a narrow spectrum of antimicrobial activity; but they are still quite useful for prophylaxis as well as for treatment of certain fulminating infections. Penicillins are potentially useful against susceptible gram-positive bacteria, including group A beta-hemolytic streptococci, gram-positive pneumococci, and staphylococci. *Treponema pallidum* and some gram-negative bacillary infections (bacteremia, empyema, endocarditis) are also eradicated by penicillins. Only the penicillinase-resistant penicillins are useful against penicillinase-producing organisms, such as indole-positive *Proteus, Escherichia coli, Pseudomonas aeruginosa,* and certain strains of *Staphylococcus aureus.* Penicillins are widely used to prevent recurrences of rheumatic fever, syphilis, and gonorrhea. They are also clinically useful in the prophylaxis of subacute bacterial endocarditis and in the preparation of clients for valvular heart surgery.

RESISTANCE

Increasingly resistant bacterial strains are surfacing due to the widespread use of penicillins. The introduction of semisynthetic penicillins in the 1960s reduced the problem of resistance, but recent evidence reports the emergence of new organisms *(Gonococcus)* resistant to both natural and semisynthetic penicillins. Culture and sensitivity tests of the throat, urine, and/or blood are a prerequisite to therapy to identify and treat the causative organism successfully. However, broad-spectrum penicillins, such as ampicillin, may be started prior to obtaining laboratory culture results as these drugs are relatively active against all organisms.

HYPERSENSITIVITY, SUPERINFECTION, AND OTHER UNTOWARD REACTIONS

Mild untoward reactions are frequently associated with the use of penicillins. Such reactions include various skin rashes, dermomucosal irritation, and mild gastrointestinal disturbances. A change in the method of administration will often relieve these symptoms; otherwise a different preparation may be indicated—for example, use of a semisynthetic derivative.

Acute anaphylaxis poses the most serious danger and is marked by histaminic constriction of the bronchioles with reduced lung vital capacity. Blood pressure may fall to shock levels and the client may experience severe gastrointestinal distress. Administration of epinephrine, corticosteroids, and supplemental oxygen is critical to recovery.

Prolonged penicillin therapy may predispose clients to superinfection by fungi and gram-negative pathogens as a result of alterations in the normal flora of the body.

Recently, a number of cases of penicillin-induced immune hemolysis have appeared in the literature. Penicillin and penicillin-type antibiotics bind to red blood cells. When high intravenous doses of penicillin are given, antibodies are produced that subsequently lyse the penicillinized cells. These antibodies can be effectively demonstrated in the direct Coombs' test. Frequent blood counts should be done for clients on penicillin therapy; the direct Coombs' test should also be done if hematocrit and hemoglobin begin to drop. Hemolysis is a hypersensitivity reaction, confirmed by a positive direct Coombs' test, and mandates discontinuation of the penicillin.

Hemolytic anemia, leukopenia, and thrombocytopenia have been associated with penicillin therapy. Nephropathy may occur in clients receiving high dosages and necessitates close observation of renal function tests. In addition, high dosages of penicillins (10 to 100 million units daily) may cause stimulation of the central nervous system and result in convulsions, stupor, and death in clients with impaired renal function.

AVAILABLE DRUG FORMS

Natural and semisynthetic penicillins are available in oral and parenteral drug forms. Preparations with prolonged action, such as penicillin G procaine, are also available and sustain blood levels over a long period of time. Dicloxacillin is reported to have better oral absorption than the other penicillinase-resistant penicillins.

NURSING MANAGEMENT

Although the nursing management of clients receiving penicillin therapy will vary according to the type, route, and purpose of administration, there are a few general considerations that apply to most penicillins.

A medical history that incorporates information on allergies and drug sensitivities is extremely important because approximately 10 to 20% of the people in the United States experience untoward reactions to penicillins. Observation for allergic and adverse reactions is crucial. If a drug reaction is observed, the medication should be stopped and the physician notified so that a different drug may be substituted and begun without sacrificing therapeutic blood levels.

Intravenous preparations should be administered slowly to prevent thrombophlebitis and electrolyte abnormalities. Administration of penicillin salts warrants close observation of the client for signs of hyperkalemia (potassium penicillins) or hypernatremia (sodium penicillins). Daily review of laboratory data is essential to identify any potential problems.

Alternate intramuscular sites should be chosen to prevent generalized soreness and sterile abscess formation. Injection sites should be carefully recorded to avoid injecting the same site twice in a short period of time.

Since oral penicillins are poorly absorbed from the gastrointestinal tract, they should be administered one hour before or two hours after meals. In addition, some penicillins decompose in a fruit juice medium; therefore, administration with fruit juice is discouraged. All penicillin preparations should be given on time and around-the-clock to sustain the level of the drug in the bloodstream.

Intrathecal administration of penicillin salts is infrequent; however, its therapeutic efficacy in the treatment of meningitis has been noted, since high levels of the drug may be achieved in the cerebrospinal fluid. The nursing responsibility is to check neurologic response and to observe for muscle twitching and other signs of central nervous system stimulation.

Care of the intravenous site is extremely important particularly when the client is receiving a course of antibiotic therapy. Dextrose solutions act as a media for growth of fungi and intravenous sites have an affinity for opportunist organisms. The insertion site should be rotated every 72 hours and the auxiliary intravenous units changed every 24 hours. Solution-saturated dressings should be removed immediately to inhibit bacterial growth.

NATURAL PENICILLINS

GENERIC NAME Penicillin G potassium (injection)

TRADE NAME Pfizerpen (RX)

CLASSIFICATION Antibiotic

Action Penicillin G potassium is a bactericidal antibiotic derived from various penicillin species *(Penicillium chrysogenum).* It is effective against gram-positive streptococci, pneumococci, nonpenicillinase-producing staphylococci, some spirochetes, and some gram-positive rods. It is particularly useful against *Diplococcus pneumoniae, Neisseria meningitidis, N. gonorrhoeae, Clostridium tetani, C. perfringens, Corynebacterium diphtheriae, Actinomyces,* group A beta-hemolytic streptococci, *Treponema pallidum,* and nonpenicillinase-producing *Staphylococcus aureus.* The drug acts by inhibiting biosynthesis of cell wall mucopeptide.

Indications for Use Severe infections caused by sensitive pathogens (syphilis, gonorrhea, hemolytic *Streptococcus* infections, diphtheria, certain pneumonias).

Contraindications Hypersensitivity to penicillins or cephalosporins.

Warnings and Precautions Use with caution in clients with a history of anaphylaxis, allergies, bronchial asthma, hay fever, and allergic reactions to other drugs, impairment of renal or hepatic function, and during pregnancy and lactation.

Untoward Reactions Allergic reactions include anaphylaxis, drug fever, maculopapular rash, urticaria, ulceration of mucous membranes, serum sickness, and eosinophilia; rashes are the most common reaction. Hyperkalemia can occur in clients receiving large dosages or prolonged therapy, particularly when renal function is impaired. Arrhythmias, CNS disturbances, and other related symptoms can occur. Blood dyscrasias, including hemolytic anemia (with a positive Coombs' test), thrombocytopenia, and agranulocytosis, can occur, particularly in clients receiving large dosages or prolonged therapy. Neurologic disturbances, including hallucinations, disorientation, convulsions, and delirium, can occur, particularly in clients receiving large dosages. Elderly clients and clients with renal insufficiency or a preexisting neurologic impairment are particularly susceptible. GI disturbances include nausea, vomiting, diarrhea, and abdominal cramps. Superinfections can occur, particularly by penicillin-resistant organisms *(Candida, Proteus, Pseudomonas).* Other untoward reactions include pain at the injection site, phlebitis, and polyarthritis.

Parameters of Use

Absorption Rapidly absorbed from intramuscular sites. About 50 to 60% bound to plasma proteins. Does not cross blood-brain barrier unless the meninges are inflamed. Half-life is 30 minutes. Peak plasma levels occur in 15 to 30 minutes. Duration of action is 2 to 5 hours.

Crosses placenta and enters breast milk.

Distribution Widely distributed to body tissues.

Excretion By the kidneys as unchanged drug and conjugates; some excreted in saliva and via bile in feces.

Drug Interactions Hyperkalemia may result if potassium-sparing diuretics (spironolactone, triamterene) are given concurrently. Hemorrhage due to heparin toxicity may result if penicillin IV is discontinued abruptly in clients receiving concurrent therapy with penicillin IV and heparin; intravenous penicillin inihibits the action of heparin. Penicillin potentiates coumarin and its derivatives; use with caution concurrently. Analgesics, particularly aspirin and pyrazolone derivatives, displace penicillin from protein-binding sites and interfere with the renal excretion of penicillin, thus potentiating the effects of penicillin. *p*-Aminohippuric acid elevates serum and cerebrospinal fluid levels of penicillin. Probenecid interferes with the renal excretion of penicillin, thus prolonging serum drug levels (duration). The following antibiotics inhibit or antagonize the bactericidal action of penicillin: actinomycin D, paromomycin, kanamycin, erythromycin. However, kanamycin and erythromycin may potentiate the action of penicillin against *Brucella abortus* and *Staphylococcus aureus,* respectively. The following antibiotics potentiate the bactericidal action of penicillin: streptomycin, sulfinpyrazone, some sulfonamides. The muscle relaxant and mild sedative chlorphenesin carbamate may reduce hypersensitivity reactions to penicillin.

Laboratory Interactions Large dosages may produce false-positive results for urinary glucose and protein with certain reagents. Clinitest, Clinistix, Tes-Tape, and Ames reagent are not affected.

Administration

Highly individualized.

- *Severe infections:* 5 to 10 million units IM or IV daily in divided doses; Dosage range: 300,000 to 20 million units for 10 days to 6 weeks.
- *Meningococcic meningitis:* Intramuscular: 1 to 2 million units q2h; Intravenous: 20 to 30 million units daily via continuous IV drip.
- *Bacteremia:* 20 to 80 million units daily via continuous IV drip.

Available Drug Forms

Multidose vials containing 1 million units for reconstitution with: 9.6 ml of diluent to yield 1 million U/ml; 4.6 ml to yield 200,000 U/ml; 3.6 ml to yield 250,000 U/ml. Multidose vials containing 5 million units for reconstitution with: 23 ml of diluent to yield 200,000 U/ml; 18 ml to yield 250,000 U/ml; 8 ml to yield 500,000 U/ml; 3 ml to yield 1 million U/ml. Multidose vials containing 10 million units for reconstitution with: 15.5 ml of diluent to yield 500,000 U/ml; 5.4 ml to yield 1 million U/ml. Multidose vials containing 20 million units for reconstitution with 31.6 ml of diluent to yield 500,000 U/ml. There is 1.7 mEq of potassium in 1 million units of penicillin potassium.

Nursing Management

Planning factors

1. Complete culture and sensitivity tests before instituting therapy.
2. Penicillin G is not penicillinase resistant.
3. Obtain complete blood cell count (CBC) and serum electrolytes prior to initiating therapy. Notify physician if serum potassium is elevated, since another penicillin (sodium penicillin G) may be preferred.
4. Check for hypersensitivity (allergy) before administering drug.
5. Clients with impaired renal function require reduced dosages.

Administration factors

1. IM injections may cause pain at injection site. Inject deep into large muscle mass and rotate sites.
2. Reconstitute with the appropriate amount of sterile water or normal saline. Label vial with date, time of reconstitution, and concentration. Refrigerate unused portion.
3. Do not use solutions reconstituted 7 or more days ago.
4. IV infusion is recommended for dosages of 10 million units/day or more.
5. When administering IV,
   (a) Add reconstituted solution to a compatible IV solution, such as sodium chloride. Penicillin G will deteriorate rapidly in alkaline dextrose solutions (5% D/W), lactated Ringer's, and IV solutions containing sodium bicarbonate, aminophylline, and vitamins B and C. Check incompatibilities.
   (b) Check patency of IV before starting infusion.
   (c) Do not give via IV bolus. Dosages of 1 million units or less can be administered over 1 hour via intermittent IV infusion; however, continuous IV drip is recommended.
   (d) Administer slowly to prevent CNS toxicity and other untoward reactions precipitated by hyperkalemia. An infusion pump is recommended, but a carefully observed IV microdrip administration set can be used.
   (e) Give each continuous IV infusion within 24 hours, since penicillin G is unstable at room temperature after that length of time.
   (f) Change the IV tubing and the in-line filter every 24 hours to ensure the elimination of endotoxin-producing bacteria that may pass through an outdated filter.

Evaluation factors

1. Observe client continuously for at least 30 minutes for hypersensitivity (allergic) reaction when therapy is first initiated. An erythema or wheal and irritation at the injection site may precede a systemic allergic reaction. If a reaction occurs, notify physician and institute measures according to agency protocol.
2. If drug is administered on an outpatient basis, retain client for at least 30 minutes. Examine client before discharging.
3. Check for CNS toxicity and hyperkalemia frequently, particularly during peak drug levels. If a reaction occurs, decrease IV rate to KVO and notify physician.
4. Determine serum electrolytes daily. If potassium is elevated, notify physician immediately.
5. Continue therapy for at least 2 days after client has become asymptomatic or cultures are negative. Therapy is usually maintained for at least 10 days.
6. Large dosages administered for a prolonged time may cause blood dyscrasias.
7. Monitor, CBC, creatinine, blood urea nitrogen, and other tests indicative of hematologic, renal, and hepatic function periodically (weekly) when prolonged therapy is required.
8. Examine client daily for superinfections. GI and vaginal infections are common. (Candidiasis may be prevented by eating yogurt.)
9. After treating a client for an allergic reaction,
   (a) Instruct client never to take any type of penicillin. Suggest the wearing of an ID band or tag (or the carrying of a card) that indicates the allergy.
   (b) Clearly indicate the allergy on the outside of the client's chart, kardex, and medication record.

GENERIC NAME Penicillin G potassium (oral)

TRADE NAMES Pentids, Pfizerpen G, SK-Penicillin G

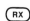

CLASSIFICATION Antibiotic (RX)

See penicillin G potassium (injection) for Contraindications and Warnings and precautions.

Action

This drug is bactericidal against penicillin-sensitive organisms during the reproduction stage. It acts by inhibiting biosynthesis of cell wall mucopeptide. It is neither stable in gastric acid or resistant to penicillinase. [See penicillin G potassium (injection).]

Indications for Use Mild to moderately severe infections; particularly effective against group A *Streptococcus* if no bacteremia is present (scarlet fever); skin and soft tissue infections; streptococcal pharyngitis; pneumococcal upper respiratory tract infections and otitis media also respond well; prophylaxis against the recurrence of rheumatic fever or chorea, bacterial endocarditis, and bacteremia following tooth extraction. (Not effective against resistant strains of *Staphylococcus aureus*, group D *Enterococcus*, meningitis, pneumonia, empyema, bacteremia, pericarditis, and septic arthritis in the acute stage.)

Untoward Reactions Less toxic than parenteral penicillin G potassium. GI disturbances, including nausea, vomiting, epigastric discomfort, diarrhea, abdominal cramps, black hairy tongue, and sore mouth and tongue, are relatively common. Most GI disturbances are due to superinfections. Although hypersensitivity reactions, including anaphylaxis, have occurred in clients on oral penicillin, the incidence is rare compared to parenteral penicillin. The most common hypersensitivity reactions after oral penicillin include skin rashes, urticaria, fever, and eosinophilia. Serum sickness reactions (chills, fever, edema, joint pains), laryngeal edema, and anaphylaxis have occurred, but rarely. [See penicillin G potassium (injection).]

Parameters of Use

Absorption About one third is absorbed from the duodenum in 30 to 60 minutes. Gastric pH of 2.0 may totally inactivate the drug (normal pH is 2.0 to 3.5). Gastric acidity, stomach emptying time, the presence of food, and other factors affect absorption. About 60% bound to serum proteins. Half-life is 30 minutes.

Crosses placenta and enters breast milk.

Distribution Tissue content varies widely. Highest in kidneys. Found in liver, skin, and intestines.

Excretion Rapidly excreted by normal functioning kidneys as unchanged drug (20%) and conjugates.

Drug Interactions Antacids decrease the absorption of oral penicillin by increasing the ionization of penicillin; do not administer concurrently. Orally administered neomycin inhibits the absorption of oral penicillin. [See penicillin G potassium (injection).]

Administration Highly individualized. Adults and children over 12 years: 500 to 1000 mg (800,000 to 1.6 million units) po daily in divided doses. Children: Under 12 years: 15 to 56 mg/kg po daily in 3 to 6 divided doses.

Available Drug Forms Uncoated scored tablets (Pentids) containing 125 mg (200,000 U), 250 mg (400,000 U), or 500 mg (800,000 U). Tablets (SK-Penicillin G) containing 400,000 or 800,000 units. Scored tablets buffered with calcium carbonate (Pfizerpen G) containing 200,000, 250,000, 400,000, or 800,000 units. Fruit-flavored powder (Pentids) for reconstitution to an oral syrup containing 125 mg (200,000 U) or 250 mg (400,000 U) in 5 ml. Oral solution containing 200,000 or 400,000 units/5 ml.

Nursing Management [See penicillin G potassium (injection).]

Planning factors

Schedule drug administration around-the-clock. Be sure that the times are at least 1 hour before meals or 2 hours after meals, so that gastric acidity will not destroy drug before it is absorbed.

Administration factors

1. Reconstitute syrup with the appropriate amount of sterile water. Label container with date, time of reconstitution, and concentration.
2. Store unused portion in refrigerator.
3. Do not use syrup reconstituted 2 weeks or more ago.
4. Give with a full glass of water, preferably on an empty stomach; avoid administering with fruit juices or food, as these alter absorption or inactivate the drug.

Evaluation factors

1. Check complete blood cell count (eosinophil count) 5 to 7 days following the onset of therapy to determine if a hypersensitivity reaction is occurring.
2. Obtain culture and sensitivity tests for clients with streptococcal pharyngitis 7 days following completion of therapy.
3. A urine culture 10 days after completion of drug therapy for a streptococcal infection is also advised to ensure eradication of the organism from the kidneys.

Client teaching factors

1. Instruct client to report the presence of rashes or other untoward reactions immediately to physician.
2. Determine the best schedule for drug administration with client.
3. Instruct client to avoid taking drug with fruit juices or food.
4. Instruct client to store tablets in a cool, dark place, and syrup in refrigerator.
5. Suggest that female clients eat yogurt at least once a day to prevent vaginitis superinfection.
6. Emphasize the need to continue therapy for the prescribed time period (10 days) even if symptoms have disappeared.

GENERIC NAME Penicillin G sodium (RX)

TRADE NAME Sodium Penicillin G

CLASSIFICATION Antibiotic

See penicillin G potassium (injection) for Indications for use, Contraindications, Warnings and precautions, and Parameters of use.

Action Bactericidal antibiotic similar to parenteral penicillin G potassium, but prepared as the sodium salt. [See penicillin G potassium (injection).]

Untoward Reactions Hypernatremia can occur in clients receiving large dosages or prolonged therapy, particularly the elderly and when cardiac, respiratory, or renal function is impaired. [See penicillin G potassium (injection).]

Drug Interactions Potassium-sparing diuretics can be used concurrently. [See penicillin G potassium (injection).]

Administration 5 to 80 million units daily IM or continuous IV drip. Dosage is highly individualized and depends on severity and type of infection.

Available Drug Forms Multidose vials containing 5 million units of crystalline powder.

Nursing Management Observe for symptoms of hypernatremia (peripheral edema, weight gain, puffy eyelids, distended hand and neck veins, ascites). A low or normal hematocrit and decreased plasma proteins may indicate a hypernatremic state. [See penicillin G potassium (injection).]

GENERIC NAME Penicillin G procaine (RX)

TRADE NAMES Abbocillin, Crysticillin A.S., Depo-Penicillin, Duracillin A.S., Lentopen, Pfizerpen A.S., Wycillin

CLASSIFICATION Antibiotic

See penicillin G potassium (injection) for Warnings and precautions and Untoward reactions.

Action This repository form of penicillin G exhibits prolonged action by providing a tissue depot from which the drug is slowly released and absorbed over a period of 12 to 24 hours to several days. Preparations of this drug have low solubility in body fluids and are dissolved in special vehicles (aqueous procaine and oily suspensions) to retard their absorption. The anesthetic effect of procaine lessens pain at injection sites. [See penicillin G potassium (injection).]

Indications for Use Mild to moderately severe infections that require continuous but low serum drug levels; prophylaxis against infection in clients with heart disease undergoing surgery or dental care; effective in the treatment of neurosyphilis when elevated blood levels are desired for 2 to 3 weeks. [See penicillin G potassium (oral).]

Contraindications Hypersensitivity to penicillins, cephalosporins, or procaine.

Parameters of Use

Absorption Very slowly absorbed from intramuscular depots. May be found in the bloodstream for as long as 4 to 5 days. Absorption rate is determined by the drug's solubility and the vehicle in which it is suspended. About 65% bound to plasma proteins. Half-life, peak plasma levels, and duration of action are determined by drug's solubility and vehicle.

Crosses placenta and enters breast milk.

Distribution Widely distributed to body tissues.

Excretion By the kidneys; some excreted in saliva and via bile in feces.

Drug Interactions Avoid current use of other bacteriostatic agents (tetracycline, sulfonamides), since penicillin is active against multiplying organisms. Aqueous penicillin may be mixed with procaine to provide immediate and prolonged effects. [See penicillin G potassium (injection).]

Administration Highly individualized. Adults: 600,000 units IM daily or bid; Dosage range: 300,000 to 1,200,000 units. Children: Up to 10,000 units/kg daily for 10 days.

Available Drug Forms Individual sterile cartridge needle units (Tubex) containing 300,000 U/ml, 600,000 U/ml, 1,200,000 U/2 ml, or 2,400,000 U/4 ml; prefilled sterile syringes containing 300,000 U/ml, 600,000 U/ml, 1,200,000 U/2 ml, or 2,400,000 U/4 ml; multidose vials containing 300,000 U/ml. The following types of penicillin G procaine are available:

1. Sterile penicillin G procaine suspension; provides a depot for long duration of effect.
2. Sterile penicillin G procaine with aluminum stearate suspended in peanut or sesame oil gelled by aluminum stearate; provides a depot for longest duration of effect.
3. Penicillin G procaine and penicillin G sodium for injection; produces rapid and high serum drug levels (from the aqueous solution) and provides a depot for prolonged duration of effect.

Nursing Management [See penicillin G potassium (injection).]

1. A test dose of procaine is recommended because a few clients are hypersensitive to this drug. Inject 0.1 ml of 1 or 2% procaine solution intradermally. Hypersensitivity is indicated if an erythema, wheal, or eruption occur at the injection site.
2. Shake multidose vials well before withdrawing dosage.
3. Before injecting, ensure that the thick suspension moves in the syringe when aspirating.
4. When administering IM, inject deep into muscle mass to facilitate deposition. Inject into the upper outer quadrant of the gluteus maximus for adults and the midlateral aspect of the thigh in children.
5. If blood is aspirated in the syringe and/or cartridge, do not inject; remove and discard drug. Choose an alternative site to administer fresh preparation.
6. Up to 2,400,000 units can be injected in one site; but no more than 1,200,000 units should be injected in one site whenever possible.
7. Store multidose vials, sterile syringes, and cartridges in refrigerator.
8. Never give intravenously. Injection into an artery or a peripheral vessel will cause neurovascular damage.

GENERIC NAME Penicillin G benzathine (RX)

TRADE NAMES Bicillin, Bicillin L-A, Permapen

CLASSIFICATION Antibiotic

See penicillin G potassium (injection) for Contraindications and Drug interactions.

Action Penicillin G benzathine is the longest acting penicillin G and has properties similar to parenteral penicillin G potassium. This diamine salt is highly insoluble in water and is converted to penicillin G by hydrolysis. Its relatively slow absorption provides low serum drug levels for a prolonged period of time. [See penicillin G potassium (injection).]

Indications for Use Mild to moderately severe infections of respiratory tract caused by penicillin G-sensitive organisms; venereal and nonvenereal diseases (syphilis, yaws, bejel, pinta); prophylaxis to prevent the recurrence of rheumatic fever and glomerulonephritis.

Warnings and Precautions Caution must be taken to prevent accidental injection into a blood vessel or nerve route as a pulmonary embolism or permanent nerve damage (paralysis) may result. [See penicillin G potassium (injection).]

Untoward Reactions Localized pain and irritation may occur at injection sites. Hypersensitivity (allergic) reactions may be severe and prolonged because of the slow release of the drug from its depot. [See penicillin G potassium (injection).]

Parameters of Use

Absorption Very slowly absorbed from intramuscular depots. Absorption rate is determined by the drug's solubility and the circulation at the injection site. May be found in bloodstream for as long as 4 weeks; Range: 1 to 4 weeks. About 60% bound to plasma proteins.

Crosses placenta and enters breast milk.

Distribution Widely distributed to body tissues.

Excretion By the kidneys; some excreted in saliva and via bile in feces.

Administration Highly individualized. Adults: Oral: 200,000 units po bid; Dosage range: 200,000 to 600,000 units bid, q4h, or q6h. Intramuscular: 1,200,000 units once a month; Dosage range: 600,000 to 1,200,000 units once a month or as often as twice a week. Children: Over 60 lb: 900,000 units as a single dose; Under 60 lb: 50,000 units/kg as a single dose; Dosage range: 300,000 to 600,000 units as a single dose.

Available Drug Forms Tablets containing 200,000 units; individual sterile cartridge needle units (Tubex) containing 600,000 U/ml; prefilled cartridges containing 1 ml (600,000 U), 1.5 ml (900,000 U), 2 ml (1,200,000 U), or 4 ml (2,400,000 U); multidose vials containing 300,000 U/ml.

Nursing Management [See penicillin G potassium (injection).]

1. Medical costs are reduced by the decreased need for repeated injections.
2. The midlateral thigh is the preferred site of injection.
3. Relatively stable at the normal pH of gastric acid. Food intake does not interfere with absorption.

GENERIC NAME Penicillin G benzathine/penicillin G procaine

TRADE NAMES Bicillin C-R, Bicillin C-R 900/300

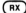

CLASSIFICATION Antibiotic (RX)

See penicillin G potassium (injection) for Action, Indications for use, Contraindications, Warnings and precautions, Untoward reactions, Drug interactions, and Nursing management.

Administration *Bicillin C-R:* Adults: 1,200,000 to 2,400,000 units as a single dose; Children: 30 to 60 lb: 900,000 units as a single dose; Under 30 lb: 600,000 units as a single dose; dose may be repeated in 2 or 3 days, as needed. *Bicillin C-R 900/300:* Adults: 1,200,000 units as a single dose; dose may be repeated in 2 or 3 days, as needed.

Available Drug Forms *Bicillin C-R:* Multidose vials containing 300,000 to 600,000 U/ml; sterile cartridge needle units. *Bicillin C-R 900/300:* Sterile cartridge needle units containing 1,200,000 U/2 ml.

ACID-RESISTANT PENICILLINS

GENERIC NAMES Penicillin V; penicillin V hydrabamine; penicillin V benzathine

TRADE NAMES Pen Vee, V-Cillin; Compocillin-V; Pen-Vee Suspension

CLASSIFICATION Antibiotic (RX)

Action Penicillin V (phenoxymethyl penicillin) inhibits the biosynthesis of cell wall mucopeptide in penicillin-sensitive organisms when they are in the stage of multiplication. Penicillin V is resistant to inactivation by gastric acid and produces higher serum drug levels than penicillin G; but is inactivated by penicillinase. Since the salts of penicillin V (penicillin V potassium) are more readily absorbed and can produce even higher serum drug levels than this parent compound, the salts are used more frequently. May be less effective than penicillin G against severe pneumonia, empyema, bacteremia, pericarditis, meningitis, and arthritis.

Indications for Use Mild to moderately severe infections caused by penicillin-sensitive organisms, including upper respiratory tract infections, scarlet fever, erysipelas, otitis media, Vincent's gingivitis, and pharyngitis; prophylaxis to prevent the recurrence of rheumatic fever; prophylaxis against bacterial endocarditis in susceptible clients (heart disease) undergoing surgery or dental care.

Contraindications Hypersensitivity to penicillins or cephalosporins.

Warnings and Precautions Use with caution in clients with a history of anaphylaxis, allergies, bronchial asthma, hay fever, and allergic reactions to other drugs and those with impaired renal or hepatic function.

Untoward Reactions GI disturbances, including nausea, vomiting, epigastric distress, diarrhea, and black hairy tongue, are common. Superinfections caused by penicillin-resistant organisms, such as *Candida, Proteus,* and *Pseudomonas,* can occur. Hypersensitivity (allergic) reactions are relatively rare with oral penicillin. Skin rashes, urticaria, serum sickness reaction, laryngeal edema, and anaphylaxis have occurred. Fever and eosinophilia may be the only symptoms of hypersensitivity. Blood dyscrasias, including hemolytic anemia, leukopenia, and thrombocytopenia, have occurred in clients receiving large dosages or prolonged therapy; but the disorders are usually associated with parenteral penicillin. Rare reactions include neuropathy and nephropathy.

Parameters of Use

Absorption Rapidly absorbed from GI tract; not affected by food or normal gastric pH (2.0 to 3.5). Up to 80% bound to serum proteins.

Distribution Widely distributed to body tissues, but only small quantities enter cerebrospinal fluid.

Excretion By the kidneys; some excreted in saliva and via bile in feces.

Drug Interactions Antacids decrease the absorption of oral penicillin by increasing the ionization of penicillin; do not administer concurrently. Orally administered neomycin inhibits the absorption of oral penicillin. Penicillin potentiates coumarin and its derivatives; use with caution concurrently. Analgesics, particularly aspirin and pyrazolone derivatives, displace penicillin from protein-binding sites and interfere with the renal excretion of penicillin, thus potentiating the effects of penicillin. *p*-Aminohippuric acid elevates serum and cerebrospinal fluid levels of penicillin. Probenecid interferes with the renal excretion of penicillin, thus prolonging serum drug levels (duration). The following antibiotics inhibit or antagonize the bactericidal action of penicillin: actinomycin D, paromomycin, kanamycin, and erythromycin. However, kanamycin and erythromycin may potentiate the action of penicillin against *Brucella abortus* and *Staphylococcus aureus* respectively. The following antibiotics potentiate the bactericidal action of penicillin: Streptomycin, sulfinpyrazone, some sulfonamides. The muscle relaxant and mild sedative chlorphenesin carbamate may reduce hypersensitivity reactions to penicillin.

Administration Highly individualized. Usual dosage: 250 mg po q6h; Dosage range: 500 to 2000 mg daily.

Available Drug Forms Tablets containing 125, 250, or 500 mg; oral suspension containing 125 mg/5 ml.

Nursing Management

Planning factors

1. Complete culture and sensitivity tests before instituting therapy.
2. Obtain complete blood cell count (CBC) and serum electrolytes prior to initiating therapy. Obtain blood urea nitrogen (BUN) and creatinine as well in geriatric clients.
3. Check for hypersensitivity (allergy) before administering drug.
4. Schedule drug administration around-the-clock to sustain therapeutic drug levels.

Administration factors

1. Reconstitute suspension with the appropriate amount of sterile water. Label container with date, time of reconstitution, and concentration.
2. Store unused suspension in refrigerator.
3. Do not use suspension reconstituted more than 2 weeks ago.
4. Shake suspension vigorously before measuring dosage.
5. Give with a full glass of water, preferably on an empty stomach, but this is not essential.

Evaluation factors

1. Check CBC (eosinophil count) 5 to 7 days after the onset of therapy to determine if a hypersensitivity reaction is occurring.
2. Obtain culture and sensitivity tests for clients with streptococcal pharyngitis 7 days following completion of therapy.
3. Check creatinine, BUN, and CBC weekly in clients on prolonged therapy.

Client teaching factors

1. Instruct client to report immediately the presence of rashes or other untoward effects.
2. Determine with client the most appropriate administration schedule.
3. Instruct client to avoid ingesting the drug with food or juices.
4. Store suspension in refrigerator.
5. Instruct female clients to eat yogurt once a day to prevent vaginal superinfections.
6. Emphasize the need to continue drug therapy for the prescribed 10 to 14 days, even though symptoms subside earlier.

GENERIC NAME Penicillin V potassium (RX)

TRADE NAMES Betapen-VK, Compocillin-VK, Ledercillin VK, Penapar VK, Penicillin VK, Pen Vee K, Pfizerpen VK, Robicillin VK, SK-Penicillin VK, Uticillin VK, V-Cillin K, Veetids

CLASSIFICATION Antibiotic

See penicillin V for Indications for use, Contraindications, Warnings and precautions, Untoward reactions, and Drug interactions.

Action The potassium salt of penicillin V is more readily absorbed from the GI tract and produces even higher serum drug levels than the parent compound. It is bactericidal against penicillin-sensitive organisms during the stage of active reproduction. The drug acts by inhibiting biosynthesis of cell wall mucopeptide. It is stable at normal gastric acidity (pH of 2.0 to 3.5); but is inactivated by penicillinase. The drug is effective against many gram-positive streptococci, pneumococci, nonpenicillinase-producing staphylococci, some spirochetes, and some gram-positive rods. May not be effective against severe pneumonia, empyema, bacteremia, pericarditis, meningitis, and arthritis. Some staphylococci are resistant to penicillin V.

Parameters of Use

Absorption Rapidly absorbed from GI tract; not affected by normal gastric acidity (pH of 2.0 to 3.5). Produces serum drug levels that are 2 to 5 times greater than those achieved by penicillin G. About 80% bound to serum proteins. Half-life is 30 minutes. Peak plasma levels occur in 30 to 60 minutes. Duration of action is about 6 hours.

Distribution Widely distributed to body tissues. Highest levels are found in the kidneys. Also found in liver, skin, and intestines. Only small amounts found in cerebrospinal fluid.

Excretion As rapid as absorption in clients with normal kidneys.

Administration Highly individualized.

- *Infections:* 125 to 500 mg po every 6 to 8 hours.
- *Prophylaxis for surgery:* Adults: 2 g po 1 hour prior to surgery; then 500 mg q6h times 8 doses after surgery. Children: 1 g po 1 hour prior to surgery; then 250 mg q6h times 8 doses after surgery.

Available Drug Forms Tablets containing 125 mg (200,000 U), 250 mg (400,000 U), or 500 mg (800,000 U); coated tablets containing 125 or 250 mg; powder for reconstitution to an oral suspension containing 125 mg/5 ml (200,000 U) or 250 mg/5 ml (400,000 U); powder for reconstitution to an oral solution containing 125 or 250 mg/5 ml; flavored granules for reconstitution to an oral solution containing 125 or 250 mg/5 ml.

Nursing Management

1. Dental care must be given concurrently in clients with Vincent's gingivitis (trench mouth) in order for therapy to be effective.
2. Oral penicillin is not recommended for prophylaxis in clients undergoing genitourinary instrumentation or surgery, lower intestinal tract surgery, sigmoidoscopy, or childbirth. (See penicillin V.)

GENERIC NAME Phenethicillin potassium (RX)

TRADE NAMES Alpen, Chemipen, Darcil, Dramcillin-250, Maxipen, Ro-Cillin, Syncillin

CLASSIFICATION Antibiotic

See penicillin V for Indications for use, Contraindications, Warnings and Precautions, Untoward reactions, and Drug interactions.

Action This semisynthetic antibiotic is similar to penicillin V in its properties, including stability in the gastric acid of the stomach. It is said to have some resistance to degradation by penicillinase and to produce very high serum drug levels, almost twice as high as an equal quantity of penicillin V after oral administration. It is active against streptococci, *Diplococcus pneumoniae, Neisseria,* and *Staphylococcus aureus.*

Parameters of Use

Absorption Incomplete from GI tract. About 40 to 50% absorbed from upper intestinal tract. Peak levels occur in 1 hour. About 80% bound to serum proteins.

Excretion About 30% excreted by normal kidneys.

Administration Adults: 125 to 250 mg po every 6 to 8 hours; Children and infants 12.5 to 50 mg/kg po daily.

Available Drug Forms Tablets containing 125 or 250 mg; powder for reconstitution to an oral solution containing 125 mg/ml.

Nursing Management Give with a full glass of water 1 hour before meals or 2 hours after meals. (See penicillin V.)

PENICILLINASE-RESISTANT PENICILLINS

GENERIC NAME Methicillin sodium (RX)

TRADE NAMES Azapen, Celbenin, Democillin, Staphcillin

CLASSIFICATION Antibiotic

Action Methicillin sodium is a semisynthetic salt of penicillin. It was the first bactericidal penicillin found to be resistant to staphylococcal penicillinase, including that produced by *Staphylococcus aureus.* However, methicillin cannot be administered orally because it is not acid resistant. It is less effective than penicillin G against streptococci and pneumococci, but is somewhat effective against pneumococcal infections. It is also effective against group A beta-hemolytic streptococci and susceptible staphylococci resistant to penicillin G. The number of methicillin-resistant strains of staphylococci has increased over the years and has prompted the limited use of methicillin to known susceptible organisms. It has also been demonstrated that methicillin-resistant strains are almost always resistant to other penicillinase-resistant penicillins and to several of the cephalosporin derivatives (cross-resistance).

Indications for Use Moderate to severe infections caused by penicillinase-producing staphylococci; initial therapy against infections that may be staphylococci in nature until results of culture and sensitivity tests are available. (General use of methicillin is not recommended.)

Contraindications Hypersensitivity to penicillins or cephalosporins.

Warnings and Precautions Use with caution in clients with a history of anaphylaxis, allergies, bronchial asthma, hay fever, and allergic reactions to other drugs and those with impairment of renal or hepatic function. Also use with caution in infants as they have incompletely developed renal functions and will excrete the drug slowly, thus resulting in abnormally high serum drug levels. Safe use during pregnancy has not been established. Not recommended for infants and during lactation.

Untoward Reactions Allergic reactions include anaphylaxis, drug fever, maculopapular rash, urticaria, ulceration of mucous membranes, serum sickness, and eosinophilia; rashes are the most common reaction. Blood dyscrasias, including hemolytic anemia, transient neutropenia, granulocytopenia, and thrombocytopenia, have been reported, particularly in clients receiving large dosages or prolonged therapy. Methicillin is more likely to cause blood dyscrasias than other penicillins. Neurologic disturbances, including hallucinations, disorientation, convulsions, and delirium, can occur, particularly in clients receiving large dosages. Elderly clients and clients with renal insufficiency or a preexisting neurologic impairment are particularly susceptible. Nephrotoxicity with resulting oliguria, albuminuria, hematuria, pyuria, or cylindruria can occur, particularly in clients receiving large dosages. Superinfections caused by fungi and penicillin-resistant bacteria, including oral and rectal monilia can occur, particularly in clients receiving prolonged therapy. Other untoward reactions include irritation and pain at intramuscular injection sites and thrombophlebitis following intravenous administration.

Parameters of Use

Absorption Readily absorbed from intramuscular sites; destroyed in gastric juices if taken orally. About 40% bound to plasma proteins. Peak plasma levels occur in: 30 to 60 minutes (IM); 15 to 30 minutes (IV). Plasma levels begin to decline in: 4 hours (IM); 2 hours (IV).

Crosses placenta and enters breast milk.

Distribution Widely distributed to body tissues. Diffuses into pleural, pericardial, and synovial fluids; little drug is found in cerebrospinal fluid unless the meninges are inflamed.

Excretion Rapidly by the kidneys as unchanged drug; small amount excreted in saliva and via bile in feces.

Drug Interactions Hemorrhage due to heparin toxicity may result if methicillin IV is discontinued abruptly in clients receiving concurrent therapy with methicillin IV and heparin; intravenous methicillin inhibits the action of heparin. Methicillin potentiates coumarin and its derivatives; use with caution concurrently. The following antibiotics inhibit or antagonize the bactericidal action of methicillin: chloramphenicol, erythromycin, kanamycin, tetracyclines. The following antibiotics potentiate the bactericidal action of methicillin: ampicillin, penicillin G potassium. Concomitant use of natural and semisynthetic penicillins produces a synergistic effect against *Streptococcus pyogenes* and *Staphylococcus aureus*. *p*-Aminohippuric acid elevates serum and cerebrospinal fluid levels of methicillin. Probenecid interferes with the renal excretion of methicillin, thus prolonging serum drug levels (duration).

Laboratory Interactions None reported.

Administration Highly individualized. Adults: Intramuscular: 1 g every 4 to 6 hours; Intravenous: 1 g q6h in 50 ml of sodium chloride given at 10 ml/min. or less. Children: 25 mg/kg IM q6h.

Available Drug Forms Vials containing 1 g for reconstitution with 1.5 ml of sterile water for injection or Sodium Chloride Injection to yield 500 mg/ml; vials containing 4 g for reconstitution with 5.7 ml of diluent to yield 500 mg/ml; vials containing 6 g for reconstitution with 8.6 ml of diluent to yield 500 mg/ml; piggyback IV packages with vials containing 1 or 4 g. There is 3.0 mEq of sodium in each gram of methicillin sodium.

Nursing Management

Planning factors

1. Complete culture and sensitivity tests before instituting therapy.
2. Obtain complete blood cell count (CBC) and serum electrolytes prior to initiating therapy.
3. Determine adequacy of renal function before instituting therapy.
4. Check for hypersensitivity (allergy) before administering drug.

Administration factors

1. Reconstitute with the appropriate amount of sterile water or normal saline. Label vial with date, time of reconstitution, and concentration. Shake vial vigorously and check to see that all powder is dissolved before withdrawing the desired amount.
2. Refrigerate unused portion.
3. Do not use solutions stored at room temperature after 24 hours. Refrigerated solutions can be used for 4 days.
4. When administering IM,
   (a) Inject deep into large muscle mass. (The intragluteal site is recommended.)
   (b) Rotate injection sites.
   (c) Observe previous injection sites for irritation prior to each administration.
   (d) The application of moist heat to previous injection sites may decrease the pain and irritation; do not apply heat to present site of injection.
5. When administering IV,
   (a) Add reconstituted solution to a compatible IV solution, such as sodium chloride or 5% D/W. Concentrated IV solutions (2 mg/ml) deteriorate within 4 hours at room temperature. Dilute solutions (10 to 30 mg/ml) are stable for 8 hours at room temperature.
   (b) Do not mix with other drugs. Methicillin is incompatible with several drugs, including aminophylline, sodium bicarbonate, antibiotics, and vitamin B-complex.

(c) Check patency of IV before starting infusion.
(d) Give intermittent infusions at a rate of 10 ml/min. or less.
(e) Administer slowly to prevent untoward reactions. An infusion pump is recommended, but a carefully observed microdrip IV administration set can be used.
(f) Rotation of IV sites every 72 hours may prevent the emergence of phlebitis.

Evaluation factors

1. Observe client continuously for hypersensitivity reaction when therapy is first initiated. If a reaction occurs, notify physician and institute measures according to agency protocol.
2. Check serum drug levels daily in infants to prevent toxicity.
3. Check adequacy of urinary output and urinalysis frequently (every 3 to 7 days). Nephrotoxicity (interstitial nephritis) may develop within 1 to 4 weeks after initiating therapy. If symptoms occur, notify physician immediately.
4. Check CBC and hepatic function frequently (once a week). If eosinophilia, anemia, or other untoward reactions occur, notify physician.
5. Continue therapy for 2 days after the client has become asymptomatic (afrebrile, negative cultures).
6. Serious systemic infections may require therapy for 1 to 2 weeks after the client has become asymptomatic (an oral penicillinase-resistant penicillin may be used).
7. Determine serum electrolytes daily. If sodium is elevated, notify physician.
8. Examine client daily for superinfections. Oral and rectal infections are relatively common.
9. After treating a client for an allergic reaction,
   (a) Instruct client never to take any type of penicillin. Suggest the wearing of an ID band or tag (or the carrying of a card) that indicates the allergy.
   (b) Clearly indicate the allergy on the outside of the client's chart, kardex and medication record.

GENERIC NAME Nafcillin sodium (RX)

TRADE NAMES Nafcil, Unipen

CLASSIFICATION Antibiotic

See methicillin sodium for Indications for use and Contraindications.

Action This semisynthetic bactericidal penicillin is resistant to acid and penicillinase. Nafcillin is used almost exclusively for penicillin G-resistant staphylococci (*Staphylococcus aureus*) and nafcillin-sensitive streptococci infections. Although it is effective against pneumococci and group A beta-hemolytic streptococci, it is seldom used for these infections.

Warnings and Precautions Oral nafcillin should not be relied upon to treat severe infections or infections in clients with hypermotility (diarrhea) or other GI disturbances. (See methicillin sodium.)

Untoward Reactions Relatively nontoxic. Untoward reactions tend to be milder and less frequent than with methicillin. (See methicillin sodium.)

Parameters of Use

Absorption Irregularly absorbed from GI tract; food interferes with absorption. Well absorbed from intramuscular sites. Often poorly absorbed in clients with GI disturbances. About 90% bound to plasma proteins. Peak serum levels occur in: 30 to 60 minutes (po); 30 to 60 minutes (IM); within 15 minutes IV. Duration of action is 4 hours (po); 4 to 6 hours (IM); 2 to 4 hours (IV).

Crosses placenta and enters breast milk.

Excretion Approximately 85% as unchanged drug via bile. Enters enterohepatic circulation and is reabsorbed. About 13% is eliminated by the kidneys unchanged; safer to use in the presence of renal impairment than methicillin.

Drug Interactions Aspirin and sulfonamides displace nafcillin from protein-binding sites, thus potentiating its action; do not give concurrently. Blood concentrations of nafcillin may be tripled with concomitant use of probenecid. (See methicillin sodium.)

Administration Highly individualized. Adults: Oral: 25 to 1000 mg every 4 to 6 hours: Intramuscular: 500 mg every 4 to 6 hours; Intravenous: 500 mg q4h. Children: Oral: 25 to 50 mg/kg in 4 divided doses; Intramuscular: 10 to 25 mg/kg bid.

Available Drug Forms Oral solution containing 250 mg/5 ml; capsules containing 250 mg buffered with calcium carbonate; tablets containing 500 mg buffered with calcium carbonate; vials containing 500 mg for reconstitution with 1.7 ml of diluent to yield 2 ml of solution; vials containing 1 g for reconstitution with 3.4 ml of diluent to yield 4 ml of solution; vials containing 2 g for reconstitution with 6.8 ml of diluent to yield 8 ml of solution. There is 2.8 mEq of sodium in each gram of nafcillin sodium.

Nursing Management (See methicillin sodium.)

1. Give oral dose 1 hour before or 2 hours after meals. Do not use oral forms for severe infections.
2. Monitor urine for potassium loss.
3. Use midlateral or anterolateral thigh sites for IM injections in children under 2 years or children with underdeveloped gluteal muscles.

GENERIC NAME Oxacillin sodium (RX)

TRADE NAMES Bactocill, Prostaphlin, Resistopen

CLASSIFICATION Antibiotic

See methicillin sodium for Indications for use, Contraindications, Warnings and precautions, and Drug interactions.

Action Oxacillin (semisynthetic isoxazolyl penicillin) is highly resistant to inactivation by penicillinase and can be administered orally, since it is relatively resistant to acid hydrolysis. It is more potent than methicillin, but the occurrence of allergic and other untoward reactions following parenteral administration has made oxacillin relatively risky to use against severe infections when compared to other penicillins. Although its therapeutic use is limited to penicillin G-resistant staphylococci infections, it is also effective against pneumococci, group A beta-hemolytic streptococci, and other staphylococci infections.

Untoward Reactions Allergic and other untoward reactions tend to be more frequent and more severe than with methicillin. (See methicillin sodium.)

Parameters of Use

Absorption Well absorbed from GI tract; food may interfere with absorption. About 90% bound to plasma proteins. Peak serum levels occur in 30 to 60 minutes. Duration of action is 4 hours. Half-life is 30 to 60 minutes.
Crosses placenta and enters breast milk.
Distribution Widely distributed to body tissues.
Excretion Rapidly by the kidneys as unchanged drug.

Administration Highly individualized. Adults: 500 mg po q4h; Dosage range: 1 to 12 g daily. Children: 50 to 100 mg/kg po daily in 6 divided doses.

Available Drug Forms Capsules containing 250 or 500 mg; oral solution containing 250 mg/5 ml. (Parenteral drug forms are no longer available.)

Nursing Management (See methicillin sodium.)

1. Observe client carefully for allergic reactions.
2. Oral solution is stable for 14 days when refrigerated and 3 days at room temperature.
3. Give 1 hour before or 2 hours after meals.

GENERIC NAME Cloxacillin sodium (RX)

TRADE NAMES Cloxapen, Tegopen

CLASSIFICATION Antibiotic

See methicillin sodium for Indications for use, Contraindications, Warnings and precautions, and Drug interactions.

Action Cloxacillin (semisynthetic isoxazolyl penicillin) is resistant to penicillinase and can be administered orally, since it is acid resistant. It produces higher serum drug levels, is less toxic, and results in fewer untoward reactions than oxacillin; but in other respects it is similar to its parent drug. (See oxacillin sodium for further details.)

Untoward Reactions GI disturbances, including nausea, epigastric discomfort, flatulence, and loose stools, have occurred. May elevate serum glutamic-oxaloacetic transaminase (less than 100 units). Hypersensitivity reactions, including wheezing, sneezing, pruritus, urticaria, rashes, and eosinophilia, have occurred occasionally. (See methicillin sodium.)

Parameters of Use

Absorption 95% bound to plasma proteins. Peak serum levels occur in 1 hour. Half-life is 30 to 60 minutes.
Crosses placenta and enters breast milk.
Distribution Widely distributed, with high concentrations in the kidneys and liver.
Excretion Primarily excreted in urine and bile as unchanged drug and metabolite.

Administration Highly individualized. Adults: 500 to 1000 mg po q6h; Children: Under 20 kg: 50 to 100 mg/kg po daily in 4 divided doses.

Available Drug Forms Capsules containing 250 or 500 mg; oral solution containing 125 mg/5 ml.

Nursing Management (See methicillin sodium.)

1. Oral solution is stable for 14 days when refrigerated and 3 days at room temperature.
2. Give 1 hour before meals or 2 hours after meals.

GENERIC NAME Dicloxacillin sodium (RX)

TRADE NAMES Dycill, Dynapen, Pathocil, Veracillin

CLASSIFICATION Antibiotic

See methicillin sodium for Indications for use, Contraindications, Warnings and precautions, and Drug interactions. See cloxacillin sodium for Parameters of use.

Action Dicloxacillin (semisynthetic isoxazolyl penicillin) is similar to cloxacillin and is resistant to both acid and penicillinase; therefore, it can be administered orally. Dicloxacillin is claimed to produce substantially higher serum drug levels than other oral penicillins. Besides being useful against penicillin G-resistant staphylococci, it is said to be effective against other commonly encountered gram-positive cocci.

Untoward Reactions GI disturbances, including nausea, vomiting, epigastric discomfort, flatulence, and loose stools have occurred. May elevate serum glutamic-oxaloacetic transaminase (less than 100 units). Hypersensitivity reactions, including wheezing, sneezing, pruritus, urticaria, rashes, and eosinophilia, have occurred. (See methicillin sodium.)

Administration Highly individualized. Adults: 125 to 250 mg po q6h; Children: Under 40 kg: 12.5 to 25 mg/kg po q6h.

Available Drug Forms Capsules containing 125, 250, or 500 mg; oral suspension containing 215 mg/5 ml.

Nursing Management (See methicillin sodium.)

1. Oral suspension is stable for 14 days when refrigerated.
2. Give 1 hour before meals or 2 hours after meals.

BROAD-SPECTRUM PENICILLINS

GENERIC NAMES Ampicillin; ampicillin sodium; ampicillin trihydrate

TRADE NAMES Amcill, Ampicillin, Omnipen, Pfizerpen-A, Polycillin, SK-Ampicillin; Omnipen-N, Polycillin-N, SK-Ampicillin-N; Ampicillin Trihydrate, Principen

CLASSIFICATION Antibiotic (RX)

Action Ampicillin (semisynthetic *D*-alpha-aminobenzyl penicillin) was the first penicillin produced with a broader spectrum of action than penicillin G. It is bactericidal against gram-positive organisms as well as some gram-negative bacteria and enterococci. It is specific for *Escherichia coli, Proteus mirabilis, Hemophilus influenzae,* non-penicillinase-producing staphylococci, *Diplococcus pneumoniae,* alpha- and beta-hemolytic streptococci, *Salmonella,* and *Shigella.* Unfortunately, several resistant organisms, particularly strains of *Salmonella* and *Shigella,* have developed since ampicillin was first released. It is also inactivated by penicillinase. Since ampicillin is relatively stable in gastric acid, it is effective when administered orally. However, severe infections caused by ampicillin-sensitive organisms require parenteral administration (ampicillin sodium).

Indications for Use Infections caused by sensitive gram-positive organisms, including streptococci, pneumococci, penicillin G-sensitive staphylococci, and enterococci; infections caused by sensitive gram-negative organisms, including *H. influenzae, E. coli, P. mirabilis, Neisseria gonorrhoeae, N. meningitidis,* and *Salmonella typhosa.* Frequently used for GI and genitourinary infections caused by gram-negative organisms.

Contraindications Hypersensitivity to penicillins or cephalosporins.

Warnings and Precautions Use with caution in clients with a history of anaphylaxis, allergies, bronchial asthma, hay fever, and allergic reactions to other drugs and those with impaired renal or hepatic function. Safe use during pregnancy has not been established. Do not use in clients with infectious mononucleosis (viral infection), since many of these clients will develop a rash.

Untoward Reactions Allergic (hypersensitivity) reactions include anaphylaxis (associated most frequently with parenteral administration), exfoliative dermatitis, erythema multiforme, skin rashes, urticaria, pseudomembranous colitis, Stevens-Johnson syndrome, and eosinophilia; rashes and urticaria are the most common reactions. A vesicular rash may develop in clients with impaired renal function; the rash does not indicate that other penicillins are contraindicated, since it may not be a true penicillin rash. GI disturbances include glossitis, stomatitis, black hairy tongue, nausea, vomiting, enterocolitis, and diarrhea; these reactions are usually associated with oral administration. Blood dyscrasias, including anemia, thrombocytopenic purpura, leukopenia, and agranulocytosis, have occurred, particularly in clients receiving large dosages or prolonged therapy; these reactions are usually reversible upon discontinuation of therapy. Superinfections can occur, particularly by penicillin-resistant organisms (*Candida, Proteus, Pseudomonas*). Moderate elevations in serum glutamic-oxaloacetic transaminase (SGOT) have occurred in infants and clients who receive intramuscular injections twice or more daily. The cause in infants is unknown, but may be related to their immature hepatic functioning. However, there is some evidence that repeated injections cause a release of SGOT from the muscles involved. Convulsions can occur if ampicillin is administered intravenously in less than 10 minutes. Other untoward reactions include pain and irritation at the injection site and phlebitis.

Parameters of Use

Absorption Fairly well absorbed from GI tract (approximately 50%). Well absorbed from intramuscular sites. About 20% bound to plasma proteins; least protein-bound drug of all the penicillins. Peak plasma levels occur in: 2 hours (po); 1 hour (IM); minutes (IV). Duration of action is: 8 hours (po); 8 hours (IM); 6 hours (IV). Half-life is about 90 minutes.

Crosses placenta and enters breast milk.

Distribution Widely distributed in body tissues. Does not enter cerebrospinal fluid unless the meninges are inflamed.

Excretion High concentrations of active drug excreted in urine and bile; about 35% of oral and 70% of intramuscular dosage are excreted in urine.

Drug Interactions *p*-Aminohippuric acid elevates serum and cerebrospinal fluid levels of ampicillin. Probenecid interferes with the renal excretion of ampicillin, thus prolonging serum drug levels (duration). The following antibiotics inhibit or antagonize the bactericidal action of ampicillin: chloramphenicol, sulfonamides, tetracyclines. Erythromycin antagonizes the action of ampicillin against all organisms (except *Staphylococcus aureus*) whereas cephalosporins antagonize its action against *Escherichia coli, Proteus,* and *Pseudomonas.* The following antibiotics potentiate the bactericidal action of ampicillin: cephalosporins, cloxacillin, methicillin, nafcillin, oxacillin, streptomycin. Ampicillin inhibits the action of carbenicillin. Hemorrhage due to heparin toxicity may result, but rarely with ampicillin, if ampicillin IV is discontinued abruptly in clients receiving concurrent therapy with ampicillin IV and heparin; intravenous ampicillin inhibits the action of heparin. Ampicillin potentiates coumarin and its derivatives; use with caution concurrently. Since ampicillin has relatively little protein binding, analgesics will have little effect. The xanthine oxidase inhibitor allopurinol should not be administered concurrently, since the client may develop a skin rash.

Laboratory Interactions Large dosages may produce false-positive results for urinary glucose with Clinitest, Benedict's solution or Fehling's solution. Clinistix, Tes-Tape, and other enzymatic glucose oxidase reactions are not affected. May increase serum creatinine phosphokinase serum glutamic-oxaloacetic transaminase due to muscle injury from intramuscular injections.

Administration Highly individualized.

- *Moderate infections:* Adults: 250 to 500 mg po, IM, or IV q6h; Children: Under 40 kg: 25 to 50 mg/kg po, IM or IV every 6 to 8 hours.

- *Bacterial meningitis and other severe infections:* Adults and Children: 150 to 200 mg/kg IM or IV daily in divided doses q4h.

Available Drug Forms Capsules containing 250 or 500 mg; oral suspension containing 125, 250, or 500 mg/5 ml; pediatric suspension with dropper calibrated at 62.5 mg ($\frac{1}{2}$ dropperful), 94 mg ($\frac{3}{4}$ dropperful), or 125 mg (1 dropperful); vials containing 125 mg for reconstitution with 1.2 ml of diluent to yield 125 mg/ml; vials containing 250 mg for reconstitution with 1.0 ml of diluent to yield 250 mg/ml; vials containing 500 mg for reconstitution with 1.8 ml of diluent to yield 250 mg/ml; vials containing 1 g for reconstitution with 3.5 ml of diluent to yield 250 mg/ml; vials containing 2 g for reconstitution with 6.8 ml of diluent to yield 250 mg/ml; piggyback vials containing 1 or 2 g. There is 2.9 mEq of sodium in each gram of ampicillin sodium.

Nursing Management

Planning factors

1. Complete culture (throat, urine) and sensitivity tests before instituting therapy.
2. Ampicillin is not penicillinase resistant.
3. Obtain complete blood cell count (CBC), serum electrolytes, renal function tests (creatinine), hepatic function tests (blood urea nitrogen, BUN), and serum enzyme levels (serum glutamic-oxaloacetic transaminase, SGOT) before instituting therapy. If any abnormalities occur, notify physician.
4. Determine adequacy of renal functioning before initiating therapy.
5. Check for hypersensitivity (allergy) before administering drug.

Administration factors

1. Give capsules with a full glass of water. Do not give with acidic juices, since ampicillin is unstable in acid solutions. For maximum absorption, give on an empty stomach.
2. Shake reconstituted oral suspension vigorously before measuring the desired dosage.
3. Oral solution is stable for 14 days when refrigerated.
4. Reconstitute parenteral solutions with the appropriate amount of sterile water or bacteriostatic water for injection. Label vial with date, time of reconstitution, and concentration. Shake vial vigorously and check to see that all powder is dissolved before withdrawing the desired amount.
5. When administering IM,
   (a) Inject deep into large muscle mass.
   (b) Rotate injection sites.
   (c) Observe previous injection sites for irritation prior to each administration.
6. When administering via intermittent IV infusion,
   (a) Add reconstituted solution to 50 or 100 ml of a compatible IV solution, such as normal saline or 5% D/W. IV solutions are stable at room temperature for 8 hours in normal saline and lactated Ringers; but only 4 hours in 5% D/0.45 NaCl.
   (b) Do not mix with other drugs. Ampicillin is incompatible with several drugs.
   (c) Check patency of IV before starting infusion. If in doubt, restart IV because ampicillin is very irritating to the vein and can cause phlebitis.
   (d) The recommended rate of drug administration is 1 hour. Convulsions may occur if the solution is administered in less than 15 minutes, particularly dosages of 2 g or more.
   (e) An infusion pump is recommended, but a carefully observed microdrip IV administration set can be used.
   (f) Rotation of IV sites every 72 hours may prevent the emergence of phlebitis.

Evaluation factors

1. Observe client continuously for at least 30 minutes for hypersensitivity reaction when therapy is first initiated. If a reaction occurs, notify physician immediately and institute measures according to agency protocol.
2. Check for the appearance of a rash daily. Ampicillin rashes occur within 3 weeks.
3. Check serum enzyme levels (SGOT) and serum electrolytes frequently (daily).
4. Check CBC, urinalysis, renal function tests (creatinine), and hepatic function tests (BUN) periodically (weekly). If untoward reactions occur, notify physician.
5. Continue therapy for at least 2 to 3 days after client has become asymptomatic with negative cultures. Therapy is usually maintained for at least 10 days for group A beta-hemolytic streptococci infections.
6. Examine client daily for suprainfections.
7. After treating a client for an allergic reaction,
   (a) Instruct client never to take any type of penicillin. Suggest the wearing of an ID band or tag (or the carrying of a card) that indicates the allergy.
   (b) Clearly indicate the allergy on the outside of the client's chart, kardex, and medication record.
   (c) Not all ampicillin rashes are thought to be allergic in nature. The client may be able to tolerate another penicillin (cloxacillin), when indicated.

GENERIC NAME Ampicillin/probenecid (RX)

TRADE NAMES Ampicillin-Probenecid Suspension, Polycillin-PRB, Principen with Probenecid

CLASSIFICATION Antibiotic

See ampicillin for Warnings and precautions, Untoward reactions, Parameters of use, and Drug interactions.

Action This is a combination of a semisynthetic penicillin and probenecid. As ampicillin is normally excreted in urine unchanged, the concurrent administration of probenecid will prolong serum ampicillin levels by inhibiting excretion. (See ampicillin.)

Indications for Use Acute *Neisseria gonorrhoeae* infections in adult males and females; severe to moderately severe infections in which high serum levels are desirable.

Contraindications Hypersensitivity to probenecid. Not recommended for clients with an acute attack of gout, a blood dyscrasia, or uric acid kidney stones. Not recommended for children. (See ampicillin.)

Administration

- *N. gonorrhoeae infection:* 3.5 g of ampicillin and 1.0 g of probenecid as a single dose.

Available Drug Forms Single-dose bottles containing 3.5 g of ampicillin and 1 g of probenecid powder.

Nursing Management (See ampicillin.)

1. Always use freshly prepared suspension.
2. Reconstitute by adding water in two portions and shaking well after each addition.
3. Reconstituted solutions are stable at room temperature for 24 hours.
4. Culture the original site 7 to 14 days after therapy. Women should have cultures from the endocervical and anal canal.

GENERIC NAMES Hetacillin; hetacillin potassium

TRADE NAMES Versapen; Versapen-K (RX)

CLASSIFICATION Antibiotic

See ampicillin for Indications for use, Contraindications, Warnings and precautions, Untoward reactions, and Drug interactions.

Action Hetacillin is a semisynthetic penicillin derived from 6-aminopenicillanic acid. The antibiotic activity of the drug is provided by its rapid conversion to ampicillin and acetone. (Hetacillin itself has no antibacterial activity.) When converted to ampicillin, its bactericidal activity is identical to ampicillin. As with ampicillin, hetacillin is not resistant to penicillinase, but it can be given orally as it is stable in gastric acid. (See ampicillin.)

Parameters of Use (See ampicillin.)

Absorption Well absorbed from GI tract; food interferes with absorption. Converted to ampicillin in 20 minutes at a pH of 7.1.

Administration Highly individualized. Adults: 225 to 450 mg po q6h; Children: Under 40 kg: 22.5 to 45 mg/kg po daily.

Available Drug Forms Capsules (Versapen-K) containing the equivalent of 225 or 450 mg of ampicillin; oral suspension (Versapen) containing the equivalent of 112.5 or 225 mg of ampicillin in 5 ml. Also available with pediatric dropper.

Nursing Management Urinary and GI infections may require several weeks of therapy. (See ampicillin.)

GENERIC NAME Amoxicillin (RX)

TRADE NAMES Amoxil, Larotid, Polymox

CLASSIFICATION Antibiotic

See ampicillin for Contraindications, Warnings and precautions, Untoward reactions, and Drug interactions.

Action Amoxicillin, a semisynthetic analog of ampicillin, has a range of antibacterial activity similar to its parent drug, but has the advantage of a longer duration of action and is often better tolerated. Although amoxicillin is stable in gastric acid, it does not resist destruction by penicillinase. (See ampicillin.)

Indications for Use Mild to moderately severe infections caused by sensitive gram-positive organisms, including *H. influenzae, E. coli, P. mirabilis,* and *N. gonorrhoeae;* mild to moderately severe infections caused by sensitive gram-negative organisms, including streptococci, *D. pneumoniae,* and nonpenicillinase-producing staphylococci. Frequently used for respiratory and genitourinary tract infections. May be used for acute uncomplicated gonorrhea.

Parameters of Use

Absorption Well absorbed from GI tract; food does not affect absorption. About 20% bound to plasma proteins. Peak serum levels occur in 1 to 2 hours. Duration of action is up to 8 hours. Half-life is 1 hour.

Distribution Widely distributed to body tissues. Does not enter cerebrospinal fluid unless the meninges are inflamed.

Excretion About 60% by the kidneys as active drug; some excreted via bile in feces.

Administration Highly individualized.

- *Infections:* Adults: 250 to 500 mg po q8h; Children: Under 20 kg: 20 to 40 mg/kg po in 3 divided doses q8h.

- *Gonorrhea:* 3 g po as a single dose.

Available Drug Forms Capsules containing 250 or 500 mg; oral suspension containing 125 or 250 mg/5 ml.

Nursing Management (See ampicillin.)

1. Unstable at room temperature; store in refrigerator.
2. May be administered with meals.

GENERIC NAME Carbenicillin disodium (RX)

TRADE NAMES Geopen, Pyopen

CLASSIFICATION Antibiotic

See ampicillin for Contraindications.

Action Carbenicillin, a semisynthetic penicillin, has one of the broadest spectrums of antimicrobial activity and is active against susceptible anaerobic bacteria and both gram-positive and gram-negative organisms. It is particularly effective against *Pseudomonas* and *Proteus* and has been used for mixed types of infections. Unfortunately, carbenicillin is not resistant to gastric acid or penicillinase; therefore, it must be administered parenterally.

Indications for Use Moderately severe to severe infections, including many ampicillin-resistant infections (meningitis, septicemia); moderately severe to severe infections caused by susceptible anaerobic bacteria, including peritonitis, empyema, lung abscess, and pelvic abscess; acute and chronic genitourinary tract infections caused by *Pseudomonas, Proteus,* or *Escherichia coli.*

Warnings and Precautions Use with caution in clients who are on sodium restriction. (See ampicillin.)

Untoward Reactions Allergic (hypersensitivity) reactions include anaphylaxis, skin rashes, pruritus, urticaria, and drug fever. Hemorrhagic manifestations associated with abnormalities of coagulation tests, such as clotting and prothrombin time, have occurred in uremic clients receiving large dosages; bleeding ceases when therapy is discontinued. As with other semisynthetic penicillins, elevations in serum glutamic-oxaloacetic transaminase and serum glutamic-pyruvic transaminase can occur, particularly in young children. Neurologic disturbances, including convulsions and neuromuscular irritability, can occur with excessively high serum levels. Blood dyscrasias, including anemia, thrombocytopenia, leukopenia, neutropenia, and eosinophilia, have occurred, particularly in clients receiving large dosages or prolonged therapy. Superinfections can occur, particularly by penicillin-resistant organisms *(Candida, Proteus, Pseudomonas).* Vein irritation and phlebitis (after intravenous administration) and pain at the injection site (after intramuscular injection) can occur. Rare reactions include nausea, temporary pain at intravenous injection sites and an unpleasant taste after intravenous infusions. Hypernatremia and hypokalemia can occur, particularly when high dosages are used. Cardiac clients may develop arrhythmias or congestive heart failure.

Parameters of Use

Absorption Rapid from intramuscular sites; poor absorption from GI tract. About 50% bound to plasma proteins. Peak serum levels occur in about 1 to 2 hours. Duration of action is 6 hours. Half-life is 1 hour.

Distribution Widely distributed to body tissues. Does not enter cerebrospinal fluid unless the meninges are inflamed.

Excretion Relatively high concentrations of active drug excreted in urine.

Drug Interactions Ampicillin inhibits carbenicillin and should not be administered concurrently. Although carbenicillin inhibits gentamicin, this combination is used for severe *Pseudomonas aeruginosa* infections. When the two drugs must be given concurrently, it is recommended that they be administered by different routes (carbenicillin IV and gentamicin IM) at different time periods. (See ampicillin.)

Administration Highly individualized.

- *Severe infections:* Adults: 200 to 500 mg/kg IV daily in divided doses; do not exceed 40 g daily. Children: 300 to 500 mg/kg IV daily in divided doses.
- *Moderately severe infections:* Adults: 1 to 2 g IM or IV q6h. Children: 50 to 200 mg/kg IM or IV in divided doses every 4 to 6 hours.
- *Infants:* Over 2 kg: Initial dosage: 100 mg/kg IM or IV; then 75 mg/kg IM or IV q6h for 3 days; then 100 mg/kg IM or IV q6h. Under 2 kg: Initial dosage: 100 mg/kg IM or IV; then 75 mg/kg IM or IV q8h.
- *Clients with renal impairment:* 1 to 2 g IV every 8 to 12 hours.
- *Gonorrhea:* 4 g IM as a single dose divided between two sites.

Available Drug Forms Vials containing 1 g for reconstitution with: 2.0 ml of diluent to yield 400 mg/ml; 3.6 ml to yield 250 mg/ml. Vials containing 2g for reconstitution with: 4.0 ml of diluent to yield 400 mg/ml; 7.2 ml to yield 250 mg/ml. Vials containing 5 g for reconstitution with: 7.0 ml of diluent to yield 500 mg/ml; 17.0 ml to yield 250 mg/ml. Piggyback units containing 2, 5, or 10 g. There is 4.7 mEq of sodium in each gram of carbenicillin disodium.

Nursing Management

Planning factors

1. Complete culture and sensitivity tests before instituting therapy. Perform a dark-field examination for syphilis in clients being treated for gonorrhea.
2. Obtain the following baseline data to avoid untoward reactions:
   (a) Creatinine clearance test—if rate is 30 ml/min. or less, notify physician. If creatinine clearance is less than 5 ml/min., probenecid 1 g may be administered 1 hour prior to carbenicillin IM to decrease rate of excretion.
   (b) Serum electrolytes—if sodium is elevated, notify physician before starting therapy.
   (c) Serum enzyme tests (serum glutamic-oxaloacetic transaminase, serum glutamic-pyruvic transaminase, creatine phosphokinase, lactate dehydrogenase).

(d) Complete blood cell count (CBC), platelet count, prothrombin time, and clotting time—if abnormal, notify physician before starting therapy.
3. Check for hypersensitivity (allergy) before administering drug.

Administration factors

1. Reconstitute parenteral solution with the appropriate amount of sterile water for injection. Label vial with date, time of reconstitution, and concentration. Shake vial vigorously and check to see that all powder is dissolved before withdrawing the desired amount.
2. When administering IM,
   (a) May be diluted with 0.5% lidocaine hydrochloride (without epinephrine) or bacteriostatic water containing 0.9% benzyl alcohol to decrease pain upon injection. Consult physician.
   (b) Do not inject more than 2 g in one site.
   (c) Inject deep into large muscle mass. Use midlateral thigh muscle in young children.
   (d) Rotate injection sites.
   (e) Observe previous injection sites for irritation prior to each administration.
   (f) Moist heat can be applied to decrease irritation at previous injection sites; do not apply heat to present site of injection.
3. When administering via intermittent IV infusion,
   (a) Add reconstituted solution to 50 or 100 ml of a compatible IV solution, such as sodium chloride or 5% D/W. The resulting concentration must be less than 1 g of drug in 10 ml of diluent (10 g must be diluted in at least 100 ml of solution). The preferred concentration is 20 ml for each gram of drug (5 g in 100 ml). Reconstituted solutions are stable for 72 hours at room temperature.
   (b) Rotation of IV sites every 72 hours may prevent the emergence of phlebitis.
   (c) Check patency of IV before starting infusion. If in doubt, restart IV because carbenicillin is very irritating to the vein and can cause phlebitis.
   (d) Do not mix with other drugs.
   (e) Run infusion for 60 minutes or more. An infusion pump is recommended to prevent rapid infusion neurotoxicity (convulsions); however, a carefully observed microdrip IV administration set can be used.
4. When administering via continuous IV infusion,
   (a) Do not mix with other drugs.
   (b) Check for compatibility of IV solution before adding drug.
   (c) Date and time IV containers upon adding the drug. Change IV solution containing drug every 24 hours.
   (d) An infusion pump is highly recommended.

Evaluation factors

1. Observe client continuously for at least 30 minutes for hypersensitivity reaction when therapy is first initiated. If a reaction occurs, notify physician immediately and institute measures according to agency protocol.
2. Watch client for neurologic reactions during IV administration. If the client demonstrates impaired thinking or has hallucinations, slow IV rate and notify physician.
3. Monitor heart rate continuously and auscultate lungs once per shift in clients with cardiac disorders.
4. Observe client for hypernatremia and hypokalemia.
5. Check serum electrolytes, creatinine, and serum enzymes frequently (daily).
6. Hemorrhagic manifestations may occur within the first day of treatment. Observe for ecchymoses, purpura, or frank bleeding before administering each dose.
7. Check, CBC, urinalysis, and hepatic function tests periodically (weekly).
8. Examine client daily for superinfections.

GENERIC NAME Carbenicillin indanyl sodium

TRADE NAME Geocillin (RX)

CLASSIFICATION Antibiotic

See ampicillin for Contraindications. See ampicillin and carbenicillin disodium for Warnings and precautions and Drug interactions.

Action This semisynthetic penicillin is the indanyl ester of carbenicillin disodium. It is rapidly converted to carbenicillin, but has the advantage of being stable in gastric acid and can therefore be administered orally. This drug is particularly useful against *Pseudomonas* and *Proteus* organisms.

Indications for Use Mild to moderately severe acute or chronic infections of the genitourinary system, including asymptomatic bacteriuria and prostatitis caused by susceptible organisms.

Untoward Reactions Common GI reactions include an unpleasant taste, nausea, vomiting, and diarrhea. Dry mouth, flatulence, and abdominal cramps have occurred. Superinfections include vaginitis and oral infections (furry tongue) caused by nonsusceptible organisms. (See carbenicillin disodium.)

Parameters of Use (See carbenicillin disodium.)

Absorption Well absorbed from GI tract; stable in gastric acid. Peak serum levels occur in 1 hour. Duration of action is up to 6 hours.

Administration Highly individualized. Adults: 1 to 2 tablets po q6h.

Available Drug Forms Coated tablets containing the equivalent of 382 mg of carbenicillin.

Nursing Management Store tablets in a cool, dry area. (See carbenicillin disodium.)

GENERIC NAME Ticarcillin disodium (RX)

TRADE NAME Ticar

CLASSIFICATION Antibiotic

See ampicillin for Contraindications. See ampicillin and carbenicillin disodium for Warnings and precautions. See carbenicillin disodium for Untoward reactions.

Action Ticarcillin is a semisynthetic penicillin derived from 6-aminopenicillanic acid. It has a wide range of antibacterial activity similar to carbenicillin. The relatively low level of toxicity of ticarcillin permits the use of large dosages for severe infections. It is particularly effective against gram-negative organisms and has been used for several anaerobic infections. Unfortunately, ticarcillin is neither resistant to gastric acid nor penicillinase.

Indications for Use Moderately severe to severe infections caused by sensitive gram-negative organisms, including *Pseudomonas, Proteus,* and *Escherichia coli;* moderately severe to severe infections caused by sensitive anaerobic bacteria, including *Bacteroides fragilis, Clostridium,* and *Peptococcus.* Frequently used for respiratory and genitourinary tract infections. May be used in septicemia, peritonitis, and intraabdominal abscesses.

Parameters of Use

Absorption Rapidly absorbed from intramuscular sites; poor absorption from GI tract. About 45% bound to plasma proteins. Peak plasma levels occur in: 30 to 60 minutes (IM); 15 minutes (IV). Duration of action is 6 hours. Half-life is about 70 minutes.

Distribution Widely distributed to body tissues. Enters cerebrospinal fluid, bile, and pleural fluid.

Excretion About 45% excreted by the kidneys as unchanged drug.

Drug Interactions Ticarcillin is synergistic with gentamicin and tobramycin against certain strains of *Pseudomonas aeruginosa.* Probenecid decreases the excretion of ticarcillin and therefore produces high and more prolonged serum drug levels. (See ampicillin.)

Administration Highly individualized.

- *Severe infections:* Adults: 200 to 300 mg/kg IV daily in divided doses q3h, q4h, or q6h. Children: Under 40 kg: 200 to 300 mg/kg IV daily in divided doses every 4 to 6 hours.

- *Moderately severe infections:* Adults: 1 to 2 g IM or IV q6h; do not exceed 2 g IM; larger dosages should be given IV. Children: Under 40 kg: 50 to 200 mg/kg IV daily in divided doses every 4 to 8 hours.

- *Infants:* Over 2 kg: Initial dosage: 75 to 100 mg/kg IV; then 75 mg/kg IV every 8 hours. Under 2 kg: 75 mg/kg IV q8h.

- *Clients with renal impairment:* Creatinine clearance: Over 30 ml/min.: 2 to 3 g IV q4h; 10 to 30 ml/min.: 2 g IV q8h; Under 10 ml/min.: 2 g IV q24h.

Available Drug Forms Vials containing 1 g for reconstitution with 2 ml of diluent to yield 400 mg/ml; vials containing 3 g for reconstitution with 7.5 ml of diluent to yield 400 mg/ml; vials containing 6 g for reconstitution with 12 ml of diluent to yield 400 mg/ml; piggyback bottles containing 3 g. There is 5.2 to 6.5 mEq of sodium in each gram of ticarcillin disodium.

Nursing Management (See carbenicillin disodium.)

1. When administering IM, dilute with sterile water, 1% lidocaine hydrochloride (without epinephrine), or bacteriostatic water containing 0.9% benzyl alcohol. The latter two diluents will decrease pain upon injection.
2. When administering IV, add reconstituted solution to a compatible IV solution, such as sodium chloride, 5% D/W, or 5% D/0.45 NaCl.
3. Reconstituted solutions are stable for 24 hours at room temperature or 72 hours when refrigerated.

GENERIC NAME Cyclacillin (RX)

TRADE NAME Cyclapen-W

CLASSIFICATION Antibiotic

See ampicillin for Contraindications, Warnings and precautions, Untoward reactions, and Drug interactions.

Action Although cyclacillin, a semisynthetic penicillin, is in the ampicillin class of penicillins, it has a more restrictive range of antibacterial activity than ampicillin. Cyclacillin is destroyed by penicillinase; but is effective against group A beta-hemolytic streptococci, *Streptococcus pneumoniae,* nonpenicillinase-producing staphylococci, *Hemophilus influenzae, Escherichia coli,* and *Proteus mirabilis.* As cyclacillin is relatively nontoxic, it can be given in reduced dosages to clients with renal insufficiency. It has the advantage of being stable in gastric acid and can therefore be administered orally. Although it may cause diarrhea, the incidence of rashes and other untoward reactions is said to be lower than with ampicillin.

Indications for Use Mild to moderately severe respiratory and urinary tract and skin infections caused by susceptible organisms. Frequently used for tonsillitis, pharyngitis, bronchitis, pneumonia, and otitis media.

Parameters of Use

Absorption Rapidly absorbed from GI tract; stable in gastric acid. About 20% bound to plasma proteins. Half-life is 30 to 40 minutes; however, it is prolonged ($3\frac{1}{2}$ hours) in renal insufficiency (creatinine clearance less than 30 ml/min.). Peak plasma levels occur in 40 to 60 minutes. Duration of action is 4 to 6 hours.

Excretion Rapidly excreted by the kidneys as unchanged drug (about 80%).

Administration Highly individualized. Adults: 250 to 500 mg po q6h; Children 50 to 100 mg/kg daily in divided doses q6h. Dosage for clients with renal insufficiency depends on creatinine clearance: 30 to 50 ml/min.: Administer full dose q12h; 15 to 30 ml/min.: Administer full dose q18h; 10 to 15 ml/min.: Administer full dose q24h.

Available Drug Forms Tablets containing 250 or 500 mg; oral suspension containing 125 or 250 mg/5 ml.

Nursing Management (See ampicillin.)

1. Refrigerate oral suspension and discard after 14 days.
2. Monitor serum creatinine levels daily in clients with renal insufficiency.

Chapter 61

Tetracyclines

TETRACYCLINES

- Tetracycline, tetracycline hydrochloride
- Chlortetracycline hydrochloride
- Demeclocycline, demeclocycline hydrochloride
- Doxycycline, doxycycline hyclate, doxycycline monohydrate
- Methacycline hydrochloride
- Minocycline hydrochloride
- Oxytetracycline hydrochloride
- Tetracycline phosphate

COMBINATION PREPARATIONS

- Azotrex
- Mysteclin
- Urobiotic–250

TETRACYCLINES WERE FIRST used in 1948 as broad-spectrum antibiotics. However, their usefulness in current antiinfective therapy is limited because of the development of a number of resistant bacterial strains. Nevertheless, tetracyclines are still the drugs of choice for rickettsial diseases.

Tetracyclines may be administered orally or parenterally. The drugs are adequately absorbed from the gastrointestinal tract; but absorption is impaired when they are taken with milk or aluminum hydroxide gels. Gastrointestinal irritation, which presents as nausea, vomiting, or diarrhea, is a common side effect of oral tetracycline preparations. However, these effects may be alleviated by giving the drugs with meals. Another cause of gastrointestinal irritation may be a superimposed gastrointestinal infection that is usually fungal in origin. For this reason, tetracycline preparations are often combined with an antifungal agent.

Young children and pregnant women are not candidates for tetracyclines. These drugs may cause yellow, gray, or brown stains in developing primary teeth. Permanent teeth may also be affected with prolonged therapy.

Since the development of superinfections is more likely with tetracyclines than with other antiinfective agents, clients should be taught that scrupulous oral and perineal hygiene is essential. They should also be instructed to be alert for early signs of monilial or fungal infections.

TETRACYCLINES

GENERIC NAME Tetracycline, tetracycline hydrochloride

TRADE NAMES Achromycin, Bristacycline, Cancycline, Panmycin, Polycycline, Robitet, Steclin, Sumycin, Tetrachel, Tetracyn, Topicycline

CLASSIFICATION Antibiotic (RX)

Action This drug is primarily bacteriostatic. It interferes with protein synthesis of infectious organisms, thereby halting growth and reproduction. It is isolated from *Streptomyces aureofaciens*, and is effective against a variety of gram-positive and gram-negative organisms, as well as some mycoplasmas, rickettsiae, and protozoa.

Indications for Use Effective against gram-positive and gram-negative organisms. Antimicrobial activity overlaps with penicillin, streptomycin, and chloramphenicol. Often effective against microbes insensitive or resistant to other antibiotics.

Contraindications Hypersensitivity to tetracyclines, hepatic or renal impairment, pregnancy, breast-feeding mothers, children under 8 years, simultaneous use of hepatotoxic drugs.

Warnings and Precautions Use with caution in clients with impaired renal function, because excessive accumulation of drug may cause hepatotoxicity. Use cautiously in undernourished clients.

Untoward Reactions GI upset can occur with oral administration. Superinfections with *staphylococcus* are the most common reaction. Fungal infections can occur and most commonly affect the mucous surfaces. Hypersensitivity reactions include skin rashes, urticaria, and increased photosensitivity. Anaphylaxis may occur if the allergic reaction is severe. Bone lesions and yellow, brown, or the gray staining of the teeth can occur in pregnant mothers, children whose mothers had taken drug during last half of pregnancy, infants, and children under 7 years. Fatty liver degeneration may occur when large dosages are administered. Fanconi-like syndrome has been reported when expired or improperly stored drug is administered. Blood dyscrasias, such as leukocytosis, atypical lymphocytes, and thrombocytopenic purpura, can occur in clients on long-term therapy. Delay in blood coagulation may also occur. Increased intracranial pressure with bulging fontanels has been reported in infants. Also possible are hepatotoxicity, nephrotoxicity, papilledema, headache, and impaired vision.

Parameters of Use

Absorption Freely soluble in water. Adequately absorbed from GI tract, particularly the upper GI tract. Absorption is increased during fasting and is impaired by milk products. Peak blood levels occur in 2 to 4 hours; half-life is 6 to 9 hours.

Distribution Removed from the blood by the liver and excreted with bile into intestine where it is partially reabsorbed. When given intravenously, drug can be detected in the cerebrospinal fluid within 6 hours. It is widely distributed to all body tissues.

Crosses placenta and enters breast milk.

Excretion In urine and feces; urine is the primary route.

Drug Interactions Tetracyclines may mask the bactericidal effect of penicillin. Oral antacids, iron preparations, and sodium bicarbonate may reduce the absorption of tetracyclines from GI tract. Tetracyclines antagonize the activity of heparin. Blood urea nitrogen may be elevated if tetracyclines are given concurrently with diuretics. Prothrombin time may be further decreased with concomitant use of tetracyclines and oral anticoagulants.

Laboratory Interactions May produce false-positive results for urinary glucose with Clinitest and Benedict's solution, and false negative results with Clinistix and Tes-Tape. May cause false increases in urinary catecholamines and false decreases in urinary urobilinogen.

Administration Adults: 250 mg po, IM, or IV q6h. Children: Oral: 10 to 20 mg/kg in divided doses; Intramuscular: 100 mg every 8 to 12 hours.

Available Drug Forms Capsules containing 50, 100, 125, or 250 mg; tablets containing 50, 100, or 250 mg; oral suspension containing 125 or 250 mg/5 ml; vials containing 100, 250, or 500 mg; powder and liquid units for topical use, to be combined to provide 2.2 mg/ml. Ointment containing 3% tetracycline.

Nursing Management

Planning factors

1. Culture and sensitivity testing should be done prior to starting drug therapy.
2. Protect all drug forms from heat, light, and humidity to prevent decomposition.
3. Store parenteral solutions at room temperature and use within 24 hours.

Administration factors

1. Check expiration date carefully. Nephrotoxicity may result from administering outdated or improperly stored tetracycline.
2. Check IV infusion site for redness, swelling, and tenderness. Infuse drug slowly. Thrombophlebitis is common, particularly with rapid infusion.
3. When administering IM, inject deep into large muscle slowly. Local irritation and pain at injection site is common.
4. Do not give orally with milk or milk products. Give on an empty stomach (1 to 2 hours after meals).
5. Antacids containing aluminum hydroxide prevent absorption of tetracycline.

Evaluation factors

1. Monitor intake and output carefully.
2. Observe client for signs of buccal, vaginal, or anal infection.

Client teaching factors

1. Advise client against unnecessary exposure to sun as skin redness can occur with minimal exposure.
2. Advise client to discard unused drug after treatment is completed, because decomposition occurs with age, resulting in a toxic product.
3. Advise client to report immediately any symptoms of superinfection (black, furry tongue; persistent diarrhea). Meticulous oral and perineal hygiene may help prevent superinfections.

GENERIC NAME Chlortetracycline hydrochloride

TRADE NAME Aureomycin (OTC) (RX)

CLASSIFICATION Antibiotic

See tetracycline for Indications for use, Contraindications, Warnings and precautions, Untoward reactions, and Drug interactions.

Action Chlortetracycline is similar to tetracycline, but may be more useful in biliary infections.

Parameters of Use (See tetracyline.)

Excretion More dependent on biliary excretion for elimination than other tetracyclines.

Administration Adults: 250 to 500 mg po, IM, or IV q6h; Children: 10 to 20 mg/kg po daily in 2 or 3 divided doses.

Available Drug Forms Capsules containing 50, 100, or 250 mg; soluble tablets containing 50 mg; oral suspension containing 125 mg/5 ml; oral powder containing 50 mg/3 ml (rounded teaspoon); IV vials containing 500 mg; topical ointment containing 3% chlortetracycline (OTC).

Nursing Management (See tetracycline.)

1. When administering more than 1 g, it is preferable to increase frequency of doses rather than giving it in a single dose.
2. Single oral dosages greater than 250 mg are not effectively absorbed.
3. Some decomposition may be expected during extended IV infusion.

GENERIC NAMES Demeclocycline; demeclocycline hydrochloride

TRADE NAMES Declomycin, DMCT; Declomycin Hydrochloride

CLASSIFICATION Antibiotic (RX)

See tetracycline for Action, Indications for use, Contraindications, Warnings and precautions, Untoward reactions, Drug interactions, and Nursing management.

Parameters of Use

Absorption More stable in acidic or basic aqueous solutions than are the hydrochlorides of chlortetracycline or tetracycline. About 50% bound to serum proteins. Peak serum levels occur in 3 to 6 hours. Therapeutic serum levels may persist for 3 days following one dose.

Distribution Concentrated in liver and excreted in bile. Enters enterohepatic circulation and is reabsorbed.

Excretion In urine and feces, but more slowly than other tetracyclines.

Administration Adults: 600 mg po daily in 2 to 4 divided doses; an initial dosage of 300 mg may be given for severe infections. Reduced dosages are required for clients with hepatic or renal impairment. Children: 6 to 12 mg/kg po daily in 2 to 4 divided doses.

Available Drug Forms Capsules containing 75 or 150 mg; oral suspension containing 60 mg/ml or 70 mg/5 ml; special coated tablets containing 150 or 300 mg.

GENERIC NAMES Doxycycline, doxycycline hyclate, doxycycline monohydrate

TRADE NAMES Doxy-Caps, Doxy-Lemmon, Vibramycin, Vibra-Tabs

CLASSIFICATION Antibiotic (RX)

See tetracycline for Indications for use, Contraindications, Warnings and precautions, Untoward reactions, and Drug interactions.

Action Similar to tetracycline, but serum levels may persist for longer periods due to the slow absorption and enterohepatic cycling of this drug. In addition, some strains of staphylococci that are resistant to tetracycline may be susceptible to doxycycline. Therapeutic dosage is less than that for other tetracyclines.

Parameters of Use

Absorption Almost completely absorbed from GI tract following oral administration. 25 to 90% bound to plasma proteins. Half-life is 15 to 22 hours.

Distribution (See tetracycline.)

Excretion 90% in bile and feces, with small amounts in urine.

Administration Adults: 100 mg po or IV q12h for first 24 hours; Maintenance dosage: 100 mg as a single dose or 50 mg q12h. Children: 4.4 mg/kg po or IV daily in 2 divided doses for first 24 hours, then 2 mg/kg daily in 2 divided doses. Dosage may be doubled for severe infections in adults and children.

Available Drug Forms Capsules containing 50 mg; oral suspension containing 25 mg/5 ml (60-ml bottles); vials of sterile powder containing 100 mg with 480 mg of ascorbic acid or 200 mg with 960 mg of ascorbic acid.

Nursing Management (See tetracycline.)

1. Protect solutions from light.
2. Reconstituted solutions are stable for 72 hours when refrigerated.

GENERIC NAME Methacycline hydrochloride

TRADE NAME Rondomycin (RX)

CLASSIFICATION Antibiotic

See tetracycline for Indications for use, Contraindications, Warnings and precautions, Untoward reactions, Drug interactions, and Nursing management.

Action Methacycline, which is derived from oxytetracycline, is similar to tetracycline; however, it is less likely to cause photosensitivity.

Parameters of Use (See tetracycline.)

Absorption Freely soluble in water. Not well absorbed from GI tract. 80% bound to plasma proteins, half-life is 16 hours.

Excretion 50% excreted in urine and 5% in feces within 72 hours.

Administration Adults: 600 mg po daily in 2 to 4 divided doses; an initial dosage of 300 mg may be given for severe infections. Children: 6 to 12 mg/kg po daily in divided doses.

Available Drug Forms Capsules containing 150 or 300 mg; oral suspension containing 75 mg/5 ml.

GENERIC NAME Minocycline hydrochloride (RX)

TRADE NAMES Minocin, Vectrin

CLASSIFICATION Antibiotic

See tetracycline for Indications for use, Contraindications, Warnings and precautions, Untoward reactions, Drug interactions, and Nursing management.

Action May be effective against staphyloccocal strains resistant to other tetracyclines. (See tetracycline.)

Parameters of Use

Absorption Rapidly absorbed from GI tract; absorption is not significantly affected by food, milk products, or antacids. Serum levels are higher and last longer than those of almost all other tetracyclines. Serum half-life is 11 to 17 hours. 70 to 75% bound to plasma proteins.

Excretion Percentage of unchanged drug excreted is one-half to one-third that of most other tetracyclines; the remainder is stored in fatty tissues.

Administration Adults: Initial dosage: 200 mg po or IV; then 100 mg q12h; do not exceed 400 mg in 24 hours. Children: Over 8 years: Initial dosage: 4 mg/kg po or IV; then 2 mg/kg q12h.

Available Drug Forms Capsules containing 100 mg; syrup containing 50 mg/5 ml; IV vials containing 100 mg.

GENERIC NAME Oxytetracycline hydrochloride

TRADE NAMES Dalimycin, Oxybiotic, Oxy-Tetrachel, Terramycin, Tetramine

CLASSIFICATION Antibiotic (RX)

See tetracycline for Action, Indications for use, Contraindications, Warnings and precautions, Untoward reactions, and Drug interactions.

Parameters of Use (See tetracycline.)

Absorption Peak plasma levels in 2 to 4 hours. Half-life is 6 to 9 hours.
Excretion In urine, bile, and feces in active form.

Administration Adults: 250 to 500 mg po, IM, or IV q6h or q12h. Children: 25 to 50 mg/kg po daily in divided doses; 15 to 25 mg/kg IM daily in 2 or 3 divided doses; 10 to 20 mg/kg IV daily in 2 divided doses.

Available Drug Forms Tablets or capsules containing 125 or 250 mg; vials for IV injection containing 250 or 500 mg; 2-ml ampules and disposable syringes containing 500 mg/ml; oral suspension containing 100 mg/ml in 10-ml dropper bottles.

Nursing Management (See tetracycline.)

1. Solutions are stable for 48 hours when stored at 4 C. Discard turbid solutions.
2. No single IM injection in children should exceed 250 mg.

GENERIC NAME Tetracycline phosphate (RX)

TRADE NAME Tetrex

CLASSIFICATION Antibiotic

See tetracycline for Action, Indications for use, Contraindications, Warnings and precautions, Untoward reactions, Drug interactions, and Nursing management.

Parameters of Use (See tetracycline.)

Absorption More rapidly and completely absorbed from GI tract than tetracycline. Produces somewhat higher blood levels after oral administration than tetracycline. Toxicity can occur more rapidly than with tetracycline.

Administration Adults: 1 g po daily in 4 divided doses; higher dosages may be required in severe infections. Children: Over 8 years: 250 mg/kg po daily in 4 divided doses.

Available Drug Forms Capsules containing 50 or 250 mg.

COMBINATION PREPARATIONS

TRADE NAME Azotrex (RX)

CLASSIFICATION Antibiotic

See tetracycline and sulfadiazene for Untoward reactions and Drug interactions.

Indications for Use Mixed urinary tract infections, cystocele, prostatitis, urethritis, prior to and following urinary tract surgery.

Contraindications Sensitivity to any ingredient; premature infants, neonates, pregnant women at term, clients with chronic glomerulonephritis, uremia, severe hepatitis, hepatic or renal failure, severe pyelitis in pregnancy.

Warnings and Precautions In renal impairment, lower doses are necessary; careful evaluation is necessary in clients with liver or kidney impairment or blood dyscrasias. Photosensitivity may occur. Use with caution in clients with history of severe allergies or asthma.

Administration 1 or 2 capsules po qid for 7 to 14 days.

Available Drug Forms Generic contents in each capsule: tetracycline phosphate: 125 mg; sulfamethizole: 250 mg; phenazopyridine hydrochloride: 50 mg.

Nursing Management (See tetracycline and sulfadiazene.)

1. Drug should be administered on an empty stomach.
2. At least 3000 ml of fluid intake per day is necessary to prevent crystalluria.

TRADE NAME Mysteclin (RX)

CLASSIFICATION Antibiotic

See tetracycline for Contraindications and Warnings and precautions.

Indications for Use Treatment of infections sensitive to tetracycline, in clients particularly susceptible to candidiasis.

Untoward Reactions Amphotericin B is usually well tolerated. (See tetracycline.)

Administration Adults: 1 or 2 capsules po qid; Children: 10 to 20 mg/lb po daily in 3 divided doses (syrup).

Available Drug Forms Generic contents in each capsule: tetracycline hydrochloride: 250 mg; amphotericin B: 50 mg. Generic contents in each 5 ml syrup: tetracycline hydrochloride: 125 mg; amphotericin B: 25 mg.

Nursing Management Drug must be given on an empty stomach. (See tetracycline.)

TRADE NAME Urobiotic-250 (RX)

CLASSIFICATION Antibiotic

Chapter 69

Anthelmintics

HELMINTHIASIS AND ITS TREATMENT

Helminthiasis, or parasitic worm disease, is the most common affliction of humankind on a worldwide basis. Although it is much more prevalent in tropical climates, it is by no means restricted to these environments and is being diagnosed with increasing frequency in temperate climates. Most infestations are confined to the gastrointestinal tract, but some worms, such as *Trichinella*, can be carried to other body organs. Trematodes are responsible for causing schistosomiasis, which is a common disease of South America, Africa, and Asia. If untreated, this disease can cause serious damage to any of the vital organs.

Effective treatment of helminthic disease depends upon accurate identification of the causative organism, which is usually accomplished by examining a stool specimen. Many anthelmintics are effective only against one specific worm, so accurate diagnosis is important.

Once helminthic disease is diagnosed, it is important to supplement pharmacologic treatment with appropriate education to avoid reinfestation. Scrupulous personal hygiene is the first line of defense, since most infestations are spread by direct transfer of the worm ova to bedding, clothing, towels, and food. Washing hands after urination and defecation is of major importance. In addition, the client's clothing and bedding should be handled separately from those of other family members. Worm eggs are destroyed by washing machines.

Anthelmintics are generally classified according to the particular helminth(s) against which they are effective. Table 69-1 identifies the common helminths that infect humans and the current drug(s) of choice in treating the infestations.

Several agents that were widely used as anthelmintics have now been replaced by newer drugs. For example, antimony potassium tartrate, hexylresorcinol, and stibophen are no longer prescribed in the United States; but may be in use in other countries. Newer drugs have a broader range of action and are generally less toxic because they are not absorbed from the gastrointestinal tract.

TABLE 69-1 Drugs Used to Treat Helminthiasis

Helminth	Drug
Nematodes	
Roundworm	Piperazine, mebendazole
Hookworm	Bephenium hydroxynaphthoate
Whipworm	Mebendazole
Threadworm	Thiabendazole, pyrvinium pamoate
Pinworm	Mebendazole, pyrantel pamoate
Pork roundworm	Corticosteroids + thiabendazole
Filarial worms	Diethylcarbamazine
Guinea worm	Thiaben-dazole
Cestodes	
Beef, pork, fish tapeworms	Quinacrine (antimalarial), Niclosamide*
Trematodes	
Blood flukes	Niridazole*
Lung fluke	Emetine (amebicide) + sulfadiazine, Bithionol*
Liver fluke	Emetine (amebicide) + sulfonamides
…uke	Tetrachloroethylene

…e only from the Parasitic Disease Drug Service, …ters for Disease Control, Atlanta, GA 30333.

ANTHELMINTICS

GENERIC NAME Bephenium hydroxynaphthoate

TRADE NAME Alcopara RX

CLASSIFICATION Anthelmintic

Action Bephenium produces contracture of nematode muscles, thus causing the parasites to be expelled.

Indications for Use Hookworm infestations, mixed hookworm and roundworm infestations.

Warnings and Precautions Use with caution in clients with hypertension, hepatic, renal, or cardiac disease, and in infants under 1 year. Safe use during pregnancy has not been established.

Untoward Reactions Incidence of toxicity is low. May cause nausea, vomiting, dizziness, abdominal cramps, diarrhea, headache, and temporary hypotension.

Parameters of Use

Absorption Poorly absorbed from GI tract.
Excretion In urine. Unabsorbed drug excreted in feces.

Drug Interactions Alcohol may reduce drug effectiveness.

Administration Adults and children: Over 22 kg: 2.5 g po bid for 1 to 3 days; Under 22 kg: $\frac{1}{2}$ dosage.

Available Drug Forms Granules in 5-g packets.

Nursing Management

Planning factors

1. No purge is required before or after therapy.
2. Appropriate diet therapy may be indicated. Clients who are debilitated, anemic, or dehydrated should be treated before initiation of therapy.

Administration factors

1. Give on an empty stomach and withhold food for 2 hours following dosage to prevent vomiting.
2. Mix with milk, orange juice, or other flavorful liquid to mask bitter taste.

Client teaching factors

1. Instruct client in appropriate methods for preventing spread of infection.
2. Advise client against ingesting alcohol.

GENERIC NAME Diethylcarbamazine (RX)

TRADE NAME Hetrazan

CLASSIFICATION Anthelmintic

Action Exact mechanism of action is not known, but diethylcarbamazine may sensitize the worms so that they are more susceptible to phagocytosis.

Indications for Use Filarial worm and roundworm infestations, tropical eosinophilia.

Contraindications Pregnancy.

Untoward Reactions Common reactions include headache, dizziness, fever, nausea, dermatoses, and weakness. Severe allergic reactions have occurred within several hours of administration; symptoms include fever, tachycardia, arthralgia, rash, pruritus, GI distress, pedal edema, and lymphadenitis.

Parameters of Use

Absorption Readily absorbed from GI tract. Peak blood levels occur in 3 to 4 hours.
Distribution Widely distributed to all body tissues.
Excretion In urine.

Administration

- *Filariasis:* 2 mg/kg po tid for 3 to 4 weeks.
- *Roundworm:* Adults: 13 mg/kg po daily for 7 days; Children: 6 to 10 mg/kg po tid for 7 to 10 days.
- *Eosinophilia:* 13 mg/kg po daily for 4 to 7 days.

Available Drug Forms Scored tablets containing 50 mg.

Nursing Management

1. If allergic reaction occurs, antihistamines, corticosteroids, and epinephrine may be given to minimize symptoms.
2. Instruct client in appropriate methods for preventing spread of infection.

GENERIC NAME Mebendazole (RX)

TRADE NAME Vermox

CLASSIFICATION Anthelmintic

Action Mebendazole blocks glucose uptake by susceptible helminths, thereby depleting their energy level until they die. It has the broadest spectrum of action of any anthelmintic. The drug is relatively safe and nontoxic, since only a minute amount is absorbed from the GI tract.

Indications for Use Whipworm, pinworm, roundworm, hookworm, single or mixed infestations.

Contraindications Hypersensitivity to mebendazole, pregnancy, children under 2 years.

Untoward Reactions In massive infestations, transient nausea, vomiting, cramps, and diarrhea may occur due to expulsion of worms.

Administration Adults and children: 100 mg po tid for 3 days.

Available Drug Forms Chewable tablets containing 100 mg.

Nursing Management

1. No purge is required before or after therapy.
2. Tablets may be swallowed whole, chewed, and/or mixed with food.
3. If client is not cured in 3 weeks, a second course of treatment may be instituted.

4. Instruct client in appropriate methods for preventing spread of infection.

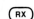

GENERIC NAME Piperazine (RX)

TRADE NAMES Antepar, Vermizine

CLASSIFICATION Anthelmintic

Action Piperazine causes muscle paralysis in worms, thus causing their expulsion.

Indications for Use Roundworm and pinworm infestations.

Contraindications Hypersensitivity to piperazine, renal or hepatic insufficiency, convulsive disorders.

Warnings and Precautions Safe use during pregnancy has not been established.

Untoward Reactions Incidence of toxicity is low. Unusually high dosages may produce the following: nausea, vomiting, diarrhea, abdominal cramps, headache, muscle weakness, visual disturbances, paresthesias, tremors, convulsions, EEG changes, exacerbation of epileptic seizures. Allergic reactions may also occur.

Parameters of Use

Absorption Some GI absorption may occur.
Excretion In urine. Unabsorbed drug is excreted in feces.

Drug Interactions May increase the extrapyramidal symptoms associated with phenothiazines.

Administration

- *Roundworm:* Adults: 3.5 g po daily for 2 days; Children: 75 mg/kg po daily for 2 days.
- *Pinworm:* 65 mg/kg po daily for 7 days. May be repeated in 7 days for severe infestation.

Available Drug Forms Tablets containing 550 mg; syrup containing 550 mg/5 ml.

Nursing Management

1. Instruct client to notify physician if any CNS, GI, or hypersensitivity reactions occur.
2. Warn client not to exceed the prescribed dosage because the risk of neurotoxicity is increased.
3. Instruct client in appropriate methods for preventing spread of infection.

NAME Pyrantel pamoate (RX)

ME Antiminth

CATION Anthelmintic

Action Pyrantel exerts a neuromuscular blocking action, thus paralyzing worms and facilitating expulsion.

Indications for Use Pinworm and roundworm infestations.

Warnings and Precautions Use with caution in clients with hepatic impairment. Safe use in children under 2 years and during pregnancy has not been established.

Untoward Reactions High dosages may cause nausea, vomiting, diarrhea, cramps, transient elevation of serum glutamic-oxaloacetic transaminase, headache, dizziness, drowsiness, insomnia, and allergic reactions.

Parameters of Use

Absorption Partially absorbed from GI tract. Peak plasma levels occur in 1 to 3 hours.
Metabolism In the liver.
Excretion Most of oral dosage excreted in feces; less than 7% in urine.

Administration 11 mg/kg po as a single dose; do not exceed a total dosage of 1 g.

Available Drug Forms Oral suspension containing 50 mg/ml.

Nursing Management

1. Laxatives or purge are not necessary before or after therapy.
2. May be given with food.
3. Instruct client in appropriate methods for preventing spread of infection.

GENERIC NAME Pyrvinium pamoate (RX)

TRADE NAME Povan

CLASSIFICATION Anthelmintic

Action Pyrvinium interferes with carbohydrate metabolism, thus causing death of worms.

Indications for Use Pinworm and dwarf threadworm infestations.

Contraindications Hypersensitivity to salicylates (as tablet coating contains tartrazine).

Warnings and Precautions Safe use during pregnancy has not been established.

Untoward Reactions Low toxicity. Nausea, vomiting, diarrhea, cramps, dizziness, and photosensitivity occur occasionally. Allergic reactions may also occur.

Parameters of Use

Absorption Not absorbed from GI tract.
Excretion In feces.

Administration 5 mg/kg po as a single dose; may be repeated in 2 to 3 weeks.

Available Drug Forms Coated tablets containing 50 mg; oral suspension containing 10 mg/ml.

Nursing Management

1. For pinworm infestations, test family members and treat accordingly.
2. Instruct client to swallow tablets whole to avoid staining teeth.
3. Warn client that drug may stain stool and vomitus a bright red color.
4. Instruct client in appropriate methods of preventing spread of infection.

GENERIC NAME Tetrachloroethylene (RX)

TRADE NAME Perchloroethylene

CLASSIFICATION Anthelmintic

Action Exact mechanism of action is not known, but tetrachloroethylene may cause paralysis of worms, thus facilitating their expulsion.

Indications for Use Hookworm infestations.

Warnings and Precautions Use with caution in severely anemic clients. Safe use during pregnancy has not been established.

Untoward Reactions Headache, vertigo, inebriation, CNS depression, giddiness, GI distress, nausea, vomiting, cardiovascular collapse (occasionally).

Parameters of Use

Absorption Not appreciably absorbed from GI tract.
Excretion In feces.

Administration 2 to 5 ml po in A.M. on an empty stomach.

Available Drug Forms Oral suspension.

Nursing Management

1. Oils, fats, and alcohol should be avoided for 24 hours before administration.
2. A saline purgative may be administered 2 hours after administration to facilitate expulsion of worms. If purgative is used, monitor client closely for signs of cardiovascular collapse.
3. Instruct client in appropriate methods for preventing spread of infection.

GENERIC NAME Thiabendazole (RX)

TRADE NAME Mintezol

CLASSIFICATION Anthelmintic

Action Thiabendazole may exert its action by interfering with metabolism in helminths. It is a broad-spectrum drug and also has analgesic and antiinflammatory properties.

Indications for Use Pinworm, threadworm, whipworm, roundworm, hookworm, guinea worm, cutaneous and visceral larva migrans, invasive trichinosis.

Contraindications Hypersensitivity to thiabendazole.

Warnings and Precautions Use with caution in clients with impaired renal or hepatic function. Safe use during pregnancy and lactation has not been established.

Untoward Reactions Common side effects include anorexia, nausea, vomiting, and dizziness. Leukopenia, crystalluria, rash, hallucinations, and olfactory disturbances occur occasionally. Rare reactions include jaundice, hypotension, bradycardia, and hyperglycemia. Allergic reactions may also occur; Stevens-Johnson syndrome may lead to fatalities.

Parameters of Use

Absorption Readily absorbed from GI tract. Peak action occurs in 1 to 2 hours.
Metabolism In the liver.
Excretion In urine within 24 hours.

Administration Adults: 25 mg/kg po bid for 1 to 4 days; Children: 22 mg/kg po bid for 1 to 4 days. Maximum total dosage: 3 g.

Available Drug Forms Chewable tablets containing 500 mg; oral suspension containing 500 mg/5 ml.

Nursing Management

1. No dietary restrictions or laxatives are necessary.
2. Give after meals.
3. Warn client that he or she may be incapacitated for several hours following administration.
4. Caution client not to drive or operate machinery for several hours after administration due to drug-induced drowsiness.
5. Instruct client in appropriate methods for preventing spread of infection.

Chapter 70

Antitubercular Agents

TUBERCULOSIS AND ITS TREATMENT

PRIMARY ANTITUBERCULAR DRUGS

- Aminosalicylic acid and salts (PAS)
- Ethambutol
- Isoniazid
- Rifampin

SECONDARY ANTITUBERCULAR DRUGS

- Capreomycin
- Cycloserine
- Ethionamide
- Pyrazinamide

TUBERCULOSIS AND ITS TREATMENT

Pulmonary tuberculosis is caused by *Mycobacterium tuberculosis,* a slow-growing, aerobic organism that is contracted by inhaling droplets from clients with active pulmonary infection. The disease can be spread to other body tissues if the organism is carried by macrophages through the lymphatic and circulatory systems.

Drug therapy for tuberculosis involves a long and often complex course of treatment because the bacillus remains active inside calcified pulmonary lesions for long periods and frequently develops resistance to one or more drugs used for treatment. For these reasons, chemotherapy almost always involves the use of two or three drugs given in the highest dosages possible in an effort to delay the development of resistant strains. The traditional course of treatment has been to administer two drugs in combination for a period of two years. A more recent approach is to use three drugs in combination for several months, followed by treatment with two of the drugs for another six to nine months. Clients receiving chemotherapy become noninfectious within the first few weeks as the living bacilli in the airways are destroyed. However, clients must understand that the bacilli remain dormant in calcified lung lesions for very long periods of time and drug therapy must be continued to prevent relapses or spread to other body tissues.

Antitubercular agents differ in effectiveness and in toxicity. The more commonly used primary drugs are the least toxic and have a broad spectrum of activity; therefore, they are generally used for clients with newly diagnosed tuberculosis. If the clinical response is not satisfactory, then secondary drugs are employed. (See Table 70-1.) The exceptions to the usual drug protocol are: (1) the need for prophylactic treatment because of high exposure to the bacillus; (2) recent conversion to a positive PPD test; and (3) the presence of another illness that would make a tubercular infection unusually serious (leukemia, diabetes, silicosis). In such cases, clients are usually treated with isoniazid alone for a period of at least one year.

TABLE 70-1 Antitubercular Agents

Primary Drugs
Aminosalicylic acid
Ethambutol
Isoniazid
Rifampin
Streptomycin (aminoglycoside)
Secondary Drugs
Capreomycin
Cycloserine
Ethionamide
Kanamycin (aminoglycoside)
Pyrazinamide

PRIMARY ANTITUBERCULAR DRUGS

GENERIC NAME Aminosalicylic acid, para-aminosalicylic acid

TRADE NAME PAS (RX)

CLASSIFICATION Antitubercular

Action Aminosalicylic acid suppresses growth and multiplication of bacilli by inhibiting folic acid synthesis. It also helps delay the development of strains resistant to isoniazid and streptomycin. The drug may compete with isoniazid for metabolism in the liver, thereby raising blood levels of isoniazid. It is never used as a sole agent, but as an adjunct to other drugs.

Indications for Use As an adjunct to isoniazid and/or streptomycin in pulmonary or extrapulmonary tuberculosis.

Contraindications Hypersensitivity to salicylates.

Warnings and Precautions Use with caution in clients with gastric ulcer or impaired renal or hepatic function. Safe use during pregnancy has not been established.

Untoward Reactions GI distress, nausea, anorexia, diarrhea, blood dyscrasias, hypokalemia, acidosis, vasculitis, encephalopathy, crystalluria, allergic reaction (fever, skin rash, jaundice, hepatitis, pancreatitis, mononucleosis symptoms).

Parameters of Use

Absorption Readily absorbed from GI tract.
Distribution Distributed to all body tissues except CNS.
Excretion In urine within 8 to 10 hours.

Drug Interactions Levels of aminosalicylic acid are increased by probenecid, salicylates, and sulfinpyrazone. May decrease the absorption of rifampin and vitamin B_{12}. May potentiate the action of oral anticoagulants. Concomitant use of urinary acidifiers increases the possibility of crystalluria.

Laboratory Interactions May cause false-positive results for urinary protein, vanilmandelic acid, and urinary glucose with Benedict's solution. Tes-Tape and Clinistix are not affected.

Administration Adults: 8 to 15 g po daily in 2 to 4 divided doses; Children: 200 to 300 mg po daily in divided doses.

Available Drug Forms Tablets, capsules, and enteric-coated pills containing 0.5 g; powder in premeasured packets of 500 mg from which solutions can be made.

Nursing Management

Administration factors

1. Give with meals. An antacid may also be prescribed to minimize gastric distress.
2. Do not use tablets, powder, or solution that have darkened in color. Drug is unstable and deteriorates rapidly; solution is stable for 24 hours when refrigerated. Protect tablets from heat and moisture.

Evaluation factors

1. Duration of therapy is generally 2 years. Dosage regime should not be interrupted, since resistant bacterial strains might develop.
2. Obtain routine sputum cultures and blood tests.

Client teaching factors

1. Instruct client in symptoms of blood dyscrasias and hypersensitivity, which may occur during the first 2 months of therapy. If symptoms occur, the drug should be discontinued to prevent hepatic or renal damage. Treatment may be resumed later with low dosages.
2. Emphasize the need of maintaining a high fluid intake and slightly alkaline urine to prevent crystalluria. Instruct client to avoid prune and cranberry juices.
3. Inform client that drug may leave a bitter aftertaste.
4. Stress the importance of maintaining a consistent dosage regime and regular medical supervision.

NAME Ethambutol (RX)

NAME Myambutol

CLASSIFICATION Antitubercular

Action Ethambutol interferes with cell metabolism, causing cell death.

Indications for Use Initial treatment of pulmonary tuberculosis (usually in combination with 1 or 2 other drugs).

Contraindications Hypersensitivity to ethambutol, optic neuritis.

Warnings and Precautions Safe use in children under 12 years and during pregnancy has not been established.

Untoward Reactions Visual changes, headache, dizziness, confusion, paresthesias, hallucinations, nausea, vomiting, abdominal pain, anorexia, elevated uric acid, acute gout, abnormal hepatic function tests, allergic reactions.

Parameters of Use

Absorption Absorbed from GI tract. Peak action occurs in 2 to 4 hours. Half-life is 3 to 4 hours.
Distribution Crosses blood-brain barrier; concentrates in erythrocytes.
Excretion About 50% in urine as unchanged drug and 25% as metabolites. About 25% is eliminated in feces (unabsorbed drug).

Laboratory Interactions Can increase serum glutamic-oxaloacetic transaminase, serum glutamic-pyruvic transaminase, and uric acid levels.

Administration Initial treatment (with isoniazid): 15 mg/kg po daily. Retreatment: 25 mg/kg po daily; decrease to 15 mg/kg after 60 days.

Available Drug Forms Tablets containing 100 or 400 mg.

Nursing Management

1. Clients with impaired renal function require lower dosages.
2. Test visual acuity prior to initiation of therapy and periodically thereafter.
3. Give with food to minimize gastric distress.
4. Since ethambutol is used in combination with other antitubercular agents, regular supervision of client is particularly important.
5. Periodic culture and sensitivity, renal, hepatic, and serum uric acid testing is recommended.

GENERIC NAME Isoniazid (RX)

TRADE NAMES Hyzyd, INH, Nydrazid, Rolazid, Teebaconin

CLASSIFICATION Antitubercular

Action Isoniazid probably acts by interfering with cellular metabolism in susceptible organisms. It can antagonize the activity of vitamin B_6. Resistance may develop rapidly when drug is used alone.

Indications for Use All forms of active tuberculosis; as a prophylactic in high-risk clients.

Contraindications Hypersensitivity to isoniazid, acute hepatic disease, pregnancy.

Warnings and Precautions Use with caution in clients with chronic hepatic disease, renal dysfunction, or convulsive disorders.

Untoward Reactions Paresthesias, peripheral neuropathy, hepatic dysfunction, visual disturbances, optic neuritis, tinnitus, vertigo, ataxia, insomnia, amnesia, euphoria, psychosis, depression, hyperreflexia, convulsions, vitamin B_6 deficiency, pellagra, gynecomastia, hyperglycemia, glycosuria, acetonuria, acidosis, proteinuria, blood dyscrasias, nausea, vomiting, constipation, headache, tachycardia, dry mouth, urinary retention, postural hypotension, rheumatic symptoms.

Parameters of Use

Absorption Absorbed from GI tract. Peak action occurs in 1 to 2 hours. Half-life is 2 to 4 hours, but is prolonged in hepatic insufficiency.

Crosses placenta and appears in breast milk.

Distribution Widely distributed to all body tissues.

Metabolism In the liver.

Excretion In urine within 24 hours; small amounts excreted in saliva and feces.

Drug Interactions Increases serum levels of phenytoin. Serum levels of isoniazid may be elevated by aminosalicylic acid. Alcohol and rifampin increase the risk of hepatotoxicity. Isoniazid may potentiate the action of sympathomimetics (leading to hypertension), anesthetics, anticoagulants, anticonvulsants, antidiabetics, antihypertensives, antiparkinsonian agents, anticholinergics, antidepressants, narcotics, and sedatives. Antacids reduce GI absorption of isoniazid.

Laboratory Interactions May give false-positive results for urinary glucose with Benedict's solution. Clinistix, Dextrostix, and Tes-Tape are not affected.

Administration

- *Treatment:* Adults: 5 mg/kg po or IM daily; up to 300 mg daily. Children: 10 to 30 mg/kg po or IM daily; up to 500 mg daily.
- *Prophylaxis:* Adults: 300 mg po daily; Children: 100 mg/kg po daily.

Available Drug Forms Tablets containing 100 or 300 mg; vials containing 100 mg/ml of solution.

Nursing Management

Planning factors

1. Complete culture and sensitivity tests prior to initiating therapy.
2. Certain clients may be slow isoniazid inactivators and are at increased risk of adverse reactions. About 50% of Caucasians and blacks are slow inactivators; most Orientals and Eskimos are rapid inactivators.
3. Store in airtight, light-resistant containers.

Administration factors

1. Oral drug form may be taken with food. When administering IM,
   a. Warm solution to room temperature to redissolve any crystals that have formed.
   b. Massage injection site following administration to alleviate pain.
   c. Rotate injection sites.

Evaluation factors

1. Schedule regular ophthalmic examinations. If visual symptoms occur, drug should be discontinued.
2. Susceptible clients (slow inactivators, undernourished, diabetic, or adolescent clients) should take supplemental vitamin B_6 (pyridoxine) to prevent neurotoxicity.
3. Complete culture and sensitivity tests periodically to detect the development of drug resistance.
4. Assist elderly clients with ambulation, especially during dosage and adjustment periods, when necessary.
5. Monitor diabetic clients closely; dosages of antidiabetic drugs may need adjustment.
6. Monitor all clients periodically for hepatotoxicity, which is most common in those over 50 years and those who drink alcohol regularly.
7. Hypersensitivity reactions generally occur with 3 to 7 weeks after beginning of therapy. If evident, drug should be discontinued.

Client teaching factors

1. Stress the importance of following prescribed drug regimen. (Duration of drug therapy is usually at least 18 months for treatment of tuberculosis.)
2. Emphasize the need of regular medical supervision for early identification of potentially serious hepatotoxicity or neurotoxicity.

GENERIC NAME Rifampin (RX)

TRADE NAMES Rifadin, Rimactane

CLASSIFICATION Antitubercular

Action Rifampin suppresses RNA synthesis in susceptible bacteria. It is effective against a variety of gram-negative and gram-positive organisms. Resistance to rifampin develops rapidly when it is used alone; hence, it is always used in combination with other agents in treating tuberculosis.

Indications for Use Pulmonary tuberculosis in conjunction with at least 1 other drug; treatment of asymptomatic carriers of meningococci when risk of meningococcal meningitis is high.

Contraindications Hypersensitivity to rifampin, concurrent use of other hepatotoxic agents, obstructive biliary disease.

Warnings and Precautions Use with caution in clients with hepatic disease or a history of alcoholism. Safe use in children under 5 years and during pregnancy has not been established.

Untoward Reactions Epigastric distress, nausea, vomiting, anorexia, cramps, diarrhea, fatigue, headache, confusion, dizziness, ataxia, numbness, auditory and visual disturbances, blood dyscrasias, abnormal hepatic function tests, renal insufficiency, acute renal failure, allergic reactions (rash, pruritus, urticaria, fever, soreness of mouth and tongue, hematuria, hemolysis, reversible renal failure).

Parameters of Use

Absorption Absorbed from GI tract. Peak action occurs in 2 to 4 hours. Half-life is 3 hours. About 90% bound to plasma proteins.

Metabolism In the liver.

Excretion In feces; some in urine.

Drug Interactions May decrease the effects of other drugs metabolized by the liver, including oral anticoagulants, estrogens, corticosteroids, oral antidiabetics, digitalis, and methadone. Concurrent use of aminosalicylic acid can impair absorption of rifampin. Action is potentiated by probenecid. Concurrent ingestion of alcohol or isoniazid increases the risk of hepatotoxicity.

Laboratory Interactions May cause retention of Bromsulphalein. May interfere with standard tests for serum folate and vitamin B_{12} and with radiopaque medium used in gall bladder x-rays.

Administration

- *Tuberculosis:* Adults: 600 mg po daily, as a single dose. Children: 10 to 20 mg/kg po daily; do not exceed 600 mg/day.
- Meningococcal carriers: Adults: 600 mg po daily for 4 days; Children: 10 to 20 mg po daily for 4 days.

Available Drug Forms Capsules containing 300 mg.

Nursing Management

1. Give on an empty stomach.
2. Obtain periodic hepatic function tests.
3. Inform client not to interrupt therapy, since hepatorenal dysfunction may result.
4. Inform client that drug may cause a harmless orange color to urine, feces, sputum, sweat, and tears.
5. Discuss with client alternative methods of birth control, since oral contraception may not be effective.
6. Inform female clients that menstrual irregularities may occur during therapy.
7. Instruct client to report hepatotoxic or hematologic symptoms.
8. Emphasize the importance of avoiding alcohol during therapy.
9. Store drug in bottle with a dessicant; moisture causes instability.

SECONDARY ANTITUBERCULAR DRUGS

GENERIC NAME Capreomycin (RX)

TRADE NAME Capastat

CLASSIFICATION Antitubercular

Action Exact mechanism of action is unknown. Capreomycin is bacteriostatic against tubercular bacillus. It has a neuromuscular blocking action in large dosages.

Indications for Use Alternative therapy for clients resistant to primary antitubercular drugs or when bacillus has developed resistance to primary drugs.

Contraindications Hypersensitivity to capreomycin, concurrent administration of streptomycin, or other ototoxic and nephrotoxic drugs.

Warnings and Precautions Use with caution in clients with renal or hepatic insufficiency. Safe use in children and during pregnancy has not been established.

Untoward Reactions Hearing loss, tinnitus, vertigo, anorexia, hematuria, proteinuria, renal tubular necrosis, pyuria, elevated blood urea nitrogen and nonprotein nitrogen, depressed phenolsulfonphthalein excretion, blood dyscrasias, hypokalemia, decreased Bromsulphalein excretion, pain and sterile abscess at injection site, headache, muscle weakness, hypersensitivity reactions.

Parameters of Use

Absorption Peak action occurs in 1 to 2 hours following intramuscular administration.

Excretion About 50% as unchanged drug in urine within 12 hours.

Drug Interactions May enhance muscle-relaxing action of neuromuscular blocking agents, antibiotics, aminoglycosides, and general anesthetics. Aminoglycosides, cephaloridine, cephalothin, ethacrynic acid, furosemide, polymyxins, and vancomycin increase the risk of nephrotoxicity. Ototoxic effects are potentiated by aminoglycosides, ethacrynic acid, furosemide, and vancomycin.

Administration 1 g IM daily for 60 to 120 days; then 1 g IM 2 to 3 times weekly; Maximum dosage: 20 mg/kg/day.

Available Drug Forms Vials containing 1 g of dry powder.

Nursing Management

Planning factors Before treatment is started, do culture and sensitivity testing and determine audiometric and vestibular functions, renal and liver functions, and serum potassium levels.

Administration factors

1. Dissolve powder in 2 ml of 0.9% sodium chloride. Allow 2 to 3 minutes for drug to go into solution. Reconstituted solution is stable for 48 hours at room temperature and 14 days when refrigerated. Solution may darken, but potency is not affected.
2. Give IM injection deep into gluteal muscle. Rotate injection sites.

Evaluation factors

1. Schedule periodic audiometric tests. Any signs of hearing loss or vertigo call for immediate discontinuation of drug.
2. Obtain renal function tests periodically. If any abnormality occurs, drug should be discontinued to prevent serious renal damage.
3. Test serum potassium levels periodically; hypokalemia may occur with prolonged treatment.

Client teaching factors Teach client importance of reporting promptly any untoward reactions.

GENERIC NAME Cycloserine (RX)

TRADE NAME Seromycin

CLASSIFICATION Antitubercular

Action Cycloserine inhibits cell wall synthesis in susceptible bacteria.

Indications for Use Alternative therapy of tuberculosis in combination with other drugs when primary therapy is ineffective; alternative therapy for acute urinary tract infections when other drugs are ineffective.

Contraindications Hypersensitivity to cycloserine, epilepsy, depression, severe anxiety, psychoses, chronic alcoholism, severe renal insufficiency.

Warnings and Precautions Safe use in children and during pregnancy has not been established.

Untoward Reactions Neurotoxicity, headache, tremors, anxiety, drowsiness, convulsions, vertigo, visual disturbances, confusion, psychoses, aggression, paresthesias, hyperreflexia, disorientation, memory loss, clonic seizures, suicidal tendencies, coma, skin rash, photosensitivity, elevated serum transaminase, vitamin B_{12} or folic acid deficiency, megaloblastic anemia.

Parameters of Use

Absorption Rapidly absorbed from GI tract. Peak action occurs in 4 to 8 hours. Half-life is 10 hours.

Distribution Distributed to all body tissues, including cerebrospinal fluid. Crosses placenta and appears in breast milk.

Excretion In urine.

Drug Interactions Neurotoxic effects are potentiated by concurrent administration of ethionamide, alcohol, and isoniazid. Cycloserine potentiates the effects of MAO inhibitors and phenytoin. May increase the excretion of vitamin B-complex.

Administration 250 mg po bid for 2 weeks; then 500 to 1000 mg daily in divided doses; do not exceed 1 g/day.

Available Drug Forms Capsules containing 250 mg.

Nursing Management

1. Complete culture and sensitivity tests periodically to detect bacterial resistance to drug.
2. Monitor blood drug levels, renal, hepatic, and hematologic tests routinely.
3. If hypersensitivity reactions or symptoms of neurotoxicity develop, drug should be discontinued.
4. Instruct client to avoid alcohol, which increases the risk of convulsions.
5. Caution client to avoid driving and operating machinery until reaction to drug is determined.

GENERIC NAME Ethionamide (RX)

TRADE NAME Trecator-SC

CLASSIFICATION Antitubercular

Action Similar to isoniazid; probably suppresses multiplication of bacillus.

Indications for Use Alternative therapy of tuberculosis in combination with other drugs when primary drug treatment is ineffective.

Contraindications Hypersensitivity to ethionamide, severe hepatic impairment.

Warnings and Precautions Safe use during pregnancy has not been established.

Untoward Reactions GI distress, peripheral and optic neuritis, rash, metallic taste, jaundice, hepatitis, thrombocytopenia, hypotension, depression, stomatitis, gynecomastia, impotence.

Parameters of Use

Absorption Readily absorbed from GI tract. Peak action occurs in 3 to 4 hours.

Distribution Distributed to all body tissues, including CNS.

Excretion In urine.

Drug Interactions Enhances neurotoxicity of cycloserine and adverse effects of other antitubercular agents. Alcohol increases the risk of neurotoxicity. May potentiate the hypotensive effects of antihypertensive agents.

Administration Adults: 0.5 to 1.0 g po daily in 1 to 3 divided doses; Children: 4 to 5 mg/kg/day po q8h.

Available Drug Forms Sugar-coated tablets containing 250 mg.

Nursing Management

1. Culture and sensitivity testing should be done prior to starting drug therapy.
2. Give with food to minimize gastric upset.
3. When used concurrently with isoniazid, vitamin B_6 supplements are necessary.
4. Antidiabetic drug dosage may need adjustment.
5. Advise client to avoid excessive alcohol intake to minimize risk of neurotoxicity.
6. Periodic renal and liver function testing and complete blood cell counts are recommended.

GENERIC NAME Pyrazinamide (RX)

TRADE NAME PZA

CLASSIFICATION Antitubercular

Action Pyrazinamide may interfere with bacterial protein synthesis. It is active only at slightly acidic pH.

Indications for Use As an adjunct with primary drugs in treatment of tuberculosis; short-term therapy before pulmonary surgery for preventing spread of infection.

Contraindications Severe hepatic damage, children.

Warnings and Precautions Use with caution in clients with a history of gout, diabetes, renal dysfunction, or peptic ulcer.

Untoward Reactions Hepatic dysfunction, fever, anorexia, malaise, hepatomegaly, splenomegaly, jaundice, yellow atrophy of liver, GI upset, anemia, dysuria, urinary retention, hyperuricemia, gout, rash, photosensitivity.

Parameters of Use

Absorption Rapidly absorbed from GI tract. Peak action occurs in 2 hours. Half-life is 9 hours.
Metabolism In the liver.
Excretion Slowly in urine.

Laboratory Interactions May produce a temporary decrease in 17-ketosteroids. May cause an increase in protein-bound iodine.

Administration 20 to 35 mg/kg po daily in 3 to 4 divided doses; Maximum dosage: 3 g/day.

Available Drug Forms Tablets containing 500 mg.

Nursing Management

1. Monitor diabetic clients closely; alteration of antidiabetic drug dosages may be necessary.
2. Aspirin or other uricosuric agents may be prescribed to control hyperuricemia.
3. Obtain hepatic function tests before and periodically during therapy. If hepatic dysfunction occurs, drug should be discontinued.
4. Emphasize the importance of regular medical supervision.
5. Teach client the importance of reporting signs and symptoms of hepatic dysfunction.
6. Instruct client to report joint pain and urinary retention, which are signs of elevated uric acid levels.

Chapter 71

Antimalarial Agents

MALARIA AND ITS TREATMENT

Malaria is still a prevalent parasitic disease endemic in South America, Africa, and southeast Asia. Human malaria is caused by four species of *Plasmodium: P. falciparum, P. vivax, P. malariae,* and *P. ovale. P. falciparum* causes malignant tertian malaria, which is usually lethal if not treated quickly. The other three plasmodia are responsible for *relapsing* malaria, as a consequence of their exoerythrocytic cycle, or secondary tissue phase. This stage is characterized by multiplication of the parasite in body tissues, where they persist for long periods, and release of erythrocyte invaders at intervals. Relapses can, therefore, occur for many years after the initial infection unless treated with appropriate drugs.

It is necessary to understand the stages of development of the *Plasmodium* in the human body in order to select appropriate drug therapy. The *Anopheles* mosquito deposits *sporozoites* (asexual forms) in humans during the bite. Sporozoites then enter the reticuloendothelial cells of the liver where they multiply for a period of 8 to 42 days, depending on the type of *Plasmodium* involved. During this primary tissue phase, the individual is asymptomatic and no parasites are found in the blood. When mature, *merozoites* enter the circulation and multiply in the erythrocytes, causing eventual rupture of the red blood cells. This stage of the disease is the familiar symptomatic one. The fever, chills, and profound sweating associated with malaria are due to the release of foreign protein and other cell products into the circulation when the erythrocytes rupture. Some merozoites are destroyed, some enter other erythrocytes and cause repeated acute attacks, and some reenter the liver and other body tissues, which is the secondary tissue phase. Still other parasites differentiate into male and female gametocytes (sexual forms) and are transferred in subsequent bites to the mosquito; thus, sexual reproduction takes place producing new sporozoites and the cycle begins again.

Drug therapy for malaria is directed at the different stages of the parasite's life cycle. Antimalarial drugs are classified into three groups as follows:

- *Prophylactic drugs*—these drugs (primaquine, chloroguanide, pyrimethamine) destroy the organism during the primary tissue phase. These drugs are so toxic in therapeutic doses that their use in prophylaxis is avoided.
- *Suppressive drugs*—these drugs (chloroquine, amodiaquine, hydroxychloroquine, pyrimethamine, quinine, tetracycline) destroy the parasites in the circulation and prevent the symptoms associated with acute attacks. They do not, however, act on the secondary tissue parasites, so acute attacks can recur when therapy is discontinued.
- *Radical cure drugs (tissue schizonticides)*—these drugs destroy the organism during the secondary tissue stage so that relapses cannot occur. Primaquine is the only drug presently used for this purpose and is often combined with chloroquine, which also suppresses the erythrocytic stage. This drug combination is used in travelers to regions where malaria is widespread and is continued for two months after return from the region.

ANTIMALARIAL AGENTS

GENERIC NAME Primaquine phosphate (RX)

CLASSIFICATION Antimalarial

Action Primaquine acts on tissue forms of *Plasmodium* by an unknown mechanism.

Indications for Use Prevention of vivax malaria relapse (radical cure).

Contraindications Rheumatoid arthritis, lupus erythematosus, concurrent use of hemolytic drugs, bone marrow depressants, or quinacrine, pregnancy.

Untoward Reactions Epigastric distress, abdominal cramps, headache, pruritus, blood dyscrasias, CNS and cardiovascular disturbances, visual accommodation disturbances, hemolytic anemia (in clients with glucose-6-phosphate dehydrogenase deficiency).

Parameters of Use

Absorption Readily absorbed from GI tract. Peak action occurs in 3 to 6 hours.

Distribution Rapidly metabolized; concentrates in liver, lungs, heart, brain, and muscles.

Excretion In urine.

Drug Interactions Primaquine toxicity is potentiated by quinacrine, hemolytic drugs, and bone marrow depressants.

Administration Adults: 26.3 mg po daily for 14 days; Children: 0.3 mg/kg po daily for 14 days.

Available Drug Forms Tablets containing 26.3 mg. Also available with chloroquine (Aralen) for prophylaxis; dosage is 1 tablet weekly.

Nursing Management

1. Dark-skinned individuals are more susceptible to hemolytic anemia because of a genetic deficiency of glucose-6-phosphate dehydrogenase.
2. Give with meals to minimize gastric upset; an antacid may be prescribed to reduce gastric distress.
3. Obtain hematologic studies periodically. A fall in hemoglobin or erythrocyte count may indicate impending hemolytic reaction.
4. Instruct client to promptly report signs of hemolytic anemia: darkened urine, chills, fever, precordial pain. Discontinue drug at once.
5. Drug should be kept in tightly closed, light-resistant containers.

GENERIC NAME Amodiaquine hydrochloride

TRADE NAME Camoquin (RX)

CLASSIFICATION Antimalarial

See chloroquine hydrochloride for Action, Indications for use, Contraindications, Warnings and precautions, Untoward reactions, Parameters of use, Drug interactions, and Nursing management.

Administration

- *Malaria, acute attack:* Adults: Initial dosage: 600 mg po; then 300 mg 6, 24, and 48 hours later. Children: 10 mg/kg po in 3 divided doses q12h.
- *Malaria, suppression:* Adults: 300 to 400 mg po once a week; Children: 5 mg/kg po once a week.

Available Drug Forms Tablets containing 200 mg.

GENERIC NAME Chloroguanide hydrochloride

TRADE NAME Paludrine (RX)

CLASSIFICATION Antimalarial

Action Chloroguanide interferes with the metabolism of plasmodia in the erythrocytic stage. It is the least toxic of the antimalarial drugs; even massive overdosage has been followed by complete recovery.

Indications for Use Prophylaxis of malaria; cure for *P. falciparum* and *P. vivax*.

Contraindications Hypersensitivity to chloroguanide.

Warnings and Precautions Safe use during pregnancy has not been established.

Untoward Reactions Nausea, vomiting, diarrhea, abdominal pain, hematuria, cells and casts in urine, megaloblastic anemia, anorexia, malaise.

Parameters of Use

Absorption Slowly absorbed from GI tract. Peak action occurs in 2 to 4 hours.
Excretion Primarily in urine; some in feces.

Administration Adults: 100 mg po daily; Children: Ages 5 to 8 years: 75 mg po daily; Ages 1 to 4 years: 50 mg po daily; Under 1 year: 25 to 50 mg po daily.

Available Drug Forms Tablets containing 25 or 50 mg.

Nursing Management

1. Inform client that drug may cause appetite suppression.
2. Give with meals or milk to minimize gastric upset.

GENERIC NAME Chloroquine hydrochloride; hydroxychloroquine sulfate

TRADE NAMES Aralen Hydrochloride, Plaquenil Sulfate

CLASSIFICATION Antimalarial (RX)

Action Exact mechanism of action is unknown, but chloroquine may interfere with nucleic acid synthesis in susceptible plasmodia. It is active against erythrocytic forms of plasmodia. Chloroquine also has amebicidal, antiinflammatory, and antihistaminic properties.

Indications for Use Suppression and treatment of acute malaria caused by all strains of plasmodia; treatment of extraintestinal amebiasis; treatment of systemic lupus erythematosus and rheumatoid arthritis.

Contraindications Hypersensitivity to chloroquine, psoriatic arthritis, retinal damage, visual field changes, pregnancy, long-term treatment in children, concurrent use of bone marrow depressants or hemolytic drugs.

Warnings and Precautions Use with caution in children; clients with hematologic, neurologic, hepatic, and gastrointestinal disorders; alcoholism; and clients with glucose-6-phosphate dehydrogenase deficiency.

Untoward Reactions Side effects usually occur with high dosages and include visual disturbances, corneal edema or opacity, retinal changes, optic atrophy, vertigo, tinnitus, ototoxicity, fatigue, convulsions, psychotic episodes, hypotension, EKG changes, dermatologic reactions, and blood dyscrasias.

Parameters of Use

Absorption Readily absorbed from GI tract. Peak action occurs in 1 to 2 hours. About 50% bound to plasma proteins.

Distribution Widely distributed to body tissues, with high concentrations in liver, kidneys, lungs, brain, spinal cord, and erythrocytes.

Metabolism Partially metabolized in the liver.

Excretion Slowly in urine; small amounts in feces. Urinary excretion is facilitated by acidification and hampered by alkalinization of urine.

Drug Interactions Other hepatotoxic drugs and MAO inhibitors increase the risk of liver toxicity. Dermatologic side effects are increased with concurrent use of gold compounds and antiinflammatory drugs. Chloroquine may antagonize the action of antipsoriatic drugs.

Administration

- *Malaria, acute attack:* Oral: Adults: Initial dosage: 600 to 620 mg base; then 300 to 310 mg base 6, 24, and 48 hours later. Children: Initial dosage: 10 mg/kg base; then 5 mg/kg base 6, 24, and 48 hours later. Intramuscular: Initial dosage: 160 to 200 mg base; repeat in 6 hours. Children: Initial dosage: 5 mg/kg; repeat in 6 hours.
- *Malaria, suppression:* Adults and children: 5 mg/kg base po once a week beginning two weeks before exposure and continuing for 8 weeks after leaving high-risk area.
- *Amebiasis:* 600 mg base po daily for 2 days; then 300 mg base daily for 2 to 3 weeks.
- *Lupus erythematosus, rheumatoid arthritis:* Initial dosage: 400 to 600 mg base po daily until clinical response; then 200 to 400 mg base daily.

Available Drug Forms *Chloroquine:* Tablets containing 250 or 500 mg (equivalent to 150 or 300 mg base); 5-ml ampules containing 40 mg base/ml. *Hydroxychloroquine:* Tablets containing 200 mg (equivalent to 155 mg base).

Nursing Management

1. May be given with meals to reduce GI distress.
2. Perform blood cell counts and eye examinations prior to treatment and periodically thereafter for clients on long-term therapy.
3. Skeletal muscle symptoms call for discontinuation of treatment.
4. Use of dark glasses in sunlight may reduce the risk of optic damage.
5. Inform client that drug may cause harmless brown discoloration of urine.
6. Instruct client to keep medication out of the reach of children; fatalities have occurred following accidental overdose.
7. Instruct client to report immediately any visual symptoms; retinal damage may be irreversible.

GENERIC NAME Pyrimethamine (RX)

TRADE NAME Daraprim

CLASSIFICATION Antimalarial

Action Pyrimethamine interferes with folic acid metabolism in the fertilized gametes carried by the mosquito, thereby preventing transmission of disease.

Indications for Use Prophylaxis of malaria due to susceptible strains; treatment of toxoplasmosis in conjunction with a sulfonamide. Usually used in conjunction with chloroquine for suppression of acute attacks.

Contraindications Chloroguanide-resistant malaria.

Warnings and Precautions Use with caution in clients with convulsive disorders. Safe use during pregnancy has not been established.

Untoward Reactions Anorexia, vomiting, rash, glossitis, blood dyscrasias, hemolytic anemia (in clients with glucose-6-phosphate dehydrogenase deficiency), convulsions (overdosage).

Parameters of Use

Absorption Readily absorbed from GI tract. Peak action occurs in 2 hours.

Distribution Concentrates in kidneys, lungs, liver, and spleen. Appears in breast milk.

Excretion Slowly in urine (30 days).

Drug Interactions Folic acid and *p*-aminobenzoic acid may inhibit the antitoxoplasmic effects of pyrimethamine. Pyrimethamine can increase blood levels of quinine by displacing it from plasma-binding sites.

Administration

- *Prophylaxis:* Adults: 250 mg po weekly; Children: Ages 4 to 10 years: 12.5 mg po weekly; Under 4 years: 6.25 mg po weekly.
- *Toxoplasmosis:* Adults: 50 to 75 mg po daily for 1 to 3 weeks; then $\frac{1}{2}$ dosage for 30 days.
- *Acute attacks:* 25 mg po daily for 2 days; then 12.5 to 25 mg weekly.

Available Drug Forms Tablets containing 25 mg.

Nursing Management

1. For malaria prophylaxis, drug therapy should begin before entering high-risk area and continue for 10 weeks after leaving area, and should be taken on the same day each week.

2. Give with meals to minimize gastric upset.
3. When administering high dosages (toxoplasmosis), monitor blood counts weekly to detect hematologic abnormalities. Leucovorin may be prescribed to prevent or treat depressed white blood cell count.
4. Instruct client to report immediately any signs of developing blood dyscrasias: fever, sore tongue, rash, diarrhea, bruising, bleeding.

GENERIC NAME Quinine sulfate (RX)

TRADE NAMES Quinamm, Quindan, Coco-Quinine

CLASSIFICATION Antimalarial

Action Exact mechanism of action is unknown, but quinine may inhibit protein synthesis and interfere with cellular metabolism. It also has analgesic, antipyretic, skeletal muscle relaxant, oxytocic, and hypoprothrombinemic properties. The use of quinine has been replaced by less toxic antimalarial drugs, but it is still useful as an adjunct in treating chloroquine-resistant falciparum malaria.

Indications for Use Chloroquine-resistant falciparum malaria; radical cure of relapsing vivax malaria in combination with other drugs.

Contraindications Hypersensitivity to quinine, pregnancy, myasthenia gravis, tinnitus, optic neuritis, glucose-6-phosphate dehydrogenase deficiency.

Untoward Reactions Cinchonism (tinnitus, dizziness, visual disturbances, headache, GI distress, fever, skin rash, flushing, asthma), confusion, excitement, syncope, convulsions, photophobia, other visual disturbances, blood dyscrasias, hypotension, respiratory depression, paralysis.

Parameters of Use

Absorption Readily absorbed from GI tract. Peak action occurs in 1 to 3 hours. About 70% bound to plasma proteins.

Crosses placenta.

Metabolism In the liver.

Excretion In urine within 24 hours; small amounts in saliva, gastric juice, bile, and feces. Alkaline urine inhibits renal excretion.

Drug Interactions Aluminum hydroxide delays absorption of quinine. Enhances the hypoprothrombinemic effects of oral anticoagulants. Decreases the effects of heparin. Concurrent use of pyrimethamine may cause elevated blood levels of quinine. Concomitant use of skeletal muscle relaxants increases the risk of respiratory depression and apnea.

Laboratory Interactions May interfere with urinary catecholamines and 17-hydroxycorticosteroids.

Administration Adults: 325 mg po qid for 7 days; Children: Do not exceed 15 mg/kg po in 24 hours.

Available Drug Forms Capsules containing 120, 200, 300, or 325 mg; tablets containing 260 mg.

Nursing Management

1. Give with meals to minimize gastric distress.
2. Do not crush capsule, since drug is irritating and has an extremely bitter taste.
3. Store in airtight, light-resistant containers.
4. Caution client to promptly report any adverse reactions.
5. Prompt treatment of overdosage is essential, since drug is rapidly absorbed. Gastric lavage is followed by supportive treatment.

Chapter 72

Amebicides

AMEBIASIS AND ITS TREATMENT

Amebic dysentery, or amebiasis, is caused by the protozoan *Entamoeba histolytica*. The disease is endemic in many tropical regions of the world, but is also found in temperate climates where environmental and sanitary conditions are unhealthy. Although the disease can be asymptomatic, clients must be treated as they are carriers and can spread the infection. Symptomatic intestinal infections present with symptoms ranging from mild diarrhea to severe bloody diarrhea, vomiting, fever, and dehydration. The most serious form of the disease occurs when protozoa escape through the traumatized intestinal wall and invade other body organs. Involvement of the liver and lungs is most common, but the organisms can also invade the heart and central nervous system.

Agents used to treat amebiasis are classified according to their site of action (see Table 72-1). Two or more drugs are generally used to treat symptomatic infections to ensure the destruction of organisms that may be encysted in bowel or other tissues. However, metronidazole is effective in both intestinal and extraintestinal amebiasis and may be used alone.

TABLE 72-1 Drugs Used to Treat Amebiasis

Asymptomatic and Symptomatic Bowel Infections
Diloxanide-furoate*
Diiodohydroxyquin
Metronidazole (miscellaneous antibiotic)
Paromomycin (aminoglycoside)
Erythromycin
Extraintestinal, or Tissue, Infections
Metronidazole
Emetine
Chloroquine (antimalarial)
Dehydroemetine*

*Available only from the Parasitic Disease Drug Service, U.S. Centers for Disease Control, Atlanta, GA 30333.

AMEBICIDES

GENERIC NAME Diiodohydroxyquin (RX)

TRADE NAMES Iodoquinol, Yodoxin

CLASSIFICATION Amebicide

Action Exact mechanism of action is unknown. However, diiodohydroxyquin has a direct amebicidal action that is restricted to the intestinal tract.

Indications for Use Asymptomatic intestinal amebiasis; symptomatic amebiasis in combination with a tissue amebicide.

Contraindications Hypersensitivity to iodides, hepatic disease.

Warnings and Precautions Use with caution during pregnancy and in clients with thyroid disorders.

Untoward Reactions Epigastric distress is the most common reaction. Nausea, vomiting, diarrhea, cramps, skin eruptions, headache, vertigo, fever, chills, optic damage, peripheral neuropathy, and thyroid hypertrophy may also occur, particularly at high dosages.

Parameters of Use

Absorption Not absorbed from GI tract. Metabolism and distribution unknown.

Laboratory Interactions Increases protein-bound iodine and can interfere with thyroid function tests.

Administration Adults: 650 mg po tid for 20 days; Children: 30 to 40 mg/kg po daily in 3 divided doses for 20 days.

Available Drug Forms Tablets containing 210 or 650 mg; powder in 25-g packets.

Nursing Management

1. Instruct client to report immediately any visual or neurologic disturbances; drug should be discontinued.
2. Hypersensitivity reactions also call for discontinuation of drug.
3. Long-term use should be avoided because of danger of ophthalmic and neurological complications.
4. Instruct client to report symptoms of iodism (sore throat, chills, fever, dermatitis, furunculosis).

GENERIC NAME Emetine hydrochloride (RX)

CLASSIFICATION Amebicide

Action Emetine causes degeneration of the cell nucleus and cytoplasm in amebae possibly by blocking protein synthesis. As the drug is cumulative, the risk of toxicity is high.

Indications for Use Acute amebiasis in combination with other amebicides; amebic hepatitis and other tissue amebiasis in combination with an intestinal amebicide.

Contraindications Pregnancy, organic cardiac or renal disease, children except those with severe amebiasis not controlled by other agents, clients who have received a course of emetine therapy within the previous 2 months.

Untoward Reactions Common reactions include pain, tenderness, soreness at injection site, nausea, diarrhea, abdominal pain, dizziness, and fainting. Vomiting, hypotension, tachycardia, EKG abnormalities, dyspnea, congestive heart failure, tremors, and skin lesions are less common.

Parameters of Use

Absorption Readily absorbed from injection site.
Distribution Widely distributed to all body tissues with highest concentrations in the liver.
Excretion Very slowly by the kidneys; may still be present in urine 60 days after last dose.

Administration Adults: 65 mg IM or subc daily for 3 to 5 days; may be given in divided doses; Children: Over 8 years: Maximum dosage: 20 mg IM or subc daily; Under 8 years: Maximum dosage: 10 mg IM or subc daily.

Available Drug Forms Vials.

Nursing Management

Planning factors

1. Hospitalize client and confine to bed during therapy and for several days after last dose.
2. Obtain an EKG before instituting therapy.
3. Protect drug from light.

Administration Factors

1. Inadvertent IV administration is dangerous; aspirate carefully before injecting dose.
2. Alternate injection sites daily. Avoid contact with eyes and mucous membranes as drug is very irritating.

Evaluation factors

1. Obtain an EKG after the fifth dose and 1 week after discontinuation of therapy.
2. Monitor vital signs at least three times daily: tachycardia may precede EKG changes.
3. Monitor neuromuscular function closely. Report any signs of weakness promptly to avoid overdosage.
4. Tachycardia, neuromuscular symptoms, or severe GI symptoms call for prompt discontinuance of drug.
5. Monitor intake and output. Report any changes immediately.
6. Treatment should never be extended beyond 10 days because of the danger of cumulative toxicity.

Client teaching factors

1. Instruct client to avoid any strenuous activities for 1 month following treatment.
2. Instruct client to report promptly any unusual symptoms during posttreatment period.

Chapter 73

Antiviral Agents

ANTIVIRAL AGENTS

- Acyclovir
- Amantadine hydrochloride
- Idoxuridine
- Trifluridine
- Vidarabine

THE DEVELOPMENT OF antiviral drugs has been very limited for several reasons. Firstly, viruses depend on the enzyme systems of the host's cells for their replication; therefore, any agent toxic to the virus is also toxic to the host cells. Secondly, viruses multiply rapidly before any symptoms develop, so that by the time the particular viral disease is symptomatic, the host's natural defenses are already active. For these reasons, viral infections are best prevented by immunization. However, there are several antiviral drugs available for limited therapeutic use, including acyclovir, amantadine, idoxuridine, trifluridine, and vidarabine.

ANTIVIRAL AGENTS

GENERIC NAME Acyclovir (RX)

TRADE NAME Zovirax

CLASSIFICATION Antiviral

Action Acyclovir inhibits viral replication by inhibiting DNA replication.

Indications for Use Initial herpes genitalis; limited mucocutaneous herpes simplex infections in clients with impaired immune responses.

Contraindications Hypersensitivity to acyclovir.

Warnings and Precautions Safe use during pregnancy has not been established.

Untoward Reactions Irritation upon application of ointment, pruritus, rash, vulvitis.

Parameters of Use

Absorption No systemic absorption has been noted following topical application.

Administration Topical: Apply to affected areas 3 to 6 times daily (q3h) for 7 days.

Available Drug Forms Ointment 5% (50 mg/g).

Nursing Management

Planning factors

1. Acyclovir is not used for prophylaxis because viral resistance may develop.
2. Initiate therapy as soon as possible after positive cultures are obtained.
3. Store ointment at room temperature in a dry place.

Administration factors

1. Use rubber gloves when applying drug to prevent transmission of infection.
2. As acyclovir is a new drug and information is limited, dosage and length of treatment should not be exceeded.

Evaluation factors

1. There is no evidence of therapeutic benefit in clients with recurrent herpes genitalis.
2. Acyclovir decreases healing time, pain, and viral shedding time, which is an important consideration in controlling transmission of genital herpes.

GENERIC NAME Amantadine hydrochloride (RX)

TRADE NAME Symmetrel

CLASSIFICATION Antiviral

Action Amantadine inhibits penetration and release of viral nucleic acids into host cells. It is specific for influenza A viruses and may be effective in relieving viral symptoms if taken early in the course of infection.

Indications for Use Prevention and management of type A influenza in high-risk clients.

Contraindications Hypersensitivity to amantadine, pregnancy, lactation.

Warnings and Precautions Use with caution in clients with congestive heart failure, epilepsy, peripheral edema, eczema, psychosis, renal impairment, elderly clients with cerebral arteriosclerosis.

Untoward Reactions Common reactions include dizziness, anxiety, irritability, confusion, depression, postural hypotension, urinary hesitancy, constipation, mild indigestion, and ankle edema. Congestive heart failure, dyspnea, headache, tremors, slurred speech, lethargy, fatigue, ataxia, psychic disturbances, dry mouth, blurred vision, anorexia, nausea, vomiting, skin rash, convulsions, and blood dyscrasias are less common.

Parameters of Use

Absorption Readily absorbed from GI tract. Peak action occurs in 2 hours.

Distribution Widely distributed to all body tissues, including red blood cells.

Excretion In urine.

Drug Interactions Concurrent use of anticholinergics, tricyclic antidepressants, and antihistamines causes additive atropine-like effects. Other CNS stimulants used concomitantly may cause excessive CNS stimulation.

Administration Adults: 200 mg po daily in 1 or 2 doses; Children: Ages 9 to 12 years: 100 mg po bid; Ages 1 to 9 years: 4.4 to 8.8 mg/kg po daily in 2 to 3 divided doses.

Available Drug Forms Capsules containing 100 mg; syrup containing 50 mg/5 ml.

Nursing Management

1. May be given in conjunction with type A influenza virus vaccine, since drug does not suppress antibody response.
2. For prophylaxis, drug is usually continued for 6 to 8 weeks.
3. Avoid giving close to bedtime to decrease the possibility of insomnia.
4. Instruct client not to operate machinery or engage in hazardous activities, since drug may cause a decrease in mental alertness.
5. Inform client that drug may cause mottling of skin, which will subside when drug is discontinued.
6. Instruct client, particularly the elderly, to change position slowly to minimize the risk of postural hypotension.

GENERIC NAME Idoxuridine (RX)

TRADE NAMES Dendrid, Herplex, Stoxil

CLASSIFICATION Antiviral

Action Idoxuridine inhibits DNA replication in herpes virus, thus blocking viral cell replication. Its use is restricted to local application to the eye, since the drug is inactivated by enzymes.

Indications for Use Treatment of herpes simplex keratitis.

Contraindications Hypersensitivity to idoxuridine.

Warnings and Precautions Use with caution during pregnancy.

Untoward Reactions Periorbital irritation, pain, pruritus, edema of eyes and surrounding area, photophobia, corneal clouding, corneal ulceration.

Drug Interactions Concurrent boric acid application will cause irritation.

Administration Ophthalmic use: Solution: Instill 1 gtt in affected eye q1h during the day and q2h at night until improvement is seen; then reduce to q2h during the day and q4h at night. Ointment: 5 applications daily with last dose at bedtime.

Available Drug Forms Solution 0.1% (1 mg/ml); ointment 0.5% (5 mg/g).

Nursing Management

1. Client should be closely supervised by ophthalmologist.
2. If topical corticosteroids are used concurrently, they should be withdrawn several days before discontinuing idoxuridine.
3. If no improvement occurs within 7 days, drug should be discontinued by physician.
4. Drug should be continued for 5 to 7 days after healing is complete.
5. Do not mix with other medications.
6. Store solution in refrigerator until dispensed.

GENERIC NAME Trifluridine (RX)

TRADE NAME Viroptic

CLASSIFICATION Antiviral

Action Exact mechanism of action is not known, but trifluridine may interfere with DNA synthesis.

Indications for Use Treatment of keratitis due to herpes simplex virus, types 1 and 2; treatment of epithelial keratitis in clients unresponsive to other drugs; ophthalmic infections due to vaccinia or adenovirus.

Contraindications Hypersensitivity to trifluridine.

Warnings and Precautions Use with caution during pregnancy and in clients with glaucoma.

Untoward Reactions Mild burning or stinging, palpebral edema, superficial punctate keratopathy, epithelial keratopathy, stromal edema, increased intraocular pressure, hypersensitivity reactions.

Parameters of Use

Absorption Intraocular penetration occurs after application. No significant systemic absorption. Half-life is 15 minutes.

Administration Ophthalmic use: Solution: Instill 1 gtt in affected eye q2h during the day; Maximum dosage: 9 gtt/day. When corneal ulcer has healed, instill 1 gtt q4h for an additional 7 days; Maximum dosage: 5 gtt/day.

Available Drug Forms 1% solution in a 7.5-ml bottle.

Nursing Management

1. Do not exceed recommended dosage. Do not use longer than 21 days under any circumstances because of the risk of ocular toxicity.
2. If no improvement occurs within 7 days, alternative treatment should be considered.
3. Inform client that stinging sensation after application will abate.
4. Store solution in refrigerator.

GENERIC NAME Vidarabine (RX)

TRADE NAME Vira-A

CLASSIFICATION Antiviral

Action Vidarabine inhibits viral DNA synthesis. It is effective against herpes simplex virus, types 1 and 2. The drug is used intravenously for herpes encephalitis secondary to immunosuppressive therapy. Ophthalmic use is often effective in clients resistant to idoxuridine.

Indications for Use Herpes simplex virus encephalitis; superficial and recurrent epithelial keratitis and acute keratoconjunctivitis due to herpes simplex virus, types 1 and 2.

Contraindications Hypersensitivity to vidarabine.

Warnings and Precautions Safe use during pregnancy has not been established.

Untoward Reactions Reactions following intravenous administration include anorexia, nausea, vomiting, diarrhea, tremors, dizziness, ataxia, confusion, hallucinations, psychosis, decreased hemoglobin and hematocrit, decreased white blood cell and platelet count, weight loss, malaise, rash, and pain at injection site. Reactions following ophthalmic administration include irritation, ocular pain, photophobia, tearing, superficial punctate keratitis, punctal occlusion, and hypersensitivity reactions.

Parameters of Use

Absorption Only negligible amounts enter the aqueous humor following ophthalmic application; there is no systemic absorption. Half-life is $3\frac{1}{2}$ hours following IV administration.

Distribution Rapidly distributed to body tissues following intravenous administration.

Excretion By the kidneys.

Administration Intravenous: 15 mg/kg daily for 10 days. Ophthalmic use: Apply $\frac{1}{2}$ inch of ointment into conjunctival sac 5 times daily at 3-hour intervals. When healing has occurred, apply bid for another 7 days.

Available Drug Forms Vials containing 200 mg/ml of suspension; ophthalmic ointment 3%.

Nursing Management

1. Do not use for trivial infections. Do not exceed recommended dosage and length of treatment, since in vivo laboratory tests indicate a mutagenic and carcinogenic potential. Diagnosis of herpes simplex is the only indication for vidarabine therapy.
2. When administering IV, infuse over 10 to 12 hours. Avoid rapid or bolus IV injections.
3. Dilute drug in appropriate IV fluid. Solubility is limited; 1 liter of IV fluid will dissolve 450 mg of drug. Warm infusion fluid to 40 C before adding drug. Agitate until solution is clear. An in-line filter may be used for administration.
4. Schedule periodic hematologic tests.
5. If complete healing does not occur within 21 days, alternative treatment should be considered.

PART XV

ANTINEOPLASTIC AGENTS

ONCOLOGY NURSING CAN be a rewarding and challenging experience for the nurse who is knowledgeable about cancer and its treatment. Since most antineoplastic agents are new, there are still many unknowns in relation to action, uses, toxic effects, dosage, and route of administration. Recent articles in appropriate periodicals and the inserts provided with drugs are currently the best sources of up-to-date information.

Many neoplasms are now treated with combinations of drugs rather than with one single agent. This combination therapy is often effective because the individual drugs act on different stages of the cell cycle. Combination chemotherapy is also less likely to cause drug resistance in neoplastic cells. Finally, by using different agents, the extent of toxicity to any one organ system is decreased. The combination drugs are usually administered in repeated cycles with dosages determined according to established protocols as well as the client's individual needs and tolerances.

Chapter 74

Antineoplastic Agents

MISCELLANEOUS CYTOTOXIC AGENTS

- Hydroxyurea
- Cisplatin
- Dacarbazine
- Etoposide
- Hexamethylmelamine
- L-Asparaginase
- Mitotane
- Procarbazine hydrochloride
- Streptozotocin

ANTIESTROGENS

- Tamoxifen

COMBINATION DRUG REGIMENS

ANTINEOPLASTICS ARE DRUGS that work to prevent the growth of abnormal cells. They have been important in the treatment of cancer for the last 30 years. Research still continues today to find new drugs that kill or attenuate cancer cells. *Antineoplastics* and *cancer chemotherapy* are used synonymously in this chapter.

In the past, cancer was treated with surgery, radiation, and then chemotherapy. However, the present trend is to use cancer chemotherapy early in the treatment of cancer to reduce and ultimately destroy all cancer cells. Adjuvant chemotherapy is also used in conjunction with surgery of the localized cancer to improve the client's chance of survival when there is a high risk of recurrence.

Antineoplastics are also being used in combination chemotherapy. When antineoplastics are used alone, the dosages and incidence of side effects are high. Furthermore, the continued use of optimal dosages may cause the tumor to become resistant to the antineoplastic, since the single drug has limited action against the neoplasm. When antineoplastics are used in combination, the dosages and the frequency of side effects of each drug are generally lower than if used singly. Combined drugs generally have different mechanisms of action and a synergistic drug interaction is achieved; that is, the total therapeutic effect is greater than the sum of the individual drugs. There is a prescribed sequence in which the drugs are used and they are repeated at precise time intervals. Common combination drug regimes are listed at the end of this chapter.

CELL CYCLE

In order to understand the action of the various antineoplastics, it is necessary to know the stages of the cell cycle and the point at which the drug acts.

Antineoplastics are either cell cycle-specific or cell cycle-nonspecific agents. Cell cycle-specific agents are more active during a specific phase of the cell cycle, whereas cell cycle-nonspecific agents are active in the proliferating and resting phases.

G_0: Resting phase—cells do not divide in this stage
G_1: Presynthetic phase—cells are preparing for DNA synthesis
S: Synthetic phase—DNA synthesis takes place with some RNA and protein synthesis
G_2: Postsynthetic phase—further RNA and protein synthesis takes place
M: Mitosis—cell division takes place (prophase, metaphase, anaphase, telophase)

Different cells in the body divide at different rates. Cells in the gastrointestinal tract, bone marrow, and skin divide frequently, whereas cells in the central nervous system and heart do not undergo division once they are formed. Various types of cancer cells also divide at different rates. Antineoplastics are more effective in the treatment of dividing cells than resting cells.

DRUG ACTION IN RELATION TO THE CELL CYCLE

Alkylating agents Alkylating agents interfere with DNA replication (synthesis), RNA synthesis, and protein synthesis. They are cell cycle-nonspecific agents, since they are equally toxic to proliferating and resting cells. The chromatin disruptive effects of alkylating agents are similar to those of radiotherapy.

Antimetabolites Antimetabolites include the folic acid, purine, and pyrimidine antagonists. They interfere with the S phase, or DNA synthesis, and are cell cycle-specific agents. Cells that absorb the antimetabolite cannot divide and so cell growth is inhibited.

Plant alkaloids Plant alkaloids, which are derived from the periwinkle, block cell division in the metaphase stage. Their action results in bizarre mitotic formations. They are cell cycle-specific agents.

Antibiotics Antibiotics prevent DNA-directed RNA synthesis. They are cell cycle-nonspecific agents, since they are active in all phases of the cell cycle.

Steroids and sex hormones Adrenocorticosteroids act on the bone marrow by destroying abnormal cells. They also affect lysis of lymphocytes and involution of lymphatic tissue. Their exact mechanism of action is not known. Androgens, estrogens, and progestins are used to treat neoplasms of reproductive organs. They slow the growth of neoplastic tissue by changing the hormonal balance. (See Chapters 21 and 25 for further details.)

DOSAGE

The dosage of antineoplastics is often determined by the weight of the client. These drugs have a narrow margin of safety because they kill both normal and cancer cells. Normal cells that reproduce rapidly, such as gastrointestinal mucosa, bone marrow, hair, and scalp, are especially prone to cytotoxic effects. This action of antineoplastics on normal cells is responsible for such side effects as alopecia, bone marrow depression, nausea, vomiting, stomatitis, and anorexia.

NURSING MANAGEMENT

In caring for a client receiving antineoplastic agents, the nurse should monitor the effectiveness of the drug. Drug treatment should cause a reduction or elimination of the tumor, which relieves some of the symptoms, such as pain, pressure, and/or edema. The nurse should also be alert for signs of drug toxicity and should try to make the client as comfortable as possible during treatment.

In assessing the client who is to receive chemotherapy, the nurse should obtain data on physical, psychologic, and social strengths and weaknesses. The newly diagnosed client is usually in a physical, psychologic, and social crisis. The treatment, whether surgery, radiation, and/or chemotherapy, may magnify that crisis, so mobilization of the client's resources is a major focus of nursing care.

Psychologic Effects

The client starting antineoplastic therapy may have many questions, fears, and anxieties. It is important for the nurse and physician to explore these concerns and feelings with the client. Some of the commonly encountered questions are: "Will this medication cure me? How long will I have to take this medicine? What side effects will I get with this drug? If the drug is stopped will the tumor return? How expensive is it? Is taking the drug worth the side effects?" Each client is unique and each will have a different set of problems and concerns. The nurse who is alert to verbal and nonverbal communication will confront different psychologic expressions of coping with cancer. The client may feel depressed, guilty, dependent, helpless, lost, or isolated. The nurse should assess the normal coping mechanisms and identify the "significant others" in the client's life. As the side effects of antineoplastic agents also include psychologic changes, the client should be informed of these prior to treatment.

Physical Effects

Nausea and vomiting Nausea and vomiting are common drug side effects. The nurse should plan the client's diet so that solid food is avoided until the nausea subsides. Deep breathing, ice chips, warm tea, or ginger ale sometimes help to reduce these symptoms. An antiemetic may be needed if symptoms are prolonged or persistent. Highly nutritious food, such as Sustogen, should be given when nausea is absent, since proteins are needed to maintain cellular function.

Anorexia An anorexic client can benefit from nursing care that creates a pleasant environment at mealtime. Mouth care given before meals may help to make meals more palatable. Smaller meals and homemade foods sometimes improve appetite. Intravenous feedings can be used to correct dehydration. Total parenteral nutrition should be instituted if anorexia is a persistent problem.

Diarrhea If the client is experiencing diarrhea, the amount of roughage in the diet should be reduced and constipating foods should be increased. Oral or intravenous fluids should be used to prevent dehydration. Anal soreness should be relieved by a lubricant.

Alopecia The client should be prepared for the possible loss of hair from the scalp, eyebrows, eyelashes, underarms, and pubic area and told that the hair usually grows back after treatment is discontinued, although it may be a different color and texture. Wigs can be purchased before treatment is initiated.

Fluid retention Fluid retention can occur in the client receiving steroid therapy. The nurse should keep an accurate record of intake and output and daily weight and assess for edema. A low-sodium diet and/or a diuretic may be ordered.

Sex characteristic changes Androgen or estrogen hormonal therapy may cause secondary sex characteristic changes. The client should be informed that these changes are temporary and will abate when therapy is discontinued.

Toxic Effects

Stomatitis Stomatitis is an early sign of toxicity. The nurse should instruct the client to use a soft toothbrush or toothettes to rub the gums. An oral anesthetic, such as Xylocaine, may help ease the pain and make eating easier. A bland diet consisting of either liquids or soft foods may be more tolerable and cold foods, such as ice cream, may be soothing.

Bone marrow depression The client on antineoplastics should be watched closely for bone marrow depression, which is manifested as leukopenia and/or thrombocytopenia. Frequent blood counts should be performed to detect any abnormalities; a bone marrow aspiration test may also be required. The nurse should explain the rationale and the procedure for all these tests.

Leukopenia If leukopenia occurs, the client's defense against infection will be reduced. Therefore, good aseptic technique is essential when caring for a client with leukopenia. The development of fever should be reported immediately, so that appropriate treatment can be initiated promptly. The client should not be exposed to anyone with an infectious or communicable disease. If the white blood count falls below 2000/mm^3, the client should be put on reverse isolation precautions and body temperature monitored frequently. Areas of the skin susceptible to infection should be inspected for breakdowns. The client should be turned frequently and be encouraged to get out of bed, when possible, to prevent skin breakdown.

Thrombocytopenia The development of thrombocytopenia results in a reduction of normal clotting ability; thus, the client should be warned to be very careful not to cut or bruise him- or herself. Parenteral injections should be stopped, if possible. Stool, urine, skin, and vomitus should be checked for bleeding.

Anemia If the client has a decreased red blood cell count, weakness, fatigue, and pallor may occur. The diet should be high in protein, vitamins, and iron. Blood transfusions may be necessary for severe blood loss. The nurse must be alert to transfusion reactions and the development of hepatitis if transfusions are frequent. The nurse should protect the client from chills and burns and encourage frequent rest periods.

ALKYLATING AGENTS

Nitrogen Mustards

GENERIC NAME Mechlorethamine hydrochloride

TRADE NAMES HN2, Mustargen, Nitrogen Mustard

CLASSIFICATION Antineoplastic (RX)

Action Mechlorethamine is a cell cycle-nonspecific agent. It alkylates nucleic acids, particularly the purine base guanine, thereby inactivating DNA and preventing mitosis. Nadir: 7 to 10 days.

Indications for Use Chronic lymphocytic leukemia, Hodgkin's disease, lymphoma, carcinoma of the lung, breast, ovary, and testicle.

Contraindications Pregnancy, myelosuppression, infectious granuloma, foci of suppurative inflammation, simultaneous treatment with other antineoplastics.

Warnings and Precautions Use with caution in women of childbearing age and clients with lymphosarcoma or chronic leukemia.

Untoward Reactions Nausea, vomiting, bone marrow depression (leukopenia, anemia, agranulocytosis, thrombocytopenia), alopecia, amenorrhea (temporary), decreased spermatogenesis, petechiae, anorexia, convulsions, stomatitis, diarrhea. Also possible are thrombophlebitis and sloughing at injection site, skin eruptions, temporary aphasia, and paralysis, peptic ulcer, jaundice, weakness, fever, drowsiness, headache, tinnitus, deafness, metallic taste following administration.

Parameters of Use

Absorption Variable absorption from GI tract; thus, administered intravenously.
Distribution Rapidly distributed to body tissues by blood.
Excretion Negligible in urine.

Drug Interactions Amphotericin B increases the possibility of blood dyscrasias.

Administration Intravenous, intracavitary, intraarterial: 0.4 mg/kg/day for 4 days or as a single dose.

Available Drug Forms Rubber-stoppered vials containing 10 mg in 90 mg of anhydrous sodium chloride.

Nursing Management (See pages 947–948 for further details.)

1. Premedicate client with sedative and/or antiemetic.
2. Padded tongue blade and padded side rails should be available in case convulsions occur.
3. Avoid contact with skin; use surgical gloves when preparing dosage.
4. Sodium thiosulfate is the antidote for skin contact or infiltrated IV.
5. Give into a rapidly flowing IV; avoid extravasation.
6. Apply cold compress for 6 to 12 hours to decrease sloughing and necrosis of IV site.
7. When given via intracavitary route, reposition client every minute for 5 minutes to distribute drug.
8. Obtain complete blood cell counts frequently.

GENERIC NAME Chlorambucil (RX)

TRADE NAME Leukeran

CLASSIFICATION Antineoplastic

See mechlorethamine for Warnings and precautions.

Action Chlorambucil is an aromatic derivative of mechlorethamine. Its action is similar to the parent drug, but is slower acting.

Indications for Use Chronic lymphocytic leukemia, Hodgkin's disease, malignant lymphoma, ovarian carcinoma, giant follicular lymphoma.

Contraindications Pregnancy, myelosuppression, infiltration of bone marrow with lymphomatous tissue.

Untoward Reactions Side effects are not common with therapeutic dosages. Bone marrow depression (thrombocytopenia) occurs with high dosages. Other reactions include nausea, vomiting, hepatotoxicity, alopecia (temporary), pulmonary fibrosis, and leukemia. (See mechlorethamine.)

Parameters of Use

Absorption Well absorbed from GI tract.
Metabolism Unknown.
Excretion Unknown.

Administration 0.1 to 0.2 mg/kg po daily for 3 to 6 weeks; Maintenance dosage: 0.03 to 0.1/mg/kg/day.

Available Drug Forms Tablets containing 2 mg.

Nursing Management (See pages 947–948 for further details.)

1. May be given before breakfast or 2 hours after supper to control nausea and vomiting.
2. Check client for infection and bleeding.
3. Check blood counts weekly.
4. Protect drug from light.

GENERIC NAME Cyclophosphamide (RX)

TRADE NAMES CTX, Cytoxan, Endoxan

CLASSIFICATION Antineoplastic

Action Similar action to mechlorethamine. Nadir: 10 to 14 days. Cyclophosphamide must be transformed to an active agent by the enzyme phosphoamidase in the liver.

Indications for Use Chronic lymphocytic leukemia, Hodgkin's disease, lymphoma, acute lymphoblastic leukemia, mycosis fungoides, multiple myeloma, carconima of the bronchus, breast, and ovary, neuroblastoma.

Contraindications Women of childbearing age; pregnancy, lactation, serious infections, myelosuppression.

Warnings and Precautions Use with caution in clients who have had recent x-ray or cytotoxic treatment, those with diabetes mellitus or hepatic or renal dysfunction, and those undergoing steroid therapy.

Untoward Reactions Anaphylaxis, nausea, vomiting, diarrhea, bone marrow depression (leukopenia, anemia, thrombocytopenia), alopecia, hemorrhagic cystitis, hepatotoxicity, darkening of nails and skin, dermatitis, amenorrhea, decreased spermatogenesis, pulmonary fibrosis, dizziness, fatigue, visual disturbances, confusion, fever, hyponatremia, hypoglycemia, hyperkalemia.

Parameters of Use

Absorption Well absorbed from GI tract following oral administration.

Metabolism In the liver and tumor cells. Accumulates in neoplastic tissues.

Excretion In urine. Also excreted in breast milk.

Drug Interactions Antagonized by allopurinol, barbiturates, and corticosteroids. Enhances the effects of insulin and succinylcholine.

Administration Oral: 50 to 200 mg/day (4 mg/kg/day). Intravenous: 20 to 40 mg/kg every 2 weeks or 2 to 8 mg/kg/day for 6 days; Maintenance dosage: 10 to 15 mg/kg every 7 to 10 days.

Available Drug Forms White tablets containing 25 or 50 mg; Vials containing 100, 200, or 500 mg of white powder.

Nursing Management (See pages 947–948 for further details.)

1. Oral dose may be given with meals if gastric upset is severe.
2. When administering IV, reconstitute 100 mg in 5 ml of sterile water. Reconstituted solution is stable for 24 hours at room temperature and 6 days when refrigerated.
3. Force fluids for 12 to 24 hours after administration. Encourage frequent voiding.

GENERIC NAME Melphalan (RX)

TRADE NAMES Alkeran, L-Pam, L-Phenylalanine Mustard, Pam

CLASSIFICATION Antineoplastic

See mechlorethamine for Contraindications and Warnings and precautions.

Action Similar to mechlorethamine. Melphalan cross-links DNA during the resting phase of mitosis.

Indications for Use Chronic lymphocytic leukemia, malignant melanoma, lymphoma, carcinoma of the ovary, breast, and testicle, multiple myeloma.

Untoward Reactions Hypersensitivity reactions, thrombocytopenia, agranulocytosis, anemia, leukopenia, nausea, vomiting (rare), sterility, leukemia, uremia, angioneurotic edema, minor neurotoxicity, thrombophlebitis at infusion site.

Parameters of Use

Absorption Well absorbed from GI tract and parenterally. Serum half-life is 2 to 6 hours.

Distribution Distributed to all body tissues.

Metabolism Unknown.

Excretion Unknown.

Administration Initial dosage: 0.15 mg/kg po daily; Maintenance dosage: 0.25 mg/kg day for 4 days every 6 weeks.

Available Drug Forms Tablets containing 2 mg.

Nursing Management (See pages 947–948 for further details.)

1. Protect client against infection and bleeding.
2. Check blood counts weekly.
3. Give with meals to reduce GI upset.
4. Protect drug from light.

GENERIC NAME Uracil mustard (RX)

CLASSIFICATION Antineoplastic

See mechlorethamine for Contraindications and Warnings and precautions.

Action Similar to mechlorethamine. Uracil mustard is incorporated into nuclear and cytoplasmic RNA, thereby preventing cell division. This drug is not widely used at the present time because it has a low therapeutic index.

Indications for Use Chronic lymphocytic leukemia, lymphoma, lymphosarcoma, reticulum cell sarcoma, carcinoma of the ovary, polycythemia vera.

Untoward Reactions Anorexia, nausea, vomiting, diarrhea, dermatitis, bone marrow depression, oral ulcerations, irritability, nervousness, increased pigmentation. Alopecia and depression occur rarely.

Parameters of Use

Absorption Variable from GI tract.

Distribution Rapidly distributed from plasma to body tissues.

Excretion Negligible in urine.

Administration 1.0 mg/kg po daily for 3 out of 4 weeks; repeat for up to 3 months.

Available Drug Forms Capsules containing 1 mg of white crystalline powder.

Nursing Management (See pages 947–948 for further details.)

1. Give at bedtime to avoid nausea and vomiting.
2. Monitor blood counts weekly.

Ethylenimides

GENERIC NAME Triethylenethiophosphoramide

TRADE NAME Thiotepa (RX)

CLASSIFICATION Antineoplastic

Action Triethylenethiophosphoramide produces nuclear changes in cells and shatters chromosomes. It has a high therapeutic index and is highly toxic.

Indications for Use Carcinoma of the ovary, breast, and lung, lymphoma, malignant effusions, Hodgkin's disease, retinoblastoma, chronic leukemias.

Contraindications Acute leukemia, pregnancy, hypersensitivity, acute infection, myelosuppression, tumor invasion of bone marrow, renal or hepatic insufficiency, concurrent treatment with other antineolastics.

Warnings and Precautions Use with caution in clients with impaired renal or hepatic function.

Untoward Reactions Nausea, vomiting, anorexia, bone marrow depression (leukopenia, thrombocytopenia), headache, amenorrhea, decreased spermatogenesis, hyperuricemia.

Parameters of Use

Absorption Slow onset of action.
Excretion By the kidneys.

Drug Interactions Potentiates the effects of succinylcholine by reducing hepatic metabolism.

Administration Intravenous intrapericardial, intraperitoneal, intrapleural; Adults and children over 12 years: 0.2 mg/kg/day at 2-week intervals.

Available Drug Forms Vials containing 15 mg of powder.

Nursing Management (See pages 947–948 for further details.)

1. Mix powder with isotonic saline and use immediately. Store powder in refrigerator.
2. Avoid contact with skin; use surgical gloves when preparing dosage.
3. Usually given to ambulatory clients.
4. When given via intracavitary route, reposition client every 15 minutes for 1 hour to distribute drug.
5. Protect client from infection and bleeding.

Alkyl Sulfonates

GENERIC NAME Busulfan (RX)

TRADE NAME Myleran

CLASSIFICATION Antineoplastic

Action Busulfan inhibits DNA, RNA, and protein synthesis. Drug-induced myelosuppression is restricted chiefly to bone marrow cells.

Indications for Use Palliative treatment of chronic myelogenous leukemia, polycythemia vera.

Contraindications First trimester of pregnancy, recent radiation or antineoplastic therapy, neutrophilia, thrombocytopenia.

Warnings and Precautions Use with caution in late pregnancy, lactation, and in women of childbearing age.

Untoward Reactions Low incidence of side effects. Reactions include bone marrow depression (leukopenia, thrombocytopenia), cataracts, amenorrhea, irreversible pulmonary fibrosis, renal damage, testicular atrophy, sterility, amenorrhea, nausea, vomiting, diarrhea, alopecia, muscle weakness, splenomegaly, Addison-like syndrome.

Parameters of Use

Absorption Well absorbed from GI tract.
Distribution Rapidly distributed to tissues by blood.
Metabolism Metabolized to methanesulfonic acid.
Excretion By the kidneys.

Administration Adults: 4 to 8 mg po daily for 2 to 3 weeks; Children: 0.06 mg/kg po daily.

Available Drug Forms Tablets containing 2 mg.

Nursing Management (See pages 947–948 for further details.)

1. Can be used in ambulatory clients.
2. Assess pulmonary function regularly.
3. White blood cell count (WBC) may drop dramatically in the second or third week of therapy. This is a serious and sometimes irreversible effect.
4. Monitor WBC weekly or biweekly.
5. Protect drug from light.

Nitrosoureas

GENERIC NAME Carmustine (RX)

TRADE NAMES BCNU, BiCNU

CLASSIFICATION Antineoplastic

Action Carmustine inhibits the synthesis of DNA, RNA, and protein in a similar manner to other alkylating agents.

Indications for Use Primary and metastatic tumors, lymphoma, Hodgkin's disease, multiple myeloma, malignant myeloma, carcinoma of the GI tract and breast, bronchogenic and renal cell carcinoma, melanoma.

Contraindications Pregnancy, myelosuppression, hepatic or renal impairment, hypersensitivity.

Warnings and Precautions Use with caution in clients with decreased platelets, leukocytes, or erythrocytes.

Untoward Reactions Diarrhea, nausea, vomiting, nephrotoxicity, bone marrow depression (leukopenia, thrombocytopenia), hepatotoxicity, pulmonary fibrosis, dyspnea, flushing, esophagitis, CNS toxicity, pain along infusion line.

Parameters of Use

Absorption Rapidly absorbed following oral and parenteral administration.
Distribution Rapidly distributed following intravenous administration. Crosses blood-brain barrier.
Metabolism Rapidly metabolized in the liver following intravenous administration. Protein-bound metabolites persist in plasma for long periods.
Excretion By the kidneys and liver.

Administration 100 to 400 mg/m^2 IV for 2 days; repeat every 6 weeks.

Available Drug Forms Vials containing 100 mg of white powder.

Nursing Management (See pages 947–948 for further details.)

1. Dilute with 3 ml of absolute alcohol, then 17 ml of water, then dilute to 100 ml with 5% D/W. Store powder in refrigerator.
2. Give antiemetic for nausea and vomiting before drug administration, if needed.
3. Infuse slowly to prevent hypotension.
4. Avoid extravasation and contact with skin.
5. Discard unused portion of diluted drug.

GENERIC NAME Lomustine (RX)

TRADE NAMES CeeNU, CCNU

CLASSIFICATION Antineoplastic

Action Lomustine inhibits the synthesis of DNA, RNA, and protein in a similar manner to other alkylating agents. Nadir: 4 to 6 weeks.

Indications for Use Hodgkin's disease, primary and metastatic tumors of the CNS, carcinoma of the stomach, kidney, and lung.

Contraindications Hypersensitivity.

Warnings and Precautions Safe use in pregnancy has not been established. Use with caution in clients with decreased platelets, leukocytes, or erythrocytes.

Untoward Reactions Stomatitis, nausea, vomiting, hepatotoxicity, nephrotoxicity, neurologic reactions, delayed myelosuppression.

Parameters of Use

Absorption Rapidly absorbed from GI tract. Serum half-life is 16 to 48 hours.
Distribution Crosses blood-brain barrier.
Excretion In urine, with 50% excreted in 24 hours.

Administration 100 to 300 mg/m^2 po every 6 weeks.

Available Drug Forms Capsules containing 10, 40, or 100 mg.

Nursing Management (See pages 947–948 for further details.)

1. Give antiemetics as necessary.
2. Give on an empty stomach with fluids.
3. Check client's temperature frequently.
4. Check for infection and bleeding.
5. Store drug in refrigerator.

GENERIC NAME Semustine (RX)

TRADE NAME MeCCNU

CLASSIFICATION Antineoplastic

See carmustine for Contraindications and Warnings and precautions.

Action Semustine inhibits the synthesis of DNA, RNA, and protein in a similar manner to other alkylating agents. Nadir: 29 to 43 days. This drug is seldom used.

Indications for Use Primary and metastatic tumors of the CNS, carcinoma of the stomach, pancreas, colon, and lung, squamous cell carcinoma, malignant melanoma.

Untoward Reactions Toxic effects include nausea, vomiting, anorexia, and bone marrow depression (leukopenia, thrombocytopenia), hepatotoxicity.

Parameters of Use

Absorption Rapidly absorbed from GI tract.
Distribution Crosses blood-brain barrier.
Metabolism Rapidly and completely metabolized.
Excretion In body tissues and fluids.

Administration 150 to 500 mg/m^2 po every 6 weeks.

Available Drug Forms Vials containing 10, 50, or 100 mg.

Nursing Management (See pages 947–948 for further details.)

1. Give antiemetic before drug administration.
2. Give on an empty stomach.
3. Check for infection and bleeding.
4. Store drug at 4 C.

ANTIMETABOLITES

Folic Acid Analogs

GENERIC NAME Methotrexate (RX)

TRADE NAMES Amethopterin, MTX

CLASSIFICATION Antineoplastic

Action Methotrexate inhibits the reduction of folic acid to tetrahydrofolic acid by reacting with folic acid reductase, thereby interfering with the synthesis of a coenzyme necessary for DNA synthesis. Nadir: 6 to 9 days. This drug is highly toxic.

Indications for Use Neoplastic diseases: acute leukemia in children, choriocarcinoma, lymphoma, trophoblastic tumor, carcinoma of the head and neck, breast, testis, and bronchus. Nonneoplastic diseases: psoriasis, immunosuppressant.

Contraindications Pregnancy, hepatic or renal impairment, women of childbearing age, concurrent use of hepatotoxic or bone-marrow depressant drugs, blood dyscrasias, alcoholism.

Warnings and Precautions Use with caution in clients with peptic ulcer, ulcerative colitis, bone marrow depression, poor nutritional status, and very young or very old clients.

Untoward Reactions Stomatitis, bone marrow depression, nausea, GI ulcerations, vomiting, diarrhea, hepatotoxicity, cirrhosis, nephrotoxicity, CNS complications (headache, drowsiness, dizziness, aphasia, visual disturbances, paralysis, convulsions), amenorrhea, azoospermia, nephrotoxicity, chills, fever, osteoporosis, pneumonitis, metabolic changes causing diabetes, dermatoses, and alopecia. Most reactions are dose-related and reversible.

Parameters of Use

Absorption Well absorbed from GI tract and after parenteral administration.

Distribution Distributed by plasma to body tissues. Remains in tissues for long periods of time. Little drug crosses blood-brain barrier.

Crosses placenta.

Excretion By the kidneys. A large portion of drug is excreted unchanged within 48 hours.

Drug Interactions Action is decreased by concurrent use of weak organic acids, such as salicylates, sulfonamides, and aminobenzoic acid. Prolonged use of vitamins, vaccines, tetracyclines, chloramphenicol, phenytoin, alcoholic beverages, and hepatotoxic drugs causes cirrhosis.

Administration Oral: 2.5 to 10 mg/day. Intramuscular, intravenous, intrathecal, intraarterial: 30 mg/m^2 twice weekly.

Available Drug Forms Tablets containing 2.5 mg; vials containing 5, 50, 500, or 1000 mg of yellow powder or liquid.

Nursing Management (See pages 947–948 for further details.)

1. Give antiemetic before drug administration. Client may also need antidiarrheal medication.
2. Dilute powder in 500 to 1000 ml of 5% dextrose for IV infusion. Store at room temperature.
3. Avoid contact with skin.
4. Provide frequent mouth care.
5. Force fluids and keep urine alkaline.
6. Assess client frequently for thrombocytopenia, GI bleeding, and oliguria.
7. The antidote for overdose is leucovorin calcium, which must be given within several hours of methotrexate administration.

GENERIC NAME 5-Azacytidine (RX)

TRADE NAME 5-Aza-C

CLASSIFICATION Antineoplastic

See methotrexate for Contraindications and Warnings and precautions.

Action Azacytidine inhibits enzymes involved in nucleic acid synthesis. It is a cell cycle-specific agent.

Indications for Use Acute granulocytic leukemia.

Untoward Reactions Severe nausea, vomiting, diarrhea, bone marrow depression, hepatotoxicity.

Parameters of Use

Distribution Data incomplete.
Excretion Rapidly by the kidneys.

Administration 150 mg/m^2 via continuous IV infusion over 5 days.

Available Drug Forms Vials for IV use only.

Nursing Management (See pages 947–948 for further details.)

1. Give antiemetics and/or antidiarrheal agents as necessary.
2. Force fluids.
3. Check blood counts weekly.

Pyrimidine Analogs

GENERIC NAME Fluorouracil (RX)

TRADE NAMES Efudex, 5-Fluorouracil, 5-FU

CLASSIFICATION Antineoplastic

Action Fluorouracil interferes with the synthesis of RNA and blocks synthesis of DNA. Nadir: 9 to 14 days. This drug is highly toxic.

Indications for Use Carcinoma of the colon, breast, liver, stomach, ovary, bladder, cervix, and pancreas. Also used topically for actinic keratoses.

Contraindications Poor nutritional state, recent surgery (2 weeks), infection, hepatic and renal dysfunction, pregnancy, myelosuppression.

Warnings and Precautions Use with caution in clients with metastases to bone marrow, hepatic or renal impairment, those with history of high-dose pelvic irradiation, and women of childbearing age.

Untoward Reactions Nausea, vomiting, diarrhea, stomatitis, GI bleeding, paralytic ileus, pharyngitis, epistaxis, bone marrow depression, dermatitis, hyperpigmentation, alopecia, darkening of veins with prolonged use, euphoria, ataxia, photosensitivity, photophobia.

Parameters of Use

Absorption Irregularly absorbed from GI tract; therefore, intravenous administration is preferred.

Distribution Rapidly disappears from circulation to tissues. Crosses blood-brain barrier.
Metabolism Converted to carbon dioxide and urea in the liver.
Excretion By the kidneys.

Administration Intravenous: 10 to 15 mg/kg weekly; Topical: Cream 1 to 5%: Apply to affected areas bid.

Available Drug Forms Vials of 10 ml containing 500 mg; solution 2 to 5% (Efudex); cream 5% (Efudex).

Nursing Management (See pages 947–948 for further details.)

1. Store drug at room temperature or in a cool place; protect from light.
2. Give slowly via IV infusion (30 minutes to 8 hours); avoid extravasation.
3. Warm vial slightly to redissolve any crystals before administration. Discard unused drug.
4. When applying topically, use gloved finger or nonmetallic applicator.
5. Topical administration causes rash and ulceration 1 to 2 minutes after treatment.
6. Monitor client for diarrhea, vomiting, and stomatitis (early signs of toxicity)
7. Adequate nutrition and careful oral hygiene are important. Weigh client weekly.
8. Advise client to avoid exposure to sunlight.

GENERIC NAME Cytarabine (RX)

TRADE NAMES Ara-C, Cytosar, Cytosine Arabinoside

CLASSIFICATION Antineoplastic

Action Cytarabine interferes with DNA synthesis by blocking the conversion of ribonucleotides to deoxyribonucleotides. The drug must be phosphorylated (activated) to exert its action and is most effective in the S phase of the cell cycle.

Indications for Use Neoplastic diseases: acute leukemia, acute myelocytic leukemia, myeloblastic leukemia. Nonneoplastic diseases: herpes simplex infection of the eye, immunosuppressant.

Contraindications Hypersensitivity, myelosuppression, pregnancy; infants, women of childbearing age.

Warnings and Precautions Use with caution in clients with renal or hepatic impairment, gout, or previous x-ray or antineoplastic therapy.

Untoward Reactions Bone marrow depression (leukopenia, thrombocytopenia), fever, rash, renal dysfunction, hepatic dysfunction, thrombophlebitis at injection site, stomatitis, nausea, vomiting, diarrhea, anorexia, weight loss, sore throat, dizziness, cellulitis, chest pain, conjunctivitis, joint pain, confusion, skin rashes or ulcerations.

Parameters of Use

Absorption Not effective after oral administration.
Distribution Appears to be taken up adequately by tumor tissue. Crosses blood-brain barrier.
Metabolism Rapidly metabolized by the liver and kidneys.
Excretion By the kidneys.

Administration 2 to 8 mg/kg IV daily for 5 to 10 days.

Available Drug Forms Vials containing 100 or 500 mg of light yellow powder.

Nursing Management (See pages 947–948 for further details.)

1. Give antiemetics and/or antidiarrheal agents as necessary.
2. Give slowly via IV infusion over a 1-hour period. Therapy should be initiated in hospital.
3. Store powder in refrigerator. Reconstituted solution is stable for 24 hours at room temperature and 7 days when refrigerated. Drug is soluble in sterile water.
4. Protect client against infection and bleeding.
5. Check blood counts frequently.

GENERIC NAME Floxuridine (RX)

TRADE NAME FUDR

CLASSIFICATION Antineoplastic

See fluorouracil for Contraindications and Warnings and precautions.

Action Floxuridine is converted by thymidine or deoxyuridine phosphorylase to fluorouracil. It inhibits thymidylic synthetase and uracil phosphatase, thereby blocking utilization of uracil in RNA. Also interferes with DNA synthesis. A comparative study is being done to see if floxuridine can be replaced by fluorouracil.

Indications for Use Carcinoma of the colon, gall bladder, and bile duct, hepatic metastasis.

Untoward Reactions Nausea, vomiting, diarrhea, stomatitis, alopecia, bone marrow depression (7 to 14 days after initiation of therapy).

Parameters of Use

Absorption Variable from GI tract; therefore, administered intravenously.
Metabolism In the liver.
Excretion By the kidneys and lungs.

Administration Intravenous: 12 mg/kg day for 3 days; Intraarterial: 0.4 to 0.6 mg/kg/day for 6 to 10 days.

Available Drug Forms Vials of 5 ml containing 500 mg of powder.

Nursing Management (See pages 947–948 for further details.)

1. Client should be hospitalized for the first course of therapy.
2. Monitor bleeding time and white blood cell count weekly.

Purine Analogs

GENERIC NAME Mercaptopurine (RX)

TRADE NAMES 6-Mercaptopurine, 6-MP, Purinethol

CLASSIFICATION Antineoplastic

Action Mercaptopurine inhibits DNA synthesis by preventing the incorporation of purine into DNA or by forming unnatural DNA.

Indications for Use Neoplastic diseases: acute lymphocytic leukemia, chronic myelocytic leukemia. Nonneoplastic diseases: immunosuppressant.

Contraindications Renal dysfunction, first trimester of pregnancy, infections.

Warnings and Precautions Use with caution in clients with renal or hepatic impairment and those taking allopurinol.

Untoward Reactions Leukopenia, thrombocytopenia, nausea, vomiting, anorexia, stomatitis, diarrhea, hepatic dysfunction (jaundice), hyperuricemia with hyperuricosuria, skin rash, drug fever.

Parameters of Use

Absorption Rapidly absorbed from GI tract. Half-life in blood is about 90 minutes.
Distribution Distributed to all body tissues. Crosses blood-brain barrier.
Metabolism In the liver.
Excretion Rapidly by the kidneys.

Drug Interactions Concurrent use of allopurinol has a synergistic effect, delaying the metabolism and increasing the potency of mercaptopurine. If used concomitantly, reduce the dosage of mercaptopurine by one-quarter.

Administration 2.5 mg/kg po daily for several weeks.

Available Drug Forms Scored tablets containing 50 mg.

Nursing Management (See pages 947–948 for further details.)

1. Give antiemetics as necessary.
2. Check blood counts weekly.
3. Force fluids and check for oliguria and hepatic dysfunction.
4. Store drug at room temperature.

GENERIC NAME Thioguanine (RX)

TRADE NAMES Tabloid, 6-Thioguanine

CLASSIFICATION Antineoplastic

See mercaptopurine for Warnings and precautions and Untoward reactions.

Action Thioguanine inhibits the synthesis of DNA by preventing purine ring biosynthesis and interconversion of purine bases.

Indications for Use Neoplastic diseases: acute leukemia. Nonneoplastic diseases: immunosuppressant.

Contraindications First trimester of pregnancy. (See mercaptopurine.)

Parameters of Use

Absorption Incompletely absorbed from GI tract.
Metabolism In the liver.
Excretion In urine.

Administration Adults and children: 2 mg/kg po daily.

Available Drug Forms Tablets containing 40 mg.

Nursing Management (See pages 947–948 for further details.)

1. Give frequent mouth care.
2. Monitor intake and output and force fluids.
3. Store drug at room temperature in airtight containers.

PLANT ALKALOIDS

GENERIC NAME Vinblastine sulfate (RX)

TRADE NAMES Velban, VLB

CLASSIFICATION Antineoplastic

Source Extracted from periwinkle plant *Vinca rosea*.

Action Vinblastine is a cell cycle-specific agent that blocks mitosis in metaphase and leads ultimately to cell death.

Indications for Use Neoplastic diseases: Hodgkin's disease, choriocarcinoma, acute lymphocytic leukemia, testicular tumor. Nonneoplastic diseases: immunosuppressant.

Contraindications Pregnancy, leukopenia, infection, women of childbearing age, elderly clients with skin ulcers or cachexia.

Warnings and Precautions Use with caution in clients with metastases to bone marrow or obstructive jaundice.

Untoward Reactions Leukopenia, nausea, vomiting, neurologic disturbances, alopecia, stomatitis, constipation, ileus, GI hemorrhage, phlebitis, cellulitis at injection site, fever, weight loss, muscle pain, weakness, urinary retention, pain in tumor site or parotid gland, sterility.

Parameters of Use

Absorption Poorly absorbed following oral administration, but rapidly removed from blood after parenteral administration. Crosses blood-brain barrier.
Metabolism Mainly in the liver.
Excretion By the liver into renal system.

Drug Interactions Glutamic acid and tryptophan inhibit the effects of vinblastine.

Administration 0.1 to 0.2 mg/kg IV weekly. Maintenance doses are individualized according to therapeutic and hematologic response.

Available Drug Forms Vials containing 10 mg of white powder.

Nursing Management (See pages 947–948 for further details.)

1. Mix powder with 10 ml of isotonic saline or sterile water. Solution is stable for 30 days when refrigerated.
2. Add to an established IV infusion. Avoid extravasation.
3. Check blood counts weekly.
4. Instruct patient to avoid exposure to infection and to avoid trauma to skin.

GENERIC NAME Vincristine sulfate (RX)

TRADE NAMES Oncovin, VCR

CLASSIFICATION Antineoplastic

Source Extracted from periwinkle plant *Vinca rosea*.

Action Vincristine is a cell cycle-specific agent that arrests mitosis in metaphase by interfering with spindle formation and leads ultimately to cell death.

Indications for Use Acute leukemia in children, Hodgkin's disease, neuroblastoma, Wilms' tumor, choriocarcinoma resistant to other agents, lymphoma.

Contraindications Pregnancy, obstructive jaundice, women of childbearing age.

Warnings and Precautions Use with caution in clients with hepatic disease, leukopenia, neuromuscular disease, hypertension, infection, clients taking neurotoxic drugs.

Untoward Reactions Nausea, vomiting, severe constipation, neurotoxicity (paresthesias, foot drop, ataxia, diplopia), alopecia, leukopenia (mild), rash, phlebitis at injection site.

Parameters of Use

Absorption Poorly absorbed following oral or intravenous administration.
Metabolism Mainly in the liver
Excretion By the liver into renal system.

Drug Interactions Vincristine is synergistic with corticosteroids; this combination is used to induce remissions in childhood leukemia. Glutamic acid inhibits the effects of vincristine. Concurrent use of methotrexate decreases blood pressure.

Administration Initial dosage: 0.05 to 0.15 mg/kg IV weekly; Maintenance dosage: 0.05 to 0.075 mg/kg/week.

Available Drug Forms Vials containing 1 or 5 mg of white powder.

Nursing Management (See pages 947–948 for further details.)

1. Mix powder with 10 ml of isotonic saline or sterile water. Stable in refrigerator for 14 days. Store powder in refrigerator and protect from light.
2. Give antiemetics as necessary.
3. Encourage high fluid intake.
4. Treat constipation with high-fiber diet, stool softeners, and suppositories.
5. Earliest sign of neurotoxicity is depression of Achilles tendon reflex. Observe client frequently for numbness and tingling of extremities.
6. Do not take rectal temperature.

ANTIBIOTICS

GENERIC NAME Dactinomycin (RX)

TRADE NAMES Actinomycin D, Cosmegen

CLASSIFICATION Antineoplastic

Action Dactinomycin, which is derived from *Streptomyces parvullus*, combines with and inactivates DNA needed for RNA synthesis, thereby inhibiting synthesis of RNA.

Indications for Use Wilms' tumor, testicular tumor, neuroblastoma, methotrexate-resistant carcinoma, osteogenic sarcoma, choriocarcinoma.

Contraindications Pregnancy, renal, hepatic, or bone marrow impairment, chickenpox, infants under 6 months, myelosuppression.

Untoward Reactions Leukopenia, agranulocytosis, GI ulcerations, stomatitis, nausea, vomiting, diarrhea, alopecia, malaise, fever, anemia, skin lesions, necrosis at injection site.

Parameters of Use

Distribution Rapidly distributed to liver, spleen, and kidneys.
Excretion About 50% unchanged in bile and 10% in urine.

Drug Interactions Dactinomycin inhibits the action of penicillin. Irradiation effects are increased by dactinomycin (erythema, desquamation, and high pigmentation in radiation area).

Administration Children and adults: 0.015 mg/kg IV daily for 5 days; Dosage and schedules are individualized according to response.

Available Drug Forms Vials containing 0.5 mg of yellow powder.

Nursing Management (See pages 947–948 for further details.)

1. Mix powder with sterile water only. Discard unused solution. Store powder at room temperature and protect from light.
2. Avoid extravasation as drug is extremely irritating to tissues.
3. Give antiemetics as necessary.
4. Force fluids.
5. Give frequent mouth care.
6. Monitor clients on radiotherapy closely as they are at greater risk of toxicity.
7. Obtain blood counts every 3 days. Toxicity may occur up to 2 weeks after discontinuation of therapy.

GENERIC NAME Bleomycin sulfate (RX)

TRADE NAME Blenoxane

CLASSIFICATION Antineoplastic

Action Bleomycin, which is derived from *Streptomyces verticillus*, inhibits mitosis and DNA synthesis by binding to DNA.

Indications for Use Lymphoma, testicular tumor, squamous cell carcinoma of the head and neck, skin, larynx, penis, cervix, and vulva.

Contraindications Hypersensitivity to bleomycin, pregnancy, women of childbearing age.

Warnings and Precautions Use with extreme caution in clients with impaired renal or pulmonary function (other than malignancy); development of pulmonary fibrosis may be fatal.

Untoward Reactions Pulmonary fibrosis, cutaneous toxicity, anorexia, nausea, weight loss, stomatitis, alopecia, fever, fatigue, hyperpigmentation, pruritic erythema, paresthesias, nail changes, hypotension, headache, cystitis, anaphylactic reaction, renal or hepatic toxicity, CNS toxicity, exacerbation of rheumatoid arthritis, pain at tumor site.

Parameters of Use

Absorption Rapid acting: half-life is 115 minutes. Seems to concentrate in skin and lungs.
Metabolism Not known.
Excretion By the kidneys as active drug.

Drug Interactions Previous radiotherapy will cause erythema and induration of radiated area.

Administration Initial dosage: 0.25 to 0.80 units/kg IM, subc, or IV once or twice weekly; maintenance dosage: 1 to 5 units/week; Maximum dosage: 400 units. Is also given by intraarterial and intrapleural routes.

Available Drug Forms Vials containing 15 units of white crystals.

Nursing Management (See pages 947–948 for further details.)

Planning factors

1. Perform a skin test 24 hours prior to initiating therapy.
2. Be prepared for anaphylactic reaction.
3. Give antiemetic before administration, if needed.

Administration factors

1. Dissolve crystals in 3 ml of saline or sterile water. Stable at room temperature for 24 hours.
2. Give IV dose slowly over a 10-minute period.

Evaluation factors

1. Observe for changes in pulmonary function. Obtain chest x-rays weekly or biweekly. Pneumonitis is a frequent complication, particularly in the elderly.
2. Monitor blood counts and renal and hepatic function tests frequently.
3. Signs of cutaneous toxicity (swollen hands, urticaria) may necessitate cessation of treatment.

GENERIC NAME Daunorubicin hydrochloride

TRADE NAME Cerubidine (RX)

CLASSIFICATION Antineoplastic

See doxorubicin hydrochloride for Contraindications, Warnings and precautions, Untoward reactions, and Parameters of use.

Action This drug inhibits synthesis of nucleic acids, but the exact mechanism of action is unknown. It also has an immunosuppressive effect.

Indications for Use Acute myelocytic leukemia, acute lymphocytic leukemia, neuroblastoma.

Administration 30 to 60 mg/m^2 IV weekly; cumulative dosage should not exceed 600 mg/m^2.

Available Drug Forms Vials containing 20 mg powder.

Nursing Management (See pages 947–948 for further details.) Reconstitute powder with 4 ml sterile water for injection, to yield 5 mg/ml. See doxorubicin.

GENERIC NAME Doxorubicin hydrochloride (RX)

TRADE NAME Adriamycin

CLASSIFICATION Antineoplastic

Action Doxorubicin, which is derived from *Streptomyces peucetius,* is similar in action to daunorubicin. It interferes with nucleic acid synthesis by binding with DNA and preventing DNA transcription and replication. Maximal cytotoxic effect occurs in S phase of cell cycle. Nadir: 7 to 10 days.

Indications for Use Osteogenic sarcoma, soft tissue sarcoma, carcinoma of the breast, lung, thyroid, and ovary, lymphoma, acute leukemia, neuroblastoma, Wilms' tumor, Hodgkin's disease.

Contraindications Bone marrow depression, heart disease, pregnancy.

Warnings and Precautions Use with caution in clients with impaired hepatic or renal function. May reactivate previous tissue radiation damage.

Untoward Reactions Severe bone marrow depression, fever, stomatitis, nausea, vomiting, cardiotoxicity, hyperpigmentation of dermal creases and nails, alopecia, rash, facial flushing, hypersensitivity reactions.

Parameters of Use

Absorption Rapidly from plasma.
Distribution Widely distributed to all tissues.
Metabolism In the liver.
Excretion About 50% in bile as unchanged drug.

Administration Adults: 60 to 75 mg/m^2 IV every 3 weeks; Total dosage should not exceed 550 mg/m^2. Children: 30 mg/m^2 IV every 3 days; repeat every 4 weeks.

Available Drug Forms Vials containing 10 or 50 mg of red-orange crystals.

Nursing Management (See pages 947–948 for further details.)

Administration factors

1. Reconstitute crystals with 0.9% sodium chloride. Shake to dissolve. (Avoid contact with skin.) Solution is stable for 24 hours at room temperature and 48 hours when refrigerated. Store crystals at room temperature and protect from light.
2. Inject directly into tubing of established IV of D/W or saline. Do not give with any other drugs.
3. Avoid extravasation. If client complains of burning at IV site, stop infusion and apply cold compress to site.

Evaluation factors

1. Obtain an EKG monthly during therapy and for several months after discontinuation.
2. Monitor vital signs, weight, and intake and output regularly to detect early signs of cardiotoxicity.

Client teaching factors

1. Inform client of red discoloration of urine for 1 to 2 days after administration.
2. Teach client importance of avoiding exposure to infections or communicable diseases.

GENERIC NAME Mithramycin (RX)

TRADE NAME Mithracin

CLASSIFICATION Antineoplastic

Action Mithramycin, which is derived from *Streptomyces plicatus,* is similar in action to dactinomycin. It inhibits RNA synthesis and probably inhibits osteoclastic activity.

Indications for Use Carcinoma of the testis, trophoblastic tumor, Paget's disease, hypercalcemia associated with cancer.

Contraindications Children under 15 years, myelosuppression, increased bleeding tendency, pregnancy, electrolyte imbalance.

Warnings and Precautions Use with caution in clients with hepatic or renal impairment or those who have had previous abdominal or mediastinal radiotherapy.

Untoward Reactions Nausea, vomiting, hypocalcemia, hypokalemia, hepatotoxicity, nephrotoxicity, fever, irritability, stomatitis, headache, drowsiness, bone marrow depression, skin rash, phlebitis.

Parameters of Use

Absorption Less potent when given orally than when given intravenously.
Distribution Incomplete data. Crosses blood-brain barrier.
Excretion Incomplete data.

Drug Interactions Concurrent use of vitamin D may potentiate hypercalcemia.

Laboratory Interactions Decreases blood calcium levels and prolongs prothrombin time.

Administration 25 to 30 mg/kg IV daily or every other day until toxicity level is reached.

Available Drug Forms Vials containing 2.5 mg of freeze-dried white powder.

Nursing Management (See pages 947–948 for further details.)

1. Mix powder with 4.9 ml of sterile water and use immediately. Store powder in refrigerator.
2. Infuse in 1000 ml of 5% D/W slowly over 4 to 6 hours.
3. Avoid extravasation. If vasculitis occurs, discontinue infusion.
4. Assess renal, hepatic, and neurologic function regularly.
5. Watch client for bleeding and fever.

GENERIC NAME Mitomycin (RX)

TRADE NAMES Mitomycin C, Mutamycin

CLASSIFICATION Antineoplastic

Action Mitomycin, which is derived from *Streptomyces caespitosus,* is similar in action to alkylating agents. It inhibits DNA synthesis. Mitomycin is highly toxic.

Indications for Use Malignant melanoma, osteogenic sarcoma, carcinoma of the breast, pancreas, lung, cervix, and head and neck in combination with other drugs.

Contraindications Hypersensitivity to mitomycin, infection, lowered platelet or white blood cell count, increased bleeding tendencies.

Warnings and Precautions Use with caution in clients with renal dysfunction.

Untoward Reactions Leukopenia, thrombocytopenia, nausea, vomiting, malaise, fever, stomatitis, pruritus, alopecia, paresthesias, renal damage.

Parameters of Use

Absorption Disappears rapidly from plasma.
Excretion In urine within 2 hours.

Laboratory Interactions Increases blood urea nitrogen and creatinine clearance.

Administration 0.05 mg/kg IV daily for 5 days; rest 2 days and repeat for 2 to 3 weeks in the absence of bone marrow toxicity.

Available Drug Forms Vials containing 5 or 20 mg of powder.

Nursing Management (See pages 947–948 for further details.)

1. Hospitalize client during therapy.
2. Reconstitute with sterile water. Stable for 7 days at room temperature or 14 days when refrigerated.
3. Avoid extravasation; give directly into running IV.
4. Give antiemetics as necessary.
5. Monitor intake and output.
6. Give frequent mouth care.
7. Check for bleeding and bone marrow toxicity.
8. Assess for fever and protect client against infection and bleeding.

MISCELLANEOUS CYTOTOXIC AGENTS

GENERIC NAME Hydroxyurea (RX)

TRADE NAME Hydrea

CLASSIFICATION Antineoplastic

Action Hydroxyurea inhibits ribonucleoside diphosphate reductase, which catalyzes the reduction of RNA to DNA. It prevents cell replication by inhibiting DNA synthesis. The drug is cell cycle–specific for the S phase. Nadir: 24 to 48 hours.

Indications for Use Chronic granulocytic leukemia, malignant melanoma, carcinoma of the ovary, prostate cancer.

Contraindications Women of childbearing age, hepatic or renal impairment, severe anemia, myelosuppression, pregnancy, children.

Warnings and Precautions Use with caution in elderly clients, clients with renal impairment, and those who have had recent cytotoxic or radiation therapy.

Untoward Reactions Bone marrow depression, nausea, vomiting, stomatitis, diarrhea, rash, alopecia, renal dysfunction, neurological symptoms.

Parameters of Use

Absorption Well absorbed from GI tract. Crosses blood-brain barrier.
Metabolism In the liver.
Excretion In urine.

Drug Interactions May cause erythema in clients who have received radiotherapy.

Administration 80 mg/kg po every 3 days or 20 to 30 mg/kg/day for 6 weeks.

Available Drug Forms Capsules containing 500 mg; vials containing 2 g of white powder.

Nursing Management (See pages 947–948 for further details.)

1. Capsule may be opened if it cannot be swallowed. Mix in glass of water, warm tea, or orange juice.
2. Dilute powder with 18.5 ml of sterile water. Stable for 2 days at 4 C.
3. Store drug at room temperature.
4. Protect client against infection and bleeding.
5. Monitor intake and output and assess renal function frequently.

GENERIC NAME Cisplatin (RX)

TRADE NAME Platinol

CLASSIFICATION Antineoplastic

Action Cisplatin inhibits DNA synthesis. It is a cell cycle-nonspecific agent.

Indications for Use Cancer of the bladder, ovary, head and neck, and testicle, usually in combination with other drugs.

Contraindications Renal impairment, myelosuppression, hearing impairment, hypersensitivity.

Warnings and Precautions Safe use in pregnancy has not been established.

Untoward Reactions Bone marrow depression, nausea, vomiting, anaphylaxis, nephrotoxicity, irreversible hearing loss (frequent), hyperuricemia, electrolyte disturbances.

Parameters of Use

Absorption Data incomplete. Half-life is 25 to 50 minutes. Concentrates in liver, kidneys, and intestines, with poor CNS penetration.
Excretion By the kidneys.

Drug Interactions Aminoglycoside antibiotics potentiate nephrotoxicity. Aluminum needles, syringes, and IV equipment react with cisplatin to form a precipitate.

Administration 20 mg/m^2 IV daily for 5 days every 3 to 4 weeks.

Available Drug Forms Vials containing 10 or 50 mg powder.

Nursing Management (See pages 947–948 for further details.)

1. Baseline blood urea nitrogen, creatinine, magnesium, calcium, and potassium levels should be assessed prior to starting therapy.
2. Give a mannitol flush (diuresis) before or concurrently with drug to prevent tubular necrosis.
3. Reconstitute powder with sterile water for injection, to yield 1 mg/ml. Solution is stable for 24 hours at room temperature. Do not refrigerate, because a precipitate will form.
4. Do not use any aluminum equipment with cisplatin.
5. If drug contacts skin, wash immediately with soap and water.
6. Lasix (40 mg) is usually administered before treatment.
7. Administer into established IV infusion line.
8. Assess client regularly for renal function, hepatic function, bone marrow depression, and hearing loss.
9. Nephotoxicity becomes more severe and prolonged with repeated drug therapy. Renal function should return to normal before each repeat dose is administered.
10. Any symptoms of neurotoxicity mandate discontinuance of drug, since peripheral neuropathy may be irreversible.

GENERIC NAME Dacarbazine (RX)

TRADE NAME DTIC

CLASSIFICATION Antineoplastic

Action Dacarbazine, which was originally thought to be an antimetabolite, has alkylating properties. It interferes with the synthesis of DNA, RNA, and protein in rapidly proliferating cells. It is a cell cycle–nonspecific agent.

Indications for Use Malignant melanoma, sarcoma, Hodgkin's disease, neuroblastoma.

Contraindications Hypersensitivity.

Warnings and Precautions Safe use in pregnancy has not been established.

Untoward Reactions Anorexia, nausea, vomiting, leukopenia, thrombocytopenia, anemia, hepatotoxicity, flushing, paresthesias, nephrotoxicity, confusion, lethargy, visual disturbances, headache, seizures, skin rash, tissue damage if drug extravasates.

Parameters of Use

Distribution Distributed by plasma. Half-life is 35 minutes.
Metabolism In the liver.
Excretion In urine.

Administration 3.5 mg/kg IV daily for a 10-day period; repeat every 28 days.

Available Drug Forms Vials containing 100 or 200 mg.

Nursing Management (See pages 947–948 for further details.)

1. Give antiemetics as necessary.
2. Avoid extravasation.
3. Protect drug from light. Solution may be stored for 24 hours under refrigeration, or for 8 hours at room temperature.
4. Protect client against infection and bleeding.
5. Evaluate client frequently for bone marrow depression, which is a common adverse effect.

GENERIC NAME Etoposide (RX)

TRADE NAMES VP-16, Vepesid

CLASSIFICATION Antineoplastic

Action Etoposide is a cell cycle–specific agent that inhibits DNA synthesis.

Indications for Use Small cell lung cancer, testicular cancer.

Contraindications Hypersensitivity, pregnancy, lactation, children.

Untoward Reactions Bone marrow depression, nausea, vomiting, diarrhea, neurotoxicity, alopecia, anaphylactic shock, hypotension, phlebitis.

Parameters of Use Data incomplete. About 90% protein-bound, with minimal CSF penetration. Excreted by the kidneys.

Administration 50 to 100 mg/m^2 IV for 5 days every 3 weeks.

Available Drug Forms Ampules containing 100 mg.

Nursing Management (See pages 947–948 for further details.)

1. Give antiemetics and antidiarrheal agents as necessary.
2. Dilute in 100 to 500 ml of isotonic saline. Infuse over 30 minutes to 6 hours. Solution is stable for 48 hours at room temperature.
3. Force fluids.
4. Assess for infection, fever, and signs of myelosuppression.

GENERIC NAME Hexamethylmelamine (RX)

TRADE NAME HMM

CLASSIFICATION Antineoplastic

Indications for Use Lung cancer, lymphoma, cervical cancer. Still under investigation.

Untoward Reactions Nausea, vomiting, bone marrow depression, neurotoxicity (peripheral neuritis).

Parameters of Use

Metabolism In the liver.
Excretion By the kidneys.

Administration 12 mg/kg po daily for 3 weeks.

Nursing Management (See pages 947–948 for further details.)

1. Give after meals.
2. Protect client against infection and bleeding.
3. Assess neurologic function regularly.
4. Visual hallucinations may occur. Instruct client to report promptly any visual changes.
5. Monitor frequently for symptoms of myelosuppression.

GENERIC NAME *L*-asparaginase (RX)

TRADE NAMES Elspar, L-ASP

CLASSIFICATION Antineoplastic

Action This drug, which is obtained from *Escherichia coli,* is cytotoxic to cells lacking the ability to synthesize *L*-asparaginase. It is a cell cycle-specific agent.

Indications for Use Acute lymphocytic leukemia, melanoma, lymphosarcoma, usually in combination with other drugs.

Contraindications Hypersensitivity to drug, history of pancreatitis.

Untoward Reactions Nausea, vomiting, confusion, hepatic and pancreatic toxicity, fever, blood dyscrasias, malaise, anaphylactic shock, allergic reactions.

Parameters of Use

Absorption Not known.
Excretion Via the reticuloendothelial system.

Drug Interactions Concurrent use of corticosteroids increases the risk of hyperglycemia, ketoacidosis, and diabetic coma. Concurrent use of vincristine increases the risk of toxicity. *L*-asparaginase diminishes the therapeutic effect of methetrexate.

Laboratory Interactions Decreases levels of coagulation factor and causes abnormal hepatic function test results.

Administration 200 to 1000 IU/kg IV for 3 to 7 days a week for 28 days.

Available Drug Forms Vials containing 10,000 units of white powder.

Nursing Management (See pages 947–948 for further details.)

1. Perform a skin test prior to initiating therapy.
2. Dilute powder with 5 ml of sterile water or saline; do not shake. Stable for 48 hours at 4 C; solution should be clear. Store powder in refrigerator.

GENERIC NAME Mitotane (RX)

TRADE NAMES Lysodren, OPDDD

CLASSIFICATION Antineoplastic

Action Mitotane inhibits adrenocortical function. Its biochemical action is unknown.

Indications for Use Inoperable adrenocortical carcinoma.

Contraindications Hypersensitivity.

Warnings and Precautions Use with caution in clients with liver disease. Safe use in pregnancy has not been established.

Untoward Reactions Adrenal insufficiency, depression, lethargy, vertigo, nausea, vomiting, diarrhea, skin rash, nephrotoxicity, hypertension, neurotoxicity.

Parameters of Use Data incomplete.

Administration 8 to 10 g po daily in divided doses.

Available Drug Forms Tablets containing 500 mg.

Nursing Management (See pages 947–948 for further details.)

1. Give antiemetics and antidiarrheal agents as necessary.
2. Assess neurologic function regularly.
3. If severe trauma or shock occur, discontinue drug and give steroids.
4. Caution client not to drive a car or operate machinery if alertness is impaired.
5. Long-term administration (2 years) may cause brain damage. Behavioral and neurological assessments should be made at regular intervals.

GENERIC NAME Procarbazine hydrochloride (RX)

TRADE NAMES Matulane, PROC

CLASSIFICATION Antineoplastic

Action Procarbazine must be metabolized before it can exert a cytotoxic effect. The drug interferes with cell metabolism by causing chromosome breaks and inhibiting mitosis. It also depolymerizes DNA and RNA. Procarbazine is a cell cycle-nonspecific agent. Nadir: 14 days.

Indications for Use Neoplastic diseases: Hodgkin's disease, lymphoma, leukemia, carcinoma of the bronchus, oat cell carcinoma. Nonneoplastic diseases: immunosuppressant.

Contraindications Hypersensitivity to procarbazine, myelosuppression, alcoholism, clients taking sympathomimetics or tricyclic antidepressants.

Warnings and Precautions Use with caution in clients with renal or hepatic impairment, clients taking CNS depressants, or those who have had radiation or chemotherapy within one month.

Untoward Reactions Bone marrow depression (leukopenia, thrombocytopenia), diarrhea, nausea, vomiting, anorexia, stomatitis, CNS dysfunction (convulsions, depression), dermatitis, alopecia, orthostatic hypotension, visual and hearing disturbances, photosensitivity, pleural effusion, tachycardia, chills, fever, and ascites.

Parameters of Use

Absorption Almost completely absorbed from GI tract. Crosses blood-brain barrier.
Metabolism In the liver.
Excretion By the kidneys.

Drug Interactions Enhances the effects of MAO inhibitors, alcohol, antihistamines, narcotics, sedatives, sympathomimetics, and tricyclic antidepressants.

Administration Initial dosage: 50 to 300 mg po daily for 1 week; Maintenance dosage: 50 to 100 mg/day.

Available Drug Forms Capsules containing 50 mg.

Nursing Management (See pages 947–948 for further details.)

Planning factors

1. Hospitalize client before initiating therapy.
2. Padded tongue blade and side rails should be available in case convulsions occur.
3. Foods with high tyramine content should be avoided.

Administration factors

1. Give antiemetics (no phenothiazines) as necessary.
2. Observe closely for CNS symptoms and orthostatic hypotension.

Evaluation factors

1. Check blood counts every 3 to 4 days.
2. Monitor vital signs and intake and output regularly.
3. Check client for bleeding and signs of infection.
4. All preparations containing sympathomimetics must be avoided because of the danger of hypertensive crisis.

Client teaching factors

1. Instruct client to avoid all OTC drugs unless prescribed by physician.
2. Caution client to avoid tyramine-rich foods (bananas, ripe cheeses, raisins, figs, chocolate, licorice, cream, yogurt, liver, aged meats, soy sauce, pickled herring, yeast), alcohol, and caffeine.
3. Instruct client to report early signs of bone marrow depression.

GENERIC NAME Streptozotocin (RX)

CLASSIFICATION Antineoplastic

Action Streptozotocin, which is an antibiotic derived from *Streptomyces*, inhibits DNA synthesis. It exerts inhibitory effects on pyridine nucleotides and certain enzymes. Streptozotocin is a cell cycle–specific toxin for the beta cells in the pancreas.

Indications for Use Metastatic pancreatic islet cell carcinoma. Other uses are still under investigation.

Contraindications Sensitivity to aminoglycosides.

Untoward Reactions Nausea, vomiting, stomatitis, nephrotoxicity, mild hepatotoxicity, diabetes (reversible).

Parameters of Use

Absorption Rapidly absorbed after parenteral administration.
Distribution Concentrates in liver and kidneys.
Excretion Negligible in urine.

Administration 500 to 1000 mg/m^2 IV; repeat every 6 to 8 weeks.

Available Drug Forms Vials containing 1 g.

Nursing Management (See pages 947–948 for further details.)

1. Infuse in established IV line over a 1-hour period. Avoid extravasation, which can cause tissue necrosis.
2. Monitor urine for glucose and protein (drug is diabetogenic).
3. Force fluids.
4. Give frequent mouth care.
5. Protect drug from light.
6. Monitor blood urea nitrogen, creatinine, and urinary protein levels frequently for early detection of nephrotoxicity.

ANTIESTROGENS

GENERIC NAME Tamoxifen (RX)

TRADE NAMES Nolvadex, TAM

CLASSIFICATION Antineoplastic

Action Tamoxifen blocks the binding of estrogen at cell receptor sites, thereby preventing estrogen from supporting the proliferation of estrogen-dependent cells.

Indications for Use Palliation for estrogen-dependent breast cancer and metastases.

Contraindications None known.

Warnings and Precautions Use with caution in clients with thrombocytopenia or leukopenia. Has been shown to be oncogenic in animals. Safe use in pregnancy has not been established.

Untoward Reactions Blood dyscrasias (mild), nausea, vomiting, hot flushes, vaginal bleeding, menstrual irregularities, skin rash, hypercalcemia in clients with bone metastases, fluid retention, retinal changes with high dosages, increased bone and tumor pain, edema, anorexia, dizziness, headache, pruritus vulvae.

Parameters of Use

Absorption From GI tract. Peak action occurs in 4 to 7 hours. Persists for days in enterohepatic circulation.
Distribution Widely distributed to body tissues.
Excretion Slowly via feces.

Administration 10 to 20 mg po bid.

Available Drug Forms Tablets containing 10 mg.

Nursing Management (See pages 947–948 for further details.)

1. Client may experience an initial increase in bone and tumor pain. This will subside with continued therapy and is not a sign that treatment is ineffective.
2. Monitor weight and blood pressure regularly to detect fluid retention.
3. Schedule annual ophthalmologic examinations.
4. Protect tablets from heat and light.

COMBINATION DRUG REGIMENS

- *Acute lymphocytic leukemia*
  POMP—prednisone, Oncovin, methotrexate, Purinethol
  VP—vincristine, prednisone

- *Acute myelogenous leukemia*
  Ara-C and TG—cytarabine, thioguanine

- *Hodgkin's disease*
  ABVD—Adriamycin, bleomycin, vinblastine, dacarbazine
  MOPP—mechlorethamine, Oncovin, procarbazine, prednisone

- *Lymphoma*
  CVP—cyclophosphamide, vincristine, prednisone
  CHOP—cyclophosphamide, doxorubicin, Oncovin, prednisone
  BACOP—bleomycin, Adriamycin, cyclophosphamide, Oncovin, prednisone

- *Breast carcinoma*
  CMF—cyclophosphamide, methotrexate, fluorouracil

PART XVI

DIGESTIVE SYSTEM AGENTS

THE MAJOR FUNCTION of the digestive system is to provide a continuous supply of nutrients to all body cells. This is accomplished within the gastrointestinal tract with the aid of the accessory exocrine gland secretions.

There are four basic physiologic processes involved in digestion and elimination; namely, muscular movement, secretion, digestion, and absorption.

Muscular movement, or motility, occurs in the mouth, pharynx, esophagus, stomach, small intestine, and large intestine. Muscular contractions are responsible for propelling food along the gastrointestinal tract, mixing the products with digestive secretions, and facilitating the transport of nutrients through the intestinal wall into the blood and lymph systems. Motility is generally enhanced by parasympathetic nervous stimulation and inhibited by sympathetic nervous stimulation. However, the various sphincter muscles respond by contracting when the sympathetic nervous system is stimulated.

Secretory activities are present in all digestive structures with the exception of the pharynx. These secretions include saliva, gastric juice, intestinal juice, pancreatic juice, bile, and mucin. The composition of secretions varies according to their intended action. For example, the presence of bile is essential for the absorption of all fat-soluble vitamins and intrinsic factor, which is normally secreted by the gastric mucosa, is essential for the absorption of vitamin B_{12}. Generally, the gastric pH is acidic and the intestinal pH is slightly alkaline.

The digestive process is designed to break down carbohydrates, fats, and proteins into molecules that can be transported across the intestinal wall. This process is aided by numerous enzymes present in saliva, gastric juice, pancreatic secretions, and intestinal secretions. Specifically, carbohydrates are chemically broken down to simple sugars, fats to fatty acids, and proteins to amino acids.

The absorptive process involves the transfer of nutrient molecules into the blood and lymph and occurs primarily in the small intestine. The intestinal villi are richly supplied with blood and lymphatic vessels and provide an appropriate surface for transport by osmosis, diffusion, active transport, and pinocytosis (see Chapter 7). Carbohydrates, in the form of monosaccharides, and amino acids are absorbed primarily from the duodenum and jejunum. Fatty acids (lipids) are absorbed mainly from the duodenum. Water absorption is highly variable and depends upon electrolyte balance and osmotic pressure. Most water is absorbed from the small intestine, but some may also be absorbed from the colon.

Research indicates that digestive activities are further controlled by hormones, histamine, serotonin, and prostaglandins. At present, however, most digestive system drugs act directly or indirectly on the muscular or glandular functions of the digestive tract. Many gastrointestinal symptoms are often caused by obscure underlying pathologic processes and pharmacologic treatment is directed at alleviating symptoms rather than curing the underlying pathology.

Chapter 75

Antacids, Deflatulents, and H_2-Receptor Antagonists

PEPTIC ULCERS CAN occur in the stomach *(gastric ulcer)* or duodenum *(duodenal ulcer)* and may be solitary *(acute)* or in groups that form a scar on healing and tend to recur *(chronic)*. Once the protective mucosal lining of the stomach has been penetrated, the acidic gastric juices begin to digest the involved stomach wall causing pain and eventual perforation. Treatment is aimed at alkalizing the gastric secretions with antacids and reducing the release of gastric juices with histamine$_2$-receptor antagonists until the ulcerated area(s) has healed.

STIMULATION OF GASTRIC SECRETIONS

The pH of gastric secretions is kept very acidic (2.0 to 3.0) to enable digestive enzymes in the stomach to function properly. For example, pepsinogen, a zymogen secreted by the chief cells of the gastric glands, is rapidly converted to the proteolytic enzyme pepsin, which functions best at a pH of 2.0; pepsin has very little activity when the pH is above 5.0. Hydrochloric acid, a caustic acid secreted by the parietal cells, helps to maintain the acid pH of the stomach. Both pepsin and hydrochloric acid are required for the digestion of dietary proteins, but they also attack unprotected ulcerative sites in the gastric wall.

Simulation of the vagus nerve (cholinergic) by the thought, smell, or sight of food stimulates the gastric glands to secrete pepsinogen and hydrochloric acid. The presence of dietary protein in the stomach also results in the secretion of the hormone gastrin, which stimulates the further release of hydrochloric acid and pepsin. Once the stomach empties into the duodenum, 30 to 60 minutes after the ingestion of food, small quantities of gastric juices continue to be secreted for as long as eight hours due to the release of duodenal hormones. The most acidic gastric pH usually occurs 60 minutes after a meal.

Certain drugs are associated with the onset of peptic ulcer disease and are considered *ulcerogenic*. Salicylates, particularly the chronic ingestion of aspirin, and the antiinflammatory agents phenylbutazone and indomethacin are considered to be ulcerogenic. Excessive ingestion of ethyl alcohol, caffeine, and nicotine (cigarette smoking) are also considered ulcerogenic and should be avoided by clients with gastric hyperacidity or a history of peptic ulcer.

CHARACTERISTICS OF ANTACIDS AND DEFLATULENTS

Aluminum, calcium, and magnesium antacids increase the pH of the stomach and thus decrease the acidic erosion of ulcerated areas. Although aluminum and calcium antacids tend to cause constipation, magnesium antacids can have the opposite effect as they form magnesium chloride, a laxative. Consequently, an aluminum or calcium compound is often combined with a magnesium antacid to neutralize these unpleasant side effects. As several of the antacids liberate carbon dioxide when they chemically combine with hydrochloric acid, the deflatulent simethicone is often added to combination antacid preparations to help prevent the entrapment of gas into pockets.

Sodium bicarbonate (baking soda) is a rapid-acting antacid; however, due to its high solubility, it leaves the stomach within 10 to 20 minutes and enters the bloodstream. Sodium bicarbonate is considered a systemic antacid because of its ability to alkalize the blood and urine. Although this agent is frequently used as a home remedy, it is seldom, if ever, prescribed by a physician for its gastric antacid effect.

Antacids are administered between meals and prevent further destruction of the gastric mucosa by maintaining an elevated pH of the gastric contents. Since the greatest hyperacidity usually occurs 60 minutes after ingestion of food, many physicians prescribe antacids to be given one hour after meals. Chewable tablets must be chewed thoroughly in order to be effective and suspensions often need to be washed into the stomach with an appropriate amount of water. Although little or no food or water should be ingested for 30 minutes following administration, fluids should be encouraged at mealtime.

CHARACTERISTICS OF H$_2$-RECEPTOR ANTAGONISTS

A new class of drugs, the histamine$_2$-receptor antagonists, were introduced following the discovery of cimetidine. Histamine, which is released from gastric mucosal cells, causes the release of hydrochloric acid. Cimetidine inhibits the action of histamine in the stomach and therefore the release of acid and the action of pepsin. Unlike antacids, cimetidine produces an increase in gastric pH that lasts for several hours. Occasionally, antacids will also be ordered to decrease ulcer pain.

SYSTEMIC ANTACIDS AND ALKALIZERS

GENERIC NAME Sodium bicarbonate (OTC)

TRADE NAME Baking soda

CLASSIFICATION Antacid and alkalizer

Action One molecule of sodium bicarbonate combines with one molecule of hydrochloric acid to form sodium chloride, water, and carbon dioxide. The pH of the gastric contents is elevated rapidly, but the release of carbon dioxide may cause belching. The drug-induced neutralization of gastric contents assists in the prevention of mucosal injury from hyperacidity and pepsin. Sodium bicarbonate is a relatively strong antacid, but it has a short duration of action and is absorbed systemically, thus prohibiting its long-term use.

Indications for Use Short-term treatment of gastric hyperacidity associated with gastritis. Has been used to alkalize the blood in short-term acidosis (parenteral sodium bicarbonate is preferred).

Contraindications Metabolic or respiratory alkalosis, severe renal impairment, severe hypertension, congestive heart failure, sodium overload (hypernatremia).

Warnings and Precautions Use with caution in the elderly and in clients with impaired renal function or those on sodium-restricted intake. Prolonged use for hyperacidity should be avoided.

Untoward Reactions Systemic alkalosis may occur with large dosages or prolonged use, particularly in clients with renal impairment. Hypernatremia and sodium overload may occur in susceptible clients, such as the elderly, hypertensive clients, and clients with a history of congestive heart failure. Rebounding hyperacidity may occur with high dosages or prolonged use. Milk-alkali syndrome may occur when sodium bicarbonate is given for a prolonged period of time with milk or a diet high in milk. This combination may cause an increase in the absorption of milk and result in hypercalcemia, metabolic alkalosis, and renal insufficiency.

Parameters of Use

Absorption Most of the sodium bicarbonate ingested is absorbed into the bloodstream. Normal serum sodium levels: 138 to 146 mEq/l.

Distribution Widely distributed to extracellular fluids.
Excretion Primarily by the kidneys.

Drug Interactions By elevating the pH, sodium bicarbonate decreases the GI absorption of barbiturates and increases their urinary excretion. Reduces the absorption of tetracyclines from the GI tract; do not use concurrently. Enhances the urinary excretion of lithium, thus inhibiting the duration of lithium action. Alkalizes the stomach contents and can therefore interfere with the absorption of numerous drugs, including penicillins, sulfonamides and other antibiotics, digitalis, salicylates, and coumarin. Do not administer sodium bicarbonate concurrently with other drugs unless specifically prescribed by physician.

Administration $\frac{1}{2}$ tsp q2h prn; Maximum daily dosage: Adults: 4 tsp; Over 60 years: 2 tsp; should not be taken longer than 2 weeks.

Available Drug Forms Boxes containing pure sodium bicarbonate powder (baking soda); each tsp contains 41.8 mEq (0.952 mg) of sodium. Also, a main ingredient of Alka-Seltzer, Bell-Ans, and Soda Mint.

Nursing Management

Planning factors

1. Obtain a description of epigastric discomfort, including location, duration, precipitating factors, and factors that relieve discomfort.
2. Schedule drug administration between meals and at bedtime.
3. Avoid administering with other drugs, since interactions may occur.
4. Obtain serum electrolytes before initiating therapy.

Administration factors

1. Dissolve powder in 4 to 6 fl oz of water before administration.
2. Encourage fluids 1 hour before or after drug administration.

Evaluation factors

1. Epigastric distress is the primary factor by which the dosage and frequency of drug administration is determined. Ask client about discomforts each time drug is administered and chart results. Persistent discomfort after 3 to 4 days of therapy may indicate perforation of ulcer, tumor, or other disease processes.
2. Obtain serum sodium level periodically.
3. Assess client for sodium overload daily.
4. Record intake and output.

Client teaching factors

1. Instruct client to dissolve powder completely in water before drinking.
2. Advise client to avoid taking antacids concurrently with any other drugs unless specifically prescribed by physician.

3. Instruct client about maximum daily dosages and urge client to notify physician if hyperacidity does not disappear within 2 to 3 days.
4. Discourage geriatric clients from using drug and explain why (sodium content).
5. Urge client to notify physician if oliguria, shortness of breath, or edema occur.

ALUMINUM ANTACIDS

GENERIC NAME Aluminum hydroxide gel (OTC)

TRADE NAMES Alterna-Gel, Amphojel, Hydroxal

CLASSIFICATION Antacid

Action One molecule of aluminum hydroxide combines with three molecules of hydrochloric acid to form aluminum chloride and water, thus raising the pH of the gastric contents. The drug-induced neutralization of gastric contents assists in the prevention of mucosal injury from hyperacidity and pepsin. Aluminum preparations are relatively weak antacids.

Indications for Use Symptomatic treatment of hyperacidity associated with gastritis, hiatal hernia, and peptic esophagitis (esophogeal reflux); as an adjunct in the treatment of peptic ulcer.

Contraindications Hypersensitivity to aluminum or aluminum preparations.

Warnings and Precautions Use with caution in clients with low serum phosphates, as high dosages or prolonged use may precipitate a phosphate deficiency syndrome; in clients with severe renal impairment, pyloric stenosis, or gastric dumping syndrome; and in clients on restricted sodium intake, since high dosages contain significant quantities of sodium.

Untoward Reactions Phosphate deficiency syndrome (hypophosphatemia) can occur, particularly with high dosages or prolonged use. Aluminum compounds interact with dietary phosphates and interfere with phosphate absorption. The symptoms include low serum phosphate levels, anorexia, and muscle weakness. Chronic hypophosphatemia may cause hypercalcemia, depressed or absent deep tendon reflexes, tremors, demineralization of bones, and the formation of kidney stones. Constipation is a common side effect, particularly in the elderly and clients with hypoactive bowels. Nausea and vomiting may also occur. Intestinal obstructions have been reported. Excessive sodium intake may precipitate congestive heart failure, hypertension, and other untoward reactions in clients with severe renal failure. Aluminum accumulates in brain tissue and may lead to death. Chronic drug ingestion may cause encephalopathy in clients with renal failure.

Parameters of Use

Absorption Little absorbed from GI tract. Alkalization of stomach contents will alter the absorption of several nutrients and drugs. Onset of action is almost immediately. Duration of action is 30 to 60 minutes and is limited by gastric emptying time.

Excretion Primarily as insoluble phosphates in feces; absorbed aluminum is excreted by the kidneys.

Drug Interactions Aluminum antacids inhibit GI absorption of isoniazid and quinidine; administer antacids 1 hour before or 2 hours after isoniazid or quinidine. Aluminum antacids form insoluble complexes with tetracyclines, thus resulting in low serum tetracycline levels. Insoluble complexes are also formed with iron; do not administer concurrently. Antacids alkalize the stomach contents and can therefore interfere with the absorption of numerous drugs, including some penicillins, nitrofurantoin, sulfonamides and other antibiotics, coumarin and its derivatives, barbiturates, digitalis, and salicylates. Do not administer aluminum antacids concurrently with other drugs unless specifically prescribed by physician. Aluminum antacids may inhibit the intestinal absorption of atropine, other belladonna alkaloids, and sodium pentobarbital; do not administer concurrently.

Administration 0.6 g or 10 ml po 5 to 6 times daily. In the presence of an active peptic ulcer, administer 0.6 g or 10 ml po q1h between meals.

Available Drug Forms Bottles containing flavored or unflavored suspension; 10 ml (640 mg) neutralizes 13 mEq of acid. Tablets containing 0.3 or 0.6 g; 0.6 g neutralizes 18 mEq of acid.

Nursing Management

Planning factors

1. Obtain a description of epigastric discomfort, including location, duration, precipitating factors, and factors that relieve discomfort.
2. Obtain history of bowel habits, including frequency and consistency of feces and last bowel movement.
3. Schedule drug administration between meals and at bedtime.
4. Avoid administering with other drugs, since interactions may occur.

Administration factors

1. Shake suspension vigorously before measuring dosage.
2. Up to 1 fl oz of water may be taken after suspension is administered (avoid ingestion of water after tablets).
3. Instruct client to chew tablets thoroughly before swallowing.
4. No food or fluids should be ingested for 30 minutes after drug administration unless otherwise prescribed by physician.
5. Encourage fluids 1 hour before or after drug administration.

Evaluation factors

1. Epigastric distress is the primary factor by which the dosage and frequency of drug administration is determined. Ask client about discomforts each time drug is administered and chart results. Persistent discomfort after 3 to 4 days of therapy may indicate perforation of ulcer, tumor, or other disease processes.
2. Check and record the number and consistency of all bowel movements. Inform physician if client has no bowel movement after 2 days.
3. Obtain serum phosphate levels periodically (weekly) in clients receiving large dosages frequently. Prescribed diets high in milk content (phosphates) assist in avoiding low serum phosphates.

Client teaching factors

1. Inform client with peptic ulcer that the objective of therapy is to avoid an empty stomach.
2. Instruct client to drink plenty of fluids to avoid constipation, but not to ingest large quantities of fluids up to 30 minutes before or 1 hour after drug administration.
3. Instruct client to shake suspension vigorously before measuring dosage or to chew tablets thoroughly.
4. Advise client to avoid taking antacids concurrently with any other drugs unless specifically prescribed by physician.

GENERIC NAME Aluminum carbonate gel (OTC)

TRADE NAME Basaljel

CLASSIFICATION Antacid

See aluminum hydroxide gel for Action, Contraindications, Warnings and precautions, Untoward reactions, and Drug interactions.

Indications for Use Antacid, lowering of serum phosphate levels in renal failure, prevention of phosphate renal calculi.

Parameters of Use

Absorption Binds with phosphates in GI tract.

Administration

- *Antacid:* 15 to 30 ml (regular strength) or 5 to 10 ml (extra strength) po qid; 2 capsules or 2 tablets (swallowed) po every 2 hours.
- *Hyperphosphatemia:* 10 ml (extra strength) po every 2 to 4 hours.
- *Maximum daily dosage:* 24 tablets, capsules, or teaspoons of regular suspension; 12 teaspoons of extra strength suspension.

Available Drug Forms 10 ml of regular suspension neutralizes 28 mEq of acid and contains 0.2 mEq of sodium; 5 ml of extra strength suspension neutralizes 22 mEq of acid and contains 1.0 mEq of sodium; 2 capsules neutralize 26 mEq of acid and contain 0.24 mEq of sodium; 2 tablets neutralize 28 mEq of acid and contain 0.18 mEq of sodium. Equivalency with aluminum hydroxide is: regular suspension, 400 mg; extra strength suspension, 1000 mg; capsules, 500 mg; tablets, 500 mg.

Nursing Management See Aluminum hydroxide gel.

1. Suspension should be taken in 4 oz of water or fruit juice.
2. Unlike aluminum hydroxide, the gel tablets are swallowed.

GENERIC NAME Aluminum phosphate gel (OTC)

TRADE NAME Phosphaljel

CLASSIFICATION Antacid

See aluminum hydroxide gel for Contraindications and Drug interactions.

Action Weak antacid action. May be used to reverse aluminum hydroxide-induced hypophosphatemia. Sometimes alternated with magnesium antacids to prevent constipation.

Indications for Use Symptomatic relief of gastric hyperacidity.

Warnings and Precautions Use with caution in the elderly and in clients with decreased bowel motility, since intestinal obstruction may occur. (See aluminum hydroxide gel.)

Untoward Reactions Constipation is a common untoward reaction. (See aluminum hydroxide gel.)

Administration 15 to 30 ml po every 2 to 4 hours.

Available Drug Forms Suspension.

Nursing Management (See aluminum hydroxide gel.)

1. Shake suspension well before measuring dose.
2. Follow with at least an ounce of water.

GENERIC NAME Dihydroxyaluminum aminoacetate

TRADE NAME Robalate (OTC)

CLASSIFICATION Antacid

See aluminum hydroxide gel for Contraindications and Nursing management.

Action Weaker antacid than aluminum hydroxide.

Indications for Use Symptomatic relief of gastric hyperacidity.

Warnings and Precautions Use with caution in the elderly and in clients with decreased bowel mobility, since intestinal obstruction may occur. (See aluminum hydroxide gel.)

Untoward Reactions May cause hypophosphatemia. Constipation is a common untoward reaction, but it is less severe than with aluminum hydroxide. (See aluminum hydroxide gel.)

Administration 500 to 1000 mg po qid.

Available Drug Forms Tablets containing 500 mg.

MAGNESIUM ANTACIDS

GENERIC NAME Magnesium hydroxide (OTC)

TRADE NAMES Milk of Magnesia, Mint-O-Mag, MOM

CLASSIFICATION Antacid

Action One molecule of magnesium hydroxide combines with two molecules of hydrochloric acid to form magnesium chloride and water. As magnesium hydroxide has a high solubility, it is an effective antacid with a rapid onset. Unfortunately, as much as one-third of the magnesium ions can be absorbed and result in hypermagnesemia with prolonged use. Unlike aluminum and calcium antacids, magnesium antacids can have a saline laxative effect and may cause diarrhea when large dosages are used. Magnesium hydroxide is seldom used alone as an antacid, but several antacid preparations contain a combination of the magnesium and either the aluminum or calcium salts, since the magnesium salts counteract the constipating effects of the aluminum and calcium salts. Magnesium hydroxide is also used to buffer the acidic effects of aspirin.

Indications for Use Symptomatic treatment of hyperacidity associated with gastritis, hiatal hernia, and peptic esophagitis (esophogeal reflux); as an adjunct in the treatment of peptic ulcer; oral supplement for mild hypomagnesemia.

Contraindications Severe renal impairment, hypermagnesemia, intestinal obstruction, fecal impaction, suspected appendicitis or intestinal perforation (nausea, vomiting, abdominal pain), diarrhea.

Warnings and Precautions Use with caution in the elderly and in clients with impaired renal function, since hypermagnesemia may occur.

Untoward Reactions Diarrhea is a common reaction to magnesium antacids. Nausea and abdominal cramps may also occur. If diarrhea occurs with antacid dosages, a combination drug is usually preferred. Hypermagnesemia may occur, particularly in clients with impaired renal function. Early symptoms include hypotension, depression of deep tendon reflexes, and absence of the knee jerk reflex. Hypermagnesemia produces a CNS depressant effect by blocking the release of acetylcholine. Aklalization of urine and precipitation may occur when large dosages are used for a prolonged period of time.

Parameters of Use

Absorption Between 10 to 30% absorbed from GI tract. Increased absorption occurs in the presence of low serum magnesium levels. Normal serum magnesium levels: 1.4 to 2.5 mg/100 ml or 1.5 to 30 mEq/l. Onset of antacid action is rapid (in minutes). Duration of action is about 60 minutes; has a longer duration of action than most antacids.

Excretion Primarily as insoluble complexes in feces; absorbed magnesium is excreted by the kidneys.

Drug Interactions Urinary excretion of weak basic drugs may be decreased by magnesium-induced alkalization of urine. Magnesium antacids may increase GI absorption of coumarin and its derivatives (dicumarol); do not administer within 2 hours of each other. Magnesium antacids may decrease GI absorption of phenothiazines; do not administer within 2 hours of each other. Antacids alkalize the stomach contents and can therefore interfere with the absorption of numerous drugs, including penicillins, sulfonamides and other antibiotics, barbiturates, and digitalis. Do not administer magnesium antacids concurrently with other drugs unless specifically prescribed by physician. Magnesium antacids form insoluble complexes with tetracyclines, thus resulting in low serum tetracycline levels. Insoluble complexes are also formed with iron; do not administer concurrently.

Administration 1 to 2 tablets or 5 to 10 ml po qid.

Available Drug Forms Bottles containing flavored and unflavored suspension (10 ml neutralizes about 27 mEq of acid); tablets containing 325 mg (1 tablet neutralizes about 11 mEq of acid).

Nursing Management

Planning factors

1. Obtain a description of epigastric discomfort, including location, duration, precipitating factors, and factors that relieve discomfort.
2. Obtain history of bowel habits, including frequency and consistency of feces and last bowel movement.
3. Schedule drug administration between meals and at bedtime.
4. Avoid administering with other drugs, since interactions may occur.
5. Obtain serum electrolytes and magnesium levels before initiating therapy.
6. Check deep tendon reflexes, including kneejerk reflex, when prolonged therapy is expected.

Administration factors

1. Shake suspension vigorously before measuring dosage.
2. Up to 1 fl oz of water may be taken after suspension is administered.
3. Instruct client to chew tablets thoroughly before swallowing.

Evaluation factors

1. Epigastric distress is the primary factor by which the dosage and frequency of drug administration is determined. Ask client about discomforts each time drug is administered and chart results. Persistent discomfort after 3 to 4 days of therapy may indicate perforation of ulcer, tumor, or other disease processes.
2. Check and record the number and consistency of all bowel movements. Inform physician if the client develops frequent loose stools.
3. Obtain serum magnesium levels periodically in clients receiving prolonged therapy.
4. Check kneejerk reflex periodically. If markedly depressed or absent, notify physician immediately.
5. Record intake and output. If oliguria occurs, notify physician.

Client teaching factors

1. Inform client with peptic ulcer that the objective of therapy is to avoid an empty stomach.
2. Instruct client to shake suspension vigorously before measuring dosage.
3. Advise client to avoid taking antacids concurrently with any other drugs unless specifically prescribed by physician.
4. Advise client to notify physician if urine becomes cloudy or scant.
5. Advise client to notify physician if frequent loose stools occur.

GENERIC NAME Magnesium carbonate (OTC)

CLASSIFICATION Antacid

See magnesium hydroxide for Contraindications, Parameters of use, and Drug interactions.

Action Neutralizes gastric acid. Formation of carbon dioxide may cause belching, abdominal distention, flatulence, and nausea. (See magnesium hydroxide.)

Indications for Use Symptomatic relief of hyperacidity.

Warnings and Precautions Not recommended for children or the elderly.

Untoward Reactions Hypermagnesemia, diarrhea. (See magnesium hydroxide.)

Administration 500 to 2000 mg po qid.

Available Drug Forms An ingredient of some antacids, such as Escot and Gaviscon.

Nursing Management Give with 4 fl oz of water. (See magnesium hydroxide.)

GENERIC NAME Magnesium oxide (OTC)

TRADE NAMES Light Magnesia, Mag-Ox, Maox

CLASSIFICATION Antacid

See magnesium hydroxide for Contraindications, Parameters of use, and Drug interactions.

Action Neutralizes gastric acid. Magnesium oxide is converted to magnesium hydroxide in the stomach. (See magnesium hydroxide.)

Indications for Use Symptomatic relief of hyperacidity.

Warnings and Precautions Not recommended for children or the elderly.

Untoward Reactions Hypermagnesemia, diarrhea. (See magnesium hydroxide.)

Administration 250 to 1000 mg po qid.

Available Drug Forms Tablets containing 500 or 1000 mg; (1000 mg neutralizes about 8 mEq of acid).

Nursing Management Give with 4 fl oz of water. (See magnesium hydroxide.)

GENERIC NAME Magnesium trisilicate (OTC)

TRADE NAME Trisomin

CLASSIFICATION Antacid

See magnesium hydroxide for Contraindications and Drug interactions.

Action Neutralizes gastric acid. Magnesium trisilicate is converted to magnesium chloride and silicon dioxide in the body. Silicon dioxide forms a gelatinous mass that may provide protection to irritated mucosa. It has a slower onset of action than magnesium hydroxide, but a long duration of action.

Indications for Use Symptomatic relief of hyperacidity.

Warnings and Precautions Not recommended for children or the elderly.

Untoward Reactions Hypermagnesemia, diarrhea, formation of silicon renal calculi with prolonged use.

Administration 1 to 4 g po qid.

Available Drug Forms An ingredient of several antacids, including Algemol, Escot, and Gaviscon.

Nursing Management Give tablets with 4 fl oz of water. (See magnesium hydroxide.)

ALUMINUM-MAGNESIUM COMPLEX ANTACIDS

GENERIC NAME Magalrate (OTC)

TRADE NAME Riopan

CLASSIFICATION Antacid

Action Magalrate is a buffering-type antacid that has a relatively high acid-consuming capacity. It is reported to eliminate the rebounding hyperacidity that can occur with other antacids. Although it contains aluminum, magalrate is not used for hyperphosphatemia associated with renal failure, since hypermagnesemia may occur.

Indications for Use Symptomatic treatment of hyperacidity associated with gastritis, hiatal hernia, and peptic esophagitis (esophageal reflux); as an adjunct in the treatment of peptic ulcer.

Contraindications Hypersensitivity to aluminum preparations, severe renal failure.

Warnings and Precautions Use with caution in the elderly, in clients with decreased intestinal mobility, since obstruction may occur, and in clients with renal failure, since hypermagnesemia may occur.

Untoward Reactions Mild constipation (aluminum) or diarrhea (magnesium) may occur when large dosages are used for a prolonged period of time. Hypermagnesemia may occur, particularly in the elderly and clients wih impaired renal function. Early symptoms include depression of deep tendon reflexes and absence of the kneejerk reflex. Phosphate deficiency syndrome (hypophosphatemia) can occur (aluminum), particularly with high dosages or prolonged use.

Parameters of Use

Absorption Little absorption occurs. Normal serum magnesium levels: 1.4 to 2.5 mg/100 ml or 1.5 to 3.0 mEq/l. Duration of buffering action is about 60 minutes.

Excretion Primarily as insoluble complexes in feces; absorbed magnesium is excreted by the kidneys.

Drug Interactions Aluminum and magnesium antacids form insoluble complexes with tetracyclines, thus resulting in low serum tetracycline levels. Antacids alkalize the stomach contents and can therefore interfere with the absorption of numerous drugs, including penicillins, sulfonamides, coumarin, barbiturates, digitalis, and salicylates. Aluminum antacids inhibit the absorption of isoniazid, quinidine, iron, atropine and other belladona alkaloids, and sodium pentobarbital.

Administration 1 to 2 tablets or 5 to 10 ml po qid.

Available Drug Forms Bottles of suspension containing 480 mg/5 ml; unit doses containing 30 ml; chewable tablets containing 480 mg; swallow tablets containing 480 mg; 5 ml or 1 tablet neutralize 13.5 mEq of acid.

Nursing Management

Planning factors

1. Obtain a description of epigastric discomfort, including location, duration, precipitating factors, and factors that relieve discomfort.
2. Obtain history of bowel habits, including frequency and consistency of feces and last bowel movement.
3. Schedule drug administration between meals and at bedtime.
4. Avoid administering with other drugs, since interactions may occur.
5. Obtain serum phosphate and magnesium levels in the elderly and clients with impaired renal function.

Administration factors

1. Shake suspension vigorously before measuring dosage.
2. Up to 1 fl oz of water may be taken after suspension is administered (avoid ingestion of water after tablets).
3. Instruct client to chew tablets thoroughly before swallowing.
4. No food or fluids should be ingested for 30 minutes after drug administration unless otherwise prescribed by physician.
5. Encourage fluids 1 hour before or after drug administration.

Evaluation factors

1. Epigastric distress is the primary factor by which the dosage and frequency of drug administration is determined. Ask client about discomforts each time drug is administered and chart results. Persistent discomfort after 3 to 4 days of therapy may indicate perforation of ulcer, tumor, or other disease processes.
2. Check and record the number and consistency of all bowel movements. Inform physician if client has no bowel movement after 2 days.
3. Obtain serum phosphate and magnesium levels periodically in the elderly and clients with renal impairment.

Client teaching factors

1. Inform client with peptic ulcer that the objective of therapy is to avoid an empty stomach.

2. Instruct client to drink plenty of fluids to avoid constipation, but not to ingest large quantities of fluids up to 30 minutes before or 1 hour after drug administration.
3. Instruct client to shake suspension vigorously before measuring dosage or to chew tablets thoroughly.
4. Advise client to avoid taking antacids concurrently with any other drugs unless specifically prescribed by physician.

CALCIUM ANTACIDS

GENERIC NAME Calcium carbonate (OTC)

TRADE NAMES Alka-2, Dicarbosil, Equilet, Titralac, Tums

CLASSIFICATION Antacid

Action One molecule of calcium carbonate combines with two molecules of hydrochloric acid to form calcium chloride, water, and carbon dioxide, thus elevating the pH of the gastric contents. The release of carbon dioxide may cause belching. The drug-induced neutralization of gastric contents assists in the prevention of mucosal injury from hyperacidity and pepsin. Calcium antacids are relatively strong antacids, but their chronic use may lead to rebounding hyperacidity and excessive calcium levels.

Indications for Use Symptomatic treatment of hyperacidity associated with gastritis, hiatal hernia, and peptic esophagitis (esophageal reflux); as an adjunct in the treatment of peptic ulcer; as a calcium supplement (multivitamin preparations) during pregnancy, lactation, and in pediatrics and geriatrics.

Contraindications Hypercalcemia, severe renal impairment and renal calculi, hypochloremic alkalosis, frank GI hemorrhage.

Warnings and Precautions Use with caution in digitalized clients, since digitalis toxicity may occur; in clients with renal insufficiency or a history of kidney stones; in clients with Addison's disease or other states of adrenocortical deficiency; in clients with hyperthyroidism or hypoparathyroidism, since hypercalcemia may develop when large dosages are used for a prolonged period of time; and in clients with dehydration or GI bleeding.

Untoward Reactions Rebounding hyperacidity may occur with prolonged use. Hypercalcemia may occur and tends to cause a variety of symptoms, including EKG changes, arrhythmias, and excitability of muscles and nerves (which may progress to tetany). Constipation and other GI disturbances may occur, including belching, anorexia, nausea, and vomiting. Renal calculi may develop, particularly after prolonged use of high dosages. Flank pain and azotemia may accompany the precipitation of calcium deposits in the kidneys. Milk-alkali syndrome may occur when calcium antacids are given with a diet high in milk (some peptic ulcer diets). This combination may cause hypercalcemia, systemic alkalosis, and renal insufficiency.

Parameters of Use

Absorption About one-third is absorbed when serum calcium levels are normal. Normal serum calcium levels: 9 to 10.5 mg/100 ml or 5 mEq/l.

Excretion About two-thirds in feces as insoluble calcium salts; absorbed calcium is excreted by the kidneys.

Drug Interactions Calcium augments the action of digitalis glycosides on the heart. Calcium antacids form insoluble complexes with tetracyclines, iron, and other compounds; do not administer concurrently. Antacids alkalize the stomach contents and can therefore interfere with the absorption of numerous drugs, including some penicillins, nitrofurantoin, sulfonamides and other antibiotics, coumarin and its derivatives, barbiturates, digitalis, and salicylates. Do not administer calcium antacids concurrently with other drugs unless specifically prescribed by physician. Vitamin D enhances the intestinal absorption of calcium.

Administration 500 to 1000 mg po qid; Maximum dosage: 8 g/day.

Available Drug Forms Tablets containing 500 or 1000 mg; (1000 mg neutralizes about 21 mEq of acid).

Nursing Management

Planning factors

1. Obtain a description of epigastric discomfort, including location, duration, precipitating factors, and factors that relieve discomfort.
2. Obtain history of bowel habits, including frequency and consistency of feces and last bowel movement.
3. Obtain history of renal disorders, including renal calculi.
4. Schedule drug administration between meals and at bedtime.
5. Avoid administering with other drugs, since interactions may occur.

Administration factors

1. Up to 4 fl oz of water may be taken following drug administration.
2. Instruct client to chew tablets thoroughly before swallowing.
3. No food or fluids should be ingested for 30 minutes after drug administration unless otherwise prescribed by physician.
4. Encourage fluids 1 hour before and after drug administration.

Evaluation factors

1. Epigastric distress is the primary factor by which dosage and frequency of drug administration is determined. Ask client about discomforts each time

drug is administered and chart results. Persistent discomfort after 3 to 4 days of therapy may indicate perforation of ulcer, tumor, or other disease processes.
2. Check and record the number and consistency of all bowel movements. Inform physician if client has no bowel movement after 2 days.
3. Monitor serum calcium levels periodically (weekly) in clients receiving large dosages frequently, since hypercalcemia may occur.
4. Record intake and output.
5. Check urine for signs of precipitation. If urine becomes cloudy, notify physician.

Client teaching factors

1. Inform client with peptic ulcer that the objective of therapy is to avoid an empty stomach.
2. Instruct client to drink plenty of fluids to avoid constipation, but not to ingest large quantities of fluids up to 30 minutes before or 1 hour after drug administration.
3. Instruct client to chew tablets thoroughly.
4. Advise client to avoid taking antacids concurrently with any other drugs unless specifically prescribed by physician.
5. Instruct client to report flank pain or any difficulty in voiding immediately.
6. Warn client to consult physician before using a home remedy for constipation.

COMBINATION ANTACIDS

Since the following drugs contain two or more antacids, the reader should refer to the individual monograph for each generic drug.

TRADE NAME Aludrox (OTC)

CLASSIFICATION Combination antacid

Indications for Use Sympomatic relief of gastric hyperacidity.

Administration 2 tablets or 10 ml po q4h prn.

Available Drug Forms Generic contents in each tablet: aluminum hydroxide dried gel: 233 mg; magnesium hydroxide: 83 mg; sodium: 0.07 mEq. Generic contents in 5 ml: aluminum hydroxide gel: 307 mg; magnesium hydroxide: 103 mg; sodium: 0.05 mEq. Two tablets neutralize 23 mEq of acid and 10 ml neutralizes 28 mEq of acid.

Nursing Management

1. Shake suspension vigorously before measuring dosage.
2. Follow suspension with a sip of water.
3. Tablets should be chewed thoroughly and may be followed with water.

TRADE NAME Camalox (OTC)

CLASSIFICATION Combination antacid

Indications for Use Symptomatic relief of gastric hyperacidity.

Warnings and Precautions Use with caution in clients with renal impairment. Prolonged use (over 2 weeks) may cause untoward reactions.

Administration 2 to 5 tablets or 10 to 20 ml po qid; Maximum daily dosage: 16 tablets or 80 ml.

Available Drug Forms Generic contents in each tablet or 5 ml; magnesium hydroxide: 200 mg; aluminum hydroxide: 225 mg; calcium carbonate: 250 mg. Sodium content: 1.5 mg per tablet; 2.5 mg per 5 ml. Two tablets or 10 ml neutralize 36 mEq of acid.

Nursing Management

1. Shake suspension vigorously before measuring dosage.
2. Tablets should be chewed thoroughly.
3. Give between meals and at bedtime.

TRADE NAME Escot Capsules (OTC)

CLASSIFICATION Combination antacid

Indications for Use Symptomatic relief of gastric hyderacidity.

Administration 1 to 2 capsules po qid.

Available Drug Forms Generic contents in each capsule: bismuth aluminate: 100 mg; aluminum hydroxide, magnesium carbonate: 130 mg; magnesium trisilicate: 160 mg.

Nursing Management Give between meals and at bedtime.

TRADE NAME Gaviscon Tablets (OTC)

CLASSIFICATION Combination antacid

Indications for Use Symptomatic relief of gastric hyperacidity. May be effective for esophageal reflux, since antacid foam is produced and rises to the top of gastric contents.

Administration 2 to 4 tablets po qid; Maximum daily dosage: 16 tablets.

Available Drug Forms Generic contents in each tablet: aluminum hydroxide dried gel: 80 mg; magnesium trisilicate: 20 mg; sodium: 0.8 mEq. Also contains sucrose, alginic acid, sodium bicarbonate, starch, calcium stearate, and flavoring.

Nursing Management

1. Tablets should be chewed thoroughly; follow with 4 fl oz of water.
2. Store at room temperature.
3. Give 1 hour after meals and at bedtime.

TRADE NAME Gaviscon Liquid (OTC)

CLASSIFICATION Combination antacid

Indications for Use Symptomatic relief of gastric hyperacidity.

Administration 15 to 30 ml po qid.

Available Drug Forms Generic contents in 15 ml: aluminum hydroxide: 95 mg; magnesium carbonate: 412 mg; sodium: 1.7 mEq. Also contains water, sorbitol, glycerin, sodium alginate, xanthan gum, edetate disodium, methylparaben, flavorings, and colors.

Nursing Management

1. Shake suspension vigorously before measuring dosage.
2. Follow suspension with 4 fl oz of water.
3. Store bottle at room temperature with cap tightly sealed.
4. Give 1 hour after meals and at bedtime.

TRADE NAME Gaviscon-2 (OTC)

CLASSIFICATION Combination antacid

Indications for Use Symptomatic relief of gastric hyperacidity.

Administration 1 to 2 tablets po qid.

Available Drug Forms Generic contents in each tablet: aluminum hydroxide dried gel: 160 mg; magnesium trisilicate: 40 mg; sodium: 1.6 mEq. Also contains sucrose, alginic acid, sodium bicarbonate, starch, calcium stearate, and flavoring.

Nursing Management

1. Tablets should be chewed thoroughly; follow with 4 fl oz of water.
2. Give 1 hour after meals and at bedtime.
3. Store at room temperature.

TRADE NAME Gelusil (OTC)

CLASSIFICATION Combination antacid

Action This preparation contains the deflatulent simethicone and two antacids.

Indications for Use Symptomatic relief of hyperacidity.

Administration 2 tablets or 10 ml po qid; Maximum daily dosage: 12 tablets or 60 ml.

Available Drug Forms Peppermint-flavored liquid and tablets. Generic contents in each tablet or 5 ml: aluminum hydroxide: 200 mg; magnesium hydroxide: 200 mg; simethicone: 25 mg. Sodium content: 0.8 mg per tablet; 0.7 mg per 5 ml. Two tablets neutralize 22 mEq of acid and 10 ml neutralizes 24 mEq of acid.

Nursing Management

1. Shake liquid vigorously before measuring dosage.
2. Follow suspension with a sip of water.
3. Tablets should be chewed thoroughly.
4. Give 1 hour after meals and at bedtime.

TRADE NAME Gelusil-M (OTC)

CLASSIFICATION Combination antacid

Action This preparation contains the deflatulent simethicone and two antacids.

Indications for Use Symptomatic relief of gastric hyperacidity.

Administration 2 tablets or 10 ml po qid; Maximum daily dosage: 10 tablets or 50 ml.

Available Drug Forms Generic contents in each tablet or 5 ml: aluminum hydroxide: 300 mg; magnesium hydroxide: 200 mg; simethicone: 25 mg. Sodium content: 1.3 mg per tablet; 1.2 mg per 5 ml. Two tablets neutralize 25 mEq of acid and 10 ml neutralizes 30 mEq of acid.

Nursing Management

1. Shake suspension vigorously before measuring dosage.
2. Follow suspension with a sip of water.
3. Tablets should be chewed thoroughly.
4. Give 1 hour after meals and at bedtime.

TRADE NAME Gelusil-II (OTC)

CLASSIFICATION Combination antacid

Action This preparation contains the deflatulent simethicone and two antacids.

Indications for Use Symptomatic relief of gastric hyperacidity.

Warnings and Precautions Use with caution in clients with renal impairment.

Administration 2 tablets or 10 ml po qid; Maximum daily dosage: 8 tablets or 40 ml.

Available Drug Forms Generic contents in each tablet or 5 ml: aluminum hydroxide: 400 mg; magnesium hydroxide: 400 mg; simethicone: 30 mg. Sodium content: 2.1 mg per tablet; 1.3 mg per 5 ml. Two tablets neutralize 42 mEq of acid and 10 ml neutralize 48 mEq of acid.

Nursing Management

1. Shake suspension vigorously before measuring dosage.
2. Follow suspension with a sip of water.
3. Tablets should be chewed thoroughly.
4. Give 1 hour after meals and at bedtime.

TRADE NAME Kudrox (OTC)

CLASSIFICATION Combination antacid

Indications for Use Symptomatic relief of gastric hyperacidity; peptic ulcer.

Administration

- *Hyperacidity:* 1 tsp po qid 30 minutes before meals and at bedtime.
- *Peptic ulcer:* 2 to 4 tsp po qid after meals and at bedtime.

Available Drug Forms Generic contents: aluminum hydroxide gel; magnesium hydroxide; sodium: 0.65 mEq per 15 mg or 5 ml. Each 5 ml neutralizes 25 mEq of acid.

Nursing Management

1. Shake suspension vigorously before measuring dosage.
2. Follow suspension with a sip of water.

TRADE NAME Maalox Suspension (OTC)

CLASSIFICATION Combination antacid

Indications for Use Symptomatic relief of gastric hyperacidity.

Administration 2 to 4 tsp po qid; Maximum daily dosage: 16 tsp.

Available Drug Forms Generic contents in 5 ml: alumininum hydroxide dried gel: 225 mg; magnesium hydroxide: 200 mg; sodium: 0.06 mEq (1.35 mg). Each 5 ml neutralizes 27 mEq of acid.

Nursing Management

1. Shake suspension vigorously before measuring dosage.
2. Give 30 to 60 minutes after meals and at bedtime.

TRADE NAME Maalox No. 1 Tablets (OTC)

CLASSIFICATION Combination antacid

Indications for Use Symptomatic relief of gastric hyperacidity.

Administration 2 to 4 tablet po qid; Maximum daily dosage: 16 tablets.

Available Drug Forms Generic contents in each tablet: aluminum hydroxide dried gel: 200 mg; magnesium hydroxide: 200 mg; sodium: 0.036 mEq (0.84 mg). Two tablets neutralize 17 mEq of acid.

Nursing Management

1. Tablets should be chewed thoroughly.
2. Give 30 to 60 minutes after meals and at bedtime.

TRADE NAME Maalox No. 2 Tablets (OTC)

CLASSIFICATION Combination antacid

Indications for Use Symptomatic relief of gastric hyperacidity.

Adminstration 1 to 2 tablets po qid; Maximum daily dosage: 8 tablets.

Available Drug Forms Generic contents in each tablet: aluminum hydroxide dried gel: 400 mg; magnesium hydroxide: 400 mg; sodium: 0.08 mEq (1.84 mg). One tablet neutralizes 18 mEq of acid.

Nursing Management

1. Tablets should be chewed thoroughly.
2. May be followed with 4 fl oz of milk or water.
3. Give 30 to 60 minutes after meals and at bedtime.

TRADE NAME Maalox Plus (OTC)

CLASSIFICATION Combination antacid

Action This preparation contains the deflatulent simethicone and two antacids.

Indications for Use Symptomatic relief of gastric hyperacidity.

Administration 2 to 4 tablets or 10 to 20 ml po qid; Maximum daily dosage: 16 tablets or 90 ml.

Available Drug Forms Generic contents in each tablet: aluminum hydroxide: 200 mg; magnesium hydroxide: 200 mg; simethicone: 25 mg; sodium: 1.0 mg; sugar: 0.55 mg. Generic contents in 5 ml: aluminum hydroxide: 225 mg; magnesium hydroxide: 200 mg; simethicone; 25 mg; sodium: 1.3 mg. Two tablets neutralize 17 mEq of acid and 10 ml neutralizes 27 mEq of acid.

Nursing Management

1. Tablets should be chewed thoroughly.
2. Shake suspension vigorously before measuring dosage.
3. Give 30 to 60 minutes after meals and at bedtime.

TRADE NAME Maalox TC (OTC)

CLASSIFICATION Combination antacid

Indications for Use Symptomatic relief of gastric hyperacidity.

Warnings and Precautions Large dosages taken for a prolonged period of time may cause renal impairment.

Administration 5 to 10 ml po qid; Maximum daily dosage: 8 tsp.

Available Drug Forms Peppermint-flavored concentrated formulation. Generic contents in 5 ml: magnesium hydroxide: 300 mg; aluminum hydroxide: 600 mg; sodium: 0.16 mg/5 ml. Each 5 ml neutralizes 28.3 mEq of acid.

Nursing Management

1. Shake suspension vigorously before measuring dosage.
2. Give between meals and at bedtime.

TRADE NAME Mylanta (OTC)

CLASSIFICATION Combination antacid

Indications for Use Symptomatic relief of gastric hyperacidity.

Administration 1 to 2 tablets or 5 to 10 ml po qid.

Available Drug Forms Generic contents in each tablet or 5 ml: aluminum hydroxide dried gel: 200 mg; magnesium hydroxide: 200 mg; simethicone: 20 mg; sodium: 0.03 mEq. One tablet neutralizes 11.5 mEq of acid and 5 ml neutralizes 12.7 mEq of acid.

Nursing Management

1. Shake suspension vigorously before measuring dosage.
2. Tablets should be chewed thoroughly.
3. Give every 2 to 4 hours between meals and at bedtime.

TRADE NAME Mylanta-II (OTC)

CLASSIFICATION Combination antacid

Action High potency antacid with a deflatulent.

Indications for Use Symptomatic relief of gastric hyperacidity.

Warnings and Precautions Prolonged use of high dosages may cause hypermagnesemia.

Administration 1 to 2 tablets or 5 to 10 ml po qid.

Available Drug Forms Generic in each tablet or 5 ml: aluminum hydroxide dried gel: 400 mg; magnesium hydroxide: 400 mg; simethicone: 30 mg. Sodium content: 0.06 mEq (1.3 mg) per tablet; 0.05 mEq (1.14 mg) per 5 ml. One tablet neutralizes 23.0 mEq of acid and 5 ml neutralizes 25.4 mEq of acid.

Nursing Management

1. Shake suspension vigorously before measuring dosage.
2. Tablets should be chewed thoroughly.
3. Give between meals and at bedtime.

TRADE NAME Riopan Plus (OTC)

CLASSIFICATION Combination antacid

Indications for Use Hyperacidity, peptic ulcer, postoperative gas, endoscopic examinations.

Administration 1 to 2 tablets or 5 to 10 ml po qid; Maximum daily dosage: 20 tablets or 100 ml.

Available Drug Forms Generic contents in each tablet or 5 ml: magaldrate: 480 mg; simethicone: 20 mg; sodium: 0.3 mg. Each tablet neutralizes 13.5 mEq of acid and 5 ml neutralizes 13.5 mEq of acid.

Nursing Management

1. Tablets should be chewed thoroughly.
2. Shake suspension vigorously before measuring dosage.
3. Give between meals and at bedtime.

TRADE NAME Simeco (OTC)

CLASSIFICATION Combination antacid

Indications for Use Symptomatic relief of gastric hyperacidity.

Administration 5 to 10 ml po qid.

Available Drug Forms Mint-flavored concentrated formulation. Generic contents in 5 ml: aluminum hydroxide gel: 365 mg; magnesium hydroxide: 300 mg; simethicone: 30 mg; sodium: 0.3 to 0.6 mEq. Each 5 ml neutralizes 22 mEq of acid.

Nursing Management

1. Shake suspension vigorously before measuring dosage.
2. May be diluted with 1 fl oz of water.
3. Give between meals and at bedtime.

DEFLATULENTS

GENERIC NAME Simethicone (OTC)

TRADE NAMES Milicon, Milicon 80

CLASSIFICATION Deflatulent

Action Simethicone disperses and prevents the formation of mucus-surrounded gas pockets in the GI tract. It changes the surface tension of gas bubbles, thus freeing the gas, which is eliminated by belching or passing flatus. Simethicone is often combined with antacid preparations to assist with the elimination of antacid-formed gas. Excessive belching and rectal flatus should be expected.

Indications for Use As an adjunct in the treatment of states in which gas retention occurs in the GI tract, including postoperative distention, air swelling, peptic ulcer, spastic or irritable colon, and diverticulitis.

Contraindications None known.

Drug Interactions None known.

Administration 40 mg po qid; Dosage range: 40 to 80 mg qid.

Available Drug Forms Dropper bottles of suspension containing 40 mg/0.6 ml; tablets containing 40 or 80 mg. An ingredient of several antacid preparations, including Gelusil, Maalox Plus, Mylanta, Riopan Plus, and Simeco.

Nursing Management

1. Tablets should be chewed thoroughly.
2. Shake suspension vigorously before measuring dosage.
3. Give 1 hour before meals and at bedtime.
4. Warn client that excessive belching or rectal flatus may occur.
5. Warn client against taking simethicone or simethicone-containing antacids indiscriminately.

H_2-RECEPTOR ANTAGONISTS

GENERIC NAME Cimetidine (RX)

TRADE NAME Tagamet

CLASSIFICATION H_2-receptor antagonist

Action Cimetidine competitively inhibits the action of histamine at H_2-receptor sites in the parietal cells of the stomach, thus inhibiting the secretion of hydrochloric acid and other gastric secretions. It inhibits the normal baseline secretion (basal acid level) of hydrochloric acid during the night and day as well as secretion of acids caused by food, histamine, pentagastin, caffeine, insulin, and other stimuli. The gastric pH of fasting clients is raised to 5 for at least $2\frac{1}{2}$ hours after drug administration, thus reducing the proteolytic action of pepsin. Unfortunately, cimetidine suppresses the secretion of intrinsic factor, which is necessary for the absorption of vitamin B_{12}; but some intrinsic factor is liberated.

Indications for Use Short-term treatment of active duodenal ulcer; prevention of duodenal ulcer and pathologic states that cause hyperacidity (Zollinger-Ellison syndrome, mastocytosis). Has been used in fasting clients being fed intravenously (clients on a respirator).

Contraindications None known.

Warnings and Precautions Use with caution in the elderly, severely ill clients, clients with hepatic or renal impairment, and clients with renal failure or chronic brain syndrome, since untoward reactions, such as confusion, may occur. Safe use in children under 16 years and during pregnancy and lactation has not been established. Drug has a weak antiandrogenic effect and may decrease fertility in males.

Untoward Reactions Transient elevations in blood urea nitrogen and serum creatinine are relatively common. GI disturbances include transient diarrhea. Perforation of chronic peptic ulcers has been reported after abrupt cessation of therapy. Confusion has been reported in susceptible clients, such as the elderly and severely ill clients. Confusion disappears upon withdrawal of drug. Dizziness and headache have also been reported. Ringing in the ears, headache, bradycardia, and confusion have occurred and may be dose related. Mild gynecomastia has been reported with prolonged drug use (over 1 month). Hepatic dysfunction has been reported, but rarely. Interstitial hepatitis, hepatic fibrosis, and jaundice have occurred. Hypersensitivity reactions include papular-type rashes, urticaria, and exfoliative dermatitis. Blood dyscrasias, including agranulocytosis, aplastic anemia, and thrombocytopenia, have been reported, but rarely. Interstitial nephritis and pancreatitis have been reported, but rarely. Animal studies indicate that tachycardia and respiratory failure may ocur with toxicity.

Parameters of Use

Absorption Rapidly absorbed from GI tract. Half-life is about 2 hours. Peak effect occurs in 45 to 90 minutes. Duration of action is 4 to 5 hours.

Crosses placenta and enters breast milk; lactating mothers should bottle-feed their babies.

Metabolism Some may be matabolized by the microsomal enzyme system of the liver.

Excretion By the kidneys as unchanged drug. About 48% is excreted within 24 hours after oral administration and 75% after parenteral administration.

Drug Interactions Cimetidine may inhibit the hepatic metabolism of warfarin, phenytoin, and theophylline, thereby increasing the blood levels of these drugs. Hypoventilation and apnea may occur when cimetidine and morphine or other opium derivatives are administered concurrently.

Administration

- *Active ulcer and pathologic hypersecretion:* Oral: 300 mg qid with meals and at bedtime; Intramuscular: 300 mg q6h; Intravenous: 300 mg q6h in 100 ml of 5% D/W infused over 30 minutes; Maximum dosage: 2400 mg/day. Usually continued for 4 to 6 weeks in clients with peptic ulcers.
- *Prophylaxis:* 400 mg po at bedtime; higher or more frequent doses do not improve effectiveness.
- *Clients with renal failure:* 300 mg po or IV q12h; should be given after dialysis.
- *Children under 16 years:* 20 to 40 mg/kg/day in divided doses.

Available Drug Forms Tablets containing 200 or 300 mg; oral liquid containing 300 mg/5 ml; single-dose injection vials containing 300 mg/2 ml; 8-ml multidose vials containing 300 mg/2 ml.

Nursing Management

Planning factors

1. Obtain baseline complete blood cell count (CBC), serum creatinine, and blood urea nitrogen (BUN). Schedule drug administration with meals and at bedtime. Give daily dose at bedtime for prophylaxis. Not recommended for children until further studies are completed.

Administration factors

1. Avoid IM injections as they are painful. If IM route is used, rotate sites frequently.
2. When administering IV,
   a. Check patency of IV before starting drug.
   b. Add drug to 100 ml of 5% D/W, sodium chloride, or Ringer's lactate.
   c. Administer medicated solution over 30 minutes. A rapid rate of administration may cause a burning sensation.

Evaluation factors

1. Check the elderly and clients with renal or hepatic failure before each dose for confusion and arrhythmias. If symptoms occur, notify physician before giving drug, since dosage may need reduction.
2. Obtain CBC, serum creatinine, and BUN periodically. Notify physician if levels are abnormal.
3. Check and record intake and output.
4. Assess the change in signs and symptoms of hyperacidity. Antacids may be given for pain, as needed.

GENERIC NAME Ranitidine hydrochloride (RX)

TRADE NAME Zantac

CLASSIFICATION H_2-receptor antagonist

See cimetidine for Indications for use.

Action Ranitidine is a potent histamine^2-blocker and is reported to be at least three times as potent as cimetidine, but induces fewer untoward reactions. It blocks H_2-receptor sites in gastric parietal cells, thus decreasing the release of hydrochloric acid and the activity of pepsin. It reduces hepatic blood flow by 20%, but is said to have no effect on hepatic microsomal enzymes. Unlike cimetidine, ranitidine is reported to have no antiandrogenic effect; however, it may affect prolactin levels.

Contraindications None known.

Warnings and Precautions Use with caution during pregnancy or lactation, or in clients with hepatic or renal impairment. Safe use in children has not been established.

Untoward Reactions Headache, malaise, dizziness, constipation, nausea, abdominal pain, and rash ziness, constipation, nausea, abdominal pain, and rash may occur. Toxicity may induce muscular tremors, vomiting, and rapid respirations. Reduction in white blood cells and platelets occur, but rarely. No agranulocytosis or aplastic anemia has been reported. May elevate serum creatinine and transaminase levels. Doubling of serum glutamic-oxaloacetic transaminase level frequently occurs.

Parameters of Use

Absorption About 50% is slowly absorbed from the GI tract. Plasma half-life is about 3 hours; peak plasma levels occur in about 2 to 3 hours. Serum protein binding is about 15%. Duration of action is about 8 hours.

Metabolism In the liver.

Excretion About 30% by the kidneys as unchanged drug and about 6% as metabolites. The remainder is excreted in feces.

Drug Interactions Propantheline increases the peak serum level of ranitidine. Significant interactions with antacids, food, and diazepam have been reported. (See cimetidine.)

Administration

- *Prevention of hypersecretion:* 100 mg bid.
- *Duodenal ulcer:* 150 mg bid.
- *Hypersecretory disorders:* 150 mg bid, tid, or qid. (Maximum daily dosage: 6000 mg.)

Available Drug Forms Tablets containing 100 or 150 mg.

Nursing Management Clients with renal insufficiency require dosage adjustments; administer drug every 12 hours. (See cimetidine.)

Chapter 76

Antidiarrheal Agents

DIARRHEA AND ITS TREATMENT

Diarrhea is considered to be a symptom of an underlying pathology and its treatment should first be directed toward eliminating the cause. Acute forms of diarrhea, which last from several hours to several weeks, are often due to the ingestion of toxic or irritating substances contained in food or drugs. Acute diarrhea is also a side effect of radiation exposure. Chronic diarrhea lasts for more than a few weeks and is usually the result of a pathologic condition, such as ulcerative colitis, bowel resection, or carcinoma. The chronic form of diarrhea can lead to many complications, including weight loss, weakness, anorexia, and electrolyte imbalance. Acute diarrhea is especially dangerous in very young infants and in the elderly and/or debilitated, since dehydration and electrolyte loss can occur within hours. Accompanying symptoms are tachycardia, fever, orthostatic hypotension, poor skin turgor, and elevated hematocrit. If the client is unable to tolerate oral fluids, hospitalization is necessary for intravenous replacement of fluids and electrolytes.

Drug treatment of diarrhea should be as conservative as possible, with primary correction of the problem aimed at treatment of the underlying cause. Table 76-1 lists the antidiarrheal agents commonly used alone or in combination with other agents.

Infectious diseases are, of course, treated with the appropriate *antibiotic.* Diarrhea caused by bacteria or other toxins can often be treated with *adsorbents,* which coat the intestinal tract, bind with the offending substances, and eliminate them in the feces. These adsorbents are also capable of binding with other substances in the gastrointestinal tract; a factor that must be kept in mind if the client is receiving other drugs by the oral route.

Antiseptics are also contained in some antidiarrheal preparations, but their effectiveness in controlling diarrhea is doubtful. *Bacterial cultures* are sometimes prescribed for clients whose diarrhea results from disruption of the normal intestinal flora by antibiotics. Although proof of their effectiveness has not been established, it is thought that these bacilli help to reestablish the normal bacterial population in the gastrointestinal tract.

TABLE 76-1 Antidiarrheal Agents

Adsorbents
Kaolin
Activated attapulgite
Activated charcoal
Bismuth subsalicylate
Antiseptics/Astringents
Phenyl salicylate
Zinc phenolsulfonate
Zinc sulfocarbolate
Bacterial Cultures
Lactobacillus acidophilus
Lactobacillus bulgaricus
Anticholinergics
Atropine sulfate
Homatropine methylbromide
Hyoscyamine
Narcotics
Codeine
Opium tincture
Camphorated opium tincture
Diphenoxylate hydrochloride
Loperamide hydrochloride

Anticholinergic drugs are also used in combination with one or more of the other antidiarrheal agents to aid in controlling spasms of the intestinal tract. However, the amount of anticholinergics contained in over-the-counter preparations is relatively ineffective for improving intestinal tone and motility. (See Chapter 42.)

The *opiates* and their derivatives are very effective in reducing intestinal motility, thereby permitting increased absorption of water and electrolytes. Opiates are contraindicated when diarrhea is caused by infectious organisms and/or toxins, since the resulting decreased bowel motility prolongs contact of the toxins with the lining of the bowel. (See Chapter 27.)

Some *bulk-forming laxatives* are also helpful in treating acute and nonspecific diarrhea. (See Chapter 77.)

NURSING MANAGEMENT

Nursing management of clients with diarrhea should be directed at ascertaining the underlying cause and giving supportive care during treatment. The following outlines some important nursing care factors.

Planning Factors

1. A complete assessment is indicated, including careful history related to recent changes in dietary intake, medications, and any exposure to sources of infection.
2. Stool tests for culture and parasites should be obtained.
3. In severe, acute diarrhea, serum electrolyte determinations are essential to determine appropriate fluid and electrolyte replacement therapy.
4. For clients who will be traveling to other countries, the nurse should provide the following information:
   (a) Avoid tap water, ice cubes, uncooked vegetables, cold foods, milk, and milk products. Fruits may be eaten if peeled first.
   (b) Commercially bottled beverages and boiled water are safe.
   (c) In the event of severe diarrhea, a drink containing replacement electrolytes can be made: $\frac{1}{2}$ tsp corn syrup or honey, pinch of table salt, $\frac{1}{4}$ tsp baking soda, 8 fl oz fruit juice (for potassium). Commercial preparations, such as Gatorade or Pedialyte, can be substituted.

Administration Factors

1. Bowel movements should be recorded.
2. If oral liquids are tolerated, intake should be 3000 ml/day to prevent fluid and electrolyte imbalance.
3. Pregnant women and nursing mothers should not use over-the-counter antidiarrheal agents without medical direction.

Evaluation Factors

1. If acute diarrhea is not self-limiting or progresses to chronic diarrhea, a more extensive diagnostic workup is indicated.
2. Antidiarrheal agents are not for long-term use because of their potential side effects and the possibility that they may mask a more serious illness.

ADSORBENTS

GENERIC NAME Kaolin (OTC)

CLASSIFICATION Antidiarrheal agent

Source An aluminum silicate obtained from clay.

Indications for Use Nonspecific diarrhea.

Contraindications Concurrent use with lincomycin, since absorption of lincomycin will be reduced by as much as 90%.

Untoward Reactions May cause constipation and obstruction because of very formed stools.

Parameters of Use

Absorption Not absorbed from GI tract.
Excretion In feces as unchanged drug.

Drug Interactions May adsorb any drug or nutrient present in the GI tract, thereby preventing absorption of medications administered concurrently.

Administration 50 to 100 g po after each loose bowel movement.

Available Drug Forms Suspension containing either 90 or 135 g in combination with pectin or magnesia.

Nursing Management

1. Give 2 hours before or after other medications.
2. Caution client to discontinue use as soon as diarrhea is controlled.
3. Instruct client not to take other medications within 2 hours of kaolin ingestion, since effectiveness of medications will be impaired.

GENERIC NAME Activated attapulgite (OTC)

TRADE NAMES Claysorb, Quintess, Rheaban

CLASSIFICATION Antidiarrheal agent

See kaolin for Parameters of use, Drug interactions, and Nursing management.

Action An inert clay compound composed primarily of magnesium oxide.

Indications for Use Nonspecific diarrhea.

Administration Initial dosage: 2 to 4 g po; then 500 to 1000 mg after each bowel movement.

Available Drug Forms An ingredient of several commercially prepared antidiarrheal mixtures.

GENERIC NAME Activated charcoal (OTC)

TRADE NAMES Charcoaid, Charcocaps, Charcodote

CLASSIFICATION Antidiarrheal agent

Action Activated vegetable charcoal is ineffective in adsorbing cyanide, ethanol, methanol, ferrous sulfate, alkalis, and mineral acids.

Indications for Use Acute poisoning; adsorption of intestinal gases. Also used investigationally in uremia.

Contraindications Clients who have ingested cyanide, ethanol, methanol, ferrous sulfate, alkalis, and mineral acids.

Parameters of Use

Absorption Not absorbed from GI tract.
Excretion In feces as unchanged drug.

Drug Interactions Do not administer with other drugs, since activated charcoal adsorbs most drugs.

Administration

- *GI disturbances:* 600 to 5000 mg po.
- *Poisoning:* 5 to 50 g po; powder form is more effective in poisoning.

Available Drug Forms Bottles of suspension (sorbitol solution) containing 30 g. Capsules containing 260 mg, tablets, granules, and power are available, but seldom used.

Nursing Management

1. If ipecac is used to induce vomiting in the treatment of poisoning, it must be administered before charcoal, since charcoal will absorb the ipecac.
2. Palatability is improved if mixed in a small amount of juice or chocolate powder.
3. Most effective if administered within 30 minutes of ingestion of poison.
4. Warn client of black discoloration of feces.
5. Instruct client to store drug in airtight containers.

GENERIC NAME Bismuth subsalicylate (OTC)

TRADE NAME Pepto-Bismol

CLASSIFICATION Antidiarrheal agent

See kaolin for Drug interactions and Nursing management.

Action This drug can be used as an adsorbent, an astringent, and an antacid.

Indications for Use Indigestion, nausea, diarrhea.

Contraindications Hypersensitivity to aspirin.

Warnings and Precautions Use with caution in clients receiving a coumarin anticoagulant.

Parameters of Use

Absorption Only slight amounts from GI tract.
Excretion In feces as unchanged drug.

Administration 0.5 to 4.0 g po; may be repeated q1h for a maximum of 8 doses.

Available Drug Forms Suspension containing 262 mg in 15 ml and tablets containing 300 mg.

BACTERIAL CULTURES

GENERIC NAMES *Lactobacillus acidophilus; Lactobacillus bulgaricus*

TRADE NAMES Bacid, DoFus, Lactinex; Novaflor

CLASSIFICATION Antidiarrheal agent (OTC) (RX)

Action These drugs help to restore normal intestinal flora and contain viable lactobacilli.

Indications for Use Uncomplicated diarrhea, after intestinal antisepsis from antibiotic therapy, fever blisters and canker sores.

Contraindications Use for more than 2 days of high concentration preparations (Bacid), high fever, infants and children under 3 years.

Administration *Bacid:* 2 capsules po bid, tid, or qid; *DoFus:* 1 tablet po daily; *Lactinex:* 4 tablets or 1 packet po tid or qid; *Novaflor:* 1 capsule po qid.

Available Drug Forms Tablets, capsules, and granules in 1-g packets.

Nursing Management

1. May initially produce an increase in flatus, but this subsides with continued use.
2. Although these are naturally occurring bacteria, excessive use of these preparations is not recommended.

NARCOTICS

GENERIC NAME Loperamide hydrochloride (CV)

TRADE NAME Imodium

CLASSIFICATION Antidiarrheal agent

Action Loperamide is related to meperidine, but has less potential for dependence. It decreases intestinal motility by a direct effect on the musculature.

Indications for Use Acute nonspecific diarrhea, chronic diarrhea secondary to inflammatory bowel disease, reduction of discharge volume from ileostomies.

Contraindications Hypersensitivity to loperamide, clients in whom constipation should be avoided, children under 12 years.

Warnings and Precautions Use with caution in clients with a history of drug abuse.

Untoward Reactions Abdominal discomfort, drowsiness, constipation, dizziness, nausea, vomiting, rash, and CNS depression may occur with long-term therapy.

Parameters of Use

Absorption Readily absorbed from GI tract. Onset of action is 30 to 60 minutes. Duration of action is 4 to 5 hours.
Metabolism In the liver.
Excretion Primarily in feces.

Drug Interactions Potentiates the effects of all other CNS depressants.

Administration Initial dosage: 4 mg po; then 2 mg after each loose stool; Maximum dosage: 16 mg/day. For chronic diarrhea, maintenance dosage is 4 to 8 mg/day.

Available Drug Forms Capsules containing 2 mg.

Nursing Management

1. Administer drug with 4 oz of water.
2. Assess the drug's effectiveness in controlling diarrhea; watch for CNS depression and other untoward effects.
3. When used to treat chronic diarrhea, instruct client to notify physician if an acute episode of diarrhea recurs or if constipation develops (no bowel movement for 48 hours or longer).
4. Emphasize the importance of frequent medical checkups when drug is used for chronic diarrhea.

COMBINATION PREPARATIONS

TRADE NAME Dia-Quel Liquid (OTC) (RX)

CLASSIFICATION Antidiarrheal agent

Indications for Use Nonspecific diarrhea, cramping, nausea.

Warnings and Precautions May be habit forming. Use with caution in the elderly, children, and in clients with glaucoma. Not for prolonged use. Discontinue use if tachycardia, dizziness, or blurred vision occur.

Administration Adults: 1 to 2 tbsp po tid or qid; Children: Over 6 years: $\frac{1}{2}$ of adult dosage.

Available Drug Forms Generic contents in 5 ml: tincture of opium: 0.03 ml; pectin: 24 mg; homatropine methylbromide: 0.15 mg; alcohol: 10%.

TRADE NAME Donnagel (RX)

CLASSIFICATION Antidiarrheal agent

Indications for Use Nonspecific diarrhea, GI upset, nausea.

Contraindications Hypersensitivity to any ingredient, glaucoma, severe renal or hepatic disease.

Untoward Reactions Common secondary reactions include blurred vision, dry mouth, and flushing of the face. Difficulty in urination may occur, particularly in elderly males. Skin dryness and a general erythema may occur with high dosages.

Administration Adults: Initial dosage: 2 tbsp po; then 1 to 2 tbsp after each stool.

Available Drug Forms Generic contents in 30 ml: kaolin: 6 g; pectin: 142.8 mg; hyoscyamine sulfate: 0.1037 mg; atropine sulfate: 0.0194 mg; hyoscine hydrobromide: 0.0065 mg; sodium benzoate: 60 mg; alcohol: 3.8%. Also available with opium 24 mg as Donnagel-PG.

TRADE NAME Kaopectate (OTC)

CLASSIFICATION Antidiarrheal agent

Indications for Use Nonspecific diarrhea.

Administration Adults: 4 to 8 tbsp po after each bowel movement. Children over 12 years: 4 tbsp po after each bowel movement. Children 6 to 12 years: 2 to 4 tbsp po after each bowel movement. Children 3 to 6 years: 1 to 2 tbsp po after each bowel movement. Children under 3 years: Consult a physician.

Available Drug Forms Generic contents in 1 fl oz: kaolin: 90 gr; pectin: 2 gr.

TRADE NAMES Parepectolin, Ru-K-N (OTC)

CLASSIFICATION Antidiarrheal agent

Indications for Use Nonspecific diarrhea, GI upset, nausea.

Contraindications Hypersensitivity to any ingredient.

Warnings and Precautions May be habit forming. Use with caution in children and in the elderly.

Administration Adults: 1 to 2 tbsp po after each stool; Maximum dosage: 4 doses/12 hours. Children: 1 to 2 tsp po after each stool; Maximum dosage: 4 doses/12 hours.

Available Drug Forms Generic contents in 1 fl oz: opium (Paregoric): 15 mg; pectin: 162 mg; kaolin: 5.5 g; alcohol: 0.69%.

Chapter 77

Laxatives and Stool Softeners

Alophen
Bilax
Carters Little Liver Pills
Casakol
Comfolax-Plus
Correctol
Dialose Plus
Dorbantyl
Dorbantyl Forte
Doxidan
Haley's M-O
Laxatyl
Milkinol
Neolax
OM-Cascara Suspension
OM-Mineral Oil Emulsion
Perdiem
Peri-Colace
Sarolax
Senokot-S
Trilax

LAXATIVES ARE THE most overused drugs in the United States. Factors that contribute to their misuse include the availability of a vast number of nonprescription preparations and extensive advertising concerning the correction of bowel irregularity. There is no scientific basis to support the necessity of daily bowel movements, since individual bowel regularity may occur several times a day, daily, every other day, or even weekly. Failure to defecate results in discomfort from bowel distention and constipation. Constipation is a condition characterized by infrequent and difficult defecation. As a symptom, constipation should be thoroughly investigated, since alterations in bowel movements may be caused by a pathologic condition, drugs, and numerous other factors.

FACTORS THAT CAN CAUSE CONSTIPATION

When feces enter the rectum, the defecation reflex is stimulated. If ignored, this reflex will slowly relax and disappear. Repeated suppression of the urge to defecate and irregular bowel habits are a primary cause of constipation. Psychotic and depressed clients who are under emotional stress, or those who experience pain upon defecation due to hemorrhoids or an anal fissure, frequently ignore the urge to defecate and develop constipation.

Tumors of the colon, abdominal adhesions, and scar tissue in the colon may obstruct the lumen of intestines and result in constipation. Paralysis of the muscles that facilitate defecation, damage to the nerve pathways to and from the rectum, and other causes of atony or spasm of the colon can also lead to constipation. In addition, conditions that disrupt the body's fluid and electrolyte balance, such as hyperparathyroidism, fever, and dehydration, may produce constipation. Drugs that affect the neurologic system, such as anticholinergic agents, central nervous system depressants, and ganglionic blocking agents can result in constipation. Other agents, such as antacids and certain mineral salts, particularly oral iron preparations, can create a problem as well. Even the habitual misuse of laxatives can result in atonic constipation.

Inadequate fluid intake and the lack of bulk in the diet can result in infrequent and hardened stools in healthy clients. Constipation may occur when a client has a change in diet, is admitted to hospital, or is placed on a special diet. Since the elderly have a lack of tone in their colon, even minor alterations in their diet can cause constipation. Pregnancy, bedrest, and environmental changes can also result in constipation.

TREATMENT OF CONSTIPATION

Constipation that lasts for several weeks may be due to an underlying pathologic condition and requires medical evaluation. The treatment for nonorganic constipation is directed toward client health education. Unless contraindicated, the client should be encouraged to enrich the diet with fresh fruits, vegetables, bulk-forming foods, whole grain cereals and bread, and bran. The ingestion of adequate quantities of fluids (soups, watery foods, water, and other beverages) and regular exercise are important considerations. Clients who are on bedrest, the elderly, and clients who are plagued with hemorrhoids that cause painful defecation, may require daily stool softeners to prevent constipation. Although temporary constipation is often self-limiting, a laxative may be required.

CLASSIFICATION OF LAXATIVES

The terms *cathartic* and *laxative* are often used interchangeably because they both relieve constipation. Historically, the classification of cathartics included the peristaltic stimulants and saline cathartics, since these substances generally caused a more intense purgative action and resulted in looser or even liquid stools. The milder substances, including bulk-forming agents and lubricants, were considered laxatives. It is now known that the distinction between cathartic and laxative is dubious as the degree of effect is directly related to the dosage and not the type of substance taken. The presently accepted classification of laxatives is listed in Table 77-1 according to the drugs' mechanism of action on the intestinal tract.

CONTRAINDICATIONS AND WARNINGS

Laxatives are contraindicated in clients with unexplained nausea, vomiting, or abdominal pain. If the underlying cause is appendicitis, rupture of the inflamed appendix or intestines may occur when intestinal peristalsis is stimulated by a laxative. For the same reason, laxatives are contraindicated in clients with intestinal obstruction, gastrointestinal hemorrhage, intestinal perforation, or fecal impaction.

Laxatives should be used with caution in clients with an inflamed or irritable colon. If rectal bleeding occurs with the use of a laxative, the physician should be notified. Although clients

TABLE 77-1 Classification of Laxatives

CLASSIFICATION	Action	Primary Uses
Peristaltic stimulants	Stimulate motor activity of the intestine by local irritation of intestinal lining or by acting on the smooth intestinal muscle	Bowel preparation prior to surgery (sigmoidoscopy) and x-ray examination (barium enema); acute resistant constipation
Saline laxatives	Slowly and incompletely absorbed from the gastrointestinal tract; osmotic properties lead to the retention of water in the large bowl; thus, feces remain soft so that passage through the colon is facilitated	Bowel preparation prior to surgery and x-ray examination; bowel cleanser following the ingestion of certain poisons and anthelmintic therapy (removes parasites); acute resistant constipation
Bulk-forming laxatives	Indigestible substances composed of natural and partially synthetic sugars and cellulose derivatives that form bulk and lubrication when they become swollen with water; peristalsis is stimulated by reflex action	Acute and chronic constipation; usually effective and safe in the elderly, postpartum clients, and clients who have misused other laxatives
Lucricant laxatives (emollients)	Lubricate feces and the intestinal tract, thus enhancing peristalsis; the absorption of water from the intestinal tract is inhibited	Prevention of straining upon defecation in clients with cardiac disorders, rectal disorders (hemorrhoids), or hernias and following abdominal surgery
Fecal softeners (wetting agents)	Lower the surface tension in the gastrointestinal tract and soften the feces by facilitating mixture of water and fecal matter	Prevention of constipation in clients on bedrest

with hemorrhoids may have a small bleed as the first hardened fecal mass is expelled, prolonged and profuse bleeding should not occur. The lack of response to adequate dosages of stimulant laxatives or enemas may indicate a pathologic state and requires medical evaluation.

PERISTALTIC STIMULANTS

GENERIC NAMES Aloe; aloin (OTC)

CLASSIFICATION Laxative

Source Dried juice of *Aloe perryi* or other *Aloe* leaves. Contains several anthraquinone glycosides, particularly barbaloin. (Chemically related to tincture of benzoine.) Aloin contains the water-soluble glycosides of *Aloe*.

Action Laxative commonly known as emodin compounds found in proprietary mixtures. The active principles are glycosides, which affect the large intestine. One of the most irritating anthraquinone laxatives. Although it is still available to the public, aloe is seldom prescribed by physicians today.

Indications for Use Temporary atonic and chronic constipation.

Contraindications Pregnancy, menstruation, hemorrhoids, appendicitis or undiagnosed abdominal disorders, active GI bleeding or ulcerations.

Warnings and Precautions Not recommended for children.

Untoward Reactions Congestion of pelvic organs, intestinal cramps, which can be severe at times, discoloration of urine (yellow in acid urine and red in alkaline urine).

Parameters of Use

Absorption Partially absorbed from intestines. Defecation response occurs in 6 to 8 hours.

Excretion Some products excreted by the kidneys.

Administration *Aloe:* 250 mg po; *Aloin:* 15 mg po; *Combination preparations:* 1 pill po.

Available Drug Forms Tablets of aloe containing 250 mg; tablets of aloin containing 15 mg. An ingredient of Podophyllin Pills, Hinkle Pills, ASBC Pills, and Alophen Pills.

Nursing Management

1. Give at bedtime because of effect on colon.
2. Instruct client to observe changes in urine color. Explain that discoloration is harmless and is due to the breakdown of products absorbed by the intestines.

GENERIC NAME Cascara sagrada (OTC)

TRADE NAMES Casanthranol, Cas-Evac, Casyllium, Cossanyl

CLASSIFICATION Laxative

Source Dried bark of *Rhamnus purshiana* (sacred bark).

Action An anthraquinone laxative that causes irritation to the large intestine. Casanthranol contains only the water-soluble glycosides, lacks the bitter taste of cascara, and softens the stools with little or no abdominal discomfort.

Indications for Use Chronic and habitual constipation, constipation in clients on bedrest.

Contraindications Symptoms of appendicitis, active GI bleeding or ulcerations, intestinal obstruction.

Untoward Reactions Discoloration of urine (yellow in acid urine and red in alkaline urine); GI disturbances (nausea, vomiting, abdominal cramps, diarrhea), particularly when large dosages are administered; fluid and electrolyte disturbances (hypokalemia, hypocalcemia).

Parameters of Use

Absorption Some glycosides absorbed from upper GI tract. Single soft or semifluid evacuation occurs in 6 to 8 hours. Clients with irritated colons may have several evacuations. Little or no efficiency is lost with repeated doses.

Administration Adults: *Aromatic cascara sagrada fluidextract:* 4 to 5 ml po; *Cascara elixir:* 5 ml po (Range: 2 to 12 ml); *Cascara sagrada fluidextract:* 1 ml po; *Cascara liquid extract:* 1 ml po (Range: 2 to 4 ml); *Cascara sagrada extract tablets, cascara tablets:* 300 mg po.

Available Drug Forms Pure fluid extracts and tablets; An ingredient of several combination laxatives (Casakol).

Nursing Management

1. Give at bedtime.
2. Unpleasant bitter taste of cascara may be disguised by the addition of sugar or volatile oils.
3. Sometimes administered with milk of magnesia and referred to as Black and White. Mix 1 dram of cascara with 30 ml of milk of magnesia.

GENERIC NAME Danthron (OTC)

TRADE NAMES Dorbane, Istizin, Modane

CLASSIFICATION Laxative

Source Although a naturally occurring substance, danthron is usually prepared synthetically from vegetables.

Action Danthron is chemically related to the anthraquinone laxatives. It does not affect the motility of the small bowel, so gripping and cramping are avoided. Similar to cascara sagrada. Frequently combined with stool softeners.

Indications for Use Relief of constipation: clients on bedrest, convalescents, cardiac disease, pregnancy and postpartum, pre- and postanorectal surgery, pediatric and geriatric management.

Contraindications Acute abdominal pain, intestinal obstruction.

Warnings and Precautions Use with extreme caution during lactation as absorbed substances may appear in milk and cause catharsis in the nursing infant.

Untoward Reactions May cause pink discoloration in alkaline urine. Overdosage may cause gripping. Prolonged use may lead to temporary brownish mucosal staining.

Parameters of Use

Absorption Small quantities absorbed from small intestine. Defecation response occurs in about 8 hours.

Excretion Absorbed substances are excreted by the kidneys.

Administration Adults: 75 to 150 mg po.

Available Drug Forms Orange scored tablets containing 75 mg.

Nursing Management

1. Give at bedtime.
2. Encourage proper diet and exercise to prevent constipation.
3. Advise client that prolonged use may cause laxative dependency.
4. Warn client that urine discoloration may occur.

GENERIC NAME Senna (OTC)

TRADE NAMES Glysennid, Senokot, X-Prep

CLASSIFICATION Laxative

Source Dried leaves of *Cassia acutifolia*.

Action Senna stimulates motor activity of the large intestine by local irritation of the intestinal lining or by acting on the intestinal smooth muscle. Its effect depends on the size and route of dosage. Gripping, intestinal cramps, increased mucus secretion, and excessive fluid evacuation may occur. Glysennid causes less cramping and gripping.

Indications for Use Constipation.

Contraindications Undiagnosed abdominal ailments, symptoms of appendicitis.

Untoward Reactions GI disturbances, including nausea, vomiting, abdominal cramps, and diarrhea, may occur, particularly when excessive dosages are administered. Fluid and electrotyte disturbances may also occur.

Parameters of Use

Absorption Some glycosides are absorbed from upper GI tract. Single soft or semifluid evacuation occurs in 6 to 8 hours. Clients with irritated colons may have several evacuations. Little or no efficiency is lost with repeated doses.

Administration Adults: Oral: *Senna fluidextract:* 2 ml; *Senna syrup:* 8 ml; *Compound senna powder:* 4 g. Rectal: 1 suppository. Children: Over 60 lb: Oral: *Senokot:* 1 tablet; Granules: $\frac{1}{2}$ level tsp; Rectal: 1 suppository.

Available Drug Forms Tablets, liquid, suppositories, capsules, extract, granules, and syrup.

Nursing Management

1. Dissolve granules in water.
2. Follow directions on label of each preparation.
3. Drug is safe for antepartum clients and nursing mothers.

GENERIC NAME Phenolphthalein (OTC) (RX)

TRADE NAMES Evac-Q-Tabs, Ex-Lax, Feen-A-Mint, Prulent

CLASSIFICATION Laxative

Action Phenolphthalein is an odorless, tasteless drug that acts on the large intestine. Its exact mode of action is unknown. It is insoluble in water, but soluble in alcohol. There is a delay of 6 to 8 hours in the cathartic action of phenolphthalein; less time may be noted in children. The drug is more often found in proprietary preparations than ordered via prescription.

Indications of Use Constipation.

Contraindications Symptoms of appendicitis, intestinal destruction, or acute abdominal pain.

Untoward Reactions Causes discoloration of urine (yellow in acid urine and red in alkaline urine). Skin eruptions and persistent discoloration may occur. Large dosages can cause a red discoloration of feces if they are made alkaline by a soap suds enema. In some cases, severe diarrhea may occur. Fluid and electrolyte disturbances are possible.

Parameters of Use

Absorption A small amount of the drug may be absorbed.
Excretion Absorbed drug is excreted in bile and urine. Drug in bile may be reabsorbed and resecreted, thus exerting a longer duration of action than most cathartics.

Administration Adults: 60 to 120 mg po. Children: Consult physician.

Available Drug Forms Tablets containing 60, 90, or 120 mg.

Nursing Management

1. Give at bedtime because of effect on colon.
2. Instruct client to observe changes in urine color. Explain that discoloration of urine and feces is harmless.
3. The disagreeable taste can be masked by having the client hold an ice cube in the mouth for 1 or 2 minutes to numb the taste buds immediately before taking drug. Eating a cracker or bland cookie can help to remove the oil from the mouth.
4. Store in refrigerator.

GENERIC NAME Castor oil (OTC)

TRADE NAME Castor Oil, Neoloid, Purge

CLASSIFICATION Laxative

Action Castor oil acts in the small intestine, where it is hydrolyzed to glycerol and recinoleic acid. Prompt bowel action results in liquid stools within 2 to 6 hours. It retards gastric emptying.

Indications for Use Acute constipation and diarrhea caused by irritants, infections, or certain types of food and drug poisoning; special preparation for x-rays of the large bowel. Rarely used for simple constipation.

Contraindications Symptoms of appendicitis, menstruation and pregnancy (as it causes congestion in the pelvic area as a result of its irritating action).

Untoward Reactions GI and electrolyte disturbances.

Parameters of Use

Absorption Poorly absorbed from small intestine.

Administration Adults: 15 to 60 ml po. Children: Consult physician.

Available Drug Forms Liquid, emulsified liquid, and aromatic and flavored castor oil.

Nursing Management

1. Give on an empty stomach.
2. Do not administer before bedtime because of rapid action.

GENERIC NAME Bisacodyl (OTC) (RX)

TRADE NAMES Dulcolax, Evac-Q-Kwik

CLASSIFICATION Laxative

Action Bisacodyl is a contact laxative that acts directly on colonic mucosa producing normal peristalsis throughout the large intestine. It initiates motility in the colon by a stimulant effect on parasympathetic nerve endings. The drug is soluble in water and alkaline solutions.

Indications for Use Bowel evacuation and constipation: preparation for surgery, delivery, proctoscopy, or radiologic examination, acute and chronic constipation, bowel retraining, antepartum constipation, postoperative constipation.

Contraindications GI fissures or ulceration (since systemic absorption of drug will be excessive), acute surgical abdomen.

Untoward Reactions No toxic effects noted. Abdominal cramps occur occasionally.

Parameters of Use

Absorption About 5% absorbed systemically. Onset of action is 15 minutes after insertion of suppository.
Excretion In urine as glucuronide.

Administration Adults: Oral: 2 to 3 tablets. Rectal: 1 suppository, as needed. Children: Oral: 1 to 2 tablets, as needed. Rectal: Over 2 years: 1 suppository; Under 2 years: $\frac{1}{2}$ suppository.

Available Drug Forms Enteric-coated tablets containing 5 mg; suppositories containing 10 mg.

Nursing Management

1. Used satisfactorily in clients with ganglionic blockade or spinal cord damage (paraplegia, poliomyelitis).
2. In colostomy care, 2 tablets at night or a suppository inserted into the colostomy opening in the morning will frequently make irrigations unnecessary; and in other cases will expedite the procedure.
3. Bisacodyl provides satisfactory cleansing of the bowel, obviating the need for an enema.
4. Instruct client to avoid chewing tablets.
5. Do not administer within 1 hour of antacids or milk.
6. Drug is safe for infants, the elderly, debilitated clients, and during pregnancy and lactation.
7. Store drug below 86 F.

SALINE LAXATIVES

GENERIC NAME Magnesium sulfate (OTC) (RX)

TRADE NAMES Epsom Salts, Mag-S

CLASSIFICATION Laxative

Action Magnesium sulfate is considered the most potent saline laxative. It increases the bulk of the intestinal contents, stimulates peristalsis, and produces frequent fluid stools.

Indications for Use Preparation of bowel for x-ray of intestines, constipation, food poisoning, with anthelmintics, induction of dehydration in clients with cerebral and cardiac edema.

Contraindications Impaired renal function, myocardial damage, heart block, digitalized clients, abdominal pain, nausea, vomiting, intestinal irritation, obstruction, perforation, fecal impaction.

Warnings and Precautions Not recommended for infants and young children.

Untoward Reactions Dehydration may occur following large dosages or after repeated use. Electrolyte imbalances, including hyperkalemia and hypermagnesemia, may occur. Excessive magnesium levels seldom occur from a single oral dose.

Parameters of Use

Absorption About 20% absorbed from upper GI tract. Defecation response in rapid, occurring within 1 to 4 hours.

Excretion Absorbed ions are excreted by the kidneys.

Drug Interactions May alter the absorption of coumarin derivatives (dicumarol); administer at least 2 hours apart. May decrease the absorption of phenothiazines; if concurrent therapy is necessary, give magnesium sulfate at least 2 hours after phenothiazines. Absorbed magnesium sulfate ions may potentiate the action of neuromuscular blocking agents and CNS depressants in clients who use magnesium sulfate repeatedly; avoid concomitant use.

Administration 15 g po; Dosage range: 5 to 15

Nursing Management

1. Add powder to 1 fl oz or more of water or citrus juice. Can be made more palatable by adding ice chips, lemon juice, or other flavorings; magnesium sulfate has an unpleasant salty taste.
2. Give on an empty stomach before breakfast or in the midafternoon.
3. Administer solution with a full glass of water to prevent nausea and net loss of body fluids.
4. Encourage client to drink a full glass of water every hour until evacuation is complete.

GENERIC NAME Milk of magnesia (OTC)

TRADE NAMES Light Magnesia, Magnesia, Magnesia Magma, MOM

CLASSIFICATION Laxative

Action Milk of magnesia is an aqueous suspension of magnesium hydroxide. It is a mild saline laxative and is less effective than magnesium sulfate. The drug has antacid properties in low dosages and a laxative action in high dosages. As much as one-third of the magnesium ions can be absorbed and can result in hypermagnesemia with prolonged use.

Indications for Use Occasional constipation, as an adjunct in the treatment of poisoning by mineral acids and arsenic, mouthwash to neutralize mouth ulcers.

Contraindications Abdominal pain, symptoms of appendicitis, intestinal obstruction, fecal impaction, severe renal dysfunction, hypermagnesemia.

Untoward Reactions Nausea, vomiting, diarrhea, alkalization of urine, electrolyte imbalances, hypermagnesemia in clients with impaired renal function (early symptoms include hypotension and absence of kneejerk reflex), rebounding hyperacidity.

Parameters of Use

Absorption As much as 10 to 30% may be absorbed. Defecation response occurs in 4 to 8 hours. Normal serum magnesium levels: 1.4 to 2.5 mg/100 ml or 1.5 to 3.0 mEq/l.

Excretion Absorbed ions are readily excreted by the kidneys. Primarily excreted as insoluble complexes in feces.

Drug Interactions Milk of magnesia may alter the absorption of coumarin derivatives (dicumarol); administer at least 2 hours apart. Insoluble complexes form if administered concurrently with tetracycline or iron; if concurrent therapy is necessary, give milk of magnesia at least 2 to 3 hours after tetracycline. May decrease the absorption of orally administered phenothiazines; if concomitant therapy is necessary, give milk of magnesia at least 2 hours after phenothiazines. May interfere with the GI absorption of penicillin, sulfonamides, barbiturates, and digitalis. Do not administer concurrently.

Administration *Light milk of magnesia:* 4 g po, as needed. *Concentrated milk of magnesia:* Adults: 30 ml po; Dosage range: 15 to 60 ml. Children: School age: Up to 30 ml po; Preschoolers: 15 ml po; Infants: 5 ml po.

Available Drug Forms *Light milk of magnesia:* Bottles containing 4 g/5 ml. *Concentrated milk of magnesia:* Bottles of flavored or unflavored magnesia suspension; unit doses containing 15 or 30 ml; unit doses containing 10, 15, or 20 ml of flavored concentrate; tablets containing 300 mg.

Nursing Management

1. Shake suspension vigorously before measuring dosage.
2. Store at room temperature or in refrigerator in airtight containers.
3. Give at bedtime or in early morning before breakfast.
4. Administer with fluid to prevent nausea.
5. Avoid administering with other drugs, since interactions may occur.
6. Instruct client to chew tablets thoroughly and to drink at least one glassful of water.
7. Check deep tendon reflexes, including kneejerk reflex, when prolonged therapy is required. If reflexes are depressed, notify physician.

GENERIC NAMES Heavy magnesium oxide; magnesium carbonate; magnesium citrate; mineral water

TRADE NAMES Heavy Magnesium; Carbonate of Magnesium; Citrate of Magnesium; Carlsbad Water, Natural Purgative Waters, Pluto Water

CLASSIFICATION Laxative (OTC)

See milk of magnesia for Indications for use, Contraindications, Untoward reactions, Parameters of use, Drug interactions, and Nursing management.

Action Similar to milk of magnesia. Magnesium citrate contains citric acid (flavoring) and sodium bicarbonate (effervescent) and is more expensive than other magnesium salts. Mineral water, both natural and commercial preparations, usually contains magnesium sulfate, sodium sulfate, or both.

Administration *Magnesium oxide:* 4 g po, as needed. *Magnesium carbonate:* 8 g po, as needed. *Magnesium citrate:* 200 to 250 ml po, as needed. *Mineral water:* 1 or more glassfuls po, as needed.

Available Drug Forms *Magnesium oxide:* Bottles containing 4 g/5 ml. *Magnesium carbonate:* Bottles containing 8 g/10 ml. *Magnesium citrate:* Bottles containing 200 to 250 ml.

GENERIC NAMES Sodium phosphate, sodium biphosphate (oral)

TRADE NAMES Fleet Phospho-Soda, Phospho-Soda

CLASSIFICATION Laxative (OTC)

Action Sodium phosphates are mild saline laxatives that cause the retention of water in the intestinal tract. Laxative action increases when the dosage is increased.

Indications for Use Constipation, preparation for intestinal diagnostic x-rays, examinations, and surgery.

Contraindications Congestive heart failure, nausea, vomiting, or abdominal pain, megacolon (as hypernatremic dehydration may occur).

Warnings and Precautions Use with caution in clients with impaired renal function, since hyperphosphatemia and hypocalcemia may occur, and in cardiac or other clients on sodium restriction. Not recommended for children under 5 years.

Untoward Reactions Dehydration can occur, particularly in geriatric and debilitated clients who ingest inadequate quantities of fluid following drug administration. Electrolyte imbalances, including hypernatremia, hyperphosphatemia, and hypocalcemia, may occur, particularly in debilitated and cardiac clients, geriatrics, and clients with impaired renal function.

Parameters of Use

Absorption Small quantities of sodium and phosphate ions are absorbed from upper GI tract. Defecation response occurs in 1 to 8 hours.

Excretion Absorbed ions are excreted by the kidneys.

Administration

- *Laxative:* Adults: 20 ml po; Teenagers: 10 ml po; Children: Ages 5 to 10 years: 5 ml po.
- *Purgative:* Adults: 40 ml po; Teenagers: 20 ml po; Children: Ages: 5 to 10 years: 10 ml po.

Available Drug Forms Multidose bottles of regular or flavored concentrated solution containing 18 g of sodium phosphate or 48 g of sodium biphosphate in each 100 ml. Each 20 ml contains 96.4 mEq of sodium.

Nursing Management

1. Give 1 hour before meals for rapid defecation or at bedtime for laxative effect in morning. Follow with a full glass of water.
2. Dilute drug in 100 to 150 ml of cold water.
3. When purgative dosage is given, instruct client to drink at least 1 full glass of water every hour to prevent dehydration.
4. Monitor intake and output to detect the development of dehydration.

GENERIC NAMES Sodium phosphate, sodium biphosphate (oral)

TRADE NAME Fleet Enema (OTC)

CLASSIFICATION Laxative

Action Fleet enemas provide complete cleansing and emptying of the descending and sigmoid colon within 2 to 5 minutes without pain or spasm.

Indications for Use Relief of constipation, routine enema, preparation for rectal examination during pregnancy and pre- and postnatally, preoperative cleansing and general postoperative care, relief of fecal and barium impaction.

Contraindications Nausea, vomiting, or abdominal pain, megacolon (as hypernatremic dehydration may occur).

Warnings and Precautions Use with caution in clients with impaired renal function, since hyperphosphatemia may occur. Frequent or prolonged use of enemas may result in dependence. Not recommended for children under 2 years.

Untoward Reactions Dehydration may occur in geriatrics and debilitated clients, but rarely. Electrolyte imbalances, including hypernatremia, hyperphosphatemia, and hypocalcemia, may occur, particularly in debilitated and cardiac clients, geriatrics, and clients with impaired renal function, but rarely.

Parameters of Use

Absorption Few ions are absorbed unless enema is retained for a prolonged period of time. Defecation response occurs in 2 to 5 minutes.

Administration Adults: 4 fl oz, as needed; Children: 2 years or older: 2 fl oz, as needed.

Available Drug Forms Ready-to-use disposable squeeze bottle containing $4\frac{1}{2}$ fl oz (adults) or $2\frac{1}{2}$ fl oz (children) with a 2-in. prelubed insertion tip. Each adult enema unit delivers 7 g of sodium phosphate and 19 g of sodium biphosphate (in 118 ml). Each delivered adult dosage contains 4.4 g of sodium.

Nursing Management

1. May be used at room temperature
2. Explain procedure to client and anticipate results, so that the client will cooperate and relax. Encourage client to hold enema fluid at least 5 minutes for best laxative effect.
3. Administer fluid slowly and evenly.

GENERIC NAME Potassium sodium tartrate (OTC)

TRADE NAMES Rochelle Salts, Seidlitz Powders

CLASSIFICATION Laxative

See sodium phosphate (oral) for Indications for use, Contraindications, Warnings and precautions, Untoward reactions, and Parameters of use.

Action Contains sodium bicarbonate and tartaric acid. Tartrate ions are poorly absorbed from GI tract.

Administration *Rochelle Salts:* 10 g po, as needed. *Seidlitz Powders:* Contents of both powder containers po, as needed.

Available Drug Forms Bottles of 15 ml containing 10 g.

Nursing Management Mix with water and swallow while still effervescing. [See sodium phosphate (oral)].

GENERIC NAME Potassium bitartrate (OTC)

TRADE NAME Cream of Tartar

CLASSIFICATION Laxative

See sodium phosphate (oral) for Indications for use, Contraindications, Warnings and precautions, Untoward reactions, Parameters of use, and Nursing management.

Administration 2 g po, as needed.

GENERIC NAME Potassium phosphate (dibasic)

CLASSIFICATION Laxative (OTC)

See sodium phosphate (oral) for Indications for use, Contraindications, Warnings and precautions, Untoward reactions, Parameters of use, and Nursing management.

Action Similar to sodium phosphate, but can be used in clients with heart disease.

Administration 4 g po, as needed.

GENERIC NAME Sodium sulfate (OTC)

TRADE NAME Glaubers Salts

CLASSIFICATION Laxative

See sodium phosphate (oral) for Indications for use, Contraindications, Warnings and precautions, Untoward reactions, Parameters of use, and Nursing management.

Action Sodium sulphate is as effective as magnesium sulfate.

Administration 15 g po, as needed.

Available Drug Forms Bottles containing 15 g/ml.

GENERIC NAME Sodium phosphate (dibasic)

TRADE NAME Sal Hepatica (OTC)

CLASSIFICATION Laxative

See sodium phosphate (oral) for Indications for use, Contraindications, Warnings and precautions, Untoward reactions, Parameters of use.

Action This salt has a less offensive taste than most salts. Also contains sodium bicarbonate, tartaric acid, and citric acid.

Administration 10 g po, as needed.

Nursing Management Mix with water and swallow while still effervescing. [See sodium phosphate (oral).]

BULK-FORMING LAXATIVES

GENERIC NAME Agar (OTC)

TRADE NAME Agar-Agar

CLASSIFICATION Laxative

Source Dried hydrophilic colloid obtained from East Indian seaweeds.

Action Agar is one of the oldest laxatives with mild action. It contains carbohydrates chemically similar to cellulose. Agar is neither absorbed nor digested by intestinal bacteria. It softens and adds bulk to the feces through water retention. Defecation response occurs in 12 to 24 hours.

Indications for Use Temporary and chronic constipation, symptomatic relief of acute diarrhea, appetite suppressant in the management of obesity.

Contraindications Intestinal obstruction or impaction.

Warnings and Precautions Clients with dysphagia should not take the dry preparation.

Untoward Reactions Hard, dry stools, fecal impaction, and possible obstruction can occur if fluid intake is inadequate.

Administration Adults: 4 g po daily or bid; Dosage range: 4 to 16 g daily.

Available Drug Forms Powder and shreds.

Nursing Management

1. Suspend in fluid or food; do not take dry.
2. Mix with cereal or add to cooked fruit. May be suspended in hot water and allowed to gel before administering. Agar can be given with milk and sugar.
3. Follow drug administration with a full glass of water or juice.
4. Instruct client to drink at least 1 glassful of fluid hourly for at least 3 hours following drug administration.

GENERIC NAME Psyllium seed (OTC)

TRADE NAME Psyllium Seeds

CLASSIFICATION Laxative

Source Dried ripe seed of *Plantago psyllium* or *Plantago indica*.

Action Psyllium seed (Plantago seed) is an old preparation, but is seldom used today. The mucilaginous seed coat swells in the presence of water, thus lubricating the intestinal tract and increasing the bulk of the intestinal contents. This action stimulates peristalsis and defecation usually occurs within 1 to 3 days.

Indications for Use Chronic and spastic constipation.

Contraindications Bowel obstruction, GI lesions (peptic ulcer, diverticulitis, tumor).

Untoward Reactions May irritate an inflamed or ulcerated bowel. Dehydration may occur in susceptible clients (geriatrics, infants, debilitated clients). If seeds are chewed, granular deposits may develop in the renal tubules.

Administration Adults: 7 to 8 g po, as needed.

Available Drug Forms Containers of whole seeds. Contained in several laxative preparations, including Casyllium and Siblin.

Nursing Management

1. Instruct client to swallow seeds whole.
2. Seeds may be steeped in a small amount of water for 3 to 5 minutes until they form a soft mass.
3. Soft mass may be mixed with honey, jelly, fruit, or other foods to increase palatability.

GENERIC NAME Psyllium hydrophilic mucilloid (regular)

TRADE NAMES Konsyl, Metamucil, Syllamalt (OTC)

CLASSIFICATION Laxative

Source Husk of the psyllium seed *(Plantago ovata)*.

Action This bulk-forming laxative contains finely ground psyllium seed husks. It is considered nonirritating to the GI tract, particularly when compared to the whole psyllium seed. Dextrose and flavorings are added to increase the drug's palatability. Each rounded teaspoon contains 3.4 g of psyllium, 3.5 g of dextrose, and 14 calories.

Indications for Use Chronic and spastic constipation, nonspecific diarrhea, irritable colon, anorectal disorders, appetite suppressant in the management of obesity, intensive bulk-producing therapy.

Contraindications Bowel obstruction (growths, adhesions), fecal impaction.

Untoward Reactions Cholesterol concentration may be increased due to a modest reduction in plasma volume. Chronic use may interfere with the reabsorption of bile salts.

Administration Adults: 1 rounded tsp (7 g) po daily, bid, or tid; Dosage range: 5 to 10 g daily. Children: Consult physician.

Available Drug Forms Multidose containers of creamy brown granular powder (flavored and unflavored); unit-dose packets of granular powder. Each rounded teaspoon contains about 7 g of drug, 1 mg of sodium, and 31 mg of potassium.

Nursing Management

1. Stir in a glass of cool fluid; do not take dry.
2. May be added to water, fruit juice, or milk; administer immediately.
3. Follow drug administration with a full glass of water.
4. Instruct client to drink 1 glassful of water hourly for at least 2 hours following drug administration.
5. Store powder in airtight containers.
6. May require repeated administration over 2 to 3 days for best effect.

GENERIC NAME Psyllium hydrophilic mucilloid (instant)

TRADE NAME Metamucil Instant Mix (OTC)

CLASSIFICATION Laxative

Action Metamucil Instant Mix effervescent requires no stirring when mixed with water or juice. The drug encourages elimination by promoting physiologic peristalsis through its soft pliant bulk. It is nonirritating to the GI tract. Each rounded teaspoon contains 3.6 g of psyllium, citric acid, sucrose, potassium bicarbonate, calcium bicarbonate, flavoring, sodium bicarbonate, and less than 4 calories.

Indications for Use Adjunctive therapy in constipation associated with a duodenal ulcer; colitis; chronic, atonic, and spastic constipation; diverticulitis; bowel management of hemorrhoids, pregnancy, convalescence, and senility; provides bulk to the stools of clients with an ileostomy or colostomy.

Contraindications Intestinal obstruction, fecal impaction, dysphagia, clients on low-sodium diets, severe renal impairment.

Untoward Reactions May cause electrolyte imbalances in susceptible clients (cardiac, geriatric, and debilitated clients).

Administration Adults: 1 packet po daily, bid, or tid. Children: Dosage varies according to age and severity of disorder.

Available Drug Forms Unit-dose packets of flavored or unflavored powder. Each packet contains about 7 mg of sodium, 60 mg of calcium, and 280 mg of potassium.

Nursing Management

1. Do not use previously opened packets.
2. May be added to tube feedings immediately after mixing.
3. Administration factors:
   a. Empty contents of packet into an empty 8-oz glass.
   b. Slowly fill glass with cool water.
   c. Drink entire contents immediately.
   d. Unless contraindicated follow with another full glass of water.
4. Observe susceptible clients frequently for electrolyte imbalances.
5. Check intake and output in clients with renal insufficiency. If oliguria occurs, notify physician.

GENERIC NAME Methylcellulose (OTC)

TRADE NAMES Cellothyl-Hydrolose Liquid, Cologel, Methocel, Saraka, Syncelose

CLASSIFICATION Laxative

Action Methylcellulose, a hydrophilic semisynthetic cellulose derivative, is a bulk laxative that swells in fluid to produce a viscous, colloidal solution. The drug increases the bulk of feces, thus simulating peristalsis. It also increases the blandness of the stool and lubricates the intestinal tract. [A highly diluted ophthalmic solution (0.25 to 1%) has also been used as a lubricant for irritated eyes.]

Indications for Use Acute and chronic constipation, bowel regulation in clients with an ileostomy or colostomy, ulcerative colitis.

Contraindications Intestinal obstruction (intestinal deformity, fecal impaction, tumor), acute abdomen, nausea, vomiting, and abdominal pain (symptoms of appendicitis).

Untoward Reactions May swell and cause obstruction of GI tract (esophageal obstruction, fecal impaction) if fluid intake is inadequate.

Administration Adults: 1 g po daily, bid, tid, or qid. Infants and children: 500 mg po bid or tid.

Available Drug Forms Tablets, powders, capsules, granules, and liquid.

Nursing Management

1. Instruct client to swallow tablets whole in order to prevent premature swelling, thus causing an esophageal obstruction.
2. Preparation for children: Mix with cereal or add to cooked fruit. Can be given with milk and sugar or stirred in a full glass of water.
3. Follow drug administration with a full glass of water or juice.
4. Instruct client to drink at least 1 glassful of fluid hourly for at least 3 hours following drug administration.
5. Check client for obstruction 30 to 60 minutes after drug administration.

TRADE NAME L. A. Formula (OTC)

CLASSIFICATION Laxative

See psyllium hydrophilic mucilloid (regular) for Indications for use, Contraindications, and Untoward reactions.

Administration 1 rounded tsp po daily, bid, or tid.

Available Drug Forms Generic contents: 50% *Plantago ovata* coating; 50% dextrose; 22 calories (1 tsp).

Nursing Management [See psyllium hydrophilic mucilloid (regular)]

1. Stir in a glass of water, fruit juice, or milk; administer immediately.
2. Follow drug administration with a full glass of water.
3. May be used for children.

TRADE NAME Syllact (OTC)

CLASSIFICATION Laxative

See psyllium hydrophilic mucilloid (regular) for Contraindications and Untoward reactions.

Indications for Use Primarily used for constipation.

Administration Adults: 1 to 9 rounded tsp po daily in divided doses. Children: 6 years and older: $\frac{1}{2}$ to $1\frac{1}{2}$ tsp po daily, bid, or tid.

Available Drug Forms Generic contents: 50% powdered psyllium seed husks; 50% dextrose; 14 calories (1 tsp).

Nursing Management [See psyllium hydrophilic mucilloid (regular).]

1. Stir in a glass of water, fruit juice, or milk; administer immediately.
2. Follow drug administration with a full glass of water.

LUBRICANT LAXATIVES

GENERIC NAMES Mineral oil; liquid petrolatum emulsion

TRADE NAMES Albolene, Agoral plain, Fleet Mineral Oil Enema, Kondremul, Mineral Oil, Mineral Oil Light, Nujol

CLASSIFICATION Laxative (OTC)

Source Hydrocarbon mixture obtained from petroleum.

Action Mineral oil (liquid paraffin) acts as a fecal softener and mechanical lubricant. The drug increases bulk in the intestinal tract by preventing the absorption of water. Emulsified preparations are more palatable, penetrate and soften stools more effectively, and induce less anal leakage than nonemulsified oils.

Indications for Use Maintenance of soft stools in chronic constipation, reduction of straining after a herniorrhaphy and in hypertensive and cardiovascular clients, retention enema when oral administration is contraindicated, fecal impaction.

Contraindications Acute abdomen, debilitated, elderly, or dysphagic clients who may aspirate the oil causing lipid pneumonia, postanal surgery, hemorrhoidectomy, pregnancy.

Untoward Reactions Can cause avitaminosis. Regular ingestion during pregnancy may reduce absorption of vitamin K and produce hypoprothrombinemia. Prolonged use may prevent the reabsorption of bile, carotene, and fat-soluble vitamins A, D, E, and K. Leakage past the anal sphincter is an annoying side effect. Normal digestion is incomplete because passage through the bowel is hastened. Interferes with the healing of postoperative anorectal wounds and may induce hemorrhage. Continuous presence of the oil in the rectum disturbs normal defecatory reflexes and prevents complete evacuation of the bowel.

Parameters of Use

Absorption Little absorbed from intestinal tract. Defecation response occurs in 8 to 24 hours.

Administration Adults: 15 to 45 ml po daily or bid.

Available Drug Forms Multidose bottles and single-dose enema.

Nursing Management

1. Store in refrigerator as drug is more palatable when given cold.
2. May be mixed with orange juice or other citrus juices to decrease the oily taste.
3. Give at bedtime to avoid interference with digestion and passage of food.
4. Warn client that repeated doses may cause unintentional seepage of oil and liquid from anus and result in anal pruritus.
5. Repeated doses may be required for several days to induce complete evacuation.
6. Keep rectal area clean and dry to prevent discomfort and pruritus.
7. Do not administer via gastric tube because of the danger of aspiration and lipid pneumonia.

GENERIC NAME Glycerin suppositories (OTC)

TRADE NAME Glycerin Suppositories

CLASSIFICATION Laxative

Action Glycerin is a lubricating substance that stimulates evacuation of the rectum. Since glycerin absorbs moisture, it can dehydrate and thus irritate the rectal mucosa, particularly after repeated use.

Indications for Use Acute constipation, postpartum constipation, recovery from hemorrhoidectomy.

Contraindications Acute abdomen, symptoms of appendicitis (nausea, vomiting, abdominal pain).

Untoward Reactions Rectal irritation and itching can occur, particularly after repeated use. Prolonged use may cause dependency.

Parameters of Use

Absorption Readily absorbed from upper GI tract; little absorption from rectum. Defecation response occurs in 5 to 30 minutes.

Metabolism Absorbed drug is metabolized in the liver to carbon dioxide and water.

Excretion Some in urine unchanged; may cause diuresis.

Administration Adults: 1 adult suppository (about 3 g) inserted deep into rectum. Children: 1 children's suppository (about 1 g) inserted deep into rectum. When using an adult suppository for a child, cut off and use the cone end.

Available Drug Forms Adult suppositories containing 3 g; children's suppositories containing 1 to 1.5 g.

Nursing Management

1. Store suppositories in cool area. Can be stored at room temperature, but keep container below 77 F.
2. Avoid touching suppository until client is prepared for insertion, since suppository melts rapidly in the hand.
3. Insert suppository deep into rectum with covered and lubricated finger.
4. Advise client to attempt to hold suppository for at least 5 minutes.
5. Inform client that defecation will continue until the rectum is empty even though the suppository has been expelled. Suppository need not melt completely to be effective.

STOOL SOFTENERS

GENERIC NAME Docusate sodium (OTC)

TRADE NAMES Bu-Lax, Colace, Comfolax, Dilax, Diomedicone, Disonate, Doxinate, Modane

CLASSIFICATION Stool softener

Action Docusate sodium (dioctyl sodium sulfosuccinate) softens the stool by lowering surface tension. It acts as a dispersing or wetting agent and appears to be inert. The effect on stools is usually apparent within 1 to 3 days.

Indications for Use Constipation due to hard stools, painful anorectal conditions, cardiac and other conditions in which ease of defecation is desired, when peristaltic stimulants are contraindicated.

Contraindications Atonic constipation, intestinal obstruction, acute abdomen, symptoms of appendicitis, fecal impaction, clients on sodium restriction.

Untoward Reactions Throat irritation and nausea are associated with the use of the syrup and liquid. Rash has occurred, but rarely.

Drug Interactions May promote the absorption of mineral oil; do not administer concurrently. May cause abdominal cramps if peristaltic laxatives are administered concomitantly. May increase the intestinal absorption of danthron, digitalis glycosides, and other orally administered compounds, thus increasing the risk of hepatotoxicity, digitalis toxicity, and other untoward reactions.

Administration Adults and older children: 50 to 200 mg po daily; Children: Ages 6 to 13 years: 40 to 120 mg po daily; Ages 3 to 6 years: 20 to 60 mg po daily; Under 3 years: 10 to 40 mg po daily.

Available Drug Forms Capsules containing 50 or 100 mg; liquid solution 1% (10 mg/ml) with calibrated dropper. Also found in combination laxative preparations.

Nursing Management

1. Store at 15 to 30 C (59 to 86 F) to prevent decomposition.
2. Give Colace liquid in half a glass of milk or fruit juice or in infant formula to mask bitter taste.
3. Colace liquid (5 to 10 ml) can be added to a retention or cleansing enema for greater effectiveness.
4. Adjust dosage according to client's response.

GENERIC NAME Docusate potassium (OTC)

TRADE NAMES Dilose, Kasof

CLASSIFICATION Stool softener

See docusate sodium for Indications for use, Contraindications, Untoward reactions, Drug interactions, and Nursing management.

Action Similar action to docusate sodium. As the drug does not contain sodium, it can be used safely in clients on sodium restriction. (See docusate sodium.)

Administration Adults: 240 mg po daily or 100 mg po tid; Children: 6 years and older: 100 mg po at bedtime.

Available Drug Forms Capsules containing 100 or 240 mg.

GENERIC NAME Docusate calcium (OTC)

TRADE NAMES Doxidan, Surfak

CLASSIFICATION Stool softener

See docusate sodium for Indications for use, Contraindications, Untoward reactions, Drug interactions, and Nursing management.

Action Similar action to docusate sodium. Docusate calcium (dioctyl calcium sulfosuccinate) may be safer for clients on sodium-restricted diets than other fecal softeners. (See docusate sodium.)

Administration Adults: 240 mg po daily or 50 mg po daily, bid, or tid; Children: Over 6 years: 50 mg po daily, bid, or tid.

Available Drug Forms Capsules containing 50 or 240 mg.

COMBINATION LAXATIVE PREPARATIONS

Complete details about the contents of the combination laxative preparations can be found by referring to the monograph for each ingredient.

TRADE NAME Agoral Plain (OTC)

CLASSIFICATION Combination laxative preparation

Administration Adults: 1 to 2 tbsp po; Children: Over 6 years: 1 to 2 tsp po.

Available Drug Forms Generic contents in 15 ml: mineral oil: 4.2 g. Also contains agar, tragacanth, acacia, egg album, glycerin, and water.

TRADE NAMES Agoral Raspberry; Agoral Marshmallow (OTC)

CLASSIFICATION Combination laxative preparation

Administration Adults: $\frac{1}{2}$ to 1 tbsp po; Children: Over 6 years: 1 to 2 tsp po.

Available Drug Forms Generic contents in 15 ml: mineral oil: 4.2 g; phenolphthalein: 0.2 g. Also contains agar, tragacanth, acacia, egg albumin, glycerin, and water.

TRADE NAME Alophen (OTC)

CLASSIFICATION Combination laxative preparation

Administration 1 pill po.

Available Drug Forms Generic contents: phenolphthalein, aloin.

TRADE NAME Bilax (OTC)

CLASSIFICATION Combination laxative preparation

Contraindications Acute hepatitis, bilary tract obstruction.

Administration 1 to 2 capsules po tid with meals.

Available Drug Form Generic contents in each capsule: docusate sodium: 100 mg; dehydrocholic acid: 50 mg.

TRADE NAME Carters Little Liver Pills (OTC)

CLASSIFICATION Combination laxative preparation

Administration 1 tablet po.

Available Drug Forms Generic contents: aloe: 16 mg; podophyllum: 4 mg.

TRADE NAME Casakol (OTC)

CLASSIFICATION Combination laxative preparation

Administration 1 tablet po daily.

Available Drug Forms Generic contents in each tablet: casanthranol: 30 mg; poloxamer: 188, 250 mg.

TRADE NAME Comfolax-Plus (OTC)

CLASSIFICATION Combination laxative preparation

Indications for Use Sluggish and irregular bowels.

Administration 1 to 2 capsules po.

Available Drug Forms Generic contents in each capsule: docusate sodium: 100 mg; casanthranol: 30 mg.

Nursing Management

1. Give at bedtime.
2. Not recommended for children under 12 years.

TRADE NAME Correctol (OTC)

CLASSIFICATION Combination laxative preparation

Administration 1 tablet po daily.

Available Drug Forms Generic contents in each tablet: docusate sodium: 100 mg; phenolphthalein: 64.8 mg.

TRADE NAME Dialose Plus (OTC)

CLASSIFICATION Combination laxative preparation

Administration 1 capsule po.

Available Drug Forms Generic contents in each capsule: docusate potassium: 100 mg; casanthranol: 30 mg.

TRADE NAME Dorbantyl (OTC)

CLASSIFICATION Combination laxative preparation

Administration 1 capsule po daily or bid.

Available Drug Forms Generic contents in each capsule: docusate sodium: 50 mg; danthron: 25 mg.

TRADE NAME Dorbantyl Forte (OTC)

CLASSIFICATION Combination laxative preparation

Administration 1 capsule po daily or bid.

Available Drug Forms Generic contents in each capsule: docusate sodium: 50 mg; danthron: 50 mg.

Nursing Management Not recommended for children under 6 years.

TRADE NAME Doxidan (OTC)

CLASSIFICATION Combination laxative preparation

Administration 1 capsule po daily or bid.

Available Drug Forms Generic contents in each capsule: docusate calcium: 60 mg; danthron: 50 mg.

Nursing Management Not recommended for children under 6 years.

TRADE NAME Haley's M-O (OTC)

CLASSIFICATION Combination laxative preparation

Administration 30 ml po daily or bid.

Available Drug Forms Generic contents: 75% milk of magnesia, 25% mineral oil.

Nursing Management Not recommended for young children or clients with dysphagia.

TRADE NAME Laxatyl (OTC)

CLASSIFICATION Combination laxative preparation

Administration 1 to 2 tablets po daily.

Available Drug Forms Generic contents in each sugar-coated tablet: docusate sodium: 60 mg; danthron: 50 mg.

TRADE NAME Milkinol (OTC)

CLASSIFICATION Combination laxative preparation

Administration Adults: 1 to 2 tbsp po; Children: Over 6 years: 1 to 2 tsp po.

Available Drug Forms Generic contents: liquid petrolatum, docusate sodium.

Nursing Management

1. Not recommended for young children, bedridden clients, and during pregnancy.
2. Mix in quarter glass of water; follow with a full glass of water.

TRADE NAME Neolax (OTC)

CLASSIFICATION Combination laxative preparation

Contraindications Acute hepatitis, biliary tract obstruction.

Administration 1 to 2 capsules po tid with meals.

Available Drug Forms Generic contents in each capsule: docusate sodium: 50 mg; dehydrocholic acid: 240 mg.

TRADE NAME MOM-Cascara Suspension (OTC)

CLASSIFICATION Combination laxative preparation

Administration 30 ml po.

Available Drug Forms Generic contents: milk of magnesia, cascara sagrada.

Nursing Management

1. Shake suspension vigorously before measuring dosage.
2. Sometimes called Black and White.

TRADE NAME MOM-Mineral Oil Emulsion (OTC)

CLASSIFICATION Combination laxative preparation

Administration 30 ml po.

Available Drug Forms Flavored and unflavored emulsion. Generic contents: milk of magnesia, emulsified mineral oil.

Nursing Management Shake emulsion thoroughly before measuring dosage.

TRADE NAME Perdiem (OTC)

CLASSIFICATION Combination laxative preparation

Administration 1 to 2 rounded tsp po at bedtime or before breakfast.

Available Drug Forms Generic contents: natural vegetable mucilage, 82% psyllium, 18% senna.

Nursing Management

1. Instruct client to swallow granules whole.
2. Follow drug administration with a full glass of water.

TRADE NAME Peri-Colace (OTC)

CLASSIFICATION Combination laxative preparation

Administration Adults: 1 to 2 capsules po; Children: 1 to 3 tsp po at bedtime.

Available Drug Forms Generic contents in each capsule or 15 ml: casanthranol: 30 mg; docusate sodium: 100 mg.

TRADE NAME Sarolax (OTC)

CLASSIFICATION Combination laxative preparation

Contraindications Acute hepatitis, biliary tract obstruction.

Administration 1 to 2 capsules po at bedtime.

Available Drug Forms Generic contents in each capsule: docusate sodium: 200 mg; phenolphthalein: 15 mg; dehydrocholic acid: 20 mg.

Nursing Management Geriatric and debilitated clients may require half of adult dosage.

TRADE NAME Senokot-S (OTC)

CLASSIFICATION Combination laxative preparation

Administration Adults: 1 to 2 tablets po daily at bedtime; Children: Over 60 lb: 1 to 2 tablets po daily or bid.

Available Drug Forms Generic contents in each tablet: senna concentrate: 187 mg; docusate sodium: 50 mg.

TRADE NAME Trilax (OTC)

CLASSIFICATION Combination laxative preparation

Contraindications Acute hepatitis, biliary tract obstruction.

Administration 1 to 2 capsules po at bedtime.

Available Drug Forms Generic contents in each capsule: docusate sodium: 200 mg; phenolphthalein: 30 mg; dehydrocholic acid: 20 mg.

Chapter 78

Emetics and Antiemetics

INDICATIONS FOR EMETICS

Emetics are indicated when a drug or poison has been ingested in larger than therapeutic amounts. Emergency treatment for such an overdose should begin with dilution and removal of as much of the offending substance from the stomach as possible. The most efficient way to accomplish this is to induce vomiting, which can be effective in removing large amounts of the toxic substance for four or more hours after ingestion. Induction of vomiting is, however, contraindicated in the client who has ingested a paraffin or petroleum product (turpentine) or any caustic (lye) or corrosive (bathroom bowl cleaner) substance, since vomiting of these substances will cause further damage to the upper gastrointestinal tract. Induction of vomiting is also contraindicated in the client who is semiconscious or convulsing because of the danger of aspiration of the stomach contents.

Several nonpharmacologic methods for inducing vomiting may be employed. First, large amounts of tepid (not hot or cold) water should be given. This dilutes the offending substance in the stomach and often induces vomiting. If vomiting does not occur, stimulating the gag reflex by tickling the back of pharynx is often effective. Other methods for inducing vomiting in the home include giving generous amounts of lukewarm mild soap (not detergent) solution, mild mustard solution (1 tsp/gal), salt water, or milk. However, salt solution and milk are contraindicated in some types of poisoning and should never be used if their safety is doubtful.

There are several effective pharmacologic methods for inducing vomiting. Ipecac syrup should be kept in the home, particularly where there are small children. It is given by mouth and is usually effective within 15 to 30 minutes. Apomorphine is administered subcutaneously and leads to vomiting within five minutes. After the client has vomited, it is advisable to administer activated charcoal to adsorb any toxin remaining in the stomach or small intestine (see Chapter 76). Activated charcoal should never be given prior to ipecac syrup, since it will adsorb a significant amount of the ipecac.

When vomiting is contraindicated, gastric aspiration and lavage may be performed in the Emergency Room. The stomach is lavaged with large amounts of tepid water, physiologic saline, starch solution, sodium bicarbonate solution, or charcoal suspension, depending upon the offending substance. This may be followed by other measures to counteract the toxic substance and to support physiologic functions when necessary.

INDICATIONS FOR ANTIEMETICS

Nausea and vomiting can occur from a variety of causes. Mild, transient vomiting can often be relieved with sips of carbonated beverages, hot tea, or locally acting agents, such as antacids. However, prolonged or serious vomiting related to drug or radiation therapy, infections, or other pathophysiology must be treated more aggressively. The choice of a particular antiemetic agent depends upon the cause of the vomiting. The most effective antiemetic drugs are those that act centrally on the chemoreceptor trigger zone in the medulla, the vomiting center, or the vestibular apparatus in the inner ear. Most of the drugs used as antiemetics are also used for various other conditions (see Table 78-1), so only those agents used specifically as antiemetics will be presented in this chapter.

EMETICS

GENERIC NAME Ipecac syrup (OTC) (RX)

CLASSIFICATION Emetic

Action Emetine is the major alkaloid. The drug acts locally on the gastric mucosa and centrally on the chemoreceptor trigger zone to induce vomiting. It also has expectorant action.

Indications for Use Induction of vomiting to eliminate unabsorbed poisons.

Contraindications Semicomatose or comatose clients, shock, ingestion of petroleum products or caustic or corrosive substances.

Untoward Reactions If drug is absorbed (not vomited) or in overdosage, bloody diarrhea, arrhythmias, cardiotoxicity, shock, convulsions, and coma may occur.

TABLE 78-1 Antiemetic Agents

Classification	Action
Anticholinergics (Chapter 42) Scopolamine	Act on vomiting center and vestibular apparatus
Antihistamines (Chapter 83) Buclizine Cyclizine Dimenhydrinate Diphenhydramine Hydroxyzine Meclizine Promethazine	Act on vestibular apparatus
Barbiturates (Chapter 29)	Act on vomiting center
Phenothiazines (Chapter 33) Chlorpromazine Fluphenazine Haloperidol Perphenazine Prochlorperazine Triflupromazine	Act on chemoreceptor trigger zone and vomiting center
Miscellaneous Agents Benzquinamide Diphenidol Thiethylperazine Trimethobenzamide	Act on chemoreceptor trigger zone

Drug Interactions Ipecac may not be effective if the ingested toxic substance was an antiemetic.

Administration Adults and children over 1 year: 15 ml po; Children: Under 1 year: 5 to 10 ml po.

Available Drug Forms OTC bottles containing 30 ml. Larger amounts require a prescription.

Nursing Management

1. Do not confuse with ipecac fluidextract, which is much stronger and can be fatal if ingested at the same dosage as ipecac syrup.
2. Follow drug administration with 1 to 3 glasses of water. Do not give milk or carbonated beverage.
3. Do not administer charcoal concurrently.

GENERIC NAME Apomorphine hydrochloride

CLASSIFICATION Emetic (Cii)

Action Apomorphine acts on the chemoreceptor trigger zone and stimulates salivation. CNS effects are dose related, but small dosages produce sedation. Vomiting occurs within 15 minutes of administration.

Indications for Use Induction of vomiting.

Contraindications Hypersensitivity to morphine, shock, ingestion of caustic or corrosive substances, overdosage with other CNS depressants.

Untoward Reactions Sedation, nausea, weakness, dizziness, postural hypotension, fainting, CNS stimulation, CNS depression.

Parameters of Use

Metabolism In the liver.
Excretion In urine.

Drug Interactions May enhance the effects of levodopa.

Administration Adults and children: 0.07 to 0.1 mg/kg subc as a single dose: adults up to 5 mg may be needed.

Available Drug Forms Soluble tablets containing 6 mg.

Nursing Management

1. A narcotic antagonist (naloxone) and other emergency equipment should be readily available.
2. Dissolve tablets in saline or other vehicle before injection.

3. Discard solutions that are discolored or contain a precipitate.
4. Protect solution from light and air.
5. Administer 2 to 3 glasses of water or other liquid immediately before injection.
6. Do not repeat dosage.

Antiemetics

GENERIC NAME Benzquinamide hydrochloride

TRADE NAME Emete-Con (RX)

CLASSIFICATION Antiemetic

Action Exact mechanism of action is unknown, but benzquinamide is thought to depress the chemoreceptor trigger zone. It also has antihistaminic, anticholinergic, and antiserotonin activities.

Indications for Use Prevention and treatment of nausea and vomiting associated with anesthesia or surgery.

Contraindications Hypersensitivity to benzquinamide, pregnancy, young children, intravenous administration in cardiac clients or those receiving cardiovascular drugs.

Untoward Reactions Drowsiness, insomnia, headache, excitement, restlessness, flushing, hiccups, dry mouth, sweating, blurred vision, hypotension, dizziness, arrhythmias, anorexia, nausea, allergic reactions.

Parameters of Use

Absorption Rapidly absorbed from injection site. Onset of action is 15 minutes. Duration of action is 3 to 4 hours. About 50% bound to plasma proteins. Half-life is 45 minutes.

Distribution Distributed to all body tissues with maximum concentrations in the liver and kidneys.

Metabolism In the liver.

Excretion In urine and feces.

Drug Interactions Other vasopressors given concurrently may cause marked hypertension. May enhance the effects of other CNS depressants.

Administration Intramuscular: Initial dosage: 0.5 to 1.0 mg/kg; may be repeated in 1 hour, then every 3 to 4 hours, as needed. Intravenous: Initial dosage: 0.2 to 0.4 mg/kg at a rate of 1 ml/min.; repeat dosages should be given intramuscularly.

Available Drug Forms Vials containing 50 mg.

Nursing Management

1. May mask signs and symptoms of overdosage from other drugs, thereby preventing accurate diagnosis.
2. When used to prevent postoperative nausea and vomiting, administer at least 15 minutes before client is expected to awaken from anesthesia.
3. Reconstitute with 2.2 ml of diluent to yield 25 mg/ml.
4. Reconstituted solution is stable for 14 days at room temperature.
5. Give IM injection deep into large muscle mass.

GENERIC NAME Diphenidol (RX)

TRADE NAME Vontrol

CLASSIFICATION Antiemetic

Action Diphenidol depresses the vestibular apparatus and inhibits the chemoreceptor trigger zone. It also has weak antihistaminic, anticholinergic, and CNS depressant activities.

Indications for Use Control of nausea and vomiting due to surgery, vestibular disturbances, infectious diseases, neoplasms, or radiation therapy.

Contraindications Hypersensitivity to diphenidol, pregnancy, infants under 25 lb, anuria, intravenous administration in clients with sinus tachycardia and in children.

Warnings and Precautions Use with caution in clients with glaucoma, pyloric stenosis, or GI or genitourinary obstructions.

Untoward Reactions Drowsiness, indigestion, dry mouth, auditory and visual hallucinations, disorientation, confusion, depression, sleep disturbances, nausea, blurred vision, headache, skin rash, hypotension, mild jaundice.

Parameters of Use

Absorption Rapidly absorbed from GI tract or injection site. Onset of action is: 30 to 45 minutes (po); 15 minutes (IM, IV). Duration of action is 3 to 6 hours.

Metabolism In the liver.

Excretion In urine.

Drug Interactions Concurrent administration of sedatives will cause additive CNS depression.

Administration Oral: Adults: 25 to 50 mg q4h. Children: 0.88 mg/kg; Maximum dosage: 5.5 mg/kg/day. Initial dosage: Intramuscular: Adults: 20 to 40 mg; then 20 mg in 1 hour if needed; then 20 to 40 mg q4h prn. Children: 0.44 mg/kg; Maximum dosage: 3.3 mg/kg/day. Intravenous: Adults: Initial dosage: 20 mg; then 20 mg in 1 hour if needed; Maximum dosage: 300 mg/24 hours.

Available Drug Forms Tablets containing 25 mg; 2-ml ampules containing 20 mg/ml.

Nursing Management

1. Administered only to hospitalized clients, since drug can cause hallucinations, disorientation, and confusion. If these effects occur, drug should be discontinued. Symptoms subside within 3 days.
2. Drug may mask signs and symptoms of other drug overdosage.
3. Monitor vital signs and intake and output.
4. Caution client against performing any hazardous activity as drowsiness is a common side effect.

GENERIC NAME Thiethylperazine (RX)

TRADE NAME Torecan

CLASSIFICATION Antiemetic

Action Thiethylperazine is thought to act on the chemoreceptor trigger zone and vomiting center. It is a phenothiazine derivative but has less tranquilizing action than other phenothiazines.

Indications for Use Relief of nausea and vomiting, treatment of vertigo.

Contraindications Hypersensitivity to phenothiazines, severe CNS depression, comatose states, pregnancy, children under 12 years, intravenous administration.

Warnings and Precautions Should not be used by clients who must operate hazardous equipment, since drowsiness frequently occurs. Safe and effective use in children under 12 years or during lactation has not been estabished. Tablets contain FD & C #5 yellow (tetrazine) and some clients may have an allergic reaction to this substance.

Untoward Reactions Drowsiness, headache, dizziness, blurred vision, restlessness, tinnitus, fever, postural hypotension, jaundice. Extrapyramidal effects have been reported, particularly in children and young adults.

Parameters of Use

Absorption Onset of action is: less than 1 hour (po, rectal); 30 minutes (IM).
Metabolism In the liver.
Excretion In urine and feces.

Drug Interactions May potentiate the effect of atropine and phosphorous insecticides and CNS depressants including anesthetics, narcotics, and alcohol.

Administration 10 to 30 mg po, IM, or rectally daily in divided doses.

Available Drug Forms Tablets containing 10 mg; rectal suppositories containing 10 mg; ampules containing 10 mg/2 ml.

Nursing Management

Administration factors

1. Discard parenteral solution if it is not clear and colorless.
2. When administering IM, instruct client to remain in bed for at least 1 hour following injection because of possibility of postural hypotension.

Evaluation factors

1. If extrapyramidal symptoms occur, dosage should be reduced or drug discontinued.
2. If client needs a vasopressor, norepinephrine or phenylephrine should be used. Epinephrine is contraindicated because it may cause further hypotension.

Client teaching factors

1. Caution client against performing any hazardous activities.
2. Warn client to report extrapyramidal symptoms immediately.

GENERIC NAME Trimethobenzamide (RX)

TRADE NAME Tigan

CLASSIFICATION Antiemetic

Action Trimethobenzamide is thought to act on the chemoreceptor trigger zone. It also has a sedative effect and weak antihistaminic activity.

Indications for Use Control of nausea and vomiting. Combined with other antiemetics in severe vomiting.

Contraindications Hypersensitivity to trimethobenzamide, benzocaine, or other local anesthetics, pregnancy, parenteral use in children, rectal administration in newborns and premature infants.

Untoward Reactions Infrequent: hypersensitivity reactions, extrapyramidal symptoms, hypotension, blurred vision, depression, diarrhea, dizziness, drowsiness, jaundice, muscle cramps, blood dyscrasias, convulsions, comas. Intramuscular administration may cause redness, stinging, and irritation at the injection site.

Parameters of Use

Absorption Onset of action is: 20 to 40 minutes (po, rectal); 15 minutes (IM). Duration of action is: 3 to 4 hours (po, rectal); 2 to 3 hours (IM).
Metabolism In the liver.
Excretion In urine.

Drug Interactions Concurrent administration of other CNS depressants can cause additive CNS depression. Concomitant use of barbiturates or phenothiazines increases the risk of extrapyramidal symptoms.

Administration Oral: Adults: 250 mg tid or qid; Children: 100 to 200 mg tid or qid. Intramuscular: Adults: 200 mg tid or qid. Rectal: Adults: 200 mg tid or qid; Children: 100 to 200 mg tid or qid.

Available Drug Forms Capsules and rectal suppositories containing 100 or 200 mg; 2-ml ampules containing 200 mg; 20-ml vials containing 100 mg/ml; 2-ml disposable prefilled syringes containing 100 mg/ml.

Nursing Management

1. When administering IM, inject deep into gluteal muscle. Avoid escape of solution along needle track.
2. Monitor blood pressure frequently following IM administration as hypotension may occur.
3. If any signs of hypersensitivity develop, drug should be discontinued.
4. CNS toxicity is characterized by disorientation, lethargy, and tremors. If symptoms occur, drug should be discontinued.
5. Abrupt onset of vomiting, lethargy, or confusion may indicate Reye's syndrome, which has been associated with the use of this and similar drugs. Prompt medical attention is a necessity if these symptoms occur.
6. Drug can mask symptoms of underlying disease and impair diagnosis.

PART XVII

OPHTHALMIC AND OTIC AGENTS

MANY OF THE medications used to treat eye and ear disorders are also used for similar disorders in other parts of the body, while some drugs are used to treat disorders specific to the sense organs. Part IV explains the special precautions required when administering medications to these delicate structures. The nurse should remember that the senses, particularly the sense of sight, are valued highly because they assist individuals to function independently. Clients who have vision or hearing disorders may fear that they will totally lose their sight or hearing and then be reliant on others for certain activities of daily living.

When administering medications to the eye or ear, the nurse must be expecially careful to apply the medication to the right structure. Medication containers for the eye and ear are similar; however, there are marked differences in the medication itself. Although the same drug may be administered to both the eye and ear, eye medications must be sterile, whereas ear medications need only be as clean as possible. In addition, the membrane of the eye is much more delicate than the surface of the ear canal. Therefore, eye medications are often given in a much more dilute form than ear medications. The inadvertent administration of an ear medication to the eye may cause infection, irritation, or even permanent damage. The nurse must take extra precautions to administer the appropriate medication to the right structure.

Chapter 79

Ophthalmic Agents

ANTIINFLAMMATORY AGENTS

- Dexamethasone sodium phosphate
- Hydrocortisone acetate
- Prednisolone sodium phosphate

COMBINATION ANTIINFECTIVE AND ANTIINFLAMMATORY PREPARATIONS

- Cortisporin
- Metimyd
- Neodecadron
- Neo-Hydeltrasol
- Optimyd

MYDRIATIC AGENTS

- Atropine sulfate
- Cyclopentolate hydrochloride
- Homatropine hydrobromide
- Hydroxyamphetamine hydrobromide
- Phenylephrine hydrochloride
- Scopolamine hydrobromide
- Tropicamide

OTHER OPHTHALMIC AGENTS

- Alpha-chymotrypsin
- Hyaluronate sodium
- Hydroxypropy cellulose

COMBINATION OPHTHALMIC PREPARATIONS

- Artificial Tears
- Clear Eyes
- Collyrium, Collyrium with Ephedrine
- Murine Eye Drops
- Murine Plus Eye Drops
- Succus Cineraria Maritina

WHEN VISION IS disrupted, humans lose a valued sense and with it an aspect of independence. Nurses are frequently involved with the diagnosis and treatment of eye injuries and disorders that have the potential for causing permanent loss of sight. Besides providing needed reassurance to the client, nursing management of clients with eye dysfunction frequently centers around the application of ophthalmic medications and teaching clients and their families to instill eye medications appropriately.

Three classes of frequently used ophthalmic agents are the *mydriatics, cycloplegics*, and *miotics*. The mydriatics induce dilation of the pupil, the cycloplegics cause paralysis of the ciliary muscle, and the miotics cause constriction of the pupil. During eye examinations, certain anticholinergic and adrenergic agents are used as mydriatics and cycloplegics in order to measure errors in refraction and to inspect the internal structure of the eye. Injuries and defects in the cornea or conjuctiva are often detected by instilling the dye fluorscein. Miotics aid the prevention of eye damage from glaucoma and are the most frequently used eye medications.

GLAUCOMA

Glaucoma is an eye disorder characterized by excessive intraocular pressure. If left untreated, blindness results. Although preventable, glaucoma is the most common cause of blindness in people over the age of 40. Aqueous humor is produced by the ciliary processes and circulates from behind the iris, through the pupil to the anterior chamber, and out the canal of Schlemm into the trabecular meshwork. Normal eye pressure is maintained at about 15 mm Hg when the amount of aqueous humor produced is equal to the amount flowing out the canal. In glaucoma, however, there is resistance to the outflow of aqueous humor, which causes the eye pressure to rise. The increased pressure eventually causes compression of the retina and optic nerve, resulting in blindness.

There are two forms of glaucoma, open-angle glaucoma and angle-closure or narrow-angle glaucoma. Open-angle glaucoma occurs in 90% of glaucoma cases. In this type of glaucoma, the outflow of aqueous humor is obstructed due to degeneration of the trabecular meshwork and/or the canal of Schlemm. Unfortunately, the client is usually asymptomatic and the damage is allowed to progress unchecked. Therefore, periodic eye examinations are recommended for all individuals over the age of 40. Screening for glaucoma includes a tonometry exam, a simple and painless office procedure that measures the intraocular pressure (normally 12 to 21 mm Hg). Angle-closure or narrow-angle glaucoma occurs in clients who have shallow anterior chambers. As the client progresses in age, the iris moves into the filtration angle. When such an individual enters a dark area, the iris can block the outflow of aqueous humor and cause a sudden increase in intraocular pressure, which produces severe pain, nausea, and vomiting. Whereas open-angle glaucoma is chronic and can easily be treated by miotics, angle-closure glaucoma is a medical emergency and usually requires surgery for long-term management.

PROPERTIES OF ANTIGLAUCOMA AGENTS

Intraocular pressure can be lowered by decreasing the formation of aqueous humor, enhancing the drainage of aqueous humor by constricting the pupil, or both. Carbonic anhydrase inhibitors (acetazolamide) and adrenergic agents with mydriatic properties (epinephrine) decrease the secretion of aqueous humor and, by means poorly understood, increase the outflow of the fluid. The beta-adrenergic blocker timolol also reduces the formation of aqueous humor and slightly increases its outflow, thus reducing intraocular pressure.

Miotics are commonly used to treat open-angle glaucoma. The cholinergic agents, such as pilocarpine, induce pupillary constriction and contraction of the ciliary body, thereby increasing outflow of aqueous humor. Unfortunately, these drugs frequenly cause blurred vision, poor accommodation, and headaches. The anticholinesterase agents are useful, but therapy for longer than 6 months creates the risk of cataract formation.

EYE INFECTIONS

Infections of the eye can occur at any age. A newborn may contract an eye infection from a pathogen in the vaginal tract of the mother. Such an infection may be so severe that blindness results. Consequently, antiinfective agents are routinely instilled in the eyes of newborns. Many individuals, particularly young children and the senile elderly, rub their eyes with their hands, creating the potential for an eye infection. Exudate from an infected eye should be cultured to determine the causative microorganism and therefore the appropriate antiinfective agent to use. Inflammation of the eye can occur in the absence of an infection; however, inflammation and infection often occur simultaneously. Consequently, several antiinfective and antiinflammatory preparations are available. Since the symptoms of an eye infection frequently disappear before the causative microorganism is completely eliminated, clients must be cautioned to use the antiinfective agent for the entire length of time prescribed by the physician.

NURSING MANAGEMENT

Most eye medications are instilled by the client or the client's family. To ensure proper results, the person administering the medication should be carefully instructed in the proper technique for instillation. Eye drops may be used during the day, but ointments are more effective for night use, since they remain in the eye longer than drops. The nurse should ascertain whether drops, ointment, or both are to be used. The purpose and frequency of drug application should be carefully explained to the client and the nurse should help the client to develop an appropriate schedule for applying the drug. The necessity of maintaining the sterility of the drug container and cap should be emphasized so that infection does not occur inadvertently. Demonstration, with a repeat demonstration at the next meeting, is usually an effective method for teaching clients and their families the proper technique for drug instillation.

When teaching clients about their eye medications, the nurse should also emphasize the necessity of regular eye examinations, follow-up visits, and the potential for adverse reactions. Untoward reactions, both secondary and adverse, should be explained so that the client knows what to expect and what to do if an untoward reaction occurs. For example, several eye medications cause temporary blurring of vision; the client should be instructed not to drive a car or operate hazardous equipment until the vision clears. Some miotics can cause the formation of cataracts after several months; the client should be warned to consult a physician immediately if changes in vision occur. It should be remembered that clients with eye disorders are often anxious and afraid that they will lose their vision. Clients should be given reassurance as needed and care should be taken to avoid raising unnecessary fears.

DIAGNOSTIC AGENTS

GENERIC NAME Fluorescein sodium (RX)

TRADE NAMES Fluorescein, Fluor-I-Strip, Ful-Glo-Strip

CLASSIFICATION Ophthalmic diagnostic aid

Action Fluorescent dye that can be seen with ultraviolet light. Outlines eye lesions and foreign bodies with yellow or green rings depending on light.

Indications for Use Diagnosis: corneal injuries, presence of foreign bodies, patency of lacrimal duct.

Untoward Reactions May cause irritation, burning sensation, or stinging.

Administration Solution: Initially instill 1 to 2 gtt 2% solution; then gently irrigate eye with normal saline. Strips: Initially moisten tips of strip and touch corner of conjunctiva or fornix; then gently irrigate eye with normal saline.

Available Drug Forms Bottles containing sterile 2% solution; ready-to-use strips coated with drug at one tip.

Nursing Management

1. Usually done in presence of physician.
2. Topical anesthetic is usually applied to eliminate discomfort from irritation.
3. If possible, have client blink 2 or 3 times to disperse medication.
4. Avoid contact with skin.
5. Store at cool room temperature in airtight containers.

GENERIC NAME Fluorescein (RX)

TRADE NAMES Fluorescite, Funduscein

CLASSIFICATION Ophthalmic diagnostic aid

Indications for Use Retinal angiography. Has been used to determine circulatory time.

Untoward Reactions Anaphylaxis, urticaria, and other hypersensitivity reactions have occurred. Nausea, vomiting, and a persistent headache are common. Urine turns bright yellow for 24 to 36 hours. Skin discoloration.

Administration Intravenous: Variable depending on purpose.

Available Drug Forms Vials containing 10 or 25% solution.

Nursing Management

1. Follow manufacturer's instructions.
2. Warn client about discoloration of urine.

GENERIC NAME Glycerin anhydrous (RX)

TRADE NAME Ophthalgan

CLASSIFICATION Ophthalmic diagnostic aid

Action Glycerin (trihydric alcohol) is a viscous liquid that is highly hygroscopic and can therefore osmotically reduce corneal edema. It is irritating to mucous membranes and may cause pain if a topical anesthetic is not instilled prior to its use.

Indications for Use Prevention and treatment of corneal edema due to ophthalmoscopy or gonioscopy. Has also been used to reduce corneal edema associated with trauma or surgery to the eye.

Administration Instill 1 to 2 gtt q3h, as needed.

Available Drug Forms Bottles containing sterile solution with a dropper. Ingredient in several OTC antiirritant eye drops, including Murine Eye Drops.

Nursing Management Store in airtight containers.

GENERIC NAME Proparacaine hydrochloride

TRADE NAME Ophthaine (RX)

CLASSIFICATION Ophthalmic diagnostic aid

Action Proparacaine is a rapid-acting local anesthetic that also contains glycerin and 0.2% chlorobutanol chloride.

Indications for Use Prevention and treatment of pain associated with tonometry, gonioscopy, and removal of foreign bodies or sutures from corneal or conjunctival scraping. Also used as a topical anesthetic to surgical procedures, including extraction of cataracts.

Contraindications Hypersensitivity to any ingredient.

Warnings and Precautions Use with caution in clients with multiple allergies, cardiac disorders, or hyperthyroidism. Anesthetized eye must be protected from irritating chemicals, foreign bodies, and mechanical injury from rubbing.

Parameters of Use

Absorption Onset of anesthesia is about 13 seconds. Duration of action is 15 minutes.

Administration

- *Surface anesthesia:* Instill 1 to 2 gtt immediately before procedure (2 to 3 minutes).
- *Deep anesthesia:* Instill 1 to 2 gtt every 5 to 10 minutes for 5 to 7 doses; then as needed.

Available Drug Forms Squeeze dropper bottles containing 15 ml of sterile 0.5% solution.

Nursing Management

1. Maintain sterility of container and cap.
2. Instill into lower conjunctival sac.
3. Application of an eye patch is recommended to prevent accidental irritation to anesthetized eye.
4. Warn client to avoid touching eyes.
5. Store unopened drug at room temperature; but when opened, refrigerate solution to retard discoloration.
6. Do not use solution if discolored.
7. Keep bottle tightly closed.

GENERIC NAME Tetracaine hydrochloride (RX)

TRADE NAME Pontocaine Hydrochloride

CLASSIFICATION Ophthalmic diagnostic aid

Action Tetracaine is a topical anesthetic related to procaine. It does not penetrate eye tissues as well as proparacaine, but tetracaine does not cause pupillary dilation or an increase in intraocular pressure.

Indications for Use Anesthesia of superficial eye structures for diagnostic procedures, removal of foreign bodies, or corneal sutures.

Untoward Reactions May cause transient stinging and irritation after instillation. Prolonged use may cause epithelial damage. Hypersensitivity reactions include urticaria and periocular rash.

Drug Interactions May interfere with the absorption of topical antiinfective agents, including sulfonamides; instill antiinfective agent 1 hour after anesthetic instillation.

Administration Instill 1 to 2 gtt every 5 to 10 minutes, as needed.

Available Drug Forms Bottles containing sterile 0.5% solution.

Nursing Management

1. Maintain sterility of container and cap.
2. Instill into lower conjunctival sac.
3. Application of an eye patch is recommended to prevent accidental irritation to anesthetized eye.
4. Do not use solution if discolored.
5. Keep bottle tightly closed.

ANTIGLAUCOMA AGENTS

Cholinergic Miotic Agents

GENERIC NAME Pilocarpine hydrochloride (RX)

TRADE NAMES Adsorbocarpine, Almocarpine, Isopto-Carpine, Miocarpine, Pilocar, Pilocel, Pilomiotin

CLASSIFICATION Cholinergic miotic agent

Source Naturally occurring alkaloid obtained from leaflets of *Pilocarpus jaborandi* or *microphyllus.*

Action Pilocarpine is a direct-acting cholinergic agent that induces constriction of the pupil and contraction of the ciliary muscle, thus facilitating the outflow of aqueous humor and a decrease in intraocular pressure. The ciliary muscle tends to contract spasmodically and may cause pain in the brow. Although the pupil becomes pinpoint in size, the pupil will still contract further when exposed to light. The drug may be absorbed systemically and cause bronchial constriction, alterations in blood pressure, and excessive respiratory and gastric secretions. Atropine antagonizes the action of pilocarpine.

Indications for Use Primary open-angle glaucoma, most types of chronic glaucoma. May be used immediately before surgery for acute narrow-angle glaucoma. Also used to counteract the effects of mydriatics and cycloplegics following eye examinations and surgery.

Contraindications Hypersensitivity to any ingredient, acute iritis, acute inflammation of anterior segment of eye.

Warnings and Precautions Use with caution in clients with bronchial asthma. Tolerance may develop with prolonged use. Drug concentrations greater than 40% provide little or no additional benefit. If therapeutic concentrations are ineffective, the miotic agent is either changed or epinephrine is added to the drug therapy (E-Carpine).

Untoward Reactions Increases respiratory tract secretions. Ciliary spasm may cause pain in the affected brow and pain upon alteration in focus, but pain tends to disappear after 1 to 2 weeks of therapy. Blurred vision may occur initially. May cause an inability to see objects in dimly lit areas. Irritation, including conjunctivitis, may occur. Hypersensitivity reactions are rare. Systemic absorption increases sweating; salivation and gastric secretions also increase and may result in nausea, vomiting, and other GI disturbances. Atropine is effective in relieving systemic symptoms.

Parameters of Use

Absorption Onset of miosis is 15 to 30 minutes. Duration of miosis is 4 to 8 hours; pupil may remain somewhat constricted for as long as 24 hours in some clients. Onset of ciliary muscle contractions (or spasm) is about 15 minutes; difficulties with accommodation will last about 24 hours. Duration of contractions is about 2 hours.

Drug Interactions Concurrent use with other direct-acting cholinergic agents, such as carbachol, will have an additive effect; do not use concurrently.

Administration Instill 2 gtt 0.5 to 4% solution daily, bid, tid, or qid depending on severity of glaucoma. Instillation of daily drops at bedtime will avoid difficulties with accommodation during the day.

Available Drug Forms Bottles containing sterile 0.5 to 4% solution.

Nursing Management

Planning factors

1. Obtain history of eye, respiratory, and cardiovascular disorders. Notify physician if client has eye infection, bronchial asthma, or severe cardiovascular disorders.
2. Complete tomometric and other eye tests prior to instituting drug.
3. Schedule once-a-day dosages at bedtime.

Administration factors

1. Double check the strength of the solution, since several concentrations are available.
2. Maintain sterility of solution and inner surfaces of dropper assembly.
3. Cleanse affected eyelid with sterile pad and normal saline before instillation. Wipe from inner to outer canthus.
4. Instill medication into lower conjunctival sac being careful to avoid touching the eye with the tip of the dropper.
5. Gently press the inner canthus over the nasolacrimal duct for 1 to 2 minutes to avoid systemic absorption.
6. Instruct client to close eye and move eye in all directions with eyelid closed to disperse the medication.

Evaluation factors

1. Examine eye for irritation or infection prior to instilling medication.
2. Record severity and duration of brow pain and nearsightedness. Inform client that symptoms will subside with continued use.
3. Schedule tonometric and other eye tests periodically, particularly when therapy is first initiated or dosage adjusted.

Client teaching factors

1. Instruct client and/or family how to administer medication. Demonstration and return demonstration are advisable. Teaching the maintenance of the solution's sterility is essential.
2. Emphasize the necessity of maintaining the dosage schedule despite the lack of symptoms in order to prevent blindness.
3. Inform client to seek medical assistance if itching, burning, or exudate develop around the eye.
4. Instruct client to avoid hazardous activities as long as drug-induced nearsightedness (about 2 hours) or brow pain persist.
5. Emphasize the need for periodic eye examinations.
6. Inform client to store drug in airtight containers away from direct light.

GENERIC NAME Pilocarpine (deposits) (RX)

TRADE NAMES Ocusert Pilo-20, Ocusert Pilo-40

CLASSIFICATION Cholinergic miotic agent

See pilocarpine hydrochloride for Contraindications, Warnings and precautions, Untoward reactions, and Drug interactions.

Action Pilocarpine deposits increase client compliance by avoiding repeated instillation of solution. They may also decrease the incidence of infection from frequent, prolonged instillation of eye drops. (See pilocarpine hydrochloride.)

Indications for Use Most types of chronic glaucoma.

Administration Insert 1 Ocusert weekly.

Available Drug Forms Clear, flexible, waferthin Ocusert with an elliptical shape filled with sterile pilocarpine solution. Ocusert Pilo-20 releases 20 mcg/hour and Ocusert Pilo-40 releases 40 mcg/hour.

Nursing Management (See pilocarpine hydrochloride.)

1. Insert at bedtime because initial effect (equal to about 1 gtt of 2% solution) may cause ciliary spasm and loss of accommodation.
2. Rinse eye with water before inserting Ocusert.
3. Insert into lower conjunctival sac. May be moved periodically (daily) from lower to upper conjunctival sac and vice versa by gentle digital movement through closed eyelid.
4. Check for presence of Ocusert daily.
5. Instruct client to mark calender to remember when to change Ocusert.
6. Watch for systemic reaction when Ocusert is changed.

GENERIC NAME Pilocarpine nitrate (RX)

TRADE NAME P.V. Carpine Liquifilm

CLASSIFICATION Cholinergic miotic agent

See pilocarpine hydrochloride for Contraindications, Warnings and precautions, Untoward reactions, Parameters of use, and Nursing management.

Action This acidic mononitrate salt of pilocarpine has action similar to pilocarpine. (See pilocarpine hydrochloride.)

Indications for Use Most types of chronic glaucoma.

Drug Interactions Incompatible with alkaline substances, including silver nitrate; check pH of other ophthalmic drugs before using. (See pilocarpine hydrochloride.)

Administration Instill 1 to 2 gtt 0.5 to 6% solution daily, bid, tid, or qid depending on severity of disorder.

Available Drug Forms Bottles containing sterile 0.5 to 6% solution with dropper.

GENERIC NAME Carbachol (RX)

TRADE NAMES Carbacel, Carbachol

CLASSIFICATION Cholinergic miotic agent

See pilocarpine hydrochloride for Contraindications, Warnings and precautions, Untoward reactions, and Nursing management.

Action Although listed as a direct-acting cholinergic agent, this drug also has mild anticholinesterase properties; therefore, it has a long duration of action. Carbachol is more potent and more stable than pilocarpine, but may be more toxic than pilocarpine.

Indications for Use Refractory glaucoma.

Parameters of Use

Absorption Erratically absorbed. Onset of miosis is 10 to 20 minutes. Duration of miosis is 4 to 8 hours.

Administration Instill 1 gtt 0.75 to 3% solution daily, bid, tid, or qid depending on severity of disorder.

Available Drug Forms Bottles containing sterile 0.75 to 3% solution with dropper.

ANTICHOLINESTERASE MIOTIC AGENTS

GENERIC NAMES Physiostigmine salicylate; physiostigmine sulfate; physiostigmine (RX)

TRADE NAMES Eserine Salicylate, Isopto Eserine; Eserine Sulfate

CLASSIFICATION Anticholinesterase miotic agent

Source Alkaloid obtained from *Physostigma venenosum*.

Action Physiostigmine is a competitive inhibitor of acetylcholinesterase at cholinergic synapses. Contraction of the pupil and ciliary body facilitates the drainage of aqueous humor through the canal of Schlemm; thus resulting in a decrease in intraocular pressure. Physiostigmine's ability to inhibit cholinesterase varies with the pH of the eye. Drug effect is greatest at a pH of 7.5 or less and neutral at a pH of 8.5 or higher. Hyoscyamine blocks the systemic effects of physiostigmine.

Indications for Use Counteracts atropine-induced mydriasis following eye examinations and surgery, acute-closure glaucoma, open-angle glaucoma.

Contraindications Secondary glaucoma, iritis, inflammatory disorders of ciliary body, bronchial asthma, severe cardiovascular disorders, obstruction of genitourinary tract, diabetes mellitus.

Warnings and Precautions Use with caution in clients with parkinsonism, bradycardia, and epilepsy. Safe use during pregnancy has not been established.

Untoward Reactions Ciliary spasm and excessive miosis may cause eyebrow pain, headache, difficulty seeing in dim light, and blurred vision. Conjunctivitis and other eye irritations may occur. Follicular cyst formation has been reported. Excessive lacrimation is common. Twitching of the eyelid is relatively common. Prolonged use may cause changes in the pigment of the iris epithelium and chronic conjunctivitis. Periocular allergic dermatitis has been reported. Systemic absorption may cause GI disturbances, bronchoconstriction, arrhythmias, bradycardia, rhinorrhea, excessive sweating, and urinary incontinence.

Parameters of Use

Absorption Readily absorbed through mucous membranes; mild systemic effects are common. Onset of miosis is 2 to 5 minutes. Duration of miosis is 12 to 24 hours; some miosis may persist for as long as 36 hours in some clients.

Drug Interactions Additive effects may occur with direct-acting cholinergic agents, such as pilocarpine. Less miosis occurs if given concurrently with isoflurophate. If concomitant therapy is required, administer topical isoflurophate 1 hour after topical physiostigmine. Organophosphate insecticides may cause a marked additive effect. Do not administer alkaline eye medications concurrently.

Administration Instill 1 to 2 gtt 0.25 or 0.5% solution daily, bid, tid, or qid depending on severity of disorder. Apply a small amount of 0.25% ointment daily, bid, tid, or qid, as needed. Solution may be used during the day and ointment at bedtime.

Available Drug Forms Bottles containing sterile 0.25 or 0.5% solution with dropper; small tubes containing sterile 0.25% ointment.

Nursing Management (See pilocarpine hydrochloride.)

1. Warn client about potential tearing and twitching of eyelid.
2. When drug is initiated, observe client closely for systemic reactions. Check vital signs periodically.
3. Place ointment (thin line about 0.5 cm long) in lower conjunctival sac.
4. Protect drug from air and light as it is oxidized and loses potency.
5. Do not use reddish solutions.

GENERIC NAME Demecarium bromide (RX)

TRADE NAME Humorsol

CLASSIFICATION Anticholinesterase miotic agent

Action Demecarium is a potent and long-acting inhibitor of cholinesterase. It allows anticholinesterase to accumulate at neuromuscular junctions. The drug is thought to also increase permeability and dilation of conjunctival vessels, thereby enhancing the reabsorption of aqueous humor. Demecarium may decrease the ability of eyeball muscles to permit convergence.

Indications for Use Glaucoma, postiridectomy, accommodative convergent.

Contraindications Narrow-angle glaucoma, history of retinal detachment, bronchial asthma, inflammatory disorders of anterior eye structures.

Warnings and Precautions Use with caution in clients with cardiovascular or GI disorders, parkinsonism, epilepsy, or myasthenia gravis. Safe use during pregnancy has not been established.

Untoward Reactions Prolonged use may cause iris cysts, lens opacity, and obstruction of nasolacrimal canal. Photosensitivity and photophobia are relatively common. (See physiostigmine salicylate.)

Drug Interactions Duration of demecarium-induced miosis is decreased if given concurrently with echothiophate iodide; adminster demecarium 1 hour before echothiophate iodide.

Administration Short-term use only. Adults: Instill 1 to 3 gtt 0.125% solution twice weekly up to as often as bid. Children: Instill 1 gtt 0.125% solution in each eye daily for 2 to 4 weeks; then 1 gtt every other day for 3 to 4 weeks; then 1 gtt twice weekly.

Available Drug Form Bottles containing sterile 0.125 or 0.25% solution.

Nursing Management (See pilocarpine hydrochloride.)

1. Physician should be present when drug is initiated, since an increase in intraocular pressure may precede desired effect.
2. Assess client frequently for systemic effects.
3. Avoid contact with skin as absorption may occur. Wash hands before and after using drug. If drug accidently comes into contact with skin, rinse area with large amounts of plain water.
4. Store in airtight containers.

GENERIC NAME Echothiophate iodide (RX)

TRADE NAMES Echodide, Phospholine Iodide

CLASSIFICATION Anticholinesterase miotic agent

See physiostigmine salicylate for Warnings and precautions and Drug interactions.

Action Echothiophate is a long-acting cholinesterase inhibitor. It also depresses plasma and erythrocyte cholinesterase levels after 2 to 8 weeks of therapy.

Indications for Use Chronic open-angle glaucoma, subacute or chronic angle-closure glaucoma, postiridectomy, glaucoma following cataract surgery, accommodative esotropia.

Contraindications Hypersensitivity to any ingredient, uveal inflammation, most cases of angle-closure glaucoma.

Untoward Reactions Activation of iritis or uveitis, stinging and burning of eyes, and iris cysts (particularly in children) may occur. Prolonged use may cause conjunctival thickening or obstruction of nasolacrimal canal.

Administration Highly individualized. Short-term use only. Instill 1 gtt 0.03 to 0.25% solution daily or bid.

Available Drug Forms Bottles containing sterile 0.03, 0.06, 0.125, or 0.25% solution.

Nursing Management (See pilocarpine hydrochloride.)

1. Physician should be present when drug is initiated, since an increase in intraocular pressure may precede desired effect.
2. Assess client frequently for systemic effects.
3. Avoid contact with skin as absorption may occur. Wash hands before and after using drug. If drug accidently comes into contact with skin, rinse area with large amounts of plain water.
4. Manual compression of inner canthus for 1 to 2 minutes after instillation is essential to minimize systemic effects.
5. Solution is stable for 1 month at room temperature and 6 months when refrigerated.

GENERIC NAME Isoflurophate (RX)

TRADE NAMES DFP, Floropryl

CLASSIFICATION Anticholinesterase miotic agent

See physiostigmine salicylate for Contraindications, Warnings and precautions, and Drug interactions.

Action Isoflurophate is a potent, long-acting cholinesterase inhibitor. It is an organophosphorous compound that induces irreversible inactivation of cholinesterase. Isoflurophate is rapidly absorbed through mucous membranes and skin.

Indications for Use Primary open-angle glaucoma, accommodative esotropia.

Untoward Reactions Prolonged use may cause lens opacities. (See physiostigmine salicylate.)

Administration

- *Glaucoma:* Apply 0.5 cm 0.025% ointment every 8 to 72 hours.
- *Strabismus, esotropia:* Apply 0.5 cm 0.025% ointment at bedtime for 2 weeks.

Available Drug Forms Small tubes containing sterile 0.025% ointment.

Nursing Management (See pilocarpine hydrochloride.)

1. Physician should be present when drug is initiated, since an increase in intraocular pressure may precede desired effect.
2. Assess client freqently for systemic effects.
3. Avoid contact with skin as absorption may occur. Wash hands before and after using drug. If drug accidently comes into contact with skin, rinse area with large amounts of plain water.
4. Place ointment in lower conjunctival sac.

ADRENERGIC AGENTS

GENERIC NAME Dipivefrin (RX)

TRADE NAME Propine

CLASSIFICATION Adrenergic agent

Action Dipivefrin is an adrenergic agent that is converted to epinephrine when instilled into the eye. The drug decreases intraocular pressure by reducing the production of aqueous humor and by increasing outflow. It also has weak mydiatric action.

Indications for Use Chronic open-angle glaucoma.

Contraindications Narrow-angle glaucoma.

Warnings and Precautions Use with caution in the elderly and in debilitated clients. Administer with extreme caution to clients who are hypersensitive to catecholamines.

Untoward Reactions May cause tearing upon instillation. Prolonged use may cause iritis or excessive dryness of the eye.

Administration Adults: Instill 1 gtt 0.1% solution every 12 hours.

Available Drug Forms Sterile 0.1% solution.

Nursing Management (See pilocarpine hydrochloride.)

1. Physician should be present when initial dose is given.
2. Assess client frequently for systemic effects.
3. Manual compression of inner canthus for 1 to 2 minutes after instillation is helpful to minimize systemic effects.

GENERIC NAMES Epinephrine bitartrate; epinephrine borate; epinephrine hydrochloride

TRADE NAMES Epitrate; Epinal, EPPY Solutions; Adrenalin Chloride, Epifrin, Glaucon

CLASSIFICATION Adrenergic agent (RX)

See dipivefrin for Warnings and precautions, Untoward reactions, and Nursing management.

Action Epinephrine is an adrenergic agent with a low surface tension. The drug has a weak mydriatic action and reduces the rate of aqueous formation. It is often used with miotics and carbonic anhydrase inhibitors.

Indications for Use Chronic open-angle glaucoma. Epinephrine hydrochloride may also be used as a 0.1% solution prior to and during eye surgery to control bleeding and conjunctivitis.

Contraindications Peripheral iridectomy, narrow-angle glaucoma.

Untoward Reactions May cause tearing upon instillation.

Administration Highly individualized. Adults: Instill 1 gtt solution as necessary (once every 2 to 3 days or tid or qid). Epinephrine bitartrate and hydrochloride are usually given bid.

Available Drug Forms Solution 0.1, 0.25, 0.5, or 1.0%.

Nursing Management Do not use solution if discolored (brown) or if a precipitate has formed.

BETA-ADRENERGIC BLOCKERS

GENERIC NAME Timolol maleate (RX)

TRADE NAME Timoptic

CLASSIFICATION Beta-adrenergic blocking agent

Action Although the precise mechanism of action is unknown, timolol decreases intraocular pressure by reducing the formation of aqueous humor and slightly increasing the outflow facility. Unlike other topical agents used in glaucoma, timolol does not alter accommodation or pupil size. The drug induces little or no depression of the myocardium. It is a well-tolerated drug that can be used for almost all types of intraocular hypertension and is said to be more effective than pilocarpine. Restrictive usage of timolol is related to its systemic absorption.

Indications for Use Chronic open-angle glaucoma, aphakic glaucoma, most types of secondary glaucoma, elevated intraocular pressure.

Contraindications Hypersensitivity to any ingredient.

Warnings and Precautions Use with caution in clients with bronchial diseases, sinus bradycardia greater than first-degree heart block, cardiogenic shock, heart failure, or severe cardiac disorders. Safe use in narrow-angle or angle-closure glaucoma, in children, and during pregnancy has not been established. Not recommended for infants with glaucoma. Tolerance may develop with prolonged use. Prolonged use has caused elevations in serum prolactin levels in mice, but no significant changes have been reported in humans.

Untoward Reactions Ocular irritation, including conjunctivitis, blepharitis, and keratitis, have been reported. A reduction in resting heart rate of about 3 beats per minute is common. Hypersensitivity reactions, including local and generalized rashes and urticaria, are rare. Aggravation or precipitation of cardiovascular and pulmonary disorders has been reported, particularly bradyarrhythmias, hypotension, syncope, and bronchospasm. Headache, dyspepsia, nausea, dizziness, hypertension, palpitations, fatigue, confusion, depression, and anxiety have been reported, but rarely.

Parameters of Use

Absorption Systemic absorption does occur and induces mild systemic beta-adrenergic blockade. Onset of action (reduction in intraocular pressure) is within 30 minutes. Peak action occurs in 1 to 2 hours and duration of action is up to 24 hours.

Drug Interactions Additive effects occur with concurrent use of systemic beta-adrenergic blocking agents, such as propranolol or metoprolol. MAO inhibitors and other psychotropic drugs known to potentiate the effects of adrenergic agents may augment the local and systemic effects of timolol. Concurrent use with topical epinephrine may cause visual disturbances.

Administration Initially instill 1 gtt 0.25% solution bid; then increase dosage to 1 gtt 0.5% solution bid if response is inadequate. Dosages above 0.5% solution bid provide little or no additional benefit.

Available Drug Forms Ophthalmic dispenser (Ocumeter) containing 5 or 10 ml of sterile 0.25 or 0.5% solution.

Nursing Management

Planning factors

1. Obtain history of eye, respiratory, and cardiovascular disorders. Notify physician if client has eye infection, bronchial asthma, or severe cardiovascular disorders.
2. Complete tonometric and other eye tests prior to instituting drug.
3. Schedule once-a-day dosages at bedtime.

Administration factors

1. Maintain sterility of solution and inner surface of dropper assembly.
2. Cleanse affected eyelid with sterile pad and normal saline before instillation. Wipe from inner to outer canthus.
3. Pressure-lowering effect stabilizes after about 4 weeks; if indicated, dosage may be reduced to 1 drop daily.
4. Instill medication into lower conjunctival sac being careful to avoid touching the eye with the tip of the dropper.

5. Gently press the inner canthus over the nasolacrimal duct for 1 to 2 minutes to avoid systemic absorption.
6. Instruct client to close eye and move eye in all directions with eyelid closed to disperse the medication.

Evaluation factors

1. Examine eye for irritation or infection prior to instilling medication.
2. Assess blood pressure, pulse, and respiration 24 hours after drug instillation or more frequently as indicated, when drug is first initiated or dosage adjusted.
3. Schedule tonometric and other eye tests periodically, particularly when therapy is first initiated or dosage adjusted.
4. Evaluate intraocular pressure frequently (every 1 to 4 weeks) when therapy is first initiated.

Client teaching factors

1. Instruct client and/or family how to administer eye medication. Demonstration and return demonstration are advisable. Teaching the maintenance of the solution's sterility is essential.
2. Emphasize the necessity of maintaining the dosage schedule despite the lack of symptoms in order to prevent blindness.
3. Inform client to seek medical assistance if itching, burning, or exudate develop around the eye.
4. Inform client to seek medical advice immediately if bradycardia or fainting occur.
5. Emphasize the need for periodic eye examinations.

ANTIINFECTIVE AGENTS

GENERIC NAME Bacitracin (RX)

TRADE NAMES Baciguent, Bacitracin

CLASSIFICATION Ophthalmic antiinfective agent

Action Bacitracin is bactericidal against most gram-positive and some gram-negative organisms. It is ineffective if used with silver nitrate.

Indications for Use Superficial infection of conjunctiva and cornea.

Warnings and Precautions Use with caution in clients with multiple antibiotic allergies.

Untoward Reactions May slow corneal healing. Temporary blurring of vision may occur initially. Irritation of conjunctiva may cause burning and itching.

Administration Apply a small amount every 4 to 6 hours until desired response.

Available Drug Forms Small tubes of sterile ointment.

Nursing Management

Planning Factors

1. Obtain history of the eye infection and any infection in other parts of the body.
2. Assess the frequency with which the client touches his or her face and eyes.
3. Young children and the senile elderly may require clean mittens or elbow restraints to prevent excessive touching of the eye area.
4. Obtain culture and sensitivity studies of the eye exudate.

Administration factors

1. Maintain sterility of container and cap.
2. Gently cleanse affected eyelid with sterile pad and normal saline solution before instillation. Wipe from inner to outer canthus. If both eyes are infected, cleanse each eye separately, using separate sterile supplies.
3. Instill medication into lower conjunctival sac, being careful to avoid touching the eye with the tip of the container.
4. Instruct client to close the eye and move eye in all directions with eyelid closed to disperse the medication.

Evaluation factors

1. Examine eye for irritation prior to instilling medication.
2. Periodically assess the degree of infection still present and record the effectiveness of the drug. Notify the physician if the infection worsens or does not respond to the drug. Another culture of the eye exudate may be required.

Client teaching factors

1. Instruct client to avoid touching or rubbing the eyes.
2. Instruct client and family how to administer eye medication. Demonstration and return demonstration are advisable. Teaching the proper cleansing of the eye and the maintenance of the drug's sterility is essential.
3. Emphasize the necessity of following the dosage schedule and completing the full course of medication, despite cessation of symptoms.
4. Inform client to seek medical assistance if itching, burning, or exudate persist.

GENERIC NAME Chloramphenicol (RX)

TRADE NAMES Chloromycetin, Ophthochlor

CLASSIFICATION Ophthalmic antiinfective agent

Action Chloromycetin ointment contains a base of petrolatum and polyethylene and Ophthochlor solution contains 5 mg/ml of chloramphenicol in boric acid-sodium borate buffer solution without a preservative. Chloramphenicol is a broad-spectrum bacteriostatic agent.

Indications for Use Superficial infection of conjunctiva and cornea.

Untoward Reactions Prolonged use of locally applied drug may cause bone marrow hypoplasia and aplastic anemia. Hypersensitivity reactions include burning, itching of eye, and periocular dermatitis.

Administration Solution: Instill 2 gtt every 2 to 3 hours for 48 hours; then every 4 to 6 hours as indicated until eye appears normal for at least 2 days. Ointment: Apply a small amount q3h for 48 hours as indicated until eye appears normal for at least 2 days.

Available Drug Forms Squeeze dropper bottles containing sterile 0.5% solution; small tubes of sterile 1% ointment.

Nursing Management (See bacitracin.)

1. After infection has subsided, drops may be used during the day and ointment at bedtime.
2. Dispose of solution after 21 days.

GENERIC NAME Erythromycin (RX)

TRADE NAME Ilotycin

CLASSIFICATION Ophthalmic antiinfective agent

Action Erythromycin is a potent antibiotic that is effective against gram-positive and gram-negative bacteria, including *Escherichia coli* and many *Pseudomonas, Klebsiella,* and *Proteus* species. Ointment base contains white petroleum with preservatives. Solution contains 3 mg/ml of erythromycin, sodium phosphates, and sodium chloride solution with benzalkonium chloride. The drug may increase the transcorneal and systemic absorption of gentamicin.

Indications for Use External ophthalmic infections.

Warnings and Precautions Use with caution in clients with hepatic disorders.

Untoward Reactions Prolonged use may cause systemic toxicity. Solution may cause transient irritation. Ointment may cause burning or stinging and retard corneal healing.

Administration Solution: Instill 1 to 2 gtt every 4 to 6 hours. Ointment: Apply a small amount daily, bid, or tid depending on severity of infection. Newborns (prophylaxis): Apply a line of ointment 0.5 to 1 cm long to each conjunctival sac at birth.

Available Drug Forms Squeeze dropper bottles containing 5 ml of sterile solution; small tubes of sterile 0.5% ointment.

Nursing Management (See bacitracin.)

1. Apply a thin line of ointment to lower conjunctival sac using aseptic technique.
2. Maintain sterility of container and cap.
3. After first few days, solution may be used during the day and ointment at bedtime.
4. Store drug at cool room temperature.

GENERIC NAME Gentamicin sulfate (RX)

TRADE NAME Garamycin

CLASSIFICATION Ophthalmic antiinfective agent

Action Gentamicin is an aminoglycoside antibiotic effective against most gram-negative and gram-positive bacteria, including some penicillin-resistant pathogens. Ointment base contains white petroleum and preservatives. Solution contains 3 mg/ml of gentamicin, disodium phosphate, monosodium phosphate, sodium chloride, and benzalkonium chloride as a preservative.

Indications for Use Infections of the external eye, including conjunctivitis, keratitis, corneal ulcers, blepharitis, and dacryocystitis caused by susceptible organisms.

Contraindications Hypersensitivity to any ingredient.

Warnings and Precautions Never inject solution below the conjunctiva or directly into the anterior chamber.

Untoward Reactions Prolonged use may cause overgrowth of nonsusceptible organisms, such as fungi. Solution may cause transient irritation. Ointment may cause occasional burning or stinging and retard corneal healing.

Administration

- *Severe infections:* Instill 2 gtt q1h for 4 to 24 hours; then 1 to 2 gtt q4h.
- *Most infections:* Instill 1 to 2 gtt q4h or apply a small amount of ointment bid or tid.

Available Drug Forms Plastic dropper bottles containing 5 ml of sterile solutions; small tubes of sterile ointment.

Nursing Management (See bacitracin.)

1. Apply a thin line of ointment to lower conjunctival sac using aseptic technique.
2. Maintain sterility of container and cap.
3. Store between 2 to 30 C (36 to 86 F). Avoid contact with heat.

GENERIC NAME Idoxuridine (RX)

TRADE NAMES Dendrid, Herplex, Stoxil

CLASSIFICATION Ophthalmic antiinfective agent

Action Idoxuridine is one of the few antiviral agents on the market. It is useful for short-term use only.

Indications for Use Effective for dendritic keratitis caused by herpes simplex.

Contraindications Hypersensitivity to idoxuridine, open ulcerations or abrasions of the eye structures.

Untoward Reactions May cause a temporary blurring of vision when drug is administered. May cause irritation to eye resulting in inflammation, burning, and edema. May cause photosensitivity. Ointment may retard corneal healing.

Administration Solution: Instill 1 gtt every 1 to 2 hours depending on severity of infection. Ointment: Apply a small amount every 4 to 6 hours depending on severity of infection.

Available Drug Forms Squeeze dropper bottles containing sterile 0.1% solution; small tube of sterile 0.5% ointment.

Nursing Management (See bacitracin.)

1. Check expiration date before using. Ointment is stable for 2 years at room temperature and solution is stable for 1 year when refrigerated.
2. Apply a thin line of ointment to lower conjunctival sac using aseptic technique.
3. Maintain sterility of container and cap.

GENERIC NAME Polymyxin B sulfate (RX)

TRADE NAME Aerosporin

CLASSIFICATION Ophthalmic antiinfective agent

Action Polymyxin is bactericidal against most gram-negative bacilli except *Proteus.*

Indications for Use Severe *Pseudomonas aeruginosa* infections of the conjunctiva or cornea.

Contraindications Hypersensitivity to polymyxins.

Untoward Reactions Mild irritation may occur. Hypersensitivity reactions may result in burning, pain, and edema in and around the eyes.

Administration Instill 1 to 3 gtt q1h until severe infection begins to subside; then gradually increase dosage and intervals; Maximum dosage: 25,000 units/kg/day. Subconjunctival injection: Up to 10,000 units/day.

Available Drug Forms Rubber-stopped multidose vials containing 500,000 units.

Nursing Management (See bacitracin.)

1. Dissolve 500,000 units in 20 to 50 ml of sterile water or saline for injection using sterile technique to yield the following:

Quantity of Added Diluent (ml)	Concentration	
	Units/ml	%
20	10,000	0.1
30	15,000	0.15
40	20,000	0.20
50	25,000	0.25

2. Date and time reconstituted solution. Store at room temperature away from light and heat and discard after 24 hours.

GENERIC NAME Silver nitrate (RX)

TRADE NAME Silver Nitrate

CLASSIFICATION Ophthalmic antiinfective agent

Action The drug contains between 0.95 to 1.05% silver nitrate in water with sodium acetate buffers. It is bactericidal against gonorrheal eye infections. Irritating germicidal and astringent to mucous membranes of eye.

Indications for Use Prevention of gonorrheal ophthalmic neonatorum.

Warnings and Precautions Use with extreme caution since cauterization of cornea with resulting blindness may occur, particularly with repeated use. Highly toxic if ingested.

Untoward Reactions Caustic and irritating to skin and mucous membranes. Chemical conjunctivitis occurs in 20% of newborns.

Administration Newborns (prophylaxis): Instill 2 gtt into each conjunctival sac.

Available Drug Forms Wax ampules containing 1% solution.

Nursing Management (See bacitracin.)

1. Cleanse eyes of newborns with sterile water and cotton. Use a different pledget for each eye and lid.
2. Pierce end of ampule with a sterile needle.
3. Press ampule to expel solution.
4. Instill drops well into conjunctival sac to prevent direct contact with eyeball. Keep in contact with conjunctival sac for 30 seconds or longer.
5. Do not irritate eyes, but wipe excess fluid with sterile pledgets. Wipe from inner to outer aspect of eye.

(Solution stronger than 1% requires irrigations to flush excess medication.)
6. Store at room temperature (59 to 86 F) away from light. Do not administer cold.
7. Drug stains clothes and utensils.

GENERIC NAME Sulfacetamide sodium (RX)

TRADE NAME Sulamyd

CLASSIFICATION Ophthalmic antiinfective agent

Action Sulfacetamide is bacteriostatic against many gram-positive and gram-negative organisms. Solution contains preservatives and sodium dihydrogen phosphate as a buffer. Ointment contains petrolatum, benzalkonium chloride, and other preservatives. Benzalkonium may increase corneal and systemic absorption.

Indications for Use Conjunctivitis, corneal ulcers, other superficial ocular infections, as an adjunct in the treatment of trachoma (may require 2 months of therapy).

Contraindications Hypersensitivity to any ingredient.

Untoward Reactions May cause burning after instilling solution (30% of clients). May slow corneal healing. Severe allergic reactions have been reported.

Drug Interactions Instill anesthetic preparations 1 hour after sulfacetamide to prevent inactivation of sulfacetamide.

Administration Strength of solution depends on the severity of the infection. Solution: Instill 1 to 2 gtt every 2 to 3 hours while awake. Around-the-clock instillation may be required in severe infections until response occurs. Ointment: Apply a small amount qid while awake and at bedtime.

Available Drug Forms Squeeze dropper bottles containing sterile 10 or 30% solution; small tube containing sterile 10% ointment.

Nursing Management (See bacitracin.)

1. Maintain sterility of container and cap.
2. Apply a thin line of ointment to conjunctival sac.
3. Do not use if discolored.
4. Solution may be used during day and ointment at bedtime.
5. Store at cool room temperature (46 to 59 F).

GENERIC NAME Sufisoxazole diolamine (RX)

TRADE NAME Gantrisin

CLASSIFICATION Ophthalmic antiinfective agent

See bacitracin for Nursing management.

Action Sulfisoxazole is bacteriostatic against many gram-positive and gram-negative organisms. Solution is isotonic with mercuric nitrate 1:1,000,000 as a preservative. Ointment base is white petrolatum, mineral oil, and phenylmercuric nitrate 1:50,000 as a preservative.

Indications for Use Conjunctivitis, corneal ulcers, other superficial ocular infections, as an adjunct in the treatment of trachoma (may require 2 months of therapy).

Contraindications Hypersensitivity to any ingredient.

Untoward Reactions May retard corneal healing. Solution may cause mild, transient burning.

Drug Interactions Instill anesthetic preparations 1 hour after sulfisoxazole to prevent inactivation of sulfisoxazole.

Administration Strength of solution depends on the severity of the infection. Solution: Instill 1 to 2 gtt every 2 to 3 hours while awake. Around-the-clock instillation may be required in severe infections until response occurs. Ointment: Apply a small amount qid while awake and at bedtime.

Available Drug Forms Bottles containing sterile 4% solution with dropper; small tubes containing sterile 4% ointment.

GENERIC NAME Tetracycline hydrochloride (RX)

TRADE NAME Achromycin

CLASSIFICATION Ophthalmic antiinfective agent

Action Tetracycline is bacteriostatic against many gram-positive and gram-negative organisms.

Indications for Use Superficial ocular infections, as an adjunct in the treatment of trachoma (may require 2 months of therapy).

Untoward Reactions May cause transient itching of eye area. Hypersensitivity reactions, including pain, edema, and dermatitis, may occur.

Administration Solution: Instill 1 to 2 gtt every 3 to 4 hours, as needed. Mild infections may need only 1 to 2 gtt bid. Ointment: Apply a small amount tid or qid.

Available Drug Forms Squeeze dropper bottles containing sterile 1% solution; small tubes containing sterile 1% ointment.

Nursing Management (See bacitracin.)

1. Maintain sterility of container and cap.
2. Apply a thin line of ointment to conjunctival sac.

3. Solution may be used during day and ointment at bedtime.
4. Store at room temperature away from heat and light.

GENERIC NAME Trifluridine (RX)

TRADE NAME Viroptic

CLASSIFICATION Ophthalmic antiinfective agent

Action Trifluridine (trifluorothymidine) is an antiviral agent effective against herpes simplex virus, types 1 and 2, vacciniavirus, and some strains of Adenovirus. Solution contains acetic acid and sodium acetate as buffers and sodium chloride. The drug is unlikely to be excreted unchanged in human milk, since drug half-life is only 12 minutes following topical administration. It is a relatively nontoxic antiviral ophthalmic agent.

Indications for Use Primary keratoconjunctivitis due to herpes simplex, recurrent epithelial keratitis due to herpes simplex, clients who are unresponsive to idoxuridine or vidarabine, stomal keratitis due to herpes simplex.

Warnings and Precautions Not effective against bacterial, fungal, or chlamydial infections of cornea or nonviral trophic lesions. Repeated use may cause viral resistance to drug. Has the potential of causing a teratogenic reaction; not used during pregnancy unless benefits outweigh risks.

Untoward Reactions Transient burning or stinging may occur upon instillation. Edema of eyelids may occur. Hyperemia and increased intraocular pressure are rare. Superficial punctate keratopathy and epithelial keratopathy have been reported.

Administration Initially instill 1 gtt q2h while awake until corneal ulcer is reepithelialized; Maximum daily dosage: 9 gtt (about 6 to 12 days); then instill 1 gtt q4h while awake for 7 more days; Maximum daily dosage: 5 gtt; Maximum duration of therapy: 21 days.

Available Drug Forms Plastic Drop-Dose dispenser containing sterile 1% solution.

Nursing Management (See bacitracin.)

1. Store in refrigerator (36 to 46 F).
2. Direct instillation into corneal ulcer may be prescribed.
3. Maintain sterility of container and cap.
4. Most ophthalmic drugs can be administered without interaction; but should be given 1 hour before or after trifluridine instillation.

GENERIC NAME Vidarabine (RX)

TRADE NAME Vira-A

CLASSIFICATION Ophthalmic antiinfective agent

Source Purine nucleoside obtained from *Streptomyces antibioticus.*

Action Vidarabine is an antiviral agent effective against herpes simplex virus, types 1 and 2, varicella zoster, and vacciniavirus. It is not effective against Adenovirus and most other RNA and DNA viruses or bacterial, fungal, or chlamydial infections. Ointment contains a petrolatum base. Excretion in breast milk is unlikely, since drug is deaminated in the GI tract.

Indications for Use Acute keratoconjunctivitis due to herpes simplex; recurrent or superficial keratitis due to herpes simplex; clients who are unresponsive to idoxuridine.

Warnings and Precautions Safe use during pregnancy has not been established.

Untoward Reactions Eye irritation, including lacrimation, sensation of presence of foreign body, burning, and photophobia are relatively common. Conjunctival infection, pain, superficial punctate keratitis, and punctal occlusion may occur. Other reactions include uveitis, stromal edema, increased intraocular pressure, trophic defects, corneal vascularization, and hyphema.

Administration Initially apply about 1 inch q3h while awake until corneal ulcer is reepithelialized; Maximum daily dosage: 5 applications; then apply 1 inch bid for 7 more days; Maximum duration of therapy: 21 days.

Available Drug Forms Small tubes containing sterile 3% ointment.

Nursing Management (See bacitracin.)

1. Maintain sterility of container and cap.
2. Store at cool room temperature.

COMBINATION ANTIINFECTIVE PREPARATIONS

TRADE NAME Chloromyxin (RX)

CLASSIFICATION Combination ophthalmic antiinfective preparation

Action Broad-spectrum antiinfective combination.

Indications for Use Superficial infections of conjunctiva or cornea.

Contraindications Hypersensitivity to any ingredient.

Untoward Reactions Bone marrow hypoplasia and aplastic anemia have occurred with local application.

Administration Initially apply a small amount q3h around-the-clock for the first 48 hours; then every 4 to 6 hours while awake; Maximum dosage: 25,000 units/kg/day.

Available Drug Forms Small tubes containing sterile ointment. Generic contents in 1g: polymyxin B sulfate: 10,000 units; chloramphenicol: 10 mg; Base contains liquid petrolatum and polyethylene.

Nursing Management (See bacitracin.)

1. Maintain sterility of container and cap.
2. Apply to lower conjunctival sac.

TRADE NAME Neosporin (RX)

CLASSIFICATION Combination ophthalmic antiinfective preparation

---

Action Neosporin is a broad-spectrum antiinfective effective against gram-negative and gram-positive organisms.

Indications for Use Superficial ocular infections.

Contraindications Hypersensitivity to any ingredient.

Warnings and Precautions Allergic cross-reactions may occur and prevent the use of kanamycin, paromomycin, streptomycin, or gentamicin. May retard corneal healing and cause the overgrowth of nonsusceptible organisms.

Untoward Reactions Neomycin is a common cutaneous sensitizer.

Administration Solution: Instill 1 to 2 gtt bid, tid, or qid. Severe infections may require 1 to 2 gtt every 15 to 30 minutes initially; then frequency of instillation is gradually reduced. Ointment: Apply a small amount every 3 to $4\frac{1}{2}$ hours depending on severity of infection.

Available Drug Forms Drop-Dose squeeze bottles containing sterile solution; small tubes containing sterile ointment. Generic contents in 1 ml: polymyxin B sulfate: 5000 units; neomycin sulfate: 2.5 mg; gramicidin: 0.025 mg; alcohol: 0.5%. Also contains thimerosal as a preservative, propylene glycol, sodium chloride, and purified water. Generic contents in 1 g: polymyxin B sulfate: 5000 units; bacitracin zinc: 400 units; neomycin sulfate: 5 mg; white petrolatum base.

Nursing Management (See bacitracin.)

1. Maintain sterility of container and cap.
2. Apply to lower conjunctival sac.
3. Reculture eye periodically during therapy.

TRADE NAME Polysporin (RX)

CLASSIFICATION Combination ophthalmic antiinfective preparation

---

Action Polysporin is effective against most gram-negative bacilli, including *Pseudomonas aeruginosa* and *Haemophilus influenzae* (polymyxin B) and most gram-positive bacilli and cocci, including hemolytic streptococci (bacitracin).

Indications for Use Superficial ocular infections involving the cornea or conjunctiva.

Contraindications Hypersensitivity to any ingredient.

Warnings and precautions May retard corneal healing and cause the overgrowth of nonsusceptible organisms.

Administration Apply a small amount every 3 to 4 hours depending on severity of infection.

Available Drug Forms Small tubes containing sterile ointment. Generic contents in 1 g: polymyxin B sulfate: 10,000 units; bacitracin zinc: 500 units; white petrolatum base.

Nursing Management (See bacitracin.)

1. Maintain sterility of container and cap.
2. Apply to lower conjunctival sac.

ANTIINFLAMMATORY AGENTS

GENERIC NAME Dexamethasone sodium phosphate

TRADE NAME Decadron (RX)

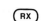

CLASSIFICATION Ophthalmic antiinflammatory agent

Action Dexamethasone is more effective as an antiinflammatory agent than hydrocortisone and induces little or no sodium retention. Solution vehicle includes creatinine, sodium citrate, sodium borate, polysorbate 80, sodium hydroxide, water for injection, and benzalkonium chloride. Ointment base contains white petrolatum and mineral oil.

Indications for Use Acute inflammatory conditions of the conjunctiva, cornea, and anterior segment of the globe, allergic conjunctivitis, keratitis, iritis, cyclitis, corneal injury due to chemical or thermal burns or penetration by foreign bodies.

Warnings and Precautions Safe use during pregnancy has not been established.

Untoward Reactions Prolonged use may caue glaucoma and damage to optic nerve, loss of visual acuity and fields of vision, or the formation of posterior subcapsular cataract. Secondary ocular infections, particularly fungal infections, may occur. Perforations may occur when there is a preexisting thinning of the cornea or sclera (steroid effect). May retard wound healing. Transient stinging and burning may occur, but rarely.

Administration Solution: Initially instill 1 to 2 gtt q1h while awake and q2h at night until favorable response. Ointment: Initially apply a small amount tid or qid until favorable response; then reduce frequency to bid, then daily.

Available Drug Forms Glass bottles containing 2.5 or 5 ml of sterile 0.1% solution with dropper; ophthalmic dispenser (Ocumeter) containing 5 ml with controlled drop tip; small tubes containing 3.5 g of sterile 0.05% ointment.

Nursing Management

1. Maintain sterility of container and cap.
2. Apply to lower conjunctival sac.
3. Eye pads may be prescribed for increased effectiveness.
4. Solution may be used during day and ointment at bedtime.
5. Check intraocular pressure prior to initiating therapy and periodically (weekly) thereafter.

GENERIC NAME Hydrocortisone acetate (RX)

TRADE NAME Hydrocortisone Acetate

CLASSIFICATION Ophthalmic antiinflammatory agent

See dexamethasone sodium phosphate for Indications for use, Warnings and precautions, Untoward reactions, and Administration.

Action Hydrocortisone acetate is an antiinflammatory agent that is more stable but less water-soluble than plain hydrocortisone.

Available Drug Forms Dropper bottles containing 5 ml of sterile 2.5% suspension; small tubes containing 3.5 g of sterile 1.5% ointment.

Nursing Management (See dexamethasone sodium phosphate.)

1. Shake suspension vigorously before measuring dosage.
2. Store at cool room temperature.

GENERIC NAME Prednisolone sodium phosphate

TRADE NAMES Hydeltrasol, Metreton (RX)

CLASSIFICATION Ophthalmic antiinflammatory agent

See dexamethasone sodium phosphate for Warnings and precautions and Untoward reactions.

Action Prednisolone sodium phosphate is an antiinflammatory agent that is a water-soluble derivative of prednisolone. It can be used for long-term therapy.

Indications for Use Usually restricted to inflammation of superficial eye structures, chronic inflammatory disorders.

Administration

- *Acute inflammation:* Initially instill 1 to 2 gtt q1h while awake and q2h at night until favorable response.
- *Chronic inflammation:* Instill 1 to 2 gtt tid or qid.

Available Drug Forms Bottles containing 5 ml with dropper; plastic dropper bottles containing 5 ml of sterile 0.5% solution.

Nursing Management (See dexamethasone sodium phosphate.)

1. Store at 36 to 86 F.
2. Protect from light.

COMBINATION ANTIINFECTIVE AND ANTIINFLAMMATORY PREPARATIONS

TRADE NAME Cortisporin (RX)

CLASSIFICATION Combination ophthalmic antiinfective and antiinflammatory preparation

---

Action Cortisporin is broad-spectrum antiinfective containing antiinflammatory agent 1% hydrocortisone.

Indications for Use Ocular inflammation when concurrent use of antibiotic is necessary.

Contraindications Hypersensitivity to any ingredient, viral infections of the cornea or conjunctiva, mycobacterial or fungal infections of the eye, uncomplicated removal of a corneal foreign body.

Untoward Reactions Prolonged use may cause glaucoma and damage to optic nerve, loss of visual acuity and fields of vision, or the formation of posterior subcapsular cataract. Secondary ocular infections, particularly fungal infections, may occur. Perforations may occur when there is a preexisting thinning of the cornea or sclera (steroid effect). May retard wound healing.

Administration Solution: Initially instill 1 to 2 gtt every 3 to 4 hours depending on severity of infection; then gradually reduce frequency. Ointment: Initially apply a small amount every 3 to 4 hours depending on severity of infection; then reduce frequency until administered once a week.

Available Drug Forms Squeeze dropper bottles containing sterile solution; small tubes containing sterile ointment. Generic contents in 1 ml: polymyxin B sulfate: 10,000 units; neomycin sulfate: 5 mg; hydrocortisone: 10 mg; thimerosal: 0.001%. Solution vehicle contains cetyl alcohol, glyceryl monostearate, mineral oil, polyoxyl 40 stearate, propylene glycol, and water for injection. Generic contents in 1 g: polymyxin B sulfate: 5000 units; bacitracin zinc: 400 units; neomycin sulfate: 5 mg; hydrocortisone: 10 mg; white petrolatum base.

Nursing Management

1. Maintain sterility of container and cap.
2. Apply to lower conjunctival sac.
3. Store at room temperature (59 to 85 F).
4. Shake suspension vigorously before measuring dosage.
5. Reexamination, including culture and measurement of intraocular pressure, should be done every 10 days or after 20 ml or 8 g of medication, whichever comes first.

TRADE NAME Metimyd (RX)

CLASSIFICATION Combination ophthalmic antiinfective and antiinflammatory preparation

---

Action Benzalkonium chloride may increase intraocular and systemic absorption.

Indications for Use Ocular inflammation when concurrent use of an antibiotic is necessary.

Contraindications Hypersensitivity to any ingredient, viral infections of the cornea or conjunctiva, mycobacterial fungal infections of the eye, uncomplicated removal of corneal foreign body.

Untoward Reactions Mydriasis, loss of accommodation, and ptosis have been reported. (See cortisporin.)

Administration Solution: Initially instill 2 to 3 gtt every 1 to 2 hours while awake and at bedtime until condition subsides; then gradually reduce frequency. Ointment: Initially apply a small amount tid or qid while awake and at bedtime until condition subsides; then gradually reduce frequency.

Available Drug Forms Dropper bottles containing 5 ml of sterile suspension; small tubes containing 3.5 g of sterile ointment. Generic contents in 1 ml: prednisolone acetate: 5 mg; sulfacetamide sodium: 100 mg. Solution vehicle contains disodium hydrogen phosphate, tyloxapol, purified water, phenylethyl alcohol, benzalkonium chloride, and sodium thiosulfate. Generic contents in 1 g: prednisolone acetate: 5 mg; sulfacetamide sodium: 100 mg. Ointment base contains mineral oil and white petrolatum.

Nursing Management

1. Shake suspension vigorously before measuring dosage.
2. Maintain sterility of container and cap.
3. Apply to lower conjunctival sac.
4. Store at cool room temperature (36 to 86 F) and protect from light.
5. Solution may be used during day, ointment at bedtime.
6. Reexamination, including culture and measurement of intraocular pressure, should be done every 10 days or after 20 ml or 8 g of medication, whichever comes first.

TRADE NAME Neodecadron (RX)

CLASSIFICATION Combination ophthalmic antiinfective and antiinflammatory preparation

---

Action Benzalkonium chloride may increase intraocular absorption.

Indications for Use Ocular inflammation when concurrent use of an antibiotic is necessary.

Contraindications Hypersensitivity to any ingredient, viral infections of the cornea or conjunctiva, mycobacterial or fungal infections of the eye, uncomplicated removal of a corneal foreign body.

Untoward Reactions Prolonged use may cause glaucoma and damage to optic nerve, loss of visual acuity and fields of vision, or the formaton of posterior subcapsular cataract. Secondary ocular infections, particularly fungal infections, may occur. Perforations may occur when there is a preexisting thinning of the cornea or sclera (steroid effect). May retard wound healing.

Administration Solution: Initially instill 1 to 2 gtt q1h while awake and q2h at night until favorable response; then gradually reduce frequency to 1 gtt q4h; then 1 gtt tid or qid. Ointment: Initially apply a small amount tid or qid until favorable response; then reduce frequency to bid, then daily.

Available Drug Forms Bottles containing 2.5 or 5 ml with dropper; ophthalmic dispenser (Ocumeter) containing 5 ml; small tubes containing 3.5 g of sterile ointment. Generic contents in 1 ml: dexamethasone sodium phosphate: 1 mg; neomycin sulfate: 3.5 mg. Solution vehicle contains creatinine, sodium citrate, sodium borate, polysorbate 80, sodium hydroxide, water for injection, benzalkonium chloride, and sodium bisulfite. Generic contents in 1 g: dexamethasone sodium phosphate: 0.5 mg; neomycin sulfate: 3.5 mg. Ointment base contains petrolatum and mineral oil.

Nursing Management

1. Maintain sterility of container and cap.
2. Apply to lower conjunctival sac.
3. Reexamination, including culture and measurement of intraocular pressure, should be done every 10 days or after 20 ml or 8 g of medication, whichever comes first.

TRADE NAME Neo-Hydeltrasol (RX)

CLASSIFICATION Combination ophthalmic antiinfective and antiinflammatory preparation

---

See neodecadron for Indications for use, Contraindications, Untoward reactions, and Nursing management.

Action Neo-Hydeltrasol is similar to Neodecadron, but probably induces more intraocular absorption of steroid.

Administration Instill 1 to 2 gtt q1h at night until favorable response; then gradually reduce frequency to 1 gtt q4h; then 1 gtt tid or qid.

Available Drug Forms Bottles containing 2.5 or 5 ml of sterile solution with dropper. Generic contents in 1 ml: prednisolone sodium phosphate: 5 mg; neomycin sulfate: 3.5 mg. Solution vehicle contains creatinine, sodium citrate, polysorbate 80, disodium edetate, potassium phosphate, hydrochloric acid, water for injection, and benzalkonium chloride.

TRADE NAME Optimyd (RX)

CLASSIFICATION Combination ophthalmic antiinfective and antiinflammatory preparation

---

See Metimyd for Action, Indications for use, Contraindications, Untoward reactions, and Nursing management.

Administration Initially instill 1 to 2 gtt q1h while awake and at bedtime; then gradually reduce frequency to 1 to 2 gtt every 3 to 4 hours and at bedtime.

Available Drug Forms Generic contents in 1 ml: prednisolone sodium phosphate: 5.5 mg; sulfacetamide sodium: 100 mg. Solution vehicle contains sodium thiosulfate, tyloxapol, sodium phosphate, sodium hydroxide, purified water, benzalkonium chloride, and phenylethyl alcohol.

Mydriatic Agents

GENERIC NAME Atropine sulfate (RX)

TRADE NAMES Atropisol, Buf-Opto Atropine, Isopto Atropine

CLASSIFICATION Mydriatic

Action Atropine is an antimuscarinic agent that competitively blocks the action of acetylcholine at muscarinic receptor sites. It has an antispasmodic effect on smooth muscle and decreases the secretions from exocrine glands, including the lacrimal glands. Atropine is the most potent mydriatic agent available, and it has a prolonged duration of action. Besides dilating of the pupil, it also has a cycloplegic effect (causes paralysis of the ciliary muscles of accommodation).

Indications for Use Acute iritis, iridocyclitis, keratitis, choroiditis, eye examinations, cycloplegic refraction.

Contraindications Narrow-angle glaucoma, urinary retention or prostatic hypertrophy, myasthenia gravis.

Warnings and Precautions Use with caution in clients with hyperthyroidism, coronary artery disease, arrhythmias, hypertension, and in debilitated clients with chronic obstructive pulmonary disease. May precipitate latent glaucoma or urinary retention in clients over 40. Children under 6 years may have an exaggerated response to the drug's action.

Untoward Reactions Elevated intraocular pressure, blurred vision, photophobia, dryness of eyes, conjunctivitis (long-term use).

Drug Interactions Antagonizes the action of anticholinesterase. Drugs that have anticholinergic activity may have additive or potentiating effects when given concurrently.

Administration

- *Inflammation:* Adults: Instill 1 to 2 gtt 1% solution bid or tid; Children: Instill 1 to 2 gtt 0.5% solution bid or tid.
- *Refraction:* Adults: Instill 1 to 2 gtt 1% solution 1 hour before examination; Children: Instill 1 to 2 gtt 0.5% solution bid for 1 to 3 days before examination and again immediately before.

Available Drug Forms Solutions and ointments.

Nursing Management

Planning factors

1. Obtain history of the eye disorder. Notify physician if client has eye infection or severe cardiovascular disorder.
2. Complete tonometric and other eye tests prior to instituting drug.

Administration factors

1. Double-check the strength of the solution, since several concentrations are available.
2. Maintain the sterility of solution and inner surfaces of dropper assembly.
3. Cleanse affected eyelid with sterile pad and normal saline solution before instillation. Wipe from inner to outer canthus.
4. Instill medication into lower conjunctival sac, being careful to avoid touching the eye with the tip of the dropper.
5. Apply gentle pressure to inner canthus of eye for at least 2 minutes after instilling medication to minimize systemic reactions.
6. Instruct client to close eye and move eye in all directions with eyelid closed to disperse the medication.

Evaluation factors

1. Examine eye for irritation or infection prior to instilling medication.
2. Some drug may be absorbed, particularly in children. Watch for secondary reactions.

Client teaching factors

1. Instruct client to avoid hazardous activities as long as drug-induced blurring of vision occurs.
2. Warn client to wear sunglasses in bright light for remainder of day.

GENERIC NAME Cyclopentolate hydrochloride

TRADE NAMES Cyclogyl, Mydplegic (RX)

CLASSIFICATION Mydriatic

See atropine sulfate for Contraindications.

Action Cyclopentolate produces cyclopegia and mydriasis rapidly, but has a short duration of action (about 24 hours or 6 hours after reversal). Heavily pigmented iritis often requires twice the normal dosage. The pH of 1% solution is 5.0 to 5.4.

Indications for Use Eye examinations, particularly refractory studies. Has been used for inflammatory eye disorders.

Warnings and Precautions Not recommended for children under 6 years.

Untoward Reactions Burning sensation upon instillation, photophobia, blurred vision, eye dryness, edema, conjunctivitis.

Administration

- *Inflammation:* Instill 1 to 3 gtt 0.5, 1, or 2% solution tid or qid.
- *Examination:* Adults: Instill 1 gtt 1% solution; repeat in 5 minutes. Children: Instill 1 gtt 0.5, 1, or 2% solution; repeat with half the initial strength in 5 minutes.

Available Drug Forms Solution 0.5, 1, or 2%.

Nursing Management (See atropine sulfate.)

1. Warn client to wear sunglasses in bright light for remainder of day.
2. Drug causes a minimal elevation in intraocular pressure, but observe elderly clients for glaucoma symptoms.

GENERIC NAME Homatropine hydrobromide

TRADE NAME Homatropine (RX)

CLASSIFICATION Mydriatic

See atropine sulfate for Nursing management.

Action Homatropine is weaker and less toxic than atropine, but is more rapid acting (15 to 20 minutes). Duration of action is about 24 hours, but can be reversed in 4 to 6 hours.

Indications for Use Eye examinations, cycloplegia, refraction, inflammatory eye disorders.

Untoward Reactions Blurred vision, photophobia, eye irritation.

Drug Interactions Solutions are incompatible with alkaline substances; precipitate will form.

Administration

- *Inflammation:* Instill 1 to 2 gtt every 3 to 4 hours while awake.
- *Examination:* Instill 1 to 2 gtt; repeat in 5 minutes.

Available Drug Forms Solution 2 or 5%.

GENERIC NAME Hydroxyamphetamine hydrobromide

TRADE NAME Paredrine (RX)

CLASSIFICATION Mydriatic

See atropine sulfate for Nursing management.

Action Hydroxyamphetamine has a more rapid onset and recovery than atropine. It is often combined with atropine to produce greater dilation of pupil. The drug produces little or no CNS stimulation, but may shrink nasal mucosa.

Indications for Use Diagnostic agent for Horner's syndrome, eye examinations.

Contraindications Narrow-angle glaucoma.

Administration Adults and children over 12 years: 1 to 2 gtt 1% solution.

Available Drug Forms Solution 0.25 or 1%.

GENERIC NAME Phenylephrine hydrochloride

TRADE NAMES Mydfrin, Neo-Synephrine (RX)

CLASSIFICATION Mydriatic

Action Phenylephrine is an effective mydriatic agent that may cause nasal dryness.

Indications for Use Eye examinations, mydriasis without cyclopegia, uveitis.

Untoward Reactions May cause transient burning or stinging upon instillation. Systemic absorption may cause hypertension and premature ventricular contractions. Elderly clients may have a systemic reaction when 10% solution is used.

- *Examination:* Instill 1 gtt 2.5 or 10% solution.
- *Adhesions of iris:* Instill 1 gtt 10% solution; do not use in infants or young children.

Available Drug Forms Solution 0.25 or 10%. An ingredient in several solutions used for eye irritation, including Isopto-Finn, Prefrin, and Tear-Efrin.

Nursing Management Check vital signs q1h. (See atropine sulfate.)

GENERIC NAME Scopolamine hydrobromide

TRADE NAME Isopto-Hyoscine (RX)

CLASSIFICATION Mydriatic

See atropine sulfate for Nursing management.

Action Similar action to atropine.

Indications for Use Eye examinations (cycloplegic refraction), inflammatory eye disorders.

Untoward Reactions Prolonged use may cause edema and conjunctivitis. Blurred vision and photophobia are common. May increase intraocular pressure and cause dryness of eyes.

Administration

- *Inflammation:* Instill 1 to 2 gtt 0.1% solution daily, bid, or tid.
- *Examination:* Adults: Instill 1 to 2 gtt 0.5 or 1% solution 1 hour before examination; Children: Instill 1 gtt 0.2 or 0.25% solution bid for 2 days before examination.

Available Drug Forms Solution 0.1, 0.2, 0.25, 0.5, or 1%.

GENERIC NAME Tropicamide (RX)

TRADE NAME Mydriacyl

CLASSIFICATION Mydriatic

See atropine sulfate for Nursing management.

Action Tropicamide has greater mydriatic effect than cycloplegic effect. It has a short duration of action (about 2 to 6 hours.)

Indications for Use Eye examinations (cycloplegic refraction, fungal infections).

Untoward Reactions Causes transient stinging sensation upon instillation, blurred vision, and photophobia.

Administration Instill 1 to 2 gtt 1% solution; repeat in 5 minutes. An additional drop may be required in 20 to 30 minutes.

Available Drug Forms Solution 0.5 or 1%.

OTHER OPHTHALMIC AGENTS

GENERIC NAME Alpha-chymotrypsin (RX)

TRADE NAMES Alpha Chymar, Alpha Chymolean

CLASSIFICATION Ophthalmic agent

Action This enzyme exerts a selective lytic action on zonule fibers of the lens, thus freeing the lens for removal.

Indications for Use As an adjunct in cataract and other ophthalmic surgical procedures.

Untoward Reactions Large dosages may cause an increase in intraocular pressure. Uveitis and corneal irritation have been reported. May delay healing of the operative site.

Drug Interactions Inactivated by alcohol and surgical detergents. Synergistic with prednisolone.

Administration Highly individualized.

Available Drug Forms Vials containing sterile powder for reconstitution.

Nursing Management

1. Reconstitute solution at time of use and discard unused portion.
2. Do not use solution if cloudy or if a precipitate has formed.
3. Injected by physician.

GENERIC NAME Hyaluronate sodium (RX)

TRADE NAME Healon

CLASSIFICATION Ophthalmic agent

Action Vehicle contains physiologic sodium chloride with a phosphate buffer. This physiologic substance is found in the extracellular matrix of connective tissue, including vitreous and aqueous humor. It also has viscoelastic properties and maintains the shape of anterior eye structures in the absence of aqueous humor, thus preventing the formation of a flat chamber during surgery. The drug is absorbed after 6 to 7 days.

Indications for Use Ophthalmic surgical aide in various anterior segment procedures (cataract surgery), vitreous replacement after vitrectomy.

Untoward Reactions Postoperative elevation in intraocular pressure may develop. May cause inflammation, but rarely.

Administration Highly individualized.

Available Drug Forms Disposable glass syringes containing 10 mg/ml.

Nursing Management

1. Store in refrigerator; but warm drug to room temperature before administering (about 30 minutes).
2. Protect from light.
3. Injected by physician.

GENERIC NAME Hydroxypropy cellulose (RX)

TRADE NAME Lacrisert

CLASSIFICATION Ophthalmic agent

Action Hydroxypropy cellulose combines with tears, stabilizes and thickens the precorneal tear film, and prolongs the tear film breakup time. It lubricates and protects the eyes.

Indications for Use Dry eye syndrome, keratoconjunctivitis sicca.

Untoward Reactions Transient blurring and matting of eyelashes are relatively common. Photophobia, ocular irritation, hyperemia, and edema of eyelids have been reported.

Administration Insert 1 Lacrisert in each eye daily or bid.

Available Drug Forms Rod-shaped water-soluble substance containing 5 mg.

Nursing Management

1. Insert Lacrisert into the inferior cul-de-sac of the eye beneath the base of the tarsus.
2. See manufacturer's instructions and illustrations.
3. Store at room temperature (below 86 F).
4. Warn client to avoid driving a car or engaging in other potentially hazardous activities.

COMBINATION OPHTHALMIC PREPARATIONS

TRADE NAMES Artificial Tears (Absorbotear, Hypotears, Isopto-Plain, Isopto-Tears, Liquifilm Tears, Lyteers, Methulose, Neotears, Tearisol, Tears Plus, Ultra Tears, Visculose) (OTC) (RX)

CLASSIFICATION Combination ophthalmic preparation

Action These preparations have a pH similar to that of the eyes. They provide moisture to prevent further drying with resulting lesions.

Indications for Use Dry eye syndrome.

Administration Instill 1 to 3 gtt tid or qid while awake. Unconscious clients: Instill 1 to 2 gtt every 2 to 4 hours.

Available Drug Forms Generic contents vary with the solution used. Many contain one or more of the following ingredients: boric acid, polyvinyl alcohol, normal saline, sodium borate, water.

Nursing Management

1. Clean eyes before using.
2. Instill into lower conjunctival sac.
3. Maintain sterility of container and cap.

TRADE NAME Clear Eyes (OTC)

CLASSIFICATION Combination ophthalmic preparation

Action Decongestant ophthalmic solution that soothes and decreases redness (vasoconstriction) of eye.

Indications for Use Minor eye irritations.

Administration Instill 1 to 2 gtt bid or tid.

Available Drug Forms Plastic dropper bottles containing 15 or 45 ml. Generic contents: naphazoline hydrochloride 0.012%, boric acid, sodium borate, water, benzalkonium chloride 0.01%, methylcellulose, edetate disodium 0.1%.

Nursing Management Keep container tightly closed.

TRADE NAMES Collyrium; Collyrium with Ephedrine

CLASSIFICATION Combination ophthalmic preparation (OTC)

Indications for Use Minor eye irritations due to smog, wind, sun glare, or excessive use of eyes for reading.

Warnings and Precautions Do not use with wetting agents containing polyvinyl alcohol.

Administration *Collyrium:* $\frac{1}{2}$ eye cupful prn. *Collyrium with Ephedrine:* Instill 2 to 3 gtt prn.

Available Drug Forms *Collyrium:* Bottles containing 6 fl oz with eye cup. *Collyrium with Ephredrine:* Bottles containing $\frac{1}{2}$ fl oz. Collyrium is a neutral solution of boric acid with antipyrine 0.4%, and thimerosal 0.002%. Collyrium with Ephedrine also contains ephedrine 0.1%.

Nursing Management

1. Instruct client in the use of an eye cup or eye drops and the prevention of eye contamination.
2. Instruct client to consult physician if irritation persists.
3. Keep container tightly closed and at room temperature.

TRADE NAME Murine Eye Drops (OTC)

CLASSIFICATION Combination ophthalmic preparation

Indication for Use Minor eye irritations.

Administration Instill 2 to 3 gtt tid or qid.

Available Drug Forms Plastic dropper bottles containing 15 or 45 ml. Generic contents: glycerin, potassium chloride, sodium chloride, sodium phosphate, water, methylcellulose, edetate disodium, benzalkonium chloride.

Nursing Management Keep container tightly closed.

TRADE NAME Murine Plus Eye Drops (OTC)

CLASSIFICATION Combination ophthalmic preparation

Action Decongestant ophthalmic solution.

Indications for Use Minor eye irritations.

Administration Instill 1 to 2 gtt bid or tid.

Available Drug Forms Plastic dropper bottles containing 15 or 45 ml. Generic contents: tetrahydrozoline hydrochloride 0.05%, boric acid, sodium borate, water, benzalkonium chloride 0.01%, edetate disodium 0.1%.

Nursing Management Keep container tightly closed.

TRADE NAME Succus Cineraria Maritima (RX)

CLASSIFICATION Combination ophthalmic preparation

Action Increases circulation in intraocular tissues and stimulates collateral circulation and normal metabolism, thus preventing further cataract formation.

Indications for Use Treatment of cataracts when detected early, certain optic opacities.

Contraindications Hypersensitivity to any ingredient.

Administration Instill 2 gtt bid.

Available Drug Forms Sterile dropper vials containing 7 ml. Aqueous and glycerin solution of senecio cineraria with witch hazel 20% and boric acid.

Chapter 80

Otic Agents

THE EXTERNAL EAR is a body cavity lined with epidermal tissue and is therefore subject to the same considerations as other dermal surfaces. The exception to this is when there is suspected or definite perforation of the tympanic membrane; in this case, the aural cavity is treated as a mucous membrane.

Medications administered to the external ear for local effect are usually instilled as drops. The container of solution should be warmed to body temperature in order to avoid dizziness from thermal stimulation of the semicircular canals. Although the ear canal is not sterile, ear medications should be kept as clean as possible in order to avoid ear infections. When a cotton plug is used to block the canal opening after applying medications, the plug will act as a wick and draw the drug solution away from the canal unless it is first moistened with one or two drops of the prescribed medication.

PROPERTIES OF CERUMENOLYTIC AGENTS

Some clients are plagued with excessive production of cerumen, which forms into clumps and plugs the ear canal. Cerumenolytic agents are used to lower the surface tension of the cerumen so that it can either drain out of the canal on its own or be easily removed by irrigation.

PROPERTIES OF ANTIINFECTIVE AGENTS

External ear infections are common in children and individuals who swim frequently. Swimmer's ear develops when contaminated water is trapped in the ear canal for a period of time. The ear canal should be cultured before an antiinfective agent is instilled to ensure that the correct drug is used for the pathogen involved. Clients with ear infections should avoid swimming or at least keep their ears out of the water until the infection is eliminated. When inflammation of the external ear accompanies an infection, a preparation containing both an antiinfective and antiinflammatory agent should be used and the ear canal should be inspected periodically for the development of a secondary infection.

NURSING MANAGEMENT

When instilling ear medications, the client should be in a sidelying position without a pillow, or with a small pillow. This position should be maintained long enough for the drug to enter deep into the external canal. Clients should be instructed in the proper technique for ear drop instillation and should be cautioned to keep the drug container at room temperature in order to avoid dizziness. If the client warms the drug container to body temperature, he or she should be warned to test the temperature of the solution on the forearm before instilling the medication so that an accidental burn to the ear canal does not occur.

CERUMENOLYTIC AGENTS

GENERIC NAME Triethanolamine polypeptide oleate-condensate

TRADE NAME Cerumenex (RX)

CLASSIFICATION Cerumenolytic agent

Action Triethanolamine 10% in propylene glycol is a surfactant that lowers the surface tension of cerumen and reduces clumps of cerumen to smaller particles. Removal of cerumen is facilitated as the cerumen particles become suspended in this aqueous-miscible solution. The drug solution has a hydrophilic property that causes it to absorb water and serous exudate. Triethanolamine is also reported to have a bacteriostatic effect.

Indications for Use Impacted cerumen, removal of cerumen prior to ear examination, audiometry, or drug therapy to the external auditory canal.

Contraindications Hypersensitivity to any ingredient, perforated eardrum, otitis media (if eardrum is in danger of perforation).

Warnings and Precautions Use with caution in clients with a history of multiple allergies.

Untoward Reactions Localized dermatitis ranging from mild erythema and pruritus to severe eczematoid reactions lasting for 2 to 10 days has been reported. Local irritation can result from prolonged exposure or too frequent use of drug. Eczema-type reactions tend to occur in clients with a history of multiple allergies. Dizziness, nausea, and vomiting may occur if the drug is instilled at a cold temperature.

Administration Adults and children: Fill ear canal with drug solution and plug opening with cotton wad. After 15 to 30 minutes irrigate ear canal with warm water or saline. Procedure can be repeated as necessary.

Available Drug Forms Bottles containing 6 or 12 ml with a blunt-end dropper.

Nursing Management

Planning factors

1. A patch test is recommended.
2. If perforation of eardrum is suspected, notify physician before instilling medication.
3. Keep drug bottle tightly closed when not in use.
4. Warm drug bottle in warm water for 30 minutes before using. Avoid using solutions that are not at or near body temperature.

Administration factors

1. Apply 1 or 2 drops of drug solution to forearm to determine if solution is at body temperature. Avoid using cold or hot solution.
2. With client lying on unaffected side, straighten ear canal and instill warm solution until canal is filled. Avoid contact with periaural tissue.
3. Place 2 or 3 drops of drug solution on inner surface of cotton plug and insert in ear canal opening.
4. Have client remain in position for 2 to 3 minutes.
5. After 15 to 30 minutes, gently irrigate ear canal with tepid saline or water. Avoid undue exposure of pinna and periaural tissue to ear drainage.
6. Wash pinna with water after irrigation.

Evaluation factors

1. Gently examine ear canal with otoscope and record amount and location of cerumen present.
2. Examine skin of canal and pinna for irritation. Notify physician of any untoward reaction.

Client teaching factors

1. Instruct client's family in the proper instillation of ear drops and ear irrigation.
2. Emphasize the importance of avoiding prolonged exposure to drug solution.
3. Instruct client to use warm solution; but to avoid excessive hot or cold solution. Medication can be administered if it is at room temperature (70 to 80 F).
4. Instruct client to store drug solution with cap tightly closed and away from moisture.

GENERIC NAME Carbamide peroxide (OTC)

TRADE NAMES Debrox, Murine Ear Wax Removal System

CLASSIFICATION Cerumenolytic agent

See triethanolamine polypeptide oleate-condensate for Contraindications, Warnings and precautions, and Untoward reactions.

Action Debrox (carbamide peroxide 6.5% in anhydrous glycerol) and Murine Ear Wax Removal System (carbamide peroxide 6.5% in anhydrous glycerin) penetrate, soften, and facilitate the removal of cerumen without causing swelling of cerumen. The peroxide releases oxygen to form a foam, which breaks up wax accumulations.

Indications for Use Prevention and treatment of ceruminosis.

Administration *Debrox:* Instill 5 to 10 gtt tid or qid, as needed. *Murine Ear Wax Removal System:* Instill 5 gtt bid for 3 to 4 days.

Available Drug Forms Squeeze dropper bottles containing 15 or 30 ml with applicator.

Nursing Management Avoid touching tip of drug bottle to ear (Debrox). (See triethanolamine polypeptide oleate-condensate.)

ANTIINFECTIVE AGENTS

GENERIC NAME Chloramphenicol (RX)

TRADE NAMES Chloromycetin Otic, Sopamycetin

CLASSIFICATION Otic antiinfective agent

Action Chloramphenicol is a broad-spectrum bacteriostatic agent that is effective against gram-positive and gram-negative organisms, including *Staphylococcus aureus, Escherichia coli, Hemophilus influenzae, Pseudomonas aeruginosa,* and *Proteus.*

Indications for Use Superficial infections of the external auditory canal.

Contraindications Hypersensitivity to any ingredient.

Warnings and Precautions Prolonged use may cause overgrowth of fungi and other nonsusceptible organisms.

Untoward Reactions Local irritation and vesicular or maculopapular dermatitis may occur. Bone marrow hypoplasia, including aplastic anemia, has been reported following local application.

Administration Instill 2 to 3 gtt tid.

Available Drug Forms Bottles containing 15 ml with a dropper. Generic contents: chloramphenicol 0.5%, propylene glycol.

Nursing Management

Planning factors

1. If perforation of eardrum is suspected, notify physician before instilling medication.
2. Warm drug bottle to at least 70°F before using.
3. Obtain history of the ear infection. Culture the ear canal before starting medication.

Administration factors

1. Apply 1 or 2 drops of drug solution to forearm to determine if solution is at body temperature. Avoid using cold or hot solution.
2. With client lying on unaffected side, instill warm solution until the ear canal is filled. Avoid contact with periaural tissue.
3. Moisten inner surface of cotton plug with 1 to 2 drops of medication before inserting.
4. Have client remain in position for 2 to 3 minutes.

Evaluation factors

1. Examine the ear canal periodically with an otoscope to monitor drug's effectiveness and to determine if a secondary infection may be present. Reculture ear periodically.
2. Examine skin of canal and pinna periodically for irritation. Notify physician of any untoward reactions.
3. Observe for sore throat and other early signs of drug toxicity.

Client teaching factors

1. Instruct client's family in the proper instillation of ear drops.
2. Instruct client to use warm solution, but to avoid excessive hot or cold solution. Medication may be administered at room temperature.

GENERIC NAME Polymyxin B/neomycin/hydrocortisone (solution)

TRADE NAMES Cortisporin, Otocort, Polymyxin B-Neomycin-Hydrocortisone

CLASSIFICATION Otic antiinfective agent (RX)

Action Bactericidal agent effective against various strains of *Bacillus polymyxa* (polymyxin), *Proteus* (neomycin), and other gram-positive and gram-negative organisms. The 1% hydrocortisone content provides antiinflammatory, antipruritic, and antiallergic activity.

Indications for Use Acute and chronic external otitis.

Contraindications Hypersensitivity to any ingredient, herpes simplex, vaccinia, varicella.

Warnings and Precautions Prolonged use may cause overgrowth of fungi and other nonsusceptible organisms and neomycin-induced ototoxicity.

Untoward Reactions Hypersensitivity to neomycin may cause erythema, swelling, dry scaling, and itchy tissue. May cause stinging and burning if drug enters middle ear.

Administration Instill 3 to 4 gtt tid or qid or insert a cotton wick moistened with 3 to 4 gtt q4h and replace at least every 24 hours.

Available Drug Forms Bottles containing 10 ml with dropper; squeeze dropper bottles containing 60 ml. Generic contents in 1 ml: polymyxin B sulfate: 10,000 units; neomycin sulfate: 5 mg; hydrocortisone: 10 mg. Solution vehicle contains cupric sulfate, glycerin, hydrochloric acid, propylene glycol, water, and potassium metabisulfite.

Nursing Management (See chloramphenicol.)

1. Client should maintain a sidelying position for 5 minutes after instillation to facilitate penetration into canal.
2. Moisten cotton plug with 1 to 2 drops before inserting.
3. Reculture ear after 1 week.

GENERIC NAME Polymyxin B/neomycin/hydrocortisone (suspension)

TRADE NAMES Cortisporin, Polymyxin B-Neomycin-Hydrocortisone

CLASSIFICATION Otic antiinfective agent (RX)

Action Similar to cortisporin solution, but less irritating to middle ear and other structures.

Indications for Use External otitis infections following mastoidectomy, otitis media when eardrum is perforated.

Contraindications Hypersensitivity to any ingredient, herpes simplex, vaccinia, varicella.

Warnings and Precautions Prolonged use may cause overgrowth of fungi and other nonsusceptible organisms and neomycin-induced ototoxicity.

Untoward Reactions Hypersensitivity to neomycin.

Administration Instill 3 to 4 gtt tid or qid; duration of treatment is usually 10 days.

Available Drug Forms Bottles containing 10 ml with dropper. Generic contents in 1 ml: polymyxin B sulfate: 10,000 units; neomycin sulfate: 5 mg; hydrocortisone: 10 mg. Suspension vehicle contains cetyl alcohol, propylene glycol, polysorbate 80, water, and thimerosal.

Nursing Management (See chloramphenicol.)

1. Shake suspension vigorously before drawing solution into dropper.
2. Client should maintain a sidelying position for 5 minutes after instillation to facilitate penetration into canal.
3. Moisten cotton plug with 1 to 2 drops before inserting.
4. Reculture ear after 1 week.

GENERIC NAME Polymyxin B/hydrocortisone

TRADE NAME Pyocidin-Otic (RX)

CLASSIFICATION Otic antiinfective agent

Action Polymyxin B is effective against *Pseudomonas aeruginosa* and other pathogens. Hydrocortisone content provides antiallergic and antiinflammatory activity.

Indications for Use External otitis.

Contraindications Hypersensitivity to any ingredient, herpes simplex, vaccinia, varicella.

Warnings and Precautions Prolonged use may cause overgrowth of fungi and other nonsusceptible organisms.

Administration Instill 3 to 4 gtt tid or qid or insert a cotton wick moistened with 3 to 4 gtt q4h and replace every 24 hours.

Available Drug Forms Bottles containing 10 ml with dropper. Generic contents in 1 ml: polymyxin B sulfate: 10,000 units; hydrocortisone: 5 mg; propylene glycol, water.

Nursing Management (See chloramphenicol.)

1. Client should maintain a sidelying position for 5 minutes after instillation to facilitate penetration into canal.
2. Moisten cotton plug with 1 to 2 drops before inserting.
3. Reculture ear after 1 week.

GENERIC NAME Polymyxin B/lidocaine/propylene glycol

TRADE NAMES Lidosporin, Polymyxin B-Lidocaine-Propylene Glycol

CLASSIFICATION Otic antiinfective agent (RX)

Action Polymyxin B is bactericidal against most gram-negative bacilli. Propylene glycol absorbs moisture, thereby drying the canal tissues. The 5% lidocaine content relieves pain and itching.

Indications for Use Relief of infection, pain, and itching associated with external otitis and furunculosis.

Contraindications Hypersensitivity to any ingredient.

Warnings and Precautions Prolonged use may cause overgrowth of nonsusceptible organisms.

Administration Instill 3 to 4 gtt tid or qid or insert a cotton wick moistened with 3 to 4 gtt every 4 to 6 hours and replace every 24 to 48 hours.

Available Drug Forms Bottles containing 10 ml with dropper. Generic contents in 1 ml: polymyxin B sulfate: 10,000 units; lidocaine hydrochloride: 50 mg; purified water: 0.022 ml; propylene glycol qs.

Nursing Management (See chloramphenicol.)

1. Client should maintain a sidelying position for 5 minutes after instillation to facilitate penetration into canal.
2. Moisten cotton plug with 1 to 2 drops before inserting.
3. Reculture ear after 1 week.

GENERIC NAME Colistin sulfate/neomycin/hydrocortisone

TRADE NAME Coly-Mycin S Otic (RX)

CLASSIFICATION Otic antiinfective agent

Action Colistin is bactericidal against most gram-negative organisms. Neomycin is bactericidal against *Staphylococcus aureus* and *Proteus*. The 1% hydrocortisone content provides antiinflammatory and antipruritic activity. Thonzonium is a surfactant that promotes penetration and dispersion of cellular debris and exudate.

Indications for Use External otitis, otitis media when eardrum is perforated, infection following mastoidectomy.

Contraindications Hypersensitivity to any ingredient, herpes simplex, vaccinia, varicella.

Warnings and Precautions Prolonged use may cause overgrowth of fungi and nonsusceptible organisms.

Untoward Reactions Hypersensitivity to neomycin.

Administration Instill 3 to 4 gtt tid or qid or insert a cotton wick moistened with 3 to 4 gtt q4h and replace at least every 24 hours.

Available Drug Forms Bottles containing 5 or 10 ml with dropper. Generic contents in 1 ml: colistin sulfate: 3 mg; neomycin sulfate: 3.3 mg; hydrocortisone acetate: 10 mg; thonzonium bromide: 0.5 mg. Also contains polysorbate 80, acetic acid, sodium acetate, and thimerosal.

Nursing Management (See chloramphenicol.)

1. Shake bottle vigorously before withdrawing suspension into dropper.
2. Have client remain at a 45° angle for 5 minutes after instillation.
3. Obliterate opening with cotton plug soaked on inside with 1 to 2 drops of drug suspension.
4. Store at room temperature (59 to 86 F); stable for 18 months.
5. Reculture ear after 1 week.

GENERIC NAME Acetic acid (OTC) (RX)

TRADE NAME Domeboro Otic

CLASSIFICATION Otic antiinfective agent

Action Acetic acid is a relatively nontoxic solution that is effective against some pathogens.

Indications for Use External otitis, prevention of swimmer's ear.

Administration

- *Infection:* Instill 4 to 6 gtt every 2 to 3 hours.
- *Prevention:* Instill 2 gtt bid, as needed.

Available Drug Forms Squeeze dropper bottles containing 60 ml. Generic contents: acetic acid 2%, aluminum acetate (modified Burrows Solution).

Nursing Management (See chloramphenicol.)

1. Client should maintain a sidelying position for 5 minutes after instillation to facilitate penetration into canal.
2. Moisten cotton plug with 1 to 2 drops before inserting.
3. Notify physician if ear irritation develops.
4. Cotton wick may be used for the first 24 hours of an acute infection.

GENERIC NAME Acetic acid/neomycin (RX)

TRADE NAME Neo-Cort-Dome Otic

CLASSIFICATION Otic antiinfective agent

Action This drug, containing 2 antiinfective agents, is effective against many pathogens. Hydrocortisone content reduces inflammation and relieves itching.

Indications for Use External otitis, otitis media when eardrum is perforated, infections following mastoidectomy.

Contraindications Hypersensitivity to any ingredient, tuberculosis, fungal lesions of the skin or ear, acute herpes simplex, vaccinia, varicella.

Administration Instill 3 to 4 gtt tid or qid.

Available Drug Forms Bottles containing 10 ml with dropper. Generic contents in 1 ml: neomycin sulfate: 0.35%; hydrocortisone: 1%; acetic acid: 2%. Also contains glycerol monostearate, stearic acid, propylene glycol, sodium acetate, and purified water.

Nursing Management (See chloramphenicol.)

1. Shake suspension vigorously before withdrawing solution into dropper.
2. Moisten cotton plug with 1 to 2 drops before inserting.
3. Cotton wick can be used, particularly during the first 24 hours.

GENERIC NAME Acetic acid/desonide (RX)

TRADE NAME Otic Tridesilon

CLASSIFICATION Otic antiinfective agent

Action Acetic acid is effective against some bacteria and fungi. Desonide is a nonfluorinated corticosteroid that has antiinflammatory, antipruritic, and vasoconstrictive actions.

Indications for Use External otitis accompanied by inflammation.

Contraindications Hypersensitivity to any ingredient, perforated eardrum.

Untoward Reactions Otic corticosteroids may cause irritation, dryness, folliculitis, decreased pigmentation, skin maceration, and secondary infection. Allergic contact dermatitis has been reported.

Administration Instill 3 to 4 gtt tid or qid or insert a cotton wick moistened with 3 to 4 gtt q4h and replace every 24 hours.

Available Drug Forms Bottles containing 10 ml with dropper. Generic contents: acetic acid: 2%; desonide: 0.05%. Also contains purified water, propylene glycol, sodium acetate, and citric acid.

Nursing Management (See chloramphenicol.)

1. Client should maintain a sidelying position for 5 minutes after instillation to facilitate penetration into canal.
2. Moisten cotton plug with 1 to 2 drops before inserting.
3. Reculture ear after 1 week.

GENERIC NAME Acetic acid/glycol (RX)

TRADE NAME VōSoL

CLASSIFICATION Otic antiinfective agent

Action Acetic acid is a relatively nontoxic solution that is effective against some organisms. Glycol is soothing to the ear canal.

Indications for Use External otitis, prevention of swimmer's ear.

Contraindications Hypersensitivity to any ingredient, perforated eardrum.

Administration

- *Infection:* Instill 4 to 6 gtt tid.
- *Prevention:* Instill 2 gtt bid.

Available Drug Forms Squeeze dropper bottles containing 15 or 30 ml. Generic contents: acetic acid: 2%; propylene glycol: 3%; benzethonium chloride: 0.02%; sodium acetate: 0.015%.

Nursing Management (See chloramphenicol.)

1. Client should maintain a sidelying position for 5 minutes after instillation to facilitate penetration into canal.
2. Moisten cotton plug with 1 to 2 drops before inserting.
3. Notify physician if ear irritation develops.
4. Cotton wick may be used for the first 24 hours of an acute infection.

GENERIC NAME Acetic acid/hydrocortisone

TRADE NAME VōSoL HC (RX)

CLASSIFICATION Otic antiinfective agent

Action Same as VōSoL, but contains hydrocortisone for its additional antiinflammatory and antipruritic effects. Prolonged use may cause systemic untoward reactions.

Indications for Use External otitis accompanied by inflammation.

Contraindications Hypersensitivity to any ingredient, perforated eardrum, vaccinia, varicella.

Administration Initially insert a cotton wick moistened with 3 to 4 gtt q4h for 24 hours; then remove wick and instill 5 gtt tid or qid with dropper.

Available Drug Forms Squeeze dropper bottles containing 10 ml. Generic contents: acetic acid: 2%; hydrocortisone: 1%; propylene glycol: 3%; benzethonium chloride: 0.02%; sodium acetate: 0.015%; citric acid: 0.2%.

Nursing Management (See chloramphenicol.)

1. Client should maintain a sidelying position for 5 minutes after instillation to facilitate penetration into canal.
2. Moisten cotton plug with 1 to 2 drops before inserting.
3. Notify physician if ear irritation develops.
4. Cotton wick may be used for the first 24 hours of an acute infection.

OTHER OTIC AGENTS

GENERIC NAME Prednisolone sodium phosphate

TRADE NAMES Hydeltrasol, Metreton (RX)

CLASSIFICATION Otic agent

Action Metreton inhibits the inflammatory response to irritation due to mechanical, chemical, or immunologic activity. It is often used as an adjunct to other agents. It is also used for ophthalmic inflammation. Hydeltrasol is similar to metreton, but contains a lower dosage and different vehicle.

Indications for Use Allergic external otitis, edema and inflammation of the ear.

Contraindications Perforation of eardrum, fungal or viral infections of the ear.

Untoward Reactions Infection may develop, particularly fungal infections. Stinging and burning may occur initially.

Administration Initially instill 3 to 4 gtt tid until inflammation subsides; then gradually reduce dosage and eventually discontinue drug.

Available Drug Forms Squeeze dropper bottles containing 5 ml. Generic contents in 1 ml of Hydeltrasol: prednisolone sodium phosphate: 5 mg; creatinine, sodium citrate, polysorbate 80, disodium edetate, potassium phosphate, water, hydrochloric acid, benzalkonium chloride, phenylethanol. Generic contents of 1 ml of Metreton: prednisolone sodium phosphate: 5.5 mg; purified water, sodium hydroxide, benzalkonium chloride, phenylethyl alcohol, tyloxapol, sodium phosphate, disodium edetate.

Nursing Management

1. Client should maintain a sidelying position for 5 minutes after instillation to facilitate penetration into canal.
2. Moisten cotton plug with 1 to 2 drops before inserting.
3. A drug-saturated cotton wick may be used for the first 12 to 24 hours.
4. Store drug between 36 and 86 F away from light.

GENERIC NAME Hydrocortisone acetate (RX)

TRADE NAME Hydrocortone

CLASSIFICATION Otic agent

See prednisolone sodium phosphate for Contraindications, Untoward reactions, and Nursing management.

Action Similar to Metreton, but contains a different steroid and vehicle.

Indications for Use Allergic external otitis, edema and inflammation of the ear.

Administration Initially instill 3 to 4 gtt tid until inflammation subsides; then gradually reduce dosage and eventually discontinue drug.

Available Drug Forms Dropper bottles containing 5 ml. Generic contents in 1 ml: hydrocortisone acetate: 25 mg; sodium citrate, sodium phosphate, sodium chloride, polyethylene glycol, polysorbate 80, water, benzyl alcohol, benzalkonium chloride.

GENERIC NAME Dexamethasone sodium phosphate

TRADE NAME Decadron Phosphate (RX)

CLASSIFICATION Otic antiinflammatory agent

See prednisolone sodium phosphate for Untoward reactions and Nursing management.

Action Decadron decreases edema and inflammation of the ear canal. It is also used in the eye.

Indications for Use Allergic external otitis, edema or inflammation of the ear.

Contraindications Perforated eardrum, herpes simplex, fungal infections of ear structures, vaccinia, varicella, localized infections of external ear structures.

Administration Initially instill 3 to 4 gtt tid or qid until inflammation subsides; then gradually reduce dosage and eventually discontinue drug.

Available Drug Forms Containers of 2.5 or 5.0 ml with dropper. Generic contents: dexamethasone sodium phosphate: 0.1%; creatinine, sodium citrate, sodium borate, polysorbate 80, and water.

GENERIC NAME Benzocaine/glycerin (RX)

TRADE NAME Americaine-Otic

CLASSIFICATION Otic analgesic agent

Action Relieves pain and itching and dries the auditory canal.

Indications for Use Pain and pruritus associated with swimmer's ear, otitis externa, and otitis media.

Contraindications Infants under 1 year, perforated eardrum.

Warnings and Precautions May mask the symptoms of a fulminating infection of the middle ear.

Administration Instill 4 to 5 gtt q4h prn; duration of therapy is usually 1 to 2 days.

Available Drug Forms Bottles containing 15 ml with dropper. Generic contents: benzocaine 20%, glycerin, polyethylene glycol-300.

Nursing Management

1. Warm drug solution to at least 70 F before using.
2. Moisten inner surface of cotton plug with 1 to 2 drops before inserting.
3. Client should maintain a sidelying position for 5 minutes after instillation to facilitate penetration into canal.

GENERIC NAME Benzocaine/antipyrine (RX)

TRADE NAME Auralgan

CLASSIFICATION Otic analgesic and decongestant agent

Action Provides decongestion (antipyrine), analgesia (benzocaine), and facilitates the removal of cerumen (glycerin).

Indications for Use Pain and congestion associated with acute otitis media, excessive or impacted cerumen.

Contraindications Hypersensitivity to any ingredient, perforated eardrum.

Warnings and Precautions Use with caution during pregnancy and lactation.

Untoward Reactions Prolonged use may cause irritation to ear canal and periaural tissues.

Administration

- *Pain:* Instill 4 to 5 gtt every 1 to 2 hours, as needed.
- *Impacted cerumen:* Instill 4 to 5 gtt tid.

Available Drug Forms Bottles containing 15 ml with dropper. Generic contents in 1 ml: antipyrine: 54 mg; benzocaine: 14 mg; glycerin (dehydrated) qs.

Nursing Management

1. Store solution in airtight containers at room temperature.
2. Warm drug solution to at least 70 F before using.
3. Moisten inner surface of cotton plug with 1 to 2 drops before inserting.
4. Client should maintain a sidelying position for 5 minutes after instillation to facilitate penetration into canal.

PART XVIII

IMMUNOLOGIC AGENTS

THE IMMUNE SYSTEM defends the body against pathogenic microorganisms and other foreign substances, as well as preventing the formation of malignancies. The two primary characteristics of the immune system are: (1) the ability to recognize "foreign" substances (microorganisms, chemicals, malignancies) and (2) memory. Exposure to an antigen (foreign substance) generates the production of a specific antibody. When exposed to mumps, chickenpox, or other infectious diseases, the body's lymphatic tissue is stimulated to produce specific antibodies against the causative microorganism. The ensuing antigen-antibody reaction eventually eliminates the invading antigen. Once established, immunity to that specific antigen continues for many years, because the newly generated lymphocytes continue to circulate in the bloodstream.

In immune disorders, the immune system can be thought of as being either underactive or overactive. When underactive (immunodeficiency), the individual is easily invaded by microorganisms. Immunodeficiency can occur when the lymphatic and other immune tissues are congenitally absent or affected by destructive agents (radiation, chemotherapy) or other overwhelming conditions (severe malnutrition, extensive burns); the immune system is then unable to adequately fight microorganisms and infection occurs. Due to the presence of maternal antibodies, newborns have immunity against some infectious diseases. This immunity is short-lived, however, and infants must soon generate their own antibodies, either by contracting the diseases or by receiving low doses of the pathogen (infant immunization).

Part of the immune system may be overactive in some individuals, causing hypersensitivity to certain substances (allergens). Bronchial asthma, hay fever, allergic rhinitis, drug allergy, and other hypersensitivity reactions may result. Certain allergic reactions induce the release of excessive amounts of histamine, normally present in the body in small quantities. Continuous low-dose exposure to an inhaled allergen, such as pollen, commonly induces allergic rhinitis, sinusitis, or even bronchial asthma in hypersensitive individuals. The body releases histamine as a by-product of the antigen-antibody reaction and the histamine causes the affected tissues to become red and inflamed. Other histamine-type reactions include hives and even anaphylactic shock. A more complete explanation of hypersensitivity reactions can be found in Chapter 8. Drugs that improve an individual's immunity and drugs used to treat histamine reactions are presented in this section.

Active immunizing agents Active immunity is the state of protection against an antigen that results from exposure to the antigen. This form of immunity can be induced by injecting or swallowing low doses of the antigen. Although active immunization can induce fever, malaise, and other reactions, immunization prevents the recipient from contracting the actual disease, with its potential for severe complications.

Diagnostic immunologic agents To determine if an individual has antibodies against a specific disease, minute quantities of a specific antigen can be injected intradermally. If redness and swelling occur at the injection site, it usually means that the individual has been exposed to the disease at some time and an antigen-antibody reaction has occurred, since antibodies are present in the bloodstream. However, if no reaction occurs, no antibodies are present, and it can be concluded that the individual has not been exposed to the disease.

Passive immunizing agents Even if an individual has been exposed to a potentially dangerous disease, the illness can still be prevented by injecting the client with serum containing antibodies against the pathogen. These antibodies are obtained from animals or humans that have active immunity to the disease. Products are also available to treat exposure to dangerous toxins and snake venom. Although passive immunity is short-lived, the individual is normally protected during the expected incubation period of the disease.

Immunosuppressive agents Occasionally it is necessary to stop the formation of unwanted antibodies. For example, clients who receive homotransplants (grafts) run the risk of rejecting the implanted foreign substance. The immunosuppressive agent azathioprine was developed to help prevent these clients from rejecting the implant. Another problem solved by an immunosuppressive agent is the rejection of future pregnancies by Rh-negative mothers who deliver Rh-positive babies. Since there are only two immunosuppressive drugs in current use, they are included in the chapter on passive immunizing agents (Chapter 82).

Antihistamines Histamine-type allergic reactions are common in humans; numerous antihistamine preparations have been developed to counteract them. Antihistamines act by competing with histamine for receptor sites, thus preventing the histamine reaction. Most of these agents are more effective in blocking H_1-receptor sites located in the respiratory and cardiovascular systems. There are also H_2-receptor sites located in the stomach. The drugs that are known to be particularly effective in blocking H_2 receptor sites can be found in Chapter 75, which explains gastric hyperacidity. Only H_1 antihistamines are presented in this section.

Chapter 81

Active Immunizing and Diagnostic Agents

ANTIGENS ARE SUBSTANCES that when perceived by the body to be "foreign" induce the formation of *antibodies*, or immune lymphocytes, with which they then react to elicit an antigen-antibody reaction. The body is able to "destroy" the antigen through agglutination, phagocytosis, or other processes. The antigen-antibody reaction is the basis of immunity. *Active immunity* is the state of protection against an antigen that results from exposure to the antigen. *Natural* active immunity occurs when an individual actually acquires and recovers from the disease; but this can be dangerous since the individual may develop complications or possibly die. *Artificial* active immunity can be provided by the injection or ingestion of an antigen. Although the individual may develop an "illness-type" reaction, such as fever and malaise, to the antigen, the individual develops antibodies without having the actual disease. When possible, the toxic properties of the antigen are destroyed without disturbing the *antigenic* ability; namely, the capability to induce the formation of antibodies.

THE ROLE OF DIAGNOSTIC AGENTS

Various agents are used to determine if an individual has antibodies against a specific disease. These biologic agents are produced from the specific antigen (bacterium, toxin) and are injected into the skin. If the injection site becomes red and swollen due to an antigen-antibody reaction, this indicates that the individual has been exposed to the antigen previously and has developed antibodies. However, some of the tests are more specific than others. For example, a false-positive result may be obtained with the tine test for tuberculosis and a negative result with the Mantoux test. Thus, the individual has not acquired immunity to tuberculosis.

TYPES OF IMMUNIZING AGENTS

Immunizing agents are substances that are injected or inoculated into the body to stimulate the production of antigens and thereby provide artificial immunity. There are two basic types: *vaccines* and *toxoids*. Vaccines are either attenuated infectious organisms (BCG, smallpox) or organisms that have been killed by physical or chemical means (rabies). Most vaccines are live infectious organisms.

The severity of a contagious disease is sometimes caused by the metabolic wastes or exotoxins excreted by the organism. Toxins retained within the body of the organism are called *endotoxins*. Toxoids are solutions of toxins, or more specifically exotoxins, modified to reduce or eliminate their toxic properties while retaining their antigenic properties. Endotoxins are present in some bacterial vaccines.

The protection provided by vaccines and toxoids is often not as effective or as lasting as natural active immunity. Injections may need to be given every few months, such as a series of DPT shots, to provide protection. As vaccines and toxoids lose their potency with time, expiration dates should be checked before administering. Refrigeration maintains the potency of some vaccines and toxoids; but freezing may destroy others. The manufacturer's instructions should be read for details. Some immunizations require periodic injections, called *boosters*, to maintain the level of protection.

OTHER ANTIGENS

Some plants and other substances can cause severe reactions in hypersensitive individuals. An unusual response to a substance that is normally nonharmful is said to be allergic. The causative antigens, which are often called *allergens*, induce the production of antibodies. However, the resulting antigen-antibody reaction often causes the liberation of either histamine or a histamine-like substance and may produce a localized or generalized reaction. Highly diluted solutions of these antigens can be injected periodically (weekly) to desensitize the individual.

IMMUNIZING CHILDREN AGAINST COMMUNICABLE DISEASES

The immunization of children is usually started at the age of 2 months. Immunization against some diseases, such as smallpox, is no longer required as these diseases have been eradicated.

Tubercular testing is sometimes done periodically, particularly in high-risk individuals. However, these tests should not be administered until some time after the live virus vaccines are given. Immunizations are available at a pediatrician's office or, at no charge to the parent, at a Well Baby Clinic. Schedules presently used for immunization are shown in Tables 81-1 and 81-2.

Immunizations may evoke an untoward reaction. Many children develop soreness or stiffness in the injected limb and fever may occur and last for 24 to 72 hours. Allowing the child to actively play will help to minimize the symptoms by promoting circulation in the affected limb. Fever and discomfort are usually well controlled by administering an appropriate analgesic/antipyretic, such as aspirin or acetaminophen. The physician should be consulted about the appropriate dosage and frequency of administration.

TABLE 81-1 Recommended Immunization Schedule for Normal Infants and Children

Age	Immunization
2 months	DPT, polio (TOPV)*
4 months	DPT, polio (TOPV)
6 months	DPT (optional)
12 months	Tuberculin test†
15 months	Measles-mumps-rubella or measles-rubella
18 months	DPT, polio (TOPV)
4 to 6 years	DPT, polio (TOPV)

*Trivalent oral poliovirus vaccine. This is suitable for breast-fed as well as bottle-fed infants.
†Tuberculin test should be done at 1 year and every 4 years thereafter.

NURSING MANAGEMENT FACTORS OF PRIMARY IMMUNIZATION AND TESTING

1. The nurse should understand that an uncomfortable procedure, such as immunization, is a real and consequential experience for a child.
2. Help the parent to be a supportive person to the child.
3. Provide an explanation of the procedure.
4. Extend support in helping restrain the child on the examining table. Most injections are given in the anterolateral thigh in children

TABLE 81-2 Recommended Immunization Schedule for Children Not Immunized before 15 Months

Time Interval	Immunization
Ages 15 Months to 5 Years	
First visit	DPT, polio, measles-mumps-rubella
3 months later, preschool	DPT
5 months later, preschool	DPT
11 to 17 months later	DPT, polio
Ages 6 Years and Older	
First visit	TD, polio (TOPV), measles-mumps-rubella
2 months later	TD (adult), polio (TOPV; optional)

After completion of immunization, each individual should receive a tetanus renewal every 10 years.

under 18 months. Children between 18 months and 5 years may continue to receive injections in the thigh or in the arm near the deltoid or subcutaneously in the upper arm. The child will be less frightened if seated on the parent's lap. It may be necessary to restrain or secure both arms and legs.

5. It is psychologically helpful to the child if the parent sits next to the child and uses restraint only when necessary. Older children may prefer to sit on a chair.
6. Inform the parents about the child's need for extra fluid intake, especially water, if fever develops and lasts for 12 hours or more.

IMMUNIZATION OF THE ELDERLY

It is recognized that the elderly are at a risk of tuberculosis, influenza, pneumococcal pneumonia, and tetanus. This increased risk is associated with the progressive decrease in the number of circulating lymphocytes. The onset of this decrease is in the middle years and the lymphocytes may be depressed by as much as 30% by the age of 60. The greatest decrease is in the number of circulating T cells, which are so necessary to elicit a cellular response. The life span of B cells remains at about 16 days with no actual change in number, but their ability to respond to stimulation from certain antigens is markedly decreased.

The elderly should be immunized against influenza, pneumococcal pneumonia, and tetanus. Due to an increase in the number of new cases among this age group, they should be skin tested for TB. There is some evidence that as a group they are anergic (a diminished reactivity to specific antigens) and caution should be exercised when performing skin tests.

DIAGNOSTIC TESTING AGENTS

GENERIC NAME Tuberculin old (RX)

TRADE NAMES Scalvo Test, Tine Test

CLASSIFICATION Tuberculin test

Action The test for tuberculin reactivity uses a device with four tines or prongs on a stainless steel disc. The tines have been dipped in a solution of old tuberculin containing 7% acacia and 8.5% lactose as stabilizers and then dried. No preservatives have been added. Cell-mediated hypersensitivity reaction begins 1 to 3 days after contact with the antigen.

Indications for Use Detecting tuberculin-sensitive individuals, screening programs to detect priorities for additional testing.

Warnings and Precautions Reaction to the test may be suppressed in clients receiving immunosuppressive agents or those recently vaccinated with live virus vaccine, such as measles.

Untoward Reactions Allergic reactions are rare and are usually due to the stabilizer acacia.

Administration 0.1 ml intradermal.

Available Drug Forms Self-contained disposable units consisting of a stainless steel disc with four tines or prongs attached to a plastic handle. Each jar contains 25 individual tests.

Nursing Management

Planning factors

1. The frequency at which an individual is tested depends on the risk of exposure and the prevalance of TB in the population. An initial test should be done at the time of or preceding the measles immunization (at about 15 months).
2. Establish if recipient has received a live virus vaccination recently.
3. Over the past century, the peak incidence of TB was among young adults. Today, however, the concern is associated with the elderly (over 65 years) and males; current incidence represents a sevenfold increase among the very low social economic group.
4. Store unrefrigerated below 30 C. This agent is stable for 5 years undiluted and 1 year diluted.

Administration factors

1. Prepare skin with alcohol, ether, acetone, or soap and water. Allow the area to dry before performing the tine test.
2. The unit remains sterile as long as the plastic cap is not removed.
3. Hold arm firmly as the sharp impact may cause the recipient to jerk, resulting in a scratch.
4. Hold test device for 1 second before removing. Four puncture sites plus a circular depression of the skin from the disc should be visible.
5. Gently circle the area around the puncture site with ink. This will facilitate identification of the puncture site when it is time to read it.
6. Never reuse the test device.

Evaluation factors Read the test in 48 to 72 hours. Palpitate the area with a gentle finger and identify the prong site. In a positive reaction, the prong site has a tendency to coalesce. Attempt to read the largest prong reaction. The interpretation of tuberculin test reactions recommended by the National Tuberculosis and Respiratory Disease Association is as follows: 5 mm induration (around one point) is considered a positive reading; 2 to 4 mm induration is doubtful; less than 2 mm induration is a negative reaction. A positive or doubtful reading should be confirmed by a standard Mantoux test.

GENERIC NAME Tuberculin purified protein derivative (Mantoux test)

TRADE NAMES Apilsol, Tubersol (RX)

CLASSIFICATION Tuberculin test

Action This aqueous solution of a purified protein fraction is isolated from culture filtrates of human-type strains of *Mycobacterium tuberculosis* by the method of F.B. Seibert.

Indications for Use The PPD (Mantoux) test is recommended by the American Lung Association as an aid in the detection of infection with *M. tuberculosis*.

Warnings and Precautions Tuberculin PPD should not be administered to known tuberculin-positive reactors because of the severity of reaction (vasiculation, ulceration, necrosis) that may occur at the test site. Avoid injecting tuberculin subcutaneously. If this occurs, no local reaction develops, but a general febrile reaction and/or acute inflammation around tuberculous lesions may occur in highly sensitive individuals. A separate, heat-sterilized syringe and needle or a sterile disposable unit should be used for each individual to prevent possible transmission of homologous serum hepatitis virus and other infectious agents from one individual to another. As with any biologic product, epinephrine should be readily available in case an anaphylactoid or acute hypersensitivity reaction occurs.

Untoward Reactions In highly sensitive individuals, strongly positive reactions, including vesiculation, ulceration, or necrosis, may occur at the test site. Cold packs or topical steroid preparations may be employed for symptomatic relief of associated pain, pruritus, and discomfort. Strongly positive reactions may result in scarring at the test site.

Administration 0.1 ml diluted tuberculin PPD intradermal.

Available Drug Forms Rubber diaphragm-capped vials containing 1 ml (10 tests/box); rubber diaphragm-capped vials containing 5 ml (50 tests/box); PPD-S (No. 49608) World Health Organization International PPD-Tuberculin Standard—this is a dried powder from which WHO and US standard tuberculin solutions are made. Heaf test is performed with Stern needle gun with disposable cartridges. Glycerinated PPD is the testing agent and is read in 3 to 5 days.

Nursing Management

Planning factors

1. Reactivity to tuberculin may be depressed or suppressed for as long as 4 weeks by viral infections, live virus vaccines (measles, smallpox, polio, rubella, mumps), or by the administration of corticosteroids. Malnutrition may also have a similar effect. When of diagnostic importance, a negative test should be accepted as proof that hypersensitivity is absent only after reaction to nonspecific irritants has been demonstrated.
2. A child who is known to have been exposed to a tuberculous adult must not be judged free of infection until a negative tuberculin reaction is obtained at least 10 weeks after contact with the tuberculous individual.

Administration factors

1. The site of the test is usually the flexor or dorsal surface of the forearm about 4 inches below the elbow.
2. Cleanse the skin at the injection site with 70% alcohol and allow to dry.
3. Administer the test material with a tuberculin syringe (0.5 or 1.0 ml) fitted with about a 26 to 27 gauge ($\frac{1}{2}$-in.)needle.
4. Sterilize the syringe and needle by autoclaving, boiling, or by the use of dry heat. Use a separate sterile unit for each individual tested.
5. Wipe the diaphragm of the vial stopper with 70% alcohol.
6. Insert the needle through the stopper diaphragm of the inverted vial. Fill the syringe with 0.1 ml, care being taken to exclude air bubbles and to maintain the lumen of the needle filled.
7. Insert the point of the needle into the most superficial layers of the skin with the needle level pointing upward. As the tuberculin solution is injected a pale bleb 6 to 10 mm in size will rise over the point of the needle. This is quickly absorbed and no dressing is required.
8. Exercise extreme caution when administering intradermal tests as the test material must be injected into, not below, the skin.
9. In the event the injection is delivered subcutaneously (no bleb will form) or a significant portion of the dosage leaks from the injection site, the test should be repeated immediately at another site at least 5 cm removed from the first site.
10. When testing a highly sensitive individual, use 1 TU (0.1 ml) instead of 5 TU.

Evaluation factors

1. Read the test 48 to 72 hours after injection. Only induration is considered when interpreting the test results.
2. Measure the diameter of the induration transversely to the long axis of the forearm and record in millimeters.
3. Disregard erythema of less than 10 mm. If the area of erythema is greater than 10 mm and induration is absent, the injection may have been made too deeply and retesting is indicated.

4. Reactions should be interpreted as follows:
   - *Positive:* Induration measuring 10 mm or more. Positive for past or present infection with *M. tuberculosis*.
   - *Doubtful:* Induration measuring 5 to 8 mm. Retesting is indicated using a different test site for injection. Evaluation to rule out cross-reactions from other mycobacterial infection should be considered.
   - *Negative:* Induration less than 5 mm. This indicates lack of hypersensitivity to tuberculoprotein and tuberculosis infection is highly unlikely.
5. Kochs' phenomenon is an inflammatory reaction at the injection site that may lead to necrosis. This focal reaction consists of inflammation and dense cellular infiltration within tuberculous lesions. Extreme caution must be exercised when performing skin tests in order to avoid this reaction.
6. Highly sensitive individuals may develop vesiculation, ulceration, or necrosis at test sites.
7. An individual who has had a primary tubercular bacillus infection will develop an induration of 10 mm in diameter within 24 to 48 hours. In most cases there is edema and erythema and in hypersensitive individuals the reactions may be accompanied by central necrosis.
8. Tuberculin test will be positive 4 to 6 weeks after infection.
9. Tests do not indicate evidence of active disease. Only isolation of the tubercule bacilli gives such proof. Never start antituberculosis chemotherapy on the basis of one positive test.
10. All positive findings should be followed through for diagnosis.

GENERIC NAME Diphtheria toxin (RX)

TRADE NAME Diagnostic Diphtheria Tox for Schick Test

CLASSIFICATION Diagnostic agent

Action The diluted toxin produced by diphtheria bacillus is injected to determine if an individual has an immunity to diphtheria. It contains a preservative approved by the National Institute of Health.

Indications for Use Determination of susceptibility to diphtheria.

Administration 0.1 ml intracutaneous.

Available Drug Forms Vials containing 1, 5, or 10 ml.

Nursing Management

1. The development of a skin reaction is an indicator of the adequacy of the number of antitoxin units present in the bloodstream.
2. Read site 4 to 7 days following injection. The time interval is determined by the solution used. Read package instructions carefully.
3. A positive Schick test indicated by a 1 cm or more inflammation and induration demonstrates susceptibility to the disease.
4. Store between 2 to 10 C, preferably at lower limits.

GENERIC NAME Scarlet fever streptococcus toxin

TRADE NAME Dick Test (RX)

CLASSIFICATION Diagnostic agent

Source Made from broth of hemolytic streptococci.

Indications for Use Determination of susceptibility of an individual to scarlet fever.

Administration 0.1 ml intradermal.

Available Drug Forms Vials containing 1 or 5 ml.

Nursing Management

1. The development of a skin reaction is an indicator of the adequacy of the number of antitoxin units present in the bloodstream.
2. Read site 4 to 7 days following injection. The time interval is determined by the solution used. Read package instructions carefully.

VACCINES

GENERIC NAME Bacille Calmette-Guérin (RX)

TRADE NAME BCG

CLASSIFICATION Vaccine

Source Attenuated *Mycobacterium bovis*.

Action BCG provides primary active immunization after one dose. Its use in the United States is limited. The World Health Organization evaluated the protective value in India. Concern has been expressed that the available studies to date have not been done in Europe and North America. It is used in 24 countries and recommended by 123 additional countries.

Indications for Use Primarily used in TB-negative individuals who are heavily exposed. Duration of protection is 10 years. Vaccination with this organism is a substitute for primary infection with virulent tubercule bacilli.

Contraindications Hypogammaglobulinemia or immunosuppression, recent smallpox, vaccinations or burns, during corticosteroid therapy.

Warnings and Precautions Use with extreme caution in individuals with chronic skin diseases. Not given to those individuals who have had a tuberculin test.

Untoward Reactions Lymphadenitis, skin abscess, local ulceration, lupus reaction, urticaria of trunk and limbs.

Drug Interactions Antagonistic with isoniazid; avoid using concurrently.

Administration 0.2 mg diluted intradermal or subcutaneous.

Nursing Management

1. Recommended in the United States only for PPD-negative contacts of ineffectively treated or persistently untreated causes and for other unusually high-risk groups.
2. Test for PPD conversion 2 months later and reimmunize if there is no conversion.
3. Do not shake bottle before reconstitution; read accompanying instructions.
4. Recommended injection site is over the insertion of the deltoid muscle.
5. Skin test 2 to 3 months after BCG vaccination to determine level of conversion to positive reactor.
6. Use freeze-dried preparation within 10 days.

GENERIC NAME Cholera vaccine (RX)

TRADE NAMES Strains OGAWA and INABA; NIH-41, NIH-35, A3

CLASSIFICATION Vaccine

Source Two strains of *Vibrio cholerae* inactivated with phenol.

Action Cholera vaccine provides short-term active immunity (tapers in 3 to 6 months). Most individuals develop antibodies following inoculation with cholera vaccine. The vaccine does not prevent transmission of infection or complete protection to all; but inoculation will prevent overt disease in most individuals. About 50% of the time, the vaccine is effective in reducing the severity of illness for 3 to 6 months.

Indications for Use Cholera prophylaxis for those traveling to or residing in epidemic areas (Asia, Middle East, Africa).

Contraindications Acute infection.

Warnings and Precautions Not recommended for the treatment of cholera or for a carrier. Does not prevent development of a carrier state.

Untoward Reactions Soreness, fever, malaise, and headache or common. Anaphylaxis and other severe allergic reactions may occur.

Parameters of Use

Absorption Antibodies are present in the lumen of the intestines (secretory IgA caproantibodies) and last a few months.

Drug Interactions Oral tetracycline tends to reduce stools in clients with cholera.

Administration Adults and children over 10 years: 0.5 to 1.0 ml IM, subc, or intradermal 1 to 4 weeks apart; Booster dose: 0.5 ml every 6 months if in cholera area. Children: Ages 5 to 10 years: First dose: 0.3 ml IM or subc followed in 1 month by a single dose of 0.5 ml; Booster dose: 0.3 ml. Under 5 years: 0.1 ml IM or subc; then 1 month later a single dose of 0.3 ml.

Available Drug Forms Vials containing 1, 1.5, or 20 ml; 1 ml contains 8 units of serotype antigen.

Nursing Management

Planning factors

1. Obtain history of immunosuppresive disorders, allergies, and all past untoward reactions to immunization.
2. Have epinephrine readily available.
3. Vaccine should be given at least 7 days prior to entering a cholera area.
4. Booster dose is advisable after 6 months when risk of exposure is still present.
5. Usually not recommended for travelers unless it is required as a condition for reentry.

Administration factors

1. Use a separate sterilized syringe and needle or a disposable unit for each individual to prevent possible transmission of homologous serum hepatitis virus and other infectious agents.
2. Inject only healthy skin.

Evaluation factors

1. Although most reactions occur within the first 48 hours, delayed reactions may occur. Notify physician if reactions occur.
2. Cold compresses may relieve pain and swelling at the injection site.
3. Aspirin is given for fever.

GENERIC NAMES Influenza virus vaccine, monovalent (Asian strain); influenza virus vaccine, trivalent A and B (whole virus)

TRADE NAMES Fluax; Fluzone-Connaught (RX)

CLASSIFICATION Vaccine

Source Sterile suspension of killed influenza virus grown in chick embryos.

Action This vaccine produces active immunity against influenza with an interval of days to several weeks before production of antibodies. Maximum antibody formation occurs during the second week following vaccination. Titer remains constant for about 1 month at peak and has a gradual decline.

Protection lasts for only a few months. It reduces the incidence and severity of influenza and it is recommended for high-risk groups. The formulation of influenza virus vaccine for use during each season is established by the Bureau of Biologics and the Food and Drug Administration. Public Health Service provides information about dosage and recommended use. Consult the product directions obtainable from the pharmaceutical house for specific details, since they may change annually.

Indications for Use Prophylaxis against influenza for those over 65 years, chronically ill children.

Contraindications Hypersensitivity to egg products, chicken, or chicken feathers.

Warnings and Precautions Prophylactic value is limited because the disease can occur with high serum antibody levels. Vaccine may not contain antigen of offending strain of virus.

Untoward Reactions Fever is common. Toxic reactions, including Guillain-Barré syndrome and anaphylaxis, may occur. Malaise and myalgia are common. Local reactions include erythema, induration, fever, and soreness. Symptoms may begin 6 to 12 hours after vaccination and may continue for 1 to 2 days. Split virus vaccine elicits fewer side effects than whole virus vaccine.

Administration Adults and children over 12 years: 0.5 ml IM whole virus vaccine; Children: Ages 3 to 12 years: 0.5 ml IM split virus; Under 3 years: 0.25 ml IM split virus.

Available Drug Forms Whole and split virus preparations.

Nursing Management

1. Obtain history of allergies, especially to eggs, chicken, and chicken feathers.
2. IM injection into deltoid or midlateral thigh may be given subcutaneously.
3. Keep epinephrine (1:1000) available for use in the event of anaphylaxis.
4. Force fluids, especially in very young children when they run a fever for more than 12 hours.
5. Cool compresses to area of induration will relieve pain.
6. On return visit, enquire about the reaction that occurred.

GENERIC NAME Measles virus vaccine (RX)

TRADE NAME Attenuvax (MSD)

CLASSIFICATION Vaccine

Source Prepared in cell cultures of chick embryo.

Action The measles (rubella) virus vaccine contains live, attenuated viruses and provides immunity against measles.

Indications for Use Produces a modified measles infection in susceptible individuals. Recommended for children with active or inactive tuberculosis. Recommended for children with chronic diseases, such as cystic fibrosis, asthma, heart disease, and chronic pulmonary diseases, to lessen the severity of the natural disease. No booster is required. May prevent natural disease if given less than 48 hours after exposure.

Contraindications Hypersensitivity to neomycin, eggs, chicken, or chicken feathers; respiratory illness, active febrile infection, or active untreated TB; individuals receiving therapy with ACTH, corticosteroids, irradiation, alkylating agents; pregnancy—when given to females, pregnancy must be ruled out at time of vaccination and prevented for 3 months.

Warnings and Precautions Defer vaccination for 3 months following blood or plasma transfusions or administration of human immune serum globulin in children 15 months or older. When given before 15 months, revaccination is required.

Untoward Reactions May cause burning or stinging at injection site. Fever (101 to 103 F) frequently occurs. A rash and fever may develop from 5 to 12 days after injection. Fever (with or without convulsions) over 103 F has been reported. Allergic reactions (wheal, flare, urticaria) at the injection site have been reported. Encephalitis, ocular palsies, Guillain-Barré syndrome, and subacute sclerosing panencephalitis have occurred, but rarely.

Drug Interactions The live virus is inactivated by detergents, antiseptic, and preservatives. Do not give human immune serum globulin concurrently with Attenuvax.

Administration Adults and children: 0.5 ml subcutaneous.

Available Drug Forms Kits containing bottles of virus and syringes.

Nursing Management

1. Protect from light.
2. Store and maintain at 10 C (50 F).
3. Fever and rash may appear within 5 to 12 days. Monitor temperature of recipient.
4. When vaccine is given at time of exposure to measles, the amount of protection is questionable. Substantial protection may be provided if the vaccine is given a few days before exposure.
5. Attenuvax may be given concurrently with monovalent or trivalent poliovirus vaccine (live, oral), rubella (Meruvax) virus vaccine, live MSD, and Mumpsvax (mumps virus live, MSD).

6. Attenuvax should not be given less than 1 month before or after administration of other live virus vaccines.
7. Recipients may complain of burning and/or stinging of short duration at the injection site due to the slightly acid pH (6.2 to 6.6).
8. Occasional moderate fever (101 to 102.9 F) may occur during the month after vaccination. Fever, rash, or both generally appear after 5 to 12 days. Rash, when it occurs, is usually minimal and not generalized.
9. High fever of 103 F is less common.

GENERIC NAME Measles, mumps, and rubella virus vaccine

TRADE NAME M-M-R II (RX)

CLASSIFICATION Vaccine

Source Mixed preparation of Attenuvax, Mumpsvax, and meruvax. Although propagated in eggs, this vaccine is essentially devoid of potentially allergic substances derived from chicken or duck embryos.

Action Antigenic agent used to produce active immunity. Hemagglutination-inhibiting antibodies are formed. Each dosage contains approximately 25 mcg of neomycin.

Indications for Use Simultaneous immunization against measles, mumps, and rubella in children from 15 months to puberty. Children less than 15 months may fail to respond to one or all three components of the vaccine due to residual circulatory measles and/or mumps and/or rubella antibody of maternal origin. Immunization of children living in inaccessible areas, since immunization programs are difficult, and population groups in which natural measles infection may occur in a significant proportion of infants before 15 months; it may be desirable to give vaccine at an earlier age then revaccinate after 15 months. Previously unimmunized children of susceptible pregnant women should receive attenuated rubella vaccine because an unimmunized child will be less likely to acquire natural rubella and introduce the virus into the household.

Contraindications Hypersensitivity to neomycin or chicken or duck eggs or feathers. Pregnancy; when postpubertal females require vaccination for sound medical reasons, pregnancy at time of vaccination must be ruled out and the possibility of pregnancy occurring in the following 3 months eliminated by medically acceptable methods. Febrile respiratory illness or other active febrile infection; active untreated tuberculosis; individuals receiving therapy with ACTH, corticosteroids, irradiation, alkylating agents, or antimetabolites. The latter contraindication does not apply to those receiving corticosteroids as replacement therapy (Addison's disease), or individuals with blood dyscrasias, leukemia, lymphoma, or other malignant neoplasms affecting the bone marrow or lymphatic system.

Warnings and Precautions Epinephrine should be available for immediate use in case of anaphylactoid reaction. M-M-R should not be given less than 1 month before or after immunization with other live virus vaccines, with the exception of monovalent or trivalent polio vaccine (live, oral), which may be administered concurrently. Use with caution in children with a history of febrile convulsions, cerebral injury, or any other condition in which stress due to fever should be avoided. Vaccination should be deferred for at least 3 months following blood or plasma tranfusions or administration of human immune serum globulin. There is no definitive evidence that the throat excretion of live, attenuated rubella virus is contagious to susceptible individuals. Although theoretically possible, it has not been regarded as a significant risk. A depression of the tuberculin skin test has been reported, therefore tuberculin tests should be done either before or simultaneously with M-M-R.

Untoward Reactions A burning and/or stinging of short duration may occur at the injection site because of the slightly acidic pH (6.2 to 6.6) of the vaccine. There may be malaise, sore throat, headache, fever and rash, mild local reactions (erythema, induration, tenderness and regional lymphadenopathy, parotitis, thrombocytopenia, purpura), and allergic reactions (wheal or flare at injected area, arthritis, arthralgia, polyneuritis or urticaria). Moderate fever (101 to 102.9 F) occurs occasionally and high fever (103 F) occurs less frequently. Rash occurs rarely and is usually minimal and not generalized. Primary immunodeficiency states, including cellular immune deficiencies, hypogammaglobulinemia and dysgammaglobulinemia, may occur.

Administration Contents of single-dose vial subc.

Available Drug Forms Single-dose vials containing a 25-gauge ($\frac{5}{8}$-in.) needle, a sterile syringe, and diluent.

Nursing Management

Planning factors

1. Obtain history of allergic reactions to chicken or duck eggs or feathers. Check recent exposure to measles, mumps, or rubella.
2. Obtain history of previous neurologic reactions at time of fever due to infections.
3. Obtain history of medications taken in the last 2 weeks.
4. Obtain history of site reactions from previous immunizations.
5. Do not give human immune serum globulin concurrently.
6. Transport at 10 C.

Administration factors

1. Before reconstitution, store at 2 to 8 C and protect from light. Store vial with vaccine in refrigerator.
2. Reconstitute with all diluent supplied. Agitate to mix and draw back into syringe if not used immediately.

3. After cleansing the immunization site, inject the total volume of reconstituted vaccine subcutaneously, preferably into the outer aspect of the upper arm. Do not inject intravenously.
4. May be given concurrently with trivalent oral polio vaccine. Antibody responses are comparable.

Evaluation factors

1. Temperature elevation may occur within 5 to 12 days following vaccination.
2. There have been reports of ocular palsies approximately 3 to 24 days after immunization with vaccines containing live, attenuated measles virus. However, no definite cause-and-effect relationship has been established.

Client teaching factors

1. Review with parent or other responsible adult the need to report temperature elevations, irritability, skin irritation, and convulsions to physician or medical center.
2. Instruct the adult in the need to increase or maintain fluid intake, especially water, to prevent dehydration.
3. Assist adult in obtaining information on appropriate antipyretics and the type and dose appropriate for the child. Instruct family in measures (tepid baths) to decrease fever. Review instructions with responsible adult.

GENERIC NAME Mumps virus vaccine (RX)

TRADE NAME Mumpsvax

CLASSIFICATION Vaccine

Source Grown in cell cultures of chick embryo.

Action Mumpsvax provides active immunization by inducing protective antibodies in essentially all nonimmune recipients. It provides protection against natural mumps in most cases. Evidence indicates that the mumps virus infection initiated by the vaccine is not contagious. The pattern of antibody levels is significantly lower than that following the natural infection. The vaccine will not offer protection when given after exposure to natural mumps. Revaccination is not required for those children vaccinated at 12 months or older. Duration of effect is permanent.

Indications for Use Active immunization against mumps in children 15 months or older. It may be given as early as 12 months, but never earlier because residual maternal mumps neutralizing antibodies may interfere with the immune response.

Contraindications Hypersensitivity to neomycin. Pregnancy; effects on fetal development have not been established. When postpubertal females require vaccination, pregnancy at the time of vaccination must be ruled out and the possibility of pregnancy occurring in the following 3 months eliminated by medically acceptable methods. Blood dyscrasias, leukemia, lymphoma, or other malignant neoplasms affecting the bone marrow or lymphatic system. Active infection; clients receiving therapy with ACTH, corticosteroids, irradiation, alkylating agents, or antimetabolites. The latter contraindication does not apply to those receiving corticosteroids as replacement therapy (Addison's disease, immunodeficiency states, including cellular immune deficiencies, hypogammaglobulinemia, and dysgammaglobulinemia).

Warnings and Precautions Hypersensitivity reactions may occur in individuals allergic to eggs, chicken, or chicken feathers. There has been widespread use of the vaccine and only rare isolated reports of minor allergic reactions. Vaccination should be deferred for at least 3 months following blood or plasma transfusions or administration of human immune serum globulin.

Untoward Reactions A burning and/or stinging of short duration may occur at the injection site because of the slightly acidic pH (6.2 to 6.6) of the vaccine. Mild fever occurs occasionally, but fever above 103 F is rare.

Administration Contents of single-dose vial subc.

Available Drug Forms Single-dose vials containing 5000 units.

Nursing Management

Planning factors

1. Take temperature and assess general health. Rule out the presence of an active infection.
2. There are no available data concerning simultaneous use of Mumpsvax with monovalent or trivalent poliovirus vaccine (live, oral) or with killed polio virus vaccine. When M-M-R is given with live polio virus vaccine, the antibody response can be expected to be comparable. Mumpsvax may be given simultaneously with monovalent or trivalent poliovirus vaccine (live or oral and attenuated) and Meruvax.
3. Mumpsvax should be given less than 1 month before or after administration of other live viruses.
4. Obtain history of immunosuppressive diseases.
5. Do not give human immune serum globulin concurrently.

Administration factors

1. Reconstitute with all diluent supplied. Agitate to mix. Draw back into syringe and inject total volume of restored vaccine subcutaneously. Do not inject intravenously.
2. Prepare solution just before using and discard all unused vials.

Evaluation factors Few side effects occur following Mumpsvax other than a brief mild fever and soreness at the injection site. Antipyretics may be prescribed.

Client teaching factors Instruct parents to notify physician immediately if a persistent high fever with obvious signs of illness occur.

GENERIC NAME Pneumococcal vaccine, polyvalent

TRADE NAME Pneumovax (RX)

CLASSIFICATION Vaccine

Source A mixture of highly purified capsular polysaccharides obtained from the 14 most prevalent or invasive pneumococcal types. This mixture accounts for at least 90% of pneumococcal disease isolates, as determined by ongoing surveillance.

Action Pneumovax provides protection against the included types of pneumococci. Antibody levels have been observed to decline over a period of 42 months.

Indications for Use Illness caused by pneumococci, such as acute exacerbations of chronic bronchitis, sinusitis, arthritis, and conjunctivitis; chronic illnesses in which there is an increased risk of pneumoccocal diseases, such as diabetes or functional impairment of cardiorespiratory, hepatic, or renal systems; closed groups of individuals who are susceptible to pneumonia, such as in residential schools, nursing homes, and other institutions; susceptible individuals in the community when there has been a generalized outbreak of pneumonia; individuals at high risk of influenza complications.

Contraindications Hypersensitivity to any ingredient, Hodgkin's disease, those receiving extensive chemotherapy and/or who have shown a depressed antibody response to a 12-valent pneumococcal vaccine (administration may depress preexisting levels to some pneumococcal types).

Warnings and Precautions The expected antibody response cannot be obtained in clients receiving immunosuppresive therapy. Pneumovax may not be effective in preventing infection resulting from basilar skull fracture or external communication with cerebrospinal fluid. Use with caution during lactation as it is not known if it can be excreted in breast milk and in clients with severely compromised cardiac or pulmonary function as a systemic reaction would pose a significant risk. Delay vaccination if a febrile illness occurs. When penicillin or another antibiotic is required prophylactically against pneumococcal infection, the antibiotic should be discontinued after vaccination with Pneumovax. Not recommended during pregnancy or in children under 2 years, since they do not respond satisfactorily.

Untoward Reactions Local erythema and soreness at the injection site frequently occur, but last for less than 48 hours. Low-grade fever (less than 100.9 F) occasionally occurs and is usually confined to the 24-hour period following vaccination. High fevers are rare.

Administration 0.5 ml IM. Revaccination should not be carried out at intervals less than 3 years.

Available Drug Forms Single-dose prefilled syringes; multidose (5) vials.

Nursing Management

1. Give IM injection into the deltoid muscle or lateral midthigh. Do not inject intravenously; avoid intradermal administration.
2. Store in refrigerator between 2 to 8 C.
3. Have epinephrine (1:1000) available for use in the event of a severe hypersensitivity reaction.
4. Pneumovax and Fluax may be given simultaneously, but in different extremities. Antibody response and untoward reactions are comparable to those when vaccines are given alone.

GENERIC NAME Poliovirus vaccine (RX)

TRADE NAME Orimune

CLASSIFICATION Vaccine

Source Mixture of three types of attenuated poliovirus propagated in cercopithecus monkey kidney cell culture. The final vaccine is diluted with a modified cell culture maintenance medium containing sorbitol.

Action The three simultaneously administered virus types in the trivalent vaccine induce permanent immunization.

The purpose of administering any live, attenuated virus vaccine is to stimulate the body mechanisms to produce an active immunity by stimulating the natural infection without producing untoward symptoms of the disease. A primary series is designed to produce an antibody response to poliovirus types 1, 2, and 3. Each dose (0.5 ml) contains less than 25 mcg of each of the antibiotics streptomycin, neomycin, and nystatin. The potency is expressed in terms of the amount of virus contained in the recommended dose as tissue culture infective doses.

This vaccine contains phenol red as a pH indicator and therefore normally has a pink coloration. Containers stored in dry ice may exhibit a yellow coloration. The red, pink, or yellow color of the vaccine has no effect on the virus or efficacy of the vaccine.

Trivalent oral poliovirus vaccine (TOPV) is often preferred to inactivated poliovirus vaccine (IPV) in the United States, since TOPV is simple to administer and induces permanent immunity.

Indications for Use Adults at increased risk of exposure due to travel to epidemic or highly endemic areas or occupational contact; individuals who have had a complete primary series may take a single booster dose if the risk of exposure is high; prevention of poliomyelitis caused by poliovirus, types 1, 2, and 3; routine immunization from 6 to 12 weeks through 18 years.

Contraindications Pregnancy; acute illness, advanced debilitated condition, persistent vomiting, or diarrhea; immunodeficiency states, such as cellular immune deficiencies, hypogammaglobulinemia, and agammaglobulinemia—it is suggested that it would be prudent to withhold vaccine from siblings of an individual known to have an immunodeficiency syndrome; altered immune status, such as in thymic abnormalities, leukemia, lymphoma, generalized malignancy, or by lowered resistance from therapy with corticosteroids, alkylating agents, antimetabolites, or irradiation.

Warnings and Precautions Individuals with an altered immune status should avoid close contact with recipients of the vaccine for at least 6 to 8 weeks, when possible. IPV is preferred when immunizing everyone in the same household or individuals with an altered immune status. Other viruses (including poliovirus and enterovirus) may interfere with the desired response to this vaccine. Although there is no convincing evidence documenting adverse effects of either TOPV or IPV on the developing fetus or pregnant woman, it is advisable not to vaccinate pregnant women. However, when immediate protection against poliomyelitis is needed, TOPV is recommended.

Drug Interactions Antibodies in the serum of whole blood may alter the response to the vaccine; do not administer vaccine within 2 to 3 months of transfusion. It is not prudent to administer TOPV shortly after human immune serum globulin unless such a procedure is unavoidable.

Administration

- *Primary series for infants:* (Suggested by Public Health Services.) First dose: 6 to 12 weeks with DPT; Second dose: not less than 6 weeks, preferably 8 weeks later; Third dose: 8 to 12 months after second dose; fourth dose before entering school is recommended for children immunized in the first and second years of life.
- *Older children and adults:* Two doses 6 to 8 or more weeks apart, followed by a third dose 8 to 12 months later. Can be given at the same time as primary DPT immunization.

Available Drug Forms Single-dose disposable pipettes; multidose (10) vials (no sorbitol) with dropper.

Nursing Management

1. To maintain the vaccine's potency, it is necessary to store it at a temperature that will maintain ice in a solid state. The vaccine may remain fluid at temperatures above 14 C because of its sorbitol content. If frozen, vaccine must be completely thawed before using. An unopened container that thaws remains stable for a maximum of 10 freeze-thaw cycles provided the temperature does not exceed 8 C during the periods of thaw and the total time period does not exceed 24 hours.
2. The vaccine can be administered directly on the tongue, mixed with distilled water or chlorine-free water, or placed on a cube of sugar or a piece of bread or cake.

GENERIC NAME Rubella virus vaccine (RX)

TRADE NAME Meruvax (MR Vax)

CLASSIFICATION Vaccine

Source Prepared in cell of duck embryo.

Action Meruvax provides active immunity by inducing hemagglutination-inhibiting antibodies. The RA 27/3 rubella strain stimulates immunity that closely resembles immunity from natural infection.

Indications for Use Routine immunization from 12 months to puberty; it is not recommended for infants under 12 months because they may retain maternal rubella neutralizing antibodies, which may interfere with the immune response. Previously immunized children of susceptible pregnant women should receive live, attenuated rubella vaccine because an immunized child will be less likely to acquire natural rubella and introduce the virus into the household. Children in kindergarten and the first grade of elementary school are often given priority for vaccination because they are the major source of virus dissemination in the community. A history of rubella illness is usually not reliable enough to exclude children from immunization. In postpubertal males, vaccination is of a much lower priority because so few are susceptible; however, the vaccine may be useful in preventing or controlling outbreaks of rubella. Postpubertal females: Women of childbearing age should not be considered for vaccination unless there is no possibility of pregnancy occurring in the next 3 months.

Contraindications Hypersensitivity to neomycin or chicken or duck eggs or feathers; pregnancy; primary immunodeficiency states, including cellular immune deficiencies, hypogammaglobulinemia, or dysgammaglobulinemia; febrile respiratory illness or other active febrile infection; individuals receiving ACTH, corticosteroids, irradiation, alkylating agents, or antimetabolites. The latter contraindication does not apply to those receiving corticosteroids as replacement therapy.

Warnings and Precautions Throat excretion of live, attenuated rubella virus has occurred in the majority of immunized susceptible individuals. There is no indication at this time that such virus is contagious to susceptible individuals. There is no evidence that live rubella virus vaccine given after exposure will prevent illness. There is no contraindication to vaccinating children already exposed to vaccinated individuals. May be given immediately in the postpartum period to those nonimmune women who have received anti-Rh_0 (D) immune globulin (human) without interfering with vaccine effectiveness. Vaccination should be deferred for at least 3 months following blood or plasma transfusions or administration of human immune serum globulin. Meruvax should not be given less than 1 month before or after immunization with other live virus vaccines, with the exception of monovalent or trivalent polio vaccine (live, oral), which may be administered simultaneously. It has been reported that live, attenuated rubella virus vaccine may result in temporary depression of tuberculin skin sensitivity; therefore, if a test is to be done, it should be administered either before or simultaneously with Meruvax.

Untoward Reactions A burning and/or stinging of short duration may occur at the injection site because of the slightly acidic pH (6.2 to 6.6) of the vaccine. Untoward reactions include regional lymphadenopathy, urticaria, wheal and flare at the injection site, rash, malaise, sore throat, fever, headache, polyneuritis, and occasionally temporary arthralgia, which is frequently associated with signs of inflammation. Moderate fever, 101 to 101.9 F, occurs occasionally and high fever, above 103 F, is rare. Transient arthritis, arthralgia, and polyneuritis are features of natural rubella and vary in frequency with age and sex. Symptoms are most common in females and least common in prepubertal children. Symptoms relating to joint pain, swelling, or stiffness and peripheral nerves (pain, numbness, tingling) that occur within approximately 2 months after immunization should be considered as possibly vaccine related. In teenage girls, the rates of these reactions probably do not exceed 5 to 10%. In women, the rates are greater and may exceed 30%. Clinical evidence in postpubertal males is very limited.

Administration Contents of a single-dose vial IM or subc.

Available Drug Forms Single-dose vials of lyophilized vaccine with a disposable syringe containing diluent and fitted with a 25 gauge ($\frac{5}{8}$-in.) needle.

Nursing Management

Planning factors

1. Obtain history, including hypersensitivity reactions and previous exposure to infections.
2. Take temperature prior to injections.

Administration factors

1. Reconstitute in dark area with all diluent supplied. Agitate to mix and draw contents back into syringe. If not used immediately after reconstitution, store in a dark place at 2 to 8 C (35.6 to 45.6 F). Discard if not used within 8 hours.
2. Vaccine should be crystal clear or reconstitution. However, the usual color after reconstitution is pinkish to red. There may be a slight color change if stored in dry ice.
3. Cleanse the immunization site and inject total volume of reconstituted vaccine into the outer aspect of the upper arm. Do not inject intravenously.
4. Have epinephrine available for immediate use in case of anaphylactoid reaction.

Client teaching factors

1. Encourage increased fluids, especially water.
2. Application of cool compresses to injection site will aid discomfort and swelling.
3. Ensure that responsible adult has and knows a suitable antipyretic.
4. Review symptoms to be reported to medical personnel.

GENERIC NAME Smallpox vaccine (RX)

TRADE NAME Dryvax

CLASSIFICATION Vaccine

Source Smallpox vaccine (calf lymph, chick embryo).

Action Provides active immunity. Duration of effect is 3 years. Revaccination is recommended if no Jennepian vesicle occurs within 6 to 8 days.

Indications for Use Limited to travelers who require a vaccination certificate. Routine smallpox vaccination has been discontinued in the United States.

Contraindications Skin disorders, pregnancy, altered immune states.

Untoward Reactions Vaccination is associated with a high risk of serious complications; immune serum globulin is available from the Communicable Disease Centers for treatment of life-threatening vaccination complications.

Administration 1 dose intradermal.

Available Drug Forms Multidose (25 or 100 vaccinations) package containing dry vaccine, diluent, and bifurcated needles.

Nursing Management

1. Obtain history of eczema, altered immune states, sensitivity to poison ivy, impetigo, acute skin lesions, or burns (until completely healed) in recipient and members of household.
2. Caution against scratching the vesicle and breaking it open. It will dry up to produce a scab resembling parchment that will fall off unassisted.
3. Caution should be exercised to prevent child from rubbing vaccine into eye.

GENERIC NAME Wistar rabies virus vaccine (RX)

TRADE NAME Rabies Vaccine

CLASSIFICATION Vaccine

Source Inactivated virus vaccine grown in human diploid cell cultures.

Action Provides active immunity. Approved by the Food and Drug Administration June 9, 1980. This vaccine may be used by individuals who are allergic to duck embryo.

Indications for Use Vaccination against rabies before or after exposure; recommended for all bite or scratch exposure to carnivores, especially bats, skunks, foxes, coyotes, or racoons, skin penetration bite of dog or cat, and for individuals at risk of exposure, such as stockbreeders, forest rangers, and veterinarians.

Contraindications No known contraindications.

Warnings and Precautions Do not give prophylactic vaccination in the presence of a developing febrile illness. Not recommended for individuals with demonstrated antibody response from previous exposure.

Untoward Reactions Swelling, erythema, induration, and slight ache at injection site; headache, nausea, slight fever.

Drug Interactions Corticosteroids and immunosuppressive agents may interfere with the development of active immunity.

Administration

- *Prophylaxis:* 1 ml IM in the arm on days 0 and 7; 1 ml IM on either day 21 or 28.
- *Postexposure:* 1 ml IM on days 0,3,7,14, and 28; given in conjunction with human rabies immune globulin (RIG) on day 0 to ensure immediate protection. RIG (50% infiltrated) is administered locally at the wound site.

Available Drug Forms Multidose vials.

Nursing Management

1. Vaccine is stable for 2 years at 2 to 8 C (35 to 47 F); do not freeze.
2. This creamy white product turns pink to red upon reconstitution. Use immediately following reconstitution.
3. Wash any animal bite immediately and thoroughly with soap and water. Wild animals that attack without provocation should be captured, killed, and tested as soon as possible. Domestic animals may be held for observation. Local and state health authorities should be notified.
4. Tetanus prophylaxis and measures to control bacterial infection may also be indicated.
5. Local reactions can be relieved with aspirin and antihistamines. Increase fluids (cola, ginger ale).
6. Test a serum sample for rabies antibodies titer at the time of the last dose when given 2 to 3 weeks later.

TOXOIDS

GENERIC NAME Diphtheria and tetanus toxoids, adsorbed

CLASSIFICATION Toxoid (RX)

Source Corynebacterium diphtheria and *clostridium tetani* prepared on a protein-free semisynthetic medium with 0.5 ml of aluminum phosphate. The antigen is adsorbed on the aluminum phosphate. Usually contains 16 flocculating units.

Action Provides active immunity that is adequate for booster response with less systemic reactions for older children. Preparation used in older children and adults has 2 flocculating units.

Indications for Use Routine immunization of infants and children up to 6 years when physician decides not to use equivalent, such as when pertussis vaccine is not tolerated.

Contraindications Acute or chronic respiratory infection, poliomyelitis outbreaks.

Warnings and Precautions Possible hypersensitivity.

Untoward Reactions Erythema and induration at injection site are common reactions. The site may be tender for a few days and a nodule may be palpable for a few weeks. Occasionally an abscess forms and should be seen by a physician. Fever (99 to 102 F) and malaise may occur for 24 to 48 hours after injection and should be treated with antipyretic agents. Rare reactions include irritability, high fever (103 F or above), convulsions, screaming episodes, focal neurological signs, shock, encephalopathy, and cardiovascular collapse.

Administration 0.5 ml IM.

Available Drug Forms Vials containing 0.5-ml unit doses and 5.0-ml multidose vials with sterile cartridge needle units.

Nursing Management

1. Obtain history concerning the occurrence of fever, local reaction, swelling, redness at site, and reactions of irritability.
2. Have epinephrine (1:1000) available for control of immediate allergic reactions.
3. Keep duplicate records as parent may move away and need documentation. Encourage parents to keep their own records.
4. Shake vial vigorously before withdrawing each dose. Do not allow solution to settle.
5. Cleanse immunization site with germicide. After skin penetration, withdraw to check position of needle. Expell antigen slowly and finish with a bubble of air. Do not give intravenously.
6. Pediatric: Insert 1-in. needle in midlateral thigh muscle. The deltoid muscle may be used in older children at time of primary immunization. Do not give more than one inoculation at a particular injection site. After primary immunization, tetanus toxoid protection persists for at least 10 years.
7. Cool injection site with witch hazel compresses. Use aspirin for fever over 102 F.

GENERIC NAME Diphtheria and tetanus toxoids and pertussis vaccine, adsorbed

TRADE NAMES DPT, Triple Antigen (RX)

CLASSIFICATION Toxoid

Action Active, primary immunization of infants.

Indications for Use Active immunization of infants and children up to 6 years against diphtheria, tetanus, and pertussis.

Contraindications Acute respiratory infection or other active infection; individuals receiving therapy with corticosteroids or other immunosuppressive agents (antimetabolites, irradiation, alkylating agents).

Warnings and Precautions The physician should take all precautions known for prevention of allergic or other untoward reaction before injecting vaccine.

Untoward Reactions Small area of erythema and induration at the site of injection may occur. A nodule may be palpable at the injection site for a few weeks. Mild to moderate elevation of temperature may occur following administration of DPT. (See diphtheria and tetanus toxoids, adsorbed.)

Administration 0.5 ml IM.

Available Drug Forms 0.5-ml unit doses in sterile cartridge needle units; multidose vials containing 7.5 ml.

Nursing Management Interruption of the recommended schedule with a delay between doses does not interfere with the final immunity achieved, nor does it necessitate starting the series over again, regardless of the length of time elapsed between doses. (See diphtheria and tetanus toxoids, adsorbed.)

GENERIC NAME Tetanus toxoid, adsorbed (RX)

CLASSIFICATION Toxoid

See diphtheria and tetanus toxoids, adsorbed for Contraindications, Warnings and precautions, Untoward reactions, and Nursing management.

Source *Clostridium tetani*, adsorbed on aluminum phosphate and detoxified by formaldehyde and heat.

Action After 2 weeks or the third injection, most individuals will have developed an antibody level sufficient to prevent tetanus. A maximum immunization level is reached in 3 to 5 months. Duration of effect is 10 years. The need for a booster after 18 years is questionable.

Indications for Use Predisposing wounds; wound prophylaxis (only with history of prior immunization); routine immunization (3 doses given 4 or more weeks apart).

Administration 0.5 ml IM times 3 doses at 3-week intervals. Booster dose is recommended every 10 years.

Available Drug Forms Vials containing 0.5 unit dose or 5.0 ml multidose; sterile cartridge needle units.

OTHER ANTIGENS

GENERIC NAME Poison ivy extract (RX)

TRADE NAME Rhus Tox Antigen

CLASSIFICATION Antigen

Action Each millimeter of sterile solution contains 40 mg of poison ivy extract in a 35% aqueous alcoholic medium with 4% benzyl alcohol to reduce pain of injection. Antigen passes the blood-brain barrier and enters amniotic fluid, breast milk, and urine.

Indications for Use Prophylaxis and treatment of Rhus dermatitis.

Contraindications None known.

Warnings and Precautions Renal complications may follow injection in clients with extensive dermatitis. In clients with severe Rhus dermatitis there may be an aggravation of symptoms following administration of poison ivy extract.

Untoward Reactions Local stinging may occur at injection site, but it disappears rapidly. Occasionally, local soreness and aching may occur, which disappears within 24 to 48 hours.

Administration

- *Prophylaxis:* Susceptible individuals can usually be protected against an attack of Rhus dermatitis for a season or longer by preseasonal injections of Rhus Tox Antigen. General dosage: 1 ml IM every 4 to 7 days times 4 or more doses. In very sensitive individuals, it may be advisable to start with a smaller dose: 0.25 to 0.5 ml IM giving a total of 4 ml or more.
- *Rhus dermatitis:* 1 ml IM every 12 to 24 hours until symptoms are controlled. A minimum of 4 injections is recommended even if symptoms are alleviated within a few hours; the tendency of future attacks will be lessened.

Available Drug Forms Vials containing 1 ml.

Nursing Management

1. Vials do not require refrigeration.
2. Instruct client to notify physician if rash appears.
3. If rash is present, instruct client to avoid scratching.
4. Clients should be informed that immunity may last only one season. Periodic reinjection is required.

GENERIC NAME Poison ivy, oak, and sumac combination

TRADE NAME Rhus All Antigen (RX)

CLASSIFICATION Antigen

See poison ivy extract for Warnings and precautions, Untoward reactions, and Nursing management.

Action A triple antigen of the active principles of poison ivy, oak, and sumac in an oil vehicle.

Indications for Use Prophylaxis for hyposensitization of Rhus dermatitis.

Contraindications Not recommended for treatment of acute Rhus dermatitis.

Administration Adults: 1 ml IM weekly for 2 to 3 weeks prior to exposure.

Available Drug Forms Multidose vials containing 5 ml.

Chapter 82

Passive Immunizing and Immunosuppressive Agents

PASSIVE IMMUNITY IS the state of protection against an antigen that results from receiving the antibodies or cells that have been produced by other individuals or animals. As antibodies are acquired *naturally* through the placenta by the fetus, the newborn has passive immunity against several of the same communicable diseases as the mother. Unfortunately, this immunity lasts only a few months and then the infant is susceptible to infectious microorganisms. Protection can be provided *artificially* by injecting biologic substances containing antibodies. Although antibiotics are available for the treatment of infectious diseases, antitoxins, gamma globulins, and other passive immunologic agents are useful in preventing and treating infectious diseases caused by viruses and other pathogens that fail to respond adequately to antibiotics.

PROPERTIES OF ANTITOXINS

Antitoxins are prepared from the blood of humans or animals, particularly horses, that have been injected with specific exotoxins, which induce the formation of antitoxins in the serum. Years ago, the proteins in horse serum could not be separated adequately and some individuals developed reactions against the animal's proteins. Today, the pseudoglobulin fraction containing the desired antitoxin can be separated with considerable precision. The antitoxins are measured in units of activity; but it should be remembered that the unit of the American or National Institute of Health may be only half as potent as the international unit. The manufacturers' guidelines for dosage should be followed.

PROPERTIES OF ANTIVENINS

Venoms are the poisonous excretions produced by certain animals, such as poisonous snakes and spiders. Venoms contain proteins with enzymatic activity and neurotoxic fractions. Snake venoms are obtained by holding the snake head over a container covered with a thin sheet of rubber. As the snake strikes the rubber cover with its fangs, the semiliquid venom is ejected into the container. The venom is then attenuated and injected into horses or other animals. Horses' serum is used to prepare the antivenin substance in a similar fashion as the antitoxins. Polyvalent antivenin preparations are solutions containing a mixture of serums against the poisonous snakes found in a particular locality or country.

PROPERTIES OF IMMUNE SERUM GLOBULINS

Immune serum globulins, or simply antiserums, are biologic agents produced from the blood of immunized humans or animals. The incidence of hypersensitivity reactions to preparations prepared from human serum is considerably less than with agents prepared from animal serums.

Antibodies are contained in the group of simple serum proteins called *globulins,* which are insoluble in water but soluble in acidic solutions. Immune serum globulin, or simply *gamma globulin,* is a solution containing the fraction of serum globulin that has most of the human antibodies. Commercially available gamma globulin is prepared from several donors so that the spectrum of antibodies present is vast.

Gamma globulin can now be separated into specific globulin fractions containing antibodies against certain diseases, such as measles, mumps, and hepatitis. These agents are used to prevent or treat the disease; however, the duration of the passive immunity is relatively short compared to that of vaccines and other active immunizing agents. One globulin preparation also has immunosuppressive properties.

PROPERTIES OF IMMUNOSUPPRESSIVE AGENTS

Immunosuppressive agents decrease the activity of all or part of the body's immune system. Technically, antimetabolites, antibiotics, alkylating agents (nitrogen mustard), and corticosteroids are all immunosuppressive agents in large enough doses. However, these products are seldom used for this purpose. There are two drugs that are presently used to suppress some aspect of the immune system; namely, anti-Rh_o (D) and azathioprine.

Anti-Rh_o (D) immune globulin is a sterile solution of globulin obtained from humans who have a high Rh antibody titer. This biologic agent neutralizes Rh-positive antigens found in the blood of Rh-negative women postpartum or those carrying a Rh-positive baby. The objective is to prevent the woman's immune system from producing antibodies against the Rh-positive antigen, thereby enabling the woman to carry a second Rh-positive baby without her body rejecting it.

Azathioprine is actually an antiinflammatory agent capable of preventing the rejection of grafts and homotransplants. It prevents the proliferation of precursors of peripheral monocytes and large lymphocytes, thus suppressing some of the antibodies that cause rejection.

ANTITOXINS AND ANTIVENINS

GENERIC NAME Botulism polyvalent antitoxin

TRADE NAME Botulism Antitoxin (Polyvalent)

CLASSIFICATION Antitoxin (RX)

Source Plasma of immunized horses containing antibodies against *Clostridium botulism.*

Action Neutralizes the toxin botulin and provides passive immunity.

Indications for Use Treatment of suspected botulism; prophylaxis is not routinely recommended, but may be given to asymptomatic, exposed individuals.

Contraindications Hypersensitivity.

Warnings and Precautions Test for sensitivity according to manufacturer's instructions before administering as anaphylaxis or serum sickness may occur in sensitive individuals.

Untoward Reactions Anaphylaxis or serum sickness can occur in sensitive clients (.25% of those given antitoxin). Clients should be tested for hypersensitivity reactions before administering drug.

Administration 1 vial IV and 1 vial IM; repeat after 2 to 4 hours if symptoms worsen and again after 12 to 24 hours.

Available Drug Forms Vials available from the U.S. Centers for Disease Control (CDC), Atlanta, GA 30333; telephone (404) 329-3311 (day); (404) 329-3644 (night). In Canada, the antitoxin can be obtained through Connaught Laboratories, Willowdale, Ontario.

Nursing Management

Planning factors

1. Obtain an accurate history of allergies, especially to horses.
2. Obtain a precise history when ingestion of contaminated food is suspected.
3. Obtain a careful history of food intake for the past 2 days; symptoms usually occur in 12 to 36 hours.
4. Determine if other family members have similar signs and symptoms and share a common food intake.
5. Prepare an emergency tray with gastric lavage, sodium bicarbonate, intravenous glucose, digitalis, and neostigmine (Prostigmin) and keep readily available.
6. Hyperbaric oxygen (oxygen under greater than normal atmospheric pressure) may be of some assistance in treating botulism.

Administration factors

1. Add contents of vial to 5% D/W, 10% D/W, or normal saline to make a 1:10 dilution.
2. Give diluted antitoxin slowly (1 ml/min.) at first. If a hypersensitivity reaction occurs, stop drug administration and treat appropriately.
3. If no reaction occurs, administer diluted antitoxin at a faster rate (2 ml/min.).

Evaluation factors

1. Observe for abnormal neurologic signs.
2. Many clients must be placed on a ventilator, since respiratory failure is the most serious symptom. Sedatives, hypnotics, and most analgesics are avoided because of their effect on respiration.
3. Watch for signs of weakness, blurred vision, and slurred speech in family members who may have contracted the disease but are without symptoms.

GENERIC NAME Diphtheria antitoxin (RX)

CLASSIFICATION Antitoxin

Source Plasma of immunized horses.

Action Erythromycin may be given to nonimmune contacts of active cases rather than antitoxin prophylaxis. Contacts should be observed for signs of illness so that antitoxin may be administered if needed.

Indications for Use Unknown or questionable immune status.

Contraindications Hypersensitivity.

Warnings and Precautions Test for hypersensitivity before administering.

Untoward Reactions Anaphylaxis may occur. Serum sickness may occur 1 to 2 weeks after administration.

Administration 20,000 to 120,000 units IM depending on severity and duration of illness.

Available Drug Forms Vials containing 10,000 units/5 ml or 20,000 units/10 ml.

Nursing Management

1. Check package insert carefully for the correct volume of each dose.
2. Refrigerate vials.
3. Check expiration date before using.

GENERIC NAME North and South American antisnakebite serum

TRADE NAME Polyvalent Crotalid Antivenin (RX)

CLASSIFICATION Antivenin

Source Prepared by injecting horses with venom. When the appropriate antibody titer reaches the desired strength, the blood serum is processed. Polyvalent antivenin contains the venoms of 4 pit vipers: Western diamondback, Florida diamondback, South American rattlesnake, South American fer-de-lance.

Action Antibodies in the drug serum interact with the venom injected by the snake.

Indications for Use Poisonous or suspected poisonous snakebite.

Contraindications Hypersensitivity.

Warnings and Precautions Perform skin or eye tests for hypersensitivity to horse serum before administering.

Untoward Reactions Anaphylaxis, laryngeal spasms.

Administration Initial dosage: 1 vial diluted in 20 ml sodium chloride solution IV; then administer as needed; Usual dosage: 3 to 5 vials.

Available Drug Forms Vials containing antivenin and diluent; a 1-ml test dose vial is also included.

Nursing Management

1. Obtain history of allergies, asthma, hay fever, infantile eczema, urticaria, and previous immunization with antivenin.
2. Recipients of antivenin are usually hospitalized for 4 to 5 days and should be closely monitored for untoward reactions involving the kidneys and the cardiovascular, respiratory, and nervous systems.
3. Have epinephrine readily available at bedside.
4. Antitetanus measures may also be required.
5. A central directory for information on use and availability of antivenins is maintained by the American Association of Zoological Parks and Aquariums at the Antivenom Index Center in Oklahoma City, OK 73126. This service is available on a 24-hour basis.

GENERIC NAME Antivenin (RX)

TRADE NAMES Polyvalent Crotalid (Crotaline Antivenin), Antivenin Polyvalent, Univalent, or Bivalent North and South American AntiSnakebite Serum (U.S.P. 1960)

CLASSIFICATION Antivenin

See North and South American antisnakebite serum for Nursing management.

Source Frozen solution of specific venom-metabolizing globulin obtained from the serum of healthy horses immunized against venoms of four species of pit vipers: Western diamondback, Florida diamondback, South American rattlesnake, South American fer-de-lance.

Action Acts as an antitoxin.

Indications for Use Treatment of snakebite caused by included species.

Contraindications Hypersensitivity.

Untoward Reactions Febrile reactions are common. Anaphylaxis and urticaria have been reported.

Available Drug Forms *Univalent:* Protection against the copperhead. *Bivalent:* Protection against the copperhead and rattlesnake in the United States; in other countries, the combinations depend on local species of snakes.

IMMUNE SERUM GLOBULINS

GENERIC NAME Immune serum globulin (RX)

TRADE NAMES Gamastan, Gammar, Immu-G, Immuglobin, Gamma Globulin

CLASSIFICATION Immune serum globulin

Source Prepared from normal blood, plasma, serum, or globulins of individuals who have recovered from a disease and retained antibodies.

Action The antibody response is suppressed due to injection of passive antibodies. These antibodies interact with invading antigens, such as infectious microorganisms, to minimize or prevent the disease process.

Indications for Use Gammaglobulinemia or hypogammaglobulinemia, serum hepatitis following transfusion, measles vaccine complications, exposure to hepatitis A, measles or measles variant, poliomyelitis, chicken pox, and rubella (in first trimester of pregnancy).

Contraindications Do not give for hepatitis after onset of symptoms or if 6 weeks or more have elapsed since exposure.

Untoward Reactions Urticaria, angioedema, anaphylaxis, local reaction at the injection site(s) (pain, erythema, muscle stiffness), headache, malaise, fever, and nephrotic syndrome have been reported.

Drug Interactions No significant interactions known.

Administration Highly individualized.

- *Postexposure:* Adults and children: 0.2 to 1.3 ml/kg IM as soon as possible after exposure.
- *Agammaglobulinemia, hypogammaglobulinemia:* Adults: 30 to 50 ml IM monthly; Children: 20 to 40 ml IM monthly.

Available Drug Forms Vials containing 10 ml.

Nursing Management

1. Obtain history of allergies and any previous reactions to immunization.
2. Have epinephrine (1:1000) available in the event of an anaphylactoid reaction.
3. Inject deep into large muscle mass. Do not exceed 5 ml per injection site.

GENERIC NAME Hepatitis B (RX)

TRADE NAMES Immune Globulin, Gammage Hep-B

CLASSIFICATION Immune serum globulin

Source Prepared from pooled plasma drawn from individuals with high titers of antibody to the hepatitis B surface antigen and who are nonreactive when tested for hepatitis B surface antigens.

Action Provides passive immunization for individuals exposed to hepatitis B virus.

Indications for Use Gammage Hep-B is indicated for prophylaxis following either parenteral exposure, direct mucous membrane contact, or oral ingestion of contaminated materials, such as blood, plasma, or serum. Such exposures might occur by accidental "needlestick," accidental splash, or a pipetting accident. Other sources of exposure continue to be evaluated, such as exposure to hepatitis B in dialysis clients, among hospital staff, and infants born to hepatitis B-positive mothers.

Contraindications Isolated immunoglobin A deficiency, severe thrombocytopenia, any coagulation disorders.

Warnings and Precautions Use with caution in clients with a history of prior systemic allergic reactions following administration of human immune globulin preparations.

Untoward Reactions Hypersensitivity reaction (rare), local pain and tenderness at injection site, urticaria, angioedema.

Drug Interactions Antibodies present in immune globulin preparations may interfere with the immune response to live virus vaccines, such as measles, mumps, and rubella; vaccination with live virus vaccines should be deferred.

Administration 0.06 ml/kg IM as soon as possible after exposure, preferably within 7 days and repeated 28 to 30 days after exposure.

Available Drug Forms Vials containing 5 ml.

Nursing Management

1. Have epinephrine available for treatment of acute allergic symptoms.
2. Check expiration date before using.
3. Inspect for particulate matter and discoloration. Gammage is a clear, very slightly amber, moderately viscous liquid.
4. Draw back on the plunger of the syringe before injection to ensure that the needle is not in a blood vessel.
5. Inject into gluteal or deltoid region. Use a separate sterile syringe and needle for each individual. Do not give intravenously.
6. Store at 2 to 8 C (35.6 to 46.4 F).

GENERIC NAME Measles immune globulin (RX)

CLASSIFICATION Immune serum globulin

See immune serum globulin for Nursing management.

Action Transfers specific antibodies with a known antibody titer into the circulation of the exposed individual, providing passive immunization.

Indications for Use Prevention of measles.

Administration 0.25 ml/kg IM within 6 days of exposure. For modification of measles, 0.05 ml/kg of globulin is given during the first week of exposure or later in the incubation period; permanent immunity usually follows. Infants and young children can obtain permanent protection by active immunization with live vaccine 8 or more weeks after the modification agent.

Available Drug Forms Vials containing 10 ml.

GENERIC NAME Tetanus immune globulin (RX)

TRADE NAMES Homo-Tet, Hyper-Tet, Immu-Tetanus

CLASSIFICATION Immune serum globulin

Action Used to provide immediate passive immunization in individuals at risk of tetanus. Tetanus toxoid may be administered concurrently to allow individual to develop active immunity to tetanus while decreasing short-term protection from immune globulin toxoid.

Indications for Use Clean, minor wounds that are less than 24 hours old; no booster dose is needed by a fully immunized child unless more than 10 years have elapsed since the last dose. Contaminated wounds that are less than 24 hours old; booster dose should be given if more than 5 years have elapsed since the last dose.

Untoward Reactions Pain, stiffness, and erythema may occur at the injection site. There is some concern over the use of boosters, even for dirty wounds. The increased incidence and severity of untoward reactions may be associated with an increased use of boosters, even for dirty wounds, more often than every 10 years. Anaphylaxis, fever, and other hypersensitivity reactions may occur.

Administration 250 units IM; this dose provides protection for several weeks.

Available Drug Forms Prefilled syringes containing 250 units; multidose vials.

Nursing Management

1. Obtain history of injury, previous tetanus immunization, allergies, and reactions to immunization.
2. The risk of sensitivity reactions with human preparations is minimal and antibodies persist longer (half-life: 3 to 4 weeks) than with equine antitoxin. When equine antitoxin is to be used, sensitivity testing should be done before injecting antitoxin.
3. Cleanse wound thoroughly and remove foreign matter.
4. When administering tetanus toxoid concurrently, use separate syringes and inject at different sites. Concomitant immunization is recommended only for major or contaminated wounds in individuals who have had fewer than 2 doses of toxoid at anytime in the past (fewer than 3 doses if wound is more than 24 hours old).
5. Store at 2 to 8 C (36 to 46 F); do not freeze.

IMMUNOSUPPRESSIVE AGENTS

GENERIC NAME Rh_o (D) immune globulin (RX)

TRADE NAME RhoGAM

CLASSIFICATION Immunosuppressive agent

Action Suppression of antibody response to the foreign RH_o (D)-positive cell by an injection of passive RH_o (D) antibody prophylactically provides immune suppressive immunization. This agent is used to prevent formation of active anti-Rh_o (D) antibodies in RH_o (D)-negative individuals.

Indications for Use Nonimmune females who have been exposed to the Rh factor: postabortion, post miscarriage, ectopic pregnancy, postpartum. When given in case of a transfusion accident, the volume of Rh-positive blood is multiplied by the hematocrit value of the donor unit. The volume of packed red blood cells is then divided by 15 ml to determine the number of vials to use. Ideally, the globulin should be given within 3 hours, but can be given up to 72 hours after delivery, termination of pregnancy, or transfusion accident.

Contraindications Infants, Rh_o (D)-positive of D^u-positive individuals, Rh_o (D)-negative and D^u-negative individuals previously sensitized to the Rh_o (D) or D^u antigen.

Untoward Reactions Side effects are extremely rare because the globulin is made from pooled homologous human serum protein; but low-grade fever or soreness at the injection site may occur.

Administration

- *Postpartum prophylaxis:* 1 vial IM within 3 days of delivery.
- *Antepartum prophylaxis:* Initial dosage: 1 vial IM over 28 weeks gestation; then, 1 vial within 3 days of delivery.
- *Miscarriage, abortion, ectopic pregnancy:* Beyond the 13th week of gestation: 1 vial.
- *Transfusion* (Rh positive cells to a Rh-negative recipient): 1 vial/15 ml of transfused red cells IM.

Available Drug Forms Single-dose and multidose vials.

Nursing Management

1. Determine infant's blood type and perform a direct Coombs' test immediately postpartum. The infant must be Rh_o (D) positive and D^u positive and have a negative Coombs' test. A positive Coombs' test must be due to antibodies other than Rh_o (D).
2. Preadministration procedure:
   - (a) Confirm lot numbers are the same for the cross-match solution and the drug to be administered: 1 vial of 1:1000 dilution of an aliquot from ramelot of Gamulin prepackaged with RhoGAM.
   - (b) Confirm mother is Rh_o (D) negative and D^u negative. If father is also Rh negative, immunosuppressive agent should not be given. Immune prophylaxis is also advisable in ABO mothers when other criteria are met.
3. Client information:
   - (a) Result of test for prior sensitivity.
   - (b) Notification to client concerning nature of medication, date, and reason for administration.
   - (c) Adequate documentation if medication is refused by client.
   - (d) Obtain history of allergies and reaction to immunization.

4. Verify all laboratory reports for both infant and mother. Check empty cross-match vial with vial of medication for same serial numbers. Complete special form that comes with package and attach to client's hospital record and/or return completed forms and empty vials to laboratory.
5. One vial can reliably inhibit the immune response to a hemomaternal bleed of 1 ml as estimated by the Betake-Kleihauser smear technique. In cases of abortion or ectopic pregnancy when Rh typing of fetus is not possible, the fetus must be assumed to be Rh_o (D) positive or D^u positive. RhoGAM is administered in transplacental hemorrhages when blood type of fetus has not been determined to be negative.
6. Do not administer intravenously.
7. Store at 2 to 8 C; do not freeze.

GENERIC NAME Azathioprine (RX)

TRADE NAME Imuran

CLASSIFICATION Immunosuppressive agent

Action Azathioprine, an imidazolyl derivative of mercaptopurine, is primarily an antiinflammatory agent that prevents the proliferation of the precursors of peripheral monocytes and large lymphocytes, thus the quantity of mononuclear cells entering an inflammed area is decreased. In large dosages, azathioprine inhibits the humoral antigen-antibody reaction; however, the drug has little or no effect on the production of antibodies. Once the body has begun to reject an organ, the drug has no therapeutic effect.

Indications for Use Preventing the rejection of renal transplants; treatment of severe, active rheumatoid arthritis that is unresponsive to traditional therapy.

Contraindications Hypersensitivity to azathioprine, pregnancy, clients previously treated with alkylating agents, since neoplasia may occur.

Warnings and Precautions Severe infections are a constant hazard. Fungal, viral, bacterial, and protozoal infections may be fatal. The drug is a known mutagen and may precipitate neoplasia. It is also known to cause teratogenic reactions in animals.

Untoward Reactions Blood dyscrasias, including leukopenia, bone marrow depression, anemia, pancytopenia, and thrombocytopenia, occur relatively frequently. GI disturbances, including nausea and vomiting, are common. Diarrhea and steatorrhea have also occurred. Toxic hepatitis with biliary stasis has occurred, particularly in clients who are homograph recipients. Elevated serum, alkaline phosphatase, and bilirubin have occurred. Pancreatitis has also been reported. The incidence of lymphoma and other neoplastic diseases is increased. Infrequent reactions include skin rashes, alopecia, fever, arthralgia, and a negative nitrogen balance.

Parameters of Use

Absorption Well absorbed. Peak serum levels occur in 1 to 2 hours. Half-life is 5 hours. About 30% bound to serum proteins.

Metabolism Primarily by xanthine oxidase in the liver. Metabolites include 6-mercaptopurine and inactive 6-theoric acid, which may disrupt RNA and DNA function.

Excretion Primarily by the kidneys as unchanged drug (50%) and metabolites.

Drug Interactions Drugs that inhibit xanthine oxidase, such as allopurinol, will interfere with the metabolism of azathioprine. If given concurrently, azathioprine should be reduced to one-third or one-quarter of the usual dosage.

Administration

- *Transplant:* Adults and children: Initial dosage: 3 to 5 mg/kg IV or in divided doses at the time of transplant; Maintenance dosage: 1 to 3 mg/kg po daily.
- *Rheumatoid arthritis:* Initial dosage: 1.0 mg/kg po daily or in 2 divided doses for 6 to 8 weeks; then increase to 0.5 mg/kg every 4 weeks until desired response; Maximum dosage: 2.5 mg/kg/day. Maximum therapeutic response may not occur for 8 to 12 weeks.

Available Drug Forms Scored tablets containing 25 or 50 mg; vials of dry lyophilized sodium salt containing 100 mg.

Nursing Management

Planning factors

1. Obtain complete blood cell count (CBC) and hepatic and renal function tests before initiating therapy.
2. Check whether client is receiving allopurinol or other drugs that inhibit metabolism.
3. Obtain history of neoplasia.
4. Client should understand the drug's untoward reactions before therapy is instituted.
5. Protect client from infection; restrict visitors; warn family about infection.

Administration factors

1. If GI disturbances occur, drug can be given in divided doses with meals.
2. Reconstitute dry powder with 10 ml of sterile water and swirl until a clear solution results. May be added to 50 to 100 ml of 5% D/W and administered over 30 to 60 minutes IV.
3. Check patency of IV site before administering. May cause irritation at IV site, particularly if extravasation occurs.
4. Avoid giving client IM injections if at all possible.

Evaluation factors

1. Obtain CBC and platelet count at least weekly. If white blood cell count is below 3000/mm^2, the drug should be discontinued immediately.
2. Reverse isolation may be required to prevent infection.
3. Inspect client's skin for bleeding periodically.

Client teaching factors

1. Warn client about serious consequences of minor infections.
2. Warn client about the potential of thinning hair.
3. Caution client to report untoward reactions, such as infections, bruising, and bleeding, immediately to health professionals.
4. Advise client to avoid conception for at least 4 months after drug therapy has been discontinued.

Chapter 83

Histamine and Antihistamines

Anamine Syrup, Anamine T.D., Brexin L.A., Cenules, Chol-Trimeton, Cordimal L.A., Deconamine Elixir and Syrup, Deconamine SR, Decongestant Repetabs, Isoclor Liquid, Isoclor Timesule

Brexin

Brocon C.R., Dimetapp Extentabs

Citra Capsules

Comhist

Co-Pyronil

Disophrol, Drixoral

Extendryl T.D., Histaspan-D, Dinovan Timed

Fedahist

Fedrazil

Histabid Duracap

Kronohist Kronocaps

Napril

Neotep Granucaps

Nolamine

Rhinex D·Lay

Rondec

Triaminic Syrup

THE ROLE OF HISTAMINE IN HYPERSENSITIVITY REACTIONS

Histamine is present naturally in the body, being produced from an amino acid called *histidine*. Histamine is found in all body tissues, with highest concentrations in the skin, lungs, and gastrointestinal tract. It is normally stored in the cytoplasm of connective tissue mast cells and circulatory basophils and is inactive, or inert, until released from the cells during a hypersensitivity reaction. Toxins and other substances, such as antigens, can alter the permeability of the cell membrane, thereby causing degranulation and the release of histamine. This freely circulating histamine is responsible for a wide range of allergic reactions (see Chapter 8).

When histamine is released it acts on two distinct receptors, namely H_1- and H_2-receptor sites. H_1-receptors are located primarily in the smooth muscle of blood vessels, bronchioles, and the gastrointestinal tract. H_2-receptors are found in the gastric mucosa and, to a lesser extent, in the myocardium and blood vessels. When these receptors are stimulated by histamine, the following physiologic reactions occur: dilation of arterioles and venules with an increase in capillary permeability; contraction of nonvascular smooth muscle of the bronchial tree, gastrointestinal tract, and other organs; stimulation of gastric acid secretions; acceleration of heart rate; release of epinephrine and norepinephrine from the adrenal medulla; central nervous system effects, such as motion sickness.

Histamine has been used clinically as an aid in the diagnosis of stomach cancer and pernicious anemia: If the client does not respond to the administration of histamine with a significant secretion of hydrochloric acid, a degenerative change in the gastric mucosa is indicated. Histamine has also been used to diagnose pheochromocytoma, a tumor of the adrenal medulla. In this condition, an injection of histamine will result in a marked increase in blood pressure. More rarely, histamine has been used in the diagnosis of asthma, since histamine will cause severe bronchospasm in asthmatics. These diagnostic uses of histamine are now generally obsolete because of the potentially dangerous consequences and the development of less toxic diagnostic agents.

PROPERTIES OF ANTIHISTAMINES

Many antihistamines have been developed over the last 40 years, but only a few are used clinically and in over-the-counter compounds. Antihistamines act by competing with histamine for receptor sites. When they bind with the receptor cells histamine is prevented from binding at the same time. Traditional antihistamines are much more effective in blocking the circulatory and bronchial effects of histamine than they are in inhibiting the gastric secretory effects. These antihistamines are therefore called *H_1-antagonists* and are classified into five major categories:

- Ethanolamine derivatives: antiemetics, CNS depression

- Ethylenediamine derivatives: antiallergic
- Phenothiazines: anti–motion sickness, CNS depression
- Propylamine derivatives: antiallergic
- Miscellaneous: anti–motion sickness/antipyretic

Pharmacologically, the action of the H_1-antihistamines is essentially the same for all five categories, with differences existing only in degree of action at various body sites.

INDICATIONS FOR USE

Antihistamines are used primarily to prevent allergic symptoms caused by histamine release. Common nasal allergies, such as hay fever, are most successfully controlled if antihistamines are taken early in the season; that is, before symptoms are manifested. These agents have no antiinflammatory action and cannot reverse the histamine reaction once it has occurred; therefore, antihistamines are not indicated for the treatment of severe allergic responses or asthmatic attacks. These conditions require a histamine antagonist, such as epinephrine. The anticholinergic properties of antihistamines make them useful for alleviating the symptoms of colds or in shortening the duration of a cold. Antihistamines are also useful for preventing motion sickness; controlling nausea and vomiting associated with anesthesia; sedating preoperative clients and insomniacs; and as an adjunct in the treatment of anaphylactic reactions, parkinsonism, and extrapyramidal symptoms associated with psychotropic drug therapy. There is no cumulative benefit from antihistamines, so their palliative effects are evident only as long as the drugs are taken.

The anticholinergic properties of antihistamines also result in some untoward reactions, namely, inhibition of secretions, blurred vision, some urinary retention, constipation, and tachycardia. Central nervous system effects include sedation and drowsiness in adults and nervousness and irritability in children. Their anticholinergic action in the vestibular pathways accounts for their usefulness in preventing motion sickness and vertigo.

PROPERTIES OF SEROTONIN ANTAGONISTS

Serotonin is a chemical substance found in mast cells, platelets, the gastrointestinal mucosa, and carcinoid tumors. Serotonin is a powerful vasoconstrictor and is thought to be a factor in sleep and sensory perception. There are several drugs that are used when serotonin activity is thought to be the causative mechanism in allergic-type reactions. These drugs possess pharmacologic actions similar to antihistamines and are subject to similar indications for use and contraindications.

DRUG INTERACTIONS

Concurrent use of any central nervous system depressant will enhance the sedative effect of antihistamines and anticholinergic agents, tricyclic antidepressants, and MAO inhibitors will enhance the anticholinergic effects of antihistamines. Furthermore, antihistamines can decrease the effects of corticosteroids, estradiol, progesterone, and testosterone.

NURSING MANAGEMENT

1. Clients receiving antihistamines should be educated about the common side effects of antihistamines and warned about the dangers of engaging in hazardous activities, such as operating machinery or driving a car. The client should be cautioned to avoid any other central nervous system depressants while taking antihistamines and to discontinue antihistamines before skin testing, since they may mask otherwise positive reactions.
2. Clients with allergies should carry an identification tag or card at all times indicating the type of allergy, the medication being used, and their physician's name.
3. Sedative effects of antihistamines usually abate with continued use. If the effects do not subside or other side effects occur, a different antihistamine is usually indicated.

Children are particularly susceptible to untoward reactions and fatalities have occurred from accidental overdosage in children.

4. Topical antihistamine preparations carry a much higher risk of hypersensitivity reactions than do oral forms. They should be discontinued at the first signs of skin sensitization and should never be applied to broken skin or draining lesions.

ETHANOLAMINE DERIVATIVES

GENERIC NAME Diphenhydramine hydrochloride

TRADE NAMES Allerdryl, Benadryl, Ben-Allergin, Benylin, Caladryl, Eldadryl, Nordryl, SK-Diphenhydramine, Valdrene, Wehdryl

CLASSIFICATION H_1 antihistamine (OTC) (RX)

Action Diphenhydramine competes with histamine at H_1-receptor sites. It also induces an atropine-like anticholinergic effect. The drug is sometimes used as a sleeping pill because of its pronounced sedative effects.

Indications for Use As an adjunct in the treatment of allergic reactions, including urticaria and anaphylaxis, rhinitis, motion sickness, sedation, temporary relief of cough. Also used as an antiparkinsonism agent.

Contraindications Neonates, premature infants, lactation, acute bronchial and other lower respiratory tract disorders, therapy with MAO inhibitors.

Warnings and Precautions Use with caution in young children and clients with hyperthyroidism, hypertension, or a history of bronchial asthma. Use with extreme caution in clients with narrow-angle glaucoma, peptic ulcer, pyloric obstruction, or urinary retention. Safe use during pregnancy has not been established.

Untoward Reactions Sedation, nausea, and epigastric distress are common. Thickening of bronchial secretions is common and may lead to the development of mucus plugs. CNS disturbances, including dizziness, disruption of balance, tremors, irritability, paresthesia, and vertigo, may occur, particularly in the elderly. Toxicity causes anticholinergic symptoms: (fixed) dilated pupils, flushing, vomiting. Hallucinations, convulsions, and death may occur in infants and children. Hypotension may occur. GI disturbances include anorexia, vomiting, diarrhea, and constipation. Genitourinary disturbances include difficulty in urination, urinary frequency, and retention. Skin rashes, photosensitivity, diaphoresis, and chills may occur. Blurred vision, diplopia, tinnitus, and acute labyrinthitis have been reported. Blood dyscrasias, including hemolytic anemia, thrombocytopenia, and agranulocytosis, may occur, particularly in the elderly and after prolonged use. Local stinging and irritation may occur at the injection site.

Parameters of Use

Absorption Readily absorbed from GI tract; pKa is 9; the pH of a 1% aqueous solution is 5. Peak action occurs in about 60 minutes. Duration of action is 4 to 6 hours.

Enters breast milk and may cross placenta.

Metabolism Mainly in the liver; some by other tissues including the kidneys and lungs.

Excretion In urine, primarily as metabolites.

Drug Interactions Anticholinergic agents and MAO inhibitors may prolong and intensify the anticholinergic effects of antihistamines; concurrent use is not recommended. Excessive sedation and other CNS disturbances may occur when alcohol, barbiturates, and CNS depressants are used concomitantly.

Administration

- *Adjunct in allergic reactions:* 10 to 50 mg IM or IV.
- *Rhinitis, motion sickness, parkinsonism:* 25 to 50 mg po tid or qid.
- *Sedation:* 25 to 50 mg po or IM hs; Maximum dosage: 400 mg/day.
- *Pediatric:* 5 mg/kg/24 hours or 150 mg/m^2/24 hours in 4 divided doses IM or IV; Maximum dosage: 300 mg/day. Over 20 lb: 12.5 to 25 mg po tid or qid.

Available Drug Forms Capsules containing 25 or 50 mg; elixir containing 12.5 mg/5 ml and 14% alcohol; cough syrup containing 12.5 mg/5 ml and 5% alcohol; multidose vials containing 10 mg/ml; prefilled syringes containing 50 mg/ml; topical cream (Caladryl) containing 1 or 2%.

Nursing Management

Planning factors

1. Obtain history of CNS, GI, and genitourinary disturbances and hypersensitivities.
2. Check for anemia or other hematologic abnormalities. Notify physician if any exist.
3. Must be used in conjunction with epinephrine for severe allergic reactions.
4. Discontinue drug for at least 72 hours prior to skin testing, since it may mask otherwise positive reactions.

Administration factors

1. Oral preparations may be given with milk or food to minimize GI disturbances.
2. Give IM injection deep into large muscle mass to avoid local irritation. Rotate injection sites.
3. Administer IV slowly to avoid irritation to vein. Flush line with normal saline.
4. Apply ointment to intact skin. Never apply to broken skin or draining lesions.

Evaluation factors

1. Observe reaction closely in elderly clients (over 60 years) and assist with ambulation as CNS disturbances are generally more pronounced in the elderly.

2. Sedative effects usually abate with continued use. If sedation and other secondary effects persist, changing the antihistamine may be helpful.
3. Perform periodic blood counts in clients on prolonged therapy.

Client teaching factors

1. Inform client about the secondary effects of drug and emphasize the dangers of driving a car or operating hazardous machinery.
2. Instruct client to avoid alcohol and CNS depressants while taking antihistamines.
3. Inform client that ice chips and sugarless gum may be helpful in relieving dry mouth.
4. Warn client to avoid direct sunlight when medicated ointment is being used because photosensitivity may occur.

GENERIC NAME Bromodiphenhydramine hydrochloride

TRADE NAME Ambodryl (RX)

CLASSIFICATION H_1-antihistamine

See diphenhydramine hydrochloride for Warnings and precautions, Untoward reactions, Parameters of Use, Drug interactions, and Nursing management.

Action Similar to diphenhydramine in action but with half the dosage.

Indications for Use Allergies, motion sickness, insomnia.

Administration 25 mg po tid; Maximum dosage: 150 mg/day.

Available Drug Forms Capsules containing 25 mg.

GENERIC NAME Carbinoxamine maleate (RX)

TRADE NAME Clistin

CLASSIFICATION H_1-antihistamine

See diphenhydramine hydrochloride for Warnings and precautions, Untoward reactions, Parameters of Use, Drug interactions, and Nursing management.

Action Carbinoxamine competes with histamine at H_1-receptor sites. Although it is an ethanolamine derivative, carbinoxamine is similar to chlorpheniramine. It induces fewer CNS and GI disturbances than diphenhydramine.

Indications for Use Allergic disorders, symptomatic treatment of bronchial asthma.

Administration Adults: 4 to 8 mg po tid or qid or 8 to 12 mg po (repeat-action form) q12h; Children: 2 to 4 mg po tid or qid.

Available Drug Forms Tablets containing 4 mg; repeat-action tablets containing 8 or 12 mg; elixir containing 4 mg/5 ml.

GENERIC NAME Dimenhydrinate (RX)

TRADE NAME Dramamine

CLASSIFICATION H_1-antihistamine

See diphenhydramine hydrochloride for Parameters of use and Drug interactions.

Action Although the exact mechanism of action is unknown, dimenhydrinate, the chlorotheophylline salt of diphenhydramine, prevents overstimulation of the labyrinth and its associated neural pathways, thus preventing nausea.

Indications for Use Prevention and treatment of motion sickness. Has also been used for hyperemesis gravidarum (nausea due to pregnancy) and nausea and dizziness associated with Meniere's syndrome and other ear disorders.

Contraindications Narrow-angle glaucoma, neonates, premature infants, urinary retention.

Warnings and Precautions Use with caution in clients with asthma, glaucoma, or prostatic enlargement. May mask ototoxic symptoms when given concurrently with antibiotics that have the potential of inducing ototoxic reactions. Tolerance may develop after prolonged use.

Untoward Reactions Drowsiness may occur, particularly when large dosages are used. (See diphenhydramine hydrochloride.)

Administration Oral, rectal suppository: Adults: 50 to 100 mg every 4 to 6 hours; Maximum dosage: 400 mg/day. Children: Ages 6 to 12 years: 25 to 50 mg every 6 to 8 hours; Maximum dosage: 150 mg/day; Ages 2 to 6 years: 25 mg every 6 to 8 hours; Maximum dosage: 75 mg/day. Intramuscular: Adults: 50 mg; Children: 1.25 mg/kg or 37.5 mg/m^2 q6h; Maximum dosage: 300 mg/day. Intravenous: Adults: 50 mg dilute IV bolus.

Available Drug Forms Scored tablets containing 50 mg; oral liquid containing 12.5 mg/4 ml and 5% ethyl alcohol; rectal suppositories containing 100 mg; ampules containing 50 mg/ml; multidose vials containing 50 mg/ml.

Nursing Management (See diphenhydramine hydrochloride.)

1. Should be taken at least 30 minutes prior to travel to prevent motion sickness.

2. When administering via IV bolus,
   (a) Dilute with at least 10 ml of sodium chloride injection.
   (b) Never mix with other drugs since numerous incompatibilities exist.
   (c) Deliver at a rate of 2.5 to 5 ml/min.
3. Give IM injection deep into large muscle mass to prevent irritation. Rotate injection sites.

GENERIC NAME Doxylamine succinate (RX)

TRADE NAME Decapryn

CLASSIFICATION H_1-antihistamine

See diphenhydramine hydrochloride for contraindications, Warnings and precautions, Untoward reactions, Parameters of use, Drug interactions, and Nursing management.

Action Similar to diphenhydramine. Doxylamine is often used in sleeping aids, such as Nyquil, since drowsiness is a common secondary effect.

Indications for Use Relief of rhinitis and other allergic symptoms.

Administration Adults: 12.5 to 25 mg po every 4 to 6 hours; Children: under 12 years: 3.75 to 6.25 mg po every 4 to 6 hours.

Available Drug Forms Tablets containing 12.5 or 25 mg; syrup containing 6.25 mg/5 ml.

ETHYLENEDIAMINE DERIVATIVES

GENERIC NAMES Tripelennamine citrate; tripelennanmine hydrochloride

TRADE NAMES Pyribenzamine Citrate; PBZ, PBZ-SR, Pyribenzamine Hydrochloride

CLASSIFICATION H_1-antihistamine (RX)

Action Tripelennamine competitively antagonizes the action of histamine at H_1-receptor sites, but does not inhibit gastric secretions from H_2-receptor sites in the stomach. Like diphenhydramine, tripelennamine induces anticholinergic and CNS effects. It frequently causes GI disturbances.

Indications for Use Allergies, transfusion reactions, as an adjunct in anaphylactic therapy, pruritus, cough, oral mucous membrane analgesia.

Contraindications Hypersensitivity to tripelennamine, neonates, premature infants, lactation, acute bronchial asthma and other lower respiratory tract disorders, narrow-angle glaucoma, stenosing peptic ulcer, prostatic hypertrophy with retention, bladder neck obstruction, pyloric stenosis, therapy with MAO inhibitors.

Warnings and Precautions Use with caution in young children and clients with hyperthyroidism, hypertension, or a history of bronchial asthma. May cause CNS disturbances in clients over 60 years. May produce excitation, particularly in young children.

Untoward Reactions Drowsiness, dry mucous membranes, dizziness, incoordination, and epigastric distress are common. Thickening of bronchial secretions is common and may lead to the development of mucus plugs. CNS disturbances, including confusion, restlessness, excitation, hysteria, irritability, euphoria, and insomnia, may occur. Convulsions have been reported. Toxicity results from CNS disturbances and anticholinergic effects. Tightness in the chest and wheezing may occur. GI disturbances, including anorexia, nausea, vomiting, diarrhea, and constipation, may occur. Urinary retention or frequency and dysuria may occur. Palpitations, tachycardia, and extrasystoles may occur. Hypotension may occur, particularly in the elderly. Photosensitivity and skin rashes may occur. Blurred vision, diplopia, vertigo, and tinnitus have been reported. Blood dyscrasias, including leukopenia, thrombocytopenia, agranulocytosis, and aplastic anemia, have been reported, particularly after prolonged drug administration.

Parameters of Use

Absorption Fairly well absorbed from GI tract. Onset of action is about 30 minutes. Duration of action is: 4 to 6 hours (regular tablet); 8 hours (sustained-release tablet). Crosses blood-brain barrier.

Excretion Primarily in urine.

Drug Interactions Cholinergic agents and MAO inhibitors may prolong and intensify the anticholinergic effects of antihistamines; concurrent use is not recommended. Excessive sedation and other CNS disturbances may occur when alcohol, barbiturates, and CNS depressants are used concomitantly.

Administration Adults: 25 to 50 mg po every 4 to 6 hours; Maximum dosage: 600 mg/day. Children: 5 mg/kg/day po in 4 to 6 divided doses; Maximum dosage: 300 mg/day.

Available Drug Forms Tablets containing 25 or 50 mg; sustained-release tablets containing 50 to 100 mg; elixir containing 37.5 mg/5 ml.

Nursing Management

Planning factors

1. Obtain history of CNS, GI, and genitourinary disturbances and hypersensitivities.
2. Check for anemia and other hematologic abnormalities. Notify physician if any exist.
3. Discontinue drug for at least 72 hours prior to skin testing, since it may mask otherwise positive reactions.

Administration factors Oral preparations may be given with milk or food to minimize GI disturbances.

Evaluation factors

1. Observe reactions closely in elderly clients (over 60 years) and assist with ambulation as CNS disturbances are generally more pronounced in the elderly.
2. Perform periodic blood counts in clients on prolonged therapy.

Client teaching factors

1. Inform client about the secondary effects of drug and emphasize the dangers of driving a car or operating hazardous machinery.
2. Instruct client to avoid alcohol and CNS depressants while taking antihistamines.
3. Inform client that ice chips and sugarless gum may be helpful in relieving dry mouth.
4. Warn client to avoid direct sunlight because photosensitivity may occur.

GENERIC NAME Methapyrilene hydrochloride

TRADE NAMES Histadyl, Semikon (OTC) (RX)

CLASSIFICATION H_1-antihistamine

See tripelennamine citrate for Warnings and precautions, Untoward reactions, Parameters of use, Drug interactions, and Nursing management.

Action Similar to tripelennamine, but causes fewer secondary effects.

Indications for Use Hay fever, allergic rhinitis, urticaria.

Administration 50 mg po qid; Maximum dosage: 400 mg/day.

Available Drug Forms Tablets containing 50 mg.

GENERIC NAME Pyrilamine maleate (OTC) (RX)

TRADE NAMES Allertoc, Neo-Antergan, Nisaval, Zem-Histine

CLASSIFICATION H_1-antihistamine

See tripelennamine citrate for Contraindications, Warnings and precautions, Untoward reactions, Parameters of use, and Drug interactions.

Action Similar to tripelennamine.

Indications for Use Allergic reactions (rhinitis, urticaria, hypersensitivity drug reactions), cough.

Administration Adults: 25 to 50 mg po every 6 to 8 hours; Children: Over 6 years: 12.5 to 25 mg po every 6 to 8 hours.

Available Drug Forms Tablets containing 25 mg. Also an ingredient of numerous OTC cough syrups and sleeping preparations.

Nursing Management (See tripelannamine citrate.)

1. Should be taken after meals or with a snack to avoid GI disturbances.
2. Warn client to avoid chewing tablets, since local anesthetic effect will result.

PHENOTHIAZINES

GENERIC NAME Promethazine hydrochloride

TRADE NAMES Histantil, K-Phen, Pentazine, Phenergan, Remsed, ZiPan

CLASSIFICATION H_1-antihistamine (RX)

Action Promethazine competes with histamine at H_1-receptor sites. The drug has marked sedative activity and will potentiate the action of analgesics and tranquilizers; therefore, it is useful as a preoperative sedative. As with other phenothiazines, large dosages of promethazine will induce extrapyramidal symptoms. Like the antihistamines, promethazine has anticholinergic and antiemetic effects, but has a longer duration of action.

Indications for Use Allergies, transfusion, motion sickness, nausea and vomiting, preoperative sedation, as an adjunct to analgesics, sedation, cough.

Contraindications Hypersensitivity to phenothiazines, epilepsy, coma, CNS depression, narrow-angle glaucoma, prostatic hypertrophy, urinary retention, intestinal obstruction, stenosing peptic ulcer, bone marrow depression, pregnancy (except during labor), newborns, lactation.

Warnings and Precautions Use with caution in clients with asthma, hepatic disorders, or hypertension. Safe use in children has not been completely established; severe untoward reactions may occur. Tolerance may develop with prolonged therapy.

Untoward Reactions Sedation is the most common secondary reaction. Excessive CNS depression may occur, particularly in the elderly. Toxicity may occur, particularly in young children. Hyperexcitability and abnormal movement may occur with normal therapeutic dosages. Respiratory depression, nightmares, delirium, and agitated behavior have been reported. Extrapyramidal symptoms may occur when large dosages are administered. Dizziness, lassitude, incoordination, fatigue, euphoria, nervousness, tremors, insomnia, hysteria, catatonic states, and convulsions may occur. Sensory disturbances include tinnitus, blurred vision, diplopia, and oculogyric crisis. Photosensitivity reactions are common. Cardiovascular disturbances include marked alterations in blood pressure and pulse, faintness, and dizziness. GI disturbances, including anorexia and dry mouth, are common. Nausea and vomiting may also occur. Blood dyscrasias, including leukopenia and agranulocytosis, have been reported. Local irritation may occur at the injection site. Accidental subcutaneous injection may cause necrosis. Venous thrombosis of the injection site has been reported.

Parameters of Use

Absorption Well absorbed from GI tract. Fairly well absorbed from muscle injection sites. Onset of action is about 4 to 6 hours and antihistamine activity may persist for 10 to 12 hours.

Crosses blood-brain barrier. Probably crosses placenta. Enters breast milk; lactating mothers should bottle-feed their babies.

Distribution Widely distributed to body tissues.

Metabolism Primarily in the liver.

Excretion Slowly by the kidneys; some in feces.

Drug Interactions Additive sedative effects occur when given concurrently with narcotics, tranquilizers, barbiturates, alcohol, and CNS depressants. Cholinergic agents and MAO inhibitors may prolong and intensify the anticholinergic effects of antihistamines.

Administration Adults: 12.5 to 50 mg po or IM as a single dose; may be repeated every 4 to 6 hours, if needed. Children: 0.25 to 0.5 mg/kg po or IM.

Available Drug Forms Tablets containing 12.5, 25, or 50 mg; syrup containing 6.25 or 25 mg/5 ml; rectal suppositories containing 12.5, 25, or 50 mg; ampules containing 25 or 50 mg/ml.

Nursing Management

Planning factors

1. Obtain history of CNS, GI, and genitourinary disturbances and hypersensitivities.
2. Check for leukopenia, anemia, or other hematologic abnormalities. Notify physician if any exist.
3. Elderly clients may require reduced dosages.
4. Discontinue drug for at least 72 hours prior to skin testing, since it may mask otherwise positive reactions.

Administration factors

1. Do not use solution if cloudy or darkened.
2. Give IM injection deep into well-vascularized, large muscle mass to avoid local irritation and necrosis. Do not give subcutaneously.
3. Administer IV slowly. Maximum IV rate is 25 mg/ml/min. Flush line with normal saline before and after administration.

Evaluation factors

1. Observe reactions closely in elderly clients (over 60 years) and assist with ambulation as CNS disturbances are generally more pronounced in the elderly.
2. Check vital signs periodically, particularly if parenteral route is used.
3. Check injection site for irritation for the first 24 hours.

Client teaching factors

1. Inform client about the secondary effects of drug and emphasize the dangers of driving a car or operating hazardous machinery.
2. Instruct client to avoid alcohol and CNS depressants while taking antihistamines.
3. Warn client to avoid direct sunlight because photosensitivity may occur.

GENERIC NAMES Methdilazine; methdilazine hydrochloride

TRADE NAMES Tacaryl; Tacaryl Hydrochloride

CLASSIFICATION H_1-antihistamine (RX)

See promethazine hydrochloride for Contraindications, Warnings and precautions, Untoward reactions, Parameters of use, Drug interactions, and Nursing management.

Action Similar to promethazine, but induces less sedation and is excreted more rapidly.

Indications for Use Pruritus.

Administration Adults: 8 mg po bid, tid, or qid; Children: 4 mg po bid, tid, or qid.

Available Drug Forms Tablets containing 4 mg; chewable tablets containing 8 mg; syrup containing 4 mg/5 ml.

PROPYLAMINE DERIVATIVES

GENERIC NAME Chlorpheniramine maleate (RX)

TRADE NAMES AL-R, Chloramate, Chlor-Trimeton, Histalon, Histaspan, Histex, Teldrin

CLASSIFICATION H_1-antihistamine

Action Chlorpheniramine competes with histamine at H_1-receptor sites. It is one of the most potent antihistamines available today; however, chlorpheniramine induces fewer secondary reactions and little if any toxicity in therapeutic dosages. Chlorpheniramine is frequently combined with a decongestant and marketed as a cold remedy.

Indications for Use Allergic rhinitis, prevention of transfusion and drug reactions, as an adjunct to epinephrine in anaphylactic reactions.

Contraindications Hypersensitivity to chlorpheniramine, neonates, premature infants, lactation, acute asthmatic episodes, therapy with MAO inhibitors.

Warnings and Precautions Use with caution in young children as toxicity may occur and in clients with a history of asthma, increased intraocular pressure, hyperthyroidism, hypertension, cardiovascular disorders, stenosing peptic ulcer, intestinal obstruction, or urinary retention. Safe use during pregnancy has not been established.

Untoward Reactions Drowsiness, dry mouth, and epigastric distress may occur, but less frequently than with other antihistamines. CNS disturbances, including dizziness, incoordination, fatigue, confusion, restlessness, excitation, tremors, irritability, insomnia, paresthesia, neuritis, and convulsions, may occur, particularly in the elderly and the very young. GI disturbances include anorexia, nausea, vomiting, diarrhea, and constipation. Genitourinary disturbances include urinary retention, frequency, and dysuria. Thickening of bronchial secretions may occur and lead to the development of mucus plugs. Wheezing, chest tightness, and nasal stuffiness have been reported. Blood dyscrasias, including thrombocytopenia, agranulocytosis, and hemolytic anemia, have been reported, particularly after prolonged administration.

Parameters of Use

Absorption Fairly well absorbed from GI tract; pKa is 9.2; pH of the aqueous drug solution is 4 to 5. Onset of action is 30 to 60 minutes. Duration of action is 3 to 6 hours.

Crosses blood-brain barrier. Enters breast milk; lactating mothers should bottle-feed their babies.

Metabolism Primarily in the liver.

Excretion By the kidneys as unchanged drug and metabolites.

Administration Adults: 2 to 4 po tid or qid or 8 to 12 mg po (timed-release form) q12h; Children: 1 to 2 mg po tid or qid.

Available Drug Forms Tablets containing 2 or 4 mg; timed-release tablets containing 8 or 12 mg; syrup containing 10, 20, or 100 mg/ml. Frequently combined with a decongestant and marketed as a cold remedy.

Nursing Management

Planning factors

1. Obtain history of CNS, GI, and genitourinary disturbances and hypersensitivities.
2. Check for anemia or other hematologic abnormalities. Notify physician if any exist.
3. Not effective for severe allergic reactions.
4. Discontinue drug for at least 72 hours prior to skin testing, since it may mask otherwise positive reactions.

Administration factors Oral preparations may be given with milk or food to minimize GI disturbances.

Evaluation factors

1. Observe reaction closely in elderly clients (over 60 years) and assist with ambulation as CNS disturbances are generally more pronounced in the elderly.
2. Sedative effects usually abate with continued use. If sedation and other secondary effects persist, changing the antihistamine may be helpful.
3. Perform periodic blood counts in clients on prolonged therapy.

Client teaching factors

1. Inform client about the secondary effects of drug and emphasize the dangers of driving a car or operating hazardous machinery.
2. Instruct client to avoid alcohol and CNS depressants while taking antihistamines.
3. Inform client that ice chips and sugarless gum may be helpful in relieving dry mouth.

GENERIC NAME Brompheniramine maleate (RX)

TRADE NAMES Bromotane, Dimetane, Puretane, Rolabromophen, Veltane

CLASSIFICATION H_1-antihistamine

See chlorpheniramine maleate for Contraindications, Warnings and precautions, Parameters of use, and Drug interactions.

Action Similar to chlorpheniramine.

Indications for Use Allergies.

Untoward Reactions Drowsiness, sweating, hypotension, and syncope may occur, particularly after intravenous administration. (See chlorpheniramine maleate.)

Administration Oral: Adults: 4 to 8 mg tid or 8 to 12 mg (sustained-release form) every 8 to 12 hours; Children: 0.5 mg/kg/24 hours in 3 to 4 divided doses. Parenteral: Adults: 5 to 20 mg as needed; Maximum dosage: 40 mg/day.

Available Drug Forms Tablets containing 4, 8, or 12 mg; sustained-release tablets and capsules containing 8 or 12 mg; elixir containing 2 mg/5 ml; vials containing 10 mg/ml. Also an ingredient of numerous cough and cold preparations.

Nursing Management (See chlorpheniramine maleate.)

1. When administering IM or subc:
   (a) Inject deep into large muscle mass.
   (b) Rotate injection sites.
2. When administering IV:
   (a) Have client in recumbent position.
   (b) Administer slowly to avoid irritation to vein. Flush line with normal saline.
   (c) May be added to IV normal saline or 5% dextrose and water solution and administered over 30 minutes.

GENERIC NAME Dexchlorpheniramine maleate

TRADE NAME Polaramine (RX)

CLASSIFICATION H_1-antihistamine

See chlorpheniramine maleate for Contraindications, Warnings and precautions, Untoward reactions, Parameters of use, and Drug interactions.

Action Dexchlorpheniramine is a potent antihistamine similar to chlorpheniramine. Drowsiness is a common side effect.

Indications for Use Allergies.

Administration Adults: 2 mg po tid or qid or 4 to 6 mg po (repeat-action form) bid; Children: ½ of adult dosage.

Available Drug Forms Tablets containing 2 mg; repeat-action tablets containing 4 or 6 mg; syrup containing 2 mg/5 ml.

Nursing Management Repeat-action tablets are not recommended for children. (See chlorpheniramine maleate.)

GENERIC NAME Pheniramine maleate (RX)

TRADE NAMES Inhiston, Trimeton

CLASSIFICATION H_1-antihistamine

See chlorpheniramine maleate for Contraindications, Warnings and precautions, Untoward reactions, Parameters of use, Drug interactions, and Nursing management.

Action Pheniramine competes with histamine for H_1-receptor sites. Although the drug has few untoward reactions, it also has a low level of antihistamine activity.

Indications for Use Allergies.

Administration Adults: 20 mg po q4H; Children: 10 mg po q4h.

Available Drug Forms Tablets containing 10 mg.

GENERIC NAME Triprolidine hydrochloride (RX)

TRADE NAME Actidil

CLASSIFICATION H_1-antihistamine

See chlorpheniramine maleate for Contraindications, Warnings and precautions, Untoward reactions, Parameters of use, Drug interactions, and Nursing management.

Action Similar to chlorpheniramine, but it has no bitter taste and a longer duration of action.

Indications for Use Allergies, transfusion reactions.

Administration Adults: 2.5 mg po tid or qid; Children: Over 6 years: ½ of adult dosage; Under 6 years: 0.3 to 0.6 mg po tid or qid.

Available Drug Forms Tablets containing 2.5 mg; syrup containing 1.25 mg/5 ml.

AGENTS WITH ANTIHISTAMINE PROPERTIES

Although they have effective antihistamine properties, most of the drugs listed in this section are used for other disorders. For example, bucilizine hydrochloride, cyclizine hydrochloride, and meclizine hydrochloride are used to treat nausea and vomiting. Further details about these drugs can be found in Chapter 78 on emetics and antiemetics. Further details about hydroxyzine hydrochloride, a tranquilizer, can be found in Chapter 35.

GENERIC NAME Azatadine maleate (RX)

TRADE NAME Optimine

CLASSIFICATION H_1-antihistamine

See diphenhydramine hydrochloride for Contraindications, Warnings and precautions, Untoward reactions, and Drug interactions.

Action Azatadine is an effective antihistamine with anticholinergic and antiserotonin properties. Drowsiness is a common side effect.

Indications for Use Allergic rhinitis, chronic urticaria.

Administration 1 to 2 mg po bid.

Available Drug Forms Tablets containing 1 mg.

Nursing Management (See diphenhydramine hydrochloride.)

1. Give with meals or a snack if GI disturbances occur.
2. Discontinue drug for 3 to 4 days before skin testing.

GENERIC NAME Buclizine hydrochloride (RX)

TRADE NAME Bucladin-S

CLASSIFICATION H_1-antihistamine

Action Although it has antihistamine properties, buclizine hydrochloride is often used as an antiemetic, since it suppresses the vomiting center in the brain.

Indications for Use Motion sickness, Meniere's syndrome, labyrinthitis.

Administration 25 to 50 mg po every 4 to 6 hours.

Available Drug Forms Tablets containing 50 mg.

GENERIC NAME Clemastine fumarate (RX)

TRADE NAME Tavist

CLASSIFICATION H_1-antihistamine

See diphenhydramine hydrochloride for Contraindications, Warnings and precautions, Untoward reactions, Drug interactions, and Nursing management.

Action Clemastine is a potent antihistamine that frequently causes sedation in the elderly. It also has anticholinergic properties. This drug is not recommended for children.

Indications for Use Rhinitis, urticaria.

Administration 1.34 to 2.68 mg po bid or tid; Maximum dosage: 8.04 mg/day.

Available Drug Forms Tablets containing 1.34 or 2.68 mg.

Nursing Management (See diphenhydramine hydrochloride.)

1. Warn client to avoid operating dangerous equipment.
2. Discontinue drug 3 to 4 days before skin testing.

GENERIC NAMES Cyclizine hydrochloride; cyclizine lactate

TRADE NAMES Marezine Hydrochloride; Marezine Lactate

CLASSIFICATION H_1-antihistamine (RX)

Action Although it is not used as an antihistamine, cyclizine is an effective antinauseant. Drowsiness is a common side effect. This drug is not recommended for children under 6 years. As the lactate salt is water soluble, it is used parenterally.

Indications for Use Motion sickness, postoperative nausea and vomiting.

Administration 50 mg po or parenterally every 4 to 6 hours; Maximum dosage: 200 mg/day.

Available Drug Forms Tablets (hydrochloride) containing 50 mg; ampules (lactate) containing 50 mg/ml.

GENERIC NAME Dimethindene maleate (RX)

TRADE NAMES Forhistal, Triten

CLASSIFICATION H_1-antihistamine

See diphenhydramine hydrochloride for Contraindications, Warnings and precautions, Untoward reactions, and Drug interactions.

Action Dimethindene is a potent antihistamine and has no bitter taste. Drowsiness is a common side effect. This drug is not recommended for children under 6 years.

Indications for Use Allergies, including respiratory and ocular allergic reactions, as an adjunct in the treatment of anaphylaxis, pruritus.

Administration 2.5 mg po bid.

Available Drug Forms Timed-release tablets containing 2.5 mg.

GENERIC NAME Diphenylpyraline hydrochloride

TRADE NAMES Diafen, Hispril (RX)

CLASSIFICATION H_1-antihistamine

See diphenhydramine hydrochloride for Contraindications, Warnings and precautions, Untoward reactions, and Drug interactions.

Action Diphenylpyraline is a potent antihistamine with a chemical structure similar to diphenhydramine, but induces few untoward reactions.

Indications for Use Allergic reactions that respond poorly to other antihistamines.

Administration Adults: 2 mg po q4h or 5 mg po (timed-release form) bid; Children: 1 to 2 mg po every 6 to 8 hours.

Available Drug Forms Tablets containing 2 mg; timed-release capsules containing 5 mg.

Nursing Management Timed-release form is not recommended for children. (See diphenhydramine hydrochloride.)

GENERIC NAME Hydroxyzine hydrochloride

TRADE NAMES Atarax, Vistaril (RX)

CLASSIFICATION H_1-antihistamine

Action Hydroxyzine, a diphenylmethane derivative, is a tranquilizing agent with antihistaminic and anticholinergic properties. It may produce marked sedation.

Indications for Use Relief of anxiety, control of emesis, sedation prior to surgery or delivery, as an adjunct in the treatment of allergies, reduction of requirements (by as much as 50%) for narcotics prior to and after surgery.

Administration Adults: 25 to 100 mg po or IM tid or qid. Children: Oral: Over 6 years: 25 to 100 mg daily in divided doses; Under 6 years: 50 mg daily in divided doses. Intramuscular: 0.5 mg/lb.

Available Drug Forms Tablets and capsules containing 10, 25, 50, or 100 mg; syrup containing 10mg/5 ml; injection containing 25 or 50 mg/ml.

Nursing Management

1. Give IM injection deep into large muscle.
2. Avoid intravenous and subcutaneous administration.

GENERIC NAME Meclizine hydrochloride (RX)

TRADE NAMES Antivert, Bonine

CLASSIFICATION H_1-antihistamine

Action Although it is an effective antihistamine, meclizine is usually used for its antinauseant properties. Drowsiness is a common side effect. This drug is not recommended for young children.

Indications for Use Motion sickness, vertigo, nausea and vomiting associated with radiation sickness.

Administration 25 to 100 mg po as a single dose or in divided doses.

Available Drug Forms Tablets, chewable tablets, and capsules containing 12.5 or 25 mg.

SEROTONIN ANTAGONISTS

GENERIC NAME Cyproheptadine hydrochloride

TRADE NAMES Periactin, Vimicon (RX)

CLASSIFICATION Serotonin antagonist

See promethazine hydrochloride for Untoward reactions, Parameters of use, Drug interactions, and Nursing management.

Action Cyproheptadine, a phenothiazine analog, has both antihistamine and antiserotonin properties. Its antihistaminic characteristics are similar to chlorpheniramine. Sedation is the primary untoward reaction, but tends to subside after 3 to 4 days of therapy. It also has anticholinergic properties.

Indications for Use Pruritus, allergic skin disorders, allergic conjunctivitis, allergic reactions.

Contraindications Neonates, premature infants, lactation, acute asthmatic episodes, glaucoma, urinary retention, therapy with MAO inhibitors.

Warnings and Precautions Use with caution in clients with a history of asthma, increased intraocular pressure, hyperthyroidism, cardiovascular disorders, or hypertension.

Administration Adults: 4 mg po tid; Children: 2 to 4 mg po bid or tid.

Available Drug Forms Tablets containing 4 mg; syrup containing 2 mg/5 ml.

GENERIC NAME Trimeprazine tartrate (RX)

TRADE NAMES Panectyl, Temaril

CLASSIFICATION Serotonin antagonist

See promethazine hydrochloride for Untoward reactions, Parameters of use, Drug interactions, and Nursing management.

Action Trimeprazine, a phenothiazine analog, is similar to cyproheptadine. It has both antihistaminic and antiserotonin properties.

Indications for Use Pruritus, allergic skin disorders.

Contraindications Neonates, premature infants, lactation, acute asthmatic episodes, glaucoma, urinary retention, therapy with MAO inhibitors.

Warnings and Precautions Use with caution in clients with a history of asthma, increased intraocular pressure, hyperthyroidism, cardiovascular disorders, or hypertension.

Administration Adults: 2.5 mg po qid or 5 mg po (Spansule) q12h; Children: 1.25 to 2.5 mg po tid.

Available Drug Forms Tablets containing 2.5 mg; Spansule capsules containing 5 mg; syrup containing 2.5 mg/5 ml.

COMBINATION ANTIHISTAMINE PREPARATIONS

Many of the antihistamines are combined with decongestant (anticholinergic) drugs and used to treat allergic rhinitis, sinusitis, and the common cold. Details concerning the decongestant ingredients can be found in Chapter 55.

TRADE NAME Actifed (RX)

CLASSIFICATION Combination antihistamine

Indications for Use Seasonal and perennial allergic rhinitis.

Contraindications Hypersensitivity to any ingredient, newborns, premature infants, lactation, lower respiratory tract symptoms, including asthma.

Warnings and Precautions Use with caution in clients with a history of increased intraocular pressure, stenosing peptic ulcer, pyloroduodenal obstruction, symptomatic prostatic hypertrophy, bladder neck obstruction, hypertension, diabetes, ischemic heart disease, or hyperthyroidism.

Untoward Reactions May induce dryness of the mouth, nose, and throat, sedation, dizziness, epigastric distress, and thickening of bronchial secretions.

Drug Interactions MAO inhibitors intensify the effects of Actifed; do not administer concurrently. Additive effects may occur if taken with other CNS depressants, such as alcohol or tranquilizers.

Administration Adults: 1 tablet po tid or qid; Children: Ages 6 to 12 years: $\frac{1}{2}$ tablet po tid or qid; Ages 4 to 6 years: 3.75 ml po tid or qid; Ages 2 to 4 years: 2.5 ml po tid or qid; Ages 4 months to 2 years: 1.25 ml po tid or qid.

Available Drug Forms Generic contents in each white, scored tablet or 10 ml: triprolidine hydrochloride: 2.5 mg; pseudoephedrine hydrochloride: 60 mg.

Nursing Management Warn client that mental and/or physical abilities may be impaired.

TRADE NAME Allerest (OTC)

CLASSIFICATION Combination antihistamine

Indications for Use Hay fever, pollen allergies, upper respiratory tract allergies, allergic colds, sinusitis, nasal passage congestion.

Warnings and Precautions Use with caution in clients with cardiac disorders, hypertension, hyperthyroidism, or diabetes.

Untoward Reactions May induce drowsiness, nervousness, and dizziness.

Administration 2 tablets po q4h prn.

Available Drug Forms Generic contents in each tablet: chlorpheniramine maleate: 2 mg; phenylpropanolamine hydrochloride: 18.7 mg.

TRADE NAMES Anamine Syrup, Anamine T.D., Brexin L.A., Cenules, Chol-Trimeton, Cordimal L.A., Deconamine Elixir and Syrup, Deconamine SR, Decongestant Repetabs, Isoclor Liquid, Isoclor Timesule (OTC) (RX)

CLASSIFICATION Combination antihistimine

Indications for Use Allergic rhinitis, rhinosinusitis, eustachian tube congestion.

Warnings and Precautions Use with caution in clients with a history of hypertension, glaucoma, cardiovascular disease, prostatic hypertrophy, diabetes, or hyperthyroidism.

Untoward Reactions May induce drowsiness, confusion, restlessness, nausea, vomiting, drug rash, anorexia, headache, anxiety, weakness, tachycardia, and sweating.

Drug Interactions MAO inhibitors and beta-adrenergic blockers increase drug effects; do not use concurrently. The antihypertensive effects of methyldopa, mecamylamine, reserpine, and veratrum may be reduced when taken concomitantly.

Administration Adults: 1 capsule po every 8 to 12 hours or 10 ml po every 4 to 6 hours; Children: Ages 6 to 12 years: 5 ml po every 4 to 6 hours; Ages 1 to 6 years: 2.5 to 5 ml po q6h; Under 1 year: 1.25 to 2.5 ml po q6h.

Available Drug Forms Generic contents in each capsule or 20 ml: chlorpheniramine maleate: 8 mg; pseudoephedrine hydrochloride: 120 mg.

TRADE NAME Brexin (RX)

CLASSIFICATION Combination antihistamine

Indications for Use Seasonal or perennial allergic rhinitis and colds.

Contraindications Narrow-angle glaucoma, urinary retention, peptic ulcer, lactation.

Warnings and Precautions Use with caution in clients with a history of hypertension, glaucoma, cardiovascular disease, prostatic hypertrophy, diabetes, or hyperthyroidism.

Untoward Reactions May induce drowsiness, nausea, dry mouth, blurred vision, cardiac palpitations, and flushing.

Drug Interactions MAO inhibitors and beta-adrenergic blockers increase drug effects; do not use concurrently. The antihypertensive effects of methyldopa, mecamylamine, reserpine, and veratrum alkaloids may be reduced when taken concomitantly. Additive effects may occur if taken with other CNS depressants, such as alcohol or tranquilizers.

Administration Adults: 1 capsule or 5 to 10 ml po tid or qid; Children: Ages: 6 to 12 years: 5 ml po q4h; Ages 2 to 6 years: 2.5 ml po q4h.

Available Drug Forms Generic contents in each capsule or 10 ml: pseudoephedrine hydrochloride: 60 mg; carbinoxamine maleate: 4 mg; guaifenesin: 100 mg (5 ml).

TRADE NAMES Brocon C.R., Dimetapp Extentabs (RX)

CLASSIFICATION Combination antihistamine

Indications for Use Possibly effective for seasonal and perennial allergic rhinitis, urticaria and pruritus due to allergens or drugs, allergic conjunctivitis.

Contraindications Pregnancy, bronchial asthma, therapy with MAO inhibitors.

Warnings and Precautions Use with caution in infants and young children and in clients with a history of cardiac or peripheral vascular disease or hypertension.

Drug Interactions Additive effects may occur if taken with other CNS depressants, such as alcohol or tranquilizers.

Administration 1 tablet po every 8 to 12 hours.

Available Drug Forms Generic contents in each tablet: brompheniramine maleate: 12 mg; phenylephrine hydrochloride: 15 mg; phenylpropanolamine hydrochloride: 15 mg.

TRADE NAME Citra Capsules (RX)

CLASSIFICATION Combination antihistamine

Indications for Use Hay fever, common pollen allergies, the common cold.

Warnings and Precautions Use with caution in clients with a history of hypertension, cardiac disease, diabetes, or hyperthyroidism.

Administration 1 capsule po q4h, as needed.

Available Drug Forms Generic contents in each capsule: phenylephrine hydrochloride: 10 mg; ascorbic acid: 50 mg; pheniramine maleate: 6.25 mg; chlorpheniramine maleate: 1 mg; pyrilamine maleate: 8.33 mg; salicylamide: 227 mg; phenacetin: 120 mg; caffeine alkaloid: 30 mg.

TRADE NAME Comhist (RX)

CLASSIFICATION Combination antihistamine

Indications for Use Allergic rhinitis, vasomotor rhinitis.

Contraindications Children under 6 years, lactation, glaucoma, asthma, severe hypertension, therapy with MAO inhibitors.

Warnings and Precautions Use with caution in clients with a history of prostatic hypertrophy, hypertension, cardiovascular disease, diabetes, thyroid disease, or peptic ulcer.

Drug Interactions Additive effects may occur if taken with other CNS depressants, such as alcohol or tranquilizers.

Administration Adults: 1 to 2 tablets po tid; Children: Ages 6 to 12 years: 1 tablet po tid or 5 to 10 ml po q4h; Ages 3 to 6 years: 5 ml po q4h.

Available Drug Forms Generic contents in each tablet or 5 ml: chlorpheniramine maleate: 2 mg; phenindamine tartrate: 5 mg; phenylephrine hydrochloride: 10 mg; hyoscyamine sulfate: 0.1037 mg; atropine sulfate: 0.0194 mg; scopolamine hydrobromide: 0.0065 mg.

TRADE NAME Co-Pyronil (RX)

CLASSIFICATION Combination antihistamine

Indications for Use Allergic rhinitis, vasomotor rhinitis.

Contraindications Neonates, premature infants, during lactation, or concurrently with MAO inhibitors.

Warnings and Precautions Use with caution in clients with a history of bronchial asthma, increased intraocular pressure, hyperthyroidism, cardiovascular or renal disorders, hypertension, or diabetes. Urinary retention may occur in the presence of prostatism. Should not be used to treat lower respiratory tract infections.

Drug Interactions Additive effects may occur if taken with other CNS depressants, such as alcohol or tranquilizers.

Administration Dosage depends on severity of symptoms. Adults: 1 to 2 pulvules or 10 to 20 ml po every 8 to 12 hours; Children: 40 to 60 lb: 5 to 10 ml po every 8 to 12 hours; 20 to 40 lb: 2.5 to 5 ml po every 8 to 12 hours.

Available Drug Forms Generic contents in each pulvule: pyrrobutamine phosphate: 15 mg; cyclopentamine hydrochloride: 12.5 mg. Generic contents in 5 ml: pyrrobutamine naphthalene disulfonate: 6.73 mg; cyclopentamine hydroxybenzoyl benzoate: 13.49 mg.

TRADE NAMES Disophrol, Drixoral (RX)

CLASSIFICATION Combination antihistamine

Indications for Use Allergies, rhinitis, eustachian tube congestion, rhinosinusitis.

Contraindications Newborns, premature infants, pregnancy at term, lower respiratory tract symptoms, therapy with MAO inhibitors or adrenergic blocking agents.

Warnings and Precautions Use with caution in clients with a history of glaucoma, stenosing peptic ulcer, pyloroduodenal obstruction, prostatic hypertrophy, or bladder neck obstruction.

Drug Interactions Additive effects may occur if taken with other CNS depressants, such as alcohol or tranquilizers. May inhibit the action of oral anticoagulants. May cause increased ectopic pacemaker activity when given concomitantly with digitalis.

Administration 1 tablet po bid.

Available Drug Forms Generic contents in each tablet: dexbrompheniramine maleate: 6 mg; pseudoephedrine sulfate: 120 mg.

TRADE NAMES Extendryl T.D., Histaspan-D, Dinovan Timed (RX)

CLASSIFICATION Combination antihistamine

Indications for Use Allergic rhinitis, allergic skin reactions, such as urticaria and angioedema.

Warnings and Precautions Use with caution in clients with a history of glaucoma, cardiac disease, hyperthyroidism, or hypertension.

Administration 1 capsule po q12h.

Available Drug Forms Generic contents in each capsule: phenylephrine hydrochloride: 20 mg; methscopolamine nitrate: 2.5 mg; chlorpheniramine maleate: 8 mg.

TRADE NAME Fedahist (RX)

CLASSIFICATION Combination antihistamine

Indications for Use Allergic rhinitis, eustachian tube congestion.

Contraindications Newborns, premature infants, lactation, severe hypertension, severe coronary artery disease.

Warnings and Precautions Use with caution in clients with a history of bronchial asthma, glaucoma, hyperthyroidism, cardiovascular disease, or hypertension.

Untoward Reactions May induce drowsiness, drug rash, hemolytic anemia, dizziness, disturbed coordination, dry mouth, photosensitivity, epigastric distress, and thickening of bronchial secretions.

Administration 1 tablet or 10 ml po q6h; Children: Ages 6 to 12 years: $\frac{1}{2}$ tablet or 5 ml po q6h; Ages 2 to 6 years: 2.5 ml po q6h.

Available Drug Forms Generic contents in each scored tablet or 10 ml: pseudoephedrine hydrochloride: 60 mg; chlorpheniramine maleate: 4 mg.

TRADE NAME Fedrazil (OTC)

CLASSIFICATION Combination antihistamine

Indications for Use Allergic rhinitis, vasomotor rhinitis, acute sinusitis.

Contraindications Pregnancy, hypertension, cardiac disease, diabetes, thyroid disease.

Administration 1 tablet po tid.

Available Drug Forms Generic contents in each tablet: pseudoephedrine hydrochloride: 30 mg; chlorcyclizine hydrochloride: 25 mg.

TRADE NAME Histabid Duracap (RX)

CLASSIFICATION Combination antihistamine

Indications for Use Allergic rhinitis, vasomotor rhinitis, allergic conjunctivitis, mild allergic skin manifestations of urticaria and angioedema.

Contraindications Therapy with MAO inhibitors.

Warnings and Precautions Use with caution during pregnancy and in clients with a history of glaucoma, peptic ulcer, hypertension, cardiac or thyroid disease, or diabetes.

Untoward Reactions May induce drug rash, photosensitivity, dry mouth, headache, hemolytic anemia, dizziness, epigastric distress, and thickening of bronchial secretions.

Drug Interactions Additive effects may occur if taken with other CNS depressants, such as alcohol or sedatives.

Administration 1 capsule po q12h.

Available Drug Forms Generic contents in each capsule: chlorpheniramine maleate: 8 mg; phenylpropanolamine hydrochloride: 75 mg.

TRADE NAME Kronohist Kronocaps (RX)

CLASSIFICATION Combination antihistamine

Indications for Use Relief of sinus and nasal congestion.

Untoward Reactions May induce drowsiness, nervousness, and tachycardia.

Warnings and Precautions Use with caution in clients with a history of hypertension, cardiac disease, diabetes, or thyrotoxicosis.

Administration 1 capsule po bid.

Available Drug Forms Generic contents in each capsule: chlorpheniramine maleate: 4 mg; pyrilamine maleate: 25 mg; phenylpropanolamine hydrochloride: 50 mg.

TRADE NAME Napril (RX)

CLASSIFICATION Combination antihistamine

Indications for Use Relief of sinus and nasal congestion.

Warnings and Precautions Use with caution in clients with a history of hypertension, cardiac disease, diabetes, or hyperthyroidism.

Untoward Reactions May induce drowsiness, nervousness, and tachycardia.

Administration 1 capsule po bid.

Available Drug Forms Generic contents in each capsule: phenylpropanolamine hydrochloride: 25 mg; pyrilamine maleate: 25 mg; chlorpheniramine maleate: 4 mg; phenylephrine hydrochloride: 15 mg.

TRADE NAME Neotep Granucaps (RX)

CLASSIFICATION Combination antihistamine

Indications for Use Hay fever, sinus congestion, the common cold.

Contraindications Therapy with MAO inhibitors.

Warnings and Precautions Use with caution in clients with a history of hypertension, cardiac or thyroid disease, diabetes, asthma, or glaucoma.

Untoward Reactions May induce drowsiness.

Drug Interactions Additive effects may occur if taken with other CNS depressants, such as alcohol or sedatives.

Administration 1 Granucap po bid.

Available Drug Forms Generic contents in each Granucap: chlorpheniramine maleate: 9 mg; phenylephrine hydrochloride: 21 mg.

TRADE NAME Nolamine (RX)

CLASSIFICATION Combination antihistamine

Indications for Use Hay fever; sinusitis, the common cold, other allergies.

Contraindications Therapy with MAO inhibitors.

Warnings and Precautions Use with caution in clients with a history of hypertension, diabetes, cardiovascular disease, hyperthyroidism, prostatic hypertrophy, or glaucoma.

Untoward Reactions May induce nervousness, insomnia, tremors, dizziness, and drowsiness.

Administration 1 tablet po q8h.

Available Drug Forms Generic contents in each timed-release tablet: phenindamine tartrate: 24 mg; chlorpheniramine maleate: 4 mg; phenylpropanolamine hydrochloride: 50 mg.

TRADE NAME Rhinex D·Lay (RX)

CLASSIFICATION Combination antihistamine

Indications for Use Vasomotor rhinitis, allergic rhinitis, the common cold.

Warnings and Precautions Use with caution in clients with a history of hypertension, cardiac or thyroid disease, or diabetes.

Administration 1 tablet po every 6 to 12 hours, as needed.

Available Drug Forms Generic contents in each tablet: acetaminophen: 300 mg; salicylamide: 300 mg; phenylpropanolamine hydrochloride: 60 mg; chlorpheniramine maleate: 4 mg.

TRADE NAME Rondec (OTC)

CLASSIFICATION Combination antihistamine

Indications for Use Allergic rhinitis, vasomotor rhinitis.

Contraindications Therapy with MAO inhibitors or beta-adrenergic blockers.

Warnings and Precautions Use with caution in clients with a history of hypertension, heart disease, hyperthyroidism, diabetes, asthma, increased intraocular pressure, or prostatic hypertrophy and during lactation.

Untoward Reactions May induce sedation, dizziness, vomiting, dry mouth, headache, tachycardia, and nervousness.

Drug Interactions May reduce the antihypertensive effects of reserpine, veratrum alkaloids, methyldopa, and mecamylamine. Additive effects may occur if taken with other CNS depressants, such as alcohol or tranquilizers.

Administration Adults and children 6 years or older: 1 tablet or 5 ml po qid; Children: Ages 18 months to 6 years: 2.5 ml po qid.

Available Drug Forms Generic contents in each tablet or 5 ml: carbinoxamine maleate: 4 mg; pseudoephedrine hydrochloride: 60 mg.

TRADE NAME Triaminic Syrup (OTC)

CLASSIFICATION Combination antihistamine

Indications for Use Upper respiratory tract allergies, the common cold.

Contraindications Therapy with MAO inhibitors.

Warnings and Precautions Use with caution in clients with a history of hypertension, cardiac disease, hyperthyroidism, diabetes, asthma, peptic ulcer, or prostatic obstruction.

Untoward Reactions May induce drowsiness, blurred vision, palpitations, GI upsets, and dizziness.

Drug Interactions Additive effects may occur if taken with other CNS depressants, such as alcohol or tranquilizers.

Administration Adults: 10 ml po q4h; Children: Ages 6 to 12 years: 5 ml po q4H; Ages 2 to 6 years: 2.5 ml po q4h.

Available Drug Forms Generic contents in 5 ml: phenylpropanolamine hydrochloride: 12.5 mg; chlorpheniramine maleate: 2 mg.

SUBJECT INDEX

DRUG INDEX